Healthcare in the United Arab Emirates

MIX
Papier aus verantwortungsvollen Quellen
Paper from responsible sources
FSC® C105338

If you have any concerns about our products,
you can contact us on
ProductSafety@springernature.com

In case Publisher is established outside the EU,
the EU authorized representative is:
**Springer Nature Customer Service Center GmbH
Europaplatz 3, 69115 Heidelberg, Germany**

Printed by Libri Plureos GmbH
in Hamburg, Germany

Humaid O. Al-Shamsi
Editor

Healthcare in the United Arab Emirates

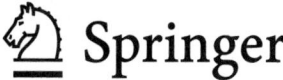

Editor
Humaid O. Al-Shamsi
Burjeel Cancer Institute, Burjeel Medical City
Abu Dhabi, United Arab Emirates

Department of Medical Oncology, Dana-Farber Cancer Institute
Harvard Medical School
Boston, MA, United States

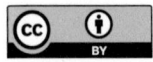

ISBN 978-981-96-0522-4   ISBN 978-981-96-0523-1   (eBook)
https://doi.org/10.1007/978-981-96-0523-1

This work was supported by Emirates Oncology Society.

© The Editor(s) (if applicable) and The Author(s), under exclusive license to Springer Nature Singapore Pte Ltd. 2025. This book is an open access publication.

Open Access This book is licensed under the terms of the Creative Commons Attribution 4.0 International License (http://creativecommons.org/licenses/by/4.0/), which permits use, sharing, adaptation, distribution and reproduction in any medium or format, as long as you give appropriate credit to the original author(s) and the source, provide a link to the Creative Commons license and indicate if changes were made.

The images or other third party material in this book are included in the book's Creative Commons license, unless indicated otherwise in a credit line to the material. If material is not included in the book's Creative Commons license and your intended use is not permitted by statutory regulation or exceeds the permitted use, you will need to obtain permission directly from the copyright holder.

The use of general descriptive names, registered names, trademarks, service marks, etc. in this publication does not imply, even in the absence of a specific statement, that such names are exempt from the relevant protective laws and regulations and therefore free for general use.

The publisher, the authors and the editors are safe to assume that the advice and information in this book are believed to be true and accurate at the date of publication. Neither the publisher nor the authors or the editors give a warranty, expressed or implied, with respect to the material contained herein or for any errors or omissions that may have been made. The publisher remains neutral with regard to jurisdictional claims in published maps and institutional affiliations.

This Springer imprint is published by the registered company Springer Nature Singapore Pte Ltd.
The registered company address is: 152 Beach Road, #21-01/04 Gateway East, Singapore 189721, Singapore

If disposing of this product, please recycle the paper.

Foreword

Healthcare is more than just a system; it is the backbone of a nation's well-being, a reflection of its priorities, and a mirror of its vision for the future. The United Arab Emirates, with its rapid development and commitment to excellence, has built a healthcare sector that not only serves its people but also inspires the world. This book, *Healthcare in the United Arab Emirates*, is a source that captures the spirit, achievements, and aspirations of this dynamic country.

In just a few decades, the UAE has transformed its healthcare landscape, evolving from humble beginnings to a thriving ecosystem characterized by advanced hospitals and inclusive, quality-focused policies. As the country continues to grow, so do its healthcare challenges, presenting opportunities for innovation, collaboration, and forward-thinking strategies.

This book is a comprehensive, multi-disciplinary exploration of the UAE's healthcare system. It dives deep into the intricacies of healthcare delivery across the seven emirates, shedding light on the interplay between public and private systems, the evolution of policy, and the pursuit of excellence in service delivery.

The UAE's healthcare story is one of collaboration, and this book showcases the collective expertise of thought leaders, practitioners, and policymakers, each bringing their unique perspectives to the table. It is an essential resource for anyone, be they a student, a physician, or an investor, seeking to understand the healthcare sector of a nation that continues to push boundaries.

As we look to the future, the coming years hold immense promises for healthcare in the UAE. With an emphasis on innovation, sustainability, and inclusivity, the sector is poised to set new benchmarks, not just regionally but globally. This book is a crucial guide to understanding where we stand today and how we can shape tomorrow.

I hope this book inspires us all to work together toward a brighter future for healthcare in the UAE.

Founder and Chairman, Burjeel Holdings   Shamsheer Vayalil
Abu Dhabi, UAE

Acknowledgments

To the two women in my life
  My Mum
  And
  My Wife
  To my mum, who has called me "Dr. Humaid" since I was six years old and pushed me to my limits as a child, shaping me into the man I am today.
  To my wife, Khadija, the mother of my beautiful kids, who supported me through the toughest challenges of my life and has been a constant source of encouragement with her words, "Always trust Allah."
  Thank you both for always being there for me.
  I love you both.

Contents

1 **History of Healthcare in the UAE**.............................. 1
   Humaid O. Al-Shamsi and Faryal Iqbal

2 **History of Kanad Hospital: The First Hospital in the UAE**........ 33
   Ralph Leo and Kaitlyn Baker

3 **Ministry of Health and Prevention in the UAE**.................. 49
   Mohammad Al-Olama and Meera Al Ali

4 **Healthcare System in the Emirate of Dubai**..................... 55
   Hamid Y. Hussein, Heba Mamdouh, and Wafa K. Alnakhi

5 **Abu Dhabi Public Health Center**............................... 71
   Omniyat Mohammed Al Hajeri,
   Sheikh Abdulla Bin Mohammed Bin Butti Al Hamed,
   and Matar Saeed Al Nuaimi

6 **An Overview of the Burden of Disease in the UAE**............... 93
   Abdulla Shehab and Asim Ahmed Elnour

7 **Health Insurances in the UAE**................................. 99
   Husam Al Majali and Mohamed Farghaly

8 **National Institute for Health Specialties (NIHS) in the UAE**....... 111
   Humaid O. Al-Shamsi, Aysha Al Dhaheri, Fouzia Shersad,
   and Mohammed Al-Houqani

9 **The Spectrum of Medical Education and Training
   in the UAE: Accomplishments and Points to Ponder**............. 123
   Salman Yousuf Guraya, Hatem Faraj Alameri, and Nabil Sulaiman

10 **Career Opportunities for Physicians and Nurses
   and the Licensing Pathways in the UAE**....................... 139
   Emilie Davies and Vivienne Mendonca

11 **UAE Medical Liability Law**................................... 153
   Ahmed Allouz, Mosaab Aly, and Amro Hassan

12	**National Vaccination Program in the UAE**......................... 163
	Dima Ibrahim and Fathima Firoz
13	**Private Healthcare in the UAE** 175
	Taha Al Hazarmerdi
14	**Health Economics in the UAE** 191
	Husam Al Majali and Maiss Ahmad
15	**Research Productivity of Health Sciences Institutions in the UAE: 20-Year-Based Bibliometric Analysis**................ 201
	Subhashini Ganesan, Humaid O. Al-Shamsi, Mohamed Mostafa, and Walid Abbas Zaher
16	**Nursing in the UAE: Reality and Future Directions** 217
	Wegdan Bani-Issa, Randa Fakhry, Mohamad Alameddine, Amina Al-Marzouqi, Jacqueline Maria Dias, Fatma Refaat Ahmed, Mini Sara Abraham, Muhammad Arsyad Subu, and Janisha Kavumpurath
17	**Advanced Practice Nursing Within the UAE**..................... 241
	Katie Hanafin
18	**Primary Health Care in the UAE** 253
	Maha Al Fahim, Ebtihal Darwish, and Farah Saeed Mohammad Al-Zaabi
19	**Obesity in the UAE** 277
	Omniyat Mohammed Al Hajeri and Omar Al Hammadi
20	**Burden and Characteristics of Diabetes and the Outcome of Care in the UAE** 293
	Khaled M. Al Dahmani, Mohamed Suliman, Khadija Hafidh, and Salem A. Beshyah
21	**Cardiovascular Healthcare in the UAE** 313
	Yosef Manla, Laszlo Göbölös, Sultan Abdulali, Azan Salem Binbrek, Arif Al Nooryani, Srinath Kidambi, and Wael Almahmeed
22	**Women's Health in the UAE** 335
	Cosette Fakih El Khoury, Jennifer Fortin, and Samantha Dumas
23	**Midwifery Care in the UAE**.................................. 351
	Saloua El Azzabi and Etab Omar Salem
24	**The Children's Health Service in the UAE: The Past, Present, and Future** 363
	Ahmed Elghoudi, Sara Awad, and Rana Ahmad Bitar
25	**Geriatric Medicine in the UAE** 373
	Salwa Alsuwaidi and Abdulla Al Ali

26	Cancer Care in the UAE	381

Humaid O. Al-Shamsi and Faryal Iqbal

27	Palliative and Hospice Medicine in the UAE	413

Neil A. Nijhawan, Humaid O. Al-Shamsi, and Halah Ibrahim

28	Pathology and Laboratory Medicine in the UAE	431

Laila Osama AbdelWareth and Annisah Binti Abdullah

29	Emergency Medicine in the UAE	439

Saleh Fares Al-Ali, Rasha Buhumaid, Khalifa Alqaydi, Muna Aljallaf, and Hind Aldhaheri

30	Intensive Care in the UAE	455

Ayesha Almemari, Saif Mohammed Alkaabi, Abdullah AlNaqbi, and Fayez Alshamsi

31	Road Traffic Collisions in the UAE	467

Hani O. Eid, Yasin J. Yasin, and Fikri M. Abu-Zidan

32	Mental Health in the UAE: Current Landscape and Future Directions	485

Ammar Albanna, Meshal A. Sultan, Faisal A. Nawaz, Hanan Derby, Mehnaz Zafar Ali, Nusrat Khan, Nahida N. Ahmed, and Omer El Rufaei

33	Rheumatic Disease History in the UAE	507

Ahmed Abogamal, Atheer Al-Ansari, and Ghita Harifi

34	Urology in the UAE	521

Humaid O. Al-Shamsi, Ali Thwaini, Faryal Iqbal, Omer Darwish, Amrith Rao, Farhad Janahi, Ahmed Abdul Rahman, Hosam Al-Qudah, and Thamer Al Kasab

35	Neurology Care in the UAE	545

U. K. D. Ajith Goonetilleke

36	Respirology in the UAE	567

Bassam Mahboub, Laila Salameh, and Mayank Vats

37	The Radiology Practice in the UAE in the Past, Present, and Future	583

Usama Albastaki

38	Postmortem Imaging in the UAE	597

Muhammad Al Shirawi

39	Evolution of Surgery in the UAE	613

Sara Al Bastaki, Zakir K. Mohamed, Nahla Al Mansoori, Ali Al Hassani, Zialyazan Sabbagh, and Hisham Hurreiz

40	Infectious Disease in the UAE Health System	629

Ahmed Abdul Kareem AlHammadi,
Fatima Ali Salem Khalfan Al Dhaheri,
Huda Sulaiman Al Dhanhani, and Jens Thomsen

41	Sports Medicine and Rehabilitation in the UAE	647

Mahesh Cirasanambati and Sabahat A. Wasti

42	Oral Health in the UAE: Current Status Within Global and Regional Perspectives	657

Nabeel H. Alsabeeha, Mohammed A. Al Shalabi,
Nada O. Al Shamsi, Shaikha A. AlSamahi, and Manal A. Awad

43	Early Childhood Caries (ECC) in the UAE	679

Anas AlSalami, Manal AlHalabi, Mawlood Kowash,
Iyad Hussein, and Mohammed Mansour

44	Safeguarding Children in UAE Healthcare Settings	699

Louise Cremonesini, Asrar Rashid, David Cremonesini,
Sara Al Marri, and Teresa Quinn

45	Genetic Diseases in the UAE	711

Mode Al Ojaimi, Rabah Almahmoud, Bashar J. Banimortada,
Abduljalil Alragheb, and Ayman W. El-Hattab

46	The Historical Perspectives, Present Status, and Future Prospects of Pharmaceutical Services in the UAE................	737

Asim Ahmed Elnour, Adel Sadeq, and Mariam Al Qahtani

47	Clinical Nutrition Specialty in the UAE	763

Rayan Daoud and Raisa Alktebi

48	Alternative Medicine in the UAE.............................	769

Khawla Mohamed Saeed binfraish Alkindi
and Kheireddine Youssef Chatra

49	Artificial Intelligence in Healthcare in the UAE	789

Khalid Shaikh and Sreelekshmi Vivek

50	Artificial Intelligence in Radiology in the UAE	817

Ahmed ElSerafi and Mohammad Rawashdeh

51	Health Media in the UAE....................................	831

Bassam Darwish

52	The Future of Healthcare in the UAE..........................	841

Vivienne Mendonca and Humaid O. Al-Shamsi

Index.. 849

History of Healthcare in the UAE

Humaid O. Al-Shamsi ⓘ and Faryal Iqbal ⓘ

1.1 Background

The information in this chapter has been compiled from various sources, including the book "History of Health Services in the Trucial States (1949–1971)" by Faisal Mohammed Abdulla Almandoos [1], "Health Services in the Trucial Coast" by Dr. Arif Al Sheikh [2], the official UAE government website's "History of Health Care in the United Arab Emirates" [3], the Arabian Gulf Digital Archive website [4], and newspaper articles titled "Health Services in the Emirates: From Traditional Medicine to International Ones" [5] and "Health Services in the Emirates: Documents and History" [6]. The information was collected and analyzed, and any discrepancies were carefully evaluated and resolved to the best of our ability, aiming to present the most evidence-based account of the history of health in the

---

H. O. Al-Shamsi (✉)
Burjeel Cancer Institute, Burjeel Medical City, Abu Dhabi, United Arab Emirates

Department of Medical Oncology, Dana-Farber Cancer Institute, Harvard Medical School, Boston, MA, United States

Harvard Medical School, Harvard University, Boston, MA, United States

College of Medicine, Ras Al Khaimah Medical and Health Sciences University, Al Juwais, Al Qusaidat, Ras Al Khaimah, United Arab Emirates

Gulf Medical University, Ajman, United Arab Emirates

Gulf Cancer Society, Alsafa, Kuwait

Emirates Oncology Society, Dubai, United Arab Emirates

College of Medicine, University of Sharjah, Sharjah, United Arab Emirates
e-mail: humaid.al-shamsi@medportal.ca

F. Iqbal
Burjeel Cancer Institute, Burjeel Medical City,
Abu Dhabi, United Arab Emirates
e-mail: Faryal.iqbal@burjeelmedicalcity.com

© The Author(s) 2025
H. O. Al-Shamsi (ed.), *Healthcare in the United Arab Emirates*,
https://doi.org/10.1007/978-981-96-0523-1_1

UAE. Please note that the titles of Arabic books have been translated into English in the references section. Consequently, these titles may not be easily found in English searches. We have included the international book standard number (ISBN) where available to assist with accurate referencing.

1.2 Introduction

This chapter focuses on the Trucial States (the United Arab Emirates (UAE)) and their division into three regions, i.e., Abu Dhabi, Dubai, and the Northern Emirates, and provides an overview of the historical development of healthcare services within these regions.

This chapter highlights the challenges and early efforts to develop healthcare in these regions, emphasizing the influence of traditional healing practices and the role of key individuals:

- *Emirate of Abu Dhabi.*
- In the 1950s, Abu Dhabi faced a lack of healthcare infrastructure and hospitals. Traditional healing methods, such as herbal medicine, Quranic healing, and traditional healers, were prevalent. Individuals like Paul Harrison and Sheikh Shakhbut bin Sultan Al Nahyan played key roles in early healthcare development [2, 7–9].
- *Emirate of Dubai.*
- In the early twentieth century, American missionaries attempted to provide medical services but faced challenges due to the strong British presence. British efforts led to the establishment of the Al Maktoum Hospital in 1943. Private clinics, including one run by Dr. Muhammad Habib al-Ridha, also contributed to healthcare [4].
- *Northern Emirates.*
- The Northern Emirates had lower income levels and fewer social services in the 1960s. Healthcare relied on traditional and herbal medicine, with traditional practitioners playing a significant role. Missionaries had a limited presence, and some clinics were established, such as the one run by Dr. Sara Hosmon in Sharjah. Notable traditional healers included Ahmed Salem bin Mazroui, Ahmed Abdulrahman Al-Nibari, Muhammad Hassan Al-Mahmoudi, and Obaid Mosbeh bin Touq [1, 6].

This history of UAE healthcare also highlights the world of missionary work, primarily focused on Christian missions aimed at converting non-Christian populations, especially within the Islamic world [1, 10]. Missionaries, who predominantly came from the Christian faith, employ various means of evangelism, both direct and indirect, to propagate their beliefs. These methods have evolved into structured disciplines taught within Christian churches, adapting to the societies they aim to impact. Direct means involve full-time missionaries and general Christian outreach, including individual missionary work and public preaching about Jesus. Additionally, auxiliary missionary aids like medical services, education, subtle methods (i.e., hidden evangelism), national contexts, and printed materials play essential roles in spreading the Christian message. This also sheds light on missionary goals in the Arabian Gulf, where the region's strategic significance attracted missionaries. They pursued both religious and political objectives, seeking religious conversion without coercion, and gaining support from Western governments, notably the United States, to secure access to the region, particularly in the context of oil exploration and concessions. This chapter provides valuable insights into the complex nature of missionary work in the Arabian Gulf [1, 2, 4].

Missionary activities in the Trucial States featured distinctive aspects, including a strong focus on education and healthcare [11, 12]. Missionaries prioritized the establishment of medical centers and educational institutions as crucial entry points for their work, capitalizing on the relative lack of infrastructure in these areas during the early days of their missionary presence [4]. Their goal was to positively influence Gulf citizens through education and healthcare services. Additionally, missionaries introduced exposure centers, originally launched in Iran, to promote modern principles of disease treatment and healthcare in the region. While full conversion to Christianity may not have always been achieved, missionaries successfully advanced modern healthcare practices in the Gulf region [1, 11].

The contributions of prominent missionaries are highlighted in the Trucial States for their evangelical efforts:

- Dr. Paul Harrison: A Johns Hopkins University graduate, Dr. Harrison went beyond medical services to promote Christian evangelization and the teachings of Christ. He focused on modernizing traditional medicine and establishing modern medical practices in the Gulf region [1, 4].
- Samuel Zwemer: A renowned missionary, Zwemer extensively worked along the Trucial States' coast and in the Gulf region. As one of the founders of the Arab mission, he spent a decade exploring regions previously unvisited by foreigners. Zwemer was well-versed in medicine and Arabic literature and authored important books about the Arabian Peninsula, including "The Arabian Peninsula, the Cradle of Islam," first published in 1921 [1, 10].
- Dr. Kennedy: Dr. Kennedy gained fame as a doctor in the Trucial States, notably in Al-Ain and the Buraimi oases. He established the Oasis Hospital in Al Ain, providing medical care alongside his wife, Marian Mayer. Dr. Kennedy also played a significant role as the medical coordinator for Sheikh Zayed bin Sultan and medical institutions, recruiting other doctors to work at Dr. Tom's Hospital [1, 10].
- Medical Staff: In some missionary hospitals, nurses held positions of equal importance to doctors due to their vital role in healthcare provision. Nurses like Gertrude Dyke (Latifa) were renowned for their contributions. Dr. Sarah Hosmon, despite eventually resigning from the mission, operated a clinic in Sharjah with the support of the Arab mission and was highly regarded in the northern regions of the Trucial States [1, 9].

The establishment of the Oasis Hospital, and many more, was one of the most important and prominent missionary hospitals in the Trucial States from 1949 to 1971:

- Al-Waha (Oasis) Hospital.
- The Oasis Hospital, a significant missionary medical institution in the Trucial States from 1949 to 1971, was established as Al-Waha (Oasis) Hospital in Al

Ain, the capital of the Eastern Region of the Emirate of Abu Dhabi [9]. Its inception was influenced by the favorable experiences of Sheikh Zayed bin Sultan, the Ruler's Representative in Al Ain, with missionary hospitals in Muscat and Bahrain. Dr. Kennedy, a missionary, was invited to explore the feasibility of establishing a comprehensive hospital offering various medical services in Al Ain. Despite the geographical distance from the capital, Abu Dhabi, the establishment of Al-Waha Hospital marked the beginning of a focus on public health in the emirate. While the hospital was affiliated with the Anglican Church (United Anglican Church), Dr. Tom, associated with the Arab Mission in Muscat, collaborated with the Abu Dhabi government in its establishment. It's worth noting that, although not directly affiliated, there was cooperation between different missionary organizations with similar goals in this endeavor [1, 2, 5].
- Collaboration with Sheikh Zayed.
- The establishment of the Oasis Hospital in Al Ain began with an invitation from Sheikh Zayed bin Sultan to Dr. Dame, aiming to create a comprehensive hospital serving Al Ain and neighboring areas. Dr. Kennedy, accompanied by Dr. Raymond, visited Sheikh Zayed, resulting in an agreement on the hospital's medical mission and establishment. Subsequent visits by doctors and the arrival of necessary equipment marked significant milestones in the hospital's development. This missionary hospital in Al Ain was established through collaborative efforts between missionaries, including Dr. Kennedy, and the local government, specifically Sheikh Zayed bin Sultan. It played a pivotal role in providing essential medical services in the region during the specified period [1, 9].

Two missionary clinics in the Trucial States were also built; details about their establishment [1, 2, 5], services, and missionary activities are given below [9]:

- Sarah Hosmon Clinic in Sharjah.
- The Sarah Hosmon Clinic in Sharjah was established by Mrs. Sarah Hosmon, a missionary from Kentucky, who faced financial and missionary challenges while working with the Arab mission in the Gulf region. She opened the clinic in Sharjah, serving patients from Sharjah and nearby Trucial States from 1926 to 1943. However, due to the challenging circumstances in the Gulf and inadequate support, the clinic temporarily closed. Mrs. Hosmon independently returned in 1952 and reopened the clinic, gaining recognition among the local population. Located near the old market in Sharjah, the clinic offered various medical services, including obstetrics, gynecological care, pediatrics, and general medical care. It collaborated with the Umm Daniel clinic in Ras Al Khaimah and Oasis Hospital in Al Ain. The clinic received some support from the Arab mission but primarily relied on patient fees and assistance from Dr. Kennedy of Oasis Hospital to sustain its operations [1, 2, 5].
- Umm Daniel Clinic in Ras Al Khaimah.
- The Umm Daniel Clinic in Ras Al Khaimah was established during the 1950s by Dr. Helen, known as Umm Daniel. This clinic primarily focused on providing obstetrics and gynecological care, and Dr. Helen played a crucial role in delivering babies in

the region, issuing birth certificates for many newborns in the coastal areas of Ras Al Khaimah. Initially constructed with fronds, the clinic received support from the Ras Al Khaimah government for upgrades. Dr. Helen managed the clinic with assistance from her husband and a small administrative staff, and the prices for medical services were kept affordable for the local population. While Dr. Helen conducted missionary work, introducing women to the Christian religion and distributing religious pamphlets, these efforts did not result in conversions [1, 6, 9].

Despite the missionary activities, the Islamic faith of the local population remained steadfast in its adherence to Islamic values and traditions. Dr. Helen eventually returned to America in the late 1970s, leaving behind a lasting medical legacy among the people of Ras Al Khaimah [5, 6].

1.3 British Health Services in the Trucial States

1.3.1 British Interest in Health Conditions in Dubai

In the initial stages, a cordial relationship existed between the British government and the Arab mission in Dubai. However, the British government developed an interest in the missionary societies' success in garnering public support and offering medical services, which were seen as a means to secure American oil concessions in the Trucial Emirates. Reports by British officials, including Mr. Latch and Mr. Fawle, underscored the significant role played by the mission in the region. These reports initiated discussions regarding the necessity of responding to these missionary activities through healthcare initiatives in the Trucial Emirates. This shift in perspective marked a change in the British government's approach to the missionary presence in the region [5].

1.3.1.1 Establishment of Al Maktoum Hospital
The establishment of the first clinic in Dubai was attributed to Dr. Muhammad Yasin, a retired Indian doctor, in 1938 [2]. Plans to create a comprehensive hospital in Dubai began in 1949, with Dr. McCauley actively involved in liaising with the British government for its establishment. This hospital featured 38 beds and was funded jointly by the British government and the Trucial States, with a notable contribution from Sheikh Saeed bin Maktoum [1, 2, 5]. Administrative guidance and financial support were provided by the British government, which also expressed keen interest in the hospital's operations and financial aspects through official communications. Discussions among members revolved around matters such as hospital equipment, medicine availability, and concerns about its remote location, which made it costly for some residents to reach [10].

1.3.1.2 Financial Matters
The British government's growing interest in healthcare services in Dubai and the establishment of Al Maktoum Hospital was evident. Initial uncertainty surrounded

the total cost required for the hospital. Due to financial constraints and insufficient local contributions, the British government considered withdrawing its support for the hospital in April 1953, as efforts to raise funds locally fell significantly short of the required budget [1, 10].

The British government recognized the financial challenges faced by Al Maktoum Hospital in Dubai and the need for increased support due to several reasons. These reasons included the necessity to expand the medical staff, especially Pakistani nurses, to handle critical cases effectively [1]. The hospital also required funds for paying salaries to two qualified nurses, purchasing an X-ray machine as previously agreed, acquiring additional medical equipment to replace an outgoing Pakistani surgeon, activating the nutrition department, and hiring a special cook to provide proper meals for patients. Dr. Mackenzie and Sir Eric, delegates from the Department of Health, Ministry of Foreign Affairs, recommended an overall increase in the hospital's requirements, prompting the need for more financial support [1, 10].

The British government emphasized the importance of local support for the hospital, suggesting that it should match or exceed British support since the hospital served all residents of the Trucial States. The goal was to encourage increased financial cooperation between the British government and local rulers, not only to sustain existing hospitals but also to promote the establishment of more healthcare facilities in the region [10]. The medical staff at Al Maktoum Hospital underwent regular changes due to the growing number of patients, primarily employing staff from Pakistan and India, facilitated by the British Colonial Office. However, local residents were not actively recruited for medical roles, and concerns arose within the British government regarding the payment of salaries to local visiting doctors and surgeons [1, 2, 5].

The British government encountered challenges in financing visiting doctors and surgeons at Al-Maktoum Hospital, and there were plans for their rehabilitation, as suggested by the British Political Resident in Bahrain through Dr. McCauley [2, 10]. Additionally, there was a proposal to increase the medical staff in anticipation of opening new medical facilities in other Trucial States similar to Al-Maktoum Hospital, involving the use of doctors from the British Royal Air Force and the hiring of qualified Pakistani nurses. However, this proposal was postponed due to potential administrative and financial burdens. This plan marked the beginning of a modest interest in British medical services in the Trucial States, especially in areas distant from Dubai and lacking transportation options. Al-Maktoum Hospital achieved success and brought significant changes to medical services in the Trucial States by introducing modern medicine and reducing reliance on traditional medical methods, as indicated by recorded numbers and statistics showing positive results [1, 2].

Since its opening, the hospital has consistently experienced an increasing daily attendance rate, with signage directing people to the facility contributing to this trend. The hospital handled a wide range of medical cases, including minor and major surgeries. In 1952, it recorded 45 operations, including 8 major surgeries and 37 medium-to-simple ones, showcasing its effectiveness in performing major operations with qualified doctors. The hospital also had rooms equipped for intensive care, with 10 beds allocated for such cases. While some patients initially left treatment after the first session due to limited awareness of the new treatment system, it was expected that this attitude would change as patients became more accustomed to the hospital's services [1].

The hospital handled general injuries, including severe cases, and a smaller percentage of patients with diarrhea, eye and skin diseases, and common ailments. Notably, in 1952, the hospital's intensive care unit treated cases ranging from double fractures, skull fractures, and lung complications to high fever, nervous spasms, and gunshot injuries. This underscores the hospital's vital role in providing healthcare in the region, particularly in addressing the widespread issue of malaria [1, 10].

Dr. McCauley attempted to collaborate with the Red Cross to provide medical supplies and establish joint clinics in the Trucial States, leveraging the Red Cross's prior involvement in the region during World War I. The Red Cross expressed willingness to cooperate but set specific conditions, including a maximum one-year commitment and the requirement for Al Maktoum Hospital to provide housing and transportation for their personnel. However, the project did not materialize due to concerns about its financial cost and logistical challenges. The British Health Office did not support the idea, leading to the Red Cross canceling all proposals to provide aid to the Trucial States [10].

During the period of British medical services at Al-Maktoum Hospital (1954–1964), there was stability in financial support, developmental initiatives, and a growing demand for hospital services from residents of Dubai, the Trucial States, and neighboring areas. The hospital's general budget experienced decisions to reduce some treatment fees and increase financial support from the rulers of the Trucial States, resulting in financial and administrative stability. In 1956, the hospital's financial gains enabled the establishment of new clinics and a library for women's rooms. Additionally, there was a proposal to hire a specialized financial accountant to ensure precise financial management, which the council agreed to [1].

The British government's direct financial support for the hospital ended in 1964, with funding responsibility shifting to the Trucial States Development Office [10].

1.3.2 Al Maktoum Hospital Administrative Matters (1954–1964)

During the period from 1954 to 1964, Al Maktoum Hospital underwent various administrative developments aimed at improving healthcare services in the Trucial Emirates. In 1954, there were attempts to abolish patient fees by the Ruler of Sharjah, but this proposal faced challenges due to the crucial role these fees played in supporting the hospital's finances. The British government expressed concern about the potential impact of fee abolition on the hospital's budget, particularly after purchasing an X-ray machine in the same year. In 1956, several new projects and constructions were planned for the hospital, including building a new residence for nurses, acquiring new medical equipment, implementing pharmacist training, exploring a public health pilot project, and requesting additional medical equipment for the following year's budget. These initiatives aimed to enhance healthcare services and infrastructure at Al Maktoum Hospital, aligning with the broader goal of providing British services in the Trucial Emirates [1, 10].

During this period, the British government initiated several improvements and collaborations to enhance Al Maktoum Hospital's facilities and services. These efforts involved constructing new housing for nurses, expanding existing hospital buildings to create additional rooms, and adding a kitchen and warehouse to enhance the hospital's capabilities. Moreover, a British company known as Dubai-B-B participated by funding four beds in one of the hospital's wards. These collaborative initiatives between the government and British businesses showcased a coordinated approach to delivering medical services, with contributions from commercial entities. The goal was to enhance access to healthcare services and facilities in the region [1, 2, 5].

In 1958, Sheikh Rashid bin Saeed issued a decision to restrict the use of unauthorized narcotic substances, impacting the hospital by limiting the use of certain medicines and narcotics by doctors and pharmacists. Dr. McCauley discussed this issue with Sheikh Rashid, and they agreed that medical narcotics could only be used by pharmacists with Dr. McCauley's approval. However, a challenge emerged when Sheikh Rashid requested a list of approved narcotic substances from Dr. McCauley. This decision had both positive and negative aspects, ensuring qualified professionals but affecting clinics and medical points within Al Maktoum Hospital. To resolve the issue, the British Political Resident in Bahrain sent Mr. Marcel W.F. Marcel to Dubai in December 1958. After discussions, the problem appeared to be resolved, with no indications of increased issues, suggesting that the decision was either canceled or amended [1].

In 1959, development work commenced at Al Maktoum Hospital, encompassing the completion of the radiology department, renovations in the operating rooms, the establishment of special rooms for hospital staff, and various other enhancements. An air-conditioning system was installed in the operating rooms, although it encountered technical issues that required assistance from the British Navy for repair. British envoys made regular visits to the hospital in the following years, producing reports that assessed the hospital's facilities and administrative processes [1]. These reports often included recommendations for expanding the hospital's buildings and improving its services. In a report authored by Mr. Hawley, several expansion recommendations were put forth for Al Maktoum Hospital [2]. These recommendations encompassed tasks such as generating a cost estimate for the expansion, reviewing the plans with reference to Mr. Harris, modelling the expansion after hospitals like the Tangier Rural Hospital in Dar es Salaam, and exploring proposed financial resources for the expansion [1, 2, 5].

In 1962, there was a significant effort to procure narcotics to prevent a potential crisis in meeting demand [1]. Substantial funds were allocated for this purpose, and the responsibility for purchasing narcotics rested with the Crown Agents. However, challenges arose related to the quality of the materials procured and the local government's adoption of these materials. Dr. McCauley's ability to address these issues was limited due to his numerous responsibilities. The year 1964 marked the final year of joint health services between the British government and the rulers of the Trucial States [1, 2]. During a 1964 meeting, it was decided to establish a new eye clinic at Al Maktoum Hospital, with an estimated cost of 23,250 pounds. Following this year, the responsibility for healthcare services would be transferred to the Development Office of the Board of Governors of the Trucial States, signifying the conclusion of the collaborative healthcare arrangement [1].

1.3.2.1 Healthcare at Al Maktoum Hospital (1954–1964)

During this period, Al Maktoum Hospital experienced a substantial rise in patient visits, drawing individuals from all the Trucial States. The hospital's growing popularity led to some patients receiving free treatment [2]. In 1957, the inpatient clinic treated 337 patients, marking an increase from 305 in 1956 and 143 in 1955. Notably, more than half of the male patients in 1954 received free treatment [1, 9].

The outpatient clinics at Al Maktoum Hospital also saw a significant increase in patients, treating a total of 14,513 individuals in 1957, compared to 10,522 in 1956. Out of those treated, 14,153 received free medical care, with 12,868 of them benefiting from free treatment. Additionally, 6511 people received vaccinations, and 95 children were born at the hospital, a notable increase from the 69 births in 1956. Most patients came from various Trucial States, with the majority originating from the Emirate of Dubai, likely due to the hospital's location in that emirate [2].

In 1959, Al Maktoum Hospital witnessed a significant surge in patient attendance across all its clinics, primarily driven by the growing population of the Trucial States, especially in Dubai. The hospital recorded a total of 2497 patients seeking medical care in its clinics [2]. Notably, a substantial number of women sought treatment, indicating an increasing awareness of the importance of hospital care among the local population. The internal clinics in 1959 admitted 485 patients, including 246 women, with 265 patients receiving free treatment [10]. This marked a significant increase in the number of inpatients compared to previous years, highlighting the hospital's expanding medical services. However, the hospital administration faced challenges with some patients not following prescribed dietary plans and medical advice regarding food choices. Malnutrition became a concern, particularly for patients without relatives to provide proper nutrition. The absence of a central hospital kitchen contributed to this issue [9].

In 1959, the outpatient clinic at Al Maktoum Hospital provided medical care to 30,375 patients in the morning period, with an additional 13,827 patients attending outpatient clinics at health points in Dubai. A significant majority, 28,782 out of 30,375 patients, received free treatment, and many of them came from economically disadvantaged backgrounds, including Pakistani and Indian students in Dubai's foreign and government schools [10]. The hospital's maternity department experienced notable growth, recording 142 births in the year, with 104 being natural deliveries and 23 requiring surgical intervention. This increase was attributed to mothers following nurses' advice and reducing certain traditional practices after childbirth. Additionally, the Operations Department conducted 21 major surgeries and 208 minor surgeries, often resulting from car accidents, which had seen an increase. The hospital also took measures to prevent the spread of infectious diseases in 1959, with the absence of major outbreaks. Some minor diseases were monitored, and the

Prevention Department conducted tests on municipal workers handling spoiled vegetables to mitigate potential health risks [10]. A few cases of influenza and bacterial infections were treated to prevent further transmission to the local population [1, 2, 5].

In the 1960s, Al-Maktoum Hospital experienced a surge in patient visits, particularly for smallpox vaccinations due to the prevalence of smallpox in the Trucial States. The outpatient clinic and affiliated medical points were busy, with a significant number of patients, especially women and children, seeking smallpox vaccinations. The year 1960 witnessed an increase in cases of appendicitis, leading to more surgical operations, including 22 major surgeries and 296 minor operations, with well-equipped and air-conditioned operating rooms [1, 10]. The presence of women in the internal clinics exceeded that of men, prompting considerations for expanding the women's wing, and the maternity department saw a rise in births, with 145 deliveries [1]. Various diseases were prevalent in 1960, including seasonal illnesses in children, a malaria epidemic, tonsil infections, ringworm, eye and ear problems, rheumatism, muscle conditions, and gastrointestinal diseases. Accidents, particularly car and construction accidents related to alcohol and drug abuse, were common [1]. Efforts were made to prevent epidemic diseases, including smallpox vaccination and pest control measures in places like the fish market and narrow lanes between homes. In 1961, cases of epidemic diseases like cholera were reported, leading to cooperation between the hospital and airport authorities to implement proper inspection and prevention measures for travellers [1, 6].

In 1962, the Political Agent in Dubai requested 50,000 doses of anti-smallpox vaccine to prevent epidemics, but only a portion of the request was fulfilled due to limited supply [1]. In 1964, the outpatient clinic recorded an attendance of 49,060 patients, with significant support from Sheikh Rashid bin Saeed, the Ruler of Dubai, who inaugurated a new outpatient clinic building. The internal clinics admitted 5492 patients, including 615 receiving free treatment. The women's section delivered 140 babies, with a total of 1094 births since 1955 [1]. The year also saw 30 major operations, 328 minor operations, and 1259 x-ray cases. These developments indicated the ongoing contributions of British Medical Services to Al-Maktoum Hospital, aligning with the growing population and healthcare needs of Dubai and the Trucial States. British support was instrumental in addressing various health challenges in the region [6].

1.3.3 British Health Services in the UAE

During the 1950s and 1960s, British medical services played a pivotal role in expanding healthcare access and services in the Trucial States, with a particular focus on Dubai and Al Maktoum Hospital [1]. This collaboration between the Council of Rulers of the Trucial States and the British government reflected a shared commitment to improving public health. In 1953, British Political Resident Robert Hay expressed a desire to enhance social services, leading to initial discussions with the Red Cross about establishing medical centers with British support. However, these plans were eventually discontinued after agreements were reached between the rulers and the British Political Agent in 1954. Subsequently, there was a growing recognition of the importance of collaboration in decision-making, resulting in significant developments in medical services. This included the opening of new clinics like the Dibba Clinic and the Khorfakkan Clinic in 1959, further contributing to improved healthcare infrastructure and access in the region [1, 2].

In 1960, the Trucial States witnessed significant advancements in healthcare accessibility and services due to the collaborative efforts of British medical services and the Council of Rulers. With ten clinics dispersed across the region, the healthcare hub of Reliance House, staffed by dedicated nurses and visiting physician Dr. Abdul Majid, played a pivotal role, attending to a substantial number of patients within a brief period [1]. In 1959 alone, the region treated over 19,000 patients, emphasizing the growing importance of healthcare services. The partnership between British medical services and the Council of Rulers led to the establishment of new clinics in 1960, where visiting doctors cared for 15,633 patients, addressing various ailments, including intestinal and respiratory conditions, malaria, skin disorders, and seasonal illnesses. This expansion involved the opening of clinics in different emirates, including Sharjah, Ras Al Khaimah, Ajman, Abu Dhabi, Al Buraimi, Dibba, and Kalba, thus significantly enhancing healthcare access. Furthermore, the establishment of 11 pharmacies further strengthened the healthcare infrastructure in the Trucial States [1, 2].

The expansion of British medical services in the Trucial States during the 1960s played a crucial role in fostering acceptance of modern medical treatment among residents. Educational publications and medical guidance were disseminated to emphasize the importance of contemporary healthcare [2]. By 1963, British clinics were treating a significant number of patients facing various ailments, including the emerging challenges of cancerous tumors and appendicitis [1]. This collaborative effort between the British government and the Trucial States resulted in substantial improvements in healthcare infrastructure and accessibility across the region. Nevertheless, the absence of female doctors capable of performing gynecological operations posed a notable challenge. In response, the British government and the Council of Rulers acknowledged the necessity of implementing future measures to integrate a female medical staff to address the healthcare needs of women attending public clinics [2].

The majority of expenses during this period were attributed to the salaries of visiting doctors in the Trucial Emirates, with the Council of Rulers of the Emirates sharing a significant portion of these costs in accordance with their prior agreement with the British government. A notable portion of the expenditure was directed toward combating malaria and procuring essential equipment, underscoring the significance of disease control measures. In 1964, visiting doctors in the Trucial States put forth recommendations stressing the importance of investing in clinics and expanding healthcare services across cities and villages in the Emirates. Their emphasis was on addressing infectious diseases, particularly in regions with abundant agricultural crops and livestock, to curb their spread. These recommendations were presented to the Political Commissioner in the region and the Council of Rulers of the Trucial States as a means to enhance healthcare services throughout the area [1].

1.3.3.1 British Health Services Ras Al Khaimah Hospital (1962–1964)

In 1961, the concept of establishing a hospital in Ras Al Khaimah was initiated by the Council of Rulers of the Trucial States, with an initial budget of £10,000 earmarked for its planning and construction. Initially, two engineers from Halcrow were tasked with the project, envisioning a small six-bed clinic and pharmacy. However, due to their other commitments, responsibility for construction was transferred to Mr. Marker's company. For the fiscal year 1962, a specific budget was allocated to meet the hospital's administrative and medical needs, including salaries for doctors, pharmacists, nurses, transportation, narcotics, emergency reserves, fuel, maintenance, office expenses, medical clothing, housing for medical staff, additional beds, washbasins, and decoration [1]. British field visits were conducted to monitor the hospital's progress, with Dr. Anderson noting issues like the informal acceptance of money by a Pakistani doctor from patients despite free treatment, leading to a recommendation for his replacement. In 1963, Ras Al Khaimah Hospital received financial support from the Council of Rulers of the Trucial States and philanthropists like Mr. Abdullah Darwish, gaining recognition as an essential component of British services in the Trucial Emirates amid competition from Kuwaiti medical services introduced in 1963 [9].

1.3.3.2 Health Services in the Emirate of Abu Dhabi and the Importance of Dr. Corksel's Report (1964)

Under the leadership of Sheikh Zayed bin Sultan, the Emirate of Abu Dhabi played a crucial role in supporting the Development Office of the Trucial States. In 1968, Sheikh Zayed made a substantial contribution of two million pounds sterling, the largest ever made by a Trucial States ruler, significantly bolstering the Development Office's treasury and enabling increased development work while settling previous project dues [1]. In 1964, Dr. Corkill conducted a comprehensive health assessment in Abu Dhabi and its dependencies, identifying various health issues such as high infant mortality rates, indigestion, anemia, malaria, and more. He recommended the establishment of an integrated hospital in Abu Dhabi, with a preliminary estimated cost of 400,000 pounds [1]. The proposed hospital was designed to offer various medical facilities but was not confirmed as realized in the available sources [2]. Dr. Corkill's recommendations encompassed a range of health initiatives, including the appointment of a health authority official, provision of first aid boxes, distribution of health guidebooks, vaccination programs, improved birth and death registration, and raising awareness of health-related issues like fish trading and marriage age restrictions [1, 2, 5, 6]. Although implementing some recommendations might have been challenging, Dr. Corkill's thorough report held the potential for positive impacts on healthcare and health awareness in the region if executed [1].

1.3.4 British Health Collateral Services in the Trucial States

1.3.4.1 British Oil Companies

The British made concerted efforts to extend healthcare assistance to the Trucial States through collaborations with British institutions and oil companies operating in the region. The Abu Dhabi Company for Onshore Oil Operations (ADCO) established a modest desert clinic in the Juwaizah area to cater to its petroleum crew and provide medical aid to the Bedouins in the Emirate of Abu Dhabi [1, 2, 5, 6]. Petroleum companies like the Abu Dhabi Petroleum Company were actively involved in delivering medical services and contributing to health development programs. They maintained clinics with dedicated doctors like Dr. Khan and Dr. Afzad, serving both company employees and local residents. Dr. Salem, affiliated with the Abu Dhabi Petroleum Company, ran a clinic in the Emirate of Abu Dhabi, offering medical services and insights into local health conditions. Dr. Salem's contributions were instrumental in shaping Dr. Corkill's final report on health conditions in Abu Dhabi [1, 2].

1.3.4.2 British Royal Forces

The British extended various auxiliary healthcare services in collaboration with the British Royal Forces in the Trucial States, involving the establishment of three small clinics across all the Trucial States [1]. The British Accreditation House in Dubai set up a clinic for the Royal Air Force. Furthermore, the British Royal Air Force facilitated the transfer of medical cases from its medical headquarters in Al Maktoum Hospital to other military medical points in locations like Bahrain, Doha, Kuwait, and Bombay. Collaborating with the Oman Coast Force, the British Royal Forces provided medical aid during health crises, including assisting the Pakistani community affected by smallpox in 1963 [1, 2, 5, 6]. They also worked alongside health offices in the UAE to combat locust infestations, manage outbreaks of diseases like smallpox, and address issues related to the proliferation of weapons. This collaborative effort led to the establishment of a military medical center in the region, contributing to the success of various development projects [2].

1.4 Kuwaiti Health Services in the Trucial States (1962–1970)

Neighboring states, including Kuwait and Saudi Arabia, played a significant role in the social development of the Trucial States, offering both government and individual aid. Governmental support came in the form of assistance from countries like Kuwait and Saudi Arabia, while social organizations, merchants, and affluent individuals from the Gulf region provided individual support. This aid covered various areas, including healthcare and social services in the Trucial States. Some notable individuals involved in providing aid include Mr. Zaki Yamani, the Saudi Minister of Petroleum, and Mr. Abdulhadi Taher, a prominent employee of the Saudi Ministry of Petroleum. In addition, Mr. Abdul Latif Al-Hamid, the Secretary of the Kuwaiti Economic Development Fund, and Mr. Suleiman Al-Mutawa, Deputy Secretary General of the Social and Economic Organization in the Middle East, were among those offering assistance from Kuwait [1, 2]. Local government aid in the Arabian Gulf region played a crucial role in the development of the Trucial States, with various offices and organizations representing different countries offering support:

- Kuwait State Office: The Kuwaiti Development Office in Dubai was instrumental in overseeing development initiatives in the Trucial States. It was involved in constructing and maintaining hospitals, clinics, and schools. Additionally, it actively contributed to the social life of the Trucial States by employing local communities in educational and healthcare facilities [1, 2].
- The Social and Economic Institute for Development in the Middle East: An independent Kuwaiti organization also played a role in the development of the Trucial States, focusing on infrastructure development [1, 2, 5, 6].
- League of Arab States: The Arab Economic Union had intentions of providing assistance to the Arab Gulf and the Trucial Emirates. Although plans were considered and funds allocated, this initiative was not implemented, partly due to opposition from Britain [1, 2, 5].
- Country Development Office: The State of Qatar expressed interest in the development of the Emirate of Dubai, driven by familial ties between ruling families. However, there is no evidence of continued interest from the Qatari government [1].
- Development Office for the Trucial States: Kuwait's government played a significant role in providing social services, including health and education, to the Trucial States, especially during the oil boom of the 1950s. Kuwait initiated support for clinics and schools in neighboring countries in 1952. In 1962, Kuwait sent specialists to assess the region's economic and social conditions and allocated part of its annual budget for social assistance to the Trucial States. This support led to the establishment of clinics across the Trucial States and significant improvements in healthcare services [1, 2, 9].

1.4.1 The Relationship of the British Government with the Kuwaiti Health Services in the Trucial States

The British government closely monitored Kuwait's efforts to provide healthcare services in the Trucial States, fearing that it might undermine British services and local public opinion regarding the modest assistance provided by the Council of Rulers of the Trucial States. Kuwait showed readiness to hire British doctors and experts for the Trucial States' medical staff, potentially diverting attention from British healthcare services [1, 2, 5, 6]. Kuwait expanded its healthcare services significantly in 1963, with hospitals and clinics in key cities [1, 10]. Although there were concerns about competition, the British government believed there was no major threat to their services and even anticipated potential cooperation between British and Kuwaiti health services. Despite aiming to reduce Kuwait health support, the balance of Arab support for the Trucial States and political differences limited broader Arab collaboration, with Kuwait remaining the primary supporter of health services in the region [1, 2].

1.4.2 The Relationship of the American Administration with the Kuwaiti Health Services in the Trucial States

The US administration was attentive to developments in the Gulf region and foreign efforts to support the Trucial States [10]. It aimed to enter the developmental movement in the area to balance domestic and foreign support and reduce competition between various actors. In 1965, the US ambassador to Kuwait engaged in talks with Kuwaiti officials, indicating US interest in understanding and potentially participating in regional development efforts. By February 1967, the American Consul in Dhahran reported on Kuwait's role in the Trucial States and its impact on American and British interests, suggesting the possibility of joint American and British support to counter Kuwait's growing role [2]. However, it is important to note that the report may have exaggerated the situation, as competition for influence among regional actors was complex, and the support from the Kuwaiti government may not have been as significant as suggested in the report. The proposed British-American partnership aimed to protect common interests, including obtaining commercial and petroleum concessions in the Gulf [1, 2].

1.4.3 The Relationship of the Trucial States Council of Rulers with the Kuwaiti Government in Providing Health Services

The relationship between the Council of Rulers of the Emirates and the Kuwaiti government was characterized by fraternity and shared goals, emphasizing Arabism. Although medical services entered the Trucial States, there was a time lag in the requests for this aid, except for Abu Dhabi. Initially, Dubai also delayed accepting Kuwaiti aid due to British involvement in development projects, including healthcare [1, 2, 5, 6]. In 1965, the ruler of Fujairah requested a clinic from the Kuwait office, highlighting Kuwaiti medical services' effectiveness. The emergence of Kuwaiti medical services coincided with the establishment of the Development Office of the Council of Rulers of the Trucial States, leading to the suggestion of joint work in public health [1]. This marked the decline of British support for health and social services in the Trucial States, as the British government saw no urgent need to compete with Kuwait, given the absence of significant involvement from other Gulf governments and the lack of British-American cooperation in the region's development [1, 2].

1.4.4 Kuwaiti Clinics: Trucial States

All Kuwaiti clinics in the Trucial States were managed by the Kuwait office, established in 1962, with its director based in Dubai overseeing their administration [1, 2, 5, 6]. The medical staff in these clinics included doctors, specialists, and other personnel, and the budget for their salaries and medical expenses was allocated by the Kuwait office. By 1967, there were nine Kuwaiti clinics spread across all the Emirates of the Trucial States [1, 2].

1.4.4.1 Kuwait Central Hospital in Dubai

The Kuwaiti Central Hospital in Dubai is a significant medical facility in the Trucial States. It started as a small clinic in 1962 but expanded and reorganized to become a central hospital with 119 beds [10]. The Emir of the State of Kuwait, Sheikh Sabah Al-Salem Al-Sabah, inaugurated this hospital during his visit to the Trucial States in May 1966. This development established the Emirate of Dubai as having access to top-tier medical services, including the Kuwaiti Hospital and the Al Maktoum Hospital, managed by the Trucial States Office for Development in 1966 [1, 2]. The Kuwaiti Hospital in Dubai includes several main departments, namely:

- The Department of General and Orthopaedic Surgery: The Department of Surgery and Orthopaedics at the Kuwaiti Hospital in Dubai has 31 beds, divided between general surgery wards for men and women, as well as orthopaedic wards for both genders. There has been a significant increase in patient visits over the years, with 1968 recording 6550 treatments, 1969 with 8212 treatments in the men's department and 1624 cases in the women's and children's ward, and 1970 seeing 8419 treatments in the men's department and 1990 cases in the women's and children's wards [1, 2]. This department primarily served men, and the increase in patient numbers in 1970 can be attributed to the accessibility of Kuwaiti clinics in the Trucial States [10].
- The Department of Obstetrics and Gynaecology: The Department of Obstetrics and Gynaecology at the Kuwaiti Hospital in Dubai played a significant role in directing women to the women's clinic in Dubai, where free medical treatment was provided. The maternity department had limited bed capacity, with just one bed dedicated to childbirth and four beds in the honor-of-birth section, while the women's wing had 19 available beds [1].
- The Ophthalmology Department: The Ophthalmology Department at the Kuwaiti Hospital has 12 beds, evenly distributed between male and female wings. However, during the months of July and August each year, the department experiences reduced activity as the ophthalmologist is on annual leave during this period. This leads to a lack of significant operations or activities during these months, as indicated by statistics from 1968 to 1970 [1, 2].
- Orthopaedics Department: The Orthopaedics Department at the hospital consists of eight beds, evenly distributed between male and female wings. This department experiences a consistent flow of patients throughout the year and operates as one of the busiest outpatient clinics in the hospital. Over the years 1968–1970, it averaged 6680 patients annually. Unlike the Eye Clinic, the Orthopaedics outpatient clinic maintains continuous activity during the summer months, despite having an equal number of specialists in both clinics. During the same period (1968–1970), the Eye Clinic performed the highest number of operations in 1970, with 273 operations, compared to the lowest recorded in 1967 with 185 operations. General anesthesia was predominantly used in these operations, accounting for 85% of all procedures each year [1, 2].
- Department of Internal Medicine: The Internal Medicine Department at the hospital consists of 18 beds, with 12 beds in the men's wing and 6 beds in the

women's wing. This department sees a higher proportion of female patients compared to male patients. Over the years 1968–1970, the department recorded a relatively high number of deaths, particularly in the "Al-Batiniyah" category, with approximately 62 deaths during this period. The highest number of deaths occurred in 1969, reaching 31. These deaths are primarily attributed to the challenge of managing internal diseases, and there may be limitations in the competence of internists in dealing with incurable illnesses [1].

- Children's Department: The Paediatrics Department at the hospital was established in March 1970 and is equipped with 12 beds and 3 incubators for underdeveloped children. It has seen a significant number of child patients, with a total of 13,043 children admitted. The month of March, when the department opened, saw the highest number of child admissions, highlighting the community's need for such a department in Al-Kuwaiti Hospital. Unfortunately, the department also witnessed child mortality cases in the same year, with a total of 40 child deaths, and the month of December recorded the highest proportion of deaths among children [1].
- The Department of Anaesthesia: The Kuwaiti Central Hospital in Dubai features an Anaesthesia Department that plays a crucial role in performing operations and procedures, particularly in the General Surgery Department and the Obstetrics Department in the women's clinic. Specialists in the Anaesthesia Department determine the appropriate type of anesthesia, whether local or general, for each operation. In 1968, the Anaesthesia Department recorded a total of 626 anesthesia cases, with the highest number of cases performed in the General Surgery Department, reaching 177 cases. The hospital's overall anesthesia cases for that year amounted to 1388 cases. This highlights the significant role played by the Anaesthesia Department in the Kuwaiti hospital in Dubai in supporting various medical procedures [1, 2].
- Laboratory Department: The Laboratory Department in the hospital is responsible for conducting examinations and analyzing patient samples, and it plays a vital role in healthcare clinics. In 1969, the department examined 20,741 samples, and the highest number of samples were examined in 1970, totaling 25,181 samples. These figures underscore the department's significance in supporting various hospital departments by providing essential examinations. The department also features a reserve blood bank, which is crucial for assisting the hospital's operating rooms. In 1970, 691 blood bags were used, with the highest consumption occurring in September, when 75 bags were utilized. Conversely, the lowest consumption of blood bags was in 1968, with 165 bags used, reflecting the reduced number of operations compared to 1970 [1, 2].
- School Health Department: The School Health Department of the Kuwait Hospital in Dubai, established in August 1970, plays a vital role in providing health services to Kuwaiti schools in the Trucial Emirates. Its responsibilities include conducting comprehensive medical examinations for first-grade students, operating school health outpatient clinics, referring students to specialists, admitting students to hospitals when necessary, and examining teachers and educational staff. Additionally, the department supervises students' nutrition, estab-

lishes health associations in schools, controls diseases, administers vaccinations, organizes laboratory visits for students, assists with age estimation for students without birth certificates, and provides health supervision for examination committees. Overall, the department significantly contributes to the health and well being of students in Kuwaiti schools in the Trucial Emirates [1, 10].
- Health Education Department: The Health Education Section in Kuwaiti hospitals, established in 1970, plays a crucial role in promoting health awareness and education among the residents of the Trucial States. This section, based in the Kuwaiti Hospital, utilizes innovative methods and visual education to raise awareness about infectious diseases and common health issues. Collaboration with Kuwait State TV in Dubai allows for the broadcasting of health documentaries, contributing to health education. Additionally, health associations in Kuwaiti schools within the Trucial Emirates work with educators to provide health guidelines, lectures, seminars, and immunization programs, offering a comprehensive approach to health education not seen in British hospitals in the region. The Kuwaiti government's support and unilateral decision-making by the Kuwait Office have been key to the success of these initiatives and the establishment of Kuwait TV in Dubai as a significant media outlet in the region during that period [1, 2, 5, 10].
- Preventive Health Department: The entry of medical services in the Trucial States coincided with the prevalence of infectious diseases like smallpox, malaria, and cholera. In 1970, a section dedicated to preventing infectious diseases was established, with collaboration between the Kuwait Office and the Development Office in the Trucial States. Significant progress was made in controlling infectious diseases, especially malaria, by 1970, thanks to joint efforts. In 1970, approximately 60,000 people across the Trucial States were vaccinated against infectious diseases, with temporary vaccination centers set up in various locations. Kuwaiti medical centers actively participated in vaccinating Kuwaiti school students in the Trucial States, focusing on diseases like smallpox, measles, and polio. These coordinated vaccination campaigns, conducted by both Kuwaiti medical centers and the Development Office, played a crucial role in rapidly reducing the incidence of infectious diseases, with a particular focus on Kuwaiti schools to streamline vaccination efforts [1, 2].

1.4.4.2 The Kuwaiti Clinic in Bur Dubai

The Kuwaiti clinic in Bur Dubai, established in 1963, primarily provided dental services, including tooth extractions, fillings, X-rays, gum treatment, denture fittings, and handling cases of jaw fractures and nerve removal [1, 5]. Tooth extractions were the most common service, with 5144 cases in 1970 alone, indicating high demand. Treatment of jaw fractures was relatively rare, with an average of just two cases per year. The clinic saw a consistent annual increase in the number of visitors, with a higher percentage of men seeking treatment compared to children and women [1, 2, 9].

1.4.4.3 Umm Suqeim Clinic for Chest Diseases

The Umm Suqeim Chest Clinic in Dubai was established in 1969 and specialized in chest diseases. It had 65 beds, with 29 for men, 16 for women, and 10 for children. The clinic predominantly served male patients, admitting 150 in 1970, while female patients numbered 48. The clinic also recorded the highest death rate among male patients, with 12 deaths in the same year [1].

1.4.4.4 The Kuwaiti Clinic in Ras Al Khaimah

The Kuwaiti clinic in Ras al-Khaimah, established in 1963 and later moving to its own building in 1967, became a significant healthcare provider in the Emirate of Ras al-Khaimah. It was managed by medical staff, including doctors, some on scholarships from Egypt and Oman, and operated as a public clinic, although it did not handle complex cases due to limited facilities and road connections to nearby hospitals. The Kuwaiti office paid salaries in Qatari-Dubai riyals, with doctors earning about 750 Qatari riyals—Dubai, and pharmacists receiving 250 Qatari riyals—Dubai in 1968 [1, 2].

A new clinic with 18 beds was established within the Kuwaiti Hospital in Ras al-Khaimah, equally divided between male and female sections. The Kuwait office also constructed three villas for the clinic's medical staff. The clinic's pharmacy played a vital role in handling medications and preparing doses according to medical standards. Despite the presence of several clinics in old Ras al-Khaimah, there was little apparent cooperation among them. However, the concentration of clinics in the area made healthcare services more accessible to the people of the emirate without the need to travel to hospitals in other emirates. The majority of patients came from the coastal areas of old Ras Al Khaimah, while residents of mountainous regions tended to prefer the British Hospital due to its location. Despite the increased patient load, the clinic reported very few deaths, with only one recorded in 1970, indicating a good record of patient care and safety [1, 2].

1.4.4.5 Kuwaiti Hospital in Sharjah

The Kuwaiti Hospital in Sharjah began as a dispensary in an old mud-built Arab house in January 1963, providing basic medical services. The dental clinic at the hospital served not only Sharjah residents but also patients from other emirates, referred from different Kuwaiti clinics in the Trucial States. The medical and administrative staff included doctors who rotated among various Kuwaiti clinics in the region, showcasing the collaborative and developmental efforts of the Kuwaiti government in nurturing national medical professionals in Dubai and Sharjah. For example, doctors like Dr. Khalil worked in multiple clinics within the same year, serving different emirates, including Ajman, Umm Al Quwain, Sharjah, and Dubai [1, 2].

The Kuwaiti Hospital in Sharjah relocated to a new building in March 1971, and this expansion included the addition of a maternity department with 10 beds [2]. While it had certain limitations and did not handle virgin birth cases, it marked a significant development for the hospital. The clinic offered various medical services, including an anesthesia department, but certain specialized services like maternity and dental procedures requiring general anesthesia were not provided.

The medical staff at the Kuwaiti Hospital in Sharjah was the largest among Kuwaiti hospitals and comprised professionals from Oman, the Trucial Emirates, and other Arab countries. They were sponsored and paid by the Kuwait office, with doctors receiving a salary of 750 Qatari-Dubai riyals or equivalent in Kuwaiti dinars or Bahraini dinars, while nurses and pharmacists received 250 Qatari riyals—Dubai. Administrative employees received 350 Qatari riyals—Dubai, and all staff members enjoyed a 30-day annual leave and an annual bonus of 30 Qatari riyals (Dubai) [1, 2, 5].

The Kuwaiti Hospital in Sharjah played a vital role in creating job opportunities for residents of the Trucial States, eliminating the need to hire medical personnel from outside the region. This approach not only accommodated local medical and administrative staff but also provided educational opportunities that could lead to job prospects [1]. In contrast, British Medical Services often imported staff from Britain, India, and Pakistan, limiting the involvement of Trucial States residents with these clinics. The dental clinic at the new hospital served patients of all ages, including men, women, and children, treating a consistent number of patients each year. Notably, the number of patients, particularly among women and children, exceeded that of men in all the years covered in the data, mainly due to the presence of a maternity department in the hospital. This reduced the percentage of women seeking treatment in other medical centers, including those in Sharjah and Dubai [1, 2].

1.4.4.6 The Kuwaiti Hospital in Ajman

The British government initially considered establishing a clinic in Ajman but abandoned the idea due to the presence and activities of Kuwaiti medical services in the area. Instead, British clinics were set up in more remote areas like Falaj Al Mualla, Masfoot, and Al Dhaid. The Kuwaiti clinic in Ajman opened in two phases [1, 2].

First Phase The Kuwaiti clinic in Ajman was established on January 19, 1963, initially as a simple dispensary located in the house of a Kuwaiti benefactor named Mr. Murshid Al-Osaimi. This house had nine rooms designated for housing teachers associated with the Kuwait office, while one room was dedicated to establishing the Kuwaiti dispensary. The clinic included essential facilities such as a doctor's room, a nursing room, a pharmacy, and an administrative room. The clinic's staff in Ajman were rotated, with doctors being assigned to different clinics across the Trucial Emirates by the Kuwait office [1, 2].

Second Phase The Kuwaiti clinic in Ajman relocated to a new building in February 1969, which included a maternity ward with seven beds. The clinic provided medical services to men, children, and women, with the highest number of new patients in 1970 being women and children, totaling 7608 patients, while men had 6217 new patients. This clinic played a crucial role in providing healthcare services to Ajman, where medical facilities were limited, and the British health services were primarily focused on other areas outside the UAE [1, 2].

1.4.4.7 Kuwaiti Hospital in Umm Al Quwain

The Kuwaiti clinic in Umm Al Quwain was established on February 11, 1963, and its presence led British medical services to focus on remote areas in the Trucial States. The clinic initially had basic facilities with a room for the doctor, a nursing room, and a pharmacy. Dr. Jaafar Al-Afghani, who also worked in the Ajman clinic, served both areas, along with other medical and administrative staff. These employees received salaries similar to those in other Kuwaiti clinics in the Trucial Emirates. The clinic operated for five hours in the morning and three hours in the evening, possibly to accommodate doctors from other Kuwaiti clinics. In January 1969, the clinic moved to a new building with 12 beds, and it saw a significant increase in the number of patients treated in 1969, with 17,254 patients compared to 13,500 in 1968, which was attributed to the new facilities and expanded services [1, 2, 5].

1.4.4.8 Kuwaiti Hospital in Khorfakkan

The Kuwaiti Hospital in Khorfakkan, which opened in 1963 and expanded in 1970, played a crucial role in providing healthcare services to the East Coast, including Omani regions in the Al Batinah Plain. In 1970, the hospital treated 38,806 patients, highlighting its strategic location and effectiveness in serving the region. The hospital also made significant efforts to address malaria cases in the area, collaborating with the development office in the Trucial States to reduce malaria outbreaks, with a peak in June and July 1970 but a subsequent decline. These efforts aimed to combat infectious diseases in areas prone to their spread due to agricultural and pastoral activities [1, 2].

1.4.4.9 The Kuwaiti Hospital in Fujairah

In 1965, at the request of the Ruler of Fujairah, a dispensary was constructed in the Trucial States, opening in 1979 to alleviate the patient load on the Kuwaiti Hospital in Khor Fakkan. In 1970, the dispensary admitted 36,910 patients, complementing the services of the Kuwaiti Hospital [1]. Kuwait made significant contributions to healthcare in the Trucial States, fostering local medical professionals in Sharjah, Ajman, and Dubai, contrasting with limited support from Britain. Kuwait's presence diminished the prominence of British health services, and their collaboration with the Development Office effectively controlled infectious diseases. These efforts highlighted Kuwait's aid and cooperation with the Trucial States in various development initiatives, leaving a positive historical legacy [1, 2].

1.5 Local Health Services in the Trucial States

1.5.1 The Health Services of the Development Office in the Trucial States Council of Rulers (1965–1971)

In 1965, the Council of Rulers in the Trucial States took over control of the Development Office, previously managed jointly with the British Accreditation House office. This transition resulted from annual meetings between the Trucial States' rulers and British authorities overseeing development services in the region

[1]. The change enhanced the efficiency of the development office and led to notable advancements in healthcare services along the coast, ensuring continued support for Al Maktoum Hospital and Ras Al Khaimah Hospital, both established in 1963 [9].

1.5.2 Contributions of the Development Office of Al Maktoum Hospital (1965–1971)

In 1965, Al Maktoum Hospital in the Trucial States experienced significant developments and changes. It expanded its facilities to accommodate a growing number of patients from Dubai and neighboring countries, reflecting the region's healthcare progress and population growth. The hospital treated a high volume of patients, with over 54,000 at the outpatient clinic. The maternity department saw an increase in births, signaling a shift away from home births. Additionally, the hospital performed numerous surgeries, radiology procedures, and administered vaccinations to combat contagious epidemics. Financially, contracts were renewed, and there were discussions about sharing health spending between Abu Dhabi and Dubai. However, debates about increasing fees for certain medical services raised concerns about the hospital's reputation, particularly among middle- and lower-income patients. In 1967, the hospital continued to serve patients from various Trucial States and neighboring countries, solidifying its reputation in the Arab Gulf region [1, 2].

In the late 1960s, Al Maktoum Hospital in the Trucial States underwent significant expansion and development. Public spending for these improvements amounted to £170,000, shared equally between the Dubai government and the Development Office in the Trucial States. Key enhancements included the creation of new clinics, expansion of medical facilities, establishment of a vaccination center, and the addition of a medical library. In 1969, plans for a special surgical suite and a new building with modern amenities were proposed. By 1970, Sheikh Rashid bin Saeed took full sponsorship of the hospital, transferring it to the Health Department in the Emirate of Dubai [10]. This marked the end of support from the Emirates Development Office, and the hospital continued to expand and improve its services under local management. The administrative responsibilities of the Development Office eventually transitioned to the Ministry of Health of the United Arab Emirates in 1971 [9].

In Dubai, there were several healthcare facilities in 1970, including the following [1, 2, 5]:

1. Al Maktoum Hospital in Deira, with approximately 134 beds and an additional 20 beds added in 1971.
2. The Kuwaiti Hospital in Deira, which had 67 beds.
3. Dubai Clinic, a children's clinic established in May 1979.
4. Al Qusais Pediatric Clinic.
5. Al Safa Children's Clinic.
6. Two hospitals were under construction in Dubai in 1970:

- The Iranian Hospital, with 100 beds, completed construction in 1971.
- Rashid Hospital, which includes 393 beds, was under construction, and its work was completed in 1972, as it was expected to be the largest hospital in the region alongside Bahrain Hospital in Bahrain and Karachi in Pakistan.

The Dubai government was keen on establishing Rashid Hospital and fostering administrative cooperation between Rashid Hospital and Al Maktoum Hospital to ensure accessibility for all citizens [10]. They also explored collaboration with the Iranian Hospital in Dubai, with plans to allocate it to the Satwa area, known for its significant Iranian community. Additionally, Dubai had a comprehensive plan to distribute ambulances and set up first aid medical points, aiming to enhance accessibility to both Al Maktoum Hospital and Rashid Hospital, ensuring easy access to medical services for the residents of Dubai [9].

1.5.3 Contributions of the Development Office of Ras Al Khaimah Hospital (1965–1970)

Despite the reduction in British financial support, Ras Al Khaimah Hospital continued to receive medical consultations from the British government through the Political Accreditation House [1, 10]. The Development Office, in collaboration with Sheikh Saqr bin Muhammad, the ruler of Ras Al Khaimah, played a significant role in supporting the hospital. In 1965, the Council allocated funds for development work, focusing on renewing medical staff and hiring new doctors. Interestingly, there were no plans to modify the hospital building, as visiting doctors found the existing facilities sufficient for accommodating patients in Ras Al Khaimah, unlike Al Maktoum Hospital, which faced a growing patient population due to Dubai's increasing population [1, 2].

In 1967, the Development Office allocated £2000 for the development of Ras Al Khaimah Hospital, and plans were made to establish a nursing institute at a cost of £110,000. By 1969, there was remarkable growth in the number of patients and visitors to the hospital, leading to increased support from the Hospital Development Office. New medical equipment was acquired, and substantial sums were allocated for development projects, totaling £146,000 in public expenditure on the hospital. Key projects included purchasing advanced medical equipment, improving medical administration, air-conditioning the hospital building, and providing housing for the growing medical staff, marking a significant milestone in the hospital's development [1].

In 1970, further development efforts at Ras Al Khaimah Hospital involved an additional £70,000 investment. This led to significant changes in the hospital's main building, the completion of air-conditioning work for specific rooms, the finalization of the medical staff building project, and the completion of the outpatient clinic's development. After the establishment of the Emirates Federation in 1971, the hospital became part of the Ministry of Health and was renamed Saif Bin Ghobash Hospital, later known as Obaid Allah Hospital, marking the end of the Development Office's role in providing health services at the hospital [1, 2].

1.5.4 Contributions of the Development Office in the Trucial States (1965–1971)

The Development Office played a significant role in providing medical services to the Trucial States, including Al Maktoum Hospital and Ras Al Khaimah Hospital. Differences in the size of the Trucial States affected the establishment of new clinics, field visits by the Development Office, and the role of visiting physicians who treated patients and assessed each clinic's operations [1]. In 1965, the Development Office allocated £200,000 for public services, including medical services in the Trucial States. A portion of this funding, £25,256, was designated for clinics within the Trucial States, and an additional £3000 was set aside for visiting doctors in Fujairah, in response to a request from the ruler of Fujairah to improve medical services in the emirate. Plans also included constructing a new clinic building in Fujairah and considering the establishment of a hospital between Kalba and Khorfakkan to enhance healthcare accessibility [1, 2, 5].

Efforts to develop medical services in the Trucial States faced challenges, particularly during the scorching summer months when doctors found it challenging to travel to remote areas due to extreme heat. To address this issue, visiting doctors like Dr. Assem Al-Jamali [1] and others played a vital role in delivering medical care during their tours, ensuring that healthcare services were still accessible to residents in those regions despite the harsh weather conditions [2].

In 1965, clinics in Al-Huwailat and Al-Faya had a good turnout despite opening earlier that year. However, the Falaj Al Mualla Clinic faced challenges, particularly in September, due to a shortage of visiting doctors. The Fujairah Clinic in October also lacked doctors because they were on summer vacation. The schedule for the last months of 1965 was not recorded due to the annual meeting of the Council of Rulers of the Trucial Emirates in November 1965. During the 1966 annual meeting, various development aspects, including a currency change and budget allocation, were discussed. Additionally, the ruler of Fujairah expressed concerns about the pharmacy in the Fujairah clinic, suggesting the need for measures to address the improper use of narcotic substances by medical staff [1].

In 1967, the Development Office continued its support for medical services in the Trucial States. During the annual meeting, administrative changes in the medical section of the Development Office were discussed, including the appointment of Mr. Horn Blow as the Chief of Public Health in the Trucial States [4]. Administrative matters, such as enacting laws to combat malaria and establishing a mental illness clinic, were also addressed. Financial matters for the year 1967 were reviewed, with significant expenditures allocated for contracts with doctors and medical staff, development work, and matters related to the medical staff of the Development Office. The highest portion of expenses went to contracts for doctors and medical staff due to the increasing presence of medical staff across the Trucial States, especially at Al Maktoum Hospital and Ras Al Khaimah Hospital, despite significant development work in these hospitals [1, 2, 5].

In 1967, development work continued in various medical centers across the Trucial States, with visiting doctors treating a significant number of patients during their tours. This indicated growing acceptance of modern treatment in clinics and facilitated the Development Office's efforts to expand health services [4]. The accession of Sheikh Zayed bin Sultan Al Nahyan to power in Abu Dhabi in 1966 strengthened the Development Office's role in the Council of Rulers of the Trucial States. Financial assistance of two million pounds from Abu Dhabi enriched the Development Office's treasury, supporting infrastructure projects. A surplus in 1968 led to additional development initiatives, including the construction of new clinics, expansion of health centers, and improvements in Al Maktoum and Ras Al Khaimah Hospitals.

In 1969, the budget for the Development Office doubled to five million pounds sterling, underscoring its effective role in the Trucial States' development. Key developments included purchasing an ambulance for Umm Al Quwain Clinic, expanding the Shaam Health Clinic, establishing the Abu Musa Island Clinic, and enhancing the surgical ward at Al Maktoum Hospital. A population increase in Dubai led to the consideration of a new hospital project, Rashid Hospital. Additionally, the Development Office expressed interest in developing medical centers in Sharjah, allocating £720,000 to projects that encompassed the Sharjah Health Center, Al Dhaid Health Center, Kalba Clinic, and Abu Musa Island Clinic in 1969 [1].

1.5.5 Sharjah Health Center

In 1969, the Development Office played a pivotal role in establishing a significant medical center in Sharjah, regarded as one of the Emirate's most important medical facilities at the time. This center was affiliated with the Sharjah Medical Center, with expenses evenly shared between the Government of Sharjah and the Development Office of the Trucial Emirates. The construction of the center occurred in multiple stages: the first phase costing £177,000 was completed in 1969, followed by the second phase amounting to £390,000, and the third phase requiring £185,000, which was allocated in a subsequent budget, marking the final stages of the center's development [1, 2, 5].

In 1970, the construction costs for both the center building and the outpatient building of Sharjah Hospital amounted to over 372,000 pounds, with the Development Office contributing half of this amount. This support allowed for the allocation of funds to other health services in Sharjah and the Trucial States. Sharjah Hospital, officially opened in 1970, featured 50 beds with the potential for future expansion to accommodate an additional 100 beds. Despite an initial agreement for the Development Office to cover half of the hospital's costs, it only contributed 400,000 Qatari riyals-Dubai, while the Government of Sharjah covered the remaining expenses. This limited contribution was attributed to the hospital's excessive purchase of medical equipment, some of which was intended for storage, despite the need for annual updates. Further expansions to Sharjah Hospital were not planned in the 1970 budget to avoid straining the Development Office's budget [1, 2].

1.5.6 Al Dhaid Health Center

The Al Dhaid Health Center was established to address the healthcare needs of the Al Dhaid area, following the experience gained from the Al Dhaid Clinic-Falaj Al Mualla. Initially, it was designed to have 30 beds, but approval was given for a smaller building with six beds, along with accommodation for the on-duty medical staff. An allocation of £65,000 was made for the center's establishment, with funds allocated for building construction (£30,000), the medical staff dormitory (£25,000), and medical equipment (£10,000) [1, 2].

1.5.7 Kalba Clinic

A new, fully equipped medical clinic was established in the city of Kalba, with the capacity to accommodate four patients. The clinic had night-shift medical staff, indicating that it operated 24/7 to provide medical services. An ambulance was also provided for the clinic's use. The total budget allocated for all activities and facilities at the clinic amounted to £15,000 [1, 2].

1.5.8 Abu Musa Island Clinic

In 1970, the final year of the Development Office's administration in the Trucial States, there was a significant increase in public spending on health services, totaling 74,605 Qatari riyals-Dubai, the second-largest allocation of funds after education. This increase was driven by efforts to expedite the completion of health clinic buildings in Sharjah, Ras Al Khaimah, and Dibba, to meet specified deadlines. Notably, Dibba Hospital was under construction, with contracts awarded to construction companies, and it was expected to open officially in 1971 following the arrival of medical equipment. Additionally, development projects on Abu Musa Island, including a medical clinic and a school, were budgeted at £15,000 and were planned to continue into the next financial year, with a combined cost of £30,000 [1–3, 5].

1.5.9 Contributions of the Development Office in the Fight Against Infectious Diseases in the UAE (1965–1970)

Since 1960, the Trucial States grappled with recurring infectious disease outbreaks, often stemming from a lack of local awareness about diseases like smallpox, cholera, and malaria. However, in 1965, the British Health Services began providing advice and guidance to the Emirates Council of Rulers on the necessity of bolstering the Health Services Department to combat these health crises. This marked a significant effort to address infectious disease issues in the Trucial States, with the Health Department of the Development Office taking charge of healthcare development initiatives in 1965 [1–3, 5].

1.5.10 The Most Important Health Crisis Faced by the Development Office in the Trucial States

1.5.10.1 Smallpox Infection

In the 1960s, smallpox posed a significant health threat in the Trucial States. To combat this outbreak, the Trucial States, in collaboration with the Emirates Council of Rulers, followed the advice of the British government and launched a vaccination campaign primarily targeting expatriate workers from Pakistan and India, especially those working in hospitals. This campaign successfully vaccinated around 31,990 individuals across the Trucial States, with Dubai recording the highest vaccination rate, covering 21,719 people [1, 2, 5, 10]. In 1965, the Development Office supplied Al Maktoum Hospital with smallpox vaccines, resulting in the vaccination of 5167 individuals against smallpox and 1171 against cholera. The hospital played a crucial role in providing vaccinations, especially to residents and travelers arriving at Dubai Airport from regions where these infectious diseases were prevalent [1–6].

In 1967, despite previous efforts to control smallpox, new cases emerged in the Trucial States. A patient from southern India was diagnosed with smallpox upon arriving in Dubai, leading to the transmission of the disease to medical staff at the hospital. A similar outbreak occurred in Sharjah, where a child was infected by a Pakistani worker who had been keeping the child at home without treatment. To address the situation, the Development Office authorized Al Maktoum Hospital to take immediate action against smallpox, distributing 112,000 boxes of smallpox vaccine across the Trucial States. Dubai received the largest share of these vaccines due to its high population density and the significant number of Indian and Pakistani workers passing through Dubai Airport. Despite the challenges posed by the crisis, the Development Office allocated funds to establish a private clinic for infectious diseases at Al Maktoum Hospital in 1978. Cooperation from the Indian and Pakistani governments was limited, prompting local authorities to take proactive measures to combat the disease [1, 2, 5, 9].

1.5.10.2 The Spread of Malaria

In the Trucial States, the malaria crisis was a significant challenge, exacerbated by stagnant water in ponds resulting from seasonal rains. In 1966, heavy rains in the Al-Munai'i and Al-Hawailiyah areas raised concerns about the spread of malaria [1, 2, 5, 6]. The Development Office, in conjunction with the Agricultural Office in Ras Al-Khaimah's Al-Daqqa area, took measures to prevent malaria's spread. They initiated a project to establish protective systems for farms in Wadi Al-Manei and Al-Hawilat, with a total cost of 10,000 pounds. To combat malaria comprehensively, the Development Office sought cooperation with international health organizations. These organizations were invited to conduct a study and develop a budget to address malaria in the eastern coastal regions, representing a modern approach to tackling epidemics in the Trucial States [5].

In May 1970, the International Malaria Organization, in collaboration with the Development Office, initiated a study to combat malaria in the Trucial Emirates. A medical team composed of specialists in infectious diseases and preventive medicine was formed, and they were given housing and administrative support. The team established a base in Khorfakkan to serve the eastern coast, which was particularly vulnerable to malaria. They conducted extensive tours across various areas of the Trucial States, equipped with necessary medical equipment, with support from the Development Office. Alongside malaria control, the World Health Organization's preventive medicine team trained local medical personnel in blood sample collection and testing. The Nursing Institute, established in 1970 with the Development Office's support, played a crucial role in enhancing healthcare services and facilitating this training in the Trucial States [1, 2, 5, 6].

1.5.11 The Council of Rulers of the Trucial States and Treatment Abroad (1963–1969)

The Emirates Development Office generally did not send patients abroad for medical treatment, but historical records show a few exceptions where individuals from the Trucial States received medical care overseas, often coinciding with rulers' visits to foreign countries. These instances include Sheikh Ahmed Al Mualla of Umm Al Quwain receiving diabetes treatment in London in 1963, Sheikh Mohammed bin Hamad Al-Fujairah seeking medical treatment in Beirut in 1963, a Dubai trader sending his son for treatment in London in 1963, Sheikh Zayed bin Sultan undergoing medical examinations in London in 1963, and Sheikh Rashid Bin Saeed's visit to observe British medical services in London in July 1969, which ultimately led to the establishment of Dubai Hospital in Dubai [1–6, 10].

1.5.12 Contributions of the Development Office for Veterinary Clinics in the Trucial States

1.5.12.1 Veterinary Clinics
The Development Office in the Trucial States expanded its efforts to include the development of veterinary clinics, recognizing the importance of maintaining livestock health for food security. Veterinary clinics were strategically established in the Digdaga area, which had a significant livestock population and was in proximity to pastoral and agricultural farms in Ras Al Khaimah. Dr. Asli, who joined in September 1970, played a key role in overseeing veterinary services, with two sections established to cover the Eastern Province and Sharjah regions, each led by a respective veterinarian. These efforts aimed to address livestock health and epidemics in the Trucial States [5].

1.6 Conclusion

The development of medical services in the Trucial States involved various actors, including American missionaries, the British government, and the Kuwaiti Development Office. While American missionaries established clinics and hospitals in the region, their efforts to promote Christianity had limited success. The British government played a modest but important role in establishing hospitals and clinics, with a focus on administrative excellence and cooperation with the Council of Rulers. Kuwait's entry into the healthcare sector led to a shift in the healthcare landscape, with Kuwaiti hospitals gaining popularity among residents and changing the dynamics of healthcare provision. The Development Office played a pivotal role in expanding medical services, with a focus on domestic treatment and controlling infectious diseases. Their unique initiative in establishing veterinary clinics addressed the healthcare needs of both humans and animals in the Trucial States. Overall, the development of healthcare services in the Trucial States was marked by diverse efforts and collaborations, with each actor contributing to the evolving healthcare landscape [1–6, 10].

Conflicts of Interest The authors have no conflicts of interest to declare.

Appendix

British Political Resident and Political Agent	The distinction between these two titles is clarified. The Political Commissioner holds a more influential position within the British political commission, typically based in one of the Trucial States, like Dubai or Abu Dhabi. These commissioners are akin to consuls in the present day. They are all part of a larger British administrative authority known as the British Political Residency, overseen by the Political Resident. This residency was originally located in Bahrain in the Persian Gulf region after relocating from Bushehr. It served as a link to the British government, specifically the British Foreign Office, and in essence, performed a role similar to that of an embassy in any other country
Trucial States	The term "Trucial States" is frequently used throughout the book chapters, referring to the region that is now recognized as the United Arab Emirates. Various alternative terms were also used historically, including "the pacified coast," "the Trucial Coast," "the Trucial Emirates Coast," or "the Omani Coast." however, the most common and earliest definition found in British documents is "the Trucial States," which remained in use until the establishment of the United Arab Emirates on December 2, 1971
Rupees	The currency circulated by the residents of the Trucial States was not an official currency, but an optional currency and served as an intermediary between the seller and the buyer. This currency was not minted by one of the rulers in the Arab Gulf, but the lack of an instrument currencies made this currency easy to trade as it came with Indian merchants coming from India to buy pearls with it, and the surplus of the currency difference remained and was used locally in that period, until the Qatar-Dubai riyal was used later in Dubai, Sharjah, and the northern regions, while the Bahraini dinar was used in the Emirate of Abu Dhabi.

References

1. History of health services in the Trucial States, 1949–1971, Faisal Mohammed Abdulla Almandoos, 1st edition, 2009. ISBN: 9789948151746.
2. Health services in the Trucial Coast, Aref Alshaikh, 2012. https://www.tawyeen.com/tword/?p=15972
3. https://atlas.fgic.gov.ae/uaeatlas/Health/HealthcareHistory. Accessed 2 Aug 2024.
4. Arabian Gulf digital archive. https://www.agda.ae/%D8%A7%D9%84%D8%B9%D8%B1%D8%A8%D9%8A%D8%A9/folder/%D8%A8%D8%AF%D8%A7%D9%8A%D8%A7%D8%AA-%D8%A7%D9%84%D8%B1%D8%B9%D8%A7%D9%8A%D8%A9-%D8%A7%D9%84%D8%B5%D8%AD%D9%8A%D8%A9-%D9%81%D9%8A-%D8%A7%D9%84%D8%A5%D9%85%D8%A7%D8%B1%D8%A7%D8%AA. Accessed 2 Aug 2024.
5. Health services in the Emirates… from traditional medicine to international ones. https://www.emaratalyoum.com/life/four-sides/2015-03-22-1.767537. Accessed 2 Aug 2024.
6. «Health services in the Emirates» documents and history. https://www.albayan.ae/culture-art/heritage/2022-12-15-1.4580248. Accessed 2 Aug 2024.
7. Children, Rafaa and Wars of Demand in the Emirates, Abu Dhabi, UAE, The Cultural Foundation, 1997, p. 53.
8. Letter of Sheikh Shakhbut bin Sultan to the British Political Resident 2 Bahrain on 11/18/1934, in Ghobash, Rafia and others, previous reference Research and Documentation Center, Abu Dhabi.
9. Ghobash R, et al. Medicine in the Emirates, United Arab Emirates Abu Dhabi. The Cultural Foundation; 1997.
10. History of health services in Dubai. https://jbhsc.ae/%D8%AA%D8%A7%D8%B1%D9%8A%D8%AE-%D8%A7%D9%84%D8%AE%D8%AF%D9%85%D8%A7%D8%AA-%D8%A7%D9%84%D8%B5%D8%AD%D9%8A%D8%A9-%D9%81%D9%8A-%D8%AF%D8%A8%D9%8A/. Accessed 2 Aug 2024.
11. Von DA. Christian presence in the Gulf region. Leicester: Islamic Foundations; 1981. p. 19.
12. Ibrahim, Okasha Ali Features of the Christianization of the Arab World. Riyadh – Kingdom of Saudi Arabia, Imam Muhammad bin Saud University Islamic, 1987, p 26.

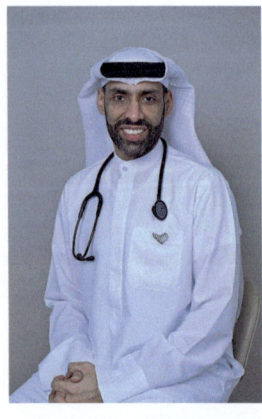

Professor Humaid Obaid Al-Shamsi is the Chief Executive Officer of Burjeel Cancer Institute in Abu Dhabi, UAE; President of the Emirates Oncology Society; Visiting Professor at Harvard Medical School at Harvard University; Visiting Scientist at Dana-Farber Cancer Center, Harvard Medical School, Boston, USA; Full Professor of Oncology at Ras Al Khaimah Medical and Health Sciences University; Ras Al Khaimah, UAE; an Adjunct Professor of Oncology at the College of Medicine, University of Sharjah; and Clinical Professor at Gulf University, Ajman, UAE. He is the first Emirati to be promoted as a professor in oncology in UAE history. He is also the Chairman for Colorectal Cancer in the MENA region, appointed by the prestigious National Comprehensive Cancer Network® in the USA. He is also the only member of the Lung Cancer Policy Network in the MENA region, which aims to advance lung cancer research and screening globally. He is the Chairman of the Oncology and Hematology Fellowship Training Program for the National Institute for Health Specialties in the United Arab Emirates. He is also the only member in the GCC in the WIN Consortium, which comprises organizations representing all stakeholders in personalized cancer medicine globally.

He is board-certified in both internal medicine and oncology from the UK, the USA (ABIM), the National Board of Physicians and Surgeons in the USA, and Canada (FRCPC). He has also been awarded the FRCP (Canada) in 2012, FRCP (London) in 2023, FRCP (Glasgow) in 2024, and FRCP (Edinburgh) in 2025. He is the only physician in the UAE with a subspecialty fellowship certification and training in gastrointestinal oncology and the first Emirati to complete a clinical post-doctoral fellowship in palliative care. He was an Assistant Professor at the University of Texas MD Anderson Cancer Center between 2014 and 2017. He has published more than 170 peer-reviewed articles in *JAMA Oncology, Lancet Oncology, Journal of Clinical Oncology, The Oncologist, BMC Cancer,* and many others. His area of expertise includes precision oncology and cancer care in the UAE. In 2016, he published with his group from MD Anderson in the *Journal of Clinical Oncology* a study describing a new distinct subgroup of colorectal cancer, NON-V600 BRAF-mutated colorectal cancer. In 2022, he published the first book about cancer research in the UAE and also the first book about cancer in the Arab world, both of which were launched at Dubai Expo 2020. *Cancer in the Arab World* has been downloaded more than 500,000 times in its first 2 years of publication and is the ultimate source of cancer data in the Arab region. He also published the first comprehensive book, *Cancer Care in the United Arab Emirates*, which is the first book in UAE history to document cancer care in the UAE, with many topics addressed for the first time. The book was also another success with over 100,000 downloads in the first 2 months of publication.

He is passionate about advancing cancer care in the UAE and the GCC and has made significant contributions to cancer awareness and early detection for the public using social media platforms. He engages actively with the public through awareness campaigns and serves on numerous national health committees, including with the UAE Ministry of Health and the Department of Health, Abu Dhabi.

He is considered the most followed oncologist in the world, with over half a million followers across his social media platforms (Instagram, Twitter, LinkedIn, and TikTok). In 2022, he was awarded the prestigious Feigenbaum Leadership Excellence Award from Sheikh Hamdan Smart University for his exceptional leadership and research, and he was also awarded the Sharjah Award for Volunteering. He was also named the Researcher of the Year in the UAE in 2020 and 2021 by the Emirates Oncology Society.

In May 2024, HH Sheikh Mansour bin Zayed Al Nahyan, Vice President of the United Arab Emirates, awarded him first place in the Emirati Talent Competitiveness Council (NAFIS) program for outstanding leadership in the private sector across all business and medical disciplines. In February 2025, he was awarded the *Sheikha Fatima bint Mubarak Family Award* for being a successful role model in UAE society.

As CEO of Burjeel Cancer Institute, he is leading the largest cancer network in the UAE with over 30 oncologists and hematologists and built the first pediatric bone marrow transplant program in the UAE. He secured the UAE's first European Society for

Medical Oncology (ESMO) accreditation for a cancer center in the UAE at Burjeel Cancer Institute.

Besides his clinical and administrative duties, he is engaged in education and various levels of research training for medical trainees to enhance their clinical and research skills. He established the UAE's first hematology and oncology fellowship training program accredited by the UAE National Institute for Health Specialties at Burjeel Cancer Institute.

His mission is to advance cancer care in the UAE and the MENA region and make cancer care accessible to everyone in need around the globe.

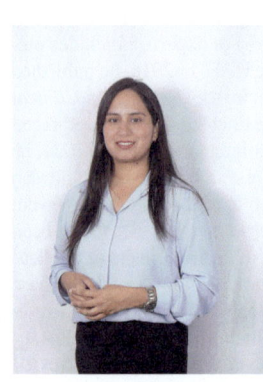

Ms. Faryal Iqbal is the Research Manager at Burjeel Cancer Institute, Burjeel Medical City in Abu Dhabi, UAE. She earned her undergraduate degree in Molecular Biology & Biotechnology, followed by a postgraduate qualification in Molecular Genetics in Pakistan, where her thesis explored the association between XRCC1 gene polymorphism and radiation exposure in healthcare workers. At Burjeel Cancer Institute, she is deeply involved in shaping the institute's research landscape. Her role extends beyond managing data and coordinating clinical studies; she mentors medical interns, supports scientific writing, and contributes significantly to the academic and editorial aspects of cancer research.

She is the co-editor of *Cancer in the Arab World*, the first comprehensive book covering cancer care across all Arab countries. The book has resonated widely across the region and beyond, gathering over half a million downloads within just two years. She has authored numerous peer-reviewed publications and contributed to at least ten book chapters, with her research interests rooted in oncology, hematology, and genetics.

In recognition of her growing contributions to the field, she was honored with the "EOS Research Award" by the Emirates Oncology Society in September 2023, an accolade that reflects both her professional excellence and her passion for advancing cancer research in the region.

Open Access This chapter is licensed under the terms of the Creative Commons Attribution 4.0 International License (http://creativecommons.org/licenses/by/4.0/), which permits use, sharing, adaptation, distribution and reproduction in any medium or format, as long as you give appropriate credit to the original author(s) and the source, provide a link to the Creative Commons license and indicate if changes were made.

The images or other third party material in this chapter are included in the chapter's Creative Commons license, unless indicated otherwise in a credit line to the material. If material is not included in the chapter's Creative Commons license and your intended use is not permitted by statutory regulation or exceeds the permitted use, you will need to obtain permission directly from the copyright holder.

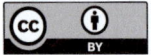

History of Kanad Hospital: The First Hospital in the UAE

2

Ralph Leo and Kaitlyn Baker

2.1 A Royal Invitation

2.1.1 First Hospital in the Emirate of Abu Dhabi

The success of Bahrain's American Mission Hospital (c. 1903) and Oman's Al-Rahma Hospital (c. 1909) was well known in Arabia in the first half of the twentieth century. The hospitals, founded by the Reformed Church in America at the invitation of local rulers, were known to treat tens of thousands of patients annually, saving countless lives [1]. In 1959, facing a desperate situation with approximately 50% infant mortality and 33% maternal mortality, Abu Dhabi's ruler, Sheikh Shakhbout bin Sultan Al Nahyan, and his brother, Sheikh Zayed, who would become the founding father of the United Arab Emirates (UAE), put out a call to bring a similar medical establishment to Al Ain. That call was answered by American physicians Dr. Burwell "Pat" Kennedy and his wife, Dr. Marian Kennedy, who had previously worked in Iraq, Lebanon, and Jordan [2]. During Dr. Pat's first scouting visit to Al Ain in December of 1959, Sheikh Zayed reportedly quipped to him, "The question is not if you will come, but when" [3].

In reply, Kennedy had more questions than answers: "Where will we practice? Where will we deliver babies? Where will we have clinics?" Everything around them was a barren desert. As the story goes, it was then that Sheikh Zayed pointed to a white, mud-block compound, which also happened to be his personal guest house, and said, "On the left side, you can live; on the right side, you can do clinics" [3].

R. Leo
Kanad Hospital Executive Board, Al Ain, United Arab Emirates

UAE University, Al Ain, United Arab Emirates
e-mail: ralphaleo@uaeu.ac.ae

K. Baker (✉)
Kanad Hospital Media Office, Al Ain, United Arab Emirates

© The Author(s) 2025
H. O. Al-Shamsi (ed.), *Healthcare in the United Arab Emirates*,
https://doi.org/10.1007/978-981-96-0523-1_2

Dr. Kennedy's initial visit was followed by a second visit in April 1960, the purpose of which was to finalize preparations for bringing his family and supplies later in the year. On that visit, however, a woman who had been in labor for two days was brought to him. She was seeking help, and it was a prime opportunity for Sheikh Shakhbout and Sheikh Zayed to observe and examine Dr. Kennedy's abilities. Not expecting to practice medicine on this preparatory trip, Dr. Kennedy did not have any medical supplies with him. However, at Sheikh Zayed's insistence, Kennedy walked over to the Land Rover that had just transported him and his colleague, Raymond Joyce, across nine hours of sand dunes from the Dubai airport. Taking out a small hose from the engine, he carefully washed it with water from a well. Kennedy was then able to use the makeshift device to deliver a healthy baby boy just moments later! Looking on in astonishment, the royal family of Abu Dhabi needed no further convincing that they had found their doctor [4] (Fig. 2.1).

And so, on November 20, 1960, the Kennedy family, accompanied by Maria Mayer, arrived in Al Ain to establish Oasis Hospital (officially renamed "Kanad Hospital" in 2019 by His Highness Sheikh Mohamed bin Zayed to perpetuate its unique legacy by acknowledging the local Arabic dialect for "Kennedy Hospital"). The first and only hospital in the entire Abu Dhabi Emirate, Oasis served not only Al Ain and its surrounding areas but also Al Buraimi, and the coastal and interior regions of Oman. It would be nearly another decade before the first government hospital was established in the Emirate, leaving Oasis as the sole provider of healthcare to those in the region [5]. Of all the births at the hospital during that first year in the desert, none would be more consequential than the tenth baby to be born. For on March 11, 1961, Sheikh Zayed and Sheikha Fatima welcomed a baby boy, born at the hands of Dr. Marian Kennedy, whom they named Mohamed. At that time, only God knew that young Mohamed would grow up to become the beloved third president of a nation that did not even exist yet, the United Arab Emirates [3]. Indeed, President Sheikh Mohamed was the first of twenty-three sons and daughters of Sheikh Zayed to be born at Kanad, which is why the hospital became known as the "birthplace of the nation's leaders." (Fig. 2.2)

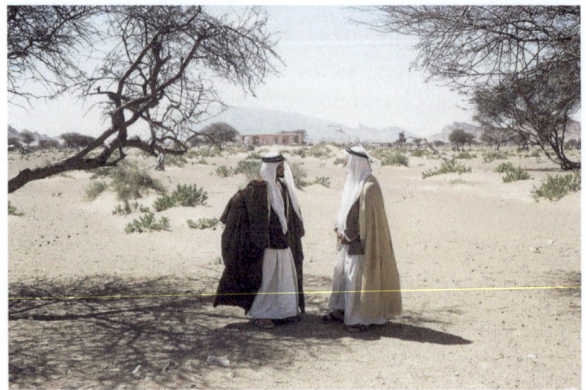

Fig. 2.1 Sheikh Zayed and Sheikh Shakhbout stand in front of the building that would become the first hospital in Abu Dhabi (April 1960). [Kanad Hospital Archives]

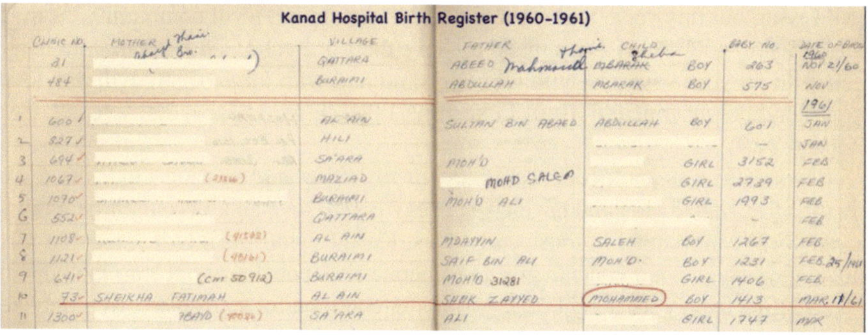

Kanad Hospital Birth Register (1960-1961)

	CLINIC NO.	MOTHER	VILLAGE	FATHER	CHILD		BABY NO.	DATE OF BIRTH
	81		GATTARA	ABEED	MBARAK	BOY	263	1960 NOV 21/60
	484		BURAIMI	ABDULLAH	MBARAK	BOY	575	NOV
								1961
1	600		AL AIN	SULTAN BIN ABAED	ABDULLAH	BOY	601	JAN
2	827		HILI				-	JAN
3	694		SA'ARA	MOH'D		GIRL	3152	FEB
4	1067	(21316)	MAZIAD	MOHD SALEM		GIRL	2739	FEB
5	1070		BURAIMI	MOH'D ALI		GIRL	1993	FEB
6	552		GATTARA				-	FEB
7	1108	(41582)	AL AIN	MDAYYIN	SALEH	BOY	1267	FEB
8	1121	(48161)	BURAIMI	SAIF BIN ALI	MOH'D	BOY	1231	FEB 25/1961
9	641	(CM 50912)	BURAIMI	MOH'D 31281		GIRL	1406	FEB
10	73	SHEIKHA FATIMAH	AL AIN	SHEIK ZAYYED	MOHAMMED	BOY	1413	MAR 11/61
11	1300	ABAYD (40024)	SA'ARA	ALI		GIRL	1747	MAR

Fig. 2.2 An original Kanad Hospital birth register listing the birth of President Sheikh Mohamed Bin Zayed on March 11, 1961. [Kanad Hospital Archives]

2.2 The Kennedys and Kanad

2.2.1 First Contact Between Muslims and Christians

In recent years, the Emirati ambassador to the United States, H.E. Yousef Al Otaiba, has fielded a plethora of questions about the roots of tolerance in UAE society. In response, he pointed to the founding of Kanad Hospital as a seminal moment in cementing the nation's fledgling DNA. Unfortunately, until the visit of the Pope in 2019 and the signing of the Abraham Accords in 2020, most Westerners were unaware of the gracious and open ethic that Sheikh Zayed worked so hard to instill in the nation throughout its early years. Al Otaiba, however, knew exactly where to turn to help people understand this dynamic. He wrote:

> In 1960, two American missionary doctors went deep into the harsh desert of the Arabian Peninsula to set up a hospital in a mud block building with dirt floors and a palm frond roof. For the Bedouins who lived there and practiced Islam, it would be their first experience with modern medicine and their first contact with Christianity. Over the next few decades, with the encouragement and support of local tribal leaders, the husband-and-wife medical team would grow the hospital, save many lives, and cement a lasting legacy of respect and admiration between Christians and Muslims in what would later become the United Arab Emirates [6].

From such a humble beginning, and with a firm belief that it was God who had called them, Drs. Pat and Marian and their four young children—Kathleen (7), Scott (5), Nancy (3), and Doug (1)—forsook the comforts of postwar America for the blessings of seeing God at work in faraway lands. As Christian missionaries in a Muslim country, they understood that they were not in Arabia to "convert" the Muslim population to the Christian religion. Rather, their purpose was to serve and honor God by loving and caring for the people in the same way that Jesus did, through self-sacrifice and unconditional love [7]. Of particular inspiration was a famous passage from the Injīl which reads, "For even the Son of Man [Jesus] did not come to be served, but to serve, and to give his life as a ransom for many" (Injīl Mark 10:45)

[8]. Living out this verse was what endeared them to the local community, as they attempted to obey Jesus's command to "love the Lord your God with all your heart and with all your soul and with all your mind and with all your strength and love your neighbor as yourself" (Injīl Luke 10:27) [8]. (Figs. 2.3, 2.4, 2.5, 2.6, 2.7, 2.8, 2.9 and 2.10)

Beyond their unapologetic commitment to loving and serving God, the team members at Kanad Hospital have also endeavored to love and serve their neighbors in the local community. In those early days, Kanad's staff quickly learned that it is not always about what you can give to someone else, but also about learning how to receive gifts from your neighbor. It was not uncommon for staff to receive gifts like donkeys, chickens, or even jewelry and precious heirlooms from the local population as a demonstration of their hospitality. Over the decades, this mutual understanding of neighborly love has blossomed into deeply rooted relationships that cross cultures, languages, and religions. In this way, Kanad helped to instill in the wider expatriate Christian community an attitude of being a blessing to the whole nation by helping its businesses, education system, and healthcare industry to flourish. For example, in Abu Dhabi, it is a well-known fact that Kanad's early staff were

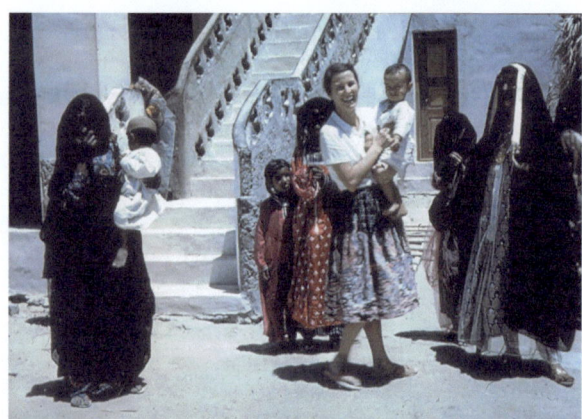

Fig. 2.3 Dr. Marian Kennedy holds young Sheikh Mohamed Bin Zayed (c. 1963). [Kanad Hospital Archives]

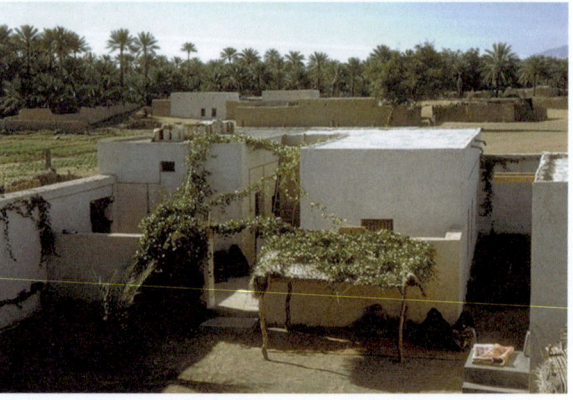

Fig. 2.4 The building where President Sheikh Mohamed Bin Zayed was born on March 11, 1961. [Kanad Hospital Archives]

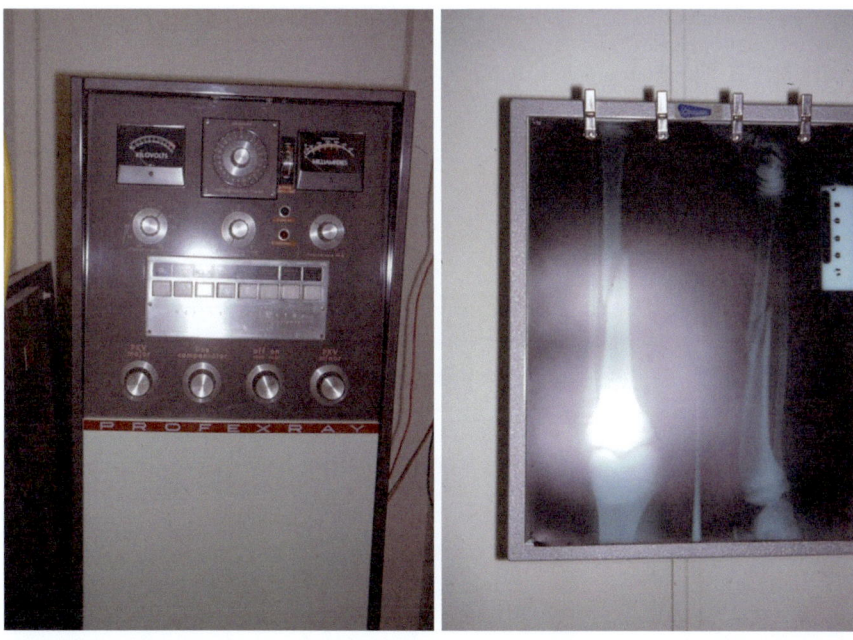

Fig. 2.5 First X-ray machine and first X-ray film taken in Abu Dhabi (1964). [Kanad Hospital Archives]

Fig. 2.6 Dr. Larry "Fouad" Liddle, Kanad's longest serving physician of over 30 years, treats Ibrahim Al Balooshi, Kanad's longest serving staff member of over 45 years. [Kanad Hospital Archives]

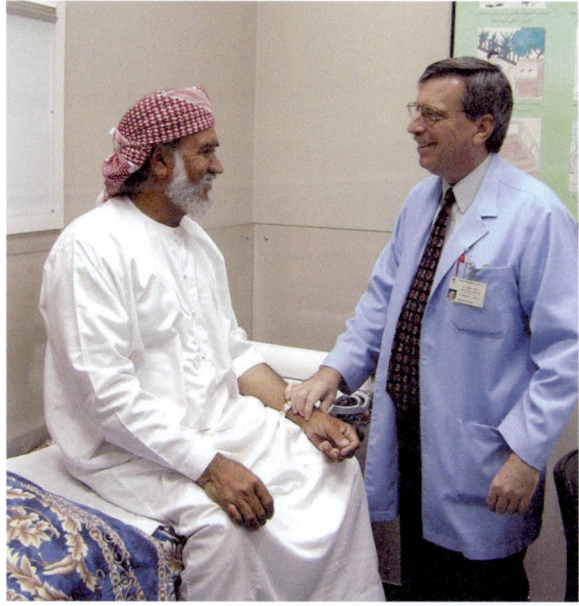

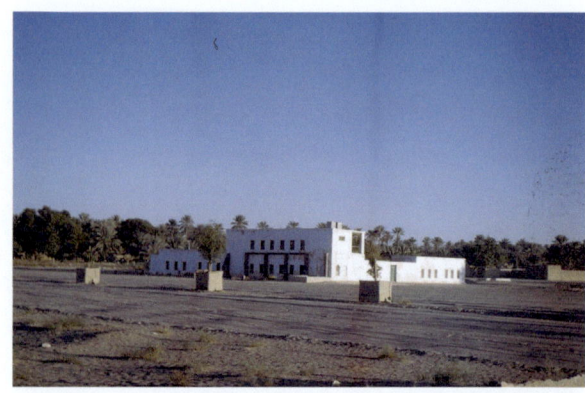

Fig. 2.7 The original hospital building given by Sheikh Zayed (1960-1963)

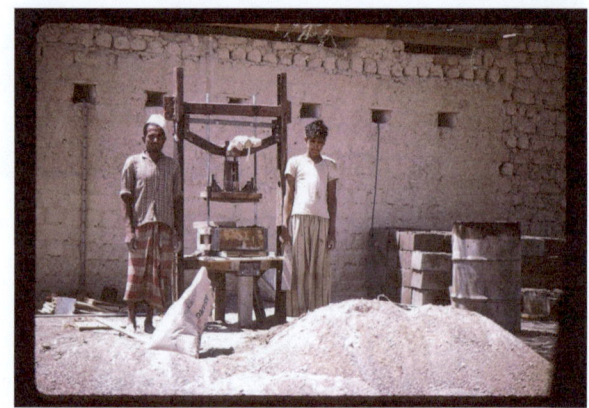

Fig. 2.8 A block machine made from a truck chassis (1964)

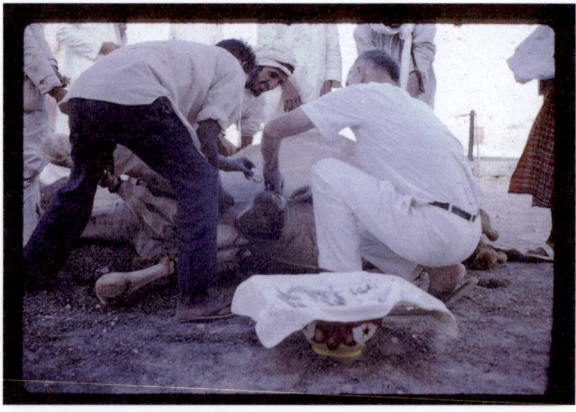

Fig. 2.9 Dr. Kennedy performs surgery on a camel (1964)

Fig. 2.10 Kanad Hospital's original majlis building (1964)

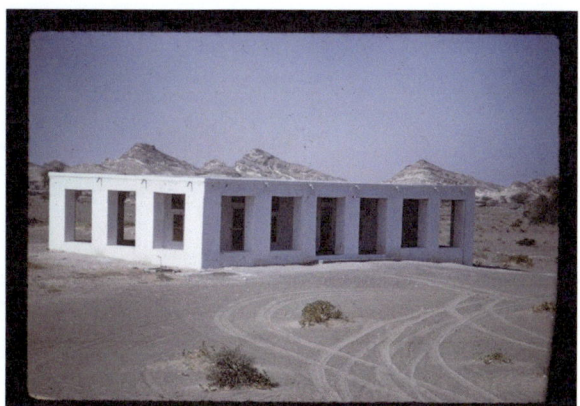

Fig. 2.11 Patients camped near Oasis Hospital (1964)

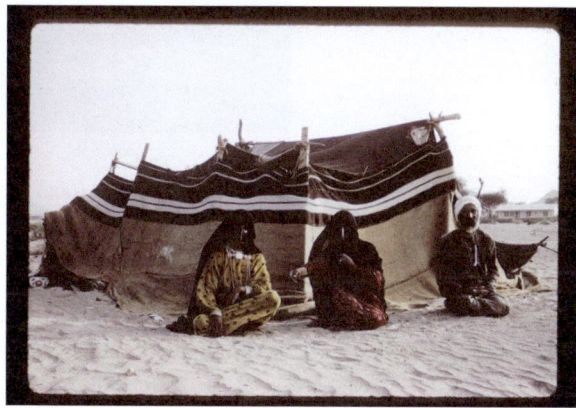

largely responsible for conceiving and developing the administrative infrastructure that would eventually become the Ministry of Health (Figs. 2.11 and 2.12).

Speaking of the relationship between the Emirati people and the hospital, President Sheikh Mohamed Bin Zayed recently noted, "You [Kanad] came before the oil, when there was nothing to gain. Many of us would not be here today if you had not come. We will always be family" [9]. *Family*. That is the word the President uses to describe the relationship between the people of the UAE and Kanad Hospital. *Family*. Muslims and Christians working together for the common good. *Family*. This is a word that goes beyond mere tolerance, cooperation, or mutual understanding. It speaks to an unconditional love that crosses the toughest of boundaries. When staff like Dr. Larry "Fouad" Liddle (Kanad's longest-serving physician) worked seemingly never-ending shifts for thirty years, religious and cultural differences faded away. Dr. Liddle was known to sleep with his work clothes turned inside out next to the bed so that he could more quickly rise and dress when the inevitable emergency calls came at 3 a.m. each night. What choice did he have, when he was the only doctor in Al Ain for years? As healthcare was

Fig. 2.12 X-ray building construction (1964)

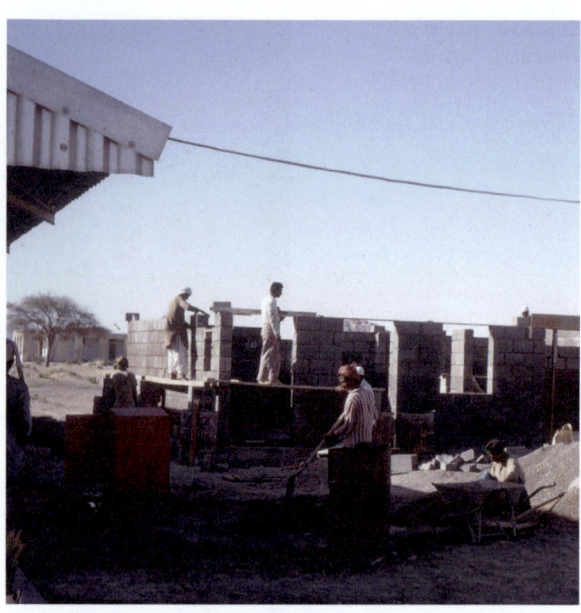

the first and, for decades, the only contact that local Muslims had with Christians, it is not surprising that familial bonds developed. Life-and-death situations have a funny way of doing that.

This religious tolerance that started on Al Ain soil has since spread to the capital city of Abu Dhabi, as well as the booming metroplex of Dubai and the entire country. Kanad Hospital continues to be perhaps the most visible example of such efforts in the country [10]. It shows not only that it is possible, but that it can also be a beautiful thing. Kanad is unashamed of its Christian mission, which is "to honor God by providing exceptional, whole-person healthcare with the love and compassion of Jesus Christ" [11]. This is what informs and equips the hospital's team members to carry out the vision—"to provide an oasis of exceptional healthcare for women and children"—and both this mission and vision fuel the hospital's core values [11]. At the heart of Kanad Hospital is one driving pulse: love God and love one another. Though Kanad's Christian identity is a minority in the community that surrounds it, from the very beginning, the Kennedys demonstrated through their medical work that people of different beliefs can still establish deep relationships as they live and work together toward a common purpose for good. With their consistent love and care, Drs. Pat and Marian Kennedy earned the trust and respect of both their patients and the nation's leaders, thereby receiving a cherished place in the heart of the community that continues to outlive them both. Their legacy continues to pave the way for the future of Kanad Hospital, thriving communal relationships, and religious tolerance in the UAE (Fig. 2.13 and 2.14).

Fig. 2.13 Dr. Marian and Joyce Melhuish (1968)

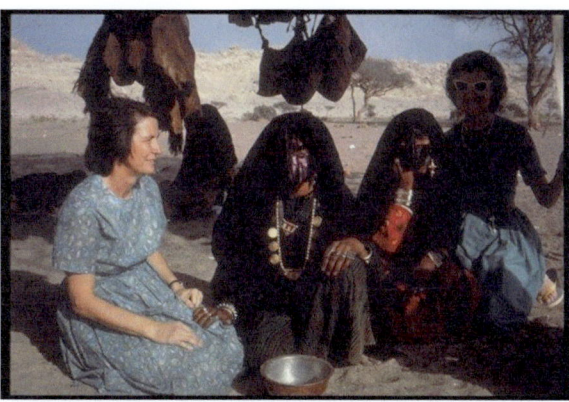

Fig. 2.14 Drs. Pat and Marian Kennedy (1968)

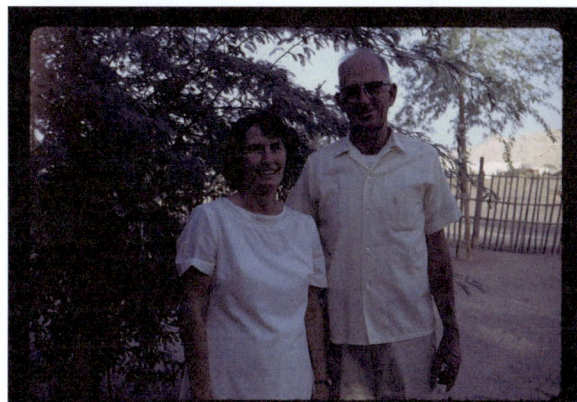

2.3 Modernizing Medicine

2.3.1 First Blood Bank and X-Ray Machine in Abu Dhabi

At Kanad Hospital's birth, it was all about saving lives. As was previously noted, when the Kennedys first arrived in Al Ain, the infant mortality rate was a striking 50%, and the maternal mortality rate was 33%. Miraculously, these brutal numbers went down sharply in the first few years following the founding of Kanad, to the point that mortality rates soon reached international standards. This incredible progress was a direct result of the Kennedys' laser focus on obstetrics, gynecology, and pediatric care. Within these fields, especially obstetrics, there is always a need for blood. At the time, however, there was no blood bank in the entire emirate of Abu Dhabi. The Kennedys and other staff always did what needed to be done, however, and they gave of themselves to make things happen. Since the hospital needed blood donations, the first blood transfusions in Al Ain used hospital staff, including the Kennedys. The first blood bank in Abu Dhabi, then, was merely a list on the wall of Oasis Hospital! Dr. Marian's blood type was O-negative, meaning she was a universal donor. Constantly donating blood made her chronically anemic for the sake of her patients. Dr. Scott Kennedy recounted how on one occasion, she was delivering a baby when the mother underwent a postpartum hemorrhage. After the engineer and lab technician had donated, still more blood was needed, so Dr. Marian scrubbed out, donated blood, then came back to complete the procedure and help the mother [3]. Incredible examples of self-sacrifice such as this would forever cement Kanad's legacy in the minds and hearts of local people [2].

Not only was Kanad the location of the first blood bank in the Emirate, but it was also where the first X-ray machine was used. Gerald "Gerry" Longjohn, who came from America with his family in 1964, worked primarily in construction and maintenance at the hospital. He was responsible for getting a machine up and running that would introduce a wholly new medical technology to Abu Dhabi. He had never received formal training as an electrical engineer, but he had worked his way through Bible college delivering motors for an electrical company in the States and had done lots of on-the-job training. When the machine was donated, Dr. Pat Kennedy tasked him first with constructing a building that could safely house an X-ray machine while also protecting the technician from radiation, and second, making the machine operational. Though he knew nothing about X-rays or building construction, Gerry set his mind to work. In the days before Google, and with no books or outside resources whatsoever to draw from, Longjohn did the best and only thing he could; he prayed to God for wisdom. After sincerely asking God to help him know what to do, he drafted some initial sketches [10].

The first step was to learn how to make concrete blocks, which had never been done in Al Ain. Step two was to figure out how to use those blocks to make double concrete walls. With lots of dedication and hard work, he successfully did both. He finished the building, and there was space for both the X-ray machine and a dark room in the basement (which he dug by hand) where film could be developed and stored [10].

Finally, Gerry opened the shipping box and laid eyes on the machine for the very first time. Then he worked slowly through the schematic and learned how to install the machine. When it came time to turn the machine on, he was supposed to look for a light inside the tube. Doug Kennedy came in and helped him, and he noticed there was no light, just a hole where it was supposed to be. The used X-ray machine was missing a crucial part, which was very expensive and would take months to arrive from the United States. One day, Sheikh Shakhbout's son came around and inquired about it. Upon learning of the situation, he paid for Gerry to fly to the United States, spend a week in training with the X-ray company, and then fly back to the UAE with the missing piece. When Gerry returned, as he was installing the part, and before he had even turned the machine on, Dr. Pat came in and asked if the machine was ready. The son of the royal family member who had donated the funds for Gerry to travel to and from the States had fallen from a camel, and the doctor needed to use the X-ray machine as soon as possible to assess the damage. Gerry finished installing the part, they took the scan, developed the film, and everyone rejoiced when they produced the first crystal-clear picture of a broken bone from this first-ever X-ray taken in Abu Dhabi [10].

2.4 Development of Facilities

2.4.1 First Mud-Block and Cement Buildings in Abu Dhabi

Kanad Hospital started with a basic facility in 1960, in the guest house donated by Sheikh Zayed. One corner of the room was dedicated to labor and delivery, another to operations, then sterilizing, and storage, plus an additional VIP patient's room, complete with its own outside door into the courtyard. There were four patient rooms made of palm branches built right outside the wall beside the delivery room. It was compact and efficient, but it was exactly what was needed at the time. There was enough space to have a separate room for each patient so that men and family could visit in private, and there was also a small communal courtyard where groups could sit and sip coffee together [4].

However, this was all destroyed by heavy rains in February and March of 1963. Typically, mud-block buildings could withstand some rain, but after seven years with no rain, the sun and wind had begun to wear down many buildings, including the guest house. The heavy rain that season simply washed away the corners of rooms, leaving them exposed to the outside world. This gave way for the hospital to make its move to a new site with prefabricated buildings. There were eight rooms made of palm branches and corrugated aluminum, but these were also destroyed just a few short months later, in October [4].

The women in the hospital were always told not to cook in the rooms, since the walls were made of palm branches and had dried leaves remaining on them inside, making them highly flammable. They could cook in the courtyard instead. Nonetheless, one day, one woman felt it was too windy outside and decided to put her primus stove in the room. The room did, in fact, catch fire [4].

Gertrude Dyck, affectionately known among locals as "Doctura Latifa," was bathing a baby in the next room when it happened. The woman came in and said, "Dhaw, dhaw!" Doctura Latifa had learned this word meant "light," so, thinking she probably just wanted to show her the sunset, she was in no hurry to go with her. She continued bathing the baby, but the lady quickly returned and repeated the message, more determined this time. At that point, Doctura Latifa went with her to see what was going on and saw the room ablaze. "Hariga!" she screamed, which was the Arabic word she had learned to say when something was on fire. Men arrived to fight the fire, but it was too late for that room and the three surrounding it. The reality is that at that time, for local Arabs, aside from the sun, the only light they had ever known was from fire. For them, the two words were one and the same; thus, the devastating miscommunication [4].

The men were immediately tasked with rebuilding the rooms. They planned to start with four mud-block rooms and hoped to continue building with cement blocks in the near future. They made the mud blocks by hand right there on the property, using clay soil. They left them in the sun to dry, and then, that night, it unexpectedly rained and washed them all away. Once again, they were faced with starting from scratch [4].

In January 1964, Leon Blosser arrived with his family, and his first assignment was to build what would be the first cement block building in Al Ain. No one had ever built using cement blocks before in Al Ain, so locals trickled in and out just to watch. The cement had to be brought from Dubai, and Leon crafted his own cement block machine using an old truck chassis and standing it on its end. He hauled gravel from the wadi and sand from the desert, then fashioned all the blocks by hand. On Gerry Longjohn's very first day at the hospital later that year, he started helping Leon complete the hospital's first inpatient building of 20 rooms. In addition, Gerry also built a *majlis* (or "meeting room") for the hospital, the first cement-block residences, and the X-ray building, which included a basement for the cool storage of pharmaceutical supplies [4] (Fig. 2.15).

In 1972, another ten patient rooms were added, which included private baths. In 1985, work started on new inpatient rooms for the obstetric, surgical, and pediatric suites, and by 1990, these were completed and in use. At the end of 1993, the original cement-block rooms were demolished, and the new outpatient building was built and opened in 1995 [4]. Further expansions took place in the early 2000s, including the Sheikh Zayed Majlis, which is a replica of the original building and is dedicated to preserving the history of Al Ain [2]. In 2015, the hospital opened its new state-of-the-art 140-bed facility, complete with the UAE's most advanced maternal and fetal medicine clinic and neonatal intensive care unit. The new building was a gracious

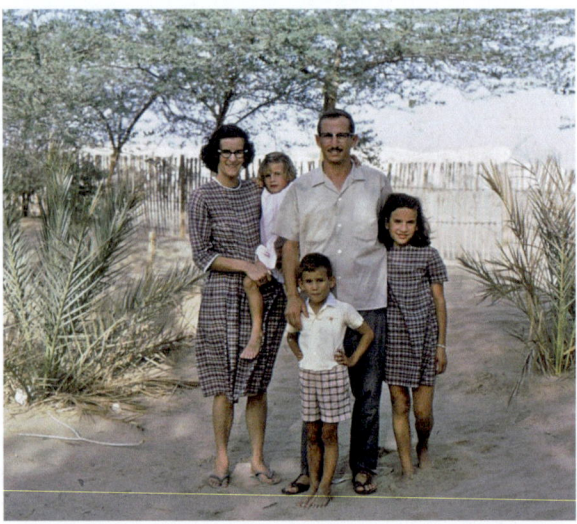

Fig. 2.15 Leon Blosser and family (1969)

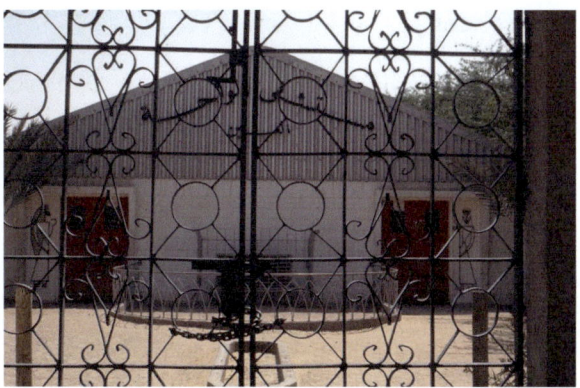

Fig. 2.16 Outpatient clinic gate, showing male and female entrances

gift from the UAE government. Its operating budget is the source of all revenue for the world-class healthcare it provides. Kanad Hospital has come a long way from its humble beginnings and continues to develop and expand alongside the community (Fig. 2.16).

2.5 Only the Beginning

2.5.1 Rich History, Bright Future

The city's history is indeed rich, and so is that of its first hospital. In many ways, Al Ain and Kanad have grown up together. Their development and growth have always run parallel, and that does not stop now. As Al Ain continues to evolve, so does Kanad Hospital. It continues to keep pace with the community it exists to serve, in the same way it has for previous decades. The future is exciting, but there are some things from the past that will always remain at Kanad, like the welcoming nature of the local people, the warm invitations into homes, the power of deep relationships, the commitment to serving God, and the mutual neighborly love [12]. Amid all the changes in medicine and facilities, these things have stayed the same. More than all the "firsts" that Kanad is known for (first hospital, first contact between Muslims and Christians, first blood bank, X-ray machine, and so on), the hospital and those who serve there long to be remembered for the way they love God and love the community, and the way they are loved in return. One might say that Kanad Hospital truly is an oasis in the desert—an oasis of exceptional healthcare, thriving community, and unconditional love. Even as the hospital embarks on the future, the people who stand on the shoulders of those who came before make every effort to remember their history and carry that same light with them as they go forth.

Conflicts of Interest The authors have no conflicts of interest to declare.

References

1. Clarke A. The American Mission Hospital Bahrain: through the changing scenes of life 1893–1993. Bahrain: American Mission Hospital Society; 1993.
2. Zaman S. Kanad Hospital: the story of the Al Ain hospital where Sheikh Mohamed was born [internet]. Abu Dhabi: Gulf News; 2021. Available from: https://gulfnews.com/uae/year-of-the-50th/kanad-hospital-the-story-of-the-al-ain-hospital-where-sheikh-mohamed-was-born-1.79714052
3. Kennedy S. Stories about Kanad's early days and growing up in Al Ain. [Personal interview, 1 September] Al Ain; 2022. (Unpublished).
4. Dyck G. The oasis: Al Ain memoirs of 'Doctora Latifa'. Dubai: Motivate Publishing; 1995.
5. Late Dr. Burwell (PAT) Kennedy and Dr. Marian Kennedy [internet]. Dubai: Sheikh Hamdan Bin Rashid Al Maktoum Award for Medical Sciences; 2005–2006. Available from: http://www.hmaward.org.ae/profile.php?id=234
6. Al Otaiba Y. Why we invited the pope to the Arabian Peninsula [internet]. Politico Magazine. 2019; Available from: https://www.politico.com/magazine/story/2019/02/02/pope-francis-visits-arabian-peninsula-224545/
7. Langton J. The inside story of two American doctors who brought medical care to Abu Dhabi [internet]. The National, UAE; 2020. Available from: https://www.thenationalnews.com/uae/heritage/the-inside-story-of-two-american-doctors-who-brought-medical-care-to-abu-dhabi-1.964261
8. The Holy Bible. Wheaton: Crossway; 2001.
9. Public remarks. November 8, 2021.
10. Longjohn G. First X-ray machine and religious tolerance in the UAE. [Personal interview, 12 September] Al Ain; 2022. (Unpublished).
11. About Kanad Hospital [Internet]. Available from: https://kanadhospital.org/about-us/
12. Missal B. Working as a nurse at Kanad Hospital. [Personal interview, 11 September] Al Ain; 2022. (Unpublished).

Ralph Leo is an assistant professor of history at the United Arab Emirates University in Al Ain. He is also the chairman of the Kanad Hospital Executive Board. Together with his wife, Tara, he co-founded True Sojourners, an American non-profit that owns and operates Kanad Hospital and various other charitable projects worldwide. He and Tara have lived in Al Ain for the past decade, raising their six children as committed "Ainawees," with a passion for camels and all things purple. A fluent Arabic speaker with a love for heritage and culture, Dr. Leo's current research focuses on the history of medicine in the region.

Kaitlyn Baker is the former content writer of the marketing team at Kanad Hospital in Al Ain, United Arab Emirates. Originally from North Carolina in the United States, she holds a B.A. in Journalism and Mass Communication from Samford University in Birmingham, Alabama. She moved to the UAE within a year of graduating to start her career and pursue her passion for storytelling in the Arab world, which she has grown to deeply cherish. Besides writing and editing (two things she truly enjoys), she loves reading, learning languages, walking in nature, making music, and connecting with people over coffee and tea.

Open Access This chapter is licensed under the terms of the Creative Commons Attribution 4.0 International License (http://creativecommons.org/licenses/by/4.0/), which permits use, sharing, adaptation, distribution and reproduction in any medium or format, as long as you give appropriate credit to the original author(s) and the source, provide a link to the Creative Commons license and indicate if changes were made.

The images or other third party material in this chapter are included in the chapter's Creative Commons license, unless indicated otherwise in a credit line to the material. If material is not included in the chapter's Creative Commons license and your intended use is not permitted by statutory regulation or exceeds the permitted use, you will need to obtain permission directly from the copyright holder.

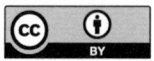

Ministry of Health and Prevention in the UAE

Mohammad Al-Olama and Meera Al Ali

3.1 Introduction

In the 1800s, travel and trade increased tremendously, which unintentionally led to outbreaks of epidemic diseases worldwide. In 1851, the first International Sanitary Conference was convened in Paris due to the epidemics of 1830 and 1847. In 1902, the International Sanitary Bureau was established, making the *Pan American Health Organization* (PAHO) the oldest international public health agency in the world. In Europe, L'Office International d'Hygiène Publique was established in 1907, and in 1919, the League of Nations established the Health Organization of the League of Nations in Geneva. In 1938, the last International Sanitary Conference was held in Paris on the eve of World War II. On the other hand, in the summer of 1948, the First World Health Assembly met in Geneva [1, 2].

Since its union on December 2, 1971, the vision of the United Arab Emirates (UAE) has been to keep pace with global developments. The health sector has witnessed great accomplishments in framing the health system and encouraging the adoption of best practices and performance targets by all healthcare services. The people in the UAE understand how important it is to have the most advanced health technologies, resources, and benefits to be able to improve that vital sector. According to Business Monitor International, healthcare costs in the UAE stood at 62.1 billion dirhams at the end of 2016 and are forecast to rise to 106 billion dirhams by 2026 [3, 4].

The health sector is one of the most developed in the UAE and ranks first worldwide across several approved health indicators. There are three health authorities in

---

M. Al-Olama (✉) · M. Al Ali
Dubai Health, Rashid Hospital, Dubai, United Arab Emirates
e-mail: mnalali@dha.gov.ae

the country. In the emirate of Abu Dhabi, the Department of Health Abu Dhabi was established in 2007. The Dubai Health Authority (DHA) was created in June 2007 in the Emirate of Dubai, and in the emirate of Sharjah, the Sharjah Health Authority was established. These entities have many similarities in their services, which include monitoring and analyzing the populations' health status and the performance of healthcare providers. They regulate and issue licenses to all healthcare providers. They also manages health insurance, health investment, and health tourism [5–8].

Public healthcare services are regulated by different authorities, which include the Ministry of Health and Prevention, the Department of Health-Abu Dhabi (formerly HAAD), the Dubai Health Authority (DHA), and the Emirates Health Authority (EHA) [3–5, 9–11].

The government of the UAE has adopted the digitalization of various governmental services. The use of artificial intelligence has become a trend. Most services in the UAE can be done through smart applications, thus saving a lot of time and effort. The use of artificial intelligence in healthcare is evident, and the Ministry of Health and Prevention has many projects and services that are integrated with artificial intelligence. By doing so, safe, high-quality, fast, and comfortable services are provided to the public [4, 12].

3.2   Projects and Initiatives

With the guidance and support of our leaders, many projects and initiatives were adopted by the Ministry of Health. As health is a priority, these innovative services were launched. They have shown success and became popular. Here are some of them [4, 13, 14]:

- *Mabrouk Ma Yak* is an integrated initiative that aims to facilitate and simplify procedures for UAE nationals to obtain the main documents for a newborn. It includes collaboration between the Federal Authority for Identity, Citizenship, Customs, and Port Security; the Ministry of Health and Prevention; the Ministry of Finance, the Dubai Health Authority, the Telecommunications and Digital Government Regulatory Authority; Emirates Post; the Federal Authority for Government Human Resources; Emirates Health Services; and other local and federal entities.
- *Tatmeen* is designed to efficiently deal with fraudulent or expired medical products and unauthorized items. The Ministry's Health Department created a digital platform based on advanced sequencing and tracking technology to track drugs from production to end-user usage.
- *The Riayati initiative for the National Unified Medical Record,* is a digitized platform integrated with the National Unified Medical Record (NUMR) program. It transforms the current UAE healthcare landscape through the centralization of medical records and the delivery of a fully integrated, innovative, digital clinical information system to enhance the quality of life for UAE citizens.

- *Public Health Management Solutions* is an advanced system designed to easily investigate, surveil, follow up on, and manage factors affecting public health to help promote health. It will help in the early detection of epidemics, monitor their spread, and determine whether the applied treatment is effective or not. In this way, it will help prevent disease by collecting and analyzing data.
- *The MA'KOM initiative* is aimed at encouraging healthier lifestyle modifications, such as increasing physical activity in Emirati society.
- *The Keep on Beating campaign* aims to detect cardiovascular disease-related risk factors early, including smoking, malnutrition, inactivity, and stress, and, in response, promote lifestyle modifications to minimize these risk factors.
- *The Heart Experts Program* aims to raise awareness of cardiovascular health, where groups of students are chosen to work as awareness ambassadors for their classmates, neighborhoods, and local communities.
- *The Healthy and Positive Work Environment Initiative* aims to build a work environment that is supportive and healthy by providing public employees with the right information and skills to help establish healthy habits and shift perceptions.
- *The Student Growth Record Initiative* aims to combat obesity in children and adolescents by providing data on dietary traditions and levels of physical activity among children between the ages of 5 and 17.
- *Ownak Initiative* This program is targeted at the elderly by developing preventive, promotional, and curative services for them. The program's goal is to facilitate and expedite the delivery of all health services to older individuals in all ministry facilities and to ensure their access to integrated healthcare.
- *Help Me Hear Initiative* aims to assist hearing-impaired children, low-income individuals, and non-citizens by facilitating cochlear implant operations.
- *Itmenan:* The National Periodic Health and Cancer Screening initiatives focus on reducing the prevalence of other non-communicable diseases, especially osteoporosis and cardiovascular disease (CVD), in the United Arab Emirates.

3.3 Smart Applications

It is a new initiative by MOHAP that allows users to follow-up on application status and reduces customer inconvenience that may be caused by physical visits to service centers. In addition, this application facilitates the reduction of paper usage and serves as a health educator. It increases health awareness by providing important information on many health topics, which helps prevent diseases or complications [4, 12].

3.4 Health Ministers

There have been a total of ten health ministers since the UAE's formation in 1971 (Table 3.1).

Table 3.1 The UAE health ministers since 1971

	Health minister	Year
1	H.E. Sheikh Sultan Bin Ahmed Al-Mualla	1971
2	H.E. Sheikh Saif Bin Mohammad Al-Nahyan	1973
3	H.E. Khalfan Al Roomi	1977
4	H.E. Hamad Abdulrahman Al Midfaa	1979
5	H.E. Ahmed Bin Saeed Al Badi	1990
6	H.E. Hamad Abdulrahman Al Midfaa	1997
7	H.E. Hamad Abdulrahman Al Midfaa	2004
8	H.E. Humaid Al Qatami	2006
9	H.E. Dr. Hanif Hassan Ali Al Qassim	2009
10	H.E. Abdul Rahman Bin Mohammed Al Owais	2011 (2013)

3.5 Minister's Message

"The United Arab Emirates (UAE) has placed a strong focus on all individuals residing in the state—both citizens and residents—aiming to provide them with comprehensive, world-class healthcare. In line with this, our role in the Ministry of Health and Prevention is to provide healthcare that is responsive to the needs of individuals, falls in line with the development and future vision of the state in all sectors and strives to be the world's best in all services.

We are all working closely, guided by a team spirit that looks towards achieving national goals and objectives aimed at maintaining the well-being of all the nationals and residents. Healthiness has been the central focus of the development and driving force of the global efforts launched by the UAE since it was founded on December 2, 1971. We are all called upon to fulfil our roles, to meet the requirements of constructive national action, to carry out national tasks and duties, and to achieve the lofty mission of the state in this vital sector" [4].

3.6 Conclusion

The Ministry of Health and Prevention in the UAE was established with the union of the country in 1971, and since then, the ministry has aimed to implement the highest health standards and technologies in the country, which has brought healthcare in the UAE to the top in a short time. Many initiatives have been implemented not only for new borns, like Mabrouk Ma Yak or for the elderly, like the *Ownak Initiative*, but for all age groups, citizens and non-citizens, like the *Help Me Hear Initiative*. The target is fast and excellent care with the best quality. The Ministry of Health and Prevention of the UAE will continue to provide the best care to all individuals in the UAE.

Conflicts of Interest The authors have no conflicts of interest to declare.

References

1. https://www.who.int/about/who-we-are/history
2. A brief history of the World Health Organization by Michael McCarthy. Lancet 360; 2002.
3. https://www.albayan.ae/across-the-uae/2001-08-10-1.1235865
4. https://mohap.gov.ae/
5. https://u.ae/en/information-and-services/health-and-fitness/health-authorities
6. https://dha.gov.ae/
7. https://www.doh.gov.ae/
8. https://sha.shj.ae/ar-ae/
9. https://www.uae-embassy.org/discover-uae/society/healthcare
10. https://gulfnews.com/uae/health/all-hospitals-will-have-international-accreditation-by-2021-1.2104886
11. https://www.almrsal.com/post/396539
12. https://www.healthcareitnews.com/
13. https://icp.gov.ae/en/service/mabrok-mayak
14. https://www.alittihad.ae/

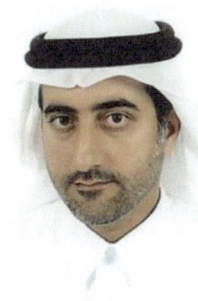

Dr. Mohammad Abdulaziz Sultan Al Olama is a consultant neurosurgeon at Rashid Hospital and also works at the University Hospital in Sharjah as a visiting doctor. He is specialized in pediatric neurosurgery, advanced neuropathic pain, and functional neurosurgery. He studied medicine in Sweden at the University of Gothenburg; trained at Frankston Hospital affiliated with Monash University in Melbourne, Australia; worked in the General Surgery Department at Al Baraha Hospital for a year; and then studied neurosurgery at Sahlgrenska University Hospital in Gothenburg, Sweden. He has trained in various fields, such as the Gamma Knife device at Karolinska Hospital in Sweden, Pittsburgh Hospital in the USA, and Johnston-Willis Hospital in Richmond, Virginia, USA. He also trained in fetal operations at Arnold Palmer Hospital in Orlando, USA. He received training on MRI-focused ultrasound in Milan, Italy, and the ZapX device in Zurich. He is also an assistant professor at Mohammed bin Rashid Medical University and holds a master's degree in executive public administration from the Mohammed bin Rashid College of Governance. He is the director of the neurosurgery residency program at Dubai Health, which is the only program in the country.

He was the first to use the endoscope for brain surgeries in Dubai Health. He was the one who introduced reprogrammable shunt devices for the treatment of hydrocephalus in the Emirates. He also introduced many advanced tools for brain operations in the country.

He was honored by Sheikh Mohammed bin Rashid as one of the pioneers in the Emirates, as he was the first to measure brain pressure in rats for weeks, having invented a method for this. It was the first time in the world that brain pressure was measured in rats that were awake and active. He was also honored by the Dubai Health Authority. As the first Emirati pediatric brain surgeon and a distinguished doctor, he was also honored by the Ministry of Health as a distinguished doctor. The Emarat Al Youm newspaper also honored him as the "Personality of November" 2015. He was the first to perform an operation on a fetus due to myelomeningocele, the first operation of its kind in the Arab world.

He is the one who founded the Emirates Society of Neurological Surgeons and is the organizer of the annual Emirates International Neurosurgery Congress. He is the General Secretary of the Arab Pediatric Neurosurgical Society, the President of the Gulf Neurosurgical Society, and the Secretary of the Asian-Australian Neurosurgical Society. He is a former member of the Emirates Council of Scientists and a former Vice President of the Emirates Medical Association. He has presented many lectures and workshops at regional and international conferences. He is a former member of the World Economic Forum's Neurotechnology Committee.

He has many research papers published in the most prestigious scientific journals, including the world's first published case of brain hemorrhage and meningitis due to the Coronavirus. He is an active member of neurosurgical journals, serving as a reviewer of scientific papers.

Finally, Dr. Mohammed Al Olama was chosen as Personality No. 4 among the 100 most powerful people in Dubai to know, according to Arabian Business magazine, published in February 2023.

Meera earned her bachelor's degree in medicine and surgery from Sharjah Medical College in 2019. After graduation, she was accepted to start her internship at one of the biggest oncology centers in the UAE, in Al Ain city, in 2019, where she spent a year working at Tawam Hospital.

In 2020, she was accepted into the neurosurgery program in the UAE and commenced her training at Rashid Hospital.

She worked at the Bahrain Defense Force Military Hospital in the neurosurgery department in 2022 and in various university and specialty hospitals in KSA, also doing neurosurgery, over the past few years. Currently, she is in her fourth year of the neurosurgery residency program and is expected to graduate in 2026.

Open Access This chapter is licensed under the terms of the Creative Commons Attribution 4.0 International License (http://creativecommons.org/licenses/by/4.0/), which permits use, sharing, adaptation, distribution and reproduction in any medium or format, as long as you give appropriate credit to the original author(s) and the source, provide a link to the Creative Commons license and indicate if changes were made.

The images or other third party material in this chapter are included in the chapter's Creative Commons license, unless indicated otherwise in a credit line to the material. If material is not included in the chapter's Creative Commons license and your intended use is not permitted by statutory regulation or exceeds the permitted use, you will need to obtain permission directly from the copyright holder.

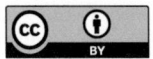

Healthcare System in the Emirate of Dubai

4

Hamid Y. Hussein , Heba Mamdouh , and Wafa K. Alnakhi

Abbreviations

AED	United Arab Emirates Dirham (currency)
AI	Artificial Intelligence
ASR	Annual Statistical Report
DHA	Dubai Health Authority
DOH	Department of Health Abu Dhabi
DHHS	Dubai Household Health Survey
DAHC	Dubai Academic Health Corporation
DOHMS	Department of Health and Medical services in Dubai
DSC	Dubai Statistics Center
EBP	Essential Benefit Plan
GDP	Gross Domestic Products
KPIs	Key Performance Indicators
MOHAP	Ministry of Health and Prevention

H. Y. Hussein
Dubai Health Authority, Dubai, United Arab Emirates
e-mail: hyhussain@dha.gov.ae

H. Mamdouh
Dubai Health Authority, Dubai, United Arab Emirates

Department of Family Health, High Institute of Public Health, Alexandria University, Alexandria, Egypt
e-mail: hmmohammed@dha.gov.ae

W. K. Alnakhi (✉)
College of Medicine, Department of Family and Community Medicine and Behavioral Sciences, The University of Sharjah (UOS), Sharjah, United Arab Emirates
e-mail: walnakhi@sharjah.ac.ae

© The Author(s) 2025
H. O. Al-Shamsi (ed.), *Healthcare in the United Arab Emirates*,
https://doi.org/10.1007/978-981-96-0523-1_4

NCEMA   National Emergency, Crisis, and Disaster Management Authority
OECD   Organization for Economic Co-operation
R and D Research and Development
UAE   The United Arab Emirates

4.1 The United Arab Emirates

The United Arab Emirates (UAE) was formed from a federation of seven emirates, consisting of Abu Dhabi (the capital), Ajman, Dubai, Fujairah, Ras Al Khaimah, Sharjah, and Umm Al Quwain. As of the 2020 Dubai Statistics Center (DSC) report, the UAE has an estimated population of roughly 9.9 million [1]. The UAE has established an infrastructure of healthcare services that is increasingly recognized as one of the best and matches international standards. The UAE healthcare sector is divided into public, private, and free zones. Public healthcare services are managed and regulated by federal/emirate level and local government entities such as the Ministry of Health and Prevention (MOHAP), the Dubai Health Authority (DHA), and the Department of Health Abu Dhabi (DOH). These entities often partner with foreign healthcare organizations to run the daily operations of hospitals and the different types of clinics through service provision arms in the UAE. The private healthcare sector and the free zone, on the other hand, are non-governmental bodies that provide high-skilled and full-spectrum care for the population. In 2018, the UAE was ranked one of the top-10 most efficient healthcare systems in the world [2].

4.2 Population and Demography of Dubai

Dubai is one of the Emirates of the UAE, occupying an area of 4114 km^2 with a population density of 754 persons per square kilometer. As per the DSC report, Dubai's population at the end of 2021 was 3.48 million; 69% of whom were males with a total of 2,400,100 individuals, and 31% of them were females (1,078,200) [3]. The higher proportion of males in Dubai (225 males per 100 females) is attributed to the fact that the majority of expatriate workers who are working in the Emirate are males who are not accompanied by their family members. Furthermore, Dubai is divided into nine geographic areas and health sectors, with each sector having a specific population mix, density, age, gender, and nationality type. These sectors assist with the planning in the Emirate by considering the distribution of infrastructure capacity, including healthcare facilities [3].

4.3 Healthcare Sectors in Dubai

The Dubai healthcare sector consists of government, private, and free zone entities that are aligned with the overall healthcare strategy of Dubai and the UAE and strive to provide quality services that are appropriate, accessible, and affordable for the community of Dubai. The Dubai Health Authority (DHA) looks after the health sector in the Emirate of Dubai, including both the private sector and the free zone at Dubai Healthcare City Authority (DHCC) and the public sector at Dubai Academic Health Corporation (DAHC). In addition, MOHAP, which is the federal ministry of health, oversees the UAE healthcare sector in general and some healthcare facilities operating in Dubai, such as Al Amal Hospital, Al Baraha Hospital, and many preventive healthcare centers [4].

4.3.1 Dubai Health Authority (DHA)

While the DHA is taking the lead in the healthcare system in Dubai, it is striving to make the population of Dubai healthier and happier by providing world-class healthcare services and fostering creativity, enhancing community engagement, and promoting innovation in alignment with the UAE Vision and Dubai Plan 2021.

4.3.2 Dubai Academic Health Corporation (DAHC)

Currently, the DAHC is operating five major hospitals (Rashid Hospital, Dubai Hospital, Latifa Hospital, Al Jalila Hospital, and Hatta Hospital), 13 primary healthcare centers, 5 specialized healthcare centers, 19 medical fitness facilities,[1] and 4 airport medical centers.

4.3.3 Private Sector

As per the 2020 DHA Annual Health Statistics Report (AHSR), there are 35 private hospitals, 46 one-day surgery centers, 1,300 clinics and healthcare centers in Dubai, about 1,000 pharmacies, and more than 1,200 other healthcare facilities [6]. The private sector in Dubai delivers the bulk of healthcare services through free zones and non-free zones, including Dubai Healthcare City, which attracts a significant number of both healthcare providers and patients in the emirate. In addition, 80% of healthcare utilization occurs in the private sector, and the remaining 20% in the

---

[1] This service enables an expatriate to obtain a certificate of good health following a fitness examination to prove that a worker is free from communicable and infectious diseases, thereby allowing or renewing a residence permit within the UAE [5].

public sector. This is in line with the estimates, which show that the public healthcare sector is used mainly by Emirati citizens. Meanwhile, expatriates make greater use of private healthcare services [6].

4.4 Healthcare in Dubai and Its Evolution

Over the years, Dubai has established an impressive health infrastructure consisting of hospitals, clinics, home care services, and diagnostic laboratories. The aim is to provide healthcare services to the growing population and establish new areas of clinical expertise in diabetes care, cancer treatment, cardiology, and other specialties. The transition from public to private sector services has been led by private sector investment, partnership with the government, and comprehensive insurance coverage [2] (Table 4.1).

Table 4.1 Historical evolution of the health system in the emirate of Dubai

Year	Evolution	Remarks
1900	Traditional medicine practice and first American Medical Mission	Traditional healers
1943	First hospital in Dubai: Al Maktoum Hospital	Government Service
1951	First outpatient Clinic: Al Maktoum Hospital	Government Service
1965	Expansion of Al Maktoum Hospital	Government Service
1952–1994	Sarah Hofmann Medical Mission/American	Private Service
1962–1971	Kuwaiti Medical Mission	Government Service
1970	Establishing Department of Health & Medical services in Dubai- (DOHMS), currently as Dubai Health Authority.	Government Service
1973	Rashid Hospital	Government Service
1983	Dubai Hospital	Government Service
1986	Dubai Blood Bank [7]	Government Service
1989	Dubai Thalassemia Centre [8]	Government Service
1991	Dubai Center for Gynecology and Infertility [9]	Government Service
1996	Al Wasel Hospital/Latifa	Government Service
1987	Primary Healthcare services (PHC)	Government Service
2003	Dubai Healthcare City	Free zone
2006	Dubai Cord Blood Centre [7]	Government Service
2006	Rashid Hospital Trauma Centre [10]	Government Service
2009	Dubai Diabetes Centre [11]	Government Service
2007	Dubai Health Authority	Reform of DOHMS
2018	DHA Restructuring and Reorganization	Reform DHA
2022	Separation of governmental Health Authorities in Dubai to Regulatory and Service Provision	Reform with division int DHA and DAHC

Source: Jamal Bin Huwaireb Center for Studies, Dubai: History of Health Services in Dubai [12]

4.5 Workforce Capacity in Dubai

The total workforce in the main health sectors in the Emirate of Dubai was 46,801, which constituted the five main healthcare workforce categories. This workforce was divided into 10,437 physicians, 2,699 dentists, 3,457 pharmacists, 19,272 nurses, and 10,936 technicians. The highest percentage of the health workforce is located in hospitals, with 20,755 employees (40%), followed by workers in health centers (29%), and the remaining employees are distributed in other types of healthcare facilities. Among the healthcare workforce, there were 11,914 were working in the DHA (23%), and 31,753 employees worked in the private sector (60.7%). In addition, 4969 employees worked in Dubai Healthcare City (9.6%), while in the Ministry of Health, there were 3438 employees, representing 6.6% of the health workforce in Dubai. As for the categories of doctors, 60.5% of doctors licensed in Dubai were specialists, followed by consultants (23.5%), and general practitioners (16.5%) [6].

4.6 The Main Healthcare Provisional Arms in Dubai

4.6.1 Operational Arm: Dubai Academic Health Corporation (DAHC)

Dubai Academic Health Corporation (DAHC) is responsible for the provision of governmental healthcare services through a network of facilities that covers the care continuum of "promotion, prevention, curing (emergency, acute, chronic, and palliative), and rehabilitation." There are 47 healthcare facilities belonging to DAHC (5 hospitals, 6 specialized healthcare centers, 13 primary healthcare centers, 19 medical fitness centers, and 4 airport medical centers). In addition, Mohamed bin Rashid Medical University, Al Jalila Hospital, and Al Jalila Research Foundation [13].

4.6.2 Delivery of Care Models In Dubai

4.6.2.1 Primary Healthcare
Primary healthcare (PHC) is defined as per the definition of WHO: it is a fundamental healthcare service made universally accessible to all individuals and their families in the community by means acceptable to them, through their full participation, and at a cost that the community and country can afford to receive the healthcare service (WHO) [14]. It is the cornerstone of all other health services; hence, DHA's objectives are to meet the World Health Organization's (WHO's) "Healthcare for Everyone" motto of the twenty-first century [15]. The PHC sector in the DHA consists of 13 health centers distributed throughout Dubai, offering a ratio of one health center or clinic for every 30,000 individuals. The geographical distribution of these centers takes into consideration the ease of accessibility for the Dubai population to the healthcare centers. Family medicine practice modules are widely applied and

fast-growing in Dubai for service provision in the private sector, and they serve as PHC services in the government sector [4].

4.6.2.2 Secondary Healthcare

Defined as the specialist treatment and support provided by physicians and health professionals for patients who have been referred to them from primary healthcare for seeking expert care, most often provided in hospitals. Almost 80% of the population's needs can be met in primary care, and 20% can be addressed at the hospital level. There are many examples of secondary care levels in Dubai, such as maternal care, dental care, and other services delivered at the hospital level [16].

4.6.2.3 Tertiary Healthcare

Defined as a level above secondary healthcare that is highly specialized medical care, usually provided over an extended period of time, and involves advanced diagnostics, procedures, and treatments. Infertility management through in vitro implantation, cord blood storage, and interventional cardiac catheterization are examples of tertiary healthcare provided in Dubai [16].

4.6.3 Regulatory Arm: Dubai Health Authority

The role of DHA is to ensure that Dubai offers an accessible, effective, and integrated healthcare system, protects population health, and improves quality of life within the emirate of Dubai. This can be achieved through a set of values, including but not limited to efficiency, excellence, accountability, integrity, patient-centricity, and a motivated workforce. DHA has been under sustainable transformation trials to provide clarity about the new paradigm. Overall, DHA covers the functions of health regulations, health insurance, health finance, public health and protection, and health policies and strategies [17].

4.6.3.1 Health Regulation

DHA is responsible for licensing healthcare professionals and healthcare facilities within the Emirate of Dubai. The health regulation department at DHA monitors the compliance of healthcare organizations—governmental and private—with the approved rules, regulations, policies, and international standards. Health regulation considers patient advocacy for any malpractice or complaints to ensure the protection of the patient's and family's rights with the Emirate of Dubai [17].

4.6.3.2 Healthcare Financing and Healthcare Insurance

The current healthcare expenditure in Dubai in 2019 was 19.27 billion AED (which is 4.7% of GDP), with 4115 AED per capita. In 2019, government healthcare expenditure accounted for 36% of total spending (6864 billion AED) and private healthcare expenditure accounted for 64% of total spending (12,410 billion AED). Employees' sources of funding were 53% from employers, 36% from government spending, and 11% from out-of-pocket spending. The share of all healthcare spending received by various providers was 42%, 26%, and 16% for hospitals, clinics, retail pharmacies, and ancillary providers, respectively. Curative care accounted for 59% of the total health expenditure. The government allocated 25% of its health expenditure to governance and administrative functions [18].

A law was introduced in 2014 by the DHA that requires all the population in Dubai to be covered by health insurance. In recent years, it has become a mandatory and legal requirement for companies in the emirate to provide a minimum level of health insurance to all employees. Both Emiratis and non-Emiratis are covered in the private sector by private insurance through the Enhanced Insurance Plans, or private health insurances. The Essential Benefit Plan (EBP) is another type of private health insurance that was developed to support expatriates who earn lower incomes and provide them with basic medical care coverage. People working for the government of Dubai are covered by government-funded employment-based schemes. In addition, Emiratis fulfilling the eligibility criteria, such as being unemployed or retired, are also covered by the government-funded social scheme. The plan also offers coverage for children, domestic worker staff, and non-working residents. Employers have the option and are free to choose a health insurance plan other than the EBP for employees earning more than 4,000 AED per month. Moreover, healthcare in Dubai is funded through taxation and the public sector; however, a small amount of funding comes from patient expenditures as co-payments [19].

4.6.3.3 Public Health Protection

Public health protection is another function of DHA and aims to develop Dubai's public health policies and services on the following levels: prevention of communicable diseases (surveillance, notification, and case-tracing systems); public health programs (non-communicable disease programs and Dubai disease registry systems); school health programs and services; and health promotion, in addition to the health education program [17].

4.6.3.4 Healthcare Policy

The existence of policies is to ensure the protection of the health and well being of individuals and to support the health system and services through a course of action [1]. Overall, Dubai Health Authority follows international standards, frameworks, and a series of processes to have the right approach and the correct end result for a policy. Monitoring and evaluation are fundamental parts of policy implementation in Dubai. In DHA, policy development starts with the direction of higher management in the government and the involvement of different stakeholders throughout the stages to fulfill the needs and requirements. In general, policies in DHA always cascade from the UAE's vision. To ensure the governance of health policy development in DHA, it is always aligned with standards, guidelines, and the usage of the right forms and documentation throughout the process. Finally, all the policies developed by DHA must be approved by the Executive Council of Dubai for authentication and execution [20].

4.7 Access to Essential Medicines in Dubai

In accordance with the WHO framework for health systems, a well-functioning health system should ensure equitable access to essential medical products, vaccines, and technologies of assured quality, safety, efficacy, and cost-effectiveness, and ensure their scientifically sound and cost-effective use [14]. In the same context, Dubai has an abundance of pharmacies, many of which are community pharmacies that dispense both over-the-counter and prescribed medications. In Dubai, there are medication policies, standards, guidelines, and regulations. In addition, policies are in place to support the rational use of medicines, commodities, and equipment through guidelines and strategies to assure adherence, reduce resistance, and maximize patient safety. However, certain medications and drugs are restricted or banned based on local policies [15].

4.8 Healthcare Information Systems

DHA has reliable and accurate health information systems that contain one of the most important sources of data and information for supporting the decision-making process. These information systems or data sources are represented in many modern electronic systems and smart applications. They all depend on the best technologies, systems, devices, and equipment that are considered the best in their field. DHA acknowledges the benefits that healthcare data can bring in terms of improving the quality of service provision, aiding in decision-making, optimizing the utilization of resources, and supporting the quality of patients' outcomes [17].

4.8.1 Availability of Data Sources

The availability of data sources at the DHA includes, but is not limited to, the following:

- Electronic Medical Record (Salama) is an integrated electronic health system that includes the data of patients treated in the facilities of the DHA and contains all information about the diseases they have previously had.
- ABIDH is Dubai's health information exchange platform for exchanging electronic medical records between healthcare facilities and providers across Dubai, both in the public and private sectors.
- The Dubai Household Health Survey (DHHS) is a field survey based on complex sampling design. It is conducted periodically, every four years. It is concerned with collecting, studying, and analyzing the social, health, and behavioral data of families in the Emirate of Dubai. It is used to describe chronic diseases and related risk factors and to utilize the data effectively.

- Satisfaction surveys (for patients, customers, and relevant partners) and follow the requesting party. These surveys are only available to all departments of the authority based on their requests.
- Specialized health surveys are specialized surveys that can be requested by the different units in DHA based on their needs. Eye surveys and dental surveys are examples of specialized surveys in DHA.
- Vital health statistics (births and deaths database) include official registered data on live births and deaths.
- The Sheryan System is an electronic system that includes comprehensive data on all healthcare provider details, including healthcare professionals and healthcare facilities. The system is fed by health facilities affiliated with the DHA.
- The Infectious Diseases Reporting System includes data on communicable diseases (defined by law) reported in the Emirate.
- Smart Salim is a medical fitness and occupational health examination system that includes medical fitness examination data.
- E-claims is an electronic claims system that contains the data of payers and health service providers in the Emirate [17].

4.9 Healthcare Research and Development

Research and development (R&D) is a top priority on the government's agenda in Dubai and the UAE, as it underpins the country's rapid growth. In Dubai, DHA has identified this priority to support medical and scientific researchers in the region by engaging them in collaborative research projects and international knowledge-exchange experiences. Funding research projects is a priority, along with having processes in place for utilizing and supporting the research and obtaining the logistics needed for research. It is important to create a culture of research and knowledge, with free-flowing dialogue between the government and research institutions on the core issue of inspiring the next generation of physicians, healthcare professionals, researchers, and all scientists in the healthcare field [2].

4.10 Healthcare Strategy

Existence of an up-to-date health strategy linked to population needs and priorities, starting with the 2016–2022 health strategy in Dubai developed by DHA and focused on health risk management, population lifestyle (smoking cessation, physical activity promotion, healthy food consumption, and mental health protection). Currently, DHA is implementing the 2022–2030 health strategy with many health initiatives and programs through an effective stakeholders' framework. Dubai has invested more in developing and applying long-term capacity planning for 2018–2030, focusing on the growth, demand, and expected shortage of supply in healthcare services for the coming 10 years and the management plan to address them. The extremely long-term plan 2071 health strategy was one of the unique vision strategies for the healthcare industry within the coming 50 years and is shaping the future of health in the emirate [4].

4.11 Responses to Crisis and Healthcare Emergencies

Dubai's response to healthcare emergencies and crises is within the context of the UAE's national response strategy. In terms of preparedness to manage an outbreak and according to the 2019 first Global Health Security Index, the UAE was placed 25th among 195 countries in commitments to improving national capacity, financing, and adherence to norms, and 56th in overall preparedness with a score of 46.7 [21]. Economically, and according to the World Economic Forum's 2019 edition of the Global Competitiveness Report, the UAE was ranked 25th in the world (gaining two positions since the last edition of the report) and second in the MENA region [22]. In terms of crisis and disaster management, the UAE established the National Emergency, Crisis, and Disaster Management Authority (NCEMA) in 2012 [23].

4.12 Collaboration Between DHA and the Organization for Economic Co-operation and Development (OECD)

As part of the Health System Performance Assessment and Data Infrastructure project, the OECD supported DHA in the development of its Academic Health System Performance Assessment (AHSPA) framework during the period of January 2021 to April 2022. A final framework that reports preliminary findings on Dubai's health system performance, based on internationally comparable data and measures, and provides an assessment of Dubai's health data infrastructure, was released internally for policy makers for better decision-making. Dubai's AHSPA framework covers 15 essential dimensions, and a substantial part of the Dubai framework aligns with the dimensions of the OECD's Health at a Glance framework. To initiate improvements in the healthcare system, an international benchmarking exercise was conducted utilizing50 key performance indicators (KPIs) of the health system that are both internationally comparable and readily accessible [19]. Table 4.2 summarizes the main dimensions of care covered and the main KPIs reported for Dubai.

Table 4.2 Dimensions of care and the main KPIs for population health and the health system's performance in Dubai: the OECD framework

Dimensions of care	Key indicators for population health and the health system performance
1. Health status	Trends in life expectancy
	Main causes of mortality (total and aggregated)
	Mortality due to respiratory diseases
	Mortality from circulatory diseases
	Cancer mortality
	Infant health
	Self-rated health
	External causes of mortality
2. Risk factors for health	Smoking among adults
	Diet and physical activity among adults
	Type I and II diabetes prevalence among adults
	Mortality due to infectious diseases
	Measured overweight (including obesity) rates among adults
3. Quality and outcomes of care	Mortality following an ischemic stroke
	Mortality following acute myocardial infarction
	Vaccinations
4. Health expenditure	Health expenditure per capita
	Health expenditure in relation to GDP
	Public funding of health spending
	Population coverage for healthcare
	Extent of healthcare coverage
	Use of primary care services
	Out-of-pocket expenditure
5. Health workforce	Health workforce total
	Practicing doctors per 1000 population
	Doctors (by age, sex, and category)
	Practicing nurses per 1000 population
	Practicing dentists per 1000 population
6. Healthcare activities	Consultations with doctors
	Hospital beds and discharge rates
	Average length of stay in hospitals
	Caesarean sections
	Occupancy rate of curative (acute) care beds

4.13 Future of Healthcare in Dubai

Dubai is aiming to have a healthy population by providing access to the highest standards of healthcare services in the world. The COVID-19 pandemic has put healthcare at the forefront of human existence, and there is no time to be lost in navigating out of the crisis and putting in place a national health strategy that will defeat COVID-19 while outlining the objectives for the healthcare sector that will support the UAE in becoming the best country in the world by 2071. Working on growing and attracting talent in the health sector in Dubai is one of the current challenges facing the future of healthcare in Dubai. The vision for 2071 is supporting the growth and development of the local talents in parallel with offering funding and grants for sending the best students overseas for the experience of working and shadowing internationally recognized physicians and healthcare professionals. Retaining quality healthcare staff remains a challenge everywhere in the world. The UAE 2071 vision is to focus on developing centers of excellence, enabling volumes of complex cases to be clustered together, supporting the development of specialists and consultants, shedding light on medical research projects, and providing the opportunity to publish research results, to deliver a higher quality of care and better patient outcomes based on evidence [24].

4.13.1 Medical Tourism

Medical tourism is a fundamental pillar of Dubai's healthcare strategy. The UAE has recently reached the top-10 list of globally ranked medical tourism destinations. According to the Medical Tourism Index, the world's most attractive countries for medical tourism are Canada, the United Kingdom, Singapore, and Costa Rica. Dubai is currently ranked sixth, and Abu Dhabi is eighth [25, 26].

4.13.2 Telemedicine

In December 2019, DHA launched a smart service titled "Doctor for Every Citizen." Under this service, individuals can take advantage of free consultations through voice and video calls 24/7. The service covers initial consultations and follow-ups with DHA-certified physicians. The physician can request laboratory and radiology tests and issue electronic prescriptions for patients who are consulting via telemedicine. Telemedicine is becoming the center of the future of healthcare delivery systems in Dubai. The benefits of telemedicine utilization include increased accessibility to healthcare, a focus on wellness and prevention, all of which result in reduced costs for certain specialties [27].

4.13.3 Artificial Intelligence

The use of artificial intelligence (AI) and machine learning in healthcare is crucial in order to support e-health delivery systems. AI data prediction tools, machine learning algorithms for image analysis, and robotics will become woven into the fabric of the future vision for healthcare. The regulators at DHA are now developing AI policy models that set out the essential requirements of AI in a healthcare framework: considering ethics, safety, role and responsibility, and security implications of AI use in healthcare [24].

4.13.4 Cloud Technology

Cloud technology offers great potential for enabling large volumes of data to be processed and managed by both regulator-controlled centralized systems and healthcare entities as end users. However, the current policy position in Dubai is for data to be hosted onshore on local servers, ensuring greater control and security. There should be a future national healthcare strategy for the use of cloud technology in association with adequate data security protections [24].

4.14 Conclusion

Developing and maintaining excellence and the continued growth of a healthcare system is not an easy task. As a result, the Dubai Health Authority is continuing to build strategies, create policies, and track key performance indicators to enable decision-makers to monitor the performance of the health system in Dubai. Overall, the healthcare system and services have greatly advanced over the years at all levels of care delivery models and across different sectors. The Government of Dubai has introduced many reforms to the Dubai Health Authority throughout the years to ensure that it addresses population needs. Since the health and well-being of the residents are a priority, the healthcare vision for 2071 shall leverage that momentum for further advancement and progress of the healthcare system. Utilizing technology, innovation, public-private partnerships, digital health, research and development, and attracting talent are all important factors supporting the healthcare system in Dubai. Building both human and machine learning technologies is essential to inspiring the next generation and enabling Dubai to be among the best healthcare systems in the world.

Acknowledgments Although the chapter was developed through the collaborative work of the co-authors, special thanks go to Dr. Eldaw Suliman, Advisor at the Strategy and Governance Department, Strategy and Corporate Sector, Dubai Health Authority, for providing feedback and insight into the flow of this chapter.

Conflicts of Interest The authors have no conflicts of interest to declare.

References

1. United Arab Emirates Population statistics (2021). Available online at: https://www.globalmediainsight.com/blog/uae-population-statistics/. Accessed 1 July 2022.
2. The U.A.E. Healthcare Sector by USA Business. Available online at: chrome-extension://efaidnbmnnnibpcajpcglclefindmkaj/. https://usuaebusiness.org/wp-content/uploads/2015/09/HealthcareReport_Update_June2014.pdf. Accessed 18 Aug 2022.
3. Population Bulletin: Emirate of Dubai, 2021. Available online at: chrome-extension://efaidnbmnnnibpcajpcglclefindmkaj/. https://www.dsc.gov.ae/Publication/Population%20Bulletin%20Emirate%20of%20Dubai%20%20-%202021.pdf. Accessed 16 July 2022.

4. Dubai Clinical Services Capacity Plan 2018–2030. Available online at: chrome-extension://efaidnbmnnnibpcajpcglclefindmkaj/. https://www.dha.gov.ae/uploads/122021/e9b6b25d-1339-4f2e-8fbf-2b8ea3217315.pdf. Accessed 16 July 2022.
5. Examination of Medical Fitness for Residency Visa. Available online at: https://www.ehs.gov.ae/en/services/services-directory/examination-of-medical-fitness-for-residency-visa. Accessed 26 Aug 2022.
6. Dubai Health Authority, Annul Health Statistical Report, 2020. Available online at: chrome-extension://efaidnbmnnnibpcajpcglclefindmkaj/. https://www.dha.gov.ae/uploads/032022/Annual%20%20Health%20Statistics%20%20Book%2020202022326320.pdf. Accessed 16 July 2022.
7. Dubai Blood Donation Center. Available online at: https://www.dha.gov.ae/en/facilities/speciality-centers/6. Accessed 18 Aug 2022.
8. Dubai Health Authority, Dubai Thalassemia Centre. Available online at: https://www.dha.gov.ae/en/facilities/speciality-centers/4. Accessed 18 Aug 2022.
9. Dubai Health Authority, Dubai Fertility Centre service catalogue. Available online at: chrome-extension://efaidnbmnnnibpcajpcglclefindmkaj/. https://www.dha.gov.ae/uploads/042022/Dubai%20Fertility%20Center%20-%20%20English2022448718.pdf. Accessed 18 Aug 2022.
10. Rashid Hospital. Available online at: https://en.wikipedia.org/wiki/Rashid_Hospital. Accessed 18 Aug 2022.
11. Dubai Diabetes Center. Available online at: https://www.dha.gov.ae/en/facilities/speciality-centers/14. Accessed 18 Aug 2022.
12. Jamal Bin Huwaireb Center for Studies, Dubai: History of health services in Dubai. Available online at: https://jbhsc.ae/%D8%AA%D8%A7%D8%B1%D9%8A%D8%AE-%D8%A7%D9%84%D8%AE%D8%AF%D9%85%D8%A7%D8%AA-%D8%A7%D9%84%D8%B5%D8%AD%D9%8A%D8%A9-%D9%81%D9%8A-%D8%AF%D8%A8%D9%8A/. Accessed 18 Aug 2022.
13. Mohammed bin Rashid issues a law establishing the Dubai Academic Health Corporation. Available online at: https://www.emaratalyoum.com/local-section/health/2021-07-17-1.1515600. Accessed 20 Aug 2022.
14. World Health Organization. Monitoring the building blocks of health systems: a handbook of indicators and their measurement strategies; 2010. Available online at: https://apps.who.int/iris/bitstream/handle/10665/258734/9789241564052-eng.pdf
15. Mohammed Bin Rashid School of Government (2018). The State of UAE Healthcare Service Delivery: Public Perceptions Preliminary Insights. Available online at: https://www.mbrsg.ae/getattachment/9e9f451a-5d2f-4080-a510-e3232e55df36/The-State-of-UAE-Healthcare-Service-Delivery.aspx. Accessed 10 June 2022.
16. Global Health Experts. Health Care Support, Training of Health Workers, Medication and Pharmaceuticals. Available online at: https://internationalmedicalcorps.org.uk/what-we-do/all-emergencies/secondary-health-care. Accessed 1 Sept 2022.
17. Dubai Health Authority. Available online at: https://www.dha.gov.ae/en. Accessed 18 Aug 2022.
18. Health Accounts System of Dubai, 2019. Available online at: chrome-extension://efaidnbmnnnibpcajpcglclefindmkaj/. https://www.isahd.ae/content/docs/HASD_2019_final.pdf. Accessed 17 Aug 2022.
19. Development of Dubai Health System Performance Assessment Framework- Dubai Health Authority – An OECD Project: Unpublished internal report, 2022.
20. Gilson, Lucy, and World Health Organization. Health policy and system research: a methodology reader: the abridged version. World Health Organization; 2013.
21. Global Health Security Index (2019). Available online at: https://www.ghsindex.org/wp-content/uploads/2019/10/2019-Global-Health-Security-Index.pdf. Accessed 18 July 2022.
22. World Economic Forum Insight Report (2019). The Global Competitiveness Report 2019. Available online at: http://www3.weforum.org/docs/WEF_TheGlobalCompetitivenessReport2019.pdf. Accessed 18 July 2022.

23. UAE Federal Law No. (2) of 2011. In Respect of the Establishment of the National Emergency, Crisis and Disasters Management Authority (NCEMA). Available online at: https://www.ncema.gov.ae/vassets/11bfa4f2. Accessed 19 June 2022.
24. Tithecott A.UAE health 2071: The future of healthcare. Al Tamimi and Co. Available online at: https://www.tamimi.com/law-update-articles/uae-health-2071-the-future-of-healthcare/. Accessed 19 June 2022.
25. Pollard K. Why Zagreb's medical tourism "strategic plan" is a sobering lesson. 2019. Available online at: https://www.imtj.com/blog/medical-tourism-strategy-where-does-it-all-go-wrong/. Accessed 19 June 2022.
26. The Medical Tourism Association: A Global Platform for the Healthcare Ecosystem (2021). Available online at: https://www.medicaltourism.com/mta/home. Accessed 19 June 2022.
27. UAE government Information and services: Telemedicine. Available online at: https://u.ae/en/information-and-services/health-and-fitness/telemedicine. Accessed 19 Aug 2020.

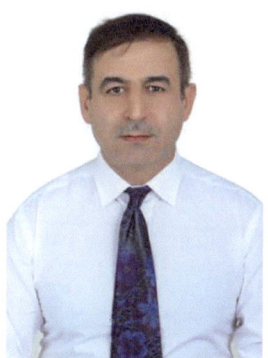

Dr. Hamid Hussein is a consultant physician and researcher in the Dubai Health Authority, WHO, and CDC; an expert consultant; and a professor at the Dubai residency training program in community and family medicine and the Arab Board for health specializations. Dr. Hussein is a professor at the Faculty of Medicine, University of Baghdad, and a member of the editorial board of 26 international medical journals worldwide. Moreover, he is a member of 33 international medical associations worldwide. He supervised more than 30 PhD theses and 25 MSc theses; published 340 articles worldwide, which were cited more than 600 times; and published 26 textbooks.

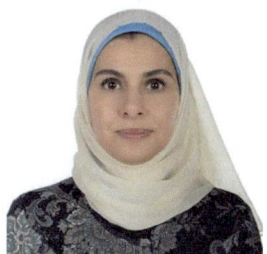

Dr. Heba Mamdouh is currently working as a research specialist in the Dubai Health Authority, UAE, and she also has two faculty appointments as adjunct associate professor in health sciences at Hamdan Bin Mohamed Smart University and Alexandria University. She graduated with a bachelor's degree in medicine, and then she earned her doctorate in public health degree from Alexandria University. With a double interest in medical research and population health, Dr. Mamdouh has more than 48 research publications and conference proceedings either internationally or regionally in the fields of population health and medical research.

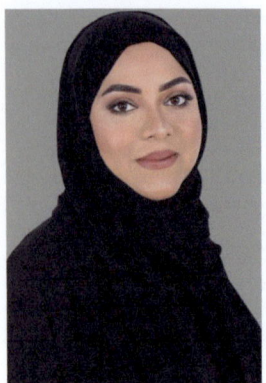

Dr. Wafa Alnakhi holds a doctorate in public health and a post-doctoral fellowship from Johns Hopkins Bloomberg School of Public Health. With 18 years of experience at Dubai Health Authority, she transitioned to academia and is currently an Assistant Professor and Director of the Clinical and Surgical Training Center at the University of Sharjah. Her research focuses on healthcare delivery, telemedicine, non-communicable diseases, and medical travel. As a published scholar, Dr. Alnakhi is committed to improving patient outcomes and health service utilization across the UAE through evidence-based policy and research.

Open Access This chapter is licensed under the terms of the Creative Commons Attribution 4.0 International License (http://creativecommons.org/licenses/by/4.0/), which permits use, sharing, adaptation, distribution and reproduction in any medium or format, as long as you give appropriate credit to the original author(s) and the source, provide a link to the Creative Commons license and indicate if changes were made.

The images or other third party material in this chapter are included in the chapter's Creative Commons license, unless indicated otherwise in a credit line to the material. If material is not included in the chapter's Creative Commons license and your intended use is not permitted by statutory regulation or exceeds the permitted use, you will need to obtain permission directly from the copyright holder.

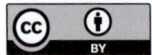

Abu Dhabi Public Health Center

Omniyat Mohammed Al Hajeri ⓘ,
Sheikh Abdulla Bin Mohammed Bin Butti Al Hamed,
and Matar Saeed Al Nuaimi

5.1 A New Horizon for Public Health

Abu Dhabi Public Health Center (ADPHC) is a newly established government entity, founded on April 23 under Law No. 14 of 2019. ADPHC is an independent entity with full legal capacity to practice its activities and follows the Department of Health-Abu Dhabi.

The center brought together, in a unique setting, both elements of public health and safety by combining and expanding the functions of the previous Abu Dhabi Occupational Safety and Health Center and the Public Health Department of the Department of Health-Abu Dhabi.

ADPHC comes with a clear vision, which is "Towards a healthy and safe society," and a mission to enhance the health of the population of Abu Dhabi and ensure the safety of its employees through the implementation of an integrated public health management system with the highest levels of innovation, excellence, and creativity. The ADPHC's work areas include:

- *Development of regulations and legislation*: Developing policies and standards related to public health and ensuring effective implementation of system requirements
- *Providing services to individuals and society*: Vaccines, awareness campaigns, early detection programs, registration of service providers, and public health practitioners

O. M. Al Hajeri (✉) · M. S. Al Nuaimi
Abu Dhabi Public Health Center, Abu Dhabi, United Arab Emirates
e-mail: ohajri@adphc.gov.ae; matalnuaimi@adphc.gov.ae

S. A. B. M. B. B. Al Hamed
Department of Health-Abu Dhabi, Abu Dhabi, United Arab Emirates

© The Author(s) 2025
H. O. Al-Shamsi (ed.), *Healthcare in the United Arab Emirates*,
https://doi.org/10.1007/978-981-96-0523-1_5

- *Building national competencies*: Public health research development, developing specialized public health courses in schools and universities, ongoing training of trainers in all sectors with a special focus on healthcare professionals to facilitate the implementation of all public health programs
- *Support for decision-makers*: Analyzing Public Health data, providing databases for public health in the Emirate of Abu Dhabi, Using innovation and Artificial Intelligence in the fields of public health to establish early warning systems, providing expert advice and consultancy services to multiple local, national, and international committees
- *Consolidation of local and international relations*: Coordination with local and international bodies to support public health projects and goals, holding strategic partnerships with internal and external parties to exchange experiences and apply best practices

5.2 Abu Dhabi Public Health Center (ADPHC)

The ADPHC has seven strategic priorities, including the governance and management of the public and preventive health system (public health system); encouraging the community to practice a healthy lifestyle; ensuring the health and safety of workers and the environment; improving the quality of life and reducing the financial burden of disease; implementing an effective system for the prevention and control of infectious diseases; building and developing sustainable national capacities in public health; and supporting decision-making with early warning, innovation, and artificial intelligence.

Priority programs are designed and selected to meet the strategic priorities of the ADPHC and fully align with the local strategies of the Abu Dhabi Government and the federal and national strategies of the country. They also ensure updating and alignment with the international World Health Organization (WHO) targets, Centers for Disease Control and Prevention (CDC) recommendations, and international agreements and commitments.

We also build the programs to target and address the main causes of mortality and morbidity in our community (Fig. 5.1), keeping in mind the importance of feasibility of implementation, maximizing the utilization of resources, building on

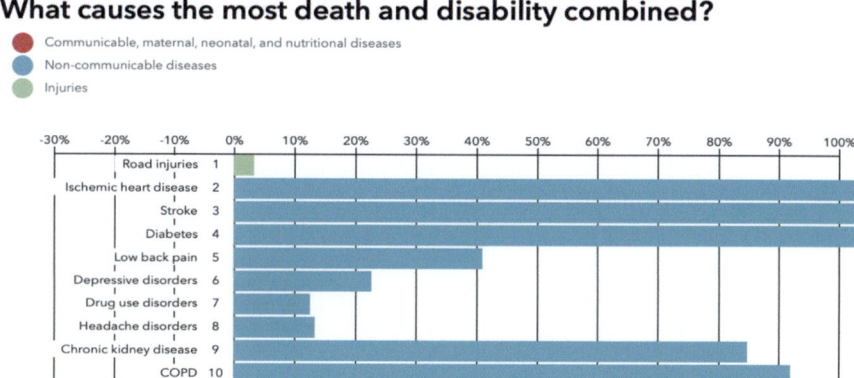

Fig. 5.1 Top ten causes of death and disability (DALYs) in 2019 and percent change 2009–2019, all ages combined

mutual synergies with partners and stakeholders, and conducting community needs assessments.

5.3 Excellence in COVID-19 Response

In the few months after the establishment of the ADPHC, the first case of COVID-19 was reported in the UAE, and the ADPHC geared up and used all its resources to play a pivotal role in the pandemic response, Supporting Decision-makers and leading many aspects of the COVID pandemic response in the health sector, educational sector and the community in general. (The details of the Abu Dhabi pandemic response are covered in Chap. 40.

The ADPHC teams worked closely with local, national, and international stakeholders and contributed positively to the success of the distinguished COVID-19 response.

Abu Dhabi was recognized globally for the high-quality COVID-19 response, which was the result of applying best-in-class operational practices, including the highest global rate of vaccination per 100 people, robust and rapid expansion in related research projects and publications, the largest single-city vaccine Phase III trial in the world, and being listed in the top 10 cities globally in safety, treatment, quality, trust, and quality of life (Bloomberg and DKG safety rankings). To ensure maintaining one of the lowest death rates associated with COVID-19 infectionInfection globally, Abu DHabi established a centralized call center with a 24/7 active hot line (ESTIJABA line) to support all the public needs related to the pandemic, enhancing the local manufacturing abilities, including extraction tests per day, highquality face masks, personal protection equipment (PPEs), vaccine needs, and opening the export market.

Abu Dhabi also managed to establish one of the largest logistics and distribution hubs globally for vaccines and played an active role in establishing the Hope consortium, serving more than 250 destinations for humanitarian missions.

Innovation led the way in Abu Dhabi, with artificial intelligence (AI) heat maps to guide testing, an online AI symptom checker, a dynamic COVID-19 website, AI-based early sensing, prediction, and management modules, 270 live COVID-19 dashboards and daily reports, and sewage early surveillance.

ADPHC also led effective contact tracing, covering more than 100% of confirmed cases within 48 hours, with a special focus on students and special groups. It pioneered efforts in promoting healthy lifestyles and raising awareness in the community through awareness-raising workshops and "Improving Immunity" campaigns. It developed educational materials and guidelines that were adopted nationally in relation to many aspects of the COVID-19 response, including return-to-work and return-to-school protocols.

5.4 Special Outreach Programs Led by ADPHC for the Abu Dhabi Community

Educational institutions and schools received special attention from ADPHC in collaboration with ADEK (Abu Dhabi Department of Education and Knowledge), ESE (Emirates Schools Establishment), and the Ministry of Education to ensure the safety and health of our students. Robust surveillance was established through routine testing in schools and in specialized centers designated for students and educational staff. Abu Dhabi was the first in the region to introduce PCR COVID-19 testing using saliva samples instead of nasal swabs as a more student-friendly testing method, which was then also expanded to people of determination and senior adults. The successful continuation of education with hybrid (virtual and in-school modules) and the successful return to schools and universities in Abu Dhabi was a result of multiple strategies that included testing, surveillance, active contact tracing with strict isolation, and quarantine, with a specialized education sector contact tracing team assigned by ADPHC to prioritize this important group. In addition to the strict cleaning, disinfection and partial or total closure guidelines and protocols in the educational institutions, we also arranged targeted vaccination visits to schools and established designated vaccination centers that give the priority to the education sector. ADPHC had also robust inspection visits to all ediucational intitutions ensuring safe environment for AD students. A special electronic data dashboard was created to track cases and vaccination numbers, with the ability to zoom down to the individual school or university and even further to a specific student or staff member using their Emirates ID. This was of great value during the pandemic.

The population-at-risk program for seniors and chronic disease patients was launched in April 2020 in response to the COVID-19 pandemic. Abu Dhabi Public Health Center (ADPHC), in collaboration with the Department of Health (DOH), worked to develop a new program to provide sustainable telehealth services to patients with chronic diseases over the age of 60. It is estimated that about 43,791 elderly people suffering from heart disease, diabetes, cancer, and other chronic diseases across Abu Dhabi benefited from the services provided by the remote care program smoothly, comfortably, and safely during the pandemic period. These services included home visits to provide health promotion advice, healthcare, and blood test services if the disease required it (phlebotomy), as well as home delivery of medicines and remote medical consultations.

This initiative harnessed the paradigm shift Abu Dhabi is taking to improve access to and quality of comprehensive care. It also supported the innovation path Abu Dhabi is taking through electronic platforms that provide access to medical support and guidance for community members in need of remote care.

It is worth noting that the telehealth program for individuals suffering from chronic diseases was started by ADPHC as a pilot program to provide care services for about 1,200 elderly patients in the Emirate of Abu Dhabi through various health facilities. After the success of the pilot phase, the program's scope, objectives, and mechanisms were expanded, and ADPHC collaborated with the DOH to include a larger segment of patients and cases.

ADPHC also published guidelines with special advice for chronic diseases during COVID-19 and circulated them to all healthcare providers. It also launched the "Towards a Healthy and Safe Community" campaign with more than 13 stakeholders and partners, targeting senior citizens and residents, in addition to patients with chronic diseases and people of determination, for general wellness and health advice.

Another iconic campaign called "We reach you wherever you are" was also launched by ADPHC[1], an initiative ensuring that all eligible senior citizens can receive the COVID-19 vaccinations, including the booster dose (when applicable), from the comfort of their own homes, thereby reducing their exposure to COVID-19 and protecting them from disease. This led to an increase in booster dose uptake of over 300%. An electronic dashboard was established with the details of all senior citizens. Individuals were called and appointments offered; if anyone was not convinced, trained staff contacted them, provided all the required information, and gave them reassurance.

The blue-collar labor outreach program was also pivotal to the COVID-19 response's success in Abu Dhabi. It ensured daily inspection missions and assessments were conducted in the labor camps and at other sites with high population density to identify positive cases for isolation and individuals for quarantine. Also, inspection visits were conducted to ensure that facilities were compatible with and appropriate for patient isolation and quarantine, that appropriate medical care was provided, and that individuals had access to medical services in the allocated isolation and quarantine accommodations. The ADPHC has collaborated with DOH, municipalities, the Abu Dhabi agriculture and food safety authority, the Abu Dhabi Police, and other stakeholders to organize medical teams, surveillance teams, and inspection teams to ensure effective logistics are in place to monitor hygiene, sanitation, food distribution, water, waste management and disposal, and security to meet the necessary standards. The teams were also responsible for educating, promoting healthy practices, and arranging for the transfer of individuals to the identified accommodations, care settings, and/or managed facilities.

5.5 Implementation of an Effective System

Implementing an effective system for the prevention and control of infectious diseases is one of the seven priority areas that ADPHC focuses on. Infectious disease in the UAE is covered in a separate chapter in this book, but it is worth highlighting some of the important elements that ADPHC works on in relation to infectious disease and emerging infections.

The effective response to the COVID-19 pandemic is a testimonial to years of ongoing training and capacity building in readiness and preparedness in general, and in infectious disease pandemic response in particular. The Emirate of Abu Dhabi, represented by DOH and ADPHC, reviews the status of the main communicable diseases in Abu Dhabi and works continuously to enhance the electronic surveillance system of communicable diseases and to create a robust early warning system for the detection of infectious diseases.

The ADPHC experts work diligently on multiple initiatives to conduct evidence-based communicable disease surveillance and response.

They should identify the yearly requirements for the vaccines for the Emirate of Abu Dhabi, as vaccination is the most effective tool for controlling and eliminating serious infectious diseases, thereby preserving public health and protecting lives. Without vaccines, diseases such as polio and measles would spread uncontrollably around the world. It is important to continue these efforts and strengthen the immunity of the community through adherence to routine vaccination and immunization campaigns when needed. ADPHC is responsible for identifying the vaccination program in the Emirate of Abu Dhabi and issuing related policies, standards, and guidelines. It is also responsible for procuring the Emirate's needs for vaccines and ensuring the safety and quality of the vaccines in use. There are different vaccination programs, including childhood, school, adult, hajj, umrah, and traveler. The vaccination service is given free of charge to eligible groups at government and semi-government healthcare facilities.

The ADPHC expert teams work closely with healthcare providers to assure safe and high-quality vaccine handling and maintain cold chain requirements through continuous monitoring, conducting periodic training for healthcare professionals involved in vaccination services, and enhancing their roles as vaccine advocates. Improving education and awareness about vaccinations is very important to reduce the impact of anti-vaccination campaigns. The vaccination register and database are important parts of the public health information system.

Prevention, early detection, and response to infectious diseases and emerging infections according to best international practices are among ADPHC's priorities. ADPHC works relentlessly to build capacity in the Emirate through training healthcare professionals and improving the diagnostic capabilities available in Abu Dhabi.

The ADPHC and DOH had previously established the first Biosafety Level 3 laboratory (BSL-3) in the country at Sheikh Khalifa Medical City and recently launched the new mobile BSL-3 lab unit, the first of its kind in the region, equipped to handle highly infectious disease agents. This will support the safe diagnosis of communicable diseases and strengthen the Emirates' pandemic preparedness.

The yearly "Stop the Spread" campaign is designed to target the public by encouraging healthy habits that prevent the spread of infectious diseases in the community, with a special emphasis on respiratory infections and seasonal influenza [2]. The campaign also highlights and raises awareness of certain infectious diseases and their common preventive measures, such as vaccination, preventive treatment, laboratory testing, and symptom control.

The center works on maintaining zero or low prevalence of infectious diseases such as diphtheria, tetanus, polio, chickenpox, measles, mumps, and rubella, and has special programs to control malaria, respiratory infections, tuberculosis, HIV, and other infectious diseases.

5.6   Public Health Agenda

During, after the pandemic, and to date, ADPHC has continued to drive forward the public health agenda in all other priority areas with multiple initiatives.

H.E. The Chairman of the Department of Health issued Decree Number 43 for the year 2022, which puts together the milestones in the development of the public health and preventive health systems in Abu Dhabi and also identifies the main responsibilities of the ADPHC in relation to other relevant entities, bodies, and individuals as necessary. This is called the public health and preventive health system for Abu Dhabi.

ADPHC launched a campaign with multiple media and communication channels to raise awareness about this system and its implications, this campaign also included the list of sanctions and penalties associated with violations of the system requirements. It also reviewed and attested to the plans for the main nine sectors regulated for occupational health and safety in the public and private sectors in the Emirate.

The center has trained and certified inspectors to audit and follow up on those plans and ensure implementation. There is also a linkage to the stakeholders through the electronic system (ADDAA) [3]. The ADPHC is notified of all serious workplace injuries and investigates those cases to ensure that appropriate measures are in place to avoid reoccurrences.

The ADPHC teams advocate and support injury prevention policies and regulations through all stages of life, with a special focus on the workplace, childhood, and the elderly, by implementing injury prevention-related programs within society in coordination with concerned stakeholders. These include multiple campaigns such as safety in the heat, preventing child injuries, drowning, weather conditions, noise awareness, height fall awareness, and elderly safety [4–6].

All those programs focus on building the capacity of the Emirate of Abu Dhabi in the relevant fields through training the trainers and experts, advocating for laws and legislation supporting the programs locally and nationally, and launching educational and awareness sessions directly and through multiple available media channels, using appropriate styles and languages for the target sub-populations.

In addition, ADPHC is working to develop and implement Abu Dhabi's occupational health and support services framework, policies, and regulations, including structural and financing models; personnel requirements (qualifications, experience, capacity, registration, etc.); support services (e.g., fitness to work, periodic medical occupational surveillance, and laboratories related to occupational and environmental sciences); reporting and data collection requirements; and mechanisms to support the implementation of world-class occupational health and the improvement of occupational health status in the Emirate of Abu Dhabi based on best international practices, ensuring excellence and sustainability in providing occupational health services.

5.7   Medical Registry Platform

ADPHC also established, in collaboration with the DOH, the Medical Registries Platform, which started with the launch of the diabetes and cancer registries and will expand progressively to cover the screening registry and several other important disease registers in Abu Dhabi [7].

In addition, the center is responsible for the continuous evaluation and improvement of death notification and mortality reports, which are essential for deciding future priorities and targeted public health interventions, and is working continuously on capacity building and team member training in the field of digital transformation and data management.

5.8   Screening Programs

As part of the initiatives targeting the improvement of quality of life and reducing the financial burden of disease, ADPHC is focusing on developing and implementing age-appropriate screening programs that serve the population starting even before they are born.

5.8.1   Premarital Screening Program

Premarital screening is part of the spectrum; it tests couples who are planning to get married soon for common chronic diseases, genetic blood disorders (e.g., sickle cell anemia and thalassemia), and infectious diseases (e.g., hepatitis B, hepatitis C, and HIV/AIDS). The program provides medical consultation on the odds of transmitting the diseases mentioned to the other partner or their future children and offers partners options that help them plan for a healthy family, including IVF and embryo selection. Pilots to expand the premarital screening genetic components are taking place to eventually link to the Emirati Genome Project and better protect future generations.

5.8.2 Maternal and Child Health Screening Program

Maternal and child health screening programs at the Abu Dhabi Public Health Center aim to reduce risk factors before, during, and after pregnancy for mothers, and to help detect any mother- and infant-related medical issues at an early stage to allow timely intervention. The screening is supported by targeted health education and advocacy, the development and revision of guidelines and standards, and relevant research projects conducted in collaboration with interested partners such as the Pregnancy Risk Assessment Survey (PRAMS) alongside early childhood authorities, and academic institutions like Khalifa University and the Mutabaa study with UAE University. These initiatives will guide policymaking and improve preventative and curative services provided to mother, children, and families [8].

5.8.3 Newborn Screening Program

Newborn screening is a highly successful public health program that identifies rare metabolic, endocrine, enzymatic, and other genetic disorders and assures early management and follow-up for those affected [8]. Finding these conditions soon after birth can help prevent some serious problems, such as brain damage and organ damage, that permanently impact the health and overall quality of life of newborns or even lead to death. This screening is followed by a structured *child visit program* and vaccination visit programs, where children are seen periodically until the age of four years.

5.8.4 School Screening Program

School Screening: A Key Component of ADPHC's School Health Programs School screening detects disease conditions that students may have, even if they appear and feel generally well. Early detection enables timely treatment and good control of the condition, and reduces the risk of serious complications and developmental delays if appropriately diagnosed.

The school screening includes multiple elements like the identification of overweight and obese children, referral of children >85th percentile for further evaluation and management, vision and hearing tests, screening for scoliosis in adolescents, dental screening, and screening for anemia. In addition to physician examinations (including growth and development assessments), school nurses should also provide health promotion guidance to students during individual and group consultations on topics including nutrition, physical activity, injury prevention, smoking prevention, oral health, and mental health [9].

This screening program is complemented by the "Eat Right and Get Active" program, which is a structured initiative driven by school nurses and teachers who are trained by ADPHC experts to implement multiple educational activities in the school setting. The goal is to help reduce the percentage of students affected by diseases and illnesses caused by poor eating habits, lack of physical activity, and inadequate sleep hygiene. The number of schools participating in the "Eat Right and Get Active" program increased from 36 schools in 2011 to 350 schools and nurseries in 2019. The participating schools included 257 government schools, 48 private schools, and 48 nurseries across the emirates of Abu Dhabi, Al Ain, and Al Dhafra. All school cycles (one, two, and three) were included in the training workshops on how to participate in the program and implement it within their schools. So far, 375 schools and nurseries have participated in the 2022–2023 cycle, and the number is expected to increase [10].

5.8.5 IFHAS Screening Program

The periodic comprehensive screening program (IFHAS) is an integrated health screening initiative that contributes to reducing the burden of the top priority chronic diseases (noncommunicable diseases, or NCDs), including cardiovascular diseases, cancer, and bone diseases, in the Emirate of Abu Dhabi among Thiqa card holders aged 18–75 years.

The IFHAS screening includes an integrated assessment of health risks through a questionnaire, in addition to a comprehensive clinical examination and tests, based on class-A evidence-based screenings identified by leading international practices, divided into screening bundles appropriate for each age group and gender [11].

The IFHAs program integrates the pre-existing Weqaya cardiovascular risk screening programs, cancer screening programs, and other new elements to enable early detection, reduce the disease burden, and prevent complications.

The new program includes screening services for the following conditions: cardiovascular disease (CVD) and risk factors such as diabetes, hypertension, dyslipidemia, and serum creatinine for renal function, obesity, and smoking history; in addition to abdominal aortic aneurysm screening for senior citizens; cancer (breast, cervical, lung, and colorectal); musculoskeletal disease (osteoporosis); mental health (depression); oral health; and senior citizens' health (including vision and hearing tests).

In the first phase, five large providers with more than 150 clinical sites between them provided services, including SEHA/ambulatory health services, VPS Group, Mediclinic, and Mubadala Health [12].

Supporting this comprehensive program, ADPHC and the involved stakeholders launched multiple awareness and educational campaigns to encourage the target population to take the test.

5.9 Emirati Genome Project

ADPHC is actively supporting the Emirati Genome Project and is currently piloting the integration of genetic analysis components into many of its screening programs to encourage personalized prevention and precision medicine initiatives. Examples of current priorities and activities in public health genomics include hereditary breast/ovarian cancer syndrome, Lynch syndrome colorectal cancer, premarital screening, rare diseases and newborn screening, familial hypercholesterolemia, and the role of pathogen genomics in infectious disease control and prevention.

5.10 Cancer Control Plan

It is important to highlight that ADPHC has a cancer control plan, providing a coordinated and comprehensive approach that addresses all aspects of the cancer continuum of care based on international best practices. The strategies include prevention, early detection, diagnosis, supportive treatment, and palliative care. ADPHC's comprehensive approach focuses on five main strategies. For example, launching an annual Cancer Wave awareness campaign that lasts for 6 months, from October to March, through social media platforms and by holding interactive community sessions to combat cancer and increase screening uptake in collaboration with more than 100 government, private organizations, and NGOs. ADPHC also participates in many different events, including international days such as World Cancer Day, oncology conferences, and national and international symposia.

ADPHC also established the cancer and screening uptake registers. Through our research arm, we are also supporting cancer-related research projects and a pilot programs that supports innovative prevention, early detection, and treatment modalities,

There have been great improvements in the early detection of cancers over the last 10 years; for example, in 2012, 50% of cervical cancer cases were diagnosed at stage four; in 2018, this dropped to 7.5% (Figs. 5.2 and 5.3) [13].

Colorectal cancer detection in late stages has improved over the years but clearly requires more focused efforts, as well as the exploration of less invasive approaches that are more acceptable within the target groups (Fig. 5.4) [14].

The fight against breast cancer started back in 2004, and the success story is a testimonial to what dedication, persistence, and collaboration can bring. The number of cases diagnosed in late stages dropped from 64% in 2007 to 15% in 2019 (Fig. 5.5) [15].

In support of the prevention and early detection of cardiovascular diseases and cancers, ADPHC focuses on a comprehensive tobacco control program. The program aims to raise overall awareness among the community about the harmful

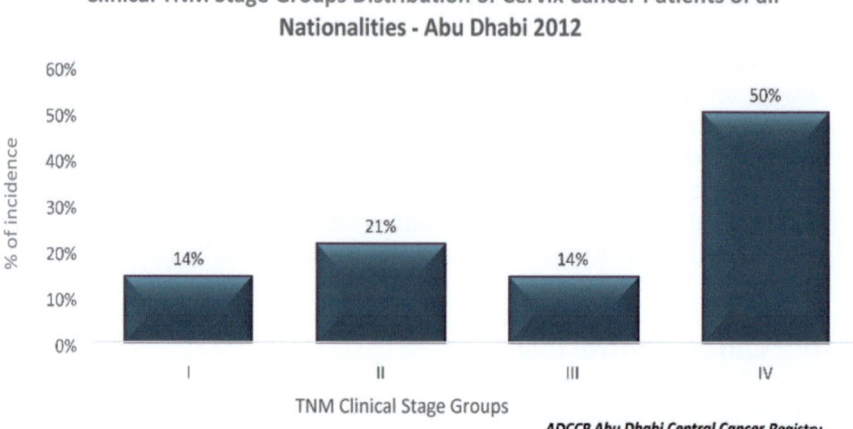

Fig. 5.2 Clinical TNM stage groups distribution of cervix cancer patients of all nationalities—Abu Dhabi 2012

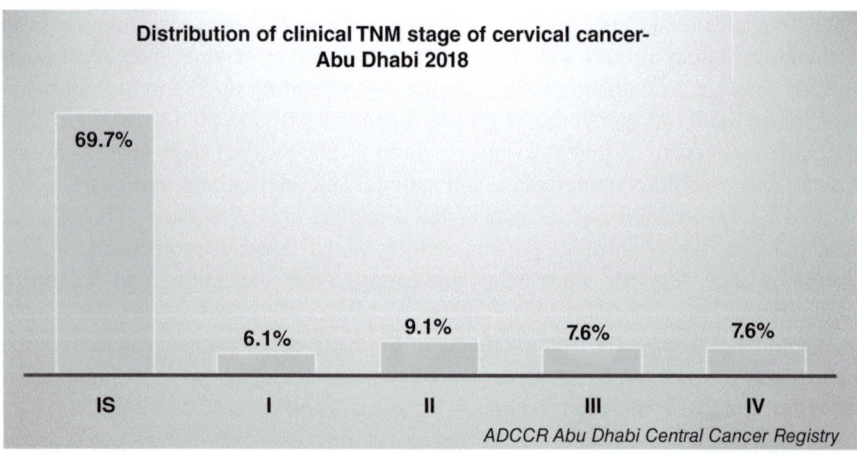

Fig. 5.3 Distribution of clinical TNM stage of cervical cancer—Abu Dhabi 2018

effects of tobacco use, secondhand smoke exposure, and the importance of leading a healthy lifestyle, as well as to advocate for the implementation of Federal Law 15 of 2009 and Executive By-Law 24 of 2013 concerning tobacco control, together with other governmental agencies and community organizations. The program also focuses on developing and empowering the healthcare workforce, establishing standards for smoking cessation, monitoring smoking cessation services, engaging partners, raising public awareness with a special focus on school kids and young adults to prevent initiation, and encouraging applied research [16].

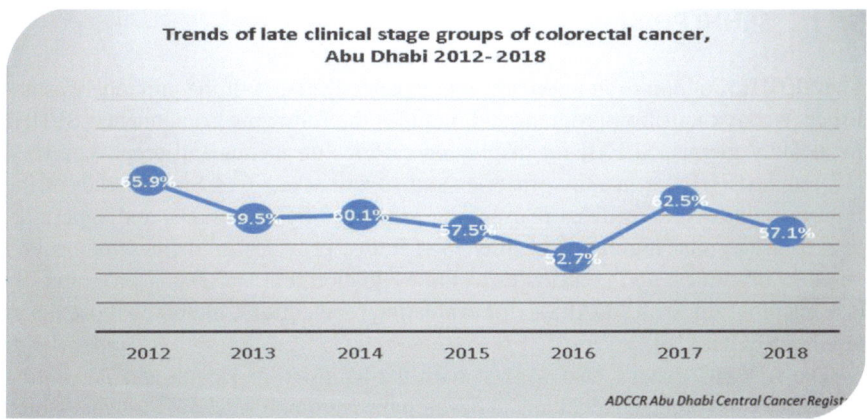

Fig. 5.4 Trends of late clinical stage groups of colorectal cancer, Abu Dhabi 2012–2018

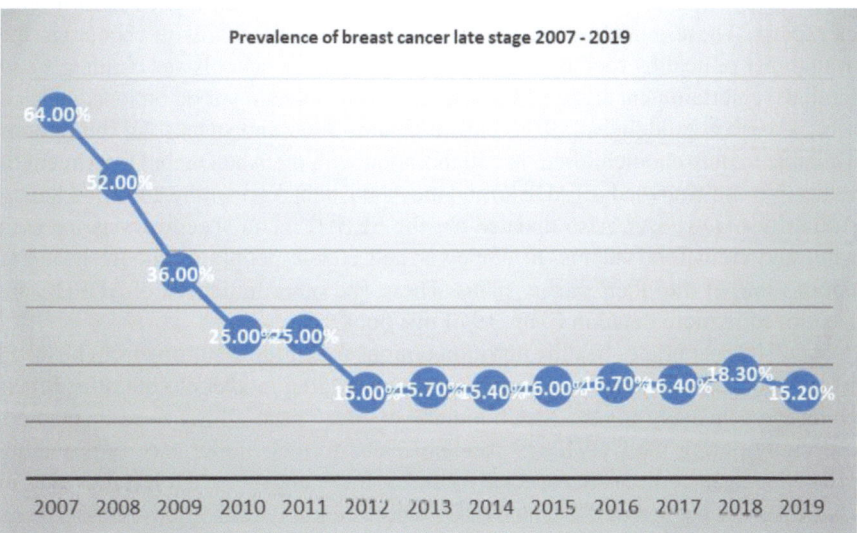

Fig. 5.5 Prevalence of breast cancer late stage 2007–2019

5.11 Prevention Programs

As part of ADPHC's priority to encourage the community to adopt a healthy lifestyle, the center oversees several large programs to support healthy nutrition and physical activity.

5.11.1 SEHHI Program

The SEHHI program is an improved and expanded version of the previously established Weqaya nutrition program and includes the following components: SEHHI for healthy menus; SEHHI for displaying calories on menus and prepacked food [17]; and SEHHI for healthy groceries and supermarkets (the Supermarket of the Future initiative). It involves rearranging groceries, hypermarkets, and supermarkets in a way that highlights healthy food items, provides guidelines for healthy vending machines, and contributes to the evaluation and star rating program, the Zaadna program, with ADAFSA, for evaluating food entities, including those registered in SEHHI [18].

The ADPHC experts also worked with the Ministry of Health and Prevention (MOHAP) and other stakeholders to develop the National Nutrition Strategy, which includes a full national strategy for fighting childhood obesity. At the Abu Dhabi Emirate level, the center worked on multiple guidelines and standards endorsed and approved by the QCC (Abu Dhabi Quality and Conformity Council) and its groups of experts. These guidelines include the Green Zone Standards to encourage the availability of healthy food options in areas surrounding schools and children's and families' entertainment areas, and to limit access to unhealthy food options; updated school canteen guidelines [19] to ensure healthy food and snacks are the options available to our schoolchildren, in collaboration with the Abu Dhabi Department of Education and Knowledge (ADEK) and the Abu Dhabi Agriculture and Food Safety Authority (ADAFSA). Also updated are the SEHHI menu specifications for both adult and child food menus, to empower and enable people to choose healthier options that fit into their dietary plans. These and other initiatives of ADPHC are mentioned in more detail in Chap. 19 of this book.

ADPHC encourages healthy nutrition options for children starting from birth via its educational and promotional activities, encouraging mothers to breastfeed their children exclusively for the first 6 months of life. These efforts were intensified, especially during the COVID-19 pandemic, due to their importance in providing protection against diseases, especially viruses, for youngsters. ADPHC provides, in collaboration with MOHAP and WHO, baby-friendly certification training to all maternity hospitals in the Emirate [20].

5.11.2 Physical Activity Programs

Physical activity is an important element of a healthy lifestyle; in addition to healthy nutrition, stress management, and good sleep hygiene, it helps maintain health and prevent disease. ADPHC has launched multiple initiatives to increase physical activity in Abu Dhabi and to integrate it as part of the daily routine for all members of the community.

ADPHC successfully hosted the ninth edition of the ISPAH (International Society for Physical Activity and Health) Congress at the Abu Dhabi National Exhibition Centre (ADNEC) in Abu Dhabi, which was co-sponsored by the World Health Organization. The congress attracted over 4,000 delegates (national, regional, and international). Around 400 abstracts were received from over 65 countries around the world, including over 100 poster presentations and more than 80 oral presentations.

As part of the countdown activities for this conference, the One Billion Steps Challenge was successfully completed in collaboration with the STEPPI application and Etihad Airways.

The physical activity enhancement initiative "Active Abu Dhabi" consists of multiple projects and programs, all of which work synergistically, complementing each other in improving levels of physical activity in the Emirate of Abu Dhabi. This includes developing technical guidelines and a code of practice for physical activity in Abu Dhabi; working together with the Abu Dhabi Quality and Conformity Council (QCC) and other stakeholders, such as the municipality and Dubai Civil Defence (DCD), to promote physical activity as part of everyday life within the infrastructure standards of Abu Dhabi (e.g., outdoor gyms, cycling lanes, and running tracks); and piloting an exercise-on-prescription project, where healthcare professionals are trained and empowered to prescribe exercise to their patients as part of their management plan to improve disease outcomes and enhance quality of life. ADPHC, in collaboration with DOH and the Abu Dhabi Tourism Authority, also launched the Citymoov application, an innovative project to promote physical activity in a fun and engaging manner using treasure hunts to explore the beautiful tourist attractions in the Emirate with the community. It was awarded as one of the top five entries in the Abu Dhabi government pavilion at GITEX 2022.

The Wellness in the Workplace program is another comprehensive health promotion program that targets employees in their workplace, starting with government entities and expanding to all workplaces in the future. The program aims to improve productivity through reduced sickness-related absenteeism, enhanced corporate image for entities, and improved work-life balance for employees through health literacy, including nutrition, exercise, stress management, good sleep, and related education and interventions.

ADPHC is also developing guidelines to standardize health promotion messages to encourage uniform, consistent communication that is scientifically accurate, in order to tackle rumors and misinformation. Appropriate systems must be put in place to ensure compliance with the guidelines.

ADPHC continued to support the successful Public Health Ambassadors Program, successfully training the eighth batch of Public Health Ambassadors. Since the program started in 2015, more than 75 organizations, including government and semi-government educational institutes in Abu Dhabi, have participated in the program, with a total of 222 Public Health Ambassadors trained. These ambassadors have significantly contributed to the volunteer workforce that helped implement the public health response to COVID-19 [21].

5.11.3 Mental Health Programs

Aligned with the WHO initiatives, mental health has been highlighted as a priority area in chronic disease prevention, and this was brought into the spotlight by the mental health impact of the COVID-19 pandemic. A number of awareness and education activities were conducted during the year to reduce the stigma around mental health and encourage the community to seek help at an early stage.

ADPHC began in 2020 to provide training programs on mental health first aid to a group of qualified volunteers, in collaboration with clinical experts in the health sector. These volunteers worked on the National Mental Health Support Line (800-HOPE). The center then launched the Estijabah Mental Help Line (800 1717) in Abu Dhabi during the pandemic. In addition, multiple educational and mental wellness promotion campaigns were conducted, targeting special groups, such as the "With You to Support You" campaign in collaboration with the Family Development Foundation, aimed at people in isolation and quarantine settings, as well as the families of those who had dead due to COVID-19 infection; the "Book Your Friend in Isolation" reading initiative with the Sheikh Mohammed Bin Khalid Foundation; and an interactive children's book to help parents support their children during the pandemic.

After the return to normal life, ADPHC collaborated with SEHA to expand and continue providing mental health support services through the ADPHC Mental Health Help Line. ADPHC also started screening for depression as part of IFHAS screening program and participated in the development of mental wellness and resilience-promoting educational messages. These were used to support anti-bullying campaigns with the Ministry of Education, resources for parents' mental well-being manuals with the Department of Community Development, and awareness and supportive messages for Abu Dhabi government employees preparing for retirement, in collaboration with the Abu Dhabi Pension Fund.

ADPHC experts contributed to multiple national and local committees responsible for mental health strategies and issues, in addition to supporting the Abu Dhabi mental health reform project. ADPHC experts also participated in multiple conferences, including the first Suicide Prevention Conference in the region; delivered several train-the-trainer workshops on school mental health; and participated with the Ministry of Interior (MOI) in the "Mental Health for a Better Quality of Life" initiative.

ADPHC also designed and organized workshops to raise awareness about mental health for people working in the fields of media and communication and Islamic affairs, and participated in the Ministry of Interior's "Health for a Better Quality of Life" initiative, reaching thousands of MOI employees.

ADPHC launched multiple mental health awareness campaigns in collaboration with stakeholders for prioritized groups such as children and youth, senior citizens, workplace professionals, frontline heroes, people of determination, and victims of substance and drug abuse [22].

5.11.4 Programs for People of Determination

ADPHC has also contributed to the development of the Abu Dhabi strategy for People of Determination, these efforts were led by Department of Community Development in collaboration with across governmental stakeholders, and launched several related initiatives that included the training of healthcare providers via the Special Olympics on proper communication and management for PODs, as well as mental health support for the caregivers of adolescents of determination in collaboration with SEDRA. In addition, multiple educational and health promotion activities have been conducted on various media platforms for children of determination and their families, in collaboration with ECA, ADEK, DCD, DOH, and Zayed Higher Organization. Awareness campaigns related to autism, Down syndrome, and rare metabolic diseases have reached more than 100,000 people [23].

ADPHC has many existing programs and standards related to the prevention and early detection of disability and developmental delay, such as premarital screening, newborn screening, maternal antenatal and postnatal screening standards, child wellness visit standards, and comprehensive school screening. In addition, these programs are linked whenever possible to the Emirati genome project, allowing even better prevention and early detection opportunities.

5.12   Research

At the end of this chapter on ADPHC and its efforts to achieve the vision of a healthy and safe Abu Dhabi, it is important to highlight the significant role of public health research, especially applied research and comparative studies that can effectively improve our public health programs and practices. COVID-19 has escalated and advanced the research agenda in Abu Dhabi, with hundreds of publications related to the pandemic. In addition, ADPHC periodically publishes the latest scientific research updates and trends on coronavirus disease (COVID-19) in one report. This scientific report provides summaries of breakthrough or updated research on COVID-19 to allow healthcare professionals and public health professionals easy and fast access to the information they need [24].

5.13   Conclusion

ADPHC works diligently on establishing a methodology for public health research and supporting and facilitating the infrastructure for public health research in the Emirate of Abu Dhabi, in alignment with the health sector research strategy in Abu Dhabi and the UAE. It aims to increase the magnitude and quality of research conducted, with a special focus on applied research and the effective translation of research findings into policies, programs, and initiatives that positively impact public health.

Conflicts of Interest   The authors have no conflicts of interest to declare.

References

1. We reach you wherever you are initiative (adphc.gov.ae).
2. Seasonal influenza (adphc.gov.ae).
3. ALADAA (adphc.gov.ae).
4. Safety in heat (adphc.gov.ae).
5. Child injury prevention (adphc.gov.ae).
6. Occupational noise program (adphc.gov.ae).
7. Electronic Disease Registry Platform (adphc.gov.ae).
8. Maternal & child health program (adphc.gov.ae).
9. School screening (adphc.gov.ae).
10. Eat right and get active program (adphc.gov.ae).
11. The periodic comprehensive periodic screening program (IFHAS), available online at: https://www.adphc.gov.ae/Public-Health-Programs/Comprehensive-screening-Program%2D%2DIFHAS.
12. Periodic comprehensive screening program – IFHAS (adphc.gov.ae).
13. Cervical cancer (adphc.gov.ae).
14. Colorectal cancer (adphc.gov.ae).
15. Breast cancer (adphc.gov.ae).
16. Tobacco control program (adphc.gov.ae).
17. Abu Dhabi guideline for implementing the declaring of calories on the menus for manufacturers and food suppliers for ready-to-eat foods in the Emirate of Abu Dhabi. Available on line at: https://qcc.gov.ae/-/media/Project/QCC/QCC/Documents/Quality-Infrastructure-Documents/Abu-Dhabi-Specification/Abu-Dhabi-Guideline/ADG-26%2D%2D-Abu-Dhabi-Guideline-for-Implementing-the-Declaring-of-Calories-on-the-Menus-for-Manufactu.pdf.
18. SEHHI program (adphc.gov.ae).
19. WHO Policy – School Canteen Guidelines of the Emirate of Abu Dhabi, Available on line at: https://extranet.who.int/nutrition/gina/en/node/63350.
20. Breastfeeding (adphc.gov.ae).
21. Public Health Ambassador Program (adphc.gov.ae).
22. Mental health (adphc.gov.ae).
23. People of determination (adphc.gov.ae).
24. COVID-19 scientific report (adphc.gov.ae).

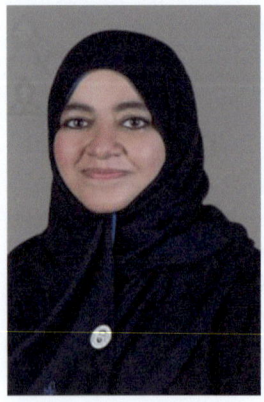

H.E. Dr. Omniyat Mohammed Al Hajeri is the Executive Director of the Community Health Division at the Abu Dhabi Public Health Center. She specializes in public health and leadership and is also a practicing consultant physician in the field of diabetes, endocrinology and metabolic diseases. She studied medicine, worked, and trained in Ireland for 10 years, and has worked around 20 years at several Abu Dhabi hospitals.

She is a member of Estijaba (the COVID response team in the Abu Dhabi health sector), with a special focus on the education sector's agile response to COVID, and also supports stakeholders involved in COVID response efforts more broadly.

Dr. Omniyat also worked at the first health authority established in Abu Dhabi and has continued to help shape the health sector and its major reforms since 2001. Before moving to the Abu Dhabi Public Health Center in 2019 as a founding member, she served in the Department of Health as Director of Public Health and Research since 2011, leading a number of departments, including communicable and non-communicable diseases, health promotion, research, and occupational and environmental health. There, she worked with her team to initiate and implement more than 20 public health programs that continue to serve the Abu Dhabi community. She also previously worked in health professional licensing (2007–2010) and human resources (2001–2007), where she served as a founding member of the licensing, examination, credentialing, continuous medical education, and postgraduate medical education services in the Emirate of Abu Dhabi.

Dr. Omniyat is a board member of the Abu Dhabi Sports Council and the Academy of Sheikha Fatima Bint Mubarak Women's Sport and was previously a board member of the Abu Dhabi National Exhibitions Company, ExCel London Exhibitions company (2016–2019), and Abu Dhabi Media Company.

She also previously served as an assistant professor of internal medicine at the University of Medicine and Health Sciences.

She was awarded the "Chairman of The Executive Council Medal" in the Executive Directors category in 2013, in addition to more than 25 academic awards and medals and 10 other recognition awards. She was elected a member of the Delta Omega Honor Society at the Johns Hopkins Bloomberg School of Public Health in May 2011 and re-elected in 2020 for lifelong membership (a U.S. national honor society that aims to encourage excellence in research, scholarship, and the practice of public health and to recognize attainments in the field of public health).

Education

- PhD/DrPH in Health Care Management and Leadership at Johns Hopkins University 2020
- Master of strategic and security studies, National Defence College, UAE, 2015
- Master of Public Health in Health Care Management, Public Health and Leadership JHSPH Bloomberg School of Public Health May 2011
- Membership of the Royal College of Physicians MRCP Ireland 2001
- MB,BCH, BAO, LRCPS NUI, the Royal College of Surgeons Ireland 1999

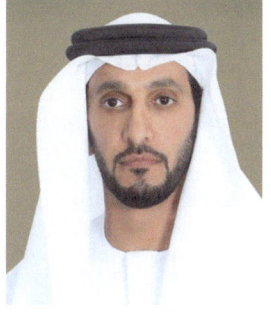

H.E. Sheikh Abdulla Bin Mohammed Bin Butti Al Hamed is currently a board member of Abu Dhabi Developmental Holding Company PJSC (ADQ), the Zayed Higher Organization for People of Determination, the board of Trustees of the Abu Dhabi Early Childhood Authority, and the Frontlines Heroes Office. He also serves as Chairman of Q Holding PJSC, a member of the Executive Committee of Al Jazira Club, chairman of the Board of Directors of Al Jazira Investment Company, and a member of the Board of Trustees of Abu Dhabi University.

H.E. has held several prominant positions, including:

Chairman of the Department of Health—Abu Dhabi where he led the Emirate's response to the COVID-19 pandemic. Member of the Abu Dhabi Executive Council, Member of the Executive Committee of the Government of Abu Dhabi, Chairman of the Energy Authority, Chairman of Regulation and Supervision Bureua, Member of the Abu

Dhabi Supreme Petroleum Council (SPC), Chairman of the Abu Dhabi Water and Electricity Authority, Undersecretary of the Ministry of Foreign Affairs, Managing Director of the European Affairs Department at the Ministry of Foreign Affairs, Chairman of the Western Region Development Council, Undersecretary of the Ruler's Representative Court House of the Western Region, and an Employee the Abu Dhabi Investment Authority.

He holds a Bachelor of Science in Business Administration the United States and a Master of Business Administration (MBA) from the New York Institute of Technology.

H.E. has participated in several prestigious training programs and leadership courses, including: Leadership Skills for Senior Executives at Harvard Business School, California, USA; "Changing the Game" Decision-Making and Negotiation Skills at Harvard Business School London, UK; "Leaders of Governance" program at the Singapore College of Civil Service, Critical circumstances Leadership programme (Antarctic Expedition), Participation, Leadership, Vision and Strategy course facilitated by Harvard Business School - Civil Service Department in Abu Dhabi; "Leadership Development" by Harvard University, USA; Abu Dhabi Executive Leadership Forum at the Singapore College of Civil Services.

His Excellency has been recognized with numerous prestigious awards for his exceptional leadership and contributions to the healthcare sector. He received the Golden Key Award, the highest honor accolade presented by the Arab Hospitals Federation, in recognition of his outstanding efforts in leading Abu Dhabi's exemplary healthcare model. He was also honored with the Pioneer Leadership Award in Healthcare at the Arab Hospitals Federation Award—Medhealth Cairo 2022". In addition, His Excellency received two prestigious awards from the Department Health—Abu Dhabi at the "2021 Middle East & North Africa Stevie® Awards", including the Gold Award for Innovative Management (Organizations with 100 or More Employees) and the "Government Hero of the year" award in the COVID-19 response category. Further cementing his reputation, His Excellency was awarded the Gold award for Executive Hero of the Year 2021 at the Globee Business Awards- CEO Awards, in recognition of his exceptional leadership in the health sector during the COVID-19 pandemic in the Emirate of Abu Dhabi.

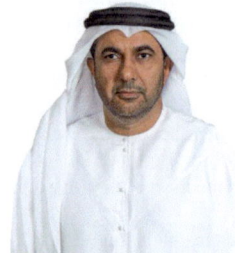

HE. Matar Saeed Al Nuaimi is the Director General of the Abu Dhabi Public Health Center (ADPHC). He started his career in the UAE military health sector in 1992 as a public health inspector and subsequently held various administrative positions until he became Commander of the Medical Services Corps in 2014. He later transitioned to the Abu Dhabi government's civil health sector, where he served as Executive Director for Emergency and Disaster Management at the Department of Health—Abu Dhabi from November 2017. In July 2019, H.E. Matar Al Nuaimi was appointed Director General of ADPHC. As Response Team Leader for the Abu Dhabi Health Sector, his strategic leadership has been instrumental in establishing the center's foundation, shaping its vision and mission, and defining the public health strategic goals in the Emirate of Abu Dhabi.

H.E. holds a Master's degree in Strategy and National Security from the National Defence College in Abu Dhabi (2014), and a Joint Command and Staff Course certificate from the Joint Command and Staff College in Abu Dhabi (2009). He also earned an Associate Degree in Health Sciences from the Kingdom of Bahrain in 1990. In addition to his

administrative and leadership roles, H.E. Al Nuaimi has led numerous medical support operations and played a key role in developing strategic plans for major national and international events and crises. Over his 30-year career, he has achieved several significant accomplishments, including:

- Chairing the Medical Committee during the Pope's visit to the UAE in 2019
- Chairing the Medical Committee at the 2018 Special Olympics MENA
- Chairing the Medical Committee at the 2019 Special Olympics World Summer Gamesin Abu Dhabi
- Serving as Response Team leader for the Abu Dhabi Health Sector from 2017 to the present

Open Access This chapter is licensed under the terms of the Creative Commons Attribution 4.0 International License (http://creativecommons.org/licenses/by/4.0/), which permits use, sharing, adaptation, distribution and reproduction in any medium or format, as long as you give appropriate credit to the original author(s) and the source, provide a link to the Creative Commons license and indicate if changes were made.

The images or other third party material in this chapter are included in the chapter's Creative Commons license, unless indicated otherwise in a credit line to the material. If material is not included in the chapter's Creative Commons license and your intended use is not permitted by statutory regulation or exceeds the permitted use, you will need to obtain permission directly from the copyright holder.

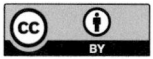

An Overview of the Burden of Disease in the UAE

6

Abdulla Shehab and Asim Ahmed Elnour

6.1 Background

Understanding the burden of diseases from diverse perspectives of their etiologies, epidemiological data, and societal, humanistic, clinical, and economic consequences enables the provision of optimal, sustainable, and excellent patient care. There are many associated facilitators, barriers, and challenges in achieving this optimum goal. The aforementioned goal could be achieved by understanding the interplay between human health, health policy, and economic development.

In the early 1990s, the World Bank and the World Health Organization (WHO) published the Global Burden of Disease (GBD) study [1]. This initiative aimed at improving critical health outcomes was preceded by an annual health assessment using standardized metrics, systematic and comparable estimates of each disease condition, and a report on the burden of each disease. The latest report on GBD published in the Lancet by several investigators covers 369 diseases and 87 attributable risk factors from 204 countries and territories.

A. Shehab
The Royal Heart Center, Burjeel Royal Hospital, and Mediclinic Hospitals, Al Ain, United Arab Emirates

Emirates Medical Association (EMA), Dubai, United Arab Emirates

New Emirates Medical Journal (NEMJ), Dubai, United Arab Emirates

Gulf Intervention Society (GIS), Dubai, United Arab Emirates

Emirates Cardiac Society (ECS), Dubai, United Arab Emirates

Asia Pacific Cardiology (APC), Dubai, United Arab Emirates

A. A. Elnour (✉)
Program of Clinical Pharmacy, College of Pharmacy, Al Ain University, Abu Dhabi Campus, Abu Dhabi, United Arab Emirates

AAU Health and Biomedical Center, Al Ain University, Abu Dhabi, United Arab Emirates
e-mail: asim.ahmed@aau.ac.ae

© The Author(s) 2025
H. O. Al-Shamsi (ed.), *Healthcare in the United Arab Emirates*,
https://doi.org/10.1007/978-981-96-0523-1_6

6.1.1 The Report's Rationale and Objective

The United Arab Emirates (UAE) results from the GBD report have provided data on the burden of disease, injuries, and risk factors in its population during the years 1990–2019. However, the report warrants further analysis of the sequential trends in mortality, health loss, risk factors, and healthcare services in the UAE from 1990 to 2019 [5].

6.2 The Findings of the Perspective

With the critical systematic evaluation of the burden of disease data in the UAE, more emphasis is placed on the health outcomes of non-communicable diseases, suggesting that efforts are required to analyze the preventable risk factors that are major contributors to the burden of disease and disability. Based on the GBD study report, the overall life expectancy of the UAE population in 2017 was 72.8 years (95% uncertainty interval: 70.9–74.7) and is projected to be 76.3 years (72.7–80.1) by 2050 and 79.6 years (74.1–84.4) by 2100, respectively [2]. The total fertility rate gradually decreased in the UAE population, reaching 1.31 (1.71–1.49) in 2017 from 4.1 (3.87–4.34) in 1990 and is predicted to reach 1.27 (1.02–1.82) by 2100 [2].

The results above suggest that 1.5 million males and more than half a million females are within the younger population aged 35–40 years. The top 10 individual causes of death in the UAE reported in 2009 were non-communicable diseases (chronic kidney disease, diabetes, chronic obstructive pulmonary disease, ischemic heart disease, stroke) and injuries (drug use disorders, falls, road injuries, self-harm). Nevertheless, the decline in all three leading injury-related mortality rates has plateaued [3].

During the 10 years between 2009 and 2019, diabetes, hypertensive heart disease, ischemic heart disease, and pancreatic cancer emerged as the fastest-growing causes of death in the UAE [4]. This represents a critical warning sign for further research and analysis of population data.

The UAE healthcare system has undergone significant transformations over the past 30 years, as measured by age-standardized death and disability-adjusted life years (DALYs) rates. The 10-year data from the GBD study (1990–2019) reported that six non-communicable diseases were among the top ten causes of mortality in the UAE in 2019: ischemic heart disease (ranked first), stroke (ranked third), chronic kidney disease (ranked fourth), diabetes (ranked fifth), COPD (ranked sixth), and hypertension (ranked seventh). Nevertheless, traffic injuries remain the second-leading cause of death, contributing to 13.5% of total deaths in the UAE. The pace of decline in the age-standardized DALY rates accelerated in age groups younger than 60 during the same time frame of 1990–2019 [5].

The impact of such a trend in non-communicable diseases and injuries exhibited a substantial reduction in age-standardized rates in congenital disabilities (64.2%) and neonatal disorders (66.2%), followed by ischemic heart disease (39%) and road injuries (35%). In the GBD report, slight progress in the percentage decrease in the DALYs rates of stroke (1.3%), diabetes (1.3%), and hypertensive heart disease (7.2%) was observed over the 10 years of data between 1990 and 2019 [5].

6.3 Discussion

The GBD2019 data provided more rigorous trends and magnitudes of exposure to 87 risk factors for 204 countries and territories [6]. The analysis of disease in the UAE provided four risk attributes for more than 50% of deaths and DALYs: high LDL cholesterol, high systolic blood pressure, high body mass index, and high fasting plasma glucose. The aforementioned metabolic attributes of risk have substantially escalated in descending order, with an average percentage change of 147% for high fasting plasma glucose, high LDL levels (141.5%), high blood pressure (140.1%), dietary risks (136.9%), smoking (136.3%), and increased body mass index (133.4%). Further, the prevalence of obesity has climbed across the UAE as a leading cause of several non-communicable diseases and premature cardiovascular disease. With respect to the UAE, the influence of each attributable risk on total DALYs remains significant as of 2019] [7, 8].

For instance, multiple diet and physical inactivity components account for 9.7% of DALYs. The burden attributed to tobacco smoking (including second-hand smoke) has remained constant (5.7% of DALYs). These changes in the burden of disease and the respective risk attributes may explain the impact on the years lived with disability and premature deaths in the UAE [7, 8].

Over the last 30 years since the forecast of the GBD study report, there has been a shift in emphasis on global health from death or premature mortality to outcomes related to morbidity and disability. In addition to estimating the incidence and prevalence of significant clinical sequelae for each disease and injury, the summary measures of fatal and non-fatal diseases have been an integral part of the GBD since the 1991 report. The recent advancements in our understanding of the GBD have suggested and implemented two key summary measures: DALY and healthy life expectancy (HLE) [7, 8].

DALYs are the sum of years of life lost due to premature mortality, plus the years lived with disability. They are estimated as the sum of the prevalence of each clinical sequela multiplied by the public's perspective of how much health loss is related to each health state. The emerging perspective of care from the summary measures (entire health outcomes) offers a holistic assessment of health, which permits a better understanding of how increased longevity can also be a mixed dividend if a large proportion of that time is spent struggling with ill health.

In summary, the GBD has thrived over the last 30 years because it has met a critical necessity in global health. The prospects of GBD remain valid with the demand for population health infomation that is regularly analyzed and aligned with the substancial influences of the current transformational changes in health issues. The role of health organizations and health authorities, particularly crucial decision-makers, is central for timely information and for translating that information into policy-relevant insights, providing enormous opportunities for health systems and population health.

6.4 Conclusion

The current article points out some of the vital estimates related to the burden of disease and its attributed risk factors. The value of the GBD 2019 report has brought new dimensions to societal and population health domains. The authors emphasized that the burden of disease imposed by the metabolic attributable risk factors deserves special attention and deemed it necessary for population health professionals to analyze the non-communicable diseases and their respective attributed risk factors. Specifically, preventive maneuvers and timely interventions directed toward the attributable risk factors require the involvement of all healthcare professionals at all levels of healthcare system. Public attention and awareness of the potentially detrimental consequences of unhealthy behaviours deserve a closer focus. The role of innovative technology such as digital health, telemedicine, data monetization, machine learning, artificial intelligence, and virtual learning, offers tremendous opportunities for improving the population's health and implementing evidence-based medicine. Further research using the technologies above remains the cornerstone of transformational changes in health strategies.

Conflicts of Interest The authors have no conflicts of interest to declare.

References

1. World Development Report 1993 — investing in health: world development indicators. Oxford: Oxford University Press; 1993.
2. Vollset SE, Goren E, Yuan CW, et al. Fertility, mortality, migration, and population scenarios for 195 countries and territories from 2017 to 2100: a forecasting analysis for the Global Burden of Disease Study. Lancet. 2020;396(10258):1285–306. https://doi.org/10.1016/S0140-6736(20)30677-2.
3. Vos T, Lim SS, Abbafati C, et al. Global burden of 369 diseases and injuries in 204 countries and territories, 1990-2019: a systematic analysis for the Global Burden of Disease Study 2019. Lancet. 2020;396(10258):1204–22. https://doi.org/10.1016/S0140-6736(20)30925-9.
4. Chen X, Yi B, Liu Z, et al. Global, regional and national burden of pancreatic cancer, 1990 to 2017: results from the Global Burden of Disease Study 2017. Pancreatology. 2020;20(3):462–9. https://doi.org/10.1016/j.pan.2020.02.011.
5. Murray CJ, Abbafati C, Abbas KM, et al. Five insights from the global burden of disease study 2019. Lancet. 2020;396(10258):1135–59. https://doi.org/10.1016/S0140-6736(20)31404-5.
6. Murray CJ, Aravkin AY, Zheng P, et al. GBD 2019 risk factors collaborators. Global burden of 87 risk factors in 204 countries and territories, 1990–2019: a systematic analysis for the Global Burden of Disease Study 2019. Lancet. 2020;396(10258):1223–49. https://doi.org/10.1016/S0140-6736(20)30752-2.

7. GBD 2019 Demographics Collaborators. Global age-sex-specific fertility, mortality, healthy life expectancy (HALE), and population estimates in 204 countries and territories, 1950–2019: a comprehensive demographic analysis for the Global Burden of Disease Study 2019. Lancet. 2020;396:1160–203.
8. GBD 2019 Diseases and Injuries Collaborators. Global burden of 369 diseases and injuries in 204 countries and territories, 1990–2019: a systematic analysis for the Global Burden of Disease Study 2019. Lancet. 2020;396:1204–22.

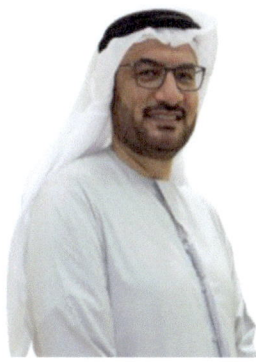

Abdulla Shehab is currently working as consultant cardiologist at the Royal Burjeel Hospital, Al Ain (UAE). He has 25 years of experience in internal medicine, cardiology and interventional cardiology, and medical education. He has several professional affiliations. He was the Immediate Past President of the Emirates Society of Cardiology. He is currently the General Secretary of the Emirates Cardiac Society and the Vice President of the Gulf Intervention Society. He is the Fellow of Royal College of Physicians, UK, a Fellow of American College of Physicians, Fellow of European Society of Cardiology, Fellow of the American College of Cardiology, Fellow of the American Society of Cardiac Intervention, and Fellow of the Heart American Association. He is the Chief Editor of Emirates Medical Journal and serves as an editor in many other regional and international journals. He published over 152 research papers in PubMed-indexed journals. His areas of particular interest include heart failure, coronary artery disease, dyslipidemia, hypertension, arrhythmia, cardiac intervention, cardiac imaging, screening for cardiac disease in sports players, and cardiovascular disease in pregnancy.

Awards and Achievements

Best Service Award from UAEU, Best Teaching and Best Clinical Research Award from UAEU.

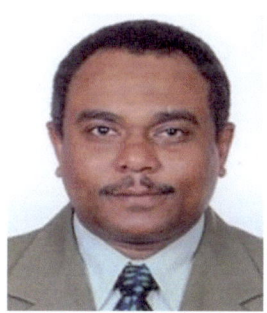

Asim Ahmed Elnour is recently working at the College of Pharmacy at Al Ain University, Abu Dhabi campus (UAE). He is author or co-author of more than 140 papers (with 1560 citations in Google Scholar h index 19 and 800 in SCOPUS h in 14 representing international peer-reviewed journals) and conference presentations. He is an editor and editorial board member for various international peer-reviewed journals in pharmacy, clinical pharmacy, medicine, nursing, clinical pharmacology, and toxicology. For instance, he is the editor-in-chief of the Journal of Pharmacy Practice (PP-Granada, Spain). He is an associate editor of the New Emirates Medical Journal (NEMJ) under the Emirates Medical Association (EMA), an editorial board member for the International Journal of Clinical Pharmacy (IJCP), a former editor for Medicine (Baltimore, USA), and an executive editor for Current Reviews in Clinical and Experimental Pharmacology Journal (CCREP). He serves as a consultant for the Association of Arab Universities and a referee for including journals in the Scopus database. He recently led a group of Sudanese pharmacy professors in free teaching, training, and research (Global Community Medical Institute).

Awards and Achievements

Best Teacher at Alain University (Abu Dhabi Campus-UAE) 2023 (Studentship survey)

Best Employee Al Ain Hospital, Alain-UAE 2012

The Award of Distinction for Continuing Professional Development for Pharmacy from Health Authority Abu Dhabi (HAAD) 2009

Open Access This chapter is licensed under the terms of the Creative Commons Attribution 4.0 International License (http://creativecommons.org/licenses/by/4.0/), which permits use, sharing, adaptation, distribution and reproduction in any medium or format, as long as you give appropriate credit to the original author(s) and the source, provide a link to the Creative Commons license and indicate if changes were made.

The images or other third party material in this chapter are included in the chapter's Creative Commons license, unless indicated otherwise in a credit line to the material. If material is not included in the chapter's Creative Commons license and your intended use is not permitted by statutory regulation or exceeds the permitted use, you will need to obtain permission directly from the copyright holder.

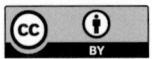

Health Insurances in the UAE

Husam Al Majali and Mohamed Farghaly

7.1 History and Current Status

Since state unification in 1971, the United Arab Emirates (UAE) has significantly improved its healthcare system's efficiency, quality, and accessibility. This advancement is evidenced by the enhancement of UAE healthcare indicators and the development of linked industries such as biomedical manufacturing and medical tourism. UAE healthcare has progressed from being fundamentally inadequate to the current situation where the health outcomes are the same or sometimes better than those in developed countries [1].

The growth in health expenditures in the UAE has been steep over the last 20–30 years. Spending continues to grow with a compound annual growth rate (CAGR) of 6%. Overall, healthcare spending accounted for 4.28% of the country's GDP in 2019, one of the highest in the region [2]. In parallel, the UAE's healthcare financing and insurance system has undergone a massive transformation and has played a vital role in restraining costs while providing affordable, accessible, and cost-effective healthcare to UAE citizens and residents. The UAE health

H. Al Majali (✉)
Emirates Health Economic Society, Dubai, United Arab Emirates

Jordan Medical Council, Amman, Jordan

Barcelona Business School, Barcelona, Spain

University of Western Ontario (UWO), London, ON, Canada
e-mail: halmajal@uwo.ca

M. Farghaly
Dubai Medical College, Dubai, United Arab Emirates

Dubai Health Insurance Corporation (DHIC) and CEO Office, Dubai, United Arab Emirates

Scientific Committee for the Emirates Family Medicine Society, WONCA EMR, Tangier, Morocco
e-mail: mnfargaly@dha.gov.ae

insurance system has been mandated, structured, and shaped to ensure that all UAE citizens and residents have equitable and efficient healthcare coverage. The UAE healthcare insurance system is a patient-centric system that prioritizes patients, offering them high standards with affordable co-payments and short wait times.

Healthcare insurance regulations and implementation in the UAE have developed gradually over the last 50 years at the federal and emirate legislative levels. Starting in 2005, the UAE commenced a large-scale strategy of health reform to advance and assemble a state-of-the-art healthcare system; it also aimed to manage the growing government healthcare expenditure and shift a significant part of the payment and provision obligations to the private sector [3]. This ambitious strategy led to universal health insurance coverage, created many other opportunities, and had positive ripple effects in enhancing public and private health services.

Historically, UAE federal authorities have considered moving toward a comprehensive health insurance system for all UAE residents [1]. The UAE Ministry of Finance (MoF) is the federal authority responsible for regulating the insurance industry related to the healthcare sector. For instance, the MoF has drafted a law mandating compulsory federal health insurance nationwide. This law is still under development and will consider all aspects of the health system's environment and dynamics in the UAE [3]. The Federal Health Insurance Authority is evolving as the federal health insurance regulator, though it is still in its developmental phase. Currently, the Ministry of Health (MOH) and emirate-level health authorities share responsibility for managing health insurance in the UAE, as well as for licensing, registration, and monitoring healthcare service providers.

7.1.1 Federal and Northern Emirates Healthcare Insurance

The UAE's Ministry of Health And Prevention (MOHAP) directs the regulations related to health insurance in the Northern Emirates, which include Sharjah, Ajman, Ras Al Khaimah, Umm al Quwain, and Fujairah. The federal healthcare network of providers extends through a vast and diverse public network of healthcare entities. The MOHAP's insurance coverage includes all UAE citizens and large segments of expatriates without private health coverage. The spectrum of MOHAP healthcare insurance includes preventive, primary, and advanced medical services, as well as palliative care.

Sharjah has no timeframe for mandatory health insurance regulations. Although Sharjah founded the Sharjah Health Authority more than 10 years ago by Sharjah Amiri Decree No. 12 of 2010, it is still not strict about enforcing many of the regulatory and health financing functions [4]. Since May 2014, the government medical insurance program has covered the families of all Sharjah government employees. However, Sharjah has not enforced a mandatory health insurance system for expatriates. This delay could be due to the reality that most of its residents are already covered through the existing Sharjah governmental insurance or through their work visa status and employment in neighboring Dubai.

Compared to other emirates, Abu Dhabi and Dubai are in the lead in terms of state-of-the-art health insurance regulations for their residents. Both Emirates have laws and regulatory bodies specific to healthcare, including health insurance regulation. All residents must have minimum medical insurance coverage [5]. Enrollment in health insurance is mandatory for non-UAE nationals and their families residing and working in both Emirates and optional in other emirates. Every individual must provide cover for those they sponsor upon their arrival date in Abu Dhabi or Dubai. Due to the growing health insurance penetration, access has markedly improved in both emirates; customer satisfaction and trust have improved, and there has been more private sector investment among service providers [6].

In the Abu Dhabi and Dubai emirates, health insurance regulations have many shared features and qualities. The law in both emirates is stringent and specifies covered and excluded services in detail. The health insurance law is committed, respectful, and aligned with the country's legal system and local cultural standards.

7.1.2 Abu Dhabi

Abu Dhabi's ambition to enforce compulsory health insurance regulations was initiated in 2005 with the Abu Dhabi Health Insurance Law (Law No. 23 of 2005). The law made it mandatory for all citizens to have basic health insurance coverage as of June 2006 [7]. Currently, the health insurance regulatory system is under the Abu Dhabi Department of Health (DOH), which is responsible for regulating, implementing, and monitoring the laws governing all aspects of health insurance in Abu Dhabi.

In Abu Dhabi, all residents should now be covered by one of three health insurance schemes, which will guarantee their access to a wide range of essential services. Abu Dhabi's laws and regulations state that health insurance is mandatory for all non-nationals who hold residence or work permits and those visiting the emirate under a tourist visa. Healthcare insurance must include coverage for primary care, emergency care, maternity care, surgeries, tests, pharmaceuticals, and other covered therapies.

There are three major categories of health insurance policies in Abu Dhabi [8]:

1. The "Thiqa Plan" is for Emirati nationals only. Abu Dhabi's government funds and provides complete medical coverage for all UAE nationals living in Abu Dhabi. Citizens get a "Thiqa" card, which gives them full access to many private and public healthcare providers registered within the semi-government insurance company Daman's network. Thiqa card holders may also choose to purchase privately a "Thiqa top-up," which is supplemental health insurance. It also includes broader geographical coverage and extra benefits.
2. Abu Dhabi's "Basic Plan" is funded by employers to insure their expatriate workers with work permits issued in Abu Dhabi who earn a salary below the AED 4000 limit. There is a DOH-regulated list of benefits, a drug formulary list,

and co-payment structures assigned to this policy. This policy is under special regulations with a risk-sharing arrangement with the Abu Dhabi government.
3. Enhanced Plan schemes. These are employer-funded schemes with diverse premiums, benefit designs, and administration policies. Enhanced schemes are priced, sold, and managed by any of the locally licensed 45–50 private health insurance companies [8].

7.1.3 Dubai

All residents of Dubai are entitled to a Dubai Health Card issued by the Dubai Health Authority (DHA), which gives them access to a network of DHA facilities, including hospitals and clinics. Additionally, the DHA regulates Dubai's health insurance, governed by Law No. 11 of 2013 [9]. The Health Insurance Law mandates that all residents have health insurance coverage meeting the minimum benefits set by the DHA. Employers sponsor private health plans, and the benefits structure ranges from the basic DHA-regulated Essential Benefits Plan (EBP) to high-end (enhanced) policies with broad designs, premiums, and benefits. Similarly, UAE nationals residing in Dubai are provided insurance coverage through the "Enaya" health insurance policy under DHA supervision [5].

Regulations issued under the Dubai Law set out the Essential Benefits Plan (EBP) for the Mandatory Insurance Scheme in Dubai [9]. The premium under the EBP is AED 600–800 per year. The coverage annual limit and services covered are limited to the essential services set by the DHA unified basic policy. However, the DHA regularly updates the cover to meet public health needs and emirate health strategies. The EBP is only available to workers with monthly salaries equal to or less than a specified AED 4000 limit. All insurers authorized under the DHA licensing power can offer enhanced insurance products to residents earning above the specified AED 4000 salary limit. These will be commercially and market-driven underwritten products, following the DHA's standard directives and policy mandates. The benefit design of enhanced policies is tailored to fit the market and customer trends and demands. These policies usually cover a broad spectrum of preventive treatments or investigations, including the most expensive new technologies [10].

"Enaya" is a government-funded health insurance program for the citizens of the emirate of Dubai. The cover also extends to expatriates employed by the Dubai government. The program provides treatment through an extensive network of healthcare providers in the private sector and DHA healthcare centers. The Enaya program is designed to complement and enhance the existing coverage for Dubai citizens in DHA's vast network of primary, secondary, and tertiary facilities.

7.2 Features of Healthcare Insurance in the UAE

The insurance system in the UAE has provided many benefits to both nationals and residents. The following features mark UAE healthcare insurance [11]:

(a) Universality: Coverage for all residents (nationals and expatriates) is an essential part of health insurance regulations across the country, at the federal and emirate levels.
(b) Affordability: UAE residents are required to pay relatively small co-payment percentages of the total care cost. The co-payment ranges between 10% and 20% of the total cost of treatment.
(c) Accessibility: The coverage conveniently extends to a continuously expanding network of different healthcare providers. Waiting times are minimal or nonexistent at most levels of care-primary or hospital care.
(d) Continuum of care: The system covers the patient through broad categories of health services across all levels of intensity of care. The UAE insurance provides "cradle-to-grave" coverage across an individual's life.
(e) Enhanced patient experience: Continuous improvement in the health insurance system ensures better patient outcomes.
(f) Generous benefit designs: Most medical services are covered, including dental, pharmaceutical, palliative care, and new innovative diagnostics and therapeutics.

7.3 Challenges for Healthcare Insurance in the UAE

The UAE healthcare insurance system endures unique country-specific challenges. Additionally, other common global challenges exist. These challenges include the following:

(a) The inherent inclination of health insurance systems toward overutilization, waste, and fraudulent activities. The misuse of health services and increased costs are traditionally fueled at many levels: induced demand by healthcare providers and patients' overuse of services due to the "moral hazard" inherent in any health insurance system [12].
(b) The growing percentage of residents living with chronic diseases and morbid conditions [13]. Global and local disease trends are directed toward more expensive and chronic conditions that mandate multifaceted, prolonged supervision, and complex care pathways.
(c) The increased complexity and cost of new, innovative technologies in the healthcare industry. Specialty and new therapy areas like gene or targeted therapies are growing and replacing the old, less-efficient technologies. The innovations are costly and add an additional burden on healthcare budgets [14].
(d) The prevailing "fee-for-service" reimbursement model challenges healthcare expenditures. This model promotes healthcare waste and the irrational utiliza-

tion of healthcare resources. However, new innovative reimbursement models have been implemented recently to transition to more efficient models of care, such as in the Diagnosis-Related Groups (DRG) system.
(e) The healthcare environment in the UAE is highly diverse, and clinicians come from a wide range of medical backgrounds and schools [15]. This diversity invites a wide variation in clinical practices and guidelines. This unwanted variation, along with the lack of standard reimbursement guidelines can create inefficiency, resource overutilization, and affect targeted improvement in clinical outcomes.

7.4   Opportunities for UAE Healthcare Insurance

The advancement in UAE healthcare insurance has created many opportunities for the whole healthcare environment in the country. The agility and innovation of the UAE health insurance regulations are responsive and steady. Additionally, the benefits extend to other economic and social aspects. The following are some of these currently existing and forecasted opportunities:

(a) Internal and external investors are growing their interest in establishing all categories of healthcare infrastructure and long-term investments in the UAE [16]. This appeal is evident as the UAE is a base for the regional offices of multinational biomedical companies. Additionally, the UAE is home to many medical facilities that are branches of or affiliated with the world's top medical centers.
(b) The medical tourism industry has witnessed vast growth in the number of inbound activities and a reduction in outbound ones [17]. This positive trend reflected further enhanced healthcare quality and the country's economy. Inbound medical tourism in the UAE is attracted by highly specialized services like specialized bone marrow transplants (BMT) and advanced cosmetic procedures.
(c) The UAE has been recognized as a regional hub for the healthcare insurance industry. Most global and regional insurance and reinsurance firms target the country's high-level infrastructure and regulations as the base for their regional operations.
(d) The wide use of international standards in claims processing, disease, and service coding has shaped the successful utilization of real-world data (RWD) in biomedical and health economic studies. The use of RWD in research and to inform health policy decision-making is a growing future trend in UAE healthcare [18].
(e) The broad utilization of health information management (HIM) technologies and systems in the healthcare industry has contributed significantly. Communicating electronic medical records and platforms, automated claims submission, and the most up-to-date disease and procedure coding all supported the advancement in healthcare quality provision and standardization. Clinical outcome measurement is used to improve medical practices and direct the

healthcare authorities toward identifying and bridging healthcare system and population health gaps.
(f) The increased adoption of initiatives toward the new concept of value-based care (VBC). This new model of VBC has the ability to transform and direct the continuum of care from a volume-based to a value-based approach. A clear example of VBC is the "EJADAH" initiative, which is explained at the end of this chapter.
(g) The health insurance regulations, policies, and advanced systems have enabled the UAE health financing system to survive the global trend of soaring healthcare expenditure. The timely and proper application of innovative payment models and benefit designs has helped the health system manage the evident medical inflation with cost-effective projects and initiatives. The Diagnosis-Related Groups (DRG) payment model is explained below as an innovative payment model.
(h) The universality feature of UAE health insurance enables the creation of fund pooling. This characteristic allows regulators to create innovative affordability and funding mechanisms for high-cost medical conditions and services.
(i) The UAE health insurance system has the potential and capabilities to build a valuable partnership model with other healthcare industries like medical devices, academia, and the pharmaceutical industry [19]. Patient Support Programs (PSP) are the most successful partnership models, helping with care coordination and cost containment. The "BASMAH" Cancer PSP is an example of this feature and is explained further at the end of this chapter.

7.5 Examples of Innovation in UAE Healthcare Insurance

7.5.1 "EJADAH" Program

EJADAH was launched by the Dubai Health Authority's Dubai Health Insurance Corporation (DHIC). This value-based model aims to enhance clinical outcomes and promote more extensive use of preventive care [20]. The model encourages the use of evidence-based guidelines and standard international medical practices. The future evaluation and payment structure will depend on the hospital's adoption of the standards and guidelines set by this initiative. It is anticipated that a significant portion of healthcare costs will shift from managing the long-term complications of noncommunicable diseases to preventive measures and care coordination, eventually reducing the total burden of the disease. Patient-centricity is at the core of the Ejadah initiative. It aims to empower patients to manage their health, apply their insights, ease access by removing barriers, and improve the overall patient experience.

The shift from volume-based care to value-based care will focus on several elements, including but not limited to the following:

(i) It is creating a cultural change focusing on managing health and quality of life rather than merely treating the illness.
(ii) It is implementing a cost model that focuses on individual episodes rather than fee-for-service.
(iii) It focuses on treatments that stem from necessity rather than prescribing patients unnecessary medical procedures, tests, and medications.
(iv) EJADAH aims to track clinical, financial, and humanistic key performance indicators (KPIs) to ensure continuous improvement and development.

7.5.2 Diagnosis-Related Groups (DRG)

As part of the UAE health insurance system reforms, DRGs were initially implemented in Abu Dhabi, followed by Dubai. This payment reform aims to reduce healthcare costs and strengthen patients' trust in the healthcare system [21]. Before the implementation of the DRG method, in-hospital admission services, surgeries, and procedures were billed and reimbursed individually under a fee-for-service model. DRGs are a bundled payment model that aims to correlate the type of patient treated with the cost incurred. Patients are categorized based on certain characteristics such as gender, age, severity, and diagnosis. DRGs will have a significant impact in many ways, including but not limited to treatment consistency, avoiding the waste or exposure of patients to unnecessary therapies, procedures, and tests; increasing the efficiency of the reimbursement process; improving clinical outcome; and reassuring patients that they will receive the best care possible.

7.5.3 "BASMAH" Cancer Patient Support Program

Cancer coverage is granted on all Dubai health insurance policies. However, the annual coverage limit in EBP is insufficient to support the costs of completing the yearly journey and course of cancer treatment. Cancer screening tests do not exist in the EBP low-end policies, and such late detection will result in delayed diagnosis and the ability to cure cancer. The "BASMAH" Dubai Health Authority's cancer initiative is based on creating a cancer fund by pooling small contributions from all current insurance policies registered with the DHA [11]. The objectives of this initiative are as follows:

(a) Implementing early detection as a critical aspect of the national cancer strategy and striving to reduce the disease mortality rate.
(b) Ensuring continuity of care for cancer patients and finance an affordable solution that will grant uninterrupted coverage and access to an immaculate treatment journey.

At the initial stage, cancer screening and extended coverage were piloted for three cancers: breast, colorectal, and cervical. However, additional cancer types will be added in subsequent stages.

In addition to the cancer initiative, DHA has also expanded coverage for HCV and HBV to Dubai's resident population. As part of this initiative, HCV and HBV screening has been mandated to improve the diagnosis rate.

7.6 Conclusion and Future Direction

The UAE boasts one of the highest-quality healthcare systems in the world. The country's health insurance system further supports this mandate, ensuring access to world-class health quality and affordable care for all UAE nationals and residents. The UAE's healthcare and insurance systems strive to protect the health of individuals by providing better access to services, securing financial stability against soaring healthcare costs, and expanding insurance coverage to new population segments with additional health benefits. With its patient-centered approach, health insurance will continue to evolve and grow to fulfill the targets assigned to the health sector in the UAE's national long-term strategies.

Conflicts of Interest The authors have no conflicts of interest to declare.

References

1. Koornneef E, Robben P, Blair I. Progress and outcomes of health systems reform in The United Arab Emirates: a systematic review. BMC Health Serv Res. 2017;17(1):1–3.
2. World Bank. Current health expenditure (% of GDP) – United Arab Emirates; 2019. Available at: https://data.worldbank.org/indicator/SH.XPD.CHEX.GD.ZS?locations=AE.
3. Blair I, Sharif A. Health and health systems performance in the United Arab Emirates. In: Papers from the 38th IHF World Hospital Congress in Oslo 2013, vol. 49(4), p. 412.
4. Bachrouch A. UAE: a new milestone for Sharjah Healthcare City-Tamimi Company. October 2021. Available at https://www.tamimi.com/law-update-articles/uae-a-new-milestone-for-sharjah-healthcare-city/.
5. Hamidi S. Evidence from the national health account: the case of Dubai. Risk Manag Healthc Policy. 2014;7:163.
6. Malaviya S, Bishai D, Soni MM, Suliman ED. Socioeconomic disparities in healthcare utilization under universal health coverage: evidence from Dubai household health survey. Int J Equity Health. 2022;21(1):1–9.
7. Vetter P, Boecker K. Benefits of a single payment system: case study of Abu Dhabi health system reforms. Health Policy. 2012;108(2–3):105–14.
8. Koornneef EJ, Robben PB, Al Seiari MB, Al Siksek Z. Health system reform in the emirate of Abu Dhabi, United Arab Emirates. Health Policy. 2012;108(2–3):115–21.
9. Dubai Health Authority. Health Insurance Law of Dubai, Employer's Information Pack. 2014. Available at: https://www.isahd.ae/content/docs/Employer%20information%20pack%20v4.4%20011014%20(1).pdf.
10. Bhardwaj K, Shetty P. Study of medical insurance market to suggest a model for a new entrant making a foray in the health insurance sector in Dubai. Available at SSRN 1452541. 14 Aug 2009. Available at: https://papers.ssrn.com/sol3/papers.cfm?abstract_id=1452541.

11. Dubai Health Authority. Cancer PSP Program Basmah Guidelines. 2020. https://www.isahd.ae/content/docs/PD%20PSP%20Program_Basmah%20Guidelines_24-11-2020.pdf. Accessed 6 Oct 2022.
12. North J. Private health insurance: history, politics and performance. Cambridge University Press; 2020.
13. Hajat C. Tackling chronic disease in the Gulf region: swings and roundabouts. Glob Heart. 2016;11(4):447–50.
14. Goyen M, Debatin JF. Healthcare costs for new technologies. Eur J Nucl Med Mol Imaging. 2009;36(1):139–43.
15. The U.S.-U.A.E. Business council. The UAE health care report. June 2021. Available at http://usuaebusiness.org/wp-content/uploads/2019/01/2021-U.A.E.-Healthcare-Report.pdf.
16. Report GN. First-of-its-kind value-based healthcare model EJADAH launched in Dubai [Internet]. UAE – Gulf News. Gulf News; 2022 [cited 2022 Oct 7]. Available at: https://gulfnews.com/uae/first-of-its-kind-value-based-healthcare-model-ejadah-launched-in-dubai-1.88881605.
17. Shukla UN, Kulshreshtha SK. United Arab Emirates as a global medical tourism destination: an explorative study. In: Global developments in healthcare and medical tourism. IGI Global; 2020. p. 277–90. https://www.igi-global.com/chapter/united-arab-emirates-as-a-global-medical-tourism-destination/241409.
18. Kozak I, Gurbaxani A, Safar A, Rao P, Masalmeh A, Assaf H, Farghaly M, Pathak P, Natarajan A, Saffar I. Treatment patterns in patients with age-related macular degeneration and diabetic macular edema: a real-world claims analysis in Dubai. PLoS One. 2021;16(7):e0254569.
19. Al-Majali H. Strategy and models for partnership for pharmaceuticals with Health Insurance Companies-UAE. Innovation Arabia 12:43.
20. Report GN. First-of-its-kind value-based healthcare model EJADAH launched in Dubai [Internet]. UAE – Gulf News Gulf News; 2022 [cited 2022 Oct 7]. Available from: https://gulfnews.com/uae/first-of-its-kind-value-based-healthcare-model-ejadah-launched-in-dubai-1.88881605.
21. Hamidi S, Akinci F. Examining the health care payment reforms in Abu Dhabi. Int J Health Plann Manag. 2015;30(2):E69–82.

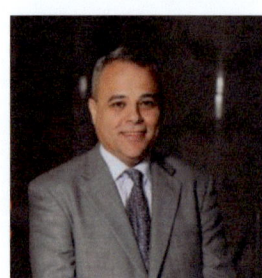

Husam Al Majali is a consultant gynecologist, health economist, and vice president of the Emirates Health Economic Society (EHES) at the Emirates Medical Association (EMA). He graduated from medical school at the University of Jordan in 1990. Later, he completed the Board Certification in Obstetrics-Gynecology consultant from Jordan Medical Council. He has completed two master's degrees: one from the Barcelona School of Management in Health Economics and Pharmacoeconomics and the second in Advanced Healthcare Practices from the University of Western Ontario (UWO) in Canada. In addition to clinical practice, he worked in various healthcare industries across different markets and countries. He is a subject-matter expert (SME) in private health insurance, equitable drug access, affordability, and universal health coverage. He is on the advisory board of leading healthcare conferences and has published papers on topics related to his expertise.

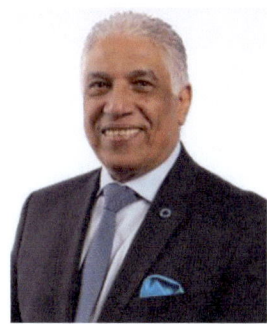

Mohamed Farghaly a professor at Dubai Medical College, is a practicing family physician and diabetologist. Additionally, he is a consultant at Dubai Health Insurance Corporation (DHIC) and CEO Office. He graduated from medical school in Egypt and completed FRCGP (UK), MRCGP (UK), DMSc (South Wales), and DIH (Ireland). He is an accredited examiner for MRCGP, General Secretary of WONCA EMR, leading many significant medical committees and scientific boards in Dubai, especially in diabetes and chronic diseases standards of care, including the EJADAH value-based care project, and chairing the scientific committee in the Emirates Family Medicine Society. In addition to his clinical practices, he is a professor and academic lead at Dubai Medical College and the Leicester University Diabetes diploma program. He published leading articles and book chapters related to clinical practice in diabetes, health economic evaluation, and health insurance.

Open Access This chapter is licensed under the terms of the Creative Commons Attribution 4.0 International License (http://creativecommons.org/licenses/by/4.0/), which permits use, sharing, adaptation, distribution and reproduction in any medium or format, as long as you give appropriate credit to the original author(s) and the source, provide a link to the Creative Commons license and indicate if changes were made.

The images or other third party material in this chapter are included in the chapter's Creative Commons license, unless indicated otherwise in a credit line to the material. If material is not included in the chapter's Creative Commons license and your intended use is not permitted by statutory regulation or exceeds the permitted use, you will need to obtain permission directly from the copyright holder.

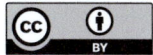

National Institute for Health Specialties (NIHS) in the UAE

8

Humaid O. Al-Shamsi, Aysha Al Dhaheri, Fouzia Shersad, and Mohammed Al-Houqani

8.1 Introduction

The National Institute for Health Specialties (NIHS) was established at the United Arab Emirates University to address the need for specialized training and professional development in the healthcare sector. Since its inception, the NIHS has played a vital role in promoting excellence and innovation in healthcare education and training in the United Arab Emirates (UAE). This manuscript provides a

---

H. O. Al-Shamsi
Burjeel Cancer Institute, Burjeel Medical City, Abu Dhabi, United Arab Emirates

Department of Medical Oncology, Dana-Farber Cancer Institute, Harvard Medical School, Boston, MA, United States

Harvard Medical School, Harvard University, Boston, MA, United States

College of Medicine, Ras Al Khaimah Medical and Health Sciences University, Al Juwais, Al Qusaidat, Ras Al Khaimah, United Arab Emirates

Gulf Medical University, Ajman, United Arab Emirates

Gulf Cancer Society, Alsafa, Kuwait

Emirates Oncology Society, Dubai, United Arab Emirates

College of Medicine, University of Sharjah, Sharjah, United Arab Emirates
e-mail: humaid.al-shamsi@medportal.ca

A. Al Dhaheri · M. Al-Houqani (✉)
National Institute for Health Specialties, United Arab Emirates University, Al Ain, United Arab Emirates

College of Medicine and Health Sciences, United Arab Emirates University, Al Ain, United Arab Emirates

International FAIMER Institute, Philadelphia, PA, USA
e-mail: a.dhaheri@uaeu.ac.ae; alhouqani@uaeu.ac.ae

© The Author(s) 2025
H. O. Al-Shamsi (ed.), *Healthcare in the United Arab Emirates*,
https://doi.org/10.1007/978-981-96-0523-1_8

comprehensive overview of the establishment, vision, achievements, and future directions of the NIHS.

8.2 Establishment of the NIHS

The NIHS was established by Cabinet Decree No. 28 of 2014, demonstrating the UAE government's commitment to enhancing healthcare education and professional development. The decree designated the NIHS as a national institution responsible for spearheading, regulating, and organizing specialty training programs for the health workforce. By establishing the NIHS, the UAE recognized the importance of specialized healthcare professionals in delivering high-quality patient care [1].

Concurrently, the landscape of postgraduate medical education in the UAE has seen a transformation. With evolving healthcare demands and the advent of novel medical technologies, there is a pressing need for advanced training modules. The NIHS, in this context, has played a key role in bridging this educational gap, ensuring that the UAE's medical professionals remain at the forefront of global healthcare standards.

8.3 Vision of NIHS

The NIHS is guided by a clear vision to become a leading institution in promoting specialized healthcare education and training in the UAE. Its vision encompasses developing a highly skilled and competent workforce that meets the multifaceted healthcare needs of the population. The NIHS envisions fostering a culture of continuous learning, research, and innovation to drive advancements in healthcare practices. The ultimate aim is to catalyze paradigm shifts in healthcare delivery, thereby ensuring enhanced patient care outcomes.

8.4 Landscape of Postgraduate Medical Education in the UAE

Since the early 1990s, the foundation of higher education in the UAE has been guided and monitored by the Ministry of Education, which established the Commission for Academic Accreditation (CAA) in 2000. The CAA has historically overseen the accreditation of all higher education programs in the country, ensuring

F. Shersad
National Institute for Health Specialties, United Arab Emirates University, Al Ain, United Arab Emirates

International FAIMER Institute, Philadelphia, PA, USA
e-mail: fshersad@uaeu.ac.ae

that they adhere to the best international standards and practices [2]. Its rigorous criteria and processes affirm the quality and relevance of education, making graduates from these institutions competitive on a global scale.

However, a discernible gap existed in medical and clinical specialty training. While the overarching education system in the UAE had an established accreditation framework, medical and clinical specialty training did not enjoy a similar national-level certification [3].

As a result, many medical professionals and graduates in the UAE sought validation from international boards. Some global entities, such as the Royal College of Physicians (UK) and the Royal College of Surgeons (UK), have recognized the depth and quality of residency training in the UAE, have established offices for registration and examination within the UAE. Many regional boards, such as the Arab Board, also maintain examination centers in the country. The reliance on international boards, while offering universally recognized validation, underscores the pressing need for the UAE to establish its own certification system for medical and clinical specialty training [4].

8.5 Achievements of the NIHS

8.5.1 Accreditation of Specialty Training Programs

One of the significant achievements of the NIHS is the development and implementation of accreditation standards for specialty training programs in the UAE. The NIHS has established rigorous evaluation processes to ensure that training programs meet internationally recognized quality benchmarks. Accreditation by the NIHS assures healthcare professionals and the public that the training programs adhere to the highest standards of education and practice. The NIHS has introduced fifty-five priority residency, fellowship, and internship programs. The signing of MOUs with organizations in the region and abroad, such as the Saudi Commission for Health Specialties, the Royal College of Physicians and Surgeons of Canada, and the Accreditation Council for Graduate Medical Education (ACGME) of the USA, represents one of the NIHS's major achievements.

8.5.2 Curriculum Development and Enhancement

The NIHS has actively collaborated with healthcare institutions and universities to develop and enhance specialty training curricula across various healthcare disciplines. By engaging experts and leveraging the latest evidence-based practices, the NIHS ensures that these curricula are relevant, comprehensive, and aligned with the evolving needs of the healthcare sector. This focus on curriculum development ensures that healthcare professionals receive the necessary knowledge and skills to excel in their respective specialties.

8.5.3 Proactive Approach Toward Optimizing the Training Methodologies for Medical Professionals

The NIHS has created a structure for continuous monitoring of competency-based training for interns, residents, and fellows undergoing postgraduate training in the country's accredited programs. Implementation of EPAs as a workplace-based assessment tool on an electronic platform is envisioned to be in place for all specialties by the end of 2024. Currently in the pilot stage of implementation, this will ensure that trainees attain their competencies at every stage of training, based on which their progression decisions are made. The governance, organization, resources required, and job descriptions for implementing such a scheme across all 55 specialties at a national level will achieve a high degree of standardization of training and motivate the creation of a safe and effective health workforce. The jurisdiction extends to medical, dentistry, nursing, pharmacy, and physiotherapy.

This initiative of NIHS has been lauded and appreciated by the specialty faculty and administrators. They have expressed relief from the pressures imposed by the diverse and sometimes conflicting requirements of various international accrediting bodies, which often fluctuate and may not align with the needs or cultural context of the UAE. The development of a unified centralized body composed of native experts and designed to meet international standards, considering the unique needs of the population and workforce of the UAE, has drawn wide acceptance and pride among the national intelligentsia.

The NIHS, recognizing the importance of feedback loops in educational training, has initiated a paradigm in which continuous monitoring of competency attainment is envisioned for all trainees, spanning from interns to fellows [5].

Entrustable professional activities (EPAs) have emerged as a promising tool for workplace-based assessments in medical education globally [6]. With an ambitious vision, the NIHS is taking strides toward digitizing this assessment methodology. Currently in the pilot phase, it is envisaged that this digital platform for EPAs will be the standard evaluative instrument across all specialties by the end of 2024. The essence of this initiative lies in ensuring that the trainees are demonstrating the competencies at each level of progression [7].

Implementing such a vast system across the nation's 55 specialties necessitates robust governance, strategic organization, and a clear demarcation of roles and responsibilities [8]. Plans are under way to implement this in a phased manner, thereby ensuring the support of stakeholders. Integration of the national strategic initiatives such as the Emirati identification and the digital UAE pass system for seamless sign-in, which are unique to the UAE, provides a compelling Emirati flavor for the national and international body of health profession trainees. The overarching ambition is to institute a gold standard for training, thereby fostering a health workforce par excellence.

8.5.4 Research and Innovation

The NIHS recognizes the importance of research and innovation in advancing healthcare practices. It encourages and supports healthcare professionals in conducting research, disseminating knowledge, and implementing evidence-based practices. The NIHS aims to contribute to the body of knowledge in various healthcare fields and facilitate the translation of research findings into improved patient care. By fostering a culture of inquiry, the NIHS encourages healthcare professionals to explore innovative solutions and drive advancements in healthcare practices.

8.5.5 Continuous Professional Development

The NIHS is committed to promoting lifelong learning and continuous professional development among healthcare practitioners. Recognizing that ongoing education is essential for maintaining and enhancing clinical competencies, the institute offers a wide range of programs, workshops, and conferences. These opportunities enable healthcare professionals to update their knowledge and skills, ensuring they stay at the forefront of their respective specialties. The continuous professional development (CPD) programs provided by the NIHS are designed to address emerging trends, advancements in technology, and changes in healthcare delivery models.

8.5.6 International Collaborations

The NIHS actively engages in international collaborations to foster knowledge exchange, promote best practices, and enhance the quality of healthcare education and training in the UAE. By partnering with renowned international institutions and organizations, the NIHS gains access to global expertise and facilitates cross-cultural learning. These collaborations enrich the educational experience of healthcare professionals and contribute to the development of a global perspective on healthcare practices.

8.6 Organizational Structure of the NIHS

The organizational structure of the NIHS is divided into academic and logistic support units, which are further subdivided into various working units.

The NIHS utilizes a multi-committee model under the aegis of the Board of Directors. Similar to the governance structures found in prominent institutions like the General Medical Council (GMC) in the UK [9] and the Accreditation Council for Graduate Medical Education (ACGME) in the USA [10], the NIHS operates under the Minister of Education, who chairs the Board of Directors (BoD). The Secretary-General leads the secretariat, which is comprised of experts and specialists dedicated to the institute's core operations. The governance model of NIHS is comprehensive and agile, designed in accordance with global best practices.

The committee structure prioritizes decentralized expertise and representative governance [11]. By harnessing the wealth of local talent, these committees are organized for specific missions, ensuring every specialty is appropriately represented by its subject matter experts. These experts, distinguished by their qualifications in their respective fields, offer invaluable insights and shape the NIHS's strategic direction.

Moreover, the NIHS's methodology of selecting surveyors and examiners from a specialized pool reflects international best practices, ensuring stringent standards and impartial evaluation [12]. The governance structure consists of the following:

- NIHS Board of Directors
- NIHS General Secretariat
- Advisory Committee
- Council of Scientific Affairs
- Specialized Scientific Committees
- Central Assessment Committee
- Central Accreditation Committee

This robust organizational framework is aimed at fostering synergy in vision, implementation, and continuous improvement, positioning the NIHS on par with internationally reputed medical accreditation and certification bodies.

8.7 Impact on the Healthcare Landscape

The NIHS has had a significant impact on the healthcare landscape in the UAE. By focusing on specialty training and professional development, the NIHS has helped bridge the gap between the growing healthcare demands of the population and the supply of highly skilled healthcare professionals. NIHS accreditation standards and curriculum development efforts have enhanced the quality of specialty training programs, ensuring that healthcare practitioners are well-prepared to provide specialized care.

Furthermore, the NIHS's emphasis on research and innovation has facilitated advancements in healthcare practices and the adoption of new treatment modalities. The institute's commitment to continuous professional development has fostered a culture of lifelong learning among healthcare professionals, enabling them to adapt to emerging technologies, evolving treatments, and modern healthcare delivery models.

The collaborations forged by the NIHS with international institutions have not only strengthened the global reputation of the UAE's healthcare sector but also facilitated the exchange of knowledge, expertise, and best practices. These partnerships have enabled healthcare professionals in the UAE to gain exposure to global healthcare trends, research innovations, and novel approaches to patient care.

8.8 Accredited Programs and Institutions by NIHS

Cleveland Clinic Abu Dhabi, a Mubadala Health partner, has received institutional accreditation from the National Institute for Health Specialties (NIHS) following the completion of the accreditation procedures. With this accreditation, aspiring doctors can advance to the consultant level of Tier 1 and earn certification from the Emirates Board [13]. The National Institute for Health Specialties officially accredited the internship and residency programs run by the Dubai Health Authority (DHA). In coordination with the DHA, several private sector hospitals obtained permits to accredit their training facilities and fall under the umbrella of the DHA as sponsors of the Excellence Program. American Hospital, Medcare Hospital, Aster Hospital, Saudi German Hospital, Dr. Sulaiman Al Habib Hospital, Fakeeh University Hospital, and Zulekha Hospital Dubai are a few of these hospitals in the UAE [13].

8.9 Future Directions

The future is based on the NIHS vision to expand specialized health programs according to the needs of the country and, in consultation with the concerned health authorities, to include nursing and allied health specialties, strengthen governance, accreditation, and evaluation systems, and ensure the highest quality standards for specialization programs in the country through policies, standards, and procedures. The NIHS's mandate also encompasses dentistry, nursing, pharmacy, and physiotherapy, underscoring its comprehensive approach to healthcare professional development [14]. It further seeks to enhance the use of technology and digital transformation to support operations and procedures, strengthen collaboration, build partnerships both internally and externally, and develop structures and capabilities to position itself among the distinguished regional and global specialized bodies.

A salient feature of the NIHS's future roadmap is the emphasis on competency-based post-graduate training [6]. Competency-based medical education, which has witnessed a global surge in recent years [15], is tailored to equip trainees with specific skills and knowledge, assessed through objective evaluations. By integrating workplace-based assessments and structured feedback on competency attainment, the NIHS ensures that training is not only comprehensive but also contextually relevant to the UAE's unique healthcare ecosystem. The NIHS is poised to leverage digitized training methods and maximize the use of artificial intelligence in assessments, making them timely, user-friendly, and error-free [16]. A feedback-driven refinement mechanism will ensure the system remains adaptive to stakeholder needs, and the resulting certifications, internationally recognized, will validate the quality of its recipients [17].

In pursuit of global excellence, the NIHS envisions being more than just a national beacon of specialized training; it aspires to be a global exemplar, a benchmark for countries to emulate. In addition to its role as a certifying body for postgraduate training, the NIHS has positioned itself as a professional licensing body, setting national standards for healthcare professionals, thereby addressing the nation's healthcare workforce needs. Major strategic directions include fostering international partnerships, optimizing digital transformation to enhance work procedures, and continuously improving its organizational structure.

8.10 Conclusion

The National Institute for Health Specialties (NIHS) in the UAE has made remarkable contributions to the advancement of specialty training and professional development in the country. Through its accreditation standards, curriculum development efforts, research initiatives, and international collaborations, the NIHS has played a central role in enhancing the quality of healthcare education and training. As the UAE's premier institution in this domain, the NIHS has positioned itself as a leading authority in shaping a highly skilled and competent healthcare workforce. Looking ahead, the NIHS must continue to address challenges, foster collaborations, and embrace emerging trends to ensure a sustainable, innovative, and prosperous future for healthcare education and training in the UAE.

Conflicts of Interest The authors have no conflicts of interest to declare.

References

1. National Institute for Health Specialties. n.d. Retrieved from https://nihs.uaeu.ac.ae/en/index.shtml.
2. Commission of Academic Accreditation. n.d. Role and functions of the CAA. [Website]. https://www.caa.ae/.
3. World Health Organization. 2019. Health workforce education and training. Regional Office for the Eastern Mediterranean. [Website]. http://www.emro.who.int/.
4. Foundation for Advancement of International Medical Education and Research (FAIMER). n.d. International Medical Education Directory (IMED). [Website]. https://imed.faimer.org/.
5. Natesan S, Jordan J, Sheng A, Carmelli G, Barbas B, King A, Gore K, Estes M, Gottlieb M. Feedback in Medical Education: An Evidence-based Guide to Best Practices from the Council of Residency Directors in Emergency Medicine. West J Emerg Med. 2023;5;24(3):479–94. https://doi.org/10.5811/westjem.56544. PMID: 37278777; PMCID: PMC10284500.
6. Ten Cate O, Scheele F. Competency-based postgraduate training: can we bridge the gap between theory and clinical practice? Acad Med. 2015;82(6):542–7.
7. Stephan A, Cheung G, van der Vleuten C. Entrustable Professional Activities and Learning: The Postgraduate Trainee Perspective. Acad Psychiatry. 2023;47(2):134–42. https://doi.org/10.1007/s40596-022-01712-2. Epub 2022 Oct 12. PMID: 36224504; PMCID: PMC10060374
8. Adams L, DeFleur M. Organizational structures in medical education: a global perspective. Int J Med Educ. 2018;9:215–23.
9. Bleakley A. Blunting Occam's razor: aligning medical education with studies of complexity. J Eval Clin Pract. 2014;20(6):849–55.
10. Nasca TJ, Philibert I, Brigham T, Flynn TC. The next GME accreditation system — rationale and benefits. N Engl J Med. 2012;366(11):1051–6.

11. Harden RM, Crosby J. AMEE guide no 20: the good teacher is more than a lecturer – the twelve roles of the teacher. Med Teach. 2019;22(4):334–47.
12. Watters DA, Green AJ. Competence and competency-based training: what the literature says. ANZ J Surg. 2016;86(5):395–9.
13. https://www.zawya.com/en/press-release/companies-news/national-institute-for-health-specialties-accredits-cleveland-clinic-abu-dhabi-x4k2k1p7. Accessed 13 June 2023.
14. https://www.dha.gov.ae/en/media/news/800. Accessed 13 June 2023.
15. Frank JR, Snell LS, Cate OT, Holmboe ES, Carraccio C, Swing SR, et al. Competency-based medical education: theory to practice. Med Teach. 2010;32(8):638–45.
16. Smith L, Lewis R. Digitized modes of training in health education: trends and challenges. J Digit Health Educ. 2018;4(1):25–31.
17. Ten Cate O, Khursigara-Slattery N, Cruess RL, Hamstra SJ, Steinert Y, Sternszus R. Medical competence as a multilayered construct. Med Educ. 2024;58(1):93–104. https://doi.org/10.1111/medu.15162.

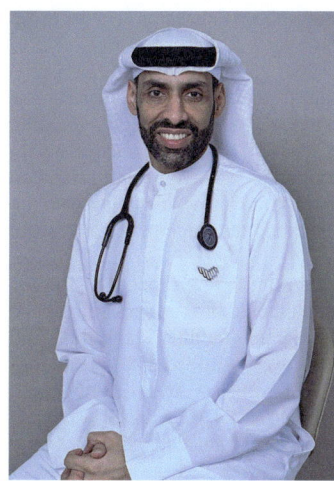

Professor Humaid Obaid Al-Shamsi is the Chief Executive Officer of Burjeel Cancer Institute in Abu Dhabi, UAE; President of the Emirates Oncology Society; Visiting Professor at Harvard Medical School at Harvard University; Visiting Scientist at Dana-Farber Cancer Center, Harvard Medical School, Boston, USA; Full Professor of Oncology at Ras Al Khaimah Medical and Health Sciences University; Ras Al Khaimah, UAE; an Adjunct Professor of Oncology at the College of Medicine, University of Sharjah; and Clinical Professor at Gulf University, Ajman, UAE. He is the first Emirati to be promoted as a professor in oncology in UAE history. He is also the Chairman for Colorectal Cancer in the MENA region, appointed by the prestigious National Comprehensive Cancer Network® in the USA. He is also the only member of the Lung Cancer Policy Network in the MENA region, which aims to advance lung cancer research and screening globally. He is the Chairman of the Oncology and Hematology Fellowship Training Program for the National Institute for Health Specialties in the United Arab Emirates. He is also the only member in the GCC in the WIN Consortium, which comprises organizations representing all stakeholders in personalized cancer medicine globally.

He is board-certified in both internal medicine and oncology from the UK, the USA (ABIM), the National Board of Physicians and Surgeons in the USA, and Canada (FRCPC). He has also been awarded the FRCP (Canada) in 2012, FRCP (London) in 2023, FRCP (Glasgow) in 2024, and FRCP (Edinburgh) in 2025. He is the only physician in the UAE with a subspecialty fellowship certification and training in gastrointestinal oncology and the first Emirati to complete a clinical post-doctoral fellowship in palliative care. He was an Assistant Professor at the University of Texas MD Anderson Cancer Center between 2014 and 2017. He has published more than 170 peer-reviewed articles in *JAMA Oncology, Lancet Oncology, Journal of Clinical Oncology, The Oncologist,*

BMC Cancer, and many others. His area of expertise includes precision oncology and cancer care in the UAE. In 2016, he published with his group from MD Anderson in the *Journal of Clinical Oncology* a study describing a new distinct subgroup of colorectal cancer, NON-V600 BRAF-mutated colorectal cancer. In 2022, he published the first book about cancer research in the UAE and also the first book about cancer in the Arab world, both of which were launched at Dubai Expo 2020. *Cancer in the Arab World* has been downloaded more than 500,000 times in its first 2 years of publication and is the ultimate source of cancer data in the Arab region. He also published the first comprehensive book, *Cancer Care in the United Arab Emirates*, which is the first book in UAE history to document cancer care in the UAE, with many topics addressed for the first time. The book was also another success with over 100,000 downloads in the first 2 months of publication.

He is passionate about advancing cancer care in the UAE and the GCC and has made significant contributions to cancer awareness and early detection for the public using social media platforms. He engages actively with the public through awareness campaigns and serves on numerous national health committees, including with the UAE Ministry of Health and the Department of Health, Abu Dhabi.

He is considered the most followed oncologist in the world, with over half a million followers across his social media platforms (Instagram, Twitter, LinkedIn, and TikTok). In 2022, he was awarded the prestigious Feigenbaum Leadership Excellence Award from Sheikh Hamdan Smart University for his exceptional leadership and research, and he was also awarded the Sharjah Award for Volunteering. He was also named the Researcher of the Year in the UAE in 2020 and 2021 by the Emirates Oncology Society.

In May 2024, HH Sheikh Mansour bin Zayed Al Nahyan, Vice President of the United Arab Emirates, awarded him first place in the Emirati Talent Competitiveness Council (NAFIS) program for outstanding leadership in the private sector across all business and medical disciplines. In February 2025, he was awarded the *Sheikha Fatima bint Mubarak Family Award* for being a successful role model in UAE society.

As CEO of Burjeel Cancer Institute, he is leading the largest cancer network in the UAE with over 30 oncologists and hematologists and built the first pediatric bone marrow transplant program in the UAE. He secured the UAE's first European Society for Medical Oncology (ESMO) accreditation for a cancer center in the UAE at Burjeel Cancer Institute.

Besides his clinical and administrative duties, he is engaged in education and various levels of research training for medical trainees to enhance their clinical and research skills. He established the UAE's first hematology and oncology fellowship training program accredited by the UAE National Institute for Health Specialties at Burjeel Cancer Institute.

His mission is to advance cancer care in the UAE and the MENA region and make cancer care accessible to everyone in need around the globe.

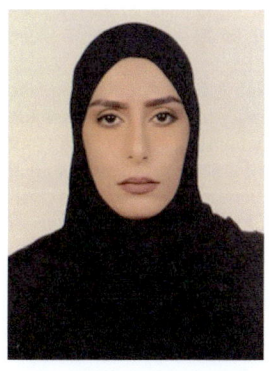

Aysha Al Dhaheri is the Senior Project Manager at the National Institute for Health Specialties, with 15 years of experience in academic administration. She previously served as the Director of the Office of the Chancellor at the United Arab Emirates University, where she managed all administrative functions and directed workflow. Throughout her career, Aysha has demonstrated expertise in overseeing projects, aligning with strategic goals, and fostering effective communication among stakeholders. Her leadership in these areas has been instrumental in enhancing organizational effectiveness and achieving objectives.

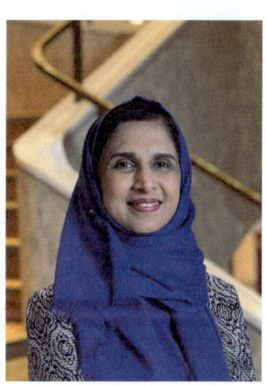

Dr. Fouzia Shersad is currently the Medical Education Expert at National Institute for Health Specialties, of UAE. She is also a project advisor of International FAIMER Institute, Philadelphia. She has over 30 years of experience as clinician, quality assessor, administrator, advisor, and medical educationist in the UAE, Oman, India, the USA, and the UK. In addition to FRCP (Glasgow), her qualifications include JMHPE, FAIMER fellowship, and PhD in Medical Education.

Dr. Fouzia has served as Associate Professor and Director of Medical Education at Dubai Medical College and as honorary lecturer of Medical Education at Keele University, UK. Dr. Fouzia led the college to win the prestigious Dubai Quality Award (DQA) and Mohammed Bin Rashid Al Maktoum Award (MRM) in 2011. After achieving training by EFQM, Dr. Fouzia was appointed as a Senior Assessor for the Dubai Quality Award.

Dr. Fouzia one of the active members in formulating the UAE National Competency Framework for medical education (EmiratesMEDs). Dr. Fouzia is one of the founding members of the planning, development, and implementation of the Emirati Board examinations of health specialties. Her special areas of research interest are quality in medical education, medical professionalism, instructional technology, competency-based assessment, and entrustable professional activities (EPAs).

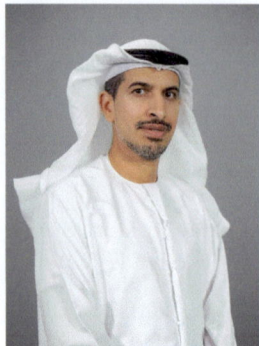

Dr. Mohammed Al-Houqani is a distinguished medical professional dedicated to advancing medical education and patient care. He currently serves as the Secretary General of the National Institute for Health Specialties (NIHS), playing a pivotal role in shaping postgraduate medical education in the UAE. Additionally, Dr. Al-Houqani is also an Associate Professor at the Department of Internal Medicine, at the College of Medicine and Health Sciences, United Arab Emirates University, and a consultant in Respiratory and Sleep Medicine.

Dr. Al-Houqani earned his MBBS degree from the United Arab Emirates University in 2003. He completed his residency in Internal Medicine at the University of Toronto in 2007, followed by a Respirology Fellowship in 2009 and Sleep Medicine Fellowship in 2010. He is certified by the Royal College of Physicians and Surgeons of Canada. Upon returning to UAE, he obtained a Master's in Public Health from UAE University.

As the inaugural Secretary General of the NIHS established by Cabinet of Ministers, Dr. Al-Houqani oversees the national institute's mandate to lead, regulate, and organize professional development for the health workforce with a focus on specialty training.

Dr. Al-Houqani's research interests include tobacco and sleep disorders, and he is a sought-after speaker at local and regional scientific meetings.

Open Access This chapter is licensed under the terms of the Creative Commons Attribution 4.0 International License (http://creativecommons.org/licenses/by/4.0/), which permits use, sharing, adaptation, distribution and reproduction in any medium or format, as long as you give appropriate credit to the original author(s) and the source, provide a link to the Creative Commons license and indicate if changes were made.

The images or other third party material in this chapter are included in the chapter's Creative Commons license, unless indicated otherwise in a credit line to the material. If material is not included in the chapter's Creative Commons license and your intended use is not permitted by statutory regulation or exceeds the permitted use, you will need to obtain permission directly from the copyright holder.

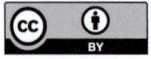

9

The Spectrum of Medical Education and Training in the UAE: Accomplishments and Points to Ponder

Salman Yousuf Guraya, Hatem Faraj Alameri, and Nabil Sulaiman

9.1 Background

The topography of medical education (MedEd) in the Middle East and North Africa (MENA), and particularly in the Arab world, embraces a diverse international community. In the Arabian context, MedEd remains at the intersection of cultural, religious, and social factors, with varying representations of knowledge, skills, and behaviors from each region. This phenomenon reflects a heterogeneous but, to some extent, shared vision of advancing the quality and delivery of healthcare systems for patient safety [1]. Likewise, there is no standardized platform for MedEd in the Arab world where leaders in academic medicine, medical students, residents, patients, and other stakeholders can convene for stewardship and health-related societal issues [2]. Although the Accreditation Council for Graduate Medical Education (ACGME) has introduced a framework of core competencies required by medical graduates [3], due to profound regional and population-specific variations in the Arab world, there is no jointly agreed upon charter for MedEd [4]. This absence of a common platform for MedEd is intensified in the United Arab Emirates

---

S. Y. Guraya
Department of Clinical Sciences, College of Medicine, University of Sharjah (UoS), Sharjah, United Arab Emirates
e-mail: sguraya@sharjah.ac.ae

H. F. Alameri
Healthcare Workforce Monitoring, Healthcare Workforce Sector, Department of Health, Abu Dhabi, United Arab Emirates

Department of Medicine, College of Medicine, Khalifa University, Abu Dhabi, United Arab Emirates

N. Sulaiman (✉)
Department of Family and Community Medicine and Behavioral Sciences, College of Medicine, University of Sharjah (UoS), Sharjah, United Arab Emirates
e-mail: nsulaiman@sharjah.ac.ae

© The Author(s) 2025
H. O. Al-Shamsi (ed.), *Healthcare in the United Arab Emirates*,
https://doi.org/10.1007/978-981-96-0523-1_9

(UAE) due to its versatile healthcare communities of patients, medical students, faculty, and healthcare professionals (HCPs). It is evident that most medical schools in the UAE have transplanted their curricula from European and North American institutions without prior "tissue matching." This situation has exacerbated an already existing blind spot in contextualized community-based medical education in the UAE. Despite these caveats in the MedEd realm in the UAE, we have witnessed the profound resilience of its federal organizations, academic institutions, decision-makers, HCPs, and communities during the COVID-19 pandemic [5]. The purpose of this chapter is to examine the status of undergraduate (UG) and postgraduate (PG) MedEd in the UAE, including residency and accreditation programs for national and international benchmarking, with a view to highlighting strengths and areas for improvement.

9.2 Undergraduate Medical Education and Training in the UAE

In the past 50 years, with the union of the seven Emirates of the UAE, the country has achieved enormous gains in the financial, economic, and educational spheres [4]. A detailed examination of the UAE's 2021 strategic plan reveals that the nation's primary objective continues to be human development through education. There are now at least eight public and private UG and PG medical institutes in the UAE, governed by a vibrant and ambitious government. These include the United Arab Emirates University (UAEU), the University of Sharjah (UoS), Dubai Medical College for Girls (DMCG), Gulf Medical University (GMU), Ras Al Khaima Medical and Health Sciences University (RAKMHSU), Mohammed Bin Rashid University of Medicine and Health Sciences (MBRU), and Ajman University (AU) and Khalifa University (KU). The United States, Canada, the United Kingdom, Australia, and certain European nations require a few years of premedical study or a premed degree in the health sciences for medical school admission. This is followed by about 4–5 years of medical school and 1–2 years of residency. This may be followed by 4-year postgraduate specialty residency programs leading to specialist privileges. Lastly, all medical graduates and experts are required to undertake continuing education in their respective fields. The same norms of conduct also apply in the UAE. Once these prerequisites are satisfied, graduates have the option of continuing their postgraduate education through master's and doctoral programs or beginning clinical residency training. Residents must complete a 1-year internship at a recognized hospital in order to be accepted into a residency program. The UAE Ministry of Education (MoE) regularly oversees the quality of medical curriculum delivery, curricular interventions, teaching and learning pedagogies, educational facilities, and educational resources. This process of quality assurance contributes to the establishment of a standard benchmark in MedEd with the objective of producing competent, qualified, and safe medical professionals [6].

As indicated in Table 9.1, the duration of the current UG MedEd culminating in a bachelor's degree is between 4 and 7 years, including a foundation year at UoS or

Table 9.1 Characteristics of undergraduate medical programs in the UAE

University	UAEU	DMCG	GMU	UoS	RAKMHS	MBRU	AU	KU
Location	Abu Dhabi	Dubai	Ajman	Sharjah	Ras Al-Khaimah	Dubai	Ajman	Abu Dhabi
Year established	1984	1986	1998	2004	2006	2016	2018	2019
Undergraduate program	MD Bachelor of Science Nutritional Science Bachelor of science dietetics Bachelor of Science of Speech-language-Pathology	Bachelor of Medicine and Surgery (MBBCh)	MD Bachelor of Biomedical Sciences Higher diploma in pre-clinical sciences	MBBS	MBBS MD	MBBS	MBBS	MD Pre-medicine bridge program
Program duration (years)	4	6	6	6	4	6	6	4

(continued)

Table 9.1 (continued)

University	UAEU	DMCG	GMU	UoS	RAKMHS	MBRU	AU	KU
Entry requirements	A minimum score of 900) in EmSAT	10 + 2 with 50% marks from the science stream (in high school EmSAT English with a minimum grade of 1100 or TOEFL above 61 or IELTS above 5	Equivalency certificate from MoE English proficiency (EmSAT/ IELTS/ TOEFL) Arabic proficiency	High school grades to enter FY Best two thirds will be promoted subject to passing the mini-interviews IELTS-6.0, TOEFL-550, EmSAT-1100	Secondary school certificate with 75% EmSAT score of 800 Admission test IELTS-5, TOEFL-500	Secondary school score of at least 85% IELTS-6, TOEFL iBT-80, EmSAT-1525 Arabic proficiency of EmSAT-800	IELTS of 6, TOEFL 550, EmSAT 1100 Arabic [proficiency] 800 in EmSAT	Bachelor's degree (STEM) Cumulative GPA 3.0 and science GPA of 3.0 MCAT score of at least 500 IELTS (6.5), TOEFL iBT (90), EmSAT English (1550)
Teaching pedagogy	PBL TBL	TBL	Student-led-seminars PBL, TBL Virtual-patient learning	PBL TBL	Integrated and PBL	PBL	TBL	PBL
Total graduated students	1287 graduates	1579 graduates	1272 graduates	1204 graduates	747 graduates	203 enrolled	49 enrolled	60 enrolled

UAEU United Arab Emirates University, *KU* Khalifa University, *RAKMHS* Ras Al-Khaimah University for Medical and Health Sciences, *MBRU* Mohammed Bin Rashid University of Medicine and Health Sciences, *GMU* Gulf Medical University, *AU* Ajman University, *UoS* University of Sharjah, *DMCG* Dubai Medical College of Girls, *MoE* Ministry of Education, *FY* Foundation Year, *MBBS* Bachelor of Medicine, Bachelor of Surgery, *MD* Doctor of Medicine, *MBBCh* Bachelor of Medicine, Bachelor of Surgery, *IELTS* International English Language Testing System, *STEM* Science, Technology, Engineering and Mathematics, *EmSAT* The Emirates Standardized Test, *TOFEL* Test of English as a Foreign Language, *TBL* Team Based Learning, *PBL* Problem Based Learning an internship at GMU. Each institution's overall study plan has been logically segmented into stages that correlate with the various curricular components.

As shown in Table 9.1, UAE MedEd is characterized by a variety of entrance criteria for UG medical programs at various universities. As mandated by the UAE Ministry of Education, an entrance exam is now required for admission to UG medical program. Currently, there is no uniform exam for admittance into medical programs across UAE medical schools, highlighting the need to develop a national curriculum and evaluation instrument for all candidates. This unified evaluation system is necessary given that many universities accept high school students from diverse educational and curriculum backgrounds. Medical school applicants may come from international school systems as well as numerous school systems within the country, including Arabic, American, British, International Baccalaureate, South Asian, European, and others. Looking into the teaching philosophies and learning paradigms, problem-based learning (PBL) remains the most popular among the UAE medical institutions, as six out of eight have adopted this student-centered, small-group teaching approach. Literature has shown the effectiveness of PBL in medical education, where student-driven learning takes place using carefully crafted clinical cases that trigger peer-assisted learning and clinical reasoning skills [7]. Though there are common strands of basic and clinical sciences across institutions, the curricula of UAE medical institutions lack horizontal and vertical integration of community-based and relevant courses in the curriculum, such as academic and physician leadership [8], interprofessional education and collaboration [9, 10], disease prevention and health promotion [11], healthcare resilience [12], medical insurance and financial matters [13], medical professionalism [14], patient safety [15], bereavement and palliative care [16], evidence-based medicine, aging and health, research, and several others. Education and training in these subjects are of paramount importance for HCPs during their clinical practice.

Since 1993–1994, when the first group of medical students graduated from the UAEU Faculty of medicine, an estimated total of 6,089 medical students have graduated from the five medical schools in the UAE, based on data collected by the authors and their colleagues. The outliers are KU, MBRU, and AU, which have not yet graduated their first cohorts of students. Even though this number of medical graduates is insufficient for a country with a population of approximately ten million that is growing steadily, many medical graduates leave the UAE after their internships due to their predetermined career destinations or the inability to gain admission to their desired residency programs. This brain drain from the UAE results in an ongoing loss of medical experts, resulting in shortages in a number of medical professions [17].

Most medical institutes in the UAE do not have affiliated teaching hospitals. This demonstrates a serious flaw in the clinical instruction of undergraduate medical students. Despite the fact that medical institutions have outsourced and organized many hospitals and healthcare facilities, clinical training and assessment remain inconsistent and heterogeneous. For successful clinical mentoring, hospital clinical faculty require intensive training and faculty development initiatives to improve their knowledge and abilities. In addition to observing and experiencing uneven training and evaluation opportunities, medical students are confronted with significant disparities between clinical and academic personnel. In recent years, the UAE has emerged as a key center for medical education and training despite these deficiencies. International progress assessments are considered the gold standard for self-evaluation and benchmarking strategies for medical schools and students. Some popular benchmarking programs include the International Foundations of Medicine (IFOM) by the National Board of Medical Examiners (NBME) [18], the European Board of Medical Assessors (EBMA), the International Database for Enhanced Assessments and Learning (IDEAL) consortium [19], the Universities Medical Assessment Partnership (UMAP), and several others. The outright advantages of these inter-institutional collaborative assessments include quality improvement and an objective comparisons of curricular effectiveness and defects in certain sections of the curriculum [20]. Currently, UoS, UAEU, and GMU are taking IFOM exams as a standard benchmark for cross-institutional evaluation.

The Commission for Academic Accreditation (CAA) UAE works with both local and national authorities across the Emirates to assure the academic quality of higher education [4]. Recognizing the value and impact of clinical training in the UAE, the CAA has recommended at least 40 hours of clinical training for UG medical training per week. At the same time, the CAA has recommended clinical training of 80 credit hours in UG MedEd across the country. This substantial emphasis on clinical training demands major curricular interventions and the availability of more stable and sustainable clinical training sites in the UAE.

9.3 Graduate, Postgraduate, and Continuous Medical Education in the UAE

9.3.1 Graduate Programs (Master's and PhDs) in Health

There are various colleges in the UAE that offer medical education graduate training programs in health-related fields. Master's and PhD programs in public health, for example, are offered by UAEU, GMU, and Hamdan bin Mohammed Smart University (HBMSU). Table 9.2 outlines a brief account of PG medical and health specialties programs in five recognized medical institutions in the UAE. Like the UG MedEd students, the PG medical and health sciences programs attract students from a wide range of regions and nationalities.

9.3.2 Residency and Fellowship Programs

Graduates of medical schools, after finishing an internship, must pass a medical examination. The Emirates Medical Residency Entry Examination (EMREE) is a multiple-choice clinical reasoning examination covering internal medicine, pediatrics, surgery, obstetrics and gynecology, family medicine, emergency care,

Table 9.2 Postgraduate programs offered by academic medical institutions in the UAE

University	UAEU	MBRU	GMU	UoS	HBMSU
Location	Abu Dhabi	Dubai	Ajman	Sharjah	Dubai
Year established	1984	2016	1998	2009	2002
Postgraduate program	Master of public health Master of Science in Genomic Medicine Master in Medical Sciences Doctor of Philosophy in public health PhD Biomedical sciences PhD Pharmacy MSc in human nutrition PhD nutritional Sciences MSc clinical psychology	MSc biomedical sciences PhD biomedical sciences	Master public health Master health professions education Executive master's in healthcare management and Economics Doctor of Philosophy in Precision Medicine	Master molecular biology Master of Science in Molecular Medicine and Transitional Research PhD molecular biology Master of Science in Leadership in Health Professions Education Master of Science in Diabetes Management Doctor of Philosophy in Molecular Medicine and Transitional Research	MSc excellence environmental management Master of Science in Public Health MSc hospital management

UAEU United Arab Emirates University, *MBRU* Mohammed Bin Rashid University of Medicine and Health Sciences, *GMU* Gulf Medical University, *UoS* University of Sharjah, *RCSI* Royal College of Surgeons Ireland, *HBMSU* Hamdan bin Mohammed Smart University

psychiatry, and public health. Due to the UAE's fragmented healthcare system, there is no centralized medical residency program under federal control. Abu Dhabi, Dubai, and the Northern Emirates implement residency programs through many authorities, including the Department of Health (DOH), Dubai Health Authority (DHA), and Ministry of Health and Prevention (MOHAP), respectively, for Abu Dhabi, Dubai, and the Northern Emirates. Each healthcare authority has recently been subdivided, further dividing and delegating responsibility to a variety of stakeholders. In addition to the PG programs provided in the UAE academic institutions, the Dubai Residency Training Program (DRTP) was launched in 2006 to improve medical training, and subsequently, the Tanseeq program (Abu Dhabi) was established in 2010. These two programs share requirements and select participants who are matched by an algorithmic system to ensure no more than one resident is selected from each institution. Through predetermined selection criteria, the DRTP manages the enrollment procedure. Prior to enrolling in one of the residency programs, residents undergo several mini-multiple interviews (MMI) to evaluate their clinical and communication skills. The Tanseeq program in Abu Dhabi, on the other hand, mandates that candidates be interviewed by a faculty panel, including the program directors, and then they are graded and matched using a robust algorithmic system in partnership with the National Residency Matching Program International (NRMP-I), the largest matching organization in the world. As it stands, the number of candidates in the 30 residency specialties of the Tanseeq program is outlined in Table 9.3. It is remarkable to note the trend of a growing number of medical specialties and residents in this program since its inception.

The majority of residency and fellowship programs have been offered in healthcare facilities managed and operated by Abu Dhabi Healthcare Service Company (SEHA) since the program's inception. However, in the last five years, the participation of other large healthcare providers (Cleveland Clinic Abu Dhabi, operated by Mubadala Health) in medical education has added a competitive spirit to the medical education movement in Abu Dhabi and the United Arab Emirates.

The Arab Board of Health Specialization (ABHS), which was founded in 1978, continues to act as the principal accreditation authority for the majority of residency and fellowship postgraduate programs in the UAE. The ABHS certification examination consists of two sections, the first of which is conducted during the first two years of residency and assesses the theoretical components of the specialty. The second component is administered in the final year and focuses on bedside clinical abilities. Certification as an expert in a certain profession requires passing both examinations. Abu Dhabi implemented the United States-based Accreditation Council for Graduate Medical Education-International (ACGME-I) for institutional and program certification in 2012 to add another layer to its accreditation system for quality improvement. In addition, the Saudi Commission for Health Specialties (internal medicine, neurology, pulmonology, anesthesia, and neurosurgery) and the German Specialty Board have accredited a variety of residency programs in Dubai, including orthopedics and trauma. In a similar fashion, the Jordanian Medical Council has accredited a number of Abu Dhabi-based resident training institutes and their specialty programs. The Cabinet Decree of 2014 established the National Institution for Health Sciences (NIHS) with the purpose of leading, regulating, and coordinating professional development for the health workforce. The NIHS is nested within the UAEU, the country's preeminent national institution of higher education. This institution's overarching mission is to promote comprehensive, high-quality specialty training in order to equip the United Arab Emirates with the necessary workforce. This was an important accomplishment for the UAE's medical education program, as it sought to ensure the quality of postgraduate specialty training, for which there is high demand but limited capacity. Currently, enrolled residents and fellows may sit for the examination(s) required by the appropriate certifying authority.

Table 9.3 Residents and fellows accepted into the Department of Health in Abu Dhabi (Tanseeq Matching Program) and the Dubai Health Authority (Dubai Residency Training Program, DRTP) between 2019 and 2022

Residency and fellowship programs	Abu Dhabi Tanseeq Program				Dubai Health Authority (DHA)			
	2019	2020	2021	2022	2019	2020	2021	2022
Anesthesia	4	6	6	7				
Cardiology	2	2	2	5	–	–	–	1
Clinical hematology	–	1	2	2				
Dermatology	2	2	2	2				
Emergency medicine	20	23	25	27	–	8	5	10
Family medicine	26	33	26	24	13	–	21	6
Gastroenterology	–	2	2	2	–	–	–	2
General pediatric	32	32	32	32				
General surgery	8	10	10	11	2	4	7	–
Hematology					–	–	2	–
Infectious disease	–	–	–	4				
Internal medicine	49	54	47	41	7	1	16	4
Medical oncology	–	2	2	1				
Mental and child health					8	9	–	6
Neonatology	4	4	4	4				
Nephrology	2	2	2	2				
Neurology	–	–	–	2	1	–	2	–
Obstetric gynecology	7	7	7	9	2	3	7	–
Ophthalmology	4	4	4	4	–	–	–	1
Orthodontics	–	3	3	3				
Otolaryngology	5	5	5	6				
Pediatrics					11	–	14	5
Pediatric dentistry	–	3	3	3				
Pediatric emergency	–	–	–	2				
Pediatric endocrine	–	–	–	1				
Pediatric gastroenterology	–	1	1	1				
Pediatric nephrology	–	–	–	1				
Pediatric rheumatology				1				
Prosthodontics	–	3	3	3				
Psychiatry	8	8	8	6	1	1	4	3
Pulmonology					–	–	1	–
Radiology	4	4	4	7	3		2	1
Rheumatology	–	2	2	2				
Urology	2	2	1	4				
Total	**179**	**215**	**203**	**219**	**48**	**26**	**81**	**39**

Source: Tanseeq Match lists (2019–2021)/Medical Education Programs Results 2022 (https://www.doh.gov.ae/en/Announcements/medical-education-2022-results, https://www.doh.gov.ae/-/media/Feature/Announcements/TANSEEQ-2021-result-list.ashx, https://www.doh.gov.ae/-/media/Feature/Announcements/TANSEEQ-2020.ashx, https://www.doh.gov.ae/-/media/Feature/Tanseeq-results-2019.ashx)
(–) no program was available in the specialty

9.3.3 Continuous Medical Education (CME)

Lifelong learning and professional development programs are important to the UAE's objective to advance and promote excellence in healthcare education. This is accomplished by enrolling practicing physicians in accredited continuous medical education programs. Continuous medical education (CME) and continuous professional development (CPD) programs are usually accredited by the main three regulatory authorities: MOHAP, DOH, and DHA. Customarily, the CME/CPD providers include medical institutions, professional organizations, and the corporate sector in conjunction with research institutes. For the renewal of a physician's license, forty CME hours per year must be completed. A few approved centers in the UAE offer high-fidelity simulation, live animals, and organs or cadavers from animals.

Actual data on the workforce and the number of graduates from undergraduate and graduate schools remain sparse. In the UAE, however, there is a clear disparity between the number of UG medical graduates and PG clinical residency positions. A medical graduate without a secure residency training location would logically depart the nation permanently. Instead of strengthening the abilities of frontline HCPs, there is always the possibility of a shortage of physicians. It is a priority for UAE healthcare policymakers to increase UG and PG medical training venues and opportunities in order to recruit and retain medical professionals in the nation.

9.4 Summary of Findings, Points to Ponder, and Proposed Corrective Remedies

To offer a community-based, relevant, and standardized medical education and training curriculum that is more relevant for UG but still applicable to PG as well, we reviewed the frameworks of several educational bodies. These included the ACGME, NBME, General Medical Council (GMC), and World Health Organization (WHO). This work identified some gaps in the curricula of UAE medical institutions. We have collected all evolving subjects in MedEd whose inclusion in the existing curricula would add value to the impact of medical training and the competency of the graduates (Fig. 9.1).

The foundation in Fig. 9.1 illustrates the existing core curricula, while the pillars signify new add-ons to the curricula that may fortify the educational and training legacy. The roof and boundary walls of Fig. 9.1 with research, medical professionalism, and technology-enhanced learning (TEL), signify a longitudinal embracement of these strands across the curricula. TEL has gained popularity during and post-COVID eras due to its perceived benefits, including addressing issues of educational equity and social exclusion, freely accessible

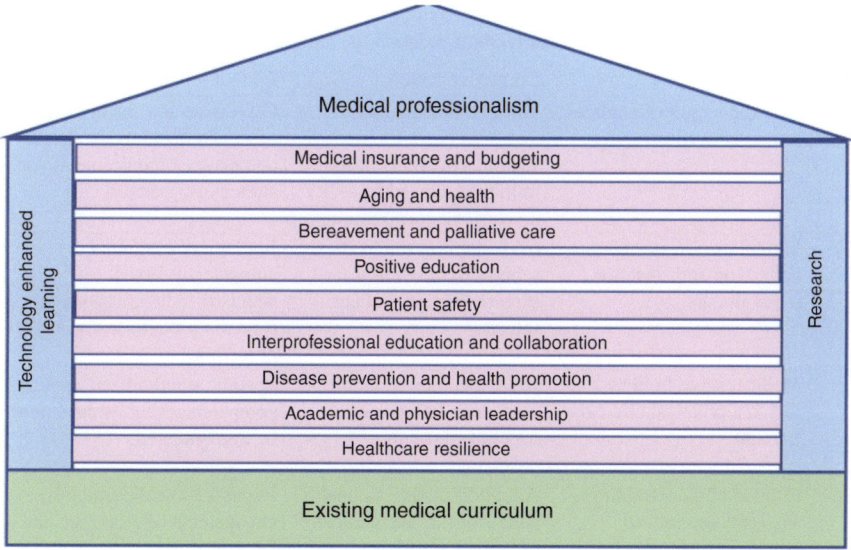

Fig. 9.1 The desired vertical and horizontal integration of medical education strands in the existing curricula of UAE medical institutions

educational opportunities, reduction in the cost of reaching, and educating a large number of students, and networking [21]. We propose to medical educators that they select the appropriate strands from this illustration and incorporate them into their curricula without disturbing the fundamental educational philosophy of the institution.

We have summarized the key findings of our research about the current realm of UG and PG medical education and training in the UAE, with some corrective remedies in Table 9.4.

Table 9.4 Summary of the challenges confronting medical education in the UAE, the UAE's response to these challenges, and our recommendation for future system improvements

	Challenges	Corrective action	Further recommendation
1	Variable length of medical school education	The CAA created a 2+4-year norm for medical school. Two years of basic training followed by 2 years of clinical training	CAA to review the application of standardized medical school competency requirements for student progression
2	Variable medical school admission and selection requirements	CAA requires the medical schools to have entry assessments for student selection	Implement a national competency-based standardized admissions test (like the MCAT) and selection procedures
3	Medical school offers variable practical clinical training	CAA specifies 80 credit hours and 40 h per week for clinical training programs	Specific standardized clinical competencies milestones must be implemented
4	Limited clinical training sites and specialized academic institutions	Adoption of various health authorities to the medical education agenda and promoting the expansion of medical education in the public sector	Expand clinical training by engagement of all public and large private healthcare facilities in the UAE
5	No National Exit or Certification Exam	Several schools utilize IFOM, IDEAL, EBMA, or EMAP as longitudinal benchmark evaluation instruments	Develop internationally benchmarked and locally driven evaluation tools and a national exit examination
6	Postgraduate medical education is exclusive to the public sector and is underdeveloped in several emirates	Expanding postgraduate medical education to semi-governmental facilities and organizations	Expand postgraduate education to all public and large private healthcare facilities in UAE
7	Multiple postgraduate international accreditation systems	The National Institute of Health Specialties established as an accreditation and certification body for the United Arab Emirates	Adoption of a national strategy for locally generated accreditation and certification standards with the eventual goal of phasing out other accrediting systems
8	Unstructured medical education financing at the postgraduate level	The initiative to create a structured funding system for postgraduate medical education is now underway	Increase funding through government grants and reimbursement packages with the alignment of medical education funding with performance and outcome metrics

(continued)

Table 9.4 (continued)

	Challenges	Corrective action	Further recommendation
9	Lack of connection between the goals of medical education and the national strategy for Emiratization and workforce planning	Work is under process to improve the alignment between the distribution of graduates of residency and fellowship programs and health system needs	Create a platform to promote local grads and increase private sector engagement in medical education
10	Due to the lack of inputs and output data in medical education, medical education research is insufficient	With the wide adoption of a medical education agenda by several regulatory authorities, more data have been collected and analyzed	The accessibility of open-source data to educators and researchers will facilitate the expansion of medical education research
11	CME's contribution to the health system is modest.	CME is utilized by regulatory authorities for licensing and relicensing of health professions.	Multiple activities are necessary to increase the quality of CME and relate it to the competencies, scope of practice, and clinical privileges of health professionals

9.5 Conclusion

This chapter acknowledges and applauds the UAE's rapid growth in medical education, training, and professional development over a short period of time. In addition, the UAE government recognizes the importance of HCPs and their professional expertise. We have seen an increase in the adoption of globally advanced medical education curricula and accrediting standards, which has led to an improvement in the quality of undergraduate and postgraduate medical education. However, the UAE's medical education system faces several obstacles. Medical education modeling lacks standards, particularly at the postgraduate level. This issue is exacerbated by the lack of HEI-dedicated teaching hospitals. Further work is required to align the organization and delivery of medical education with the needs of the community.

Acknowledgements The authors would like to acknowledge Dr.S. Gurumadhva Rao, President of RAKMHSU; Dr. Yousif El Tayab, Clinical Dean of DCMG; and Dr. Wadeia Mohammad Sharief Abdul Rahim, Director of Medical Education and Research Department, Dubai Health Authority, for providing the data for Table 9.3. Thanks to Dr. Hossam Hamdy, Chancellor of Gulf Medical University, Ajman, for his generous help with this chapter. Additionally, we thank Dr. Phyu Hnin Hlaing, postdoctoral researcher at CoM, UoS, for her contributions to data collection.

Conflicts of Interest The authors have no conflicts of interest to declare.

References

1. Letaief M, Leatherman S, Tawfik L, Alboksmaty A, Neilson M, Horemans D. Quality of health care and patient safety in extreme adversity settings in the Eastern Mediterranean region: a qualitative multicountry assessment. East Mediterr Health J. 2021;27(2):167–76.
2. Albejaidi F, Nair KS. Building the health workforce: Saudi Arabia's challenges in achieving vision 2030. Int J Health Plann Manag. 2019;34(4):e1405–e16.
3. Kang D, Siddiqui S, Weiss H, Sifri Z, Krishnaswami S, Nwomeh B, et al. Are we meeting ACGME core competencies? A systematic review of literature on international surgical rotations. Am J Surg. 2018;216(4):782–6.
4. Alameri H, Hamdy H, Sims D. Medical education in The United Arab Emirates: challenges and opportunities. Med Teach. 2021;43(6):625–32.
5. Guraya S. Combating the COVID-19 outbreak with a technology-driven e-flipped classroom model of educational transformation. J Taibah Univ Med Sci. 2020;15(4):253.
6. Goldie J. Integrating professionalism teaching into undergraduate medical education in the UK setting. Med Teach. 2008;30(5):513–27.
7. Liu Y, Pásztor A. Effects of problem-based learning instructional intervention on critical thinking in higher education: a meta-analysis. Think Skills Creat. 2022;45:101069.
8. Montgomery BL. Academic leadership: gatekeeping or groundskeeping? J Values Based Leadersh. 2020;13(2):16.
9. Guraya SY, Barr H. The effectiveness of interprofessional education in healthcare: a systematic review and meta-analysis. Kaohsiung J Med Sci. 2018;34(3):160–5.
10. Zhang X-Q, Zhang B-S, Wang M-D. Application of a classroom-based positive psychology education course for Chinese medical students to increase their psychological well-being: a pilot study. BMC Med Educ. 2020;20(1):1–9.
11. Madjar B, Shachaf S, Zlotnick C. Changing the current health system's vision for disease prevention and health promotion. Int Nurs Rev. 2019;66(4):490–7.
12. Wiig S, Aase K, Billett S, Canfield C, Røise O, Njå O, et al. Defining the boundaries and operational concepts of resilience in the resilience in healthcare research program. BMC Health Serv Res. 2020;20(1):1–9.
13. Chisholm D, Docrat S, Abdulmalik J, Alem A, Gureje O, Gurung D, et al. Mental health financing challenges, opportunities and strategies in low-and middle-income countries: findings from the Emerald project. BJPsych Open. 2019;5(5):e68.
14. Goddard AF, Patel M. The changing face of medical professionalism and the impact of COVID-19. Lancet. 2021;397(10278):950–2.
15. Garcia CL, Abreu LC, Ramos JLS, Castro CFD, Smiderle FRN, Santos JA, et al. Influence of burnout on patient safety: systematic review and meta-analysis. Medicina. 2019;55(9):553.
16. El-Jawahri A, Nelson AM, Gray TF, Lee SJ, LeBlanc TW. Palliative and end-of-life care for patients with hematologic malignancies. J Clin Oncol. 2020;38(9):944.
17. Abdel-Razig S, Alameri H. Restructuring graduate medical education to meet the health care needs of Emirati citizens. J Grad Med Educ. 2013;5(2):195–200.
18. Chandramouli R, Gopakumar A, Venkatramana M, Hamdy H. Impact of NBME international foundations of medicine "IFOM" examination on students' academic achievement. Health Prof Educ. 2019;5(4):345–51.
19. Prideaux D, Gordon J. Can global co-operation enhance quality in medical education? Some lessons from an international assessment consortium. Wiley Online Library; 2002. p. 404–5.
20. Muijtjens AM, Schuwirth LW, Cohen-Schotanus J, Thoben AJ, Vleuten CPVD. Benchmarking by cross-institutional comparison of student achievement in a progress test. Med Educ. 2008;42(1):82–8.
21. Karunathilake I. Technology enhanced learning with limited resources-transforming limitations into advantages. South Asian J Med Educ. 2017;11(1):1–2.

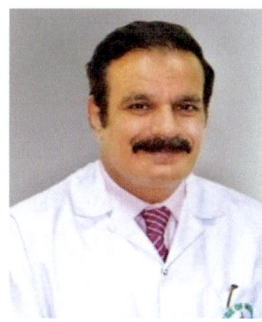

Prof. Salman Yousuf Guraya is an internationally recognized academic surgeon and educator, World top 2% Scientists by Stanford/Elsevier 2020-2024, and sits on the WHO Academy Advisory Group for Lifelong Learning. Currently, he is serving University of Sharjah as lead clinical training, simulation and assessment and chair of the interprofessional education. Holding senior academic leadership positions, Prof. Guraya has led national and international reforms in healthcare education, postgraduate surgical and medical training, and institutional strategies. His affiliations include academic leadership roles with the Royal College of Surgeons of England and Ireland, AAMC, MedBiquitous, and AMEE. A prolific scholar, Prof. Guraya has extensively published as principal investigator in the world leading journals on digital professionalism, patient safety, interprofessional collaboration, surgical oncology, and weight loss and transoral thyroidectomy. Prof. Guraya has conceptualized transformative educational models, and has championed interprofessional collaboration, leadership development, and digital identity formation. Beyond academia, Prof. Guraya has played a strategic role in enhancing institutional branding and rankings, leading national KPIs, NIHS surveys, and academic reputation initiatives. He is also a Founding Editor and Editor-in-Chief of several international journals under Springer Nature, Wolters Kluwer, Frontiers, and contributes to global networks in surgical education and medical scholarship.

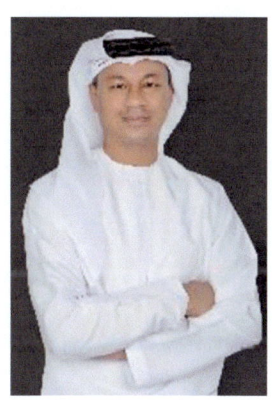

Dr. Hatem Faraj Alameri is the division director of the Department of Health Abu Dhabi's Healthcare Workforce Monitoring division, an adjunct clinical professor of medicine at Khalifa University's College of Medicine and a visiting consultant of pulmonary medicine at Shaikh Khalifa Medical City. Over the last two decades, he has conceived and promoted projects to improve healthcare and health professions education in the Emirate through his roles at several academic and regulatory organizations and authorities. He was instrumental in the establishment of the First National Residency Matching System in Abu Dhabi (Tanseeq) in 2011, which was followed by the accreditation of the Abu Dhabi Residency Programs by the Accreditation Council for Graduate Medical Education International (ACGME-I) in 2013. He also established the first Medical Education Funding Program in support of the Emirates' medical education agenda. For his long-renowned contribution to regional and worldwide medical education, he received the ACGME-I Physician Leader Award in 2020.

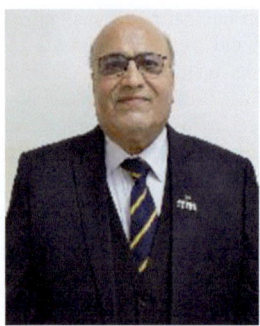

Nabil Sulaiman is a professor of family and community medicine. He was born in Iraq and trained in Iraq and the UK. He served as a leader in medical education and research for about 40 years, working at several universities in the UK, Australia, and the Middle East. He has been a founding member of the College of Medicine at the University of Sharjah since 2005 and the founding Head of the Department of Family and Community Medicine and Behavioral Sciences, as well as the founding director of the Sharjah Clinical and Surgical Training Centre. Nabil's research interests are diabetes, medical education, and family and community medicine. He has published over 100 papers in high-impact-factor (IF) journals.

Open Access This chapter is licensed under the terms of the Creative Commons Attribution 4.0 International License (http://creativecommons.org/licenses/by/4.0/), which permits use, sharing, adaptation, distribution and reproduction in any medium or format, as long as you give appropriate credit to the original author(s) and the source, provide a link to the Creative Commons license and indicate if changes were made.

The images or other third party material in this chapter are included in the chapter's Creative Commons license, unless indicated otherwise in a credit line to the material. If material is not included in the chapter's Creative Commons license and your intended use is not permitted by statutory regulation or exceeds the permitted use, you will need to obtain permission directly from the copyright holder.

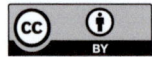

Career Opportunities for Physicians and Nurses and the Licensing Pathways in the UAE

Emilie Davies and Vivienne Mendonca

10.1 The Healthcare System in the UAE

The healthcare sector in the United Arab Emirates (UAE) is one of the most rapidly expanding in the region [1], with the highest number of Joint Commission International (JCI)—accredited hospitals in the Gulf Cooperation Council (GCC) [2]. Remarkable growth in recent decades has been driven by the UAE government's vision to provide access to high-quality medical services that are on par with international standards for all citizens and residents [3]. Population growth and the increasing prevalence of chronic lifestyle-related diseases, such as diabetes and obesity, have lead to increased demand for health services [4]. The UAE is also a popular medical tourism destination for patients seeking high-quality, accessible medical care. The Medical Tourism Index 2020–2021 ranked Dubai sixth as the top destination in the Middle East, with Abu Dhabi also in ninth place [5].

The UAE is seeking to become a global leader in high-tech medical applications and digital innovation. There have been major investments in telemedicine [4], robotic-assisted surgery [6], and 3D printing techniques for surgical specialties including oncology, cardiology, and orthopedics [4]. Significant investment has also been made in medical research and the expansion of medical education in the UAE [7]. The establishment of the new Dubai Academic Health Corporation is part of a broader strategy to advance health services in Dubai by integrating healthcare, medical education, and scientific research [8]. The UAE is developing its medical education and training capacity and encouraging more Emirati nationals to enter the healthcare sector. However, it still relies heavily on skilled and experienced healthcare professionals from abroad [4].

E. Davies (✉)
CEO and Founder of Allocation Assist, Dubai, United Arab Emirates
e-mail: emilie@allocationassist.com

V. Mendonca
Professional Medical Writer, Dubai, United Arab Emirates

The government oversees health insurance coverage for UAE nationals within each emirate. Citizens may access free or subsidized care either through the comprehensive government-funded health service or in private hospitals covered by their insurance network [9]. Expatriate residents, who make up approximately 88% of the population [10], mainly receive care in the rapidly expanding private sector, which is mostly insurance-based. In Abu Dhabi and Dubai, it is mandatory for employers to provide health insurance to their employees, although coverage for their dependents can vary [9].

The healthcare sector in the UAE is regulated by the Ministry of Health and Prevention (MOHAP). Healthcare facilities and professionals are regulated by the Department of Health (DOH) in the emirate of Abu Dhabi and the Dubai Health Authority (DHA) in Dubai. In the Northern emirates, medical licensing is regulated by MOHAP.

The strength of the UAE's healthcare sector was demonstrated during the COVID-19 pandemic. UAE authorities issued a national alert even before COVID-19 was declared a public health emergency of international concern by the World Health Organization. The government and private healthcare sectors worked together in an efficient, coordinated response managed by the National Crisis and Emergency Management Authority (NCEMA) [11].

10.2 Opportunities, Benefits, and Challenges for Healthcare Professionals in the UAE

The growing healthcare sector in Dubai and the wider UAE requires additional skilled and experienced doctors, nurses, and allied health professionals. There is a high demand for specialties such as medical oncology, orthopedics, and pediatrics. The increasing prevalence of chronic diseases requires professionals skilled in managing conditions such as cardiovascular disease and diabetes [12]. Western-trained doctors, especially those with advanced fellowships post-specialization, are sought after to bring new skills and techniques to the region.

As there is no set salary scale for doctors or other health professionals in the UAE, salaries are negotiable, depending on the specialty, grade, qualifications, and experience. However, salaries are often considerably higher than in their country of origin, and there is no income tax. Private hospitals often offer extra performance-based or revenue-sharing incentives. Although government hospitals do not offer performance-based incentives, they usually provide allowances for accommodation, children's education, and annual flights home. Other benefits for expatriate health professionals relocating to the UAE include 30 days of paid annual leave, employer-provided medical insurance, and a one-month salary bonus paid at the end of the employment contract for each year worked.

In addition to financial incentives, the UAE is an attractive location for expatriate healthcare professionals to live. Expatriates from over 200 countries make up around 88% of the total population of approximately 10 million [9]. The Expat City Ranking 2021 named Dubai as the best city for expats to live and work in the Middle East and the third best city globally, with Abu Dhabi being the third best in the Middle East and 16th globally [13]. The UAE is a strategically located travel hub where east meets west, leading to a vibrant, international, and family-friendly culture. Doctors licensed by UAE health regulatory bodies can apply for a 10-year, easily renewable "Golden Visa" as an added incentive to remain in the Emirates for the long term [14].

The UAE healthcare market is dynamic and competitive, and those relocating may face challenges such as adapting to a different culture and healthcare system. Doctors need to be proactive in networking and marketing to build their referral network and establish a patient base.

Medical licensing in the UAE can be a lengthy process, depending on the country where qualifications and training were obtained. As employers often aim to fill positions quickly, it is strongly recommended to review the specific requirements and begin the licensing process as early as possible.

10.3 Medical Licensing in the UAE

The United Arab Emirates recruits healthcare professionals from around the globe and has established rigorous systems to verify their identity, qualifications, skills, and experience. These measures ensure that healthcare professionals are licensed to practice safely in accordance with UAE law and international best practices. To be eligible, candidates must hold a valid professional license to practice in their home country and/or their most recent country of employment. Non-UAE nationals must also meet the experience requirements outlined in the Unified Healthcare Professional Qualification Requirements (PQR). The required post-qualification experience depends on the profession and professional grade [15].

10.3.1 Medical Licensing Authorities in the UAE

There are three different authorities that regulate the licensing of medical professionals within different emirates:

- The Department of Health (DOH) for Abu Dhabi (previously known as the Health Authority of Abu Dhabi (HAAD).
- Dubai Health Authority (DHA) for Dubai.
- Ministry of Health and Prevention (MOHAP) for all other emirates: Sharjah and Fujairah, Umm Al Quwain, Ras Al Khaimah, and Ajman.

For all health professionals, the process starts with creating an account with a username and password on the relevant medical licensing authority's platform. The required documents are then uploaded for primary source verification (PSV). This is the process of confirming the accuracy and authenticity of academic, professional, and legal credentials, and is outsourced to DataFlow, a leading global provider of specialized PSV solutions [16].

All healthcare regulatory authorities in the UAE (DOH, DHA, and MOHAP) comply with the same Unified Healthcare Professional Qualification Requirements, which list the licensing titles and the requirements and specifications for each of those titles [15]. The DataFlow (PSV) report is transferable between the three licensing authorities. However, as some aspects of the licensing process and examination requirements may differ, it is advisable for an applicant to plan which emirate they wish to work in before applying for licensure with the corresponding authority.

10.3.2 UAE Medical Licensing Pathways

The following are the common steps for the licensing process, with discussion of differences between the licensing authorities.

1. Create a new application
   Applicants need to register on the Department of Health—Abu Dhabi (DOH) [17], Dubai Health Authority (DHA) [18], or Ministry of Health and Prevention (MOHAP) [19] website before initiating the "New License" process. The DHA has a self-assessment tool that allows applicants to assess whether they meet the Unified Healthcare Professional Qualification Requirements (PQR) before starting the application [20]. Online forms must then be completed with comprehensive personal and professional details. The requirements vary according to the healthcare profession, qualifications, country of training, specialty, and grade [21].
2. Upload documents, as set out by the PQR [15]. This may include, but are not limited to:

   - Educational certificates.
   - Professional qualification certificates.
   - Recent professional and employment experience.
   - For dental and surgical specialties: a logbook for the last 2 years with hospital stamp(s) and signature of the medical director or other authorized person.
   - Valid license or registration from the medical licensing body of the country of recent employment.
   - Valid good standing certificate, not older than 6 months.
   - Valid passport copy.
   - Recent photo.
   - Academic transcripts.

3. Primary Source Verification (PSV) by DataFlow, which verifies documents directly from the original or primary source, usually takes between 6 and 12 weeks. For MOHAP, initial approval of the uploaded documents is required before primary source verification can start.

   Once the PSV is completed, a positive DataFlow report is issued, which must be linked to the DHA/DOH/MOHAP application. The DataFlow report can also

be used for other UAE emirates and many other Gulf countries, and the verifications never expire.
4. Verification Examinations (if required)
   The PQR has a tier system that recognizes postgraduate qualifications and training programs from specific countries [15]. According to the exam equivalency criteria, healthcare professionals who have successfully completed international examinations and/or hold an active registration or license to practice with certain regulatory bodies (allocated to Tier 1) will be exempt from the assessment. Those allocated to Tiers 2 and 3 are required to pass an assessment before obtaining a license to practice in the UAE [21]. Tier 2 trained doctors may be exempt from the required exam if they fulfill certain conditions relating to experience, seniority, and research or publications [15]. Assessment exemption criteria do not apply to healthcare professionals with more than two years of gap in practice (excluding UAE nationals and children of Emirati women after providing the discontinuity of practice requirements) [15].

   There are two types of assessment: computer-based testing (CBT) and oral assessment. The mode of assessment depends on the healthcare professional's title and training [21]. Oral examinations, usually taken in the UAE, involve a panel of senior consultants from the applicant's field asking scenario-based clinical questions to assess their knowledge and competency. Computer-based tests (CBTs) on a healthcare professional's specialty are outsourced to globally recognized companies: Prometric for the DHA and MOHAP [22, 23], and Pearson for the DOH (Abu Dhabi) [24]. They can be taken at many testing centers around the world. Table 10.1 shows the examination equivalency criteria.

An examination is usually not required for consultant physicians who have completed their specialist training in Austria, Australia, Belgium, Canada, Denmark, Finland, France, Germany, Iceland, Ireland, Luxembourg, the Netherlands, New Zealand, Norway, Singapore, South Africa, Sweden, Switzerland, the UK, or the USA [15].

For general practitioners, those who have completed recognized training in Australia, Canada, Ireland, New Zealand, the UAE, the UK, or the USA are exempt from the licensure examination [15].

Nurses and midwives who have a valid license and a good standing certificate (GSC) issued by the following countries can be exempted from licensure examination: Austria, Australia, Belgium, Canada, Denmark, Finland, France, Germany, Iceland, Ireland, Luxembourg, the Netherlands, New Zealand, Norway, Singapore, South Africa, Sweden, Switzerland, the UK, and the USA [15]. Additional equivalency criteria may be applied at the discretion of each individual authority. UAE nationals and children of Emirati women who meet the PQR requirements for the applied title are exempt from the authority examinations [15, 21].

For the DOH (Abu Dhabi), the DataFlow report must be completed before booking examinations (Fig. 10.1). For the DHA and MOHAP, these exams may be booked while waiting for the DataFlow report. However, for the DHA, the DataFlow

Table 10.1 Exam equivalency criteria

Profession	Exempted (Tier 1) countries	Note:
Consultant or specialist physician	Austria, Australia, Belgium, Canada, Denmark, Finland, France, Germany, Iceland, Ireland, Luxembourg, the Netherlands, New Zealand, Norway, Singapore, South Africa, Sweden, Switzerland, the UK, the USA	Applicants from these countries are exempted from licensing exams if they have completed recognized international exams and/or hold an active license to practice with certain regulatory bodies (Tier 1) and meet experience requirements, as defined by the PQR
General practitioners	Australia, Canada, Ireland, New Zealand, the UAE, the UK, or the USA	Applicants with other qualifications or licenses (Tier 2 or 3) may be required to pass a licensing examination
Nurses and midwives	Austria, Australia, Belgium, Canada, Denmark, Finland, France, Germany, Iceland, Ireland, Luxembourg, the Netherlands, New Zealand, Norway, Singapore, South Africa, Sweden, Switzerland, the UK, the USA	

NB: Applicants should check the current requirements with the licensing authority, as these vary according to specialty and are subject to change

Sources: Unified Healthcare Professional Qualification Requirements (The Ministry of Health—UAE; Department of Health—Abu Dhabi; Dubai Health Authority; Sharjah Health Authority) [15]

must be completed before any oral examination (Figs. 10.2 and 10.3). The time frame for assessments depends on the specialist panel's or test center's availability.

Three attempts are allowed to pass either the CBT or oral exams. Applicants may be granted one final attempt with a different authority after failing three attempts with another authority [15]. If still unsuccessful, the professional may only apply for a different specialty or a higher title with a new qualification, provided they fulfill the relevant PQR criteria [25].

5. Registration and Licensing

    The DHA and MOHAP issue a registration certificate, which can be shown to potential employers as proof of eligibility to practice in the UAE. Once the Data Flow and any examination are successfully completed, an application for registration can be submitted (Figs. 10.2 and 10.3). The DHA or MOHAP usually responds within 1–2 weeks and may ask for additional information if required. The registration is activated as a license once the candidate successfully secures a job. Registration is valid for one year for the DHA or five years for the MOHAP and can be easily renewed, provided there is no discontinuity in practice.

    For the DOH (Abu Dhabi), no registration certificate is issued. The applicant must have an employer sponsorship letter in order to complete the licensing process (Fig. 10.1).

    Once a professional obtains their license, they must comply with continuing medical education (CME) requirements for their specialty in order for it to be

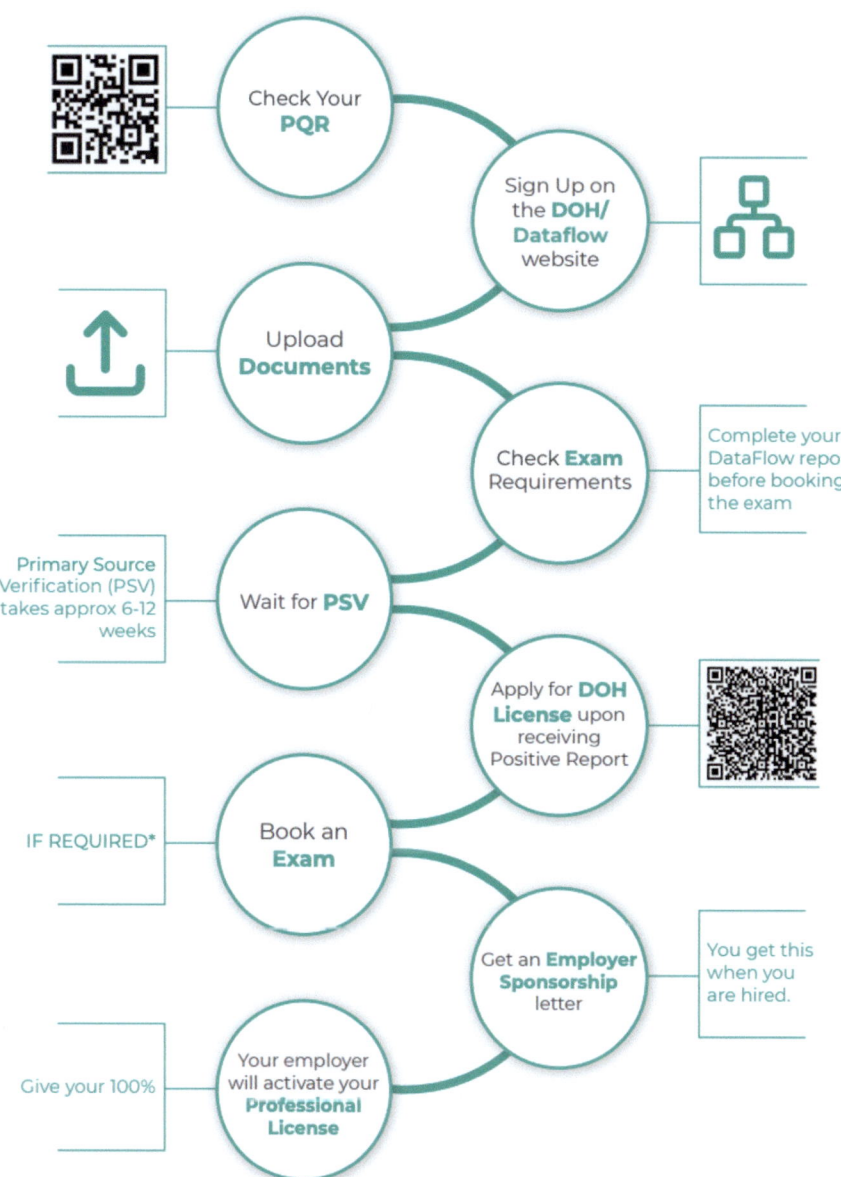

Fig. 10.1 Flowchart for the Department of Health licensing process. (Source: Allocation Assist, Dubai, United Arab Emirates)

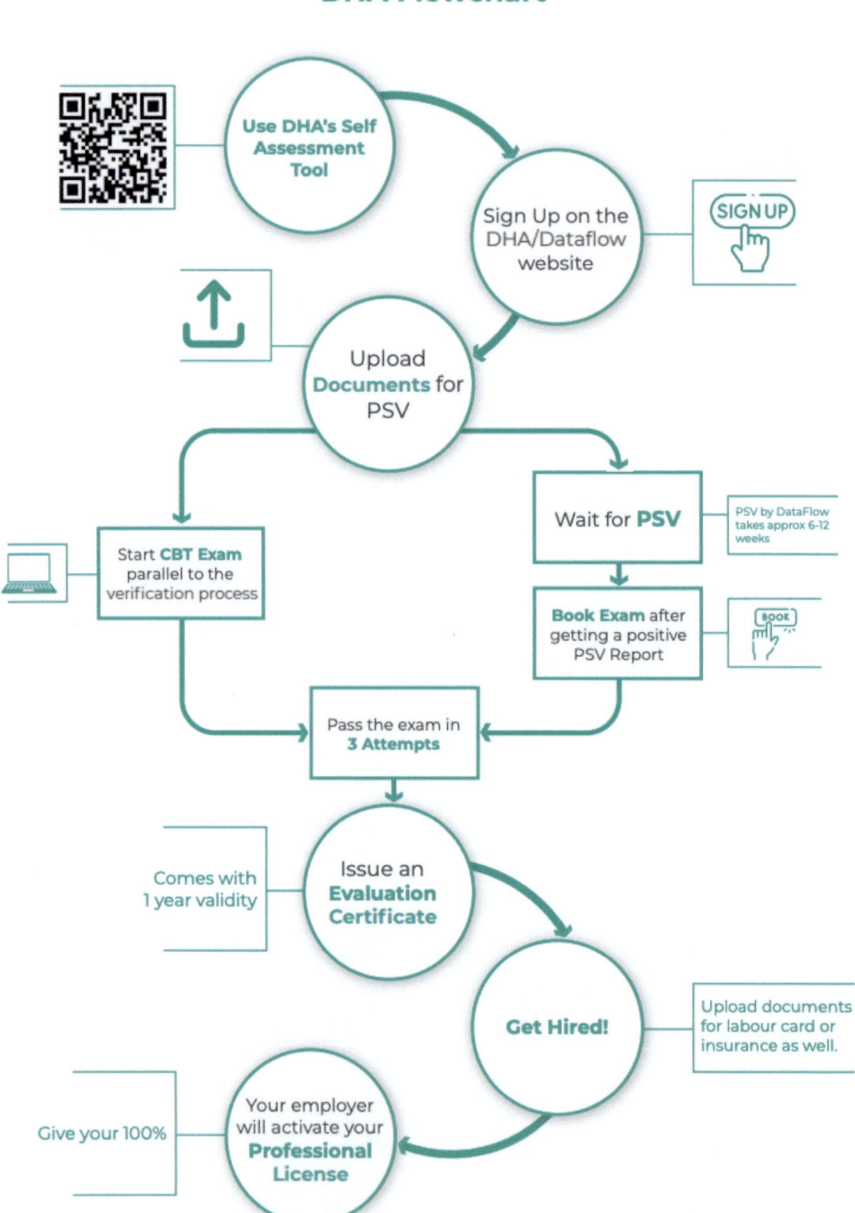

Fig. 10.2 Flowchart for the Dubai Health Authority licensing process. (Source: Allocation Assist, Dubai, United Arab Emirates)

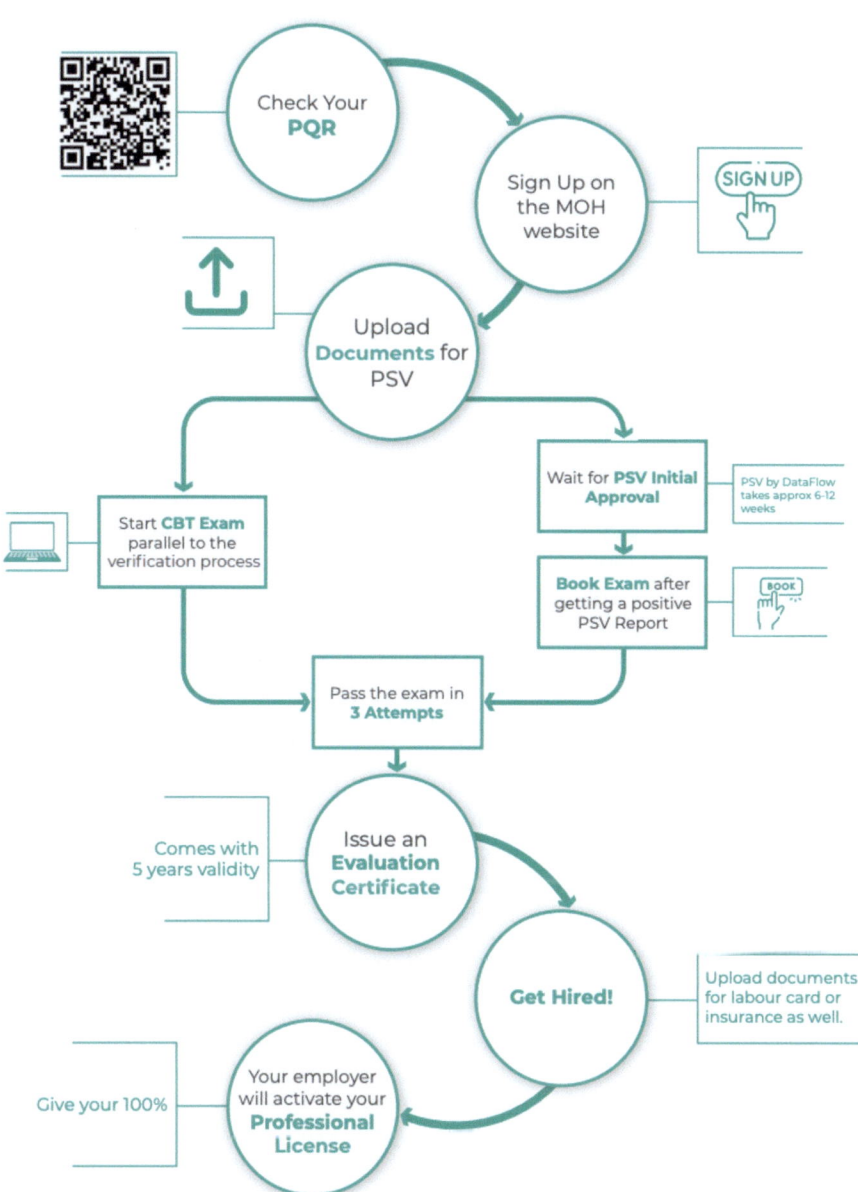

Fig. 10.3 Flowchart for the Ministry of Health's licensing process. (Source: Allocation Assist, Dubai, United Arab Emirates)

renewed on an annual basis [15]. Physicians and dentists in surgical specialties should also provide logbook(s) as a prerequisite for renewing the license [15].

Professional licensing fees are payable at different stages of the process and are subject to change. See the relevant websites for the current fees [17–19].

10.4 Frequently Asked Questions About the UAE Medical Licensing Process

Q. *How long does the licensing process take?*
The time required for the licensing process can vary. Unexpected delays can occur, such as requests for additional documents or issues with verifying documents in their country of origin. From past experience, for professionals from Tier 1 countries whose training programs are recognized by the UAE licensing authorities, the process may take between 3 and 6 months on average. However, when examinations are required, it may take up to 12 months.

Q. *Is it necessary to obtain a medical license before applying for jobs in the UAE?*
The UAE healthcare recruitment market is dynamic and competitive. Hospitals looking to fill vacancies as soon as possible prefer candidates who have already proven their eligibility to work in the country. For the DHA and MOHAP, it is advisable to obtain your registration before applying for jobs. For the DOH—Abu Dhabi, there is no registration step before obtaining a license, but you can start the process and obtain the DataFlow report to expedite the licensing process.

Q. *What are the main differences between the DOH, DHA, and MOHAP licensing processes?*
The MOHAP (the licensing authority for all emirates except Abu Dhabi and Dubai) requires initial approval of the uploaded documents before the primary source verification by DataFlow can begin.

The DOH (Abu Dhabi) sometimes asks for additional documents, such as privilege certificates, proof of residency, vaccination records, or academic transcripts.

Examination exemptions vary between the Ministry of Health and Prevention, the Department of Health, and the Dubai Health Authority (Table 10.1). It is also important to check the updated Professional Qualification Requirements (PQR) [15].

For the DOH (Abu Dhabi), the DataFlow report must be completed before booking assessments (Fig. 10.1). For the DHA and MOHAP, these tests may be booked while waiting for the primary source verification. However, for the DHA, the DataFlow must be completed before any oral examination (Figs. 10.2 and 10.3).

The DHA and MOHAP issue a registration certificate, which can be shown to potential employers as proof that a candidate meets the licensing requirements. The registration is activated as a license once a job is secured (Figs. 10.2 and 10.3).

For the DOH (Abu Dhabi), no registration certificate is issued. The applicant must have an employer sponsorship letter in order to apply for a license (Fig. 10.1).

Q. *What is the applicant's responsibility during the licensing process?*
The licensing process is necessarily exacting, with strict attention to detail. Applicants are required to be cooperative and patient. They should provide factual, accurate information to the best of their ability and must never forge, misinterpret, or elaborate on any details.

Q. *Can I apply for a medical license if I have a gap in practice?*
If you have a gap in practice exceeding 2 years, continuing medical education (CME) requirements must be fulfilled, and additional training may be required. In general, non-UAE nationals will not be able to apply for a license if they have had a clinical practice gap of more than 5 years (or more than 10 years for UAE nationals) [15].

Q. *What happens if I fail the examination?*
You are allowed three attempts to pass the examination. A final attempt may be granted by a different authority after failing three attempts with another authority [15]. If you are still unsuccessful, you may only apply for a different specialty or a higher title, after obtaining a new qualification, provided you fulfill the relevant PQR criteria [25].

Q. *If I have a DOH—Abu Dhabi license, can I work in Dubai?*
No. You need to apply for a DHA license to work in Dubai. However, the DataFlow report is transferable. In addition, once a healthcare professional has worked for at least 6 months in the UAE, they can apply for a license with a different UAE health authority without having to repeat a licensing examination.

Q. *If I have a registration certificate for the Dubai Health Authority (DHA), can I activate this into a medical license to work in Abu Dhabi or one of the other emirates?*
No. Although the Dataflow report is transferable [26], you need to apply individually to the licensing authority that has jurisdiction over the emirate where you want to work.

Q. *What is attestation for documents? Is it needed for the licensing process?*
Attestation is the process of obtaining legal authentication from a country's embassy, for a document that has been issued in another country. This is a legal process and different from the DataFlow Primary Source Verification.

Attestation is not routinely required for the licensing process. However, it is often necessary to have documents such as professional qualifications and birth or marriage certificates attested for a UAE employment visa application. It is usually quicker and less expensive to have your documents attested in your home country before moving to the UAE.

10.5 Conclusion

There are opportunities within the dynamic and growing UAE healthcare sector for doctors, nurses, and other healthcare professionals with the right qualifications, skills, and experience. Even as the government's Emiratization strategy [27] encourages more citizens to train and work in the healthcare sector, the UAE is currently still reliant on expatriate healthcare professionals to meet workforce demands. A rigorous process ensures that all credentials are thoroughly checked before a license to practice can be obtained. This exacting process can appear daunting and requires cooperation and patience. Many candidates choose to submit their applications with the help of a company specializing in medical licensing. Such companies can guide candidates on the requirements, check and upload documents, and follow up on the progress of the application. This support throughout the medical licensing process can save busy healthcare professionals time and stress.

Conflicts of Interest The authors have no conflicts of interest to declare.

References

1. ITA, U.S. Department of Commerce, UAE – Country Commercial Guide. https://www.trade.gov/country-commercial-guides/united-arab-emirates-healthcare-services. Accessed 16/10/23.
2. Joint Commission International, JCI-Accredited Organizations. https://www.jointcommissioninternational.org/who-we-are/accredited-organizations/#sort=%40aoname%20ascending. Accessed 16/10/23.
3. UAE Government, Vision 2021 and health, https://www.vision2021.ae/en/uae-vision. Accessed 16/10/23.
4. US-UAE Business Council, The UAE Healthcare Sector, June 2021, http://usuaebusiness.org/wp-content/uploads/2019/01/2021-U.A.E.-Healthcare-Report.pdf. Accessed 16/10/23.
5. Medical Tourism Index 2021–22. https://www.medicaltourism.com/mti/home. Accessed 16/10/23.
6. Duphat, Robotic Surgery Landscape in the UAE. https://duphat.ae/robotic-surgery-landscape-in-the-uae/. Accessed 16/10/23.
7. Alameri H, Hamdy H, Sims D. Medical education in The United Arab Emirates: challenges and opportunities. Med Teach. 2021;43(6):625–32. https://doi.org/10.1080/0142159X.2021.1908978. https://www.tandfonline.com/doi/figure/10.1080/0142159X.2021.1908978?scroll=top&needAccess=true. Accessed 16/06/22
8. Arabian Business (17/07/21), Dubai healthcare shake-up as ruler issues law to raise global status. https://www.arabianbusiness.com/healthcare/466221-dubai-healthcare-shake-up-as-ruler-issues-law-to-raise-global-status. Accessed 16/10/23.
9. UAE Government, Health Insurance. https://u.ae/en/information-and-services/health-and-fitness/health-insurance. Accessed 16/10/23.
10. CIA, The World Factbook, United Arab Emirates. https://www.cia.gov/the-world-factbook/countries/united-arab-emirates. Accessed 16/10/23.

11. Al Hosany F, Ganesan S, Al Memari S, et al. Response to COVID-19 pandemic in the UAE: a public health perspective. J Glob Health. 2021;11:03050. https://doi.org/10.7189/jogh.11.03050. https://www.ncbi.nlm.nih.gov/pmc/articles/PMC8005306/#R2. Accessed 16/10/23
12. KPMG, UAE Healthcare Perspectives (Sept 2020). https://assets.kpmg/content/dam/kpmg/ae/pdf-2020/09/uae-healthcare-perspectives.pdf. Accessed 16/10/23.
13. Internations, Expat Insider 2021. https://www.internations.org/expat-insider/2021/the-best-worst-cities-for-expats-40189. Accessed 16/10/23.
14. Allocation Assist, UAE opens 10-year 'Golden Visa' scheme to all resident doctors. https://www.allocationassist.com/uae-opens-10-year-golden-visa-scheme-to-all-resident-doctors/. Accessed 16/10/23.
15. Unified Healthcare Professionals Qualification Requirements (PQR) 3rd Version (The Ministry of Health – UAE, Department of Health –Abu Dhabi, Dubai Health Authority, Sharjah Health Authority). Downloaded from https://www.dha.gov.ae/uploads/072022/Unified%20Healthcare%20Professional%20Qualification202273235.pdf. Accessed 15/10/23.
16. DataFlow, Who We Are, DataFlow. https://corp.dataflowgroup.com/about-us/who-we-are/. Accessed 16/10/23.
17. DOH – Abu Dhabi Government Services, Register a New License for a Healthcare Professional. https://www.tamm.abudhabi/en/aspects-of-life/healthsafety/healthcareprofessionals/LicensingandCertificates/requestregistrationofnewlicenceforahealthcareprofessional. Accessed 16/10/23.
18. DHA, Get Registered. https://www.dha.gov.ae/en/services/details?id=245&segment=professional_services. Accessed 16/10/23.
19. MOHAP, Licensing of a Doctor. https://mohap.gov.ae/en/services/licensing-of-a-doctor. Accessed 16/10/23.
20. DHA, Self-Assessment Tool. https://services.dha.gov.ae/sheryan/wps/portal/home/services-professional/service-description?scode=MPQR&CATALOGUE_TYPE=PROFESSIONAL. Accessed 16/10/23.
21. DOH, Introduction to Professional Qualification Requirement. https://www.doh.gov.ae/en/pqr. Accessed 16/10/23.
22. Prometric, Dubai Health Authority. https://www.prometric.com/test-takers/search/dha. Accessed 16/06/22.
23. Prometric, Ministry of Health and Prevention. https://www.prometric.com/test-takers/search/emoh. Accessed 16/06/22.
24. Pearson Vue, Abu Dhabi DOH. https://home.pearsonvue.com/doh. Accessed 16/06/22.
25. Dubai Health Authority, Health Regulation Sector Service Catalogue, p. 79. https://www.dha.gov.ae/uploads/062022/health_regulation_5-12-19202263580.pdf. Accessed 9/11/23.
26. DHA, FAQs. https://services.dha.gov.ae/sheryan/wps/portal/home/faq. Accessed 16/06/22.
27. The National, Abu Dhabi healthcare sector given new Emiratisation target for 2025. https://www.thenationalnews.com/uae/2023/07/10/abu-dhabi-healthcare-sector-given-new-emiratisation-target-for-2025/. Accessed 16/10/23.

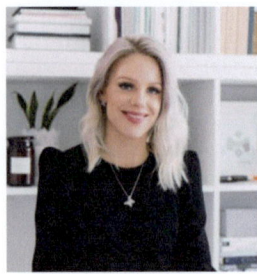

Emilie Davies is the CEO and founder of Allocation Assist Middle East, a UAE medical recruitment and licensing company based in Dubai. Allocation Assist has a proven track record of connecting highly skilled doctors and other healthcare professionals with opportunities in the UAE that match their training and experience. Over the years, Allocation Assist has developed strong working relationships with the most prestigious and advanced hospitals in the UAE. Prior to founding Allocation Assist in 2015, Emilie worked as an emergency nurse in the NHS in London, UK. Emilie's strengths lie in networking and building trust to establish long-term relationships with high-caliber doctors and leaders in the UAE healthcare sector.

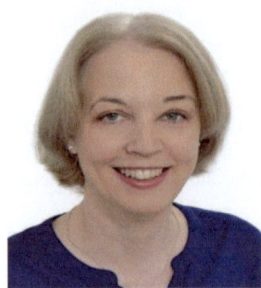

Vivienne Mendonca is a British dental surgeon and professional medical writer, based in Dubai. After graduating from the University of Liverpool in 1998, she worked for 12 years in general dental practice and the NHS Community Dental Service, as well as for one year in an Oral and Maxillofacial Surgery Hospital Department. She gained her MFDS from the Royal College of Surgeons of England in 2005 and her Master's in Public Health with merit from the University of Liverpool in 2018. Her MPH dissertation research was published in the *Cleft Palate-Craniofacial Journal* in 2020. Vivienne enjoys researching and writing on a wide variety of medical and healthcare topics. Her experience of living and working in the UK, USA, India, and UAE has given her a broad insight into challenges and solutions in healthcare systems. Vivienne's writing is concise, clear, and tailored for the target audience. She is skilled in both scientific writing and explaining health information and research in plain language.

Open Access This chapter is licensed under the terms of the Creative Commons Attribution 4.0 International License (http://creativecommons.org/licenses/by/4.0/), which permits use, sharing, adaptation, distribution and reproduction in any medium or format, as long as you give appropriate credit to the original author(s) and the source, provide a link to the Creative Commons license and indicate if changes were made.

The images or other third party material in this chapter are included in the chapter's Creative Commons license, unless indicated otherwise in a credit line to the material. If material is not included in the chapter's Creative Commons license and your intended use is not permitted by statutory regulation or exceeds the permitted use, you will need to obtain permission directly from the copyright holder.

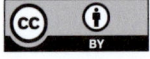

UAE Medical Liability Law

11

Ahmed Allouz, Mosaab Aly, and Amro Hassan

11.1 Introduction

The main federal law that currently regulates medical liability in the United Arab Emirates (UAE) is Federal Decree Law No. 4 of 2016 Concerning Medical Liability (as amended) (hereinafter referred to as the "*MLL*"). Prior to the MLL, medical liability was regulated by Federal Decree Law No. 10 of 2008 Concerning Medical Liability (the "*Previous MLL*"). The MLL came into effect on 15 August 2016 and is still in force.

The MLL is supplemented by the UAE Cabinet Resolution No. 40 of 2019 Concerning the Executive Regulations of the MLL (the "*MLL Executive Regulations*"), which came into force on 16 July 2019, superseding the executive regulations of the previous MLL.

The MLL generally sets out the duties of medical practitioners and the standards, procedures, and principles that they must follow. It also defines what acts constitute a medical error, regulates certain medical practices (e.g., the regulation of natural death, gender reassignment procedures, and abortion), and outlines the framework for complaints against medical practitioners and the scope of their civil and criminal liability. On the other hand, the MLL Executive Regulations supplement the MLL and implement its provisions.

In the following sections, we will highlight the key features of the provisions of the MLL (as supplemented by the MLL Executive Regulations).

A. Allouz · M. Aly · A. Hassan (✉)
Dispute Resolution Department and Healthcare Practice Group, Al Tamimi & Company, Dubai, United Arab Emirates
e-mail: a.allouz@tamimi.com; m.aly@tamimi.com; a.hassan@tamimi.com

11.2 Duties of Medical Practitioners

The MLL places responsibility on everyone who practices the medical profession in the UAE to observe both general and specific duties and standards. The MLL, therefore, aims to ensure that medical practitioners fulfil their duties with the level of accuracy and honesty required by the profession, in accordance with recognized scientific and technical standards, and in a way that guarantees the due care of patients [1].

Examples of the specific duties placed on medical practitioners under the MLL include the requirements to follow the rules and standards depending on their grade and field of specialization, to keep patients informed of treatment options, and to inform patients of possible complications. The MLL also prohibits, among other things, abstaining from treating a patient or providing first aid to an injured person, using unauthorized or illegal methods in the treatment of the patient's medical condition, disclosing patients' secrets, and prescribing any treatment before carrying out a clinical examination of the patient [2].

11.3 Medical Error

The MLL places legal responsibility on physicians to perform their duties with the level of accuracy and honesty required by the medical profession, in accordance with recognized scientific and technical standards, and in a way that guarantees the due care of the patient without exploiting the patient's need to achieve illegal interests, whether for themselves or for any other party, and without discrimination between patients [3]. According to the MLL, a medical error is committed when a practitioner:

(a) Is ignorant of the technical issues that every practitioner of the same degree and specialization should be aware of
(b) Fails to follow recognized professional and medical standards
(c) Fails to act with the necessary due diligence
(d) Is negligent and fails to act carefully and with precaution [4]

11.3.1 Examples of Certain Medical Practices Regulated by the MLL

11.3.1.1 Natural Death
Natural death provisions under the MLL grant medical professionals the discretion to allow the natural course of passing for terminally ill patients. Nonetheless, this is governed by certain conditions that must be fulfilled to allow such practice. These conditions are as follows:

- The patient suffers from an irreversible medical condition.
- All medical treatment options have been approached and explored.
- Treatment futility has been established within the context of the specific medical condition.
- The attending doctor advises against preforming CPR.
- A minimum of three consulting doctors must testify that the patient's best interest is best served by refraining from CPR to allow a natural death. It is important to note that obtaining the patient's, guardian's, or custodian's consent is not obligatory for this condition.

Once all these conditions are satisfied, medical professionals will abstain from preforming cardiopulmonary resuscitation (CPR), leading to a natural death. However, it is essential to note that if the patient explicitly requests resuscitation, even if such efforts would not contribute to treatment efficacy, it cannot be refused [5].

11.3.1.2 Gender-Reassignment Surgery

The MLL provides for certain cases in which gender-reassignment surgeries become permissible. These instances arise when an individual's physiological, biological, and genetic characteristics are counterproductive to their sexual orientation and attributes. However, this surgical procedure is contingent upon the verification of these circumstances through medical documentation and the endorsement of the reassignment procedure by a medical committee designated by the health regulatory body. Once the medical committee approves, there is an additional requirement of referring the patient to a psychologist to facilitate the necessary psychological adjustments they might face [6].

11.4   Consent for Surgical Procedures

Consent is a standard prerequisite that is practiced in the UAE healthcare system when performing surgical procedures; however, there are certain exceptions where consent can be overlooked/exempted. Firstly, in emergency cases that necessitate an immediate and imperative surgical procedure to mitigate the life-threatening risk the patient is undergoing, consent is not required. Similarly, this applies to an unborn fetus. Secondly, the MLL includes a provision that allows for surgical intervention when the patient lacks the capacity to provide consent, and securing consent from their spouse or family members up to the fourth degree is not feasible/attainable. However, this is conditional upon obtaining a report that confirms the necessity of the surgery executed by the attending doctor, another doctor from the same hospital, and the hospital's director [7].

11.5 Disclosure

The MLL has introduced modifications to previous provisions regarding disclosure. These amendments are driven by the objective of safeguarding public health; thus, the provision allows the release of patient information at the request of the health authority subject to conditions specified by the MLL Executive Regulations. This provision applies in cases where a physician discloses information as a means of self-defense before the investigation authority or judicial entities. Additionally, this provision empowers healthcare practitioners by allowing them to disclose a patient's medical records to support their defense in legal claims [8].

11.6 Medical Complaints and Medical Liability Committees [9]

The Medical Liability Committee (MLC) is an institution that the MLL has adopted to undertake the responsibility of scrutinizing medical complaints and malpractice while ensuring that the standard of care is maintained. It is governed by the provisions of Federal Law No.7 of 2012 to the extent it does not conflict with MLL provisions. The process commences with filing a complaint through the Ministry of Health and Prevention or through any of the local authorities within whose jurisdiction the incident took place. The relevant authority then directs the complaint to its designated MLC. Alternatively, the Ministry or health authority might also receive a complaint through channels such as a court or the Public Prosecution, which can initiate the referral to an MLC for further consideration. When the complaint is brought before the MLC, the committee's role involves ascertaining whether a medical error has occurred and evaluating its severity. This determination relies on a thorough examination of the available facts, medical records, investigations, and other relevant information such as the disability of the affected organ. However, in instances involving several liabilities, the MLC aims to ascertain the proportion of each individual's involvement in the error as a means of providing a fair decision and allocating appropriate damages.

11.7 Higher Committee for Medical Liability

Medical reports produced by the MLC can be contested through an appeal process to a higher committee known as the Higher Committee for Medical Liability (HCML) within 30 days of the report's service to the relevant medical facility or practitioners. The HCML is entrusted with the duty of examining grievances submitted by both healthcare professionals and patients concerning reports issued by the MLC. Decisions made by the HCML carry conclusive weight and are not subject to further challenges or appeals before any governing body according to the MLL. It is important to highlight that an MLC medical report becomes final if not contested within the stipulated appeal timeframe [10].

11.8 Civil Liability

Patients who suffered any medical malpractice are eligible to pursue civil claims for financial compensation. However, according to the MLL, in order to be compensated, the civil claim must be preceded by the process of filing a medical claim with the Ministry or local authority and then by the referral of the claim to the MLC, which will then provide a medical report [11]. Courts will utilize the medical report, once it becomes final, to establish the compensation to be awarded, evaluated based on the criteria of civil liability. The compensation amount is determined by the trial court, factoring in various considerations, including the extent and severity of the harm endured by the patient.

11.9 Criminal Liability

Contrary to civil liability, criminal liability under the MLL is typically limited to cases where a doctor commits gross medical error. The law in this area grants patients the right to submit complaints related to medical malpractice to the Public Prosecution. Furthermore, it mandates the prosecution to directly forward these medical malpractice complaints to the appropriate health authority. This step is taken to initiate the essential investigative procedure, starting with the evaluation of the complaints through the MLC and subsequently through the HCML. Despite a complaint being filed, the MLL seeks to strike a balance between the rights of the patient and the rights of healthcare professionals, specifically in the context of criminal liability. Thus, it contains a provision that prohibits the scrutiny of healthcare professionals and their detainment or temporary confinement until a conclusive medical report verifying that gross medical error has been committed is officially issued [12].

As stipulated in the MLL Executive Regulations, a medical error that is gross in nature is categorized as resulting in the demise of the patient or fetus, the inadvertent removal or impairment of a human organ, or any other significant harm. In order for a gross medical error to be established, the foregoing results must be accompanied by one of the following criteria:

(a) Demonstrating an inexcusable lack of familiarity with established medical standards that align with the practitioner's level and specialization.
(b) Implementing medical methods that lack recognition.
(c) Departing from medical norms and regulations without justification.
(d) Providing medical care under the influence of drugs, alcohol, or psychotropic substances.
(e) Deliberately practicing beyond the scope of specialization or clinical privileges conferred by the professional license.
(f) Employing diagnostic or therapeutic techniques without prior training or experience and without medical supervision.

(g) Lack of awareness or incompetence resulting in gross negligence when carrying out established medical procedures. Examples include administering the wrong dose or the wrong medication to a patient [13].

However, should the HCML or MLC establish that a medical practitioner is not accountable for a significant medical error, they may not be subject to criminal medical negligence charges [14].

11.10 Penalties

As set out by the MLL, below is a list of examples highlighting the penalties medical practitioners are subject to facing in the case of violating the set provisions, and the applicable laws in each case. The penalties and laws follow as such [15]:

- Physicians administering sex-change procedures can face a maximum sentence of 10 years; with the minimum being a 3-year prison sentence.
- Physicians refusing to provide treatment for emergency patients or interceding the patient's treatment will be subject to a minimum fine of AED 10,000 if it has affected the safety of the patient's body. In cases where unnecessary medical or surgical procedures are carried out without a patient's informed consent, the medical practitioner responsible will be subject to an identical penalty; a minimum fine of AED 10,000.
- In cases of gross medical errors, a minimum penalty of one year in prison and/or a minimum fine of AED 200,000 will be imposed on the medical practitioner. If the gross medical error results in death, the maximum penalty of imprisonment is two years; the minimum fine is AED 500,000. In the event that the gross medical error results in death and is committed under the influence of alcohol or drugs, the penalties are as follows: a maximum sentence of 2 years in prison, and/or a minimum fine of AED 500,000 with a maximum of AED 1,000,000.

These are penalties medical practitioners risk facing in the event of violating the regulations determined by the MLL; however, they can also be subject to disciplinary penalties set out in other legislation for identical violations, such as a warning or a temporary suspension of the license, and in rare cases, a permanent revocation of the UAE license.

11.11 Option of Settlement in Legal Proceedings

In accordance with the regulations of the MLL, a settlement between a patient and a medical practitioner can be facilitated by the patient's heirs and/or attorney. Moreover, in cases where gross medical errors are committed by medical practitioners, it is permitted for the settlement between the victim and the medical practitioners to be filed or submitted at any point after the complaint is made, regardless of the status of the action; this includes the time prior to the public prosecution as well as the period after the judgment is passed.

The settlement option acts as a protective barrier for medical practitioners, as it seeks to encourage rectification between the parties in the hopes of terminating the criminal case against the medical practitioner that is likely to lead to the imposition of criminal liability. Once an agreement is reached, and both parties have settled, the immediate withdrawal of the criminal case ensues. The withdrawal means the suspension of the criminal action and penalty against the health practitioner; this applies even if the execution of the penalty is already underway. However, the patient is still free to persist in claiming compensation in civil court. As long as the settlement does not extend to the waiver of civil actions against the medical practitioner, the victim is allowed to pursue civil proceedings for compensation [16].

11.12 Conclusion

The MLL sets out general and specific duties to be observed by medical practitioners. It also defines medical errors, explains the process of medical complaints against practitioners, and outlines the consequences of medical errors. The procedures established in the MLL aim to ensure that healthcare professionals accused of malpractice are not prosecuted until the MLC or the HCML issues a final report, and they mandate that patients submit their claims to the health authority to be reviewed by the MLC in order for civil claims for compensation to be admissible to the courts. The MLL also provides a grievance process that protects both patients and doctors by affording them the right to have their appeals thoroughly reviewed by the HCML.

The MLL also introduced new provisions that regulate certain medical practices (such as natural death and gender-reassignment surgeries). The provisions of the MLL clarify the circumstances under which CPR may be withheld, give patients the right to undergo gender-reassignment procedures (subject to certain conditions), and prohibit physicians from undertaking unnecessary medical or surgical procedures on patients without their informed consent.

The provisions of the MLL safeguard the legal interests of both patients and medical practitioners, thus serving to enhance the quality and delivery of healthcare in the UAE and the manner in which medical malpractice cases are managed before the judicial authorities. The MLL also promotes the amicable resolution of legal proceedings and makes it possible for patients and medical practitioners to settle criminal cases at any stage of the proceedings.

Conflicts of Interest The authors have no conflicts of interest to declare.

References

1. Medical Liability Law 2016 (UAE) Art. 3.
2. Medical Liability Law 2016 (UAE) Art. 4 & 5.
3. Medical Liability Law 2016 (UAE) Art. Article 3.
4. Medical Liability Law 2016 (UAE) Art. 6.
5. Medical Liability Law 2016 (UAE) Art. 11.
6. Medical Liability Law 2016 (UAE) Art. 7.
7. Medical Liability Law 2016 (UAE) Art. 8.
8. Medical Liability Law 2016 (UAE) Art. 5.6.
9. Medical Liability Law 2016 (UAE) Art. 18 & 19.
10. Medical Liability Law 2016 (UAE) Art. 20 & 21.
11. Cassation Appeal 97 Civil (2022) (Dubai Court of Cassation).
12. Medical Liability Law 2016 (UAE) Art. 24.
13. Article (5) of the MLL Executive Regulations.
14. Cassation Appeals 776, 780, 784 and 785 Criminal (2020) (Dubai Court of Cassation).
15. Medical Liability Law 2016 (UAE) Art. 28–34.
16. Medical Liability Law 2016 (UAE) Art. 35.

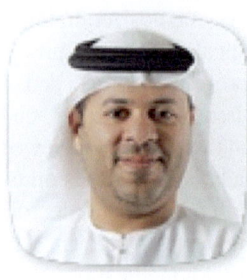

Ahmed Allouz is a Partner at Al Tamimi and Company and the regional co-head of the firm's Dispute Resolution Department. He also leads the firm's medical malpractice sector.

As an Emirati national, Ahmed has full rights of audience before the UAE courts. He represents a wide range of domestic and international clients in contentious matters and has developed particular expertise in the field of medical negligence. Ahmed has secured numerous favorable judgments for clients in medical negligence claims, where he has represented medical professionals and hospitals.

Ahmed also regularly advises clients in other types of litigation, including commercial, corporate, civil, rental, and real estate disputes. In addition, Ahmed routinely deals with criminal cases with particular expertise in medical negligence criminal-related complaints. In all these areas, Ahmed has achieved notable successes for clients in court cases and represented clients in negotiating settlements for complex litigation cases.

Ahmed regularly delivers workshops and seminars to clients in relation to various litigation topics, particularly in relation to medical negligence claims. He also publishes articles in the firm's *Law Update* magazine.

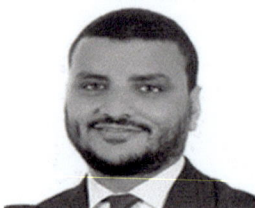

Mosaab Aly besides being qualified as a lawyer by the Egyptian Bar Association, Mosaab is also an English solicitor (SRA qualified) and a registered practitioner (Part II) with full right of audience before the DIFC Courts. He is also admitted by the Legal Affairs Department of the Government of Dubai to practice in the UAE as a legal consultant.

Since early 2009, Mosaab has been heavily involved in dispute resolution practice and contentious matters, whether in the form of litigation before the UAE courts, including the DIFC courts, or in form of domestic and international arbitration proceedings before different arbitral forums, including DIAC, DIFC-LCIA, ICC, ADCCAC, and other ad hoc arbitral tribunals.

Mosaab is a core member of the medical malpractice team. He acted and successfully defended clients on very high-profile claims related to professional negligence and malpractice. In this regard, he defended multinational auditing firms in claims that exceeded one billion US dollars and is regularly defending major healthcare providers in the region in medical malpractice litigation. Mosaab has also advised governmental entities on the restructuring and governance of the local healthcare system.

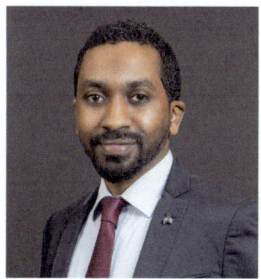

Amro Hassan is a senior associate in the firm's dispute resolution department and a member of the healthcare practice team.

Amro specializes in handling a wide variety of disputes, including complex and high-value civil, real estate, and commercial disputes, before all courts and special committees in the UAE. Amro has particular expertise in relation to medical malpractice disputes. He has advised and acted for several well-known medical institutions and medical practitioners in the UAE in various complex multi-million-dirham medical malpractice claims brought before the UAE Courts. Amro also handles criminal medical malpractice disputes and has experience handling and advising on medical complaints filed before health authorities. Amro has also been regularly involved in advising health facilities on the management and reporting of medical incidents since their early stages.

In addition, Amro has experience in real estate and commercial arbitration disputes and is a member of various regional arbitral institutions and associations.

Prior to joining Al Tamimi Amro worked in the arbitration and litigation departments of two leading law firms in the UAE, where he represented local and multinational companies in several contentious and non-contentious real estate, civil, and commercial matters.

Open Access This chapter is licensed under the terms of the Creative Commons Attribution 4.0 International License (http://creativecommons.org/licenses/by/4.0/), which permits use, sharing, adaptation, distribution and reproduction in any medium or format, as long as you give appropriate credit to the original author(s) and the source, provide a link to the Creative Commons license and indicate if changes were made.

The images or other third party material in this chapter are included in the chapter's Creative Commons license, unless indicated otherwise in a credit line to the material. If material is not included in the chapter's Creative Commons license and your intended use is not permitted by statutory regulation or exceeds the permitted use, you will need to obtain permission directly from the copyright holder.

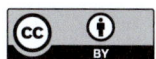

National Vaccination Program in the UAE

12

Dima Ibrahim and Fathima Firoz

12.1 Introduction

Vaccination is a proven preventive tool for controlling life-threatening infectious diseases and is estimated to avert approximately between 1.5 to 3 million deaths each year [1].

The United Arab Emirates (UAE) guidelines for immunization are based on international guidelines to include World Health Organization (WHO) immunization recommendations, Centre for Disease Control and Prevention (CDC) immunization resources, and UK immunization guidelines.

Vaccines are administered at all the ministry's preventive medicine centers in accordance with international standards of safety and precautionary measures to prevent infection [2].

12.2 Vaccination for Children

The UAE government mandates vaccinations for children from birth until Grade 11. Pediatric mandatory vaccination is given to decrease the burden of tuberculosis, diphtheria, pertussis, tetanus, hepatitis B, Hemophilus Influenzae type B, poliovirus, pneumococcus, measles, mumps, rubella, rotavirus, and papillomavirus infections [3].

In 2019, the Ministry of Health and Prevention (MoHAP) updated the National Immunization Program in accordance with the latest scientific recommendations [4].

D. Ibrahim (✉)
College of Medicine and Health Sciences, Khalifa University,
Abu Dhabi, United Arab Emirates

Burjeel Medical City, Abu Dhabi, United Arab Emirates
e-mail: dima.ibrahim@burjeelmedicalcity.com

F. Firoz
Dubai Pharmacy College for Girls, Dubai, United Arab Emirates

© The Author(s) 2025
H. O. Al-Shamsi (ed.), *Healthcare in the United Arab Emirates*,
https://doi.org/10.1007/978-981-96-0523-1_12

Based on UAE vaccination results and vaccine coverage, it was decided to decrease the number of pneumococcal doses from 4 to 3.

The National Immunization Program, in concordance with the Global Polio Eradication Initiative and global strategy, introduced the Infanrix-Hexa vaccine (Combined Diphtheria-Tetanus-acellular Pertussis (DTPa), Hepatitis B, Inactivated Poliovirus, and Haemophilus influenzae type B vaccine), which should be taken at the age of 4 months.

On another note, meningitis vaccine has been added to the 11th-grade school students' vaccination schedule. Below is a briefing on childhood vaccination as per the latest Dubai Health Authority (DHA) recommendations and WHO childhood vaccination schedule for the UAE [5, 6]:

I. *BCG vaccine*: Given after birth. Infants older than 6 months should undergo a tuberculin skin test (TST) before vaccination. Immunocompetent persons who have an induration <5 mm on the TST should receive the BCG vaccine (Australian handbook of immunization 2017).
II. *DTaP (Diphtheria and tetanus toxoids and acellular pertussis)/DTP (Diphtheria, Tetanus Toxoids and Pertussis) vaccines*: Administered as part of a hexavalent or pentavalent vaccine at 2, 4, 6, and 18 months, and again at 5–6 years.
III. *Poliovirus Vaccine (IPV/OPV)*: Administered as part of a hexavalent or pentavalent vaccine at 2, 4, 6, and 18 months, and again at 4–6 years.
IV. *Measles, Mumps, Rubella (MMR)*: The first dose of the vaccine should not be given before 1 year of age. A total of two doses are recommended for all children at least 4 weeks apart.
V. *Hemophilus Influenza B (HiB) vaccine*: Administered at 2, 4, 6, and 18 months as part of the pentavalent, hexavalent, and pentaxim vaccines.
VI. *Hepatitis B vaccine*: Administered at birth, 2, 4, and 6 months.
VII. *Varicella vaccine*: Given in 2 doses starting at 12 months of age, second dose to be given between 4-6 years of age.
VIII. *Rotavirus vaccine*: Administered at 2, 4, and 6 months.
IX. *Pneumococcal Conjugate vaccine (PCV)*: Administered at 2, 4, and 6 months. DHA also provides clear guidance on catch-up schedules for missed immunizations.
X. *Meningococcal vaccination*:
    Meningococcal conjugate vaccine (Menactra/Menveo): Approved for ages 2 months to 55 years, based on seasonal and geographic mandates (e.g., for travelers to Hajj, Umrah, or the African meningitis belt from Senegal to Ethiopia).
    Meningococcal Polysaccharide vaccine (MPSV4): Approved for ages 2 years and above, with the same mandates as conjugate vaccine. Administered as a single dose, with revaccination every 3 years recommended for individuals at continuous risk.
XI. *Human Papillomavirus (HPV) vaccine*: Recommended for individuals aged 11 or 12 years, and for all persons through age 26 if not previously vaccinated.

12.3 Vaccination for Adults

Protection from some childhood vaccines wanes over time. Adults need immunization to reduce their risk of acquiring infectious doseases that may have substantial social, professional, and financial impacts.

Adult vaccination should be tailored to the patient's age, medical conditions, and risk factors. Despite its importance, adult vaccination remains underutilized in the UAE.

Hiba J. Barqawi et al. published a study highlighting physicians' knowledge regarding adult vaccination in the UAE and concluded that knowledge in this field is poor, emphasizing issues with accessibility to local guidelines [7].

DHA recently updated its immunization guidelines, and for the first time, included immunization guidance for some growing high-risk populations in the UAE, such as hematopoietic stem cell and solid organ transplant patients [6].

Below is a briefing on general adult immunization guidance as well as immunization for special populations.

12.3.1 General Adult Vaccination

I. *Influenza (flu) vaccine*: Recommended annually for all adults.
II. *Td or Tdap vaccine*: Every adult should receive a Tdap vaccine, followed by a booster every 10 years. In addition, one dose is recommended during each pregnancy.
III. *HPV vaccination*:
   HPV vaccination is recommended for all preteen women at age 11 or 12 and for all individuals through age 26 if not previously.

   An HPV vaccination program for females was introduced by Abu Dhabi's Health Authority (HAAD) in 2008. Abu Dhabi, making Abu Dhabi the first in the Middle East and Arab region to implement HPV vaccination [8].

   Although it is of utmost importance for the prevention of cervical cancer, a cross-sectional survey showed that knowledge of the HPV vaccine and infection among women is generally low in the UAE. Increasing age and higher levels of the husband's education were associated with better knowledge of HPV infection [9]. Another cross-sectional study evaluating Emirati men's knowledge of HPV vaccination showed that they had a limited understanding of HPV infection and were generally against vaccination [8]. These two studies highlight the importance of increasing education among both men and women regarding this cancer-preventing immunization.

   Since HPV is transmitted to women sexually and is also associated with male cancers such as anal, rectal, and throat cancers, the latest clinical guidelines for best practice in immunization published by the DHA recommended HPV vaccination for both females and males from 11 years up to 45 years of age. Vaccination beyond 26 years should be decided in consultation with physicians, based on the individual patient's risk status [6].

IV. *Shingles' vaccine*: Recommended for healthy adults aged 50 years and older.
V. *Pneumococcal vaccination*:

   polysaccharide vaccine (PPSV23): Recommended for all adults aged 65 years and older, and for adults younger than 65 years with certain chronic health conditions.

   Conjugate vaccine: Recommended for all adults with specific conditions such as cerebrospinal fluid leak or cochlear implant.

   Recent update: As of 2023, CDC recommends PCV 20 for adults aged 19–64 years with chronic medical conditions or immunosuppressive conditions, and for all adults aged 65 years and older. Further details regarding indications by age and risk factors are available through the *PneumoRecs VaxAdvisor* (mobile app or web version) [10].

   In alignment with CDC updates, the DHA recently incorporated PCV 20 and 15 into its adult vaccination guidance [6]. Details regarding administration are outlined in Appendix 11 of the DHA guidelines.

   In one study published by Mostafa Zayed et al. among Dubai residents, PCV20 was found to reduce the economic cost of pneumococcal infection among Dubai expatriates compared with the previous pneumococcal regimen [7].

VI. *Hepatitis B vaccination* for high-risk groups to include the following:
   - Healthcare workers without hepatitis B immunity
   - Patients with chronic kidney disease on dialysis or with chronic liver disease
   - HIV-infected persons or patients with high-risk sexual behavior
   - Injection drug users
   - Travelers to high-endemic countries

VII. *Hepatitis A vaccination* for high-risk groups should include the following:
   - Persons with chronic liver disease
   - HIV-infected patients
   - Men who have sex with men
   - Drug users (injection or no injection)
   - Persons working in research laboratories that handle hepatitis A infections.
   - Travelers to countries endemic for hepatitis A, or close contacts of persons coming from endemic areas.
   - Persons working with high-risk populations for hepatitis A, including centers caring for drug users, developmentally disabled persons, or in nursing home facilities.

VIII. *MMR vaccination* for the following categories:
   - HIV-infected persons with no evidence of immunity to measles, mumps, or rubella (who maintain a CD4 count ≥ 200 cells/mm3 for at least 6 months).
   - Non-vaccinated healthcare workers (born in 1957 or later).
   - Students in post-high school institutions
   - International travelers

IX. *Meningococcal vaccination*:
   Conjugate vaccine MenACWY: Recommended for:
   - Individuals with Asplenia (anatomical or functional)
   - HIV - infected persons
   - Individuals with primary complement component deficiency or secondary deficiency due to medication (e.g., eculizumab, ravulizumab) use
   - Travelers to endemic countries
   - Microbiologists
   - College students living in residential housing
   - Military personnel

   Serogroup B meningococcal (MenB) vaccination: Recommended for:
   - Individuals with Asplenia
   - Individuals with primary complement component deficiency or secondary deficiency due to medication (e.g., eculizumab, ravulizumab) use
   - Microbiologists

X. *Varicella (Chickenpox) vaccine*:
   Recommended for healthcare workers with no history of chickenpox infection or no serological evidence of prior varicella infection

12.3.2 Special Population Vaccinations

I. *Asplenia/splenectomy and sickle cell disease patients*:
   - Pneumococcal 13-valent vaccine (PCV13)
   - 23-valent pneumococcal polysaccharide vaccine (PPSV23), administered at least 8 weeks after PCV13, and a second dose of PPSV23 should be administered 5 years later
   - PPSV23-naive patients aged 2 years or older who are scheduled for splenectomy should receive PPSV23 at least 2 weeks before or after surgery
   - A single dose of the Hib vaccine is recommended
   - Meningococcal conjugate vaccines, including Bexsero and Menactra, should be administered

II. *Patients with cancer*
   - Newly diagnosed adults with hematological or solid malignancies and children with malignancies should receive PCV13 vaccination. PPSV23 should be administered at least 8 weeks after PCV13. PCV 20 can be also used as an alternative, replacing PCV13 and PPSV23. Immunization should be delayed for at least 6 months in individuals receiving Rituximab or other anti-B cell therapies.

III. *Hematopoietic stem cell transplant (HSCT) population.*
   Prior to HSCT:
   - Candidates should receive vaccines recommended for their age group, with an interval of at least 4 weeks for live vaccines and at least 2 weeks for inactivated vaccines before starting the conditioning regimen

Table 12.1 Vaccines needed after HSCT, timing of immunization, and number of doses

Vaccines	Time post-HSCT to vaccine administration	Number of doses
Influenza-inactivated	6 months (for patients aged ≥6 months)	1, annually
PCV13	3–6 months	3[a]
PPSV23	≥12 months post-transplant if no GVHD	1
Hib	6–12 months	3
Tetanus/diphtheria	6 months	3
Hepatitis B	6–12 months[b]	3
Polio-inactivated	6–12 months	3
MMR	24 months[c]	2
Varicella (VAR)	24 months[c]	2

[a]Patients with chronic GVHD may receive a fourth dose of PCV13 12 months after hematopoietic stem cell transplantation (HSCT)
[b]If the post-vaccination anti-HBs concentration is not at least 10 mIU/mL, a second 3-dose series of HepB vaccine, using a high dose for adolescents and adults, should be given
[c]For patients without chronic GVHD or ongoing immunosuppression VAR or MMR can be given at 24 months. Recombinant zoster vaccine (inactivated vaccine) can be given for shingles prevention starting 3-6 months after transplant

After HSCT:
- Basic vaccinations needed after HSCT are summarized in Table 12.1. Additional vaccinations include COVID-19 vaccination and recombinant zoster vaccines

Travelers
- In Dubai, respiratory diseases are the fourth-leading cause of death among the elderly, with a significant portion (80%) attributed to pneumonia-related deaths in individuals aged 60 and above [11].
- Travelers, particularly the elderly, are advised to follow the vaccination recommendations provided by the Centers for Disease Control (CDC) based on their age.
- The Dubai Health Authority (DHA) recommends vaccination based on the specific destination, which can be found in the CDC's Travel Destination, which is available at the following link: CDC Travel Destinations List

IV. *HIV population*
- HIV-infected patients should receive vaccinations according to the CDC's annual schedule based on their age, including hepatitis A and quadrivalent human papillomavirus (HPV4) vaccines.
- Additional considerations for HIV-infected patients include:
  - Meningococcal conjugate vaccination for HIV-infected children aged 11–18 years.
  - Hepatitis B (HepB) vaccine series, for HIV-infected patients, with a potential high-dose HepB vaccine (40 μg/dose) for adults and adolescents.
  - HIV-infected patients should not receive live-attenuated influenza vaccines

- MMR vaccine should be administered to HIV-infected patients with a CD4 T-cell lymphocyte count of 200/mm^3 or higher.
- Varicella vaccine can be given to clinically stable, non-immune HIV-infected children with CD4 T-lymphocyte counts greater than 15%, and to adults with CD4 cell counts >200 cells/mm^3.

V. *Solid organ transplant population*
- Vaccination should be avoided in solid organ transplant (SOT) recipients during intensified immunosuppression, particularly within the first 2 months after transplant, due to the potential for an inadequate immune response.
- A standard inactivated vaccine series, appropriate for the recipient's age, should be administered 2–6 months after the transplant. The specific timing depends on the level of immunosuppression and includes recommendations for pneumonia, hepatitis B, and annual influenza vaccination.
- Live-attenuated vaccines, such as MMR and varicella (chickenpox), are generally avoided after transplant, especially during the first year and when the patient is under high-level immunosuppression. Pre-transplant vaccination can be given to non-immune individuals and should be administered at least 4 weeks before transplantation.
- Recombinant Zoster vaccine (RZV) should preferably be administered at least 2 weeks before initiating immunosuppression (2 doses, 1-2 months apart).

VI. *Pregnancy*.
- Tdap: Pregnant women should receive one dose of Tdap during each pregnancy, ideally between gestational weeks 27 and 36, regardless of previous Tdap vaccination history. New recommendations regarding Respiratory Syncytial Virus vaccination during pregnancy have emerged. RSVpreF is recommended between 32 and 36 weeks of gestation to optimize the transfer of protective antibodies to the infant.
- Inactivated influenza vaccine (IIV) is recommended for pregnant women.
- MMR: Pregnant women without evidence of rubella immunity should receive one dose of MMR after completing the pregnancy. Non-pregnant women of childbearing age without evidence of rubella immunity should also receive one dose of MMR.

12.4 COVID-19 Vaccination

The UAE has implemented a proactive and comprehensive approach to combat COVID-19, including a strong focus on vaccination. The country has been at the forefront globally in terms of the number of COVID-19 tests conducted and vaccination coverage relative to its population [8].

In September 2020, the Ministry of Health and Prevention authorized the emergency use of COVID-19 vaccines, prioritizing frontline healthcare workers who were at higher risk of infection. The Pfizer and Sinopharm vaccines received emergency registration from the Ministry of Health and Prevention in December 2020.

These vaccines were made available free of charge to adult residents and citizens of the UAE.

In May 2021, the Ministry of Health and Prevention approved the emergency use of the Pfizer vaccine for children aged 12–15, expanding the eligible population for vaccination.

Further progress was made in November 2021, when the Ministry of Health and Prevention approved the emergency use of the Pfizer vaccine for children aged 5 and 11, providing vaccination options for a younger age group [12].

12.4.1 ALHOSN UAE Application

ALHOSN UAE is a modern, multilingual national digital application launched by the UAE government since the COVID-19 outbreak. It provides information about COVID-19 testing, vaccination certificates, and exemptions and has gained high levels of confidence, credibility, and reliability inside and outside the country.

This application was awarded the US-based Global Excellence Award (GEA) as "App of the Year 2021" in the COVID-19 Response category, reflecting the advanced level of the UAE's health system in curbing the spread of the pandemic [13].

12.4.2 COVID-19 Vaccination Research

The UAE government has been a strong supporter of COVID-19 research and has actively participated in various initiatives to combat the pandemic.

The Mohammed bin Rashid Medical Research Institute, established as part of Al Jalila Foundation, serves as the UAE's first independent biomedical research center. Inaugurated in August 2020, its primary focus is conducting research to address the COVID-19 pandemic and other viral diseases [14].

The UAE has also been actively involved in COVID-19 vaccine clinical trials, including Sinopharm's Phase III clinical trial and Russia's Sputnik V Phase III clinical trial since July 2020.

Currently, numerous COVID-19 vaccine trials are ongoing, exploring different vaccination options for primary and booster immunizations.

As part of the Department of Health's ongoing efforts to provide the best services during the COVID-19 pandemic, especially for the most vulnerable population, Evusheld (a combination of two monoclonal antibodies) was approved in January 2022 for use as pre-exposure prophylaxis in patients with weakened immune systems due to immunosuppressive health conditions or treatments. This approval was based on the Food and Drug Administration's (FDA) emergency use authorization of this drug for patients with moderate-to-severe immunosuppressive conditions [15].

To gather critical real-world data on the safety and effectiveness of AstraZeneca's long-acting antibody combination, Evusheld, in protecting immunocompromised patients from symptomatic COVID-19, the Emirate of Abu Dhabi launched the

EVOLVE study in August 2022. The study is being conducted across multiple centers in the UAE, including Sheikh Khalifa Medical City and Burjeel Medical City. Its aim is to provide valuable insights into the use of Evusheld among the immunocompromised population in the UAE [16].

12.4.3 Hayat-Vax

In March 2021, the UAE announced that it had begun manufacturing a COVID-19 vaccine called Hayat-Vax. This vaccine is significant as it is the first COVID-19 vaccine produced in the region. The manufacturing of Hayat-Vax is the result of a joint venture between Sinopharm, a pharmaceutical company, and G42, a leading technology company based in Abu Dhabi. The development and production of Hayat-Vax align with the UAE's commitment to joining global efforts in combating the COVID-19 pandemic [17].

12.5 Conclusion

The UAE healthcare authorities update their immunization guidance periodically according to international recommendations. National immunization guidelines mandate vaccination for children from birth until Grade 11. Adult immunization, despite the growing elderly population, remains underutilized in the UAE and may require greater focus in future implementation. Local guidance has been developed to include immunization for high-risk populations, including transplant and cancer patients. COVID-19 vaccination has been of utmost importance for UAE authorities, who have taken remarkable actions not only in providing and mandating immunization but also in supporting COVID-19 vaccination-based research.

Conflicts of Interest The authors have no conflicts of interest to declare.

References

1. Immunization [Internet]. [cited 2022 Nov 26]. Available from: https://www.who.int/news-room/facts-in-pictures/detail/immunization
2. Emirates News Agency – Cabinet approves "National Policy on Vaccinations" [Internet]. [cited 2022 Nov 26]. Available from: https://wam.ae/en/details/1395302868000
3. Children's health – The Official Portal of the UAE Government [Internet]. [cited 2022 Nov 26]. Available from: https://u.ae/en/information-and-services/health-and-fitness/health-of-vulnerable-groups/childrenshealth
4. Ministry of Health and Prevention adopted 4 Updates on the National Immunization Program | News | Media Hub | Ministry of Health and Prevention – UAE [Internet]. [cited 2022 Nov 26]. Available from: https://mohap.gov.ae/en/media-center/news/16/10/2019/ministry-of-health-and-prevention-adopted-4-updates-on-the-national-immunization-program

5. Vaccination schedule for United Arab Emirates [Internet]. [cited 2022 Nov 26]. Available from: https://immunizationdata.who.int/pages/schedule-by-country/are.html?DISEASECODE=&TARGETPOP_GENERAL=
6. CLINICAL GUIDELINES FOR BEST PRACTICE IN IMMUNIZATION Version 2.0 Health Policies and Standards Department Health Regulation Sector (2023) Guidelines for Best Practice in Immunization.
7. Barqawi HJ, Samara KA, Hassan MS, Amawi FB. Adult vaccination in The United Arab Emirates – a physicians' knowledge and knowledge sources study. Front Public Health. 2022;10:678.
8. Al Shdefat S, Al Awar S, Osman N, Khair H, Sallam G, Elbiss H. Health care system view of human papilloma virus (HPV) vaccine acceptability by Emirati Men. Comput Math Methods Med. 2022;2022
9. Ortashi O, Raheel H, Shalal M, Osman N. Awareness and knowledge about human papillomavirus infection and vaccination among women in UAE. Asian Pac J Cancer Prev [Internet]. 2013;14(10):6077–80. Available from: https://pubmed.ncbi.nlm.nih.gov/24289628/
10. Pneumococcal Vaccination: Who and When to Vaccinate | CDC [Internet]. [cited 2023 Jul 5]. Available from: https://www.cdc.gov/vaccines/vpd/pneumo/hcp/who-when-to-vaccinate.html
11. Al Dallal SAM, Farghaly M, Ghorab A, Elaassar M, Haridy H, Awad N, et al. Real-world evaluation of costs of illness for pneumonia in adult patients in Dubai – a claims database study. PLoS One. 2021;16(9):e0256856. https://doi.org/10.1371/journal.pone.0256856.
12. Vaccines against COVID-19 in the UAE – The Official Portal of the UAE Government [Internet]. [cited 2022 Nov 26]. Available from: https://u.ae/en/information-and-services/justice-safety-and-the-law/handling-the-covid-19-outbreak/vaccines-against-covid-19-in-the-uae
13. Al Hosn App awarded Global Excellence Award in Covid-19 Response category | News | Media Hub | Ministry of Health and Prevention - UAE [Internet]. [cited 2022 Nov 26]. Available from: https://mohap.gov.ae/en/media-center/news/1/2/2022/al-hosn-app-awarded-global-excellence-award-in-covid-19-response-category
14. Scientific research on prevention and treatment of COVID-19 – The Official Portal of the UAE Government [Internet]. [cited 2022 Nov 26]. Available from: https://u.ae/en/information-and-services/justice-safety-and-the-law/handling-the-covid-19-outbreak/scientific-research-on-prevention-and-treatment-of-covid-19
15. FACT SHEET FOR HEALTHCARE PROVIDERS: EMERGENCY USE AUTHORIZATION FOR EVUSHELD™ (tixagevimab co-packaged with cilgavimab) HIGHLIGHTS OF EMERGENCY USE AUTHORIZATION (EUA) these highlights of the EUA do not include all the information needed to use EVUSHELD™ under the EUA. See the Full Fact Sheet for healthcare providers for EVUSHELD.
16. Emirates News Agency – Abu Dhabi witnesses launch of real-world evidence study to assess AstraZeneca's Evusheld [Internet]. [cited 2022 Nov 26]. Available from: https://wam.ae/en/details/1395303078665
17. News Details | UAE Coronavirus (COVID-19) Updates [Internet]. [cited 2022 Nov 26]. Available from: https://covid19.ncema.gov.ae/EN/News/Details/1832

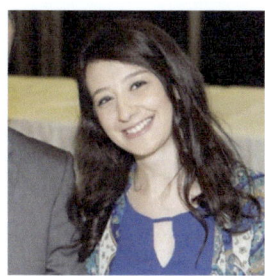

Dr. Dima Ibrahim is a transplant infectious diseases doctor. She completed her internal medicine and infectious diseases specialization at the American University of Beirut. After that, she completed a transplant infectious diseases fellowship at Duke University Medical Center, NC, USA. Currently, she is based in Abu Dhabi and works at Burjeel Medical City. She is the clinical lead of Infectious Disease, chairperson of the infection control committee and medical quality lead. She covers outpatient and inpatient infectious diseases and consults for transplant and non-transplant populations.

Academically, she has been appointed as an assistant professor at Khalifa University, College of Medicine and Health Sciences, in June 2023.

She has been the principal investigator for many COVID-19 vaccination and prophylaxis trials. She is the author of several articles published in indexed journals. Her research interest is mainly the treatment of infections in the transplant population, especially CMV and fungal infections.

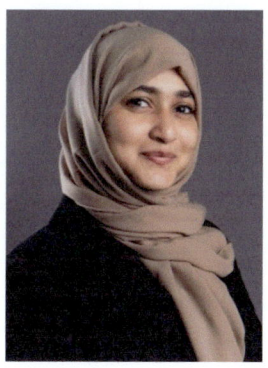

Fathima Firoz is a driven and dedicated pharmacy graduate with a keen interest in research. She completed her pharmacy degree with excellence, showcasing her strong academic foundation and passion for exploring innovative pharmaceutical solutions. Currently, she is actively involved in a research project titled "Thermo-activated in situ rectal gel preparation for ibuprofen using eutectic mixture with menthol," demonstrating her commitment to advancing drug delivery methods.

In addition to her project work, she has contributed to survey-based research focused on the mental health of UAE students. Recognizing the significance of mental well-being, she is dedicated to shedding light on this critical topic and improving support for students in the UAE.

With her combined theoretical knowledge and practical experience, Fathima is poised to make valuable contributions to the fields of pharmacy and research. Her determination, curiosity, and passion for learning set her apart as a promising professional in the pharmaceutical industry.

Open Access This chapter is licensed under the terms of the Creative Commons Attribution 4.0 International License (http://creativecommons.org/licenses/by/4.0/), which permits use, sharing, adaptation, distribution and reproduction in any medium or format, as long as you give appropriate credit to the original author(s) and the source, provide a link to the Creative Commons license and indicate if changes were made.

The images or other third party material in this chapter are included in the chapter's Creative Commons license, unless indicated otherwise in a credit line to the material. If material is not included in the chapter's Creative Commons license and your intended use is not permitted by statutory regulation or exceeds the permitted use, you will need to obtain permission directly from the copyright holder.

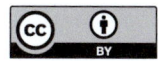

Private Healthcare in the UAE

13

Taha Al Hazarmerdi

13.1 Historical Background

When we look back to the start of the modern healthcare system in the United Arab Emirates (UAE), the first health facility was established in Dubai in 1943 [1].

In 1951, the first phase of Al Maktoum Hospital was built and expanded over succeeding years until a 157-bed hospital was completed [2].

In 1966, Pat and Marian Kennedy started a clinic in Al Ain [3]; this later became officially known as Oasis Hospital, and unofficially as the "Kennedy Hospital" to locals.

Also, in 1966, a small outpatient department opened in Abu Dhabi, which led the then ruler of Abu Dhabi, Sheikh Zayed, to open a new hospital, Central Hospital, in 1968 [4].

13.2 Introduction

The healthcare sector in the UAE has witnessed rapid expansion, positioning itself as a global center for healthcare services. Private healthcare has played a pivotal role in this growth, although it faces various challenges that necessitate attention. This chapter explores the benefits, barriers, and future prospects of private healthcare in the UAE.

Private healthcare in the UAE offers a wide range of medical services and treatments. Private hospitals and clinics are equipped with cutting-edge facilities and advanced medical technologies, enabling them to deliver exceptional care. Moreover, the presence of internationally trained doctors, specialists, and medical

T. Al Hazarmerdi (✉)
American University in the Emirates, Dubai, United Arab Emirates

University of Sharjah, Sharjah, United Arab Emirates
e-mail: Taha1957@hotmail.com

© The Author(s) 2025
H. O. Al-Shamsi (ed.), *Healthcare in the United Arab Emirates*,
https://doi.org/10.1007/978-981-96-0523-1_13

staff enhances the level of expertise and specialization available in private healthcare institutions. Patients have access to diverse treatment options and receive personalized healthcare tailored to their specific needs.

Additionally, private healthcare in the UAE boasts shorter waiting times compared to public healthcare facilities, which often face overcrowding and long waiting lists due to high demand. In contrast, private healthcare facilities efficiently manage patient flow, ensuring individuals receive timely and prompt medical attention. This is particularly critical in emergency cases, where quick access to healthcare services can be a matter of life and death.

Furthermore, the private healthcare sector has significantly contributed to medical tourism in the UAE. People from around the world visit the country in search of top-notch medical care. The UAE has gained a reputation for its world-class healthcare services, advanced technologies, and highly trained medical professionals. The presence of private healthcare institutions has fueled the growth of medical tourism, attracting patients seeking specialized treatments, cosmetic procedures, and advanced surgeries. Medical tourism not only stimulates the economy but also promotes cross-cultural exchange, enhancing the country's reputation as a leading healthcare destination.

Despite its numerous advantages, private healthcare in the UAE faces challenges, including the high cost of healthcare services, which is generally higher compared to public healthcare. This disparity in accessibility and affordability raises concerns about equitable access to quality healthcare services. Efforts should be made to address this issue through the implementation of insurance schemes, price regulation, and subsidies, ensuring that healthcare remains accessible to all segments of the population [4].

The UAE has demonstrated a commitment to improving its healthcare system. Between 2011 and 2015, healthcare spending in the country increased by 10%, reaching US$11 billion [5]. In 2014, His Highness Sheikh Mohammed bin Rashid Al Maktoum launched the UAE National Agenda 2021, aiming to make the UAE one of the world's top countries by its 50th anniversary [6]. The agenda includes specific targets and pathways for enhancing the health of citizens and the performance of the healthcare system. The UAE aspires to rank among the top 20 countries globally according to the International Prosperity Indicator. Notably, the UAE achieved a global ranking of 34th in 2015, an improvement from 37th place in 2014 [7].

In recent decades, the UAE has made progress, but it has also embarked on a health system reform program since the early 2000s to further enhance health and healthcare services, addressing quality and cost challenges. These reform efforts have focused on the introduction of private health insurance, encouraging the growth of the private health sector, and addressing rapid population growth, as well as the increasing prevalence of chronic diseases and risk factors such as obesity, low physical activity levels, and diabetes [8].

13.3 Current Level of Private Healthcare in the UAE

The population composition of the UAE is predominantly comprised of expatriates rather than Emirati nationals. As a result, there is a higher number of private hospitals and healthcare facilities compared to public ones. As of 2021, the UAE had a total of 121 hospitals, with 34 being government-funded and 87 privately funded [9].

Abu Dhabi is home to 14 government hospitals and 25 private hospitals. In Dubai, there are 6 government hospitals and 48 private hospitals. Sharjah has five government hospitals and 10 private hospitals. Ras Al Khaimah has four government hospitals and one private hospital. Ajman has one government hospital and two private hospitals. Fujairah has two government hospitals and one private hospital. Lastly, Umm Al Quwain has two government hospitals and no private hospitals (Table 13.1) [9].

For instance, the healthcare facilities in Dubai have witnessed significant growth in recent years to cater to the needs of both the local population and the medical tourism strategy. The Dubai Health Authority website provides a snapshot. Table 13.2 illustrates the expanding number of healthcare providers in Dubai [9]. Figure 13.1 shows the facility growth in Dubai from 2020 to 2022. Table 13.3 shows the total growth of healthcare professionals in Dubai.

Figure 13.2 shows the number of healthcare professionals in Dubai [9].

Abu Dhabi, the capital city of the UAE, is home to 39 hospitals, of which 14 are government-funded and 25 are privately funded. Among these, 26 hospitals have received accreditation from the Joint Commission International (JCI). The total number of beds available is 4,226, resulting in a ratio of 2.7 beds for every 1500 individuals. These hospitals cater to a population of approximately 2.5 million people [10]. Figure 13.3 shows the JCI-accredited healthcare facilities in the UAE [11].

Dubai, a major city in the UAE, has a larger number of hospitals compared to Abu Dhabi. There are 54 hospitals in Dubai, including 6 government hospitals and 48 private hospitals. Among the private hospitals, 20 have received JCI

Table 13.1 Distribution of hospitals in various Emirates [9]

Emirates	Govt. hospital	Private hospital
Abu Dhabi	14	25
Dubai	6	48
Sharjah	5	10
Ras Al Khaimah	4	1
Ajman	1	2
Fujairah	2	1
Umm Al Quwain	2	0

Table 13.2 Healthcare facility growth in Dubai [9]

Year	Hospitals	DCS	OPDs	Pharmacies	Total
2022	54	58	2100	2007	4219

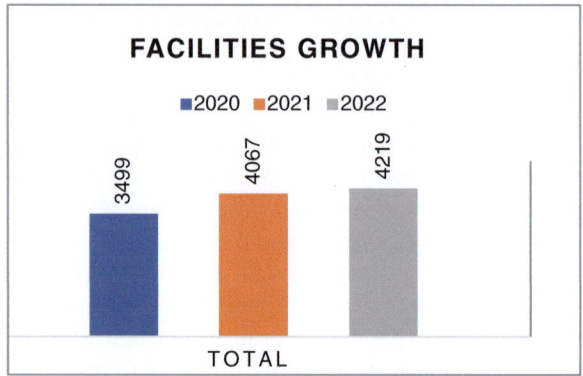

Fig. 13.1 Shows the facility growth in Dubai from 2020 to 2022

Table 13.3 Total growth of healthcare professionals in Dubai

Year	Total healthcare professional
	39,611
2021	47,895
2022	51,764

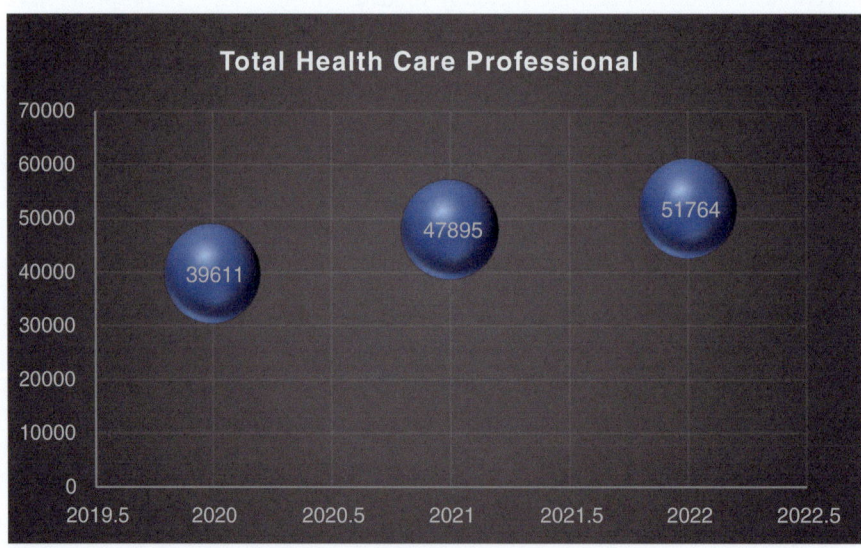

Fig. 13.2 Healthcare professionals in Dubai [9]

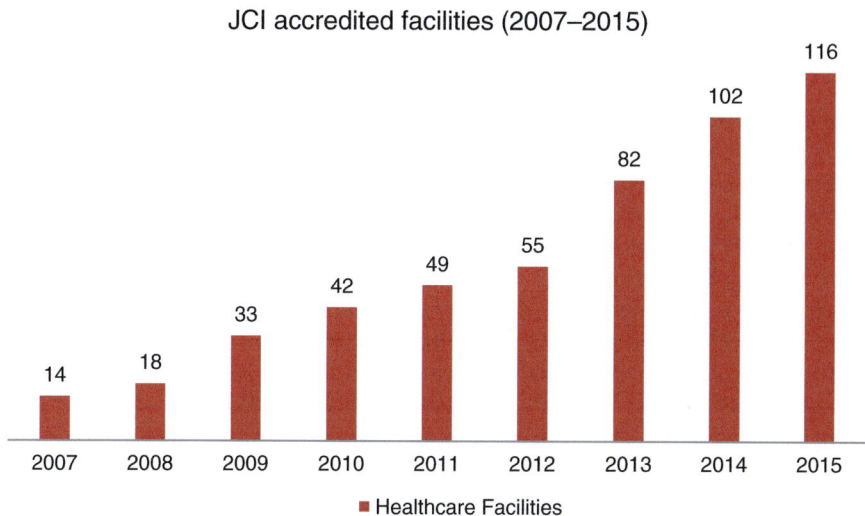

Fig. 13.3 Joint Commission International accredited facilities, UAE, 2007–2015 [11]

accreditation. The total number of beds in Dubai is 3857, resulting in a ratio of 1 bed for every 532 individuals. These hospitals provide healthcare services to a population of approximately 2.1 million people [12].

In *Sharjah*, there are 15 hospitals, with 5 being government-funded and 10 privately funded. Only one hospital in Sharjah has received JCI accreditation. The total number of beds available is 808, resulting in a ratio of 1 bed for every 1670 individuals. These hospitals serve a population of approximately 1.5 million people [13].

Ras Al Khaimah has 5 hospitals, with 4 being government-funded and 1 privately funded. Among these, one hospital has received JCI accreditation. The total number of beds available is 562, resulting in a ratio of 1 bed for every 533 individuals. These hospitals cater to a population of approximately 300,000 people [14].

Ajman has 3 hospitals, including 1 government hospital and 2 private hospitals. One hospital in Ajman has received JCI accreditation. The total number of beds available is 189, resulting in a ratio of 1 bed for every 1,269 individuals. These hospitals provide healthcare services to a population of approximately 240,000 people [14].

In *Fujairah*, there are 3 hospitals, including 2 government hospitals and 1 private hospital. No JCI accreditation is mentioned for these hospitals. The total number of beds available is 358, resulting in a ratio of 1 bed for every 558 individuals. These hospitals serve a population of approximately 200,000 people [14].

Lastly, Umm Al Quwain has one government hospital with 165 beds. The ratio of beds is 1 bed for every 606 individuals. This hospital provides healthcare services to a population of approximately 100,000 people [14].

13.4 Healthcare Infrastructure and Workforce

After conducting a thorough review of numerous articles, it has been observed that over the past decade, there has been a significant increase in the number of hospital beds, physicians, and nurses. These numbers have generally kept pace with population growth, ensuring adequate healthcare provision.

Specifically, the total number of beds in hospitals has more than doubled, indicating a substantial expansion in healthcare infrastructure. Furthermore, there has been a nearly five-fold increase in the number of clinical staff, demonstrating the efforts made to meet the growing demand for healthcare services [15].

Several in-depth case scenarios have thoroughly examined the existing demand and supply dynamics, providing valuable insights and suggestions for future configuration and capacity planning. These studies have utilized data specific to Abu Dhabi [16].

To evaluate the current healthcare system, we need to have new strategies built on more studies to focus on optimising resources and addressing potential challenges. The aim is to ensure that healthcare services are aligned with the evolving demands of the population and that adequate capacity is available to meet future requirements [16].

According to recent studies, there is a justified need to increase hospital beds and manpower numbers [16, 17]. The Health Authority of Abu Dhabi has projected that Abu Dhabi alone would require an additional 4,800 physicians and 13,000 nurses by 2022 to meet the projected demand [16]. It is important to note that this estimation has been revised upward following the impact of the COVID-19 pandemic [17].

The objective is to elevate the level of clinical manpower to the international standard, which entails nearly doubling the number of nurses and increasing the number of physicians by 20% [16]. However, several studies and a report from the regulatory authority in Abu Dhabi have also indicated the possibility of a potential oversupply in certain areas [17, 18].

An additional significant challenge is the low retention rate of clinical staff. A report suggests that approximately 13% of nurses and 15% of physicians left their posts and jobs in the UAE in 2012 alone [19]. To mitigate this impact, the government has implemented various measures, including issuing golden visas to medical and nursing staff, particularly in response to the COVID-19 pandemic. These efforts aim to establish sustainable growth in the healthcare workerforce to meet the increasing demand from the UAE community.

13.5 Current Status of Regulators

The Dubai Health Authority (DHA) and the Department of Health–Abu Dhabi (DoH0 are the respective health authorities responsible for licensing, regulation, and quality assurance in their emirates in the UAE.

In the other five emirates, i.e., Sharjah, Ajman, Um Al Quwain, Fujairah, and Ras Al Khaimah, these functions are carried out by the Federal Ministry of Health and

Prevention (MOHAP), which also performs certain high-level functions for all Emirates [18, 19].

Approximately 70% of outpatient visits in both Dubai and Abu Dhabi are made to private healthcare facilities. In Abu Dhabi, 40% of inpatient activity takes place in private facilities, while in Dubai, the proportion is 60% [14, 15]. The MOHAP acts as both the regulator and the provider of most healthcare services in the remaining five emirates, i.e., Sharjah, Ajman, Umm Al Quwain, Fujairah, and Ras Al Khaimah. As of 2021, the UAE had a total of 34 government hospitals and 87 private hospitals, representing a 25% increase since 2009 [16].

There was a major health system reform program introduced by the government of Abu Dhabi in 2006. The program primarily targeted healthcare financing and the regulatory system [20]. As part of this initiative, the regulatory function was separated and placed under the oversight of the Health Authority Abu Dhabi, while service provision was entrusted to the Abu Dhabi health services company (SEHA). Another key aspect of the new system was the requirement for every individual to have private health insurance. Additionally, a centralized platform was established to automate claims processing with the goal of improving accountability, transparency, and market regulation [19].

A study found significant differences in healthcare utilization rates between UAE nationals and expatriates. On average, UAE nationals utilized outpatient clinical services once per month, while expatriates had usage rates that were three to four times lower [19].

Dubai introduced mandatory health insurance for all residents in 2017. According to a recent assessment of the Dubai health system, a recommendation was made to transition from focusing primarily on curative services to emphasizing preventive healthcare [20]. The review also highlighted the problem of excessive hospital usage and proposed a shift towards outpatient care, home-based services, and day surgery. It is anticipated that the rest of the UAE will adopt a similar approach by implementing mandatory private health insurance, although an exact timeline for its implementation has not been determined [21].

Currently, the Ministry of Health is contemplating the implementation of health insurance, but it has not yet been put into effect. In some emirates, the private sector is not as developed as in Abu Dhabi and Dubai. Furthermore, there are significant variations in the cost and quality of services between these regions and the rest of the country [21].

Several studies have examined the UAE's health system and highlighted challenges such as fragmentation, lack of control by regulators, and competition between health insurance players, which hinder cost efficiency in the market [19, 22]. However, studies evaluating the UAE's regulatory system for healthcare professionals have noted significant progress in implementing best–practice regulations [22].

Research studies examining healthcare service regulation in Abu Dhabi have identified specific difficulties concerning quality enhancement. The existing healthcare model in Abu Dhabi lacks adequate support for self-care, prevention, screening, and integrated diagnostic services within care plans [22]. Furthermore, patients in Abu Dhabi have unrestricted access to services and specialized care, resulting in inappropriate utilization and an oversupply of services [19].

13.6 Population at Risk

The population of the UAE can be described as young and rapidly increasing. The analysis of the UAE population reveals a significant proportion of young individuals and a high concentration of male expatriates [22]. The median age is close to 30, but among UAE nationals, they account for nearly 11% of the population; 79% are under the age of 35 [3, 16]. Expatriates, although typically of working age, also tend to be aged 35 or younger.

The population growth rate in the UAE is remarkable. For instance, in 1950, the population was 70,000, which grew to 180,000 by 1968. Currently, the population stands at 9.16 million [23]. Over the past decade, the population has more than doubled, primarily due to the significant influx of expatriates to meet the demands of the workforce market.

Due to the relatively small proportion of UAE nationals in the overall population, their birth rate has a limited impact on population growth. From 2010 to 2014, the UAE population increased by over one million people. However, during this period, the national population only grew by 126,609 individuals, based on births minus deaths. This means that population growth among UAE nationals accounted for only 11.7% of the total population growth. In contrast, natural growth among expatriates contributed 19% of the total population growth, while the remaining 70% was attributed to net immigration [23].

The expat population in the UAE is predominantly composed of young males, primarily originating from Asian countries. It is estimated that around 2.6 million Indian nationals are residing in the UAE [24]. Over time, there has been a decline in the total fertility rate, representing the average number of children a woman would have in her lifetime, from 4.4 in 1990 to 2.4 in 2010 [24]. Simultaneously, there has been an improvement in average life expectancy, increasing from 72 years to 77 years during the same period [24]. These distinctive characteristics of the UAE population should be taken into account when formulating and implementing health strategies and policies. Key areas of focus should encompass the delivery of child and maternal health services, tailored services for youth, health promotion and preventive measures, as well as occupational health services [18].

In recent years, the UAE has undergone a second health transition, known as an epidemiological transition. The healthcare landscape has witnessed a shift from communicable diseases to noncommunicable, or chronic, diseases such as heart disease, diabetes, and cancer [24].

13.7 Disease Pattern

Extensive research has been conducted on mortality, morbidity, and risk factors in the UAE, focusing on the patterns of both communicable and noncommunicable diseases. The UAE government has set ambitious targets through its Vision 2021 strategy [5]. These targets include reducing cardiovascular-related deaths, decreasing the prevalence of diabetes among adults, reducing obesity rates among children, and increasing healthy life expectancy.

Since 1971, the UAE has made remarkable strides in improving life expectancy and decreasing maternal and infant mortality rates [24]. Nevertheless, the nation continues to grapple with the challenge of addressing the growing prevalence of noncommunicable diseases, such as diabetes, cardiovascular diseases, and cancer [24].

The UAE has made significant advancements in controlling and preventing communicable diseases through measures such as surveillance, mandatory immunization, mandatory reporting to authorities and providers, and effective treatment. The mandatory screening of expat workers as part of the visa application and renewal process has also had a positive impact [24]. The national neonatal screening program implemented has been successful in the early detection, treatment, and follow-up of newborn babies, with coverage increasing from 50% in 1998 to 95% in 2010 [24]. Similar to global trends, noncommunicable diseases are now the leading causes of death in the UAE, particularly among individuals aged 60 years or younger. Road injuries, cardiovascular diseases, and respiratory illnesses are the primary causes of premature death in the country [24].

Numerous articles have identified unhealthy lifestyles and a lack of focus on prevention, chronic disease management, and early interventions as contributing factors to this health burden. Proposed solutions include establishing reliable surveillance and monitoring programs, improving training and education for healthcare professionals, and enhancing treatment options for chronic diseases and their complications [17, 18, 24].

To address the burden of noncommunicable diseases in Abu Dhabi, the Health Authority established the Weqaya program in 2011. The objective of this program is to screen adults for risk factors associated with cardiovascular disease and offer specific follow-up, treatment, and secondary prevention measures [19]. Through the Weqaya program, a significant prevalence of risk factors related to cardiovascular disease has been identified among the adult population. It has also been recommended that a national diabetes screening program be implemented [22]. Studies examining the economic burden of diseases such as asthma and diabetes have found significant costs, but relatively lower per capita costs compared to European or North American benchmarks [14, 24]. The direct medical costs of diabetes care were found to be substantial, particularly in cases with complications [23].

Several studies analyzing the economic costs associated with high-burden diseases have consistently recommended improvements in disease management. These recommendations encompass the implementation of universal screening programs and the prompt adoption of best-practice clinical guidelines. These measures aim to improve patient outcomes while effectively managing costs.

13.8 Impact of Healthcare Costs

Through an analysis of multiple studies on healthcare financing, it is evident that the UAE has witnessed a significant increase in total health expenditure as a percentage of the gross domestic product (GDP) over the past 12 years. According to published WHO data, healthcare spending rose from 2.2% of GDP in 2000 to 3.0% in 2012, reflecting a growth of over 36%. In absolute terms, the UAE's GDP increased from US$101.3 billion in 2000 to US$372.3 billion in 2012, resulting in health spending rising from US$2.3 billion to US$11.2 billion. Recent reports indicate an additional increase to US$13.6 billion in 2014, with a projected estimate of US$25.7 billion by 2024 [24].

In Abu Dhabi, the implementation of mandatory health insurance for both nationals and expatriates has been a key driver of healthcare changes since 2006 [23]. The insurance schemes consist of two categories for expatriates (Basic and Enhanced) and one for UAE nationals (Thiqa). The number of insurance claims has steadily risen, reaching over 22 million claims and US$2.9 billion in costs by 2014 [15]. This increase is seen as appropriate due to the overall expansion of health insurance coverage, transparent payment regulations, and standardized rules that ensure cost control, meet healthcare needs, and provide patients with the freedom to choose their healthcare providers [8, 17]. However, some studies have indicated that the rising number of claims and costs necessitate further changes to ensure long-term financial sustainability [19].

It is estimated that the UAE government allocated almost a quarter of its total healthcare expenditure in 2010 to fund medical treatments abroad for its citizens [17, 22]. For instance, the Dubai Health Authority sponsored 2717 patients for treatment abroad in 2014, reflecting a substantial increase over the decade [11, 24]. Similarly, the Health Authority Abu Dhabi sponsored over 1400 patients in 2013 [11, 25] (Table 13.4).

The UAE has been actively working to attract medical tourists to its highly specialized hospitals and healthcare facilities. For instance, in 2012, Dubai alone welcomed over 500,000 medical tourists, and this number was projected to grow annually by 10–15% [24]. Compared to other countries in the region and worldwide, the level of out-of-pocket (OOP) healthcare expenses in the UAE is relatively low, with an average of 20%, and levels ranging from 4% to 15%, indicating a reasonable degree of financial protection [14]. However, several studies have noted the low rates of generic prescribing (ranging from 4% to 15%) and the high utilization of branded pharmaceuticals, which inevitably leads to increased costs [19, 22].

Table 13.4 Funding of international patient care by Dubai Health Authority (2004–2014) [11, 26]

No.	Year	No. of UAE patients who received medical treatment outside UAE	Average cost per patient (US $)	Total (US $)
1	2004	808	40,436.00	32,672,262.00
2	2005	679	54,768.00	37,187,738.00
3	2006	863	57,221.00	49,381,471.00
4	2007	946	51,499.00	48,717,711.00
5	2008	850	75,204.00	63,923,706.00
6	2009	1073	59,128.00	63,444414.00
7	2010	975	68,392.00	66,682,561.00
8	2011	1428	57,766.00	82,489,373.00
9	2012	1819	50,681.00	92,189,101.00
10	2013	2010	46,921.00	94,311,172.00
11	2014	2717	44,142.00	119,932,970.00

13.9 The Impact of Changes in the Healthcare System on Quality

JCI accreditation has experienced significant growth in the UAE, with an increasing number of healthcare providers seeking and obtaining accreditation. Currently, it is estimated that 47% of healthcare facilities in the UAE hold JCI accreditation, highlighting its growing importance [24]. The UAE government aimed to achieve 100% accreditation by 2021, emphasizing its commitment to upholding quality standards [5].

In a study conducted in Dubai, researchers assessed the quality of care for diabetic patients and identified variations compared to the benchmark set in the United States. The study recommended the implementation of a nationwide benchmarking program to enhance the quality of care [14, 22]. Another study examined the impact of JCI accreditation on a private hospital and found that, while the hospital maintained its performance following accreditation, there was no significant overall improvement [14, 22].

Furthermore, when evaluating patient satisfaction, the UAE consistently demonstrates high levels compared to other countries, as indicated by various studies [8, 25]. This suggests a positive patient experience and a high level of satisfaction with healthcare services in the UAE.

13.10 Conclusion

The UAE has demonstrated a strong commitment to building a world-class healthcare system through major reforms implemented over the past two decades. The objectives of these reforms include the following:

1. Ensuring high patient satisfaction through comprehensive transformations in the healthcare system, with an increased role for the private sector.
2. Implementing mandatory requirements for quality improvement across all facilities through the gradual implementation of legislation related to facility standards, qualifications of healthcare workers, malpractice insurance, and licensing standards.
3. Acknowledging that the healthcare system in the UAE comprises many systems, the major ones being under the supervision of the health authorities of the Northern Emirates, i.e., Dubai and Abu Dhabi, along with the Ministry of Health and Prevention (MOHAP).
4. Expanding these systems in line with population growth and increased national income, with significant changes aimed at improving public health and quality of care while maintaining sustainable costs, thereby achieving a world-class health service.
5. The implementation of mandatory private health insurance for all citizens and expatriates has been a key element of these revolutionary changes.
6. The growth of the private sector in healthcare services and the separation of planning and regulatory roles from provider functions have attracted substantial investments in the healthcare industry, prompting significant reforms in the United Arab Emirates' healthcare system.
7. The implementation of these changes has varied across emirates, with Abu Dhabi and Dubai taking significant steps towards the privatization of healthcare facilities, while other emirates are still in the development phase or just beginning.
8. This uneven implementation has resulted in variable outcomes in terms of access, affordability, and quality of healthcare services across the different emirates.
9. The UAE has a rapidly growing population with unique age and sex distributions, including a high proportion of young people and expatriates of working age. The planning and implementation of healthcare services should take these unique characteristics into account.
10. Child and maternal health services are well developed and continue to experience increasing demands.
11. The UAE has made significant progress in managing preventable diseases, as evidenced by impressive reductions in health loss from infections, including the successful response to the COVID-19 pandemic.
12. The burden of noncommunicable diseases, particularly cardiovascular diseases, diabetes, and road injuries, is increasing in the UAE. The country has demonstrated a high level of commitment to managing these diseases based on international best practices.
13. Total healthcare expenditure has increased in absolute terms and as a percentage of national income, driven by population growth, aging, advances in technology, price inflation, and the need to meet new healthcare demands.
14. The private sector faces challenges such as overuse, waste, and fraud, raising concerns about the sustainability of increased activity and costs. Stricter legis-

lation and increased awareness among healthcare workers and communities are necessary.
15. Measures are being taken to reduce high staff turnover, especially among nurses and physicians, through initiatives like the Golden Visa, which provides long-term plans for settlement and career growth.
16. Disease management programs, such as the Abu Dhabi Weqaya program, aim to identify and manage individual cardiovascular disease risk factors, but further actions are needed to evaluate outcomes, assess effectiveness, and make recommendations for extending such programs to the entire adult population.
17. There is a significant need for increased involvement of the private sector in preventive medicine programs for communicable diseases, cancer screening, and chronic illness prevention.
18. Regulators play a crucial role in streamlining relations with payers to ensure cost-effective services and promote pay-for-quality schemes.

Through these extensive efforts and ongoing improvements, the UAE aims to establish a comprehensive, efficient, and high-quality healthcare system that effectively meets the diverse needs of its population.

Conflicts of Interest The authors have no conflicts of interest to declare.

References

1. "Archived copy". Archived from the original on 2015-12-22. Retrieved 2015-12-22.
2. "Our History – Dubai Health Authority" Archived 2013-03-24 at the Way back Machine.
3. "Oasis Hospital History" Archived 2014-02-09 at the Way back Machine.
4. Beshyah, Salem, Anas. "Central Hospital of Abu Dhabi: forty years of service to the community (1968–2008)"; Kazi, Nazir Mohammad, "Early days of Health Service in Abu Dhabi, United Arab Emirates: a personal perspective". Ibnosina J Med Biomed Sci. 2013;5(2):99–13. [1]
5. United Arab Emirates country profile. Library of Congress Federal Research Division (July 2007). This article incorporates text from this source, which is in the public domain.
6. DHA web site. private health care in Dubai.
7. "OxHA Summit '10—Video". 3FOUR50. Archived from the original on 26 February 2012. Retrieved 4 September 2013.
8. Seha, Abu Dhabi Health services Co. (12 October 2008), Electronic Patient Care Reporting System Issue date (PDF). Retrieved January 23, 2009.
9. Malzahn M. Mapping the United Arab Emirates. In: Lévy C, Westphal B, editors.
10. Géocritique: Etat Des lieux/Geocriticism: a survey. Limoges: Pulim PressUniversitaires de Limoges; 2014. p. 259–265.
11. Koornneef E, Robben P, Blair I. Progress and outcomes of health systems reform in the United Arab Emirates: a systematic review. BMC Health Serv Res. 2017;17:672. https://doi.org/10.1186/s12913-017-2597-1.
12. Bell J. Modern UAE health care: from a mud hut to skyscraper hospitals.
13. National UAE [Internet] 2013 [cited 2016 Aug 11]. Available from: http://www.thenational.ae/news/uae-news/health/modern-uae-health-care-from-a-mud-hutto
14. World Health Organization. World health statistics 2015. Geneva: World Health Organization; 2015. [cited 2016 Aug 11]. Available at: http://apps.who.int/iris/

15. Mahate A, Hamidi S. Frontier efficiency of hospitals in United Arab Emirates: an application of data envelopment analysis. J Hosp Admit. 2015;5(1):7–17.
16. Vision 2021 [internet]. Dubai: UAE Prime Minister's Office; 2014. National Agenda [cited 2016 Aug 11]. Available at: https://www.vision2021.ae/en/
17. BBC News [Internet]. United Kingdom: BBC; 2016. UAE creates ministers for happiness and tolerance; 2016 Feb 09 [cited 2016 Aug 11].
18. The Legatum Institute. The Legatum prosperity index 2015 [internet]. United Kingdom: Legatum Institute; 2015 [cited 2016 Aug 11].
19. Koornneef EJ, Robben PBM, Al Seiari MB, et al. Health system reform in the emirate of Abu Dhabi. Health Policy. 2012;108(2–3):115–21. https://doi.org/10.1016/j.healthpol.2012.08.026.
20. Okma KGH, Cheng T, Chinitz D, et al. Six countries, six health reform models?
21. Gwatkin DR. The need for equity-oriented health sector reforms. Int J Epidemiol. 2001;30(4):720–3. https://doi.org/10.1093/ije/30.4.720.
22. Moher D, Liberati A, Tetzlaff J, The PRISMA Group, et al. Preferred reporting items for systematic reviews and meta-analyses: the PRISMA statement. PLoS Med. 2009;6(6):e1000097. https://doi.org/10.1371/journal.pmed1000097.
23. Brownie SM, Hunter LH, Aqtash S, et al. Establishing policy foundations and regulatory systems to enhance nursing practice in The United Arab Emirates. Policy Polit Nurse Practice. 2015;16(1–2):38–50. https://doi.org/10.1177/1527154415583396.DHA.
24. Dubai Health Authority. Dubai Annual Health Statistical Report 2015. Dubai: Dubai Health Authority; 2016 [cited 2016 Aug 11]. Available at: https://www.dha.gov.ae/DHAOpenData/Annual%20Statistical%20Books/DHADoc768681140-28-07-2016.pdf
25. Health Authority Abu Dhabi. Health statistics 2014. Abu Dhabi: Health Authority Abu Dhabi; 2015 [cited 2016 Aug 11]. Available at: http://www.haad.ae/HAAD/LinkClick.aspx?fileticket=KeJK5ZsIuns%3d&tabid=1516
26. Dubai Health Authority's Annual Reports [Dubai Health Authority. Health Accounts System of Dubai First update 2013–14. Dubai: Dubai Health Authority, Government of Dubai; 2016 [cited 2016 Aug 11]. Available at: http://www.isahd.ae/content/docs/4th%20Report%20-%20HASD%202013-2014.pdf

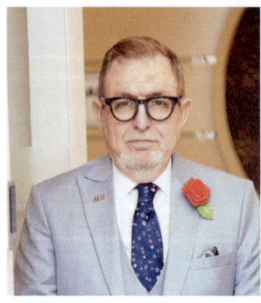

Dr. Taha is a highly accomplished medical professional with over 42 years of experience in the healthcare industry, including 20 years spent in senior executive management positions. He is passionate about quality and has successfully led JCIA accreditation of three hospitals and a medical center with flying colors. He has been recognized for practicing at the top level as a general surgeon, combined with significant management experience in leading large hospital organizations. He is an expert in leading multifunctional teams, utilizing industry-specific knowledge to achieve organizational objectives, with an outstanding track record of providing strategic advice to governmental entities (MOH–UAE), resulting in system transformation in the healthcare industry, especially in emergency and disaster management. Dr. Taha is currently leading the transformation of medical services in remote areas of a major oil company in Abu Dhabi, with state-of-the-art hospitals and eight clinics.

Open Access This chapter is licensed under the terms of the Creative Commons Attribution 4.0 International License (http://creativecommons.org/licenses/by/4.0/), which permits use, sharing, adaptation, distribution and reproduction in any medium or format, as long as you give appropriate credit to the original author(s) and the source, provide a link to the Creative Commons license and indicate if changes were made.

The images or other third party material in this chapter are included in the chapter's Creative Commons license, unless indicated otherwise in a credit line to the material. If material is not included in the chapter's Creative Commons license and your intended use is not permitted by statutory regulation or exceeds the permitted use, you will need to obtain permission directly from the copyright holder.

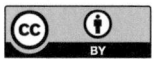

Health Economics in the UAE

14

Husam Al Majali and Maiss Ahmad

14.1 Introduction to Health Economics

Health economics (HE) is one of the leading interdisciplinary sciences that links economic advances with healthcare practices. Its roots date back almost six decades, and since then, it has undergone massive development in terms of research and applications [1]. For decades, health economics has served the health sector worldwide. It has supported governments, healthcare providers, and the health industry by facilitating rational resource allocation and making medical services far more accessible and affordable to people than ever before [2].

Economics is a social science that studies human behavior when challenged by scarcity. Health economics is a branch of economics that applies economic theory, models, and techniques to the analysis of decision-making by health systems (governments, providers, and individuals) concerning health and healthcare. In other words, HE is an applied scientific discipline that enables health systems to conduct a systematic and rigorous evaluation in order to make the right decisions in health

---

H. Al Majali (✉)
Vice President of Emirates Health Economic Society, Dubai, United Arab Emirates

Board Certified Gynecologist-Jordan Medical Council, Amman, Jordan

Master of Health Economy - Barcelona Business School, Barcelona, Spain

Master of Advanced Health Care Practice, University of Western Ontario (UWO), London, ON, Canada
e-mail: halmajal@uwo.ca

M. Ahmad
The British University in Dubai, Dubai, United Arab Emirates

Master of Quality Management, University of Poitiers, Poitiers, France

Bachelor of Pharmacy, Damascus university, Damascus, Syria

© The Author(s) 2025
H. O. Al-Shamsi (ed.), *Healthcare in the United Arab Emirates*,
https://doi.org/10.1007/978-981-96-0523-1_14

policy. For this reason, HE is considered one of the most vital economic disciplines in terms of its impact on policy, professional practice, and people's lives [1, 3].

In the last two to three decades, the increased complexity of healthcare systems and delivery has motivated the growth of a specialized healthcare discipline that tackles specific aspects and domains in health economics. Nowadays, health economics is a thriving sub-specialty of economics. Health economics insights help analyze the healthcare market, find cost-effective ways to eradicate diseases, prioritize medical care, and manage healthcare expenditures [1]. HE has specialized journals, textbooks, research centers, and academic postgraduate programs.

Currently, around two-thirds of health systems worldwide systematically use HE models under the Health Technology Assessment (HTA) umbrella. HTA is a policy process that follows a multidisciplinary evaluation approach to assess health technologies' clinical, ethical, legal, and economic aspects [4].

Real-world data (RWD) is a new and significant HE concept defined as health-linked information generated and reported in real-world medical settings, independent of standard randomized controlled trials [5]. The growing tendency to digitalize our daily activities, health transactions, and environmental interactions has created a new data source that can be used to study healthcare in more real-world settings. The sources include electronic health records (EHRs), administrative insurance electronic claims, disease registries, smartphone apps, prescription data, and observational studies. The most important source of RWD is patient-reported outcomes research, which is generated by collecting patients' inputs regarding the disease or the treatment provided. RWD helps conduct a more real-life analysis of disease burden, intervention outcome, and health system efficiencies.

14.2 Domains of Health Economics

There are two main subdivisions of the health economy in any health system: first, macroeconomics, which focuses on large-scale aspects such as the governance of the health system, sociopolitical aspects, business dynamics of the market, and so on; second, microeconomics, which focuses on the components of the health system such as the behaviors and interactions of health policy stakeholders, operational aspects of healthcare services, and so on [6]. In the same way, macro-allocation of health resources refers to the amount and type of resources allocated for each sector or category of the health system, while micro-allocation refers to the operations and procedures by which these allocated resources are delivered to the population in need of these healthcare services [7]. Health economics knowledge and theories can support findings on a wide range of services and goods, ranging from national health financing plans to the level of economic suitability for changing medication dosing [8].

14.3 Health Economics in the UAE

The United Arab Emirates (UAE) has achieved remarkable advancement in many sectors, and the healthcare system is one of them [10]. The UAE has made noticeable progress toward implementing specific HEs models across the health system, such as external reference pricing for out-patent medications, cost-effectiveness models, and others [11, 12]. Yet, the UAE still has a long way to go in standardizing the application of HE models across its entire health system [13, 14].

The adequate and wise utilization of available resources at the level of the health system or government is a core part of the health economy. In the early days of the UAE's unification, the UAE's health system leaders, budget holders, and public health experts practiced health economics concepts. The health economic principles were valuable for studying and making decisions on the topics at the intersection of medicine and economics: health policy setting and implementation, and the proper allocation of financial resources to meet the rapid and substantial growth of the country's health services [15].

The health economy in the UAE has been developing rapidly in the last two decades. The stakeholders that supported and participated in this growth are found in both the public and private sectors. Nowadays, public health regulators and providers have dedicated departments and high-level specialized health economists who work closely to apply proper economic evaluation for public funding or financing decisions [10]. The private sector has also advanced the practice of health economics and incorporated economic evaluation across the domains of healthcare [16]. The health economy plays an essential role in the planning, execution, and operational management of healthcare investments and private institutions.

14.4 The Outlines of the UAE's Health System

Health governance in the UAE is a symbol of the country's overall political structure, which is federal in certain aspects and central in others. Accordingly, the decision-making process in the UAE's health system has two pathways: top-down in certain elements and bottom-up in others [15, 16]. Figure 14.1 demonstrates the macrostructure of the UAE's health system, which has several regulators and operators.

The healthcare expenditure rate in the UAE is around 4.2% of the gross domestic product (GDP) [18]. The expenditure on healthcare is almost equally divided between the public and private sectors (including out-of-pocket costs). The demand for high-level health services, demographic changes in age, and noncommunicable diseases will consequently escalate the expenditures steeply in all health domains. It is forecasted that health spending will increase further in the next 10 years [19]. The growing investment in the private sector, health insurance, and the government's expanding coverage mandates broader adoption of health economic strategies, better utilization of the current resources, and efficient adoption of complex and rapidly advancing therapies and technologies.

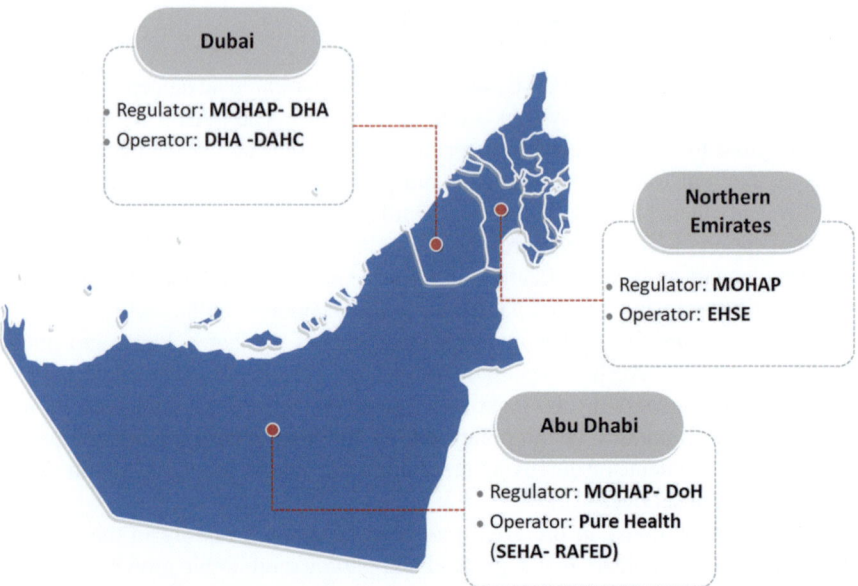

Fig. 14.1 The macrostructure of the UAE's health system. *MOHAP* The Ministry of Health and Prevention, *DoH* Department of Health Abu Dhabi, *Pure Health* The most prominent integrated healthcare network in the UAE, *SEHA* The operational network in the UAE responsible for managing healthcare operations in Abu Dhabi, *RAFED* is a Group Purchasing Organization in Abu Dhabi, *DHA* Dubai Health Authority, *DAHC* Dubai Academic Health Corporation, *EHSE* Emirates Health Services Establishment

Health funds in the UAE are operated by a hybrid public-private system; the public part is governmental and allocated for UAE nationals, who constitute around 12% of the UAE population—noting that some government health spending is also directed toward expatriates with no or limited private health insurance [9]. Additionally, the basic health insurance scheme for low-income workers in Abu Dhabi (AD) is subsidized and supported by the AD government [9]. Health coverage for expatriates is mainly funded by their employers and managed through private insurance companies. The majority (88%) of the population in the UAE are expatriates [17], so private health insurance plays a vital role in the UAE's efforts toward universal health coverage.

14.5 Health Economics in the UAE's Public Sector

Before 2007, the Ministry of Health and Prevention (MOHAP) was the country's primary regulator and service provider. The MOHAP financial executives and hospital leaders were the stakeholders responsible for making decisions across different levels of budget allocations, healthcare financing, purchasing, and procurement. Since 2000, and with the establishment of the Abu Dhabi Department of Health

(DOH) and Dubai Health Authority in 2007, both emirates' local healthcare financing and health economic decisions have been reallocated accordingly. While MOHAP is still the principal regulator in the northern emirates, it is the exclusive authority for pharmaceutical registrations and pricing across the UAE [20].

The public health regulator in the UAE has established and developed dedicated departments to implement and apply health economic and pharmacoeconomic concepts across their different activities, future planning, and resource investments. These departments include the Center for Research and Innovation in DOH and the Health Economics Department in DHA [21]. MOHAP has also supported and employed the pharmacoeconomic aspects of health economics in its drug registration and pricing decisions in the UAE [22].

14.6 Health Economics in the UAE's Private Sector

The introduction of mandatory private health insurance regulation in Abu Dhabi (2005) and Dubai (2011) [20] has boosted interest in and the practice of health economic principles that can serve the efficiency and sustainability of the growing health insurance industry. The booming UAE health insurance industry benefited from the drafting and implementation of up-to-date and robust protocols by the industry's regulators (DOH and DHA). The regulations included the early adoption of efficient electronic claim structures, updated unified disease and procedure coding systems, cost-containment strategies, and utilization review mechanisms [22]. Another significant enhancement in health economics implementation was the enforcement of major healthcare reforms like the mandated Pharmacy Benefits Management (PBM) and Diagnosis-Related Groups (DRGs) in Abu Dhabi and Dubai [23]. The health insurance industry has also introduced significant innovations and health economic interventions focused on cost containment, enhancing efficiency, and optimizing the use of healthcare resources. These interventions are evident in many tactics, such as rigorous utilization review for providers' claims, the application of user charges to mitigate moral hazard, drug management policies, and stringent pre-authorization systems [23]. The embrace of innovative health economic approaches is evident in the implementation of multicriteria decision analysis (MCDA) in healthcare. MCDA is used efficiently by health insurance regulators, as in the DHA, to support health insurance coverage decisions based on multiple objectives [24].

Private biomedical manufacturers, such as the pharmaceutical and medical device industries, are also actively participating in the UAE's health economic development and growth. Multinational and local manufacturers focus on the practice, training, and education of health economics among their employees and partners in the healthcare industry. Partnering with UAE regulators in the value demonstration of biomedical innovation is becoming essential for access decisions and reimbursement in the UAE [25]. An increasing number of health economic studies are conducted in the UAE; these studies utilize the growing availability of

RWD generated through administrative claims data and other locally sourced data [26, 27].

Specialized scientific societies in HE are significant in advancing health economy science in the UAE. Researchers from these reputable organizations have been vital in conducting high-impact studies and training programs that enhance HE adoption and the overall environment in the UAE [9, 14]. The Emirates Health Economic Society (EHES) was established in 2020 as an active member of the Emirates Medical Association. EHES scientific programs and its annual conference bring leading HE local, regional, and international researchers and scientists together to share and present the most up-to-date knowledge and studies in the HE. The workshops and plenary sessions address the regional and local challenges and opportunities for all stakeholders in the healthcare industry [28]. The UAE local chapter of the International Society for Pharmacoeconomics and Outcomes Research (ISPOR) was established in 2011. Its main activities focus on conducting educational activities, participating in international and regional conferences, and representing the UAE in all activities and functions of the global ISPOR [29].

Academic institutions are contributing to knowledge by introducing HE courses into the undergraduate curriculum. A study has found that seven out of eight UAE pharmacy schools offer pharmacoeconomics in their undergraduate programs [30]. Many postgraduate healthcare programs have also included basic and advanced HE components in their curricula. A reputable postgraduate master's program in HE is offered on a part-time basis in one of the higher education schools in the UAE [31].

14.7 The Future of Health Economics in the UAE

There are several opportunities and challenges in the UAE's journey to optimize the application and, consequently, the benefits of HEs models. These factors are either contextually related to the governance and structure, technical in association with HE's science, or social and political in relation to stakeholders' characteristics, interests, and interactions [13, 14, 32].

First, the UAE is an ambitious country. Its leadership has a clear vision for distinction, quality, and sustainability in all sectors, including healthcare and related sectors [32–34]. The UAE's innovative environment is an excellent opportunity for HE experts to work through and promote the use of HEs to improve the efficiency and sustainability of UAE health systems. Second, there is a wide range of health expertise in the UAE, with multinational scientific, professional, and cultural backgrounds and qualifications. This unique feature of the UAE's health system creates a scientifically and professionally conducive environment for integrating HE models and applications into the system [14, 35]. Another significant opportunity is the remarkable evolution of HE research and applications across various health systems worldwide [1, 36, 37]. The global expansion of HE science supports a solid scientific and technical base for expanding the use of HE models in the UAE's health system.

Nonetheless, there may be some hurdles along the way. First, the macrostructure of the health system (multiple regulators and operators) can create complexities for payers and manufacturers when applying different HE models. However, many other similar systems have successfully standardized the use of HE applications. Many other similar systems worldwide have successfully standardized the use of HE applications across their entire systems [1, 38]. Thus, the UAE's health system can draw on their experience with a diligent outlook that respects the unique characteristics of the UAE and serves the UAE's future strategy.

The second challenge is the need for a centralized data warehouse and health records, the partial absence of disease registries, and constrained access to payer databases [39, 40]. Since data is a crucial component for RWD studies, local modeling and adaptation emphasize the importance of addressing this gap to advance HE applications in the UAE.

Other inherent challenges are not specific to the UAE's context. They exist across all global health systems, including unpredictable and irregular demand and conflicting priorities between stakeholders and partners in healthcare provision and reimbursement [8]. The uncertainty in demand can be mitigated by building a resilient and robust health system [41], while the tension between stakeholders can be addressed by creating a collaborative policy dialogue [12].

In conclusion, the vitality of health needs is universal; yet the needs of each healthcare system and population are significantly unique. In a pioneering country with an aspirational future such as the UAE, those needs are distinct, advanced, and dynamic, which highlights the importance and value of applying HE models as one of the components to achieve the national aspiration in the health system. Health economics is one of the essential tools to measure, plan, prioritize, and sustain the delivery of those distinct needs.

14.8 Conclusion

The UAE is witnessing marked advancements in the field of health economics and its application to rapidly growing healthcare expenditures. Health economic evaluation is constantly used for efficient budget allocation and resource utilization in the public sector. The growing private health insurance industry significantly enhances and adopts new health-economic policies and strategies. Public-private partnerships accelerates the country's progress toward strong health-economic science adoption. The specialized scientific societies and academic institutions are supporting the UAE's efforts for capability building and the implementation of evidence-based health economic evaluation. There are great opportunities and potential for further growth of health economic science and practice in the UAE.

Conflicts of Interest The authors have no conflicts of interest to declare.

References

1. Jakovljevic M, Ogura S. Health economics at the crossroads of centuries–from the past to the future. Front Public Health. 2016 Jun;9(4):115.
2. Fuchs VR. The future of health economics. J Health Econ. 2000 Mar 1;19(2):141–57.
3. Torbica A, Tarricone R, Drummond M. Does the approach to economic evaluation in health care depend on culture, values, and institutional context? Eur J Health Econ. 2018 Jul;19:769–74.
4. O'Rourke B, Oortwijn W, Schuller T. Announcing the new definition of health technology assessment. Value Health. 2020 Jun 1;23(6):824–5.
5. Center HS, Schedule HT, Plan S, Roundtable PR, Advancing HE, Framework HC, Kit M. About real-world evidence. Signals. 2022;08
6. Culyer AJ. Encyclopedia of health economics. Newnes; 2014 Feb 21.
7. Igoumenidis M, Kiekkas P, Papastavrou E. The gap between macroeconomic and microeconomic health resources allocation decisions: the case of nurses. Nurs Philos. 2020 Jan;21(1):e12283.
8. Hjelmgren J, Berggren F, Andersson F. Health economic guidelines—similarities, differences and some implications. Value Health. 2001 May 1;4(3):225–50.
9. Hamidi S, Akinci F. Examining the health care payment reforms in Abu Dhabi. Int J Health Plann Manag. 2015 Apr;30(2):E69–82.
10. Verma VS. UAE National Health Workforce Account (NHWA) Report 2019–2020 [Internet]. Mohap.ae. MOHAP UAE; [cited 2023 Feb 7]. Available from: https://mohap.gov.ae/assets/download/d70898b/NHWA%20UAE%20Report%202019-2020.pdf.aspx
11. AlAujan SS, Almazrou SH, Al-Aqeel SA. A systematic review of sources of outcomes and cost data utilized in economic evaluation research conducted in the Gulf Cooperation Council. Risk Manag Healthc Policy. 2021 Jan;20:209–20.
12. Kanavos P, Tzouma V, Fontrier AM, Kamphuis B, Parkin GC, Saleh S. Pharmaceutical pricing and reimbursement in the Middle East and North Africa region. London School of Economics. 2018 Nov. Available online: http://www.Lseacuk/business-and consultancy/consulting/consulting-reports/pharmaceutical-pricing-andreimbursement-in-the-middle east-and-north-africaregion. Accessed on 26 Nov 2020.
13. Kanavos P, Kamphuis BW, Fontrier AM, Parkin GC, Saleh S, Akhras KS. Pricing of in-patent pharmaceuticals in the Middle East and North Africa: Is external reference pricing implemented optimally? Health Policy. 2020 Dec 1;124(12):1297–309.
14. Ahmad M, Akhras KS, Saleh S. Genuine policy learning is fundamental: the journey of The United Arab Emirates toward the establishment of health technology assessment. Int J Technol Assess Health Care. 2023;39(1):e3.
15. Koornneef E, Robben P, Blair I. Progress and outcomes of health systems reform in The United Arab Emirates: a systematic review. BMC Health Serv Res. 2017 Dec;17:1–3.
16. The U.A.E Healthcare Sector Updates [Internet]. US-U.A.E Buisness; [cited 2023 Feb 7]. Available from: https://usuaebusiness.org/wp-content/uploads/2019/01/2019-Healthcare-Report.pdf
17. Al-Khouri AM. The challenge of identity in a changing world: the case of GCC countries. In Conference proceedings, the 21st-century Gulf: the challenge of identity 2010 Jun 30 (vol. 30).
18. Current health expenditure per capita (current US$)—United Arab Emirates. Data. [cited 2023 Feb 11]. https://data.worldbank.org/indicator/SH.XPD.CHEX.PC.CD?locations=AE
19. Khoja T, Rawaf S, Qidwai W, Rawaf D, Nanji K, Hamad A. Health care in Gulf Cooperation Council countries: a review of challenges and opportunities. Cureus. 2017 Aug 21;9(8):e1586.
20. Blair I, Sharif A. Health and health systems performance in the United Arab Emirates. In Papers from the 38th IHF world hospital congress in Oslo 2013 (vol. 49, no. 4, p 412).
21. Department of Health. Research and innovation center [Internet]. Dubai Government Media Office. [cited 2023 Feb 11]. Available from: https://www.doh.gov.ae/en/research/landing-page.

22. Koçkaya G, Wertheimer A, editors. Pharmaceutical market access in developed markets. SEEd; 2018.
23. Al-Majali H. Strategy and models for partnership for pharmaceuticals with health insurance companies-UAE. Innov Arabia 12:43.
24. Farghaly MN, Al Dallal SA, Fasseeh AN, Monsef NA, Suliman EA, Tahoun MA, Abaza S, Kaló Z. Recommendation for a Pilot MCDA tool to support the value-based purchasing of generic medicines in the UAE. Front Pharmacol. 2021 Jun 8;12:680737.
25. Al Dallal S, Pitts PJ. Value over volume: maximizing resources by prioritizing value: the Dubai healthcare experience. J Commer Biotechnol. 2021;26(3):5–4.
26. Al Hammadi A, Pakran J, Farghaly M, Ahmed HM, Cha A, Balkan D, Afifi S, Ramachandrachar BC, Natarajan A, Linga S, Al JK. Healthcare resource utilization and direct cost of patients with atopic dermatitis in Dubai, United Arab Emirates: a retrospective cohort study. dermatol Ther. 2022 Aug;12(8):1859–83.
27. Al Dallal SA, Farghaly M, Ghorab A, Elaassar M, Haridy H, Awad N, Chickballapur Ramachandrachar B, Natarajan A. Real-world evaluation of costs of illness for pneumonia in adult patients in Dubai—A claims database study. PLoS One. 2021 Sep 1;16(9):e0256856.
28. Emirates News Agency. EHES highlights scientific, economic innovations in Regional Health Ecosystem. Wam. 2022, February 14. Retrieved February 11, 2023, from https://www.wam.ae/en/details/1395302997505
29. ISPOR UAE Chapter Annual Report 2013. ISPOR regional chapters. Retrieved February 15, 2023. From https://www.ispor.org/docs/default-source/regional-chapters/united-arab-emirates/annual-report-2013.pdf?sfvrsn=f79f287f_0
30. Farid S, Baines D. Pharmacoeconomics education in the middle east and North Africa Region: a web-based research project. Value Health Reg Issues. 2021 Sep 1;25:182–8.
31. Master in Health Economics. Sorbonne Abu Dhabi. 2023, February 13. Retrieved February 15, 2023, from https://www.sorbonne.ae/study/postgraduate-study/master-in-health-economics/
32. Bulatovic I, Iankova K. Barriers to medical tourism development in The United Arab Emirates (UAE). Int J Environ Res Public Health. 2021 Feb;18(3):1365.
33. Al-Utaibi G, Albloush A, Taha S, Nassoura A, Albasheer O, Masoud N, Mohamed MA. Predicting future health demands in United Arab Emirates. Int J Psychosoc Rehabil. 2020;24(5):3385–90.
34. Al Badi FK, Alhosani KA, Jabeen F, Stachowicz-Stanusch A, Shehzad N, Amann W. Challenges of AI adoption in the UAE healthcare. Vision. 2022 Jun;26(2):193–207.
35. Paulo MS, Loney T, Lapão LV. How do we strengthen the health workforce in a rapidly developing high-income country? A case study of Abu Dhabi's health system in The United Arab Emirates. Hum Resour Health. 2019 Dec;17:1–8.
36. Zrubka Z, Rashdan O, Gulácsi L. Health economic publications from the Middle East and North Africa Region: a scoping review of the volume and methods of research. Glob J Qual Saf Healthcare. 2020 May;3(2):44–54.
37. O'Rourke B, Oortwijn W, Schuller T. The new definition of health technology assessment: A milestone in international collaboration. Int J Technol Assess Health Care. 2020 Jun;36(3):187–90.
38. Teerawattananon Y, Painter C, Dabak S, Ottersen T, Gopinathan U, Chola L, Chalkidou K, Culyer AJ. Avoiding health technology assessment: a global survey of reasons for not using health technology assessment in decision making. Cost Eff Res Alloc. 2021 Dec;19(1).1–8.
39. Kapar H, Mukadam M, Mohamed O. Health technology assessment in MEA, pharmaceutical perspective. Dubai; 2018.
40. Fasseeh A, Karam R, Jameleddine M, George M, Kristensen FB, Al-Rabayah AA, Alsaggabi AH, El Rabbat M, Alowayesh MS, Chamova J, Ismail A. Implementation of health technology assessment in the Middle East and North Africa: comparison between the current and preferred status. Front Pharmacol. 2020 Feb 21;11:15.
41. Najib D. COVID-19 and the Arab world–between a rock and hard place. Sci Dip. 2021 Jan;10.

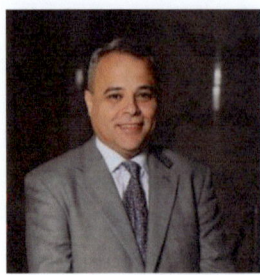

Husam Al Majali is a consultant gynecologist, health economist, and vice president of the Emirates Health Economic Society (EHES) at the Emirates Medical Association (EMA). He graduated from medical school at the University of Jordan in 1990. Later, he completed the Board Certification in Obstetrics-Gynecology consultant from Jordan Medical Council. He has completed two master's degrees, one from the Barcelona School of Management in Health Economics and Pharmacoeconomics and the second in Advanced Healthcare Practices from the University of Western Ontario (UWO) in Canada. In addition to clinical practice, he worked in various healthcare industries across different markets and countries. He is a subject-matter expert (SME) in private health insurance, equitable drug access, affordability, and universal health coverage. He is on the advisory board of leading healthcare conferences and has published papers on topics related to his expertise.

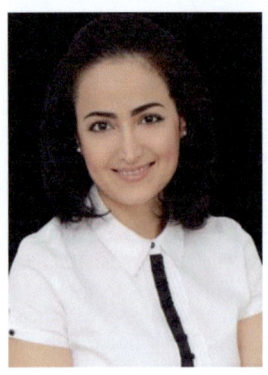

Maiss Ahmad a pharmacist, holds a Ph.D. degree in health policy science–Business Management program from the British University in Dubai (2022). She also holds a diploma in analytical food chemistry and a master's degree in quality, safety, and environmental management from the University of Poitiers-France (2011). Maiss has 15 years of diversified professional experience in the health industry; this experience has accumulated from 9 years of national and regional experience at GSK, taking on different responsibilities in sales, account management, and marketing, and 6 years of leading the regulatory department at one of the principal distributors in the UAE.

Maiss currently works as a researcher at the College of Health Sciences, the University of Sharjah, as she is a part-time lecturer in the healthcare leadership postgraduate program.

Maiss' academic aspiration is to contribute to the policy and management discipline in the healthcare field, namely, in the topics that are of current and future value for our region, community, and people.

Open Access This chapter is licensed under the terms of the Creative Commons Attribution 4.0 International License (http://creativecommons.org/licenses/by/4.0/), which permits use, sharing, adaptation, distribution and reproduction in any medium or format, as long as you give appropriate credit to the original author(s) and the source, provide a link to the Creative Commons license and indicate if changes were made.

The images or other third party material in this chapter are included in the chapter's Creative Commons license, unless indicated otherwise in a credit line to the material. If material is not included in the chapter's Creative Commons license and your intended use is not permitted by statutory regulation or exceeds the permitted use, you will need to obtain permission directly from the copyright holder.

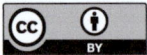

Research Productivity of Health Sciences Institutions in the UAE: 20-Year-Based Bibliometric Analysis

15

Subhashini Ganesan, Humaid O. Al-Shamsi ⓘ, Mohamed Mostafa, and Walid Abbas Zaher

15.1 Introduction

The United Arab Emirates (UAE), comprising seven different Emirates, has undergone rapid economic growth over the past 20 years, with the fast-growing population reaching close to ten million. The population of the UAE has doubled in the past 10 years and has an 85% expat population that belongs to more than 200 different nationalities [1]. This rapid population growth has led to a federal government policy shift toward a diversified, knowledge-based economy. This growth has also resulted in a high demand for educational services. To cater to these needs, an

---

S. Ganesan
IROS (Insights Research Organization & Solutions), Masdar City, Abu Dhabi, United Arab Emirates

IROS, Abu Dhabi, United Arab Emirates

H. O. Al-Shamsi
Burjeel Cancer Institute, Burjeel Medical City, Abu Dhabi, United Arab Emirates

Department of Medical Oncology, Dana-Farber Cancer Institute, Harvard Medical School, Boston, MA, United States

Harvard Medical School, Harvard University, Boston, MA, United States

College of Medicine, Ras Al Khaimah Medical and Health Sciences University, Al Juwais, Al Qusaidat, Ras Al Khaimah, United Arab Emirates

Gulf Medical University, Ajman, United Arab Emirates

Gulf Cancer Society, Alsafa, Kuwait

Emirates Oncology Society, Dubai, United Arab Emirates

College of Medicine, University of Sharjah, Sharjah, United Arab Emirates
e-mail: humaid.al-shamsi@medportal.ca

M. Mostafa
PDC-CRO, Science Park, Dubai, United Arab Emirates
e-mail: mohamed.mostafa@pdc-cro.com

© The Author(s) 2025
H. O. Al-Shamsi (ed.), *Healthcare in the United Arab Emirates*,
https://doi.org/10.1007/978-981-96-0523-1_15

increasing number of educational institutions, including branch campuses of foreign universities, have been established across various Emirates of the UAE.

In order to achieve the transition toward a knowledge-based economy that relies on research and innovation, in 2015 the UAE Ministry of Economy focused on strategies to establish research centers, link education with development, and turn it into a source of research and innovation through universities and research institutes. Hence, the higher education landscape grew in the UAE along with the fast-growing economy. The higher education sector in the UAE comprises three federal government institutions, which include the United Arab Emirates University (UAEU), Zayed University, and the Higher Colleges of Technology; the rest of the providers are nonfederal or private institutes. The UAEU was established in 1976 and enrolls approximately 11,000 students, while Zayed University, which was established in 1998, enrolls approximately 9,000 students. The Higher Colleges of Technology operate 17 campuses in different emirates, enrolling over 23,000 students. The UAE hosts 31 international branch campuses, which is one of the highest concentrations of international branch campuses in the world [2].

The Department of Health (DOH) in the UAE has established a research and innovation center with a vision to be a leading regional center for healthcare and life sciences research aimed at achieving a healthier population [3]. Recently, the UAE government also launched the R&D governance policy in 2021, which resulted in the establishment of the Emirates Research and Development Council. These initiatives were launched to support R&D and expand international partnerships to boost research capacity [4]. The national strategy for innovation was also launched by the UAE government, with the aim of making the UAE one of the most innovative nations in the world, and health research is one of the key sectors under this initiative [5].

Based on such initiatives, research outputs from the UAE have increased over the past few years, and this chapter aims to present a bibliometric analysis of medical research publications, which involves the application of statistical methods to analyze research productivity and evaluate the outcomes and quality of research conducted in the UAE.

15.2 Bibliometric Analysis

A bibliometric analysis was conducted using the Web of Science (WOS) and InCites databases. The WOS is considered a gold-standard source of scientific outputs and analytics on research publications, citations, and indexed journals. The analysis was

W. A. Zaher (✉)
Carexso, Science Park, Dubai, United Arab Emirates

College of Medicine and Health Sciences, Khalifa University,
Abu Dhabi, United Arab Emirates

College of Medicine and Health Sciences, United Arab Emirates University,
Al Ain, United Arab Emirates
e-mail: walid.zaher@carexso.com

based on the following research topics defined by the OECD in InCites: medical and health sciences, including clinical medicine, basic medicine, health sciences, medical biotechnology, and medical engineering. The study focused on WOS core collections of publications by the name of the country as "United Arab Emirates" and the time period from 2000 to the end of 2022. The subject category analysis focused on "medicine and allied health" and highlighted information on bibliometric indicators such as area of research, study designs, and the total number of publications, including indicators broken down by institution and year in medical and allied health sciences.

15.3 Research Outputs

15.3.1 Publications Based on Medical and Health Sciences

The total publications from the WOS core collections based on medical and health sciences, including clinical medicine, basic medicine, health sciences, medical biotechnology, and medical engineering, were 18,936 globally. The year-wise publications of UAE entities show that the number of publications has increased steadily over the years from 2000 to 2022, with exponential growth seen in the last 5 years. About 55% of the 18,936 publications were published in the last 5 years, with 14% published in 2022 alone (Fig. 15.1).

Fig. 15.1 Year-wise publications (2000–2022) by the UAE research entities

Publication Years	Record Count	% of 18,936
2022	2692	14.216
2021	2571	13.577
2020	2040	10.773
2019	1674	8.84
2018	1441	7.61
2017	1136	5.999
2016	986	5.207
2015	902	4.763
2014	718	3.792
2013	624	3.295
2012	600	3.169
2010	522	2.757
2011	491	2.593
2009	451	2.382
2008	408	2.155
2007	281	1.484
2006	271	1.431
2005	236	1.246
2004	211	1.114
2003	189	0.998
2001	176	0.929
2002	173	0.914
2000	143	0.755

15.3.2 Publications from Major Institutions in the UAE

The InCites WOS search classified the following 17 organizations as UAE entities that focused on our research topic of interest. These include Abu Dhabi University, Ajman University, American University in Dubai (AUD), American University of Ras Al Khaimah, American University of Sharjah, Canadian University Dubai, Dubai Hospital, GlaxoSmithKline–United Arab Emirates, Higher Colleges of Technology–United Arab Emirates, Khalifa University of Science & Technology, Mohamed Bin Zayed University of Artificial Intelligence, Sanofi-Aventis–United Arab Emirates, Technology Innovation Institute, United Arab Emirates University, University of Dubai, University of Sharjah, and Zayed University.

The results based on Table 15.1 summarize the total year-wise publications for the time period from 2000 to 2022 from the selected 17 organizations in the UAE. The United Arab Emirates University (UAEU) had the highest number of publications, followed by the University of Sharjah and Khalifa University. The UAEU has a Research and Innovation Center, and one of the key strengths of the UAEU is its research domain, which focuses on the research activities of its faculty and students. This could have paved the way for an increased number of publications from this university.

15.3.3 International Collaborations in Research

The tree map presents publications by entities in the UAE in collaboration with global entities, and UAE research institutes have collaborated with more than 20

Table 15.1 Publication and citation reports of major institutions in the UAE

S. No	Organization	Organization type	WOS total publications	International collaborations (%)	Number of citations
1	United Arab Emirates University	Academic	4540	2981 (65.7)	110,525
2	University of Sharjah	Academic	1987	1682 (84.7)	37,752
3	Khalifa University of Science & Technology	Academic	779	651 (83.6)	6701
4	Dubai Hospital	Health organization	560	402 (71.8)	9886
5	Ajman University	Academic	502	415 (82.7)	3416
6	Zayed University	Academic	418	358 (85.7)	9457
7	American University of Sharjah	Academic	331	195 (58.9)	3696

different countries. The highest number of collaborations was with the United States of America (USA), with 4550 (24%) publications (Fig. 15.2). The number of publications with international collaborations has increased over the years, and in recent years, about 50% of the research output has been in collaboration with international counterparts (Fig. 15.3). This shows that the UAE has turned the focus of international scientifically advanced countries like the USA, England, Germany, and Canada, and more opportunities for such collaborations have been created by the UAE government as part of its efforts to the country at the forefront of scientific advancements.

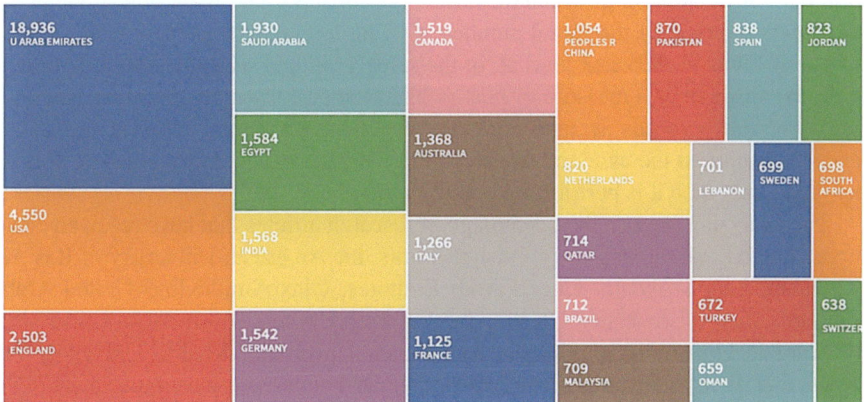

Fig. 15.2 The tree map presents publications by entities in the UAE in collaboration with global entities

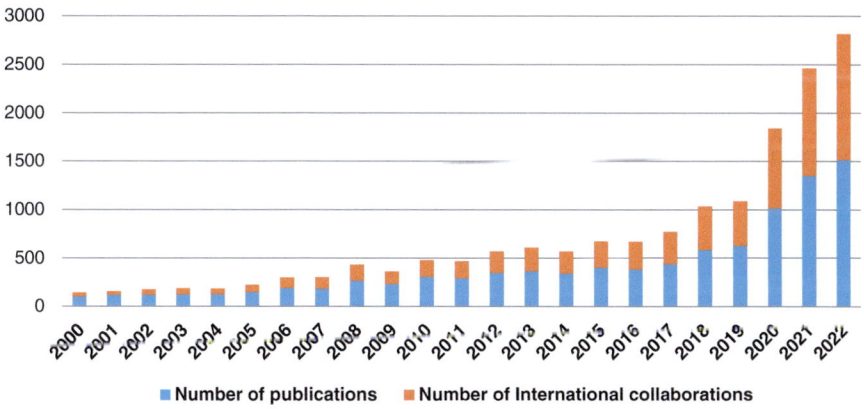

Fig. 15.3 Publications and international collaborations in research year-wise from 2000 to 2022

15.3.4 Citation Impact of Publications

Citation impact refers to the number of times a publication or article is cited by subsequent publications. It can serve as a tool to track the evolution of research ideas and to monitor or validate the impact of the published research paper. The impact of a research publication is measured by how many citations the paper has received. While the number of publications says a lot about the volume of research being conducted at an institution, the percentage of research publications that have received citations indicates how much of an impact the research has had on science. The Journal Normalized Citation Impact (JNCI) is an indicator that shows the citation rate for the journal in which the article is published. The JNCI of a single publication is the ratio of the actual number of citing items to the average citation rate of publications in the same journal, in the same year, and with the same document type. It can serve as a measure of post-publication performance, revealing how the research work exceeds average performance. If the numerical value of the JNCI exceeds one, then the assessed research entity is performing above average. If it is less than one, then it is performing below average.

The analysis based on the percentage of research articles that have received citations showed that, among the published works, the American University of Ras Al Khaimah, Sanofi-Aventis–United Arab Emirates, GlaxoSmithKline–United Arab Emirates, Zayed University, United Arab Emirates University, American University of Sharjah, University of Sharjah, Abu Dhabi University, Khalifa University of Science & Technology, and Canadian University Dubai each have more than 70% of their publications cited.

Figure 15.4 shows the top institutions that had the highest citation impact based on their published works. The American University of Ras Al Khaimah, United

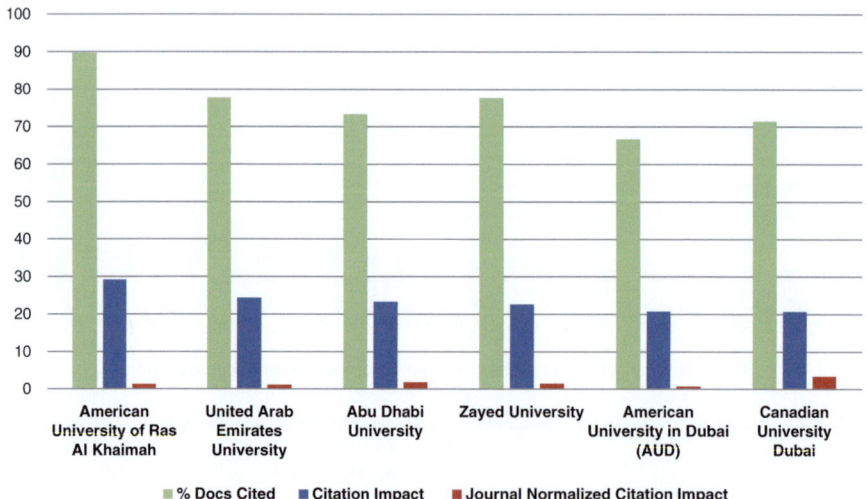

Fig. 15.4 Citation impact of publications

Arab Emirates University, Abu Dhabi University, Zayed University, American University in Dubai (AUD), and Canadian University Dubai have a citation impact of 20 and above. The JNCI was the highest (3.5) for Canadian University Dubai.

15.3.5 Journal-Based Analysis

A journal-based analysis was done among the total 18,936 publications that were published in the last two decades to understand the primary focus of journals and the prioritized areas of research. The top two journals are *Obesity Surgery* and *PLOS ONE*, where 349 (2%) and 250 (1.3%) articles, respectively, of the total 18,936 were published.

Obesity Surgery is the official journal of the International Federation for the Surgery of Obesity and Metabolic Disorders (IFSO) and an official journal of the British Obesity and Metabolic Surgery Society (BOMSS), with an impact factor of 3.3. The journal provides an international, interdisciplinary forum for research regarding surgical and laparoscopic techniques for treating obesity and metabolic disorders [6].

PLOS ONE is a peer-reviewed open-access journal published by the Public Library of Science (PLOS). It is a multidisciplinary journal covering science, engineering, medicine, and the related social sciences and humanities. It has an impact factor (IF) of 3.7 [7].

These two journals are followed by the *International Journal of Environmental Research and Public Health* (IF: 4.6), *Scientific Reports* (IF: 4.6), *Medicine* (IF: 1.5), *Saudi Medical Journal* (IF: 1.4), *Journal of the Neurological Sciences* (IF: 4.5), *Diabetes Research and Clinical Practice* (IF: 8.1), and *Value in Health* (IF: 4.5); in each of these journals, more than 100 articles have been published.

15.3.6 Publications by Areas of Research

The publications were analyzed based on the area of research, and the WOS search identified 3,948 articles that focused on 15 different research areas based on the classification of the InCites system. The major focused research area was cancer, which included 1,188 publications, followed by infection with 722 publications, cardiovascular with 416 publications, and other major research focus areas were toxicity/intoxication, endocrine/metabolic, inflammatory, respiratory, and immune, each with more than 200 publications (Fig. 15.5).

15.3.7 Publications Identified by Study Designs

The analysis identified 1,969 published studies based on study designs. Among them, there were 617 randomized controlled trials (RCTs), 472 epidemiological studies, 458 observational studies, and 422 clinical trials.

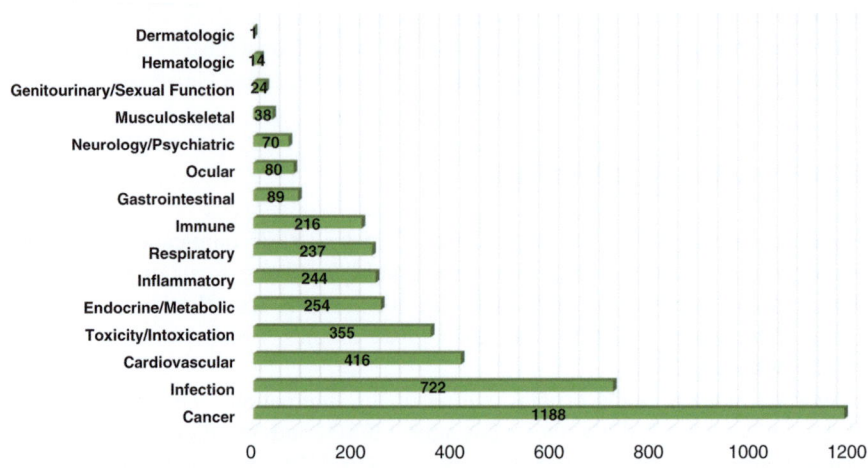

Fig. 15.5 Publications based on subject areas of research

15.4 Discussion

The bibliometric review of the past 20 years of research in medical and health sciences showed that research productivity in the UAE has increased 18-fold over the past two decades. The number of international collaborations in research has also increased over the years, with the highest number of collaborations identified with research-advanced nations like the United States of America (USA) and England. This tremendous growth in medical and health sciences research is a result of the nation's vision to position the UAE at the forefront of health research, and the various initiatives launched to achieve that goal.

15.4.1 Research Departments

The Department of Health (DOH) in Abu Dhabi has launched the Research and Innovation Center, under which there are 73 authorized facilities to carry out research on human subjects and 56 active healthcare research ethics committees working on healthcare research [3].

Similarly, the Medical Research sector under the Dubai Health Authority (DHA) encourages medical research on diagnosing and treating various diseases, and the Dubai Scientific Research Ethics Committee (DSREC) acts as the Central Ethics Committee for the Emirate of Dubai. The committee reviews and provides approval for research planned at DHA-licensed facilities. The Medical Research section further supports researchers by providing free consultations with specialists in preparing a research proposal, research designs, sample sizes, and statistical analysis [8].

15.4.2 Research Initiatives by the UAE Government

15.4.2.1 Research Repository
In mid-2016, the Ministry of Health and Prevention (MOHAP) in Dubai established the first-ever health-related research bank in the UAE. It is a digital repository that has a collection of UAE-based health research articles, and this online resource is freely accessible [9]. Researcher.ae is the first national scientific research-funding platform that provides the UAE's researchers with the funding and support required to collaborate with local and international networks of researchers for their innovative research projects [10].

15.4.2.2 Research Centers and Foundations
Al Jalila Foundation, a global healthcare philanthropic organization, was founded by His Highness Sheikh Mohammed Bin Rashid Al Maktoum, Ruler of Dubai, in April 2013 with a vision to position the UAE at the forefront of medical research and innovation. The foundation supports research that addresses major health challenges particular to the UAE region, like cancer, cardiovascular diseases, diabetes, obesity, and mental health [11].

The Emirate of Abu Dhabi launched the Public Health Center to improve the health of the population in the UAE through scientific research that mainly focuses on diseases of concern among the Emirati population, such as diabetes and obesity, including smoking cessation [12].

The Al Qasimi Foundation provides funding opportunities that support academic research and has grant programs that are open to local and internationally based applicants. It provides doctoral research grants and faculty research grants for a wide range of disciplines and professional fields to undertake research to inform policymaking in the UAE [13].

15.4.3 Research Grants and Awards

15.4.3.1 Sandooq Al Watan Fellowship Program
The Sandooq Al Watan Fellowship program supports students and innovators in implementing small-scale applied scientific research. This program aims to create a cadre of young researchers, and funding is available in three categories: independent projects, undergraduate projects, and graduate projects. This program is open to all UAE nationals [10].

15.4.3.2 SWARD Program
The SWARD program aims to bridge the gap between academia and industry in the UAE to deliver tangible social and economic outcomes for the country. This program supports medium- to large-scale projects across four areas of interest, one of which is healthcare and genomics [10].

15.4.3.3 Grants Program

The grants program serves as a one-stop shop where announcements of various funding opportunities offered to researchers by other entities in the UAE can be found [10].

15.4.3.4 Abu Dhabi Award for Research Excellence (AARE)

The Department of Knowledge and Education in Abu Dhabi launched the Abu Dhabi Award for Research Excellence (AARE), the Abu Dhabi Young Investigator Award (AYIA), and the Visiting International Professorships (ViPs). From 2015 to 2019, over 150 research projects were funded under this program, including those in health and life sciences [14].

15.4.4 Research Facilities and Institutions

The UAE government has established research institutions and facilities to promote research and innovation. Dubai Science Park facilitates research and development for companies working in the field of life sciences. It is the first free zone in the Middle East for meeting the needs of the science sector, providing excellent laboratories and other ancillary services needed for research. Similarly, Abu Dhabi's Masdar City, Mohammed bin Rashid Solar Park, the Arab Institute for Science and Technology in Sharjah, the Technology and Innovation Center in Ras Al Khaimah, and the Centre of Excellence for Applied Research and Training (CERT) were established to promote research aimed at an innovation-driven economy [15, 16].

15.4.5 Research Policy and Programs

The UAE, along with the National Institutes of Health (NIH) in the USA, created the Collaborative Research Initiative (UAE-NIH-CRI). This initiative was created with a vision of capacity building in biomedical research and to foster cooperative research between the UAE and the USA on common priorities in the fields of infections, immunology, and allergic diseases. The Mohammed Bin Rashid University of Medicine and Health Sciences, Khalifa University, and UAE University are partnering universities for this research initiative [17].

The Arab Youth Research Platform and Arab Youth Research Council were launched to support Arab youth's efforts in research. The Arab Youth Research Platform is an online portal that publishes findings of research conducted by Arab youth, assists in managing the platform, and supports scientific research [18].

The UAE government also launched the R&D governance policy in 2021, which resulted in the establishment of the Emirates Research and Development Council. These initiatives were launched to support R&D and expand international R&D partnerships to boost research capacity. Under this initiative, 4 billion dollars have been allotted by the Abu Dhabi government to boost R&D [19].

The Dubai Research and Development Program was launched in 2022 with the aim of developing a comprehensive framework for research across the emirate, and one of its key priorities was health and well-being [20].

15.5 Limitations

The bibliometric analysis using WOS/InCites has some limitations; the software could identify only a few studies based on study design classification, such as randomized controlled trials (RCTs), epidemiological studies, observational studies, or clinical trials, while other publications were not classified based on study designs. Similarly, the major therapy areas or areas of research were identified using an automated keyword-based theme capture technique. Publications that were not related to these themes may include general health, digital health, etc., which were not reviewed in this analysis. These limitations might have caused some differences from the actual number of research findings; however, this does not affect the observations made from the analysis.

15.6 Conclusion

Tremendous growth in medical and health sciences research has been observed over the past two decades in the UAE. Growth in the international sphere is also well reflected in the increased international collaborations with scientifically advanced nations. This is the product of various research initiatives and new research-supportive policies from the UAE government. The UAE has significant potential, and the strategic approach of the government would expedite the attainment of its goal of positioning the UAE at the forefront of scientific research.

Conflicts of Interest The authors have no conflicts of interest to declare.

References

1. UAE Statistical Annual Report. 2020 [cited 2023 15 September]; Available from: https://mohap.gov.ae/assets/download/53ceb061/UAE%20Statistical%20Annual%20Report%202020.pdf.aspx
2. QAA. Quality Assurance Agency for Higher Education. Country Report; United Arab Emirates 2016 [cited 2023 22 September]; Available from: https://www.qaa.ac.uk/docs/qaa/international/country-report-uae-2017.pdf?sfvrsn=25caf781_6
3. Department of Health (DOH). Research and Innovative centre. Research activities [cited 2023 19 September]; Available from: https://www.doh.gov.ae/en/research/Dashboard/Research-Activities
4. The Research and Development Governance Policy. 1 Feb 2023 [cited 2023 22 September]; Available from: https://u.ae/en/about-the-uae/science-and-technology/the-research-and-development-governance-policy#:~:text=Launched%20in%20September%202021%2C%20the,and%20development%20in%20the%20UAE

5. United Arab Emirates. Ministry of Cabinet Affairs. UAE National Innovation Strategy 2015 [cited 2023 22 September]; Available from: https://u.ae/en/about-the-uae/strategies-initiatives-and-awards/strategies-plans-and-visions/strategies-plans-and-visions-untill-2021/national-innovation-strategy#:~:text=The%20strategy%20seeks%20to%20develop,availability%20of%20investments%20and%20incentives
6. Obesity surgery. The Journal of Metabolic Surgery and Allied Care. Springer Nature. [cited 2023 19 September]; Available from: https://www.springer.com/journal/11695
7. PLOS ONE. Journal Information. [cited 2023 19 September]; Available from: https://journals.plos.org/plosone/s/journal-information#loc-journal-impact
8. Dubai Health Authority (DHA). Medical Research. [cited 2023 21 September]; Available from: https://www.dha.gov.ae/en/MedicalEducationandResearch/MedicalResearch
9. United Arab Emirates. Ministry of Health and prevention (MOHAP). Health Research Bank 2016 [cited 2023 21 September]; Available from: https://mohap.gov.ae/en/open-data/health-research-bank
10. The United Arab Emirates' Governmental Portal. Research Platform. [cited 2023 21 September]; Available from: https://u.ae/en/about-the-uae/science-and-technology/scientific-research/researcher-platform
11. Al Jalila Foundation. [cited 2023 25 September]; Available from: https://www.aljalilafoundation.ae/who-we-are/about-us/
12. NYU Abu Dhabi. Public Health Research Centre. [cited 2023 25 September]; Available from: https://nyuad.nyu.edu/en/research/faculty-labs-and-projects/public-health-research-center.html
13. Sheikh Saud Bin Saqr Al Qasimi. Foundation for Policy Research. Grants. [cited 2023 25 September]; Available from: https://www.alqasimifoundation.com/grants
14. Department of Education and Knowledge (ADEK). Research and Development. [cited 2023 25 September]; Available from: https://www.adek.gov.ae/Abu-Dhabi-Research-Awards
15. United Arab Emirates. Information and Services. Research in the field of health. [cited 2023 25 September]; Available from: https://u.ae/en/information-and-services/health-and-fitness/research-in-the-field-of-health
16. United Arab Emirates. Innovation. Key achievements in innovation. [cited 2023 25 September]; Available from: https://u.ae/en/about-the-uae/the-uae-government/government-of-future/innovation-in-the-uae#:~:text=The%20UAE's%20key%20achievements%20in%20innovation%20include%3A&text=Dubai%20Science%20Park,Center%20in%20Ras%20Al%20Khaimah
17. Al Jalila Foundation. Research. UAE-NIH-CRI. [cited 2023 25 September]; Available from: https://www.aljalilafoundation.ae/what-we-do/research/uae-nih-cri/
18. United Arab Emirates. Scientific Research. The UAE's support to youth's efforts in research. [cited 2023 25 September]; Available from: https://u.ae/en/about-the-uae/science-and-technology/scientific-research/the-uaes-support-to-youths-efforts-in-research
19. Invest Emirates. R&D. [cited 2023. 25 September]; Available from: https://www.investemirates.ae/en/r-and-d
20. United Arab Emirates. Strategies and Visions. Dubai Research and Development Programme. [cited 2023 25 September]; Available from: https://u.ae/en/about-the-uae/strategies-initiatives-and-awards/strategies-plans-and-visions/industry-science-and-technology/dubai-research-and-development-programme

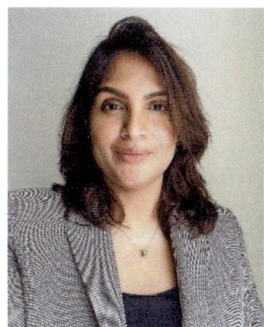

Dr. Subhashini Ganesan is a senior researcher at IROS, a clinical research organization, where she consults on conducts and manages various clinical research studies. She has contributed significantly to research on various aspects of the COVID-19 pandemic and published her findings in well-reputed journals, supporting the company's efforts in fighting the COVID-19 pandemic. Conducts and manages various clinical research studies. Dr. Subhashini has earlier worked as an assistant professor at the PSG Institute of Medical Sciences and Research, India, and was an active member of the Research and Ethics committee. She has more than 25 scientific publications in peer-reviewed journals, including *Nature*. She has worked as a consultant on various community-based research projects in India. She is trained at the World Health Organization (WHO), Geneva, in adolescent and reproductive health research. She graduated with a Bachelor of Medicine and Surgery (MBBS) and Doctor of Medicine (MD) in Public Health from the PSG Institute of Medical Sciences and Research, India. She also holds a PG Diploma in Research and Bioethics.

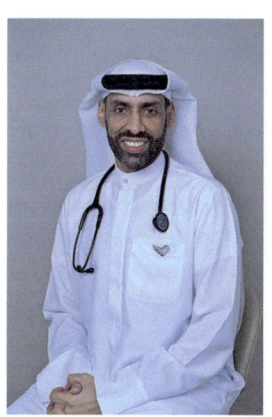

Professor Humaid Obaid Al-Shamsi is the Chief Executive Officer of Burjeel Cancer Institute in Abu Dhabi, UAE; President of the Emirates Oncology Society; Visiting Professor at Harvard Medical School at Harvard University; Visiting Scientist at Dana-Farber Cancer Center, Harvard Medical School, Boston, USA; Full Professor of Oncology at Ras Al Khaimah Medical and Health Sciences University; Ras Al Khaimah, UAE; an Adjunct Professor of Oncology at the College of Medicine, University of Sharjah; and Clinical Professor at Gulf University, Ajman, UAE. He is the first Emirati to be promoted as a professor in oncology in UAE history. He is also the Chairman for Colorectal Cancer in the MENA region, appointed by the prestigious National Comprehensive Cancer Network® in the USA. He is also the only member of the Lung Cancer Policy Network in the MENA region, which aims to advance lung cancer research and screening globally. He is the Chairman of the Oncology and Hematology Fellowship Training Program for the National Institute for Health Specialties in the United Arab Emirates. He is also the only member in the GCC in the WIN Consortium, which comprises organizations representing all stakeholders in personalized cancer medicine globally.

He is board-certified in both internal medicine and oncology from the UK, the USA (ABIM), the National Board of Physicians and Surgeons in the USA, and Canada (FRCPC). He has also been awarded the FRCP (Canada) in 2012, FRCP (London) in 2023, FRCP (Glasgow) in 2024, and FRCP (Edinburgh) in 2025. He is the only physician in the UAE with a subspecialty fellowship certification and training in gastrointestinal oncology and the first Emirati to complete a clinical post-doctoral fellowship in palliative care. He was an Assistant Professor at the University of Texas MD Anderson Cancer Center between 2014 and 2017. He has published more than 170 peer-reviewed articles in *JAMA Oncology*, *Lancet Oncology*, *Journal of Clinical Oncology*, *The Oncologist*, *BMC Cancer*, and many others. His area of expertise includes precision oncology and cancer care in the UAE. In 2016, he published with his group from MD Anderson in the *Journal of Clinical Oncology* a study describing a new distinct subgroup of colorectal cancer, NON-V600 BRAF-mutated colorectal cancer. In 2022, he published the first book about cancer research in the UAE and also the first book about cancer in the Arab world, both of which were launched at Dubai Expo 2020. *Cancer in the Arab World* has been downloaded more than 500,000 times in its first 2 years of publication and is the ultimate source of cancer data in the Arab region. He also published the first comprehensive book, *Cancer Care in the United Arab Emirates*, which is the first book in UAE history to document cancer care in the UAE, with many topics addressed for the first time. The book was also another success with over 100,000 downloads in the first 2 months of publication.

He is passionate about advancing cancer care in the UAE and the GCC and has made significant contributions to cancer awareness and early detection for the public using social media platforms. He engages actively with the public through awareness campaigns and serves on numerous national health committees, including with the UAE Ministry of Health and the Department of Health, Abu Dhabi.

He is considered the most followed oncologist in the world, with over half a million followers across his social media platforms (Instagram, Twitter, LinkedIn, and TikTok). In 2022, he was awarded the prestigious Feigenbaum Leadership Excellence Award from Sheikh Hamdan Smart University for his exceptional leadership and research, and he was also awarded the Sharjah Award for Volunteering. He was also named the Researcher of the Year in the UAE in 2020 and 2021 by the Emirates Oncology Society.

In May 2024, HH Sheikh Mansour bin Zayed Al Nahyan, Vice President of the United Arab Emirates, awarded him first place in the Emirati Talent Competitiveness Council (NAFIS) program for outstanding leadership in the private sector across all business and medical disciplines. In February 2025, he was awarded the *Sheikha Fatima bint Mubarak Family Award* for being a successful role model in UAE society.

Besides his clinical and administrative duties, he is engaged in education and various levels of research training for medical trainees to enhance their clinical and research skills. He established the UAE's first hematology and oncology fellowship training program accredited by the UAE National Institute for Health Specialties at Burjeel Cancer Institute.

Besides his clinical and administrative duties, he is engaged in education and various levels of research training for medical trainees to enhance their clinical and research skills. He established the UAE's first hematology and oncology fellowship training program accredited by the UAE National Institute for Health Specialties at Burjeel Cancer Institute.

His mission is to advance cancer care in the UAE and the MENA region and make cancer care accessible to everyone in need around the globe.

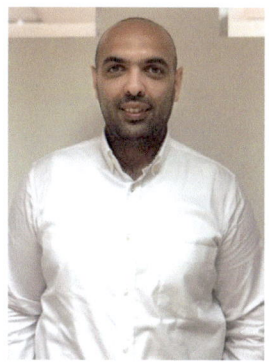

Mohamed Mostafa has been the Chief Executive Officer at PDC CRO since 2020. As such, he is responsible for overall management and strategic initiatives within the organization. Mohamed holds a bachelor's degree in Pharmaceutical Science, with more than 15 years' experience in the Pharma/CRO industry in the MEA region. He has led various scientific initiatives with local and international partners and worked closely with regulatory agencies across the region on guidelines and strategic plans. Mohamed has a solid understanding of the MEA region's Pharma, Biotech, and Healthcare markets and continues to work closely with colleagues to further develop clinical research capabilities within the MEA region.

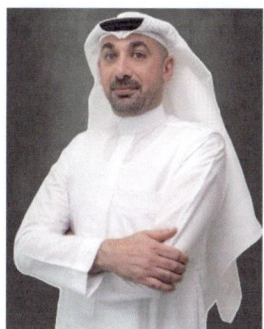

Dr. Walid Abbas Zaher is a highly awarded scientist, medical doctor, and businessman from the Kingdom of Saudi Arabia. He is the current CEO of Carexso, the MENA region's first site management organization for biotech and medical research. He previously founded and served as CEO of the UAE's first contract research organization, as well as Chief Research Officer (CRO) of G42 Healthcare, and, before that, was Corporate Group R&D Director at SEHA in Abu Dhabi. He was instrumental in revamping the clinical and R&D ecosystem in Abu Dhabi, as exemplified by his leadership of 4Humanity, the Middle East's largest clinical trial, the empowerment of COVID-19 vaccine manufacturing, and spearheaded the Emirati Genome Program, one of the most ambitious population genomics and precision medicine programs to date. He also helped achieve over 100x company growth in two years. He has driven innovative health technology platforms, regenerative medicine, and longevity initiatives. Dr. Zaher has authored over 78 publications in peer-reviewed journals and book chapters, including papers in *Nature* and *JAMA*. He holds a degree in medicine from King Saud University with a residency in Obstetrics and Gynecology, followed by two MScs and a PhD in Regenerative Medicine from Odense University Hospital in Denmark, with a visiting research period at Harvard Medical School. He is known for his work in transformative genomics, pioneering health and longevity, and next-generation implementation of research and innovation.

Open Access This chapter is licensed under the terms of the Creative Commons Attribution 4.0 International License (http://creativecommons.org/licenses/by/4.0/), which permits use, sharing, adaptation, distribution and reproduction in any medium or format, as long as you give appropriate credit to the original author(s) and the source, provide a link to the Creative Commons license and indicate if changes were made.

The images or other third party material in this chapter are included in the chapter's Creative Commons license, unless indicated otherwise in a credit line to the material. If material is not included in the chapter's Creative Commons license and your intended use is not permitted by statutory regulation or exceeds the permitted use, you will need to obtain permission directly from the copyright holder.

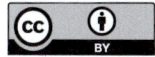

Nursing in the UAE: Reality and Future Directions

16

Wegdan Bani-Issa, Randa Fakhry, Mohamad Alameddine, Amina Al-Marzouqi, Jacqueline Maria Dias, Fatma Refaat Ahmed, Mini Sara Abraham, Muhammad Arsyad Subu, and Janisha Kavumpurath

16.1 The Nursing Profession: What Is Nursing?

"Nurses are a unique kind. They have this insatiable need to care for others, which is both their strength and a fatal flaw." Jean Watson, American nurse theorist and nursing professor. Nursing is an integral part of the healthcare system. It involves the independent and interdisciplinary care of individuals, families, and communities, both sick and well, in all types of settings [1]. Nurses function alongside other members of the healthcare team to help promote health, prevent disease, and care for sick people across all age groups. Nurses' scope of practice includes providing direct patient care as well as health promotion, health education, research, and healthcare decisions [1]. According to the World Health Organization (WHO), the global nursing and midwifery workforce comprises approximately 27 million men and women, accounting for nearly 50% of the overall health workforce [2].

Nursing care has existed in some form for millennia. The nursing profession as it is known today originated in the eighteenth and nineteenth centuries and has changed considerably from hospital-based training to formalized education, specialization, and certification. The development of the nursing profession in each country is influenced by the healthcare needs of the population as well as economic, social, technological, and political factors. This chapter provides insights into the nursing profession in the United Arab Emirates (UAE), starting with the status of nursing and highlighting challenges facing nursing practice, education, and research. We conclude by presenting a collective vision for the future of nursing in the UAE, where nurses fully participate in healthcare reform.

16.2 Nursing Practice in the UAE

The UAE is a vital member of the Gulf Cooperation Council and the Arab world. Today, the UAE represents a strategic hub for global investment and modernization and offers an attractive work environment with rapid development across all sectors [3, 4]. The healthcare sector in the UAE has witnessed rapid transformation since the formation of the federation, from only 7 hospitals in 1971 to more than 200 hospitals [5]. The expansion of the healthcare system required the nursing taskforce to be scaled up to meet the growing healthcare needs of the UAE population. This increasing demand for qualified nurses to provide care has driven leaders and decision-makers to refocus resources on supporting the growth of the profession. However, nursing in the UAE was not well established before the 1970s [6, 7]. The poor image of nursing and the reluctance or unwillingness of Emirati nationals to enter the profession were major barriers to the advancement of the profession at that time [6, 7]. The first Emirati nurse was Salma Salim Al Sharhan (1933–2014), who was known as the "Florence of the UAE." Salma was an inspiration for Emiratis, as she delivered an extraordinary message to nurses about being part of saving lives and serving the country.

"*Nursing is one of the fine arts: I had almost said the finest of fine arts.*" Florence Nightingale, founder of modern nursing. In the 1970s, most nurses received hospital-based training to function as bedside nurses without an academic degree or license to practice [6]. There were few Emirati nurses, with the majority recruited from abroad, including India, the Philippines, Egypt, and Jordan. The first school of nursing in the UAE was established in 1975 in the Emirate of Abu Dhabi. This school, which was funded and administered by the federal government, offered an 18-month assistant nursing program. In 1977, a 3-year diploma nursing program was added, and by 1983, the school had graduated 247 nurses from both programs (15% Emirati nationals) [5]. Two additional nursing schools were established in the UAE to train nurses, one in Dubai under the sponsorship of the Dubai Department of Health and Medical Services and the other run by the UAE Armed Forces. Other nursing institutes followed in Sharjah, Ras Al Khaimah, and Fujairah [4, 6, 7]. After the launch of the Department of Nursing at Emirates Health Services (EHS) and the Emirates Nursing Association (ENA) in 2003, the nursing profession became more robust, and national nurses started providing nursing services across hospitals in different Emirates.

The UAE Nursing and Midwifery Council (NMC) was established by a Cabinet Decree in 2009 to regulate the nursing and midwifery professions and ensure the provision of health services at the highest standards [7]. The Council was formed with representatives from all nursing stakeholders in the UAE, including Emirates Health services (EHS), Ministry of Higher Education and Scientific Research, SEHA (Abu Dhabi Health Services Company), the Dubai Health Authority (DHA), the Ministry of Interior-Medical Services, nursing educational institutions, the ENA, and the private sector.

The Council aimed to regulate the profession and set standards for nursing education, research, and practice. *The* Council further raised the profile of nursing, both in the UAE and abroad, and worked on strengthening ties with international organizations, including the International Council of Nurses (ICN) and the WHO. Core priorities for the Council included developing a unified scope of practice for various nursing and midwifery specializations and setting standards for registration and licensure for these specializations. Importantly, the Council issued a national plan for nursing and midwifery education with standards that applied to all programs offered in the UAE. The Council also promoted the Emiratization of nursing and midwifery by encouraging Emirati men and women to pursue nursing and midwifery as career options and by retaining those already in the field. Finally, the Council attempted to build national capacity in research through the establishment of the UAE Nursing and Midwifery Council Research Center (n.d.; for more information, visit the Council's website at: https://www.who.int/news-room/fact-sheets/detail/nursing-and-midwifery).

16.3   Nursing Education in the UAE

Nursing education in the UAE has evolved rapidly over the past few years. The driving force behind establishing undergraduate nursing education in the UAE was the persistent demand for a larger number of qualified registered nurses to function within complex modern healthcare settings. In addition, there was an urgent need to comply with the requirements of international regulatory bodies (e.g., the ICN) that mandate baccalaureate education as the minimum requirement for entry into nursing practice [6, 8].

Several academic programs were launched around the UAE to provide quality nursing education and prepare graduates to meet the needs of various practice settings. The first university-based baccalaureate program in nursing was established in 1999 at the University of Sharjah (UOS) in affiliation with McMaster University in Canada. The program had two streams: a basic stream for high school graduates and a bridging stream for diploma-prepared nurses. The former stream gained ground in 2002, and the bridging stream attracted diploma-prepared nurses who were required to obtain a bachelor's degree in nursing to retain their jobs, as mandated by the Federal Department of Nursing [4, 9].

Economic and social changes in the UAE, including extensive economic growth, diversified population health needs, an improved image of nursing, and an enhanced digital footprint of nursing in social media, have led to the launch of several baccalaureate programs in nursing to provide formal nursing education. Most programs offered student funding or scholarships from different entities, including the UOS, Sharjah Electricity Water and Gas Authority, DHA, and EHS [7, 10]. To date, there are seven programs that offer Bachelor of Science in Nursing programs in the UAE. These include the UOS, Ras Al Khaimah Medical and Health Sciences University, Gulf Medical University, Fatima College of Health Sciences, Higher Colleges of Technology, the University of Wollongong, and the University of Fujairah. Table 16.1 presents information about nursing programs in the UAE.

All of these nursing programs continue to attract students of all nationalities and genders. For example, in 2017–2018, the UOS had 201 female and 19 male nursing students, which increased to 395 female and 162 male students in 2022. Strategies to attract more UAE nationals to nursing at the UOS have shown promise, with 23% of students from the UAE in 2017–2018 compared to 31% in 2022.

Nursing education in the UAE was further strengthened by stringent local accreditation processes and standards. All baccalaureate nursing programs in the UAE are accredited by the local accreditation body, the Council for Academic Accreditation (CAA), within the Ministry of Education and Higher Education Affairs (previously known as the Ministry of Higher Education and Scientific Research). The CAA established a robust framework and standards to ensure that nursing education in the UAE is accredited and comparable with similar programs in the region and globally. To maintain accreditation, nursing programs are required to incorporate modern teaching strategies that are appropriate for adult learners, such as problem-based learning, team-based learning, flip classes, simulation in teaching and learning, and the incorporation of sufficient clinical practice hours [11].

In response to the demand for uniformity of nursing educational curricula and professional core expectations of baccalaureate nurses, a national consensus-based framework addressing core domains was developed in 2021 by external educational experts and stakeholders, including the Ministry of Education, nursing leaders from higher education institutions, EHS, the Department of Health-Abu Dhabi, SEHA, DHA, and the UAE NMC. This framework is entitled "UAE National Competency and Professional Practice Framework for Undergraduate Nursing Programs." The framework articulates core expectations and captures the most salient elements of the nursing programs offered across all academic institutions in the UAE.

National and international educational experts worked through four phases to develop the framework. These phases involved: reviewing the existing UAE NMC framework; identifying basic domains essential for baccalaureate education; drafting, consulting, and revising degree-level expectations; and formulating all expected core competencies for undergraduate education into an all-inclusive UAE Professional Practice Framework for the Bachelor of Science in Nursing. An important event in this process was the international conference held over 2 days in February 2022, entitled "Quality Measurement in Health Professional Education—Revisiting the Metrics." All educational entities in the UAE were invited to this forum, where competencies were vigorously reviewed to reform nursing curricula

16 Nursing in the UAE: Reality and Future Directions

Table 16.1 Summary of nursing programs in the UAE

Institution	Program	Admissions criteria	Language	Study mode	Total credits	Theory credits	Clinical/Lab credits	Duration of study (years)	Accreditation status
University of Sharjah	Undergraduate	Completion of secondary education or an equivalent level with the required average no earlier than 3 years prior to joining the university. The applicant should not have been expelled from the university or any other institution for academic or disciplinary reasons. The applicant should be medically, physically, and mentally fit to be admitted to the university in accordance with the desired major. Applicants should indicate their order of preference for majors on the application form. Applicants are accepted in different majors according to the student's preference and her/his grade average and depending on the capacity of each college.	English	Full time	137 credits	106 credits	31 credits	4	Accredited
	Postgraduate	The student must hold a bachelor's degree from a recognized university from the MOHE in the UAE with a minimum grade of good and a CGPA of 3 on a 4-point scale. Students with a CGPA of 2.5 to 2.99 may be admitted conditionally provided that they register up to 6–9 credit hours in the first semester of their study and obtain a "B" average. The degree must be in a major that enables the student to study the master's program, and students from majors different from the master's program may be admitted upon the recommendation of the department and the college and the approval of the college council and after studying the prerequisite courses assigned by the department. Attendance for the bachelor's degree must not be less than 75% of the total hours required for graduation. The student must obtain 550 points on the TOEFL test or 6 on the IELTS. A student may be admitted conditionally if he/she obtains 530 points or better on the TOEFL, provided that the student enrolls in an English language course and receives a TOEFL score of 550 at the end of his/her first semester of study. The student will be expelled from the program if these two conditions are not met. The student must submit a letter of approval by his/her employer if he/she is employed.	English	Full time/part time	36 credits	26 credits	10 Credits	2	Initial accreditation

(continued)

Table 16.1 (continued)

Institution	Program	Admissions criteria	Language	Study mode	Total credits	Theory credits	Clinical/Lab credits	Duration of study (years)	Accreditation status
Ras Al Khaimah medical and health sciences university	Undergraduate	An EmSAT score of six hundred for Arabic language. Alternatively, the international students can register for a non-credited basic Arabic language course at the institution. An EmSAT score of seven hundred in mathematics or equivalent, plus scores of seven hundred in two of the three science subjects (chemistry, biology, or physics). (students who studied within UAE are required to submit the score).In the case that EmSAT scores in mathematics and two science subjects are not available, a candidate shall sit an equivalent admission/entrance exam designed by the college which includes chemistry, biology, physics, and mathematics. (this is applicable only for international students who studied outside UAE). Passing a personal interview set by the college.	English	Full time	120 credits	71 credits	29 credits	4	Accredited
	Postgraduate	Bachelor of science in nursing degree with minimum CGPA (cumulative grade point average) of 3.0 on a 4.0 scale or equivalent. Proficiency in English equivalent to a TOEFL score of 550 in paper-based test OR 79 in internet-based test OR academic IELTS score of 6 OR EmSAT achieve-English score of 1400 OR equivalent tests prescribed by the ministry is required. 1 year of clinical experience around specialty for BSN applicants. They are as follows: Either adult or community experience is necessary for the adult specialization. Either adult or community experience is necessary for the community specialization. Either pediatric or community experience with evidence that this has included pediatrics is necessary for the pediatric specialization. Psychiatric mental Health experience is necessary for the psychiatric mental health specialization. Midwifery experience is necessary for the master of science in midwifery or 2-years post-diploma for the RN-BSN-qualified applicants. RN-licensure from country of origin.	English	Full time/part time	43 credits	28 credits	15 credits	2 years	Accredited

		English	Full time	127 credits	97	30	4 years	Accredited
Fatima College of health sciences	Undergraduate	UAE *national* and children of Emirati *mothers*, emirates, a completed NAPO application form. For all applicants, a filled-out college application form. Original or attested high school Certificate from Ministry of Education. If the secondary high school curriculum studied is an international one, then an equivalency must be obtained from the Ministry of Education in UAE and submitted along with the transcript. The high school Certificate should not be more than 3 years old for Emiratis and for the same year for international students. Applicants' maximum age is 24 years old. Copy of the EmSAT English score, or an IELTS overall score or equivalent certificate, as pertinent to program/degree applied for. Medical fitness certificate (to be submitted upon enrolment). For Emiratis, copy of identity card, passport, and family book issued by the United Arab Emirates and his/her father and mother For international students, copy of identity card and valid passport with residence visa for applicant and his/her father and mother (family book is required for National Mother). Copy of birth certificate. Certificate of good conduct (from MOI). (4) personal photos For Emiratis IBAN letter is required from the bank (applicant's account). Applicants to the bridging program for nursing must further have a diploma in nursing and provide the following: A minimum EmSAT English score of 1400 or a minimum IELTS academic overall 6.0 or equivalent. A certificate of experience no less than 2 years. A no objection letter from the workplace.							

(continued)

Table 16.1 (continued)

Institution	Program	Admissions criteria	Language	Study mode	Total credits	Theory credits	Clinical/Lab credits	Duration of study (years)	Accreditation status
Higher colleges of technology	Undergraduate	Minimum GSC overall average of 80% for general stream; minimum of 70% for advanced stream and a minimum of 65% for elite stream, or equivalent. EmSAT-Arabic > = 600 or equivalent. EmSAT-math> = 700 or equivalent. 700 or higher in two of three science subjects (EmSAT-chemistry, EmSAT-biology or EmSAT-physics) or equivalent Minimum EmSAT-English score of 1100 or equivalent. Pass the personal interview. In certain cases, and upon directives from the HCT senior management, applicants who don't meet any of the aforementioned criteria can be considered for admission in certain programs. To enter a bachelor's program at the HCT, students must have achieved an EmSAT English score of at least 1100, or a band of 5.0 in Academic IELTS. Students who have not achieved the equivalent of EmSAT 1100 may be admitted conditionally to certain programs. To be considered for their final admission, they must successfully complete 1–2 prerequisite English communication courses, within one academic year, before enrolling in program courses.	English	Full time	134 credits	106	28	4 years	Accredited

		English	Full time	120 credits	59	61	4 years	Accredited
Gulf Medical University	Undergraduate	The applicant must have completed a minimum of 12 years of school. The applicant must complete 18 years of age on or before the December 31 in the year of admission for student visa purpose. The applicant must have passed any one of the following English language proficiency tests with a minimum score as follows: 1100 in Emirates standardized language test (EmSAT) Five hundred in TOEFL (CBT 173—iBT 61). 5.0 in IELTS for academic Valid English proficiency minimum requirement is mandatory before admission. EmSAT Arabic is mandatory. UAE applicant for the BSN program must score EmSAT Arabic of six hundred minimum and all international students shall register for a non-credit based basic Arabic language course in the institution. Those who have not completed Arabic will be on conditional admission and on successful completion of Arabic course, the admission is regularized. EmSAT Maths and EmSAT biology are mandatory with EmSAT chemistry or EmSAT physics with a minimum score of seven hundred for all UAE nationals and students passing from UAE education system. UAE resident applications with international curriculum are also required to complete EmSAT requirements. All international students are required to pass the EmSAT equivalent admission exam set by the College of Nursing that includes Sect. 16.1 with MCQ'S in the subjects: Mathematics and biology mandatory, chemistry or physics and Sect. 16.2 with multiple mini interviews (MMIs). Applicants from any other non-UAE educational systems not listed above must have secured a minimum aggregate score equivalent to UAE advanced track 70% as per international grade conversion table published by world education system (WES). Applicants from any other non-UAE educational systems must submit an equivalency Certificate of their high school Certificate from Ministry of Education, UAE. Student should complete science subjects (biology, chemistry, in tenth and 11th or 12th grades). Applicants who lack sufficient background in mathematics and science subjects (biology or chemistry or physics) may register for the non-credit remedial course offered by the university. All applicants shall be evaluated for cognitive and non-cognitive traits demonstrating their aptitude for the chosen area of study by the admissions committee. On successful completion of the EmSAT or the admission exam, the applicant shall meet the GMU admissions committee for a personal interview. The decision of the admission committee shall be final and binding.						

(continued)

Table 16.1 (continued)

Institution	Program	Admissions criteria	Language	Study mode	Total credits	Theory credits	Clinical/Lab credits	Duration of study (years)	Accreditation status
Mohamed bin Rashed university	Master of science in cardiovascular nursing	Hold a registered nurse license as certified by the appropriate nursing licensing authority. Have at least 1-year (full time equivalent) post-registration experience specific to the area of specialist practice being undertaken. Hold a bachelor of nursing degree or equivalent with a minimum GPA of 3 for admission. Are permitted and potentially supported by their employer. Available to undertake the course on the date of commencement. Have evidence of meeting the good health and character requirements. Applicants whose first language is not English are required to have a minimum IELTS band of 6 (with minimum 5.5 in each skill) or TOEFL iBT 80 with writing score of 20 or an equivalent qualification acceptable to the university and achieved within the last 2 years.	English	Full time Part time	30 credits	24	6	1 years (full time) 2 years (part time)	Accredited
University of Wilmington Dubai (credit point system)	Bridging/conversion	To be eligible for this degree you need to be a registered nurse who holds a recognized diploma in nursing and also meet the admission requirements based on the type of high school curriculum you have followed. All students applying for these programs are required to have an EmSAT in mathematics with a score of 600 or equivalent.	English	Full time	72 credit points (6 credit points = 3 credit hours	5–6 semesters each 10 weeks (2 years)	0 clinical hours	2 years	Accredited

across all institutions (n.d.; for more information on the forum, visit https://qmhpe-gmuconference.com/).

The UAE Professional Practice Framework for the Bachelor of Science in Nursing (2021) aims to support the UAE National Strategy for Nursing and Midwifery: A Roadmap to 2025 and its fourth strategic pillar, "Quality, Innovation, Education, and Professional Development." The framework embraces the futuristic directions shared by the leaders at multiple levels through the adoption of healthcare technology, nursing informatics specialty inclusion, and capacity building in disaster preparedness, leadership, and research. This competency-based framework aims to produce competent nurse graduates prepared to transition into professional roles as registered nurses or midwives and contribute to the evolution, advancement, and sustainability of the UAE healthcare system. The framework presents a meta-paradigm of the nursing profession through its seven domains. These seven domains are illustrated in Fig. 16.1.

The framework was recently reviewed, endorsed, and published to serve as a standard document for all nursing bodies, which will eventually guide the transformation of nursing education and the nursing profession. It is expected that academic institutions will conduct a thorough curriculum revision to integrate the new competencies and begin implementing this framework.

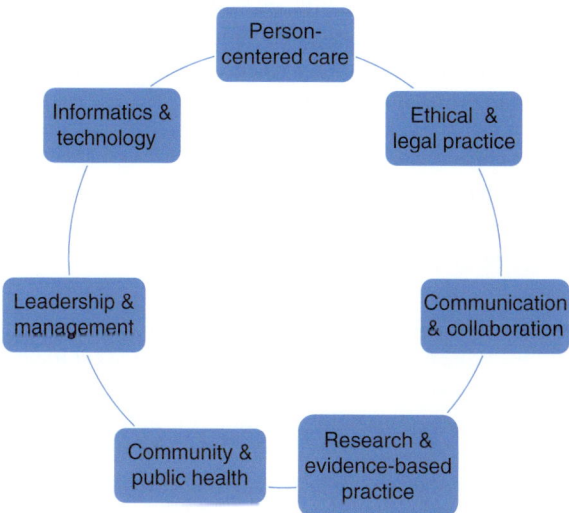

Fig. 16.1 The UAE professional practice framework for the bachelor of science in nursing. (Source: UAE Competency and Professional Practice Framework for Undergraduate Nursing Programs. (2021). Available at: https://www.caa.ae/PORTALGUIDELINES/2022-08-09%20 UAE%20Professional%20Practice%20Framework%20for%20Bachelor%20of%20Sciences%20 in%20Nursing%20(BSN)%20Graduates.pdf)

16.4 Nursing Research in the UAE

Nursing research is a domain that has not evolved or received as much attention as nursing practice or education. Most nursing and healthcare research in the UAE has been conducted by academic researchers, with little involvement from practicing nurses. Research is not a requirement for nurses' professional development or job advancement, and, therefore, most nurses avoid being involved in nursing research. Identified barriers to participation in nursing research include insufficient time to read research articles or implement new research ideas, insufficient preparation to critically appraise research, and competing work demands [12].

Nurse leaders acknowledge that practicing nurses in the UAE have inadequate preparation and skills to conduct scientific research. The UAE NMC established a research center with specific units: fundraising, *research projects, grants programs, capacity building, and research dissemination and research funding* [12]. The overall aim of the Research Center is to define strategic directions for nursing and midwifery research and provide structure and support mechanisms for the continued expansion and advancement of nursing and midwifery research and researchers.

Nursing has grown significantly in the UAE, as evidenced by the above discussion. However, in the context of an increasingly globalized world, healthcare system challenges continue to evolve. These challenges are, to a great extent, similar to those facing nurses worldwide and need to be tackled to allow further growth of the profession as the backbone of the healthcare system. The following section considers the major challenges confronting three overlapping nursing domains (nursing practice, nursing education, and nursing research) in the UAE and suggests future directions to move the profession forward.

16.5 Existing Challenges and Future Directions

16.5.1 Nursing Practice

16.5.1.1 Nursing Shortage

The nursing shortage represents a major challenge that is accentuated by substantial population growth with diverse health needs and a major rise in chronic and emerging communicable diseases. According to the EHS, the UAE had 5.68 nurses for every 1,000 people in 2017, which was lower than the ratio in Western countries [13]. Increasing the number of nurses is an essential component of the UAE's vision to provide world-class healthcare.

The reliance on foreign nurses to fill this gap carries its own challenges, including cultural and linguistic barriers, a high turnover rate, and a delay in replacing nurses in some specialties [14], resulting in reduced contribution to the stability and progression of the profession [14, 15]. The solution to the nursing shortage is to build a more sustainable nursing workforce with reduced reliance on expatriate nurses and improved retention of national nurses in the healthcare system.

Recruitment campaigns were initiated by the EHS Department of Nursing to attract young male and female Emiratis to the profession and boost the public image of nursing [15]. However, more action is needed to enhance the Emiratization of the nursing profession. This requires coordination and collaboration across all sectors to change the public image of nursing. Having nursing role models and stories of successful nurses in the media may motivate young people to join the profession. Nurses are in the best position to promote nursing as competent, ethical, and trusted healthcare professionals [16].

The use of artificial intelligence, machine learning, and greater adoption of electronic health records should also be explored to reduce repetitive nursing tasks contributing to burnout and turnover [17]. The integration of healthcare technology can substantially reduce administrative burdens on nurses and facilitate the assessment process and workflow, resulting in time savings for nurses [17]. The nursing shortage in the UAE must be closely monitored by a responsible federal entity that advises decision-makers across the healthcare and education sectors. Such an entity can examine strategies to attract and retain Emirati nurses by improving their working conditions. The nursing shortage must be taken seriously as it significantly impacts patient outcomes, including increased adverse events, longer hospital stays, and increased mortality and morbidity [18]. Improved patient outcomes can bring significant cost savings to healthcare institutions and the UAE as a whole.

16.5.1.2 Lack of Advanced Nursing Practice and Specialization

To date, nurses in the UAE are still functioning under general nursing roles, with an absence of advanced practice nursing (APN) roles such as nurse practitioners, certified nurse-midwives, certified registered nurse anesthetists, and clinical nurse specialists [19]. Nurses in APN roles must have sufficient competencies, education, and preparation to enable them to make clinical decisions, evaluate clinical cases, diagnose diseases, and prescribe medications without physician oversight [20]. Establishing APN roles relies on academic institutions with agreed-upon competencies and a scope of practice. Recruiting experienced nurse faculty with APN preparation, interprofessional collaboration between healthcare organizations and academic institutions, updating teaching practices, and conducting curriculum revisions are some strategies that academic institutions can adopt to facilitate the preparation of nurses for APN roles [21]. A clear strategy to open APN academic programs that focus on the direct involvement of the UAE is essential for the successful development and implementation of this extended nursing role.

The APN role must be coupled with increased diversity in nursing specialization to meet rising population needs. With the changing profile of the population and the emergence of pandemics, there is an urgent need for specialties in nursing, such as pediatric nurses, home nurses, geriatric nurses, community nurses, public health nurses, and critical care nurses. With the necessary education and training, these specialized nurses can practice autonomously and independently [22, 23]. Nurses should also be encouraged to join local and international committees to advance their specializations and certifications, such as the American Nurses Association and the International Council of Nurses (ICN).

16.5.1.3 Lack of Involvement in Healthcare Decisions

Nurses in the UAE are still underrepresented in healthcare decisions, which puts patient care quality and healthcare reform at risk. This can be attributed to decision-makers' lack of trust and confidence in nurses' abilities to make such decisions. Nurses' involvement in strategic health decisions requires them to have the relevant qualifications and advanced preparation so they can be trusted by policymakers [24]. Advancing nursing practice aligns with the call of the ICN to support the global effort to enhance nurses' readiness to participate in health policy development [25]. Clear career paths must also be in place to encourage and motivate nurses to pursue APN roles and specializations in nursing. Advancing levels of practice and specialization must therefore be a top priority for the EHS and UAE NMC and are essential for the viability of the profession. Barriers that contribute to nurses' lack of participation in policy decision-making include nursing-related factors and organization-related factors, all of which need to be addressed [26].

The EHS governance or leadership structure should include the official representation of nurses in healthcare-related decisions. Nurses should be represented in healthcare committees at local, regional, and international levels to ensure their participation and involvement in decision-making in areas such as ethics, healthcare informatics, disease prevention, and health promotion.

16.5.2 Nursing Education

16.5.2.1 Inconsistent Nursing Curriculum and Revision

Although the national competency framework has been published, no clear roadmap exists to ensure the implementation of the new competencies in nursing curricula. Mechanisms to follow up on implementation are critical and must be standardized and closely monitored. Furthermore, nursing educational curricula must be ready to incorporate innovative teaching practices such as debates, simulation, problem-solving, team-based learning, informatics, self-directed learning, computer-assisted teaching and learning, reflective journals, and concept mapping [27]. These authentic teaching approaches are essential for preparing nurses for reflective practice, critical thinking, problem-solving, and clinical judgment, which are essential components of the nursing profession.

The COVID-19 pandemic highlighted the importance of integrating social responsibility competencies into nursing educational curricula. This integration ensures that nurses are accountable and responsive to community healthcare needs [28] and better equips nursing students to deal with future health crises without physical and mental burnout [29, 30].

16.5.2.2 Limited Postgraduate Nursing Programs

The development of postgraduate nursing programs to match growing population needs and national and international standards for providing quality healthcare is essential [31, 32]. Few master's-level programs are currently open and remain insufficient to accommodate the educational needs of nursing graduates. Available programs include the Master of Science in Adult Critical Care Nursing program at the UOS; Master of Science in Nursing programs in Adult Health and Gerontology Nursing, Pediatric Nursing, Psychiatric Mental Health, and Community Health Nursing at RAK College of Nursing; Master of Nursing at the University of Wollongong in Dubai; and Master of Science programs in Cardiovascular Nursing and Pediatric Nursing at the College of Nursing and Midwifery at the Mohammed Bin Rashid University of Medicine and Health Sciences. Opening higher-level programs remains a challenge given the shortage of qualified nursing faculty with specialized clinical practice to teach and lead new graduate programs. There is a need to attract qualified faculty with the necessary specializations who can contribute to program development and accreditation processes. Seeking affiliation and support from well-established universities may facilitate the process of establishing high-quality graduate programs in the UAE.

16.5.2.3 Limited Clinical Training Sites

Academic institutions are challenged by the limited number of clinical training sites that meet the training needs of the increased number of students. The limited number of clinical training sites mean students' clinical training is compromised until large teaching and specialty hospitals can be established with a core mission of training health professionals—first and foremost, nurses [33]. These futuristic teaching hospitals should be equipped with state-of-the-art technology to ensure that quality graduates can function in high-tech healthcare settings. A partnership model between academia and clinical practice is important to serve the needs of both academic institutions and clinical practice. This can be achieved through an expanded memorandum of understanding (MOU) that includes international training opportunities for students through exchange programs. For example, the UOS signed an MOU with University College Dublin for an exchange program that will provide students with exceptional training opportunities. All academic institutions should initiate such MOUs with other well-established institutions that allow students exposure to different healthcare systems and therefore equip them with the new skills needed to affect positive change in nursing practice.

16.5.3 Research

16.5.3.1 Limited Acquisition of Scientific Research Competencies

Limited progress has been made in boosting nursing research and motivating nurses to be involved in scientific research in the UAE. The heavy workloads, nursing shortage, poor research knowledge and skills, negative attitudes toward research, and lack of awareness of the importance of research for clinical practice are obstacles to nurses' involvement in conducting research [34].

Research knowledge is the key strategy to build research capacity for nurses working in healthcare settings [35]. Educating nurses to conduct research relies on support from academic institutions with nurse scientists and research faculty. This can be accomplished through establishing global partnership initiatives that motivate nurses to be involved in scientific research [36]. As nurses in clinical practice have limited knowledge about research, nursing faculty and researchers need to partner with nurses in clinical practice to identify clinical research priorities and facilitate data collection. Practitioners and academic researchers complement each other and must work together to improve nursing research skills and build capacity [37].

Impactful nursing research requires time and attention that often compete with organizational interests. Nurse leaders must therefore be proactive in supporting nurses' involvement in healthcare research. Healthcare organizations must prioritize resources and invest in nursing research by expanding research databases and resources providing research funding and training opportunities for nurses [37].

To improve patient outcomes, health services, and the profession's long-term viability, the UAE needs a robust nursing research agenda that sets out a clear road map for futuristic nursing research. This agenda must determine prioritized areas of research and enable nurse leaders to use their collective energies to build nursing research capacity. The agenda should be clinically based and focus on strengthening patient clinical outcomes, such as falls, pressure ulcers, catheter-related infections, electronic healthcare records, medication safety, and adverse nursing events [37]. Furthermore, factors contributing to better staffing and nurses' satisfaction (e.g., caseloads, shift patterns, nurses' competencies, and professional development needs) must be addressed in the future research agenda.

The research agenda should target a range of population and community health issues. Optimizing quality of care and meeting population health needs must be the major goals of the new research agenda [38]. Disseminating and publishing research findings would motivate nurse leaders to participate in research to achieve better-quality healthcare. Nurse-led research is critical for producing high-quality evidence that addresses priority research questions for patients, families, and the wider community.

16.5.3.2 Inadequate Knowledge and Implementation of Evidence-Based Practice

Evidence-based practice (EBP) is a cornerstone of nursing that ensures patient safety and quality of care. It refers to translating research into routine clinical practice [39]. In the UAE, nursing practice is challenged by inadequate preparation and integration of EBP. A recent national cross-sectional survey of 1602 nurses showed that nurses had an intermediate level of EBP knowledge and reported the need for training in EBP skills and knowledge [40]. A mixed-methods study using a questionnaire and focus groups to collect data revealed low knowledge and low self-confidence in implementing EBP processes among nurses in UAE hospitals [41].

The EHS has worked on improving nurses' EBP skills in clinical practice and has recently adopted the John Hopkins Nursing Evidence-Based Practice Model in clinical practice settings across the organization. The model uses a problem-solving approach to clinical questions and appraises the best available scientific evidence to bring about a transformative change in clinical practice.

Greater efforts must be implemented to improve nurses' skills in EBP. Stakeholders and nurse leaders must offer extensive training in EBP and provide sufficient resources to enable nurses to implement EBP in their working units. A partnership between researchers from academia and practice settings is critical to improving practice and knowledge related to EBP. Academic institutions must adopt innovative teaching methods that integrate EBP into education curricula to prepare nurses with EBP skills. Distance learning, on-the-job training, and evening classes that suit nurses' working conditions are suggested strategies to train nurses in EBP. Facilities are also encouraged to create a new position entitled "research nurse" for candidates with adequate training in EBP to assist practicing nurses in the application and dissemination of clinical evidence. Implementation of EBP puts nurses in the best position to influence healthcare decisions and contribute to healthcare reform.

16.6 Conclusion

"...I salute those who dedicate their lives to this profession. While medicines may treat, it is their support and care that gives us the hope for a healthier tomorrow." His Highness Sheikh Mohamed Bin Zayed Al Nahyan, Abu Dhabi Crown Prince and Deputy Supreme Commander of the UAE Armed Forces. This chapter highlights important milestones facing nurses in the UAE, discusses existing challenges, and envisions the future of the profession. Today, nurses in the UAE are at a paradigm-shifting moment that requires reflection, transformative leadership, EBP knowledge, and skills to impact and lead healthcare reform. There is a need for an action-oriented blueprint that strengthens the nursing taskforce in the UAE to meet the growing population's needs for quality care.

Conflicts of Interest The authors have no conflicts of interest to declare.

References

1. Nursing Definitions | ICN - International Council of Nurses [2002]. Available from: https://www.icn.ch/nursing-policy/nursing-definitions
2. World Health Organization. Nursing and Midwifery. https://www.who.int/news-room/fact-sheets/detail/nursing-and-midwifery#:~:text=Key%20facts,current%20shortage%20in%20health%20workers
3. The official portal of the UAE government, 2022. Available at: https://uaecabinet.ae/en/details/prime-ministers-initiatives/the-united-arab-emirates-government-portal
4. Al-Yateem N, Almarzouqi A, Dias JM, Saifan A, Timmins F. Nursing in The United Arab Emirates: current challenges and opportunities. J Nurs Manag. 2021;29(2):109–12. Available from: https://pubmed.ncbi.nlm.nih.gov/32100891/
5. Kronfol NM, Athique MM. Nursing education in The United Arab Emirates. Int J Nurs Stud 1986 Jan 1;23(1):1–10. Available from: https://doi.org/10.1016/0020-7489(86)90033-7.

6. El-Haddad M. Nursing in The United Arab Emirates: an historical background. Int Nurs Rev. 2006;53(4):284–9. Available from: https://onlinelibrary.wiley.com/doi/full/10.1111/j.1466-7657.2006.00497.x
7. Brownie SM, Hunter LH, Aqtash S, Day GE. Establishing policy foundations and regulatory systems to enhance nursing practice in The United Arab Emirates. Policy Polit Nurs Pract. 2015;16(1–2):38–50. Available from: https://journals.sagepub.com/doi/10.1177/1527154415583396
8. Oulton JA. A final word. Int Nurs Rev. 2008;55(3):251. Available from: https://onlinelibrary.wiley.com/doi/full/10.1111/j.1466-7657.2008.00678.x
9. Swan M. Nursing schools seek to entice Emiratis 2010 Nov 3.; Available from: https://www.thenationalnews.com/uae/health/nursing-schools-seek-to-entice-emiratis-1.541327
10. Brownie SM, Rossiter RC, Hamad AO, Aqtash S. The role and value of nurses in care provision: views and expectations of Emirati nationals in the western region of Abu Dhabi, United Arab Emirates. J Hosp Adm. 2017;6(6):42. Available from: https://www.sciedupress.com/journal/index.php/jha/article/view/12392
11. Bani-issa W, Al Tamimi M, Fakhry R, Al Tawil H. Experiences of nursing students and examiners with the objective structured clinical examination method in physical assessment education: a mixed methods study. Nurse Educ Pract. 2019;35:83–9. Available from: https://pubmed.ncbi.nlm.nih.gov/30739050/
12. Al-Yateem N, Al-Tamimi M, Brenner M, Al Tawil H, Ahmad A, Brownie S, et al. Nurse-identified patient care and health services research priorities in The United Arab Emirates: a Delphi study. BMC Health Serv Res. 2019;19(1):1–8. Available from: https://bmchealthservres.biomedcentral.com/articles/10.1186/s12913-019-3888-5
13. Number of Nurses per 1,000 Population. Available from: https://www.vision2021.ae/en/national-agenda-2021/list/card/number-of-nurses-per-1-000-population
14. Paulo MS, Loney T, Lapão LV. How do we strengthen the health workforce in a rapidly developing high-income country? A case study of Abu Dhabi's health system in The United Arab Emirates. Hum Resour Health. 2019;17(1):1–8. Available from: https://human-resources-health.biomedcentral.com/articles/10.1186/s12960-019-0345-9
15. Almansour H, Gobbi M, Prichard J. Home and expatriate nurses' perceptions of job satisfaction: qualitative findings. Int Nurs Rev. 2022;69(2):125–31. Available from: https://onlinelibrary.wiley.com/doi/full/10.1111/inr.12699
16. Godsey JA, Houghton DM, Hayes T. Registered nurse perceptions of factors contributing to the inconsistent brand image of the nursing profession. Nurs Outlook. 2020;68(6):808–21. Available from: https://pubmed.ncbi.nlm.nih.gov/32763085/
17. Hazarika I. Artificial intelligence: opportunities and implications for the health workforce. Int Health. 2020;12(4):241–5. Available from: https://pubmed.ncbi.nlm.nih.gov/32300794/
18. Haddad LM, Annamaraju P, Toney-Butler TJ. Nursing shortage. Br Med J. 2022;3(5669):534–5. Available from: https://www.ncbi.nlm.nih.gov/books/NBK493175/
19. Fitzgerald C, Kantrowitz-Gordon I, Katz J, Hirsch A. Advanced practice nursing education: challenges and strategies. Nurs Res Pract. 2012;2012:1–8. Available from: https://pubmed.ncbi.nlm.nih.gov/22220273/
20. Lopes-Júnior LC. Advanced practice nursing and the expansion of the role of nurses in primary health care in the Americas. 2021 May 24;7. Available from: https://journals.sagepub.com/doi/full/10.1177/23779608211019491
21. Oermann MH. Is nursing education an advanced practice specialty? Nurse Educ. 2021;46(5):267. Available from: https://pubmed.ncbi.nlm.nih.gov/34435759/
22. Ryskina KL, Lam C, Jung HY. Association between clinician specialization in nursing home care and nursing home clinical quality scores. J Am Med Dir Assoc. 2019;20(8):1007–1012.e2. Available from: https://pubmed.ncbi.nlm.nih.gov/30745174/
23. Mueller C, Burggraf V, Crogan NL. Growth and specialization of gerontological nursing. Geriatr Nurs (Minneap). 2020;41(1):14–5. Available from: https://linkinghub.elsevier.com/retrieve/pii/S0197457220300136

24. Maier CB, Barnes H, Aiken LH, Busse R. Descriptive, cross-country analysis of the nurse practitioner workforce in six countries: size, growth, physician substitution potential. BMJ Open. 2016;6(9):e011901. Available from: https://bmjopen.bmj.com/lookup/doi/10.1136/bmjopen-2016-011901
25. Smith S. Participation of nurses in health services decision-making and policy development. Int J Evid Based Healthc. 2014;12(3):193. Available from: https://journals.lww.com/ijebh/Fulltext/2014/09000/Participation_of_nurses_in_health_services.71.aspx
26. Shariff N. Factors that act as facilitators and barriers to nurse leaders' participation in health policy development. BMC Nurs. 2014;13(1):1–13. Available from: https://bmcnurs.biomedcentral.com/articles/10.1186/1472-6955-13-20
27. Kumar SR. Emerging innovative teaching strategies in nursing. JOJ Nurse Heal Care. 2017;1. Available from: https://juniperpublishers.com/online-submission.php
28. Schaffer M, Hargate C. Moving toward reconciliation: community engagement in nursing education. J Community Engagem Scholarsh. 2015;8(1) Available from: https://jces.ua.edu/articles/10.54656/PFQK9362
29. Ajab S, Ádam B, Hammadi MAL, Bastaki NAL, Al Junaibi M, Al Zubaidi A, et al. Occupational health of frontline healthcare workers in the United Arab Emirates during the COVID-19 pandemic: a snapshot of summer 2020. Int J Environ Res Public Heal. 2021;18(21):11410. Available from: https://www.mdpi.com/1660-4601/18/21/11410/htm
30. Bani Issa W, Professor A, Al Nusair H, Rababa M, Saqan MPHR, Assistant R, et al. Posttraumatic stress disorders and influencing factors during the COVID-19 pandemic: a cross-sectional study of frontline nurses. Int Nurs Rev. 2022;69(3):285–93. Available from: https://onlinelibrary.wiley.com/doi/full/10.1111/inr.12734
31. Al-Yateem N, Ahmed FR, Alameddine M, Dias JM, Saifan AR, Subu MA, et al. Psychological distress among the nursing workforce in The United Arab Emirates: comparing levels before and during the COVID-19 pandemic. Nurs Forum. 2022;57:1314. Available from: https://onlinelibrary.wiley.com/doi/full/10.1111/nuf.12808
32. Alameddine M, Clinton M, Bou-Karroum K, Richa N, Doumit MAA. Factors associated with the resilience of nurses during the COVID-19 pandemic. Worldv Evid-Based Nurs. 2021;18(6):320–31. Available from: https://onlinelibrary.wiley.com/doi/full/10.1111/wvn.12544
33. Yanarico DMI, Balsanelli AP, Gasparino RC, Bohomol E. Classification and evaluation of the environment of the professional nursing practice in a teaching hospital. Rev Lat Am Enfermagem. 2020;28:e3376. Available from: https://pubmed.ncbi.nlm.nih.gov/33084777/
34. Hendricks J, Cope V. Research is not a 'scary' word: Registered nurses and the barriers to research utilisation. Nord. J. Nurs. Res. 2016;37(1):44–50. Available from: https://journals.sagepub.com/doi/10.1177/2057158516679581
35. King O, West E, Lee S, Glenister K, Quilliam C, Wong Shee A, et al. Research education and training for nurses and allied health professionals: a systematic scoping review. BMC Med Educ. 2022;22(1):1–55. Available from: https://bmcmededuc.biomedcentral.com/articles/10.1186/s12909-022-03406-7
36. Al Nusair H, Bani-issa W, Alnjadat R, Fonbuena M, Perinchery S, AlAzza R. The effect of multicomponent approach in enhancing the level of confidence with evidence-based practice activities and promoting evidence-based practice culture among nurses in a clinical setting in The United Arab Emirates. J Nurs Manag. 2022;30:4285. Available from: https://pubmed.ncbi.nlm.nih.gov/36190519/
37. Hughes TL, George M, Shah R, Dias BM, Dohrn JE, De Bortoli Cassiani SH. Nursing engagement in research priorities focused on health systems and services in Latin America countries. Hum Resour Health. 2022;20(1):1–9. Available from: https://human-resources-health.biomedcentral.com/articles/10.1186/s12960-022-00746-9
38. Evans CJ, Bone AE, Yi D, Gao W, Morgan M, Taherzadeh S, et al. Community-based short-term integrated palliative and supportive care reduces symptom distress for older people with chronic noncancer conditions compared with usual care: a randomised controlled single-blind

mixed method trial. Int J Nurs Stud. 2021;120:103978. Available from: https://linkinghub.elsevier.com/retrieve/pii/S0020748921001231
39. Katowa-Mukwato P, Mwiinga-Kalusopa V, Chitundu K, Kanyanta M, Chanda D, Mbewe Mwelwa M, et al. Implementing evidence based practice nursing using the PDSA model: process, lessons and implications. Int J Afr Nurs Sci. 2021;14:100261. Available from: https://linkinghub.elsevier.com/retrieve/pii/S2214139120301384
40. Alblooshi SM, Abdul Razzak H, Hijji FHR, Wishah AM Alkarbi M, Zaid Harbi A. Knowledge, attitude and implementation of evidence-based practice among nurses; a national survey. 2022; Available from: https://doi.org/10.21203/rs.3.rs-2113129/v1
41. Ramukumba MM, El Amouri S. Nurses' perspectives of the nursing documentation audit process. Heal SA = SA Gesondheid. 2019;24. Available from: https://pubmed.ncbi.nlm.nih.gov/31934421/

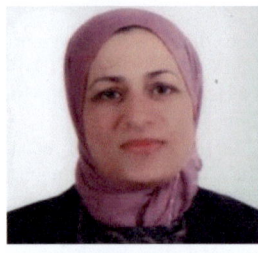

Prof. Wegdan Bani-Issa is a distinguished full professor at the University of Sharjah's College of Health Sciences/Nursing Department/UAE. She received her bachelor's degree in nursing science from Jordan University of Science and Technology, her master's degree in nursing science from the University of Windsor in Ontario, Canada, and her PhD from the University of Kansas Medical Center in the United States. Her research findings have been published in a number of scientific journals, and she has received numerous grants and funding to conduct research in the disciplines of women's health, geriatrics, and health promotion techniques. Her involvement in the nursing profession was demonstrated by a number of professional affiliations, her teaching, and her intellectual endeavors.

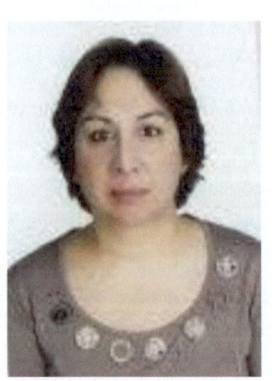

Ms. Randa Fakhry is a lecturer at the University of Sharjah's College of Health Sciences/Nursing Department/UAE. She received her bachelor's degree in nursing and her master's degree in public health from the American University of Beirut. Her research findings have been published in a number of peer-reviewed journals with an emphasis on women's health, breastfeeding practices, mental health, geriatrics, and health promotion techniques. Her involvement in the nursing profession was demonstrated by her teaching, research, and community involvement.

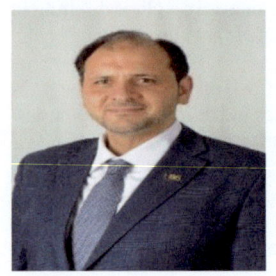

Professor Mohamad Alameddine is the Dean of the College of Health Sciences and a Professor of Health Management and Policy at the University of Sharjah. Professor Alameddine holds a PhD in Health Policy from the University of Toronto and a Masters of Public Health from the American University of Beirut. He has led multiple programs and initiatives supporting the planning, organization, and management of human capital in the health sector in public, private, and non-governmental entities in the GCC and beyond. Professor Alameddine is highly published in his field and is regarded as a regional expert on health systems, human resources planning, management and development, and the quality of work environments.

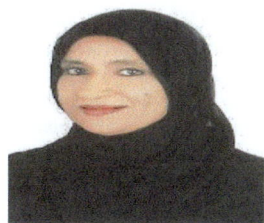

Amina Al-Marzouqi is an experienced associate professor with more than 30 years of experience in the fields of education, community, leadership, and management. She gained her master's degree in Health Management, Planning, and Policy from the Nuffield Institute, Leeds University, UK, and her PhD from the University of South Carolina, Columbia, USA in Healthcare Management and Planning. Her current position as the Vice Chancellor for Branches and Students at the University of Sharjah showcases her leadership skills and her dedication to the development of higher education in the country.

Dr. Amina served as a dean and faculty member at the College of Health Sciences at the same university and contributed to shaping the health sciences education and training future of healthcare professionals. She led and contributed to curriculum development, faculty development, accreditation, research integration, clinical and practical training, quality assurance, and interdisciplinary and international collaborations.

In addition to her teaching and administrative duties, Dr. Amina excelled in research, as she is the recipient of several research grants and has produced several publications in healthcare-related disciplines. Her passion for improving the healthcare system in the UAE through the integration of innovative practice strategies speaks to her visionary mindset and her drive to make a positive impact on society.

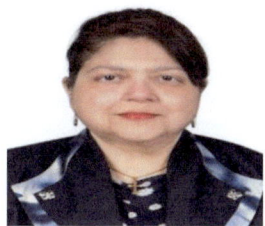

Dr. Jacqueline Maria Dias is the Chair and Associate Professor, a TEIG scholar, and a Faculty Advising Champion at the University of Sharjah, College of Health Sciences, and Department of Nursing, UAE. She heads the BSN program and Bridging Post-RN and has commissioned the first Masters in Adult Critical Care Program in the UAE in September 2020. She is recognized as one of the leads in the UAE who has developed the National Competency and Professional Practice Framework for Undergraduate Nursing Program in 2022. In addition, she is a senior fellow with the Higher Education Academy (HEA), UK, as well as an AnneMarie Schimmel Scholar. She has acquired an Advanced Diploma in Health Professions Education and a Professional Diploma in Health Professions.

She has over 30 years' experience in medical and nursing education, simulation, e-learning, administration, and international consultation. Her former appointments include Nurudin Jivraj Professor and Chair, founding director of Blended Learning, director of the Bachelor of Science in Nursing, director of the Post-RN BScN program, director of International Programs, and founding director of the Centre of Innovation in Medical Education. She is the recipient of several grants and awards and has numerous publications to her credit.

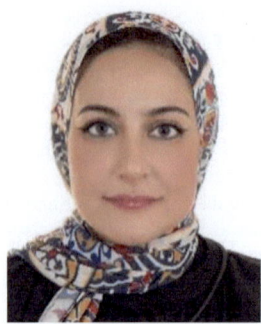

Dr. Fatma Refaat Ahmed is an assistant professor at the University of Sharjah's College of Health Sciences/Nursing Department/UAE. She got her MSc in 2013 and her PhD in 2016 from Alexandria University, Egypt. She has around 15 years of experience in academia. She participated in more than 20 international conferences and published articles in well-respected international journals. She is a BLS, ACLS, ETC, and HIS instructor. She was an advisor and co-advisor for around 20 doctoral dissertations and a master's thesis. Fatma is also an academic editor for *PLOS ONE* and *BMC Nursing Journal*. She is also an editorial board member of the *Journal of Emergency Nursing* and the *Journal of Nursing Management*.

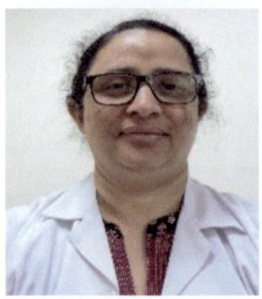

Ms. Mini Sara Abraham is a lecturer working at the College of Health Sciences/Nursing Department/University of Sharjah, UAE. She attained her bachelor's degree from SNDT University Bombay, followed by her master's degree from Trivandrum Medical College, University of Kerala. She has vast clinical experience in the capacity of nurse manager in critical care settings and around 22 years of teaching experience. Mini is enthusiastic about implementing innovative teaching strategies in clinical settings and she reflects on the findings of her research. Mini has published articles in reputed international journals, and her research interests are in the fields of education, management, simulation, and mental health.

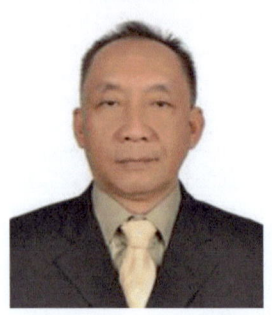

Dr. Muhammad Arsyad Subu is an assistant professor at the University of Sharjah's College of Health Sciences/Nursing Department/UAE. His specialization is psychiatric—mental health nursing and qualitative research methods. Dr. Subu got his MSN in nursing education in 2003 from Villanova University, Philadelphia, Pennsylvania, USA. He completed his PhD in 2015 from the nursing program at the College of Health Sciences at the University of Ottawa, Canada. He has around 35 years of experience in academia. He participated in more than 50 international conferences and published articles in well-respected international journals. Dr. Muhammad Arsyad Subu is also an academic editor for *PLOS ONE* and *BMC Nursing Journal*. His research interests are related to psychiatric—mental health nursing, community/public health nursing, stigma and mental illness, nursing education, and students with disabilities.

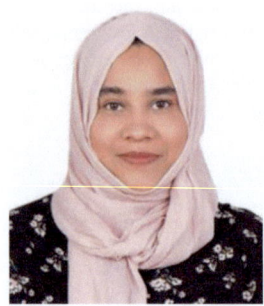

Ms. Janisha Kavumpurath is a clinical instructor at the University of Sharjah's College of Health Sciences in the Nursing Department, UAE. She earned her bachelor's and master's degrees in nursing science from Rajiv Gandhi University of Health Sciences and is presently pursuing a PhD from the University Putra Malaysia. Her research interests include critical care nursing, cardiothoracic nursing, adult health, innovative nursing education, and simulation education.

Open Access This chapter is licensed under the terms of the Creative Commons Attribution 4.0 International License (http://creativecommons.org/licenses/by/4.0/), which permits use, sharing, adaptation, distribution and reproduction in any medium or format, as long as you give appropriate credit to the original author(s) and the source, provide a link to the Creative Commons license and indicate if changes were made.

The images or other third party material in this chapter are included in the chapter's Creative Commons license, unless indicated otherwise in a credit line to the material. If material is not included in the chapter's Creative Commons license and your intended use is not permitted by statutory regulation or exceeds the permitted use, you will need to obtain permission directly from the copyright holder.

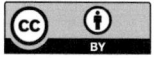

Advanced Practice Nursing Within the UAE

17

Katie Hanafin

17.1 Introduction

The last 30 years have seen a significant rise in the role of advanced practice nurses. This has come about because of several factors; the two biggest drivers have been a shortage of medical professionals and an increasing number of patients with complex health problems. It is estimated that by 2030, there will be a shortage of up to 18 million healthcare workers worldwide [1]. The United Arab Emirates (UAE), like many other countries, is not exempt from these issues. In addition to an ongoing need for more hospital beds and medical and nursing staff, there is a constant rise in non-communicable diseases and a developing obesity crisis. The World Obesity Federation [2] has shown that 70% of men and 64% of women in the UAE are either overweight or obese [2]. This ultimately leads to an increase in the incidence of cancer, diabetes, and heart disease, all of which put further strain on the health system.

The healthcare workforce in the UAE is unlike most other countries in the world, in that it is mostly expats, with only 18% of physicians and 4% of nurses being Emiratis [3]. This was previously due to a lack of medical and nursing education in the UAE, but this is now changing, with several universities now offering medical and nursing education in an effort to retain Emiratis within the UAE healthcare workforce once qualified.

The Abu Dhabi Economic Vision 2030 plan was released with a goal of long-term economic progress; as part of this, there is a focus on not only attracting qualified health professionals from other countries but also training local medical and nursing staff in order to develop the sector sufficiently [4]. Many countries around the globe have tried to combat the issue of a shortage of medical personnel by training their nursing staff to an advanced practice level in order to provide quality and cost-effective healthcare in a manner that suits their healthcare system.

K. Hanafin (✉)
Burjeel Medical City, Abu Dhabi, United Arab Emirates
e-mail: katie.hanafin@burjeelmedicalcity.com

© The Author(s) 2025
H. O. Al-Shamsi (ed.), *Healthcare in the United Arab Emirates*,
https://doi.org/10.1007/978-981-96-0523-1_17

The International Council for Nurses [5] defines advanced practice nursing as "A nurse practitioner (NP) or advanced practice nurse (APN) is a registered nurse who has acquired an expert knowledge base, complex decision-making skills, and clinical competencies for expanded practice, the characteristics of which are shaped by the context and/or country in which s/he is credentialed to practice". An APN should be educated to the master's or doctorate level in their specific area of practice, with graded assessments of knowledge and clinical skills. This level of training and assessment gives them the freedom and authority to act autonomously for their patients, making decisions on assessment, diagnosis, and treatment [6].

Within advanced practice nursing, there are two main job profiles in the UK and UAE: the advanced nurse practitioner (ANP) and clinical nurse specialist (CNS). In the USA, there are also nurse midwives and nurse anaesthetists who are considered advanced practice nurses. The ANP and CNS roles require a master's-level qualification to be licensed as an NP or CNS, but there are some differences in their day-to-day practice. A nurse practitioner can practice both autonomously and collaboratively with members of the multidisciplinary team; they perform assessments and diagnoses, order laboratory tests and radiology examinations, prescribe medications and clinical treatments, and perform procedures within their authorised scope of practice. An NP will often work as part of the physician rota in acute hospital settings.

Clinical nurse specialists manage the care of complex and vulnerable populations in specific areas such as diabetes care, oncology, paediatrics, wound care, and gastroenterology. As well as patient-focused care, they provide evidence-based education and support to patients and staff to ensure a culture of safety within the healthcare system. The context of the practice setting and the characteristics of the patient population define the exact needs of the role. A CNS will remain within the nursing workforce and can work with or without prescribing privileges in the UK and USA; however, in the UAE, a CNS is not given prescribing privileges at this time. Currently, the Professional Qualification Requirements (PQR) set by the NMC include only specialty nurse and nurse practitioner within the PQR table.

See Table 17.1 for a description of the levels of specialization and their varying educational requirements, as defined by the UAE Nursing and Midwifery Council Specialization Committee.

Advanced practice nurses (APNs) are innovative leaders who pave the way for high-level, excellent quality of care while educating and guiding the next generation of nurses to reach their career goals. Despite NPs often working within physician rotas, there are many other aspects to the NP role that are not typically seen in the physician role. These include being a researcher, a nurse leader and innovator who demonstrates best practice, a local and national policymaker, and an educator to nurses, junior physicians, and patients.

NPs are also extremely cost-effective in comparison to physicians, with research demonstrating this in primary, secondary, and long-term care settings. It has been shown that NPs are able to provide the same level of care as physicians with equal outcomes, yet their salary can be up to half that of a physician [8]. If a team of NPs is employed in a department, the internal cost savings can be significant for the

Table 17.1 Levels of RN specialisation in the UAE

Qualification/Job title	Description	Education
Registered Nurse (RN)	A nurse with experience in a certain area of nursing who is recognised by the employer or licensing authority as "specialised" in their field	Bachelor's degree in Nursing
RN	Specialty-specific certificate short courses	One month wound care course
Speciality RN	Post-RN graduate specialty programmes focusing on a patient population (e.g. paediatrics, neonatal, critical care), OR a nurse that completed a 3-year degree in a specialised area	Qualification as Registered Nurse and Postgraduate certificate in one of the nursing specialties with minimum 1 year full-time course duration OR Bachelor's degree in one of the nursing specialties (minimum 3 years course duration
Speciality RN or Advanced Practice RN/Nurse practitioner or clinical nurse specialist	Specialised in a specific patient population or disease process (e.g. cardiology or paediatric clinical nurse specialist) or in a functional field of nursing (quality, education, etc.)	Qualification as an RN plus a master's level programme
Advanced Practice RN/Nurse practitioner	"Advanced practice" nurse training results in autonomous practitioners (nurse practitioner)	Clinical Master or Doctorate degree in nursing including: Pharmacology for prescribing drugs as a nurse practitioner; differential diagnosis, ordering, and interpretation of diagnostic tests (Radiological and pathological tests); Advanced Health Assessment

Source: Adapted from Machon with permission [7]

employer. UAE healthcare expenditure is one of the highest per capita in the world; it was estimated there would be $104.6 billion in healthcare expenditure in 2022, with the National Health Agency report in 2018 stating that 19% of healthcare expenditure is spent on medicines. Multiple studies have shown that NP-led care can lead to an overall lower cost of drugs during inpatient stays [9, 10].

There is a growing emphasis on community-based healthcare services, which is in part due to the increasing level of chronic health needs of the population and the consequential ever rising expenditure on chronic disease management. Non-communicable diseases (principally cardiovascular disease (CVD), cancer, diabetes, and chronic respiratory disease) are responsible for 77% of all deaths in the UAE, and the probability of dying prematurely (before the age of 70) from one of these diseases is 17%. The role of family nurse practitioners (FNPs) is to provide primary care services for patients ranging from infants to seniors. They conduct well-checks, screen for disease symptoms, administer treatments, and order tests under the premise of enhancing a patient's overall well-being [11]. It is a positive sign that the UAE now has several hospitals and primary care clinics that have licensed FNPs independently seeing patients; this will not only help to provide high-quality care with easier access to services for patients but will also save money.

Within traditional healthcare in the past, nurses had one role and doctors had another; there was no cross-over between the specialities. Then, in the 1930s in the USA, the role of some nurses began to change with the development of the clinical nurse specialist role. In 1965, Loretta Ford, EdD, PNP, and Henry Silver, MD, at the University of Colorado established the first nurse practitioner training course. The role was founded on the principles of the extended role of specialist nurses, but it also openly incorporated traditional medical diagnostic skills. Initially a certificate programme, it became a master's degree programme in the 1970s as the role became more established. By 2015, over 205,000 nurse practitioners had been trained and registered to work in the USA. The UK was somewhat later, with Barbara Stillwell establishing the first nurse practitioner course in 1992. Each of these innovative leaders has enhanced the role of nursing to heighten consumer value, reduce costs, and improve outcomes.

Despite advanced practice nursing being utilized in the USA, UK, and Australia for many years, the UAE has only recently begun to recognise the discipline of advanced practice nursing. The Health Authority of Abu Dhabi (HAAD) first agreed in 2015 to provide licenses for NPs to work specifically at Cleveland Clinic Abu Dhabi (CCAD) [12].

17.2 Timeline of Events Leading to the Development of APN Within the UAE

The World Health Organization (WHO) groups the UAE as part of the Eastern Mediterranean Region (EMR), which comprises 21 member states and the occupied Palestinian territory (West Bank and Gaza Strip). In 1990, the WHO formed a regional advisory panel on nursing with the aim of providing a mechanism for nurse leaders in the region to identify needs and priorities requiring action by the WHO. The panel also assisted the regional office with action plans on how to support and strengthen nursing and midwifery in the region.

In June 2001, the regional advisory panel held their fifth meeting in Pakistan. The meeting was arranged to consult on the development of advanced practice nursing and nurse prescribing within the EMR [13]. This was the first time that the idea of developing a new role in the region had been openly debated. They discussed the scope of professional roles and responsibilities, the regulation of advanced practice nursing, and the implications for nursing education and practice. The meeting was a milestone in the future development of the APN role in the Eastern Mediterranean region (EMR); it was held over three days and attended by chief nurses, deans of schools of nursing, presidents of national nursing organisations, regional and international nursing experts, as well as physicians and pharmacists from across the EMR, including the UAE, with Mr. Mark Fielding representing the Emirates [14].

A year prior to the panel meeting, the International Council of Nurses launched the Nurse Practitioner/Advanced Practice Nursing Network. The idea of this network was to provide international leadership and guidance to countries that had not already developed the concept of advanced practice nursing. Through the expertise of members of the Network, international guidelines were developed in 2002 for the definition, scope of practice, professional standards, and competencies for advanced practice nursing [15].

The next important stage in the development of APN in the region was in 2008, when the WHO regional office committee produced a technical paper (EM/RC55/R.5) on promoting nursing and midwifery development in the Eastern Mediterranean Region. This paper advocated for specialized roles and advanced practice nursing development within primary, secondary, and tertiary care [16].

Following on from this, in 2014, the WHO regional panel sent a nursing and midwifery survey to the 22 member countries of the EMR. The survey was designed to identify key challenges and assess the current status of nursing and midwifery within the EMR. The results helped guide the development of the Framework for Action on Strengthening Nursing and Midwifery in the Region 2015–2025 [17]. The majority of EMR members that responded to the survey believed that there is a place for the development of APN, especially its integration into primary care and chronic illness management. Concerns and possible barriers to implementation include physician dominance and opposition, role ambiguity, a lack of understanding of the role by both the public and other healthcare professionals, a lack of highly educated nurses, and a lack of support at the governmental and local levels.

Recommendations from the survey that relate to APN:

- Nurses and midwives should practice to the full extent of their education, scope, and standards of practice to ensure safe and quality health and nursing services for all populations. As part of this, expanded or advanced practice nursing and midwifery roles should be introduced.
- Increase access to quality nursing and midwifery education. Integral to this is the development of the capacity of those in educator roles and those engaged in educational planning, management, and leadership.
- Nurses and midwives should be engaged in research that is responsive to health priorities and that informs health, nursing, and midwifery policies. A significant part of the role of an APN is to assist in policy writing and participate in research.

These recommendations fit well within the UAE Nursing and Midwifery Council (NMC) Nursing and Midwifery Education Strategy [18] that was published in 2013 and has five clear goals. Goal three is to expand the educational programmes available within the UAE to include post-RN specialisation programmes, master's degrees for advanced practice, and/or expanded roles in clinical, education, or management, and doctoral programmes. Goal five is to ensure there are enough qualified faculty for nursing and midwifery education programmes in the UAE.

In 2023 there are three nursing master's courses available in the UAE: a Paediatric Nursing MSc and Cardiovascular MSc at Mohammed Bin Rashid University of

Medicine and Health Sciences (MBRU), and an Adult Critical Care Nursing MSc at University of Sharjah. These courses are already in their third cohort of students, with the first cohort now completing the course and able to work as clinical nurse specialists in their specialised areas, yet at this present time there is no separate title of CNS within nursing licensure. The Master of Science courses offer the theoretical knowledge and practical skills to enable a growing specialist nurse workforce that is 'fit for purpose', knowledgeable, clinically competent, thoughtful, critical, and articulate [19].

Going back to 2015, we see the first licenses granted for Nurse Practitioners in the UAE. HAAD agreed to grant NP licenses exclusively at CCAD as a 'trial' development of this new role [20]. To start with, just two NPs began working at CCAD: a family nurse practitioner (FNP) based in the outpatient clinic and an adult acute care NP who was based in the urgent care department [21]. In the two years following the arrival of the first two NPs at CCAD, the team began to grow with NPs in other departments such as pulmonary and transplant, the intensive care unit, and the emergency room. I The team of NPs at CCAD continues to expand and demonstrates how well-advanced practice nursing can be successfully integrated into UAE healthcare.

As there was no agreed scope of practice for NPs in the UAE when the first NPs arrived, a framework based on the Ohio APN scope of practice, minus prescribing privileges, was used to develop the programme. Although the early NP licenses did not include full prescribing authority, the NPs were able to prescribe from specified order sets, which were then countersigned by doctors before prescriptions could be administered. Restrictions on the ability of NPs to practice to the full extent of their training not only limit access to care for patients but also have a negative effect on job satisfaction, as APNs find themselves unable to embrace and practice to the fullest extent of their scope of practice [22]. This is possibly one of the reasons for the relatively quick turnover of NPs in the first few years of practice in the UAE.

In April 2018, the UAE Nursing and Midwifery Council released a report titled 'Model for Nursing and Midwifery Specialisation in the United Arab Emirates' [23]. The framework identified nursing roles for specialisation that include the nurse specialist, advanced practice nurse, and advanced practice midwifery, with recommendations made to establish speciality roles in acute and ambulatory settings. It is also the first time it has been documented that advanced practice nurses and midwives should have the authority to prescribe. The ICN's [24] scope of practice for specialty nurses was used to help guide this document.

The release of this document led to changes in scope of practice and prescribing authority within CCAD.

Following the successful development of NPs in several adult-based areas of CCAD, in October 2019, Danat al Emarat (DAE) Women's and Children's Hospital in Abu Dhabi became the first hospital in the UAE to employ an ANNP. This was the first hospital outside of CCAD to be granted an NP license. The ANNP role within DAE, like the early NPs in CCAD, faced some challenges to overcome, largely due to the lack of prescribing privileges that stunted the growth of the role. Not being able to prescribe had a significant negative effect on role progression as well as the understanding of the role by healthcare professionals. It leads to a reduction in autonomy for the APN when he or she is required to always seek assistance from a physician to prescribe after making a clinical treatment decision. Ultimately, this causes a reduction in job satisfaction due to the inability to practice to their full capabilities [25].

One of the first NPs in CCAD wrote her thesis on the development of the APN role within CCAD [26]. Questionnaires sent out to nurses and physicians working in CCAD showed a lack of understanding of the role and the privileges NPs should have. Prescribing authority, specifically prescribing controlled medications, caused a lot of different opinions. Ambiguity over role capabilities and a lack of understanding and agreement about what the role entails create barriers to the successful development of the APN role. These findings were similar to those of a systematic review completed in 2016, which was undertaken to generate evidence based on the experiences of doctors, nurses, and patients who had contact with advanced practice nurses working in general practice [27].

In 2021, during the Dubai Expo, a nursing leadership forum was held with senior nurse leaders, educators, and regulators from across the UAE Healthcare system. The challenges faced in developing the APN role in the UAE were discussed at length, with an agreement that leadership collaboration across all healthcare sectors is required to enable the successful development of the APN role.

Burjeel Medical City (BMC), a quaternary care facility within the Burjeel Holdings healthcare group, was the next hospital to employ an ANNP in 2021. This has been a significant success in the extended development of the APN role, with prescribing privileges granted to enable the NP to practice to their full abilities, work as an autonomous practitioner, and provide full holistic care to the most vulnerable patients. The neonatal intensive care unit is now planning to expand its team of ANNPs following the initial success of the role. The only challenge to full role development within BMC has been the inability to see patients in outpatient clinics due to holding a GN (nurses) license number instead of a GD (doctors) license number. This again reflects a lack of understanding of the role and privileging by the UAE insurance market. The same challenge has been encountered in other hospitals employing NPs in the UAE. To move forward and enable NPs to see patients in clinic, it may require input from higher leadership levels to change practices and adapt billing processes.

Within the primary care arena, the role of family nurse practitioner has been a success not just in Abu Dhabi but also in Dubai, with several clinics employing FNPs. This is currently the only NP role within Dubai. There are many clinical nurse specialists in areas such as diabetes care, paediatrics, wound care, and theatres. Now, with the first cohorts of paediatric and intensive care nursing MSc programs completed, we should expect to see a significant rise in CNSs within these areas across the UAE. With the current drive to expand community-based care provision across the UAE, having more FNPs available can only be an advantage for the Emirates, as they are able to effectively manage a multitude of chronic conditions in a safe and cost-effective manner (Fig. 17.1).

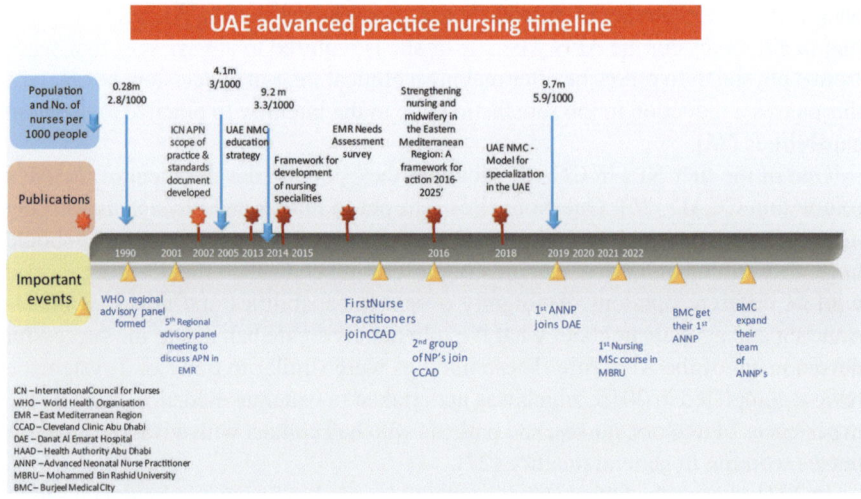

Fig. 17.1 Timeline of advanced practice nursing [13–15, 17, 23]

17.3 The Future of Advanced Practice Nursing in the UAE

The hard work has been done by many organisations to get to this point, where we can now license APNs within the UAE. Now that this is possible, it is the responsibility of nurse and physician leaders across the country to advocate for the role to be developed within their institutions. For those institutions that choose to develop the role of APN within their services, they must take responsibility for defining the role requirements from the beginning, as well as continuing to review the role as it progresses to ensure that it is fit for purpose in the desired areas. If barriers to role progression can be identified before they happen, then their occurrence can be avoided. Evaluation of role development should be shared at a regional level to assist other institutions in their journey toward advanced practice nursing. The International Council of Nurses [5] provides a clear list of considerations to help develop the role effectively with minimal obstacles along the way. These include the provision of a uniform scope of practice, a licencing authority, specific certification requirements, and country-specific regulations. The Department of Health (DOH) in Abu Dhabi has recently produced a Standard on Collaborative Practice Agreement between Physician and Advanced Healthcare Professionals [28]. The purpose of the standard is for NPs and consultant physicians to agree on and sign an agreement detailing the responsibilities of both parties regarding the role of an NP, to ensure the assigned tasks are within the NP's scope of practice, and to streamline the duties and obligations in alignment with the healthcare facility's scope. This is an excellent process when used correctly to support the autonomous working of the NP.

In November 2022, the DOH released the updated scope of practice for nursing; this now includes APNs, with examples given of (but not limited to) nurse practitioners and certified anaesthesia nurses. This document helps to ensure that the role is clear not only to the advanced practitioners but also to other multidisciplinary team members.

Moving forward, despite prescriptive authority now being in the PQR and scope of practice, it is still not being granted across all facilities; this should be a uniform authority for all NPs. The DOH agrees that NPs can prescribe; however, narcotics, psychotropic drugs, and semi-controlled substances are currently not allowed to be prescribed by anyone other than a Physician [29].

Developing a better understanding of the APN role among all stakeholders is vital. A team of nurse leaders and educators, including three nurse practitioners, working in the UAE, began to undertake a research project in 2023 that will survey over 350 senior healthcare leaders, licencing authority administrators, educators, nurse faculty, and medical directors. Field observations of practicing APNs will also be performed. This study aims to identify the challenges confronting APNs integrating into the UAE health system and determine what changes are needed to successfully integrate APNs into the structure or process of care. This should play a significant role in the future development of the APN role within the UAE.

The lack of access to APN courses in the UAE, combined with the license requirement of two years of experience at the APN level, has hindered the number of APNs as hospitals have to rely on bringing experienced staff from abroad to fill posts. Expanding access to nursing master's courses within the UAE will help retain staff and increase the number of APNs working within the region.

Universities have taken the first steps in providing MSc nursing courses, but these will need a non-medical prescribing course to be included as part of the programme in order for students to be licensed as Nurse Practitioners upon completion. This again points to the need for appropriately qualified educators in universities to provide the level of education required. MBRU in Dubai is currently partnered with Queen's University in Ireland to provide the Paediatric MSc course with fully qualified educators; this partnership could provide a pathway for introducing the prescribing module, using educators from Ireland to run the module.

As a country, the UAE has started making some positive steps towards the integration of APN into private healthcare. It is now important to build momentum, with new posts being made available not only across private facilities but also in government facilities. The future of advanced practice nursing is bright, but there will be undoubtedly be challenges to overcome each time a new facility begins its path toward role development.

17.4 Conclusion

The role of the advanced practice nurse within the UAE is still very much in its infancy, but there are notable positive changes now, not only within healthcare institutions employing advanced-level nurses, but also in educational institutions within the Emirates, which are now beginning to offer MSc courses.

For the nurse practitioner role to become more widely accepted as part of healthcare in the UAE, it will take forward-thinking physicians and hospital leaders to change the way they approach medical provisioning. This requires a team approach because simply employing a nurse practitioner does not guarantee the role will flourish; it requires support, guidance, and acceptance of the role from the physicians alongside whom the NP will be working.

The DOH publishing a scope of practice for nursing is an excellent start, especially with the scope including advanced practice nursing with prescriptive authority for all medications other than narcotics and semi-controlled substances. This will hopefully change in time to cover all aspects of prescribing, enabling full autonomy for practitioners working in acute areas such as NICU, ICU, and emergency rooms. Other elements that will require change to further increase the number of nurse practitioners in the UAE include incorporating non-medical prescribing into MSc nursing courses and reviewing the current licencing requirement of two years post-qualified experience at the nurse practitioner level. This will encourage nurses not only to study for advanced qualifications within the UAE but also to stay and work here to build the advanced practice nursing workforce.

Conflicts of Interest The author has no conflicts of interest to declare.

References

1. World Health Organization. Addressing the 18 million health worker shortfall—35 concrete actions and 6 key messages. 2019. Retrieved from https://www.who.int/hrh/news/2019/addressing-18million-hwshortfall-6-key-messages/en/
2. World obesity federation. Global obesity observatory 2022. Retrieved from https://data.worldobesity.org/country/united-arab-emirates-225/
3. British Centres for Business. Education and the UAE's healthcare workforce. 2022. Retrieved from https://bcbuae.com/2022/01/16/education-and-the-uaes-healthcare-workforce/#:~:text=As%20the%20global%20shortage%20of,roughly%2018%20million%20healthcare%20workers
4. Abu Dhabi Government. The Abu Dhabi economic vision. 2009. Retrieved from https://www.actvet.gov.ae/en/Media/Lists/ELibraryLD/economic-vision-2030-full-versionEn.pdf
5. Schober M. International council of nurses, guidelines on advanced practice nursing. 2020. Retrieved from https://ICN_APNReport_EN_WEB.pdf
6. Royal College of Nursing. Advanced Level Nursing Practice: Introduction. 2018. Retrieved from https://www.rcn.org.uk/Professional-Development/publications/pub-006894
7. Machon M. Nursing specialization in the UAE. Conference presentation 2013. Retrieved from http://uaenmc.gov.ae/Data/Conferences/March%202013/Conference/11%20Michelle%20Machon_Nursing%20Specialization%20in%20the%20UAE.pdf
8. AANP. Position paper: Nurse practitioner cost effectiveness. American Association of Nurse Practitioners 2013. Retrieved from https://www.aanp.org/advocacy/advocacy-resource/position-statements/nurse-practitioner-cost-effectiveness
9. Chen C. McNeese-Smith D. Cowan M. Upenieks V. Afifi A. Nursing economics; Pitman. vol. 27, iss. 3, May/Jun 2009;160–8. Retrieved from https://pubmed.ncbi.nlm.nih.gov/19558076/
10. Paez K.A. and Allen J.K. Cost-effectiveness of nurse practitioner management of hypercholesterolemia following coronary revascularization. J Am Acad Nurse Pract, 2006. 18: 436-444. Retrieved from doi:https://doi.org/10.1111/j.1745-7599.2006.00159.x
11. Norwich University Online. The role of the family nurse practitioner in primary care. 2020. Retrieved from https://online.norwich.edu/academic-programs/resources/family-nurse-practitionerrole#:~:text=What%20Does%20a%20Family%20Nurse,a%20patient's%20overall%20well%2Dbeing

12. Murray J. Chief of emergency operations, personal communication, November 12, 2015.
13. Regional Advisory Panel on Nursing. Fifth Meeting of the Regional Advisory Panel on Nursing and consultation on advanced practice nursing and nurse prescribing: Implications for regulation, nursing education and practice in the eastern Mediterranean. 24–26 June 2001. Retrieved from https://apps.who.int/iris/bitstream/handle/10665/254928/who_em_nur_348_e_l_en.pdf?sequence=1&isAllowed=y
14. Al-Darazi F, Advanced A-MM. Practice nursing in the eastern Mediterranean region. Chapter 8. In: Hassmiller SB, Pulcini J, editors. Advanced practice nursing leadership: a global perspective. Springer; 2020.
15. ICN. Definition and characteristics of the role. 2008. Retrieved from https://international.aanp.org/Practice/APNRoles
16. World Health Organization-Eastern Mediterranean Region. Promoting nursing and midwifery development in the Eastern Mediterranean Region. Technical Paper, EM/RC55/5. 2008. Cairo: Regional Office of the Eastern Mediterranean. Retrieved from https://apps.who.int/iris/handle/10665/122665
17. World Health Organization-Eastern Mediterranean Regional Office. Strengthening nursing and midwifery in the Eastern Mediterranean Region—a framework for action 2016–2025. Cairo: World Health Organization; 2016. Retrieved from https://apps.who.int/iris/handle/10665/250372
18. UAE Nursing and Midwifery Council. UAE nursing and midwifery education strategy 2013. Retrieved from http://uaenmc.gov.ae/Data/Files/Education%20Strategy.pdf
19. MBRU. Master of science in pediatric nursing. 2022. Retrieved from https://www.mbru.ac.ae/programs/master-of-science-in-pediatric-nursing/
20. CCAD. Innovative roles attract UAE nationals to nursing careers. 2017. Retrieved from https://www.clevelandclinicabudhabi.ae/en/media-center/news/innovative-roles-attract-uae-national-to-nursing-careers
21. Miller N, NP in Cleveland Clinic Abu Dhabi. Personal email correspondence, 6th October 2022.
22. Steinke MK. Rogers M. Lehwaldt D. Lamarche K. An examination of advanced practice nurses' job satisfaction internationally. Int Nurs Rev 2018 65(2):162–172. Retrieved from https://pubmed.ncbi.nlm.nih.gov/28657146/
23. UAE Nursing and Midwifery Council. Model for Nursing and Midwifery specialization in the UAE. 2018. Retrieved from http://www.uaenmc.gov.ae/Data/Files/MODEL%20FOR%20NURSING%20AND%20MIDWIFERY%20SPECIALIZATION%20IN%20THE%20UNITED%20ARAB%20EMIRATES.pdf
24. International Council of Nurses. Scope of practice for a specialty nurse: ICN framework of competencies for the nurse specialist. Geneva: International Council of Nurses. 2009. Retrieved from https://siga-fsia.ch/files/user_upload/08_ICN_Framework_for_the_nurse_specialist.pdf
25. De Milt D.G. Fitzpatrick J.J. and McNulty S.R. (2011) Nurse practitioners' job satisfaction and intent to leave current positions, the nursing profession, and the nurse practitioner role as a direct care provider. J Am Acad Nurse Pract, 23: 42–50. Retrieved from https://onlinelibrary.wiley.com/doi/10.1111/j.1745-7599.2010.00570.x.
26. Miller N. Establishing an evidence-based educational framework for the implementation of the role of the APN-NP into Abu Dhabi. Thesis, Vanderbilt University School of Nursing.
27. Jakimowicz M, Williams D, Stankiewicz G. A systematic review of experiences of advanced practice nursing in general practice. BMC Nurs. 2017;16(1):1–12.
28. DOH (2023) Standard on collaborative practice agreement between physician and advanced healthcare professionals. Department of Health. Retrieved from https://www.doh.gov.ae/en/resources/standards.
29. DOH Standard for the management of narcotics, psychotropic and semi controlled medicinal products. June 2021. Retrieved from https://www.doh.gov.ae/-/media/8F268D5B4B074905AF42644F6D08DC17.ashx

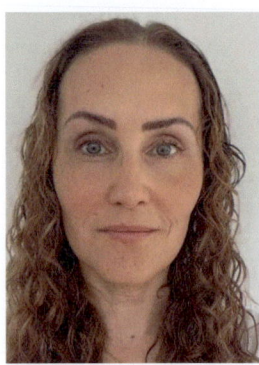

Katie Hanafin is an Advanced Neonatal Nurse Practitioner. After qualifying as a paediatric nurse at City University London, she began her career in a Special Care Baby Unit in the Northeast of England, working as a staff nurse. A year later, she moved to a busy Neonatal Intensive Care Unit in North Tees Hospital, where she worked as a bedside NICU nurse for 10 years. During this time, she completed many university courses, including the Neonatal Intensive Care degree module, Mentorship in Practice, and Independent Non-medical Prescribing, before pursuing her dream of becoming an advanced nurse practitioner in 2014 at Southampton University.

After successful completion of an MSc in Advanced Neonatal Care, Katie began to work within the medical roster at North Tees NICU, where she stayed until 2019, when she moved, along with her family, to Abu Dhabi to become the first neonatal nurse practitioner in the UAE.

Carving out a new role in a private healthcare system has been very successful. Katie not only enjoys the clinical side of her role but also nursing education, and participating in and leading research studies.

Open Access This chapter is licensed under the terms of the Creative Commons Attribution 4.0 International License (http://creativecommons.org/licenses/by/4.0/), which permits use, sharing, adaptation, distribution and reproduction in any medium or format, as long as you give appropriate credit to the original author(s) and the source, provide a link to the Creative Commons license and indicate if changes were made.

The images or other third party material in this chapter are included in the chapter's Creative Commons license, unless indicated otherwise in a credit line to the material. If material is not included in the chapter's Creative Commons license and your intended use is not permitted by statutory regulation or exceeds the permitted use, you will need to obtain permission directly from the copyright holder.

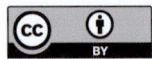

Primary Health Care in the UAE

18

Maha Al Fahim, Ebtihal Darwish,
and Farah Saeed Mohammad Al-Zaabi

18.1 Introduction

Primary health care (PHC) provides integrated preventive, health promotion, curative, and palliative healthcare services, addressing individuals' physical, mental, and social health across the lifespan [1]. In contrast to specialist-focused health services, primary health care encompasses a generalist, patient- or family-centered approach that includes the treatment of common illnesses and conditions, preventive care, health promotion, chronic disease management, and coordinated care with specialty and adjunct health services [2]. In keeping with evidence demonstrating the association between a strong primary healthcare system and better patient and population health outcomes, as well as increased health equity and greater cost efficiency in healthcare systems, the World Health Organization and many governments around the world have advocated for the development of a primary health care-driven health system [1–6]. The United Arab Emirates' (UAE) Ministry of Health and Prevention, Abu Dhabi's Department of Health, and the Dubai Health

---

M. Al Fahim (✉)
Family Medicine & Chair, Education Institute, Abu Dhabi, United Arab Emirates

Khalifa University, Abu Dhabi, United Arab Emirates
e-mail: maalfahim@seha.ae

E. Darwish
Ethraa for Consultation and Training, Dubai, United Arab Emirates

Unilabs Middle East, Dubai, United Arab Emirates
e-mail: ebtihal.darwish@gmail.com

F. S. M. Al-Zaabi
Abu Dhabi, United Arab Emirates

UAEU College of Medicine, Al Ain, United Arab Emirates
e-mail: farah.alzaabi@mod.gov.ae

Authority have all formally stated that primary health care is the cornerstone model upon which the healthcare system and healthcare policy are built [7–9].

This chapter profiles PHC in the UAE. Following a brief overview of relevant demographics in the UAE, major primary care statistics and a history of PHC in the UAE are presented. The Donabedian Model [10] provides a framework for evaluating the quality of the PHC system by examining its structure, process, and outcomes in the UAE. Primary care research, as well as primary care education and training, are discussed. Challenges and advantages related to PHC are analyzed. Finally, the chapter addresses the likely future of PHC in the UAE.

18.2 Demographics

The current population of the UAE is 9,441,990 (Table 18.1), based on projections of the latest United Nations data (2022) [78]. Driven by rapid economic expansion and labor migration, the UAE population expanded rapidly in the first few decades following its formation in 1971, with annual growth rates reaching double digits in the 1970s and 1980s, and reaching a robust 7.92% annual growth rate as recently as 2005 [11] (Table 18.2).

Fig. 18.1 shows the UAE population pyramid for 2022 [79]. The UAE has an unusual demographic profile and population pyramid, as the majority of the population falls in the adult (20–65 years) male group, which represents the immigration of labor into the country. According to most estimates, UAE nationals comprise only 10–12% of the total population [11]. The UAE has one of the highest net migration rates in the world, with the majority of new migrants being young and male. The UAE has the world's highest male/female gender imbalance of 2.2 male:female overall and 2.75 male: female in the 15- to 65-year-old age group, which also accounts for nearly 80% of the total population [11] (Figs. 18.1 and 18.2).

The UAE's fertility rate is relatively low, at 1.42 births per woman [78]. The fertility rate in the UAE has been declining rapidly, causing concern for the

Table 18.1 The UAE's important demographic indicators

Total population	9,441,990
Population rank	97
Growth rate	0.81%
World percentage	0.12%
Land area	83,600 km^2
Density	113/km^2
Birth per day	51
Death per day	10
Total male[a]	6,826,000
Total female[a]	3,054,000
Life expectancy at birth, average, years[a]	78.1
Life expectancy at birth, male, years[a]	77.4
Life expectancy at birth, female, years[a]	79.5

[a] [12] estimated in 2020
Source: World population review [78]

Table 18.2 Population number based on city

City	Population
Dubai	2,956,587
Sharjah	1,324,473
Abu Dhabi	603,492
Ajman City	490,035
Ras Al Khaimah City	351,943
Musaffah	243,341
Al Fujairah City	86,512
Khalifah A City	85,374
Reef Al Fujairah City	82,310
Bani Yas City	80,498

Source: World population review [78]

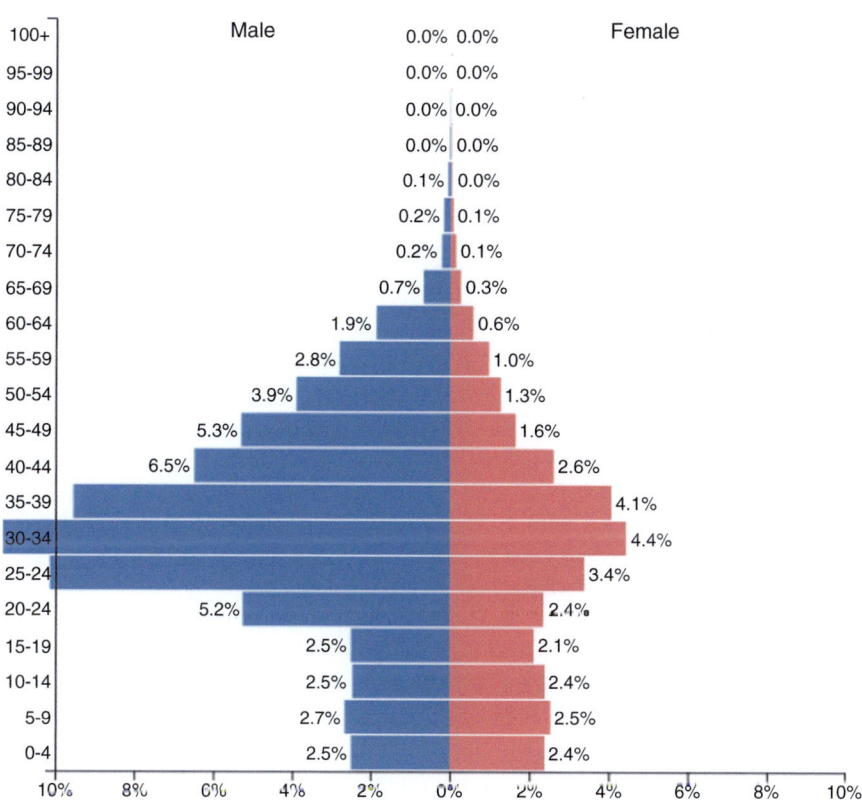

Fig. 18.1 The UAE's population pyramid 2022. (Source: Population Pyramids of the World from 1950 to 2100 [79])

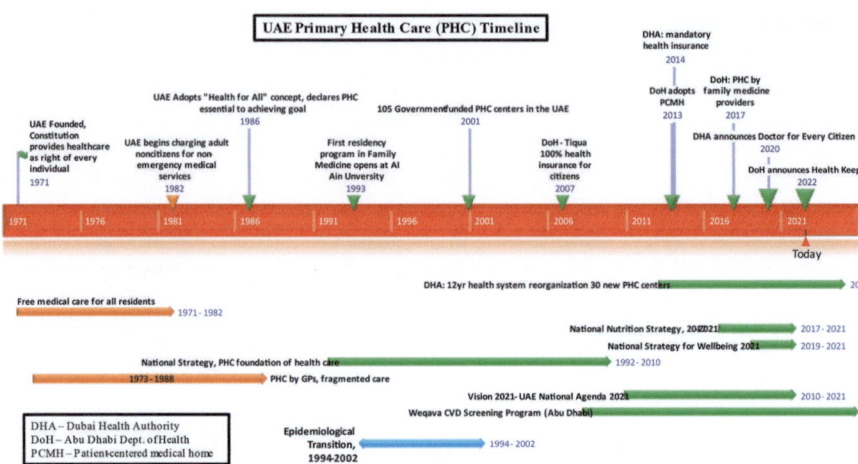

Fig. 18.2 Timeline of primary health care in the UAE. The figure illustrates major milestones, strategies, policies, and programs in the history and development of PHC in the UAE. Author-created figure. Sources of information included in the figure are cited within the discussion of PHC history in the UAE

government. The UAE government has adopted policies, such as helping young married people financially, to encourage childbearing among its citizens. The median age was 32.6 for 2020, but it is expected to increase if the fertility rate does not rise [78].

The UAE witnessed a significant increase in the population of foreigners during the past decade because of major growth in various economic sectors. More than 200 nationalities live in the UAE for work and/or education. After growing by over five million people from 2000 to 2010, population growth in the UAE has slowed significantly. The population currently stands at nine million people, and is projected to continue growing until 2033, when it will reach its peak at 10.7 million people. The population is then expected to decline very slowly and plateau, ending the twenty-first century with about nine million people [78].

18.3 Primary Healthcare Statistics

Primary health care in the UAE provides the first point of contact with the national healthcare system for individuals, families, and the community. PHC, as it was first established in the early years of UAE independence, focused on the provision of basic vaccination- and screening-oriented preventive health care, as well as immediate, repeat, and regular care related to infections, injuries, and chronic conditions [15]. After 1986 and the decision to endorse the World Health Organization's "Health for All" mandate, PHC in the UAE moved toward a more comprehensive model of primary care that envisioned PHC as the foundation of the national health system and the access point for individuals, families, and communities to obtain preventive, curative, promotive, and rehabilitative health services [16].

By the late twentieth century, the UAE was counted among the world's high-income countries. The rates of parasitic and other common infectious diseases had fallen dramatically, as had key health indicators such as those pertaining to child and infant mortality [17]. For example, between 1990 and 2019, deaths per 1000 live births for infants under age one dropped from 16.8 to 3.9, while deaths per 1000 for children under age five dropped from 21.6 in 1990 to 5.3 in 2019 [13]. Instead of infectious diseases, the primary cause of death and disability in the UAE was, like in the rest of the developed world, non-communicable diseases [18]. The UAE had completed its epidemiological transition [6, 19]. As of 2020, non-communicable diseases (NCDs) accounted for 77% of deaths in the UAE [20]. By 2012, the total burden of disease attributable to NCDs was 65.2%, while communicable diseases accounted for 11.5% of the burden of disease, and injuries (with road injuries being the largest single category in this group) accounted for the remaining 23.2% of the disease burden [21]. More recent studies indicate that NCDs now account for nearly 70% of the total burden of disease in the UAE [18].

The PHC sector in the UAE provides preventive, curative, promotional, rehabilitative, and coordinated health care services for patients with conditions across the entire disease burden spectrum. Based on comprehensive data through 2019, no communicable or infectious diseases rank in the UAE's top ten causes of death or top ten causes of death and disability (DALYs) [13, 18]. PHC plays an important role in ensuring that the total disease burden from communicable and infectious illnesses remains less than 10%. The PHC sector coordinates with public health authorities and government-based population health policies and measures related to surveillance, immunization, and post-exposure treatment to prevent infectious disease outbreaks or re-emergence and to respond to newly emerging infectious diseases, including COVID-19 [19, 22]. The UAE has a national control program for major infectious diseases, including HIV, viral hepatitis, and tuberculosis [21]. Screening for communicable diseases is typically required for expatriate workers seeking employment in the UAE, individuals seeking residency status, and all persons in certain occupational categories, including healthcare workers, cooks, maids, and drivers [19]. The UAE's national immunization program for children targeting vaccine-preventable diseases has historically been very successful in achieving immunization rates in excess of 90% [21].

Although communicable and parasitic diseases are no longer a major health concern in the UAE, the UAE health authorities and the PHC sector must be alert to threats from new and emerging communicable diseases. In the wake of the COVID-19 pandemic, coronavirus disease became a leading cause of death and disability in some subpopulations. It is unlikely that COVID-19 will account for a significant portion of the UAE population's disease burden in the period 2020–2022. On January 29, 2020, the UAE became the first country in the Middle East to register a case of COVID-19, and in March 2020, the UAE became one of the first countries in the world to implement strict measures (e.g., travel bans, curfews, school closures, mask requirements) to control the pandemic [23]. To date, the number of cases has been low, and with only a small number of deaths so far, the UAE has one of the lowest COVID-19 case-fatality rates (0.26) in the world [24]. With 248 cases per million population (versus 601 in Kuwait, 1023 in Oman, 2718 in the UK, and 2045 in the USA), the UAE has the lowest COVID case rate in the region and one of the lowest rates in the world [25]. At the same time, high rates of obesity and diabetes among the UAE population have raised concerns that UAE COVID-19 patients may have a high risk of disease severity [23, 26]. The availability of effective treatments and an aggressive national vaccination program administered through the UAE National Emergency Crisis and Disaster Management Authority relies on the support of the PHC sector to help manage the UAE's ongoing response to the threat posed by COVID-19 [22, 27].

Injuries, which once accounted for about 23% of the UAE's burden of disease [21], now account for an estimated 12–14% of the disease burden in the UAE [18]. Road injuries account for about two-thirds of injury-related deaths in the UAE [19]. In 2009, road injuries were the leading cause of death in the UAE [13]. Between 2009 and 2019, the total number of road injury-related deaths in the UAE increased by 18.2%, a percentage change slightly above the 16.4% increase in the UAE population during that decade but not sufficient to outpace ischemic heart disease, which replaced road injuries as the leading cause of death in the UAE in 2019 [13]. Other major causes of injury-related death in the UAE include suicide, which ranked as the seventh leading cause of death in 2009 and the tenth leading cause of death in 2019, and falls, which ranked as the ninth leading cause of death in 2009 and the twelfth leading cause of death in 2019 [13]. Other injury-related causes of death included drowning, fire-related, poisoning, occupational injuries, medical injuries, environmental-related accidents, and homicide [19]. Across all injury categories, males in the UAE are much more likely to suffer an injury-related death, with the male:female injury ratio reported at 1.78 [19].

Non-communicable diseases and conditions currently account for almost 77% of all deaths and the majority of the death and disability (DALY) burden in the UAE [20]. The list of leading non-communicable disease causes of death and disability in the UAE is dominated by cardiovascular disease (CVD) and, to a somewhat lesser extent, metabolic disorders [17]. CVD, which is the biggest contributor to non-communicable diseases worldwide, includes a range of conditions affecting the heart and blood vessels, including ischemic heart disease or coronary artery disease (CAD), stroke, hypertensive heart disease, inflammatory heart diseases, and heart failure [28]. CVD emerged as a major health problem in the UAE as soon as the country completed its epidemiological transition, with rates of CVD burden significantly outpacing those in other Gulf Cooperative Council Countries (GCC) as well as those in the USA and the UK [29]. As of 2019, three CVD diseases—ischemic heart disease, stroke, and hypertensive heart disease—ranked as the first, third, and seventh leading causes of death in the UAE [13]. Ischemic heart disease and stroke ranked as the second and third leading causes of all-age combined death and disability in the UAE in 2019, while ischemic heart disease, stroke, and hypertensive heart disease ranked as the first, third, and seventh leading causes, respectively, of age-standardized death and disability in 2019 [13].

Diabetes and chronic kidney disease (CKD), which are often comorbid with CVD, also figure prominently in the UAE's disease burden. Diabetes was the fifth leading cause of death and the second leading cause of age-standardized death and disability in 2019, while CKD was the fourth leading cause of death and the fifth leading cause of age-standardized death and disability in 2019 [13]. Pancreatic cancer, which ranked as the 17th leading cause of death in the UAE in 2009, was the ninth leading cause of death in 2019 and the only cancer to make the top ten leading causes of death [13]. Alarmingly, according to UAE epidemiologists, deaths from pancreatic cancer increased by 241% between 2009 and 2019 [17]. Deaths from pancreatic cancer, which is a particularly deadly form of cancer, have been increasing globally over the past two decades, with the rise in cases and deaths especially noticeable in high-income countries [30]. There is a well-established association between diabetes and pancreatic cancer, and recent research studies have provided high-quality evidence that pancreatic cancer deaths can be mainly attributed to smoking, high fasting plasma glucose, and obesity [30]. Chronic obstructive pulmonary disease (COPD) was the fifth leading cause of death in both 2009 and 2019, while drug use disorders ranked as the eighth leading cause of death in 2009 and 2019 [13]. Other disorders that were not included among the leading causes of death in the UAE in 2019 but were included among the leading causes of death and disability were depressive disorders, headache disorders, and low-back pain [17].

The preventive care and health promotion mandate of PHC requires the identification of risk factors associated with the leading causes of death and disability. Risks may be behavioral, metabolic, or environmental and may be modifiable or non-modifiable. Globally, risk factors for disease and/or injury-related deaths vary based on social and economic development as well as the socio-demographic characteristics of the population [18, 20]. The top four risk factors driving the most death and disability combined in the UAE in both 2009 and 2019 were obesity, high blood pressure, tobacco use, and high fasting blood glucose [13] (Table 18.3).

Table 18.3 Leading causes of death, death and disability, and risk factors for death and disability in the UAE in 2019

Rank	Cause of death	Cause of death/disability combined (all age)	Risk factors
1	Ischemic heart disease	Road injuries	Obesity (high BMI)
2	Road injuries	Ischemic heart disease	High blood pressure
3	Stroke	Stroke	Tobacco use
4	Chronic kidney disease	Diabetes	High fasting blood glucose
5	Diabetes	Low back pain	High LDL cholesterol
6	COPD	Depressive disorders	Air pollution
7	Hypertensive heart disease	Drug use disorders	Dietary risks
8	Drug use disorders	Headache disorders	Kidney dysfunction
9	Pancreatic cancer	Chronic kidney disease	Drug use
10	Self-harm/suicide	COPD	Occupational risk

Source: Author-created table, compiled from Institute of Health Metrics Evaluation global burden of disease data analytics [13]

18.4 History and Timeline of PHC in the UAE

The UAE's Constitution established health care as a right of every individual and conferred on the government the responsibility to provide healthcare facilities that would offer free medical care to all UAE residents [15, 31]. While free, medical care during the first decades after the country's founding was fragmented and of varying quality, with primary care delivered mainly by general practitioners who were trained in non-Western medical schools [31]. The rapid expansion of the expatriate population and the rising demand for services overwhelmed government resources, and in 1982, the UAE government announced that it would begin charging non-citizens for medical services, except for emergency and child and maternal services, which would continue to be provided at no charge [31].

The UAE government made a significant commitment to the PHC model in 1986. Ministerial decree no. 139/86 declared the UAE's adoption of the World Health Organization's (WHO) "Health for All" declaration from the 1978 Alma-Ata Conference that supported primary health care as a human right [15]. In 1992, the UAE National Strategy formalized the foundational role of PHC in the UAE health system, defining PHC as a comprehensive and integrated health service and requiring individuals to receive referrals from PHC to receive secondary or tertiary services [15]. In 1993, the UAE's first residency program in Family Medicine was established at Al Ain University [5]. The UAE's deliberate strategy to develop a strong PHC system as the foundation of its healthcare infrastructure included a plan to rely on certified family medicine practitioners rather than general practitioners (GPs), and a vision of PHC as an integrated, comprehensive service providing preventive, curative, promotive, and rehabilitative care [5]. By 2001, the UAE had established 105 dedicated PHC centers across the country [31] (Fig. 18.2).

The drive to develop and improve the quality and coverage of the PHC was fueled by rising expectations amid rapid economic development and increasing wealth [32]. PHC system development also occurred in conjunction with the UAE's epidemiological transition and the increasing need to address healthcare needs associated with non-communicable diseases [19, 33]. In 2006, the Abu Dhabi Ministry of Health (MoH) mandated health insurance coverage, thus guaranteeing access to healthcare for all expatriates [34]. The following year, the MoH introduced *Thiqa* (Trust), a health insurance system providing 100% coverage to all UAE nationals in the Emirate [34]. Significant advances in integrating preventive health in PHC occurred in April 2008 with the inauguration of the Abu Dhabi-based *Weqaya* (prevention) Program that provides screening for cardiovascular disease risk factors [29]. In 2010, the UAE national government announced its Vision 2021 strategy, which was further developed and combined in 2014 into the Vision 2021/UAE National Agenda 2021 strategy. This strategy included the objective of achieving a globally competitive health system by the year 2021 [6].

From 2010 to 2022, national and Emirate-level health authorities took several steps to further strengthen the UAE's PHC system [7]. In 2013, Dubai Health Authority (DHA) announced a 12-year plan to reorganize the health system and create 40 new PHC centers [14]. Also in 2013, the Abu Dhabi MoH announced the system-wide adoption of the patient-centered medical home (PCMH) model [35,

36]. In 2014, the DHA announced mandatory health insurance [14]. A number of prevention-focused initiatives were launched in the late 2010s, including the 2017–2021 National Nutrition Strategy and the National Strategy for Wellbeing 2021 that was initiated in 2019 [34]. In December 2017, the Abu Dhabi DoH announced that in the future, primary care would be offered only by licensed family medicine departments and clinics [37]. Furthering the advancement of health informatics, in July 2019, the DoH announced the establishment of an electronic medical records central database [34]. In 2020, responding to the challenges of delivering health care during the COVID-19 pandemic and taking advantage of advances in telemedicine technologies, the DHA announced the launch of its Doctor for Every Citizen mobile health app for UAE nationals to receive free, remote telemedicine consultations from qualified health experts 24/7 [38]. Finally, in July 2022, the Abu Dhabi DoH announced the introduction of a New Primary Care Model to be implemented over the next 5 years [8]. The new patient-centered model will include a "Health Keeper" component that allows individuals to select a primary healthcare provider and receive ongoing care from that provider.

18.5 Structure of Primary Health Care

The structure of PHC in the UAE, while much more defined than in the twentieth century, is still developing and varies between emirates, reflecting the fact that it is not a single system but instead a national system combined with emirate-based systems, with Dubai and Abu Dhabi exerting primary authority over their health systems [6]. PHC is delivered at government-based PHC centers as well as hundreds of private clinics and departments. Throughout the UAE, there is adherence to a model that places PHC at the center of an integrated, holistic system. While there are an insufficient number of certified family medicine doctors to provide PHC at all clinics and centers, UAE health authorities have endorsed the family medicine doctor rather than the GP doctor as the appropriate provider of PHC (Table 18.4).

Table 18.4 Structure of PHC in the UAE health system

PHC element or aspect	Description
Healthcare authorities [39, 40]	Ministry of Health and Prevention (MoHAP) (federal): (primary responsibility for the five northern emirates, national oversight, emirates health services establishment (EHS), national preventive health programs, public health oversight, research, and statistics).
	Dubai Health Authority (DHA) (emirate) (regulates 2 health insurance companies, health policy, and health services in Dubai, including in 2 free zones).
	Health Authority of Abu Dhabi (HAAD) (Abu Dhabi Department of Health) (emirate) (regulates 3 health insurance companies, healthcare services in the emirate, oversight for SEHA, a public joint stock company that operates public healthcare assets, health policies).
	Sharjah Health Authority (SHA) (emirate) (manages Sharjah Healthcare City (SHCC), manages health insurance for Sharjah government employees and dependents; coordinates with WHO on Sharjah healthy City).

(continued)

Table 18.4 (continued)

PHC element or aspect	Description
Where PHC delivered [7, 9, 33, 37, 41]	Government primary health Care centers, private clinics, primary care departments of hospitals (private/public), ambulatory healthcare services, school-based clinics, occupational clinics
Number of UAE PHC centers and providers, 2019 [7]	Government PHC Centers: 149 UAE-wide (66 Abu Dhabi, 20 Dubai, 23 Sharjah, 5 Ajman, 4 U.A.Q., 18 R.A.K., 13 Fujairah). Private PHC clinics: 4547 UAE-wide (1152 Abu Dhabi, 1963 Dubai, 801 Sharjah, 231 Ajman, 41 U.A.Q, 224 R.A.K., 135 Fujairah).
Who delivers PHC [7, 8, 34, 42–44]	Family Medicine physicians, general practitioners (GPs), some internal medicine, pediatric physicians; nurses (mainly assisting or supervised)
Physicians per 10,000 population, various categories, recent estimates	Medical doctors (MDs) per 10,000 UAE population, 2019: 27.0 [45] (comparator: UK, 58.23 per 10,000; USA, 26.1; Saudi Arabia, 27.3) MDs per 10,000 population, Dubai Emirate, 2018: 29.0 [14] Primary care MDs per 10,000 UAE population, 2017: 2.3 [3] Family medicine MDs per 10,000 UAE population, 2015: 0.16 [46]
PHC services	Core full PHC services (at most government PHC centers): Maternal and child care, preventive care (risk and disease screening, immunizations, preventive treatments), acute care, chronic care, diabetes clinics, patient education, health and wellness, consultation on complex conditions, referrals to specialty care as needed, care coordination, laboratory, pharmacy, nutrition/dietary [8, 9, 36, 37, 47–49] Expanded/specialty PHC services (at limited number of PHC centers): Geriatric care, substance use screening/treatment, behavioral/mental health, adolescent health, complementary and alternative medicine, 24-h and emergency services [7, 34, 50–54]
Model of care (planned/ideal) [7, 8, 33, 39, 46]	PHC as foundation for health system and integrated care Patient-centered care Family Medicine versus GP directed Patient-centered medical home Health and wellness focused
Healthcare information technology	Limited health information technology regulatory system, including patient privacy protections [55, 56] Progress in implementing electronic medical record in Abu Dhabi [34, 57] Telemedicine widespread and expanding, including m-health [38, 58, 59]

Funding	UAE healthcare expenditure, 5.4% of GDP in 2020, forecast 6.4% by 2030 [12]
	Primary care-related targeted spending areas in National Strategy [7]:
	    Tobacco use reduction and prevention
	    Obesity control and prevention
	    Wellness promotion and happiness
	    Workforce development
	    Quality improvement

18.6 Processes of Primary Care in the UAE

PHC, as it has developed in the UAE, has moved firmly toward a patient-centered, integrative care model that includes a family medicine primary care physician (PCP) serving as the care coordinator, gatekeeper, and primary caregiver/care director who takes into account not only evidence-based medicine but also patient preferences and input in medical decision-making [6, 18, 33, 48]. The processes in contemporary PHC in the UAE derive from the objectives and components of the patient-centered integrative model and the health needs and preferences of the UAE population. Moreover, the processes are affected by factors such as available resources, the structure of care, budget or funding, and supportive infrastructure, including regulatory frameworks [14, 48].

In the aftermath of the completion of the epidemiological transition in the UAE, the PHC health services processes increasingly focus on chronic care, chronic disease management, and prevention and health promotion services. These services focus on the diseases and conditions that are the leading causes of death and disability, and thus there is a focus on chronic care services for diabetes, cardiovascular diseases, COPD, depressive disorders, chronic kidney disease, and others [29, 49, 60–63]. In addition to direct care and management for chronic diseases, processes associated with chronic disease management include patient education in disease self-management, such as glucose monitoring, diet, weight, and exercise for diabetes control [49]. Prevention and risk reduction processes are closely related to chronic disease management processes. These processes include patient screening for disease and disease risk, as well as focused risk reduction, disease prevention, and health promotion programs [28, 29, 64, 65]. A number of recent preventive health and risk reduction programs in the UAE have focused on reducing and preventing obesity in population groups with high obesity rates, including women and adolescents [53, 66–68]. Another major risk reduction, health promotion, and disease prevention effort has focused on reducing tobacco smoking in the population, particularly among the two groups with the highest smoking rates: adult males (15.7% versus 2.4% of adult females) and adolescent males (11.3%) [69]. The PHC sector works closely with public health authorities in the UAE to implement primary prevention programs, including childhood, adolescent, and adult vaccination and immunization programs [7, 14]. The COVID-19 pandemic was also associated with a range of preventive health processes for PHC, including efforts to promote COVID-19 vaccination and COVID-19 prevention and mitigation processes for vulnerable groups, such as the elderly [27, 70].

Although many PHC direct care processes involve chronic diseases and chronic disease prevention, PHC in the UAE remains the first response and contact for population needs related to acute care, including care for routine injuries and illnesses, rapid response to symptom emergence and referral to appropriate specialist care, and response to new and emerging diseases, including COVID-19 and Monkeypox. By the end of 2020, UAE primary care providers were conducting the majority of COVID-19 testing, care, and follow-up [22, 26, 71]. As a result of the COVID-19 pandemic and the need to take mitigating steps to prevent transmission, PHC dramatically expanded its involvement in processes related to telemedicine [59].

In addition to preventive, curative, promotive, and rehabilitative care processes, PHC is also involved in processes related to quality improvement and system development within the PHC sector. Quality improvement processes include efforts to improve the quality and efficiency of physician-patient communications, the examination of factors affecting patient satisfaction and dissatisfaction, and various process improvement projects [32, 51, 60, 72, 73]. Other process improvement efforts have involved physician use of electronic medical records systems, physician overprescribing practices, and physician knowledge and practice concerning COVID-19 among PHC workers [14, 57, 59, 71].

18.7 Primary Care Research

Policies, strategies, and operational plans should be informed by the best available evidence of what works and what does not; operational research is key to providing this. This includes research on interventions that support all components of the PHC approach, strategies to engage people in their own care and in service design, self-management of common health problems, the substitution of professionals, and the transfer of care responsibilities along integrated care pathways. By its very nature, PHC research will need to consider complex interventions involving multiple policies and services [1].

Several UAE institutes have placed significant emphasis on PHC-based research to guide PHC policies and strategies, including health authorities, research foundations, and universities. In order to promote the culture of research among PHC doctors, health institutes have made it mandatory for family and community medicine residents to conduct and publish research during their training years.

UAE universities are increasingly conducting innovative medical research. For instance, the University of Sharjah created the Research Institute of Medical and Health Sciences, which seeks to help make the university a national and international leader in biomedical and health sciences. Its research focuses on many aspects of medicine, including clinical epidemiology and health policy. Moreover, NYU Abu Dhabi has created the Public Health Research Center (PHRC), which seeks to identify environmental and genetic determinants of health problems in Abu Dhabi and develop and test new public health interventions to promote wellness in the emirate [14].

Meanwhile, several dedicated medical research centers have emerged in the country. In March 2017, the Thumbay Research Institute for Precision Medicine and Translational Research opened on the site of Gulf Medical University to conduct postgraduate research, particularly on diabetes and cancer. The Thumbay Institute of Population Health focuses on research in the fields of public health, epidemiology, evidence-based medicine, big data analysis, and global health [14].

The Mohammed Bin Rashid Medical Research Institute, an initiative of the Al Jalila Foundation, is a world-class biomedical research institute strategically located in the heart of Dubai Healthcare City next to the Mohammed Bin Rashid Academic

Medical Center, which houses the Mohammed Bin Rashid University of Medicine and Health Sciences, ensuring seamless collaboration in the academic, healthcare, and scientific communities. It is the UAE's first independent multidisciplinary medical research center and aims to bring together leading local and international scientists to work together to discover solutions for the region's biggest health challenges: cancer, cardiovascular disease, diabetes, obesity, and mental health. In April 2020, the Al Jalila Foundation expanded its research portfolio in response to the novel coronavirus (COVID-19) outbreak with dedicated research grants to address the pandemic and infectious diseases [14].

In addition, the UAE was one of the 26 participating countries in the PURE study (PROSPECTIVE URBAN AND RURAL EPIDEMIOLOGICAL STUDY), which has been ongoing since 2005, aiming to examine the impact of urbanization on the development of primordial risk factors (e.g., physical activity and nutrition changes), primary risk factors (e.g., obesity, hypertension, dysglycemia, and dyslipidemia, smoking), and cardiovascular diseases. It is an observational 20-year study that has involved many family physicians in the Dubai Health Authority. As of 2022, The PURE study had 66 international publications in several PURE study areas.

The UAE adopted several research collaborations to improve clinical research in the country, including:

- *Harvard International Medicine* and the government of Dubai founded the Dubai Harvard Foundation for Medical Research to support cutting-edge collaborative research and establish sustainable research and education programs focused on diseases relevant to the MENA region. In January 2015, it formed the Harvard Medical School Center for Global Health Delivery-Dubai in Dubai Healthcare City. This institution is mandated to address regional health issues through research, medical education, and training, through which hundreds of family physicians and public health specialists have been trained in clinical research [14].
- *New York University Abu Dhabi (NYU Abu Dhabi)* announced the launch of the "UAE Healthy Future Study" in early 2017, which is a long-term study of 20,000 Emiratis to better understand the risk factors of obesity, diabetes, and heart disease. The study is being conducted in collaboration with SEHA, Zayed Military Hospital, UAE University, Zayed University, Khalifa University, EBTIC, Healthpoint, Capital Health Screening Center, and Daman [14].
- *The Medtronic Foundation* gave a two-year $100,000 Health Access Grant to the Al Jalila Foundation in February 2017 to fund a local research program focusing on Vitamin D deficiency across the country. The grant allowed the Al Jalila Foundation to promote early detection and prevention of the disease [14].

18.8 Education and Training

Family medicine has been recognized as an essential specialty to improve the quality of primary health care, which has led to the evolution of family medicine residency training programs across different emirates in the UAE. The UAE's education program for family medicine began in 1993 with the launch of the Family Medicine

Residency Program, first in Dubai (through the Dubai Health Authority's residency training program) and then extended to Al Ain (1994), Abu Dhabi (1997), Sharjah, and the Northern Emirates [5]. The family medicine program was the UAE's first post-graduate medical residency program [75] and is recognized by the Arab Board of Medical Specializations. There are currently 34 centers that are accredited by the Arab Board of Medical Specializations in the UAE. Four of these centers are in Abu Dhabi, nine in Al Ain, ten in Dubai, four in Sharjah, three in Ras Al Khaimah, one in Ajman, and three in Fujairah. This accreditation allows the centers to train a specified number of physicians who will eventually be eligible to take the Family Medicine Board examinations after successfully completing the required training.

The program is 4 years in duration; residents spend the first 3 years of the program primarily in hospital rotations through various specialties, and the final year in PHC centers and clinics. However, residents are required to spend at least 1 day per week in a PHC clinic throughout the first 3 years of training to establish their family medicine continuity clinics. The Arab Board examinations consist of two parts: a written component (Part I) and a clinical skills examination (Part II). The examination is prepared by the Arab Council of Medical Specializations and is unified and then taken at the same time across all Arab countries in accredited centers. This qualification allows the graduates to practice across the UAE as Family Medicine Specialists. After completing the required years of practice, which differ according to the Emirate, specialist physicians can apply for consultant licenses. The goal of these residency programs is to provide UAE self-sufficiency through skilled family physicians who practice with high professionalism and proper ethical standards. Graduates of these programs are primary healthcare specialists who are capable of practicing medicine independently according to international standards. Moreover, the programs aim to train family physicians who can successfully compete for advanced fellowship training positions. These well-structured family medicine programs enabled the graduates to reach high clinical, administrative, leadership, and academic positions. During its first 25 years, the family medicine residency training programs in the UAE produced more than 300 UAE citizen-certified family practitioners to work in UAE PHC [76]. The residency programs in Abu Dhabi and Al Ain managed by Sheikh Khalifa Medical City and Ambulatory Healthcare Services further achieved accreditation through the Accreditation Council for Graduate Medical Education International (ACGME-I) in 2013. The program at Zayed Military Hospital archived the same accreditation in 2021.

In 2020, the emerging need to create the UAE National Board Examination materialized through the National Institute of Health Specialization (NIHS)—Emirati Board, which is aligned with the competency-based medical education model and is a significant step toward improving quality and outcomes in residency education.

Interest in further education and fellowships among primary care physicians has grown over the past decade. This increased demand has encouraged various local universities and international organizations to provide a range of programs. iHeed, an Irish-based organization operating in the UAE, has become the frontrunner in providing further training for primary care physicians in the country. They offer access to a full range of online postgraduate qualifications that are accredited by prestigious UK and Irish universities. These include master's and diplomas across Diabetes Care, Public Health, Medical Education, Healthcare Leadership, and Clinical Research with the University of Warwick, and Pediatrics, Women's Health, Medicine for the Older Person, Dermatology, and Infectious Diseases with the Royal College of Physicians of Ireland (RCPI). Over the last five years, over 180 physicians have enrolled from across the UAE. Furthermore, in collaboration with the Dubai Health Authority and the Irish College of General Practitioners (ICGP), iHeed established a clinical fellowship for family Medicine in the UAE on Maternal and Child Health. This Dubai-based clinical fellowship has graduated 24 physicians to date.

18.9 Challenges and Advantages

The single biggest challenge facing the UAE primary healthcare sector now and for the next few decades concerns the shortage of primary care providers, particularly family medicine practitioners [45, 46]. Each year, the UAE's family practitioner (FP) residency training programs graduate about 16 physicians, and even if 100% of them take up positions in the nation's PHC centers, they will not begin to fill the growing need of the nation's expanding network of PHC centers [5]. The UAE has struggled with a shortage of qualified physicians, along with an even more dire shortage of qualified nurses, for many years [14, 45]. The overwhelming majority (85% or more in most sectors) of the UAE healthcare workforce is comprised of expatriates, whose professional qualifications may not fully meet the emerging UAE quality and certification standards and who often view their UAE posting as a temporary position. While turnover among expatriate healthcare professionals is very high, there is a profound shortage of Emirati medical professionals, and the mismatch between supply and demand in the primary care sector is particularly dire [14, 39, 46]. The UAE is not alone in facing a primary care practitioner shortage, as the USA, the UK, and other nations have struggled with this problem for many years. The decision to place primacy on the family practitioner distinguishes the UAE PHC model from that found in the USA, where primary care is delivered not only by family practitioners but also by internal medicine physicians, pediatricians, obstetricians-gynecologists, and geriatricians, as well as by non-physician providers including nurse practitioners and physician assistants. As they look toward filling healthcare workforce shortages, the UAE health authorities may consider the merits of adjusting their current commitment to the family practitioner model to allow for other medical specialties.

Changing the model does not necessarily ensure that applicants will follow, however. A recent survey of UAE internal medicine residents found that only about 25% of them had any interest in working in primary care [46]. Increased reliance on physician assistants and advanced practice nurses, such as certified family nurse practitioners (FNPs), could potentially help address the shortage, although at present the shortage of nurses at all levels is even greater than that of physicians, and an estimated 98% of the UAE nursing workforce is expatriates [45]. Other possible ways to help address the problem include offering incentives to the Emiratis to train as family practitioners, significantly expanding training and education programs, partnering with foreign universities, and offering incentives to UAE nationals to obtain training abroad and return to practice in the UAE [39, 41, 77].

Over the longer term, another challenge facing the UAE PHC sector is the aging of the UAE population [11, 17]. While the UAE population is still quite young, demographic projections indicate that the population will age significantly over the next century, a process that may be hastened by deliberate efforts to increase the ratio of nationals to expatriates and the low fertility rate [13, 14]. As the population ages, the burden of disease associated with chronic illnesses such as diabetes and cardiovascular diseases will only increase [13, 33, 62]. Currently, the patient-centered model within the UAE PHC system contains several elements that align well with the chronic care model [48]. Further enhancing and developing system-wide capacity to address chronic care needs as well as expanding system capacity to respond to the specific healthcare needs and risks of older adults and the elderly will be needed in the future. As the UAE PHC sector navigates these and other challenges, it will enjoy the advantages of a stable and growing economy and a government that has championed and supported the development and expansion of PHC. The PHC system will be able to draw on these resources as it develops a strong professional healthcare workforce and meets the needs of a growing population with changing demographics. Moreover, the existing patient-centered model will serve as an advantage as the primary care sector continues to make quality improvements, expand service offerings, and integrate new health information technologies [35, 72].

18.10 The Future of Primary Care

The future of primary care in the UAE is very much the future of healthcare in the UAE. The Ministry of Health and Prevention, the Dubai Health Authority, the Department of Health of Abu Dhabi, and the UAE government, through its national strategy, have prioritized the achievement of a world-class healthcare system that rests on a foundation of patient-centered primary care. In the coming years, the number of PHC centers and the range of services provided at these centers will continue to expand to ensure that all residents have access to state-of-the-art healthcare. There will be increased attention focused on preventive care and health promotion, as well as expanded services related to chronic disease management and the health needs of older adults [6, 48]. In recent years, increasing efforts have been made to improve the quality of care, and it is anticipated that these efforts will continue and expand, with particular attention to patient satisfaction, patient safety, evidence-based medicine, and the cost-effectiveness of care [72, 74]. The PHC sector in Abu Dhabi has made progress in the implementation of the electronic medical record, and nationwide, there has been widespread implementation of telemedicine technologies [34, 38]. In the future, the PHC sector will benefit from the full adoption of the electronic medical record as well as many other health information technologies that can improve efficiencies and enhance the quality and scope of patient care [55].

18.11 Conclusion

In 1986, nearly four decades ago, the UAE leadership made the decision to adopt the World Health Organization's "Health for All" mandate and declared primary health care essential to achieving those objectives. The national government, the federal health authority, and the health authorities of the emirates of Abu Dhabi and Dubai have never wavered in their commitment to developing and implementing a primary healthcare system that fully meet the needs of the individuals, communities, and population health in the UAE. Today, the PHC system stands out as the foundation and driving force behind a booming, world-class health system.

Conflicts of Interest The authors have no conflicts of interest to declare.

References

1. (WHO), W.H.O. and U.N.C.s.F. (UNICEF), A vision for primary health care in the 21st century: towards universal health coverage and the sustainable development goals, in technical series on primary health care. Geneva: World Health Organization; 2018. pp. 1–46.
2. Hansen J, et al. Living in a country with a strong primary care system is beneficial to people with chronic conditions. Health Aff (Millwood). 2015;34(9):1531–7.
3. Irving G, et al. International variations in primary care physician consultation time: a systematic review of 67 countries. BMJ Open. 2017;7(10):e017902.
4. Mate K et al. Review of health systems of the middle east and North Africa Region, in International Encyclopedia of Public Health. 2017. pp. 347–356.
5. van Weel C, et al. Primary healthcare policy implementation in the Eastern Mediterranean region: experiences of six countries. Eur J Gen Pract. 2018;24(1):39–44.
6. Koornneef E, Robben P, Blair I. Progress and outcomes of health systems reform in The United Arab Emirates: a systematic review. BMC Health Serv Res. 2017;17(1):672.
7. UAE Ministry of Health & Prevention. Ministry of Health & prevention – home page. [web, multimedia] 2022 July 2022 [cited 2022 July 15, 2022]; Home page of UAE Ministry of Health & Prevention]. Available from: https://mohap.gov.ae/en/home.
8. Department of Health Abu Dhabi. Introducing primary care in Abu Dhabi. 2022 [cited 2022 July 12, 2022]; Description of the Emirate's primary care model]. Available from: https://www.doh.gov.ae/en/programs-initiatives/Primary-Care
9. Dubai Health Authority. Primary health centres 2022. 2022 [cited 2022 July 14, 2022]. Available from: https://www.dha.gov.ae/en/facilities/health-centers
10. Berwick D, Fox DM. "Evaluating the quality of medical care": Donabedian's classic article 50 years later. Milbank Q. 2016;94(2):237–41.
11. World population review United Arab Emirates population 2022 (live). World Population Reviewcom, 2022.
12. Fitch Solutions Group Limited, United Arab Emirates pharmaceuticals and healthcare report: includes 10-year forecasts to 2030. London; 2021.

13. (IHME), I.f.H.M.a.E., Country profile: United Arab Emirates. IHME, Seattle: University of Washington; 2021.
14. US-UAE Business Council, The U.A.E. healthcare sector. Washington DC.; 2021.
15. Bener A, Abdullah S, Murdoch JC. Primary health care in The United Arab Emirates. Fam Pract. 1983;10(4):444–8.
16. Hasan S, et al. Patient expectations and willingness to use primary care pharmacy services in The United Arab Emirates. Int J Pharm Pract. 2015;23(5):340–8.
17. Bhagavathula AS, Shehab A. Measuring the burden of disease in the United Arab Emirates, 1990–2019: a road to future. New Emir Med J. 2021;2(1):2–5.
18. Murray CJL, et al. Global burden of 87 risk factors in 204 countries and territories, 1990–2019: a systematic analysis for the global burden of disease study 2019. Lancet. 2020;396(10258):1223–49.
19. Loney T, et al. An analysis of the health status of The United Arab Emirates: the 'Big 4' public health issues. Glob Health Action. 2013;6:20100.
20. Alnakhi WK, et al. The socio-demographic characteristics associated with non-communicable diseases among the adult population of Dubai: results from Dubai household survey 2019. Healthcare (Basel). 2021;9(9)
21. Mediterranean, W.H.O.R.O.f.t.E., United Arab Emirates health profile 2015. Cairo: WHO, Regional Office for the Eastern Mediterranean; 2016. pp. 1–38.
22. Al Falasi RJ, Khan MA. The impact of COVID-19 on Abu Dhabi and its primary care response. J Gen Pract. 2020:49.
23. Al Zahmi F, et al. Ethnicity-specific features of COVID-19 among Arabs, Africans, south Asians, East Asians, and Caucasians in The United Arab Emirates. Front Cell Infect Microbiol. 2021;11:773141.
24. Authority, N.E.C.a.D.M. UAE coronavirus (COVID-19) updates. [Internet, multimedia] 2022 July 21, 2022 [cited 2022 July 22, 2022]; UAE Government COVID-19 dashboard]. Available from: https://covid19.ncema.gov.ae/en
25. Ritchie H, et al. United Arab Emirates: Coronavirus pandemic country profile. Our World in Data COVID-19 dataset, 2022.
26. Radwan H, et al. Indirect health effects of COVID-19: unhealthy lifestyle behaviors during the lockdown in The United Arab Emirates. Int J Environ Res Public Health. 2021;18(4):1964.
27. Alshaali A, et al. Preventive steps implemented on geriatric services in the primary health care centers during COVID-19 pandemic. J Public Health Res. 2022:11.
28. Dalibalta S, Davison G. Exercise and cardiovascular health in the UAE, in handbook of healthcare in the arab world; 2021. p. 1661–80.
29. Hajat C, Harrison O. The Abu Dhabi cardiovascular program: the continuation of Framingham. Prog Cardiovasc Dis. 2010;53(1):28–38.
30. Pourshams A, et al. The global, regional, and national burden of pancreatic cancer and its attributable risk factors in 195 countries and territories, 1990–2017: a systematic analysis for the global burden of disease study 2017. Lancet Gastroenterol Hepatol. 2019;4(12):934–47.
31. Margolis SA, et al. Patient satisfaction with primary health care services in The United Arab Emirates. Int J Qual Health Care. 2003;15(3):241–9.
32. Badri MA, Attia S, Ustadi AM. Healthcare quality and moderators of patient satisfaction: testing for causality. Int J Health Care Qual Assur. 2009;22(4):382–410.
33. Paulo MS, Loney T, Lapao LV. The primary health care in the emirate of Abu Dhabi: are they aligned with the chronic care model elements? BMC Health Serv Res. 2017;17(1):725.
34. Oxford Business Group. How Abu Dhabi is revitalising its medical offerings. Abu Dhabi; 2020.
35. Paulo MS, Loney T, Lapao LV. Pushing chronic care forward in Abu Dhabi by identifying priorities and addressing barriers: a modified Delphi technique. BMJ Open. 2018;8(6):e020189.
36. Baynouna Al Ketbi LM, et al. Integration of a patient-centered medical home into ambulatory health care services centers in Abu Dhabi. J Ambul Care Manage. 2018;41(3):158–70.
37. Zaman S. 49 providers currently offer quality primary care, in gulf news. Dubai: SyndiGate Media; 2018.

38. Dubai Health Authority, Doctor for every citizen: service catalogue, G.o.D. Dubai Health Authority, Editor. Dubai: Dubai Health Authority; 2020. pp. 1–14.
39. Rafeea SJ, et al. Healthcare industry challenges and potential opportunities in the UAE, a review paper. Acad Strateg Manag. 2021;20:1–9.
40. United Arab Emirates' Government Portal. Health regulatory authorities. [Internet, multimedia] 2022 April 22, 2022; Office UAE government web portal]. Available from: https://u.ae/en/information-and-services/health-and-fitness/health-authorities
41. Paulo MS, Loney T, Lapao LV. How do we strengthen the health workforce in a rapidly developing high-income country? A case study of Abu Dhabi's health system in The United Arab Emirates. Hum Resour Health. 2019;17(1):9.
42. Chaudhary SB. 4 new primary health care centres to open in 2019 beginning, in gulf news. Dubai: SundiGate Media Inc.; 2018.
43. Dubai Health Authority's new organizational structure approved, In Gulf News. Dubai: SyndiGate Media; 2018.
44. Yeboah DA. Impact of population variables on health services demand and provision in The United Arab Emirates. Arab Stud Q. 2007;29(1):61–70.
45. Verma VS, UAE National health Workforce Account (NHWA) Report 2019–2020. Dubai: Ministry of Health & Prevention (MOHAP) Statistics and Research Centre; 2021.
46. Schiess N, et al. Career choice and primary Care in The United Arab Emirates. J Grad Med Educ. 2015;7(4):663–6.
47. KPMG, Who cares, wins: UAE healthcare perspectives. 2020.
48. Paulo MS, Loney T, Lapao LV. Improving primary health care in Abu Dhabi towards patient centeredness with chronic care model, in European health management association EHMA. Budapest: EHMA; 2018.
49. Reed RL, et al. A clinical care trial of chronic care diabetic clinics in general practice in The United Arab Emirates: a preliminary analysis. Arch Physiol Biochem. 2001;109(3):272–80.
50. Ramadan M, Butt A. Health systems for the elderly in the Arabian Gulf Region, in handbook of healthcare in the arab world; 2021. p. 1773–87.
51. Matheson C, et al. A controlled trial of screening, brief intervention and referral for treatment (SBIRT) implementation in primary care in The United Arab Emirates. Prim Health Care Res Dev. 2018;19(2):165–75.
52. Chowdhury N. Integration between mental health-care providers and traditional spiritual healers: Contextualising Islam in the twenty-first century. J Relig Health. 2016;55(5):1665–71.
53. Khansaheb HH, et al. Quantitative assessment of some preventive health services provided for adolescent individuals in Dubai. J Health Hum Serv Adm. 2016;39(1):95–121.
54. Shirwaikar A, Govindarajan R, Rawat AK. Integrating complementary and alternative medicine with primary health care. Evid Based Complement Alternat Med. 2013;2013:948308.
55. El Jabari C, Adwan L. Health informatics in the arab world, in handbook of healthcare in the arab world; 2021. p. 1681–92.
56. Sarabdeen J, Moonesar IA. Privacy protection laws and public perception of data privacy. BIJ. 2018;25(6):1883–902.
57. Al Alawi S, et al. Physician user satisfaction with an electronic medical records system in primary healthcare centres in Al Ain: a qualitative study. BMJ Open. 2014;4(11):e005569.
58. AbdulRahman M, et al. Digital health Technology for Remote Care in primary care during the COVID-19 pandemic: experience from Dubai. Telemed J E Health. 2022;28:1100.
59. Alhajri N, et al. Exploring quality differences in telemedicine between hospital outpatient departments and community clinics: cross-sectional study. JMIR Med Inform. 2022;10(2):e32373.
60. Baynouna LM, et al. A successful chronic care program in Al Ain-United Arab Emirates. BMC Health Serv Res. 2010;10:47.
61. Khan S, et al. Exploratory study into the awareness of heart diseases among Emirati women (UAE) and their health seeking behaviour- a qualitative study. BMC Womens Health. 2016;16(1):71.

62. Al Awadi F, et al. Prevalence of diabetes and associated health risk factors among adults in Dubai, United Arab Emirates: results from Dubai household survey 2019. Dubai Diabetes Endocrinol J. 2020;26(4):164–73.
63. Saadi H, et al. Prevalence of undiagnosed diabetes and quality of care in diabetic patients followed at primary and tertiary clinics in Abu Dhabi, United Arab Emirates. Rev Diabet Stud. 2010;7(4):293–302.
64. Badrinath P, et al. A study of knowledge, attitude, and practice of cervical screening among female primary care physicians in The United Arab Emirates. Health Care Women Int. 2004;25(7):663–70.
65. Alawadi F, et al. The prevalence of diabetes and pre-diabetes among the Dubai population: findings from Dubai household health surveys, 2014 and 2017. Dubai Diabetes Endocrinol J. 2020;26(2):78–84.
66. Samara A, Andersen PT, Aro AR. Health promotion for preventing obesity in the arab gulf states, in handbook of healthcare in the arab world; 2021. p. 893–1002.
67. Abouchacra S, et al. Adolescent eating behaviors in the UAE: time to intervene. J Family Med Prim Care. 2021;10(8):2998–3004.
68. Ali HI, Baynouna LM, Bernsen RM. Barriers and facilitators of weight management: perspectives of Arab women at risk for type 2 diabetes. Health Soc Care Community. 2010;18(2):219–28.
69. Alraeesi FH, et al. Smoking behavior, knowledge, attitude, and practice among patients attending primary healthcare clinics in Dubai, United Arab Emirates. J Family Med Prim Care. 2020;9(1):315–20.
70. Suliman DM, et al. UAE efforts in promoting COVID-19 vaccination and building vaccine confidence. Vaccine. 2021;39(43):6341–5.
71. Albahri AH, et al. Knowledge, attitude, and practice regarding COVID-19 among healthcare workers in primary healthcare centers in Dubai: a cross-sectional survey, 2020. Front Public Health. 2021;9:617679.
72. Fadlallah R, et al. Quality, safety and performance management in primary health care: from scoping review to research priority setting and implementation plan in the eastern Mediterranean region. BMJ Glob Health. 2019;4(Suppl 8):e001477.
73. Pflanz-Sinclair C, et al. Physicians' experiences of SBIRT training and implementation for SUD management in primary care in the UAE: a qualitative study. Prim Health Care Res Dev. 2018;19(4):344–54.
74. Albarrak AI, Ali Abbdulrahim SA, Mohammed R. Evaluating factors affecting the implementation of evidence based medicine in primary healthcare centers in Dubai. Saudi Pharm J. 2014;22(3):207–12.
75. Abyad A, et al. Development of family medicine in the Middle East. Fam Med. 2007;39(10):736–9.
76. Ahmed A, Abdulrahman M, Withnall R. Evolution of the Dubai health authority's residency training program: a 25-year review, challenges and outcomes. J Family Med Prim Care. 2018;7(2):319–23.
77. Sheikh JI, et al. Capacity building in health care professions within the Gulf cooperation council countries: paving the way forward. BMC Med Educ. 2019;19(1):83.
78. United Arab Emirates Population 2022 (Live). Available from: https://worldpopulationreview.com/countries/united-arab-emirates-population
79. Population Pyramids of the World from 1950 to 2100. Available from: https://www.populationpyramid.net/united-arab-emirates/2022/

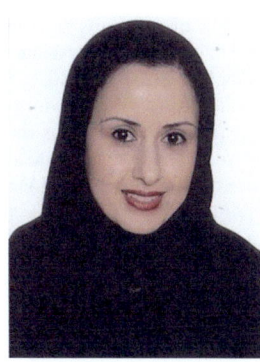

Dr. Maha Al Fahim is a consultant in family medicine, family medicine residency program director, as well as the Chair of Education and DIO (designated institutional official) at Sheikh Khalifa Medical City in Abu Dhabi. She received her MD from the Royal College of Surgeons in Ireland and went on to do her residency training in family medicine at McGill University in Montreal, Canada. She received a Master's degree in Leadership in Healthcare Management from the Royal College of Surgeons in Ireland (2008), followed by another Master's degree in Leadership in Health Professions Education from the Royal College of Surgeons in Ireland (2013).

Dr. Maha was a member of the original Sheikh Khalifa Medical City (SKMC) Graduate Medical Education Committee and played an integral role in leading SKMC through an extensive award-winning medical education transformation for its initial ACGME-I accreditation in 2011. She was instrumental in implementing change across the institution and, as Program Director, entirely restructured the SKMC Family Medicine Residency Program as it prepared for its initial accreditation in 2012 and all subsequent re-accreditations over the last 10 years. Dr. Maha's dedication and passion for medical education at SKMC led to her selection as the Deputy Chair of Education at SKMC in 2014 and eventually into the full-time Chair of the SKMC Education Institute position in April 2016. Dr. Maha recently also accepted leadership of all Corniche Hospital training programs under the umbrella of the SKMC Education Institute.

In her role as Chair of the SKMC Education Institute, Dr. Maha has consistently maintained ACGME-I accreditation at SKMC across the institute and all programs and led SKMC to be the first institute to achieve NIHS accreditation, the new Emirati national board accreditation, and more recently, Royal College of Physicians of Canada accreditation. She has worked hard to expand the existing programs and increase opportunities through the addition of fellowship programs. She has dedicated her career to advocating and improving medical education in the UAE as a whole, not only through her activities as DIO but also through additional contributions she has made as an active member of the Arab Board Family Medicine Training & Accreditation Committee, as both an Arab Board and Jordanian Board Examiner, as a member of the Curriculum Working group at Khalifa University Medical School, in her former capacity as a member of the ACGME-I Review Committee, and more recently as an active member of the newly formed UAE National Institute for Health Specialties (NIHS) Scientific Committee working on establishing an effective and credible Emirati Board for UAE programs, she was also the original Chair of the Family Medicine Specialty Review Committee for the NIHS.

In addition to the extensive amount of time she dedicates to the above activities, Dr. Maha also actively participates in research and publications and regularly provides teaching lectures to both her own and other programs across the hospital system. She also regularly chairs structured internal reviews of programs in both Abu Dhabi and Dubai and has been an Adjunct Clinical Associate Professor at Khalifa University, Abu Dhabi, UAE, since 2020.

Dr. Maha remains a steadfast leader in quality medical education in the UAE, as illustrated by the quality of the programs she manages. She is also a determined and vocal resident advocate at all levels of management and governance of programs in the UAE.

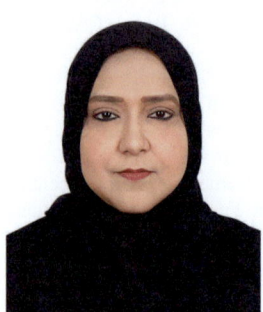

Dr. Ebtihal Darwish consultant family physician, currently working as director of Research and Academic Department at Unilabs Middle East, Dubai. She is the founder and the CEO of Ethraa for consultancies and training, a firm established to empower health professionals in the region. She is also Adjunct Clinical Assistant Professor in Family Medicine Department, Sharjah University and Former Vice Chairperson of MRCGP Int. Examination Board in Dubai. In addition, Dr. Darwish has a long experience in healthcare management and occupied several managerial jobs at DHA.

Dr. Darwish had several qualifications and certifications including MSc in Health Care Management, DHA Leadership Development Program by Harvard School of Public Health, HR Diploma, Excellence in Training by RCGP, Arab Board Family Medicine, MD AGU, and Bachelor of Basic Medical Science, AGU, Bahrain.

During her professional life, Dr Ebtihal contributed effectively in the development of health sector in UAE. She received lots of certificate of recognitions and awards including: Shaikh. Mohammed Bin Rashid Award for SMEs, distinguish female staff award in DHA, Sheikh Rashid Award for Distinguish Academic achievement - PhD holders, Sheikh Rashid award for Distinguish Academic achievement - secondary school, Distinguish trainer in the health sector and Fourth Future Day appreciation letter and many others.

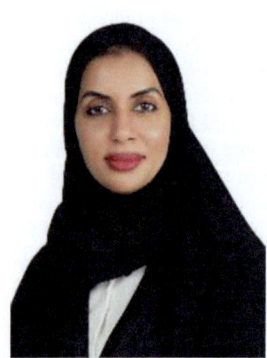

Dr. Farah Saeed Mohammad Al-Zaabi began working at Zayed Military Hospital in 2006 as a consultant in family medicine and chronic pain management after receiving her Canadian Certificate in Family Medicine. She then completed two fellowships, one in chronic pain and addiction and the second in medical education, from the University of Toronto in 2006. In 2011, to improve her administrative and leadership skills, she earned her Executive Masters in Health Administration from Zayed University in Abu Dhabi.

In January 2010–June 2021, Dr. Farah was appointed Designated Institutional Official and Medical Education Director to oversee the residency programs at Zayed Military Hospital. Immediately, she began instituting a variety of additional trainings, educational programs, and activities within the hospital and achieving international accreditation for these programs. In addition, Dr. Farah is a member of several national and international committees, serves as adjunct faculty at a couple of local medical schools, and speaks at national and international conferences. Dr. Farah created a multi-disciplinary team approach in the clinical treatment of chronic pain to provide a more effective outcome for patients. Currently, she is the head of the medical education and training division in the millinery health executive directorate at MOD. Dr. Farah has always been eager to improve the UAE healthcare system, enhance the care provided by healthcare workers at all levels, and spread and share knowledge nationally, regionally, and internationally.

Open Access This chapter is licensed under the terms of the Creative Commons Attribution 4.0 International License (http://creativecommons.org/licenses/by/4.0/), which permits use, sharing, adaptation, distribution and reproduction in any medium or format, as long as you give appropriate credit to the original author(s) and the source, provide a link to the Creative Commons license and indicate if changes were made.

The images or other third party material in this chapter are included in the chapter's Creative Commons license, unless indicated otherwise in a credit line to the material. If material is not included in the chapter's Creative Commons license and your intended use is not permitted by statutory regulation or exceeds the permitted use, you will need to obtain permission directly from the copyright holder.

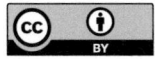

Obesity in the UAE

19

Omniyat Mohammed Al Hajeri and Omar Al Hammadi

19.1 Introduction

Obesity is viewed as a long-lasting and recurrent condition that profoundly affects one's overall well-being and quality of life [1]. Several medical conditions, including cardiovascular disease, hypertension, diabetes, sleep apnea, degenerative joint disease, digestive tract disease, thrombo-embolic diseases, dermatologic diseases, and cancer (particularly breast, gynecologic, prostate, kidney, liver, gallbladder, and colon malignancies), have been acknowledged to consider obesity as a risk factor [2, 5, 13]. It is linked to a diminished quality of life and a decreased life expectancy [3, 4].

The fundamental cause of obesity and overweight is an energy imbalance, where the calories consumed exceed the calories expended. Increased intake comes from the large consumption of energy-dense foods rich in fat and sugar, and increased physical inactivity comes from a sedentary lifestyle resulting from the nature of work, the environment, food processing, marketing, education, transportation, and urbanization [13, 16]. Obesity is considered a global epidemic; the development of obesity is influenced by a multitude of factors, including genetic, epigenetic, physiological, iatrogenic, environmental, and sociocultural factors [5, 10].

The presence of obesity during adolescence is linked to an elevated risk of experiencing severe obesity in adulthood; obese adults who have a history of childhood obesity are at increased risk of having dyslipidemia, diabetes, and carotid artery atherosclerosis [2]. Despite significant investments, many countries have been unable to reduce the rate of obesity in children.

O. M. Al Hajeri
Abu Dhabi Public Health Centre, Abu Dhabi, United Arab Emirates
e-mail: ohajri@adphc.gov.ae

O. Al Hammadi (✉)
ADNOC Group, Abu Dhabi, United Arab Emirates

Table 19.1 Adult body mass index (BMI) [9]

BMI	Considered
Below 18.5	Underweight
18.5–24.9	Healthy weight
25.0–29.9	Overweight
30 or higher	Obesity, Class 1: BMI of 30 to < 35, Class 2: BMI of 35 to <40
40 or higher	Class 3 or severe obesity

Source: CDC, C., n.d. Defining Adult Overweight & Obesity. [online] Available at: https://www.cdc.gov/obesity/basics/adult-defining.html

19.2 Classifications

Body Mass Index (BMI) is considered an indicator of body fatness, where the risk of non-communicable diseases increases with increased BMI [9, 13]. It is a screening tool for obesity and overweight; however, it does not diagnose fatness or health. It must be used carefully by trained healthcare workers to determine an individual's health status and risks. It seems to be strongly correlated with health outcomes and is calculated by dividing weight in kilograms by the square of height in meters ($BMI=Kg/m^2$). See Table 19.1 [9].

19.3 Epidemiology

The sedentary lifestyle prevalent in recent decades, especially in the Middle East region, has been identified as a contributing factor to the global increase in the prevalence of diabetes, metabolic syndrome, and obesity [6]. The World Obesity Federation has predicted that the consequences of obesity will lead to an annual expenditure of $1.2 trillion starting in 2025. The World Health Organization (WHO) predicts that 2.7 billion adults will be overweight or obese by 2025 [7].

Since 1975, the global prevalence of obesity has tripled. In 2016, over 1.9 billion adults aged 18 years and older were overweight, with 650 million of them being obese. Among adults, 39% were classified as overweight, with 39% of men and 40% of women falling into this category. Additionally, 13% of adults were considered obese, with 11% of men and 15% of women affected. The majority of individuals live in countries where overweight and obesity contribute to a higher mortality rate compared to underweight conditions [13].

The United Arab Emirates (UAE) has witnessed rapid urbanization and an increasing number of expatriate workforce, which has resulted in a modern, fast-paced, and technology-driven lifestyle. This has resulted in a notable decline in physical activity levels in various aspects of life, including occupation, domestic tasks, and leisure-time activities, in addition to increased consumption of unhealthy diets, including calorie-dense, processed, and pre-packaged food with poor nutritional benefits [6, 16].

According to the national health survey 2017–2018, the prevalence of obesity in the UAE among adults was reported to be 27.8%, and it reached 17.35% among children and adolescents [8, 16]. The prevalence of obesity was higher among female respondents, especially among the Emirati population; 41.8% of Emirati females were estimated to have obesity [8]. According to the same report, the prevalence of overweight was 67.9%, and males were more overweight than females. The age group of 33–44 years exhibited the highest prevalence of obesity and overweight [7, 8].

In a previous study conducted as part of a population-wide cardiovascular screening program in Abu Dhabi, involving 50,138 adults aged 18 years and older, similar prevalence rates were observed. The study reported rates of overweight at 32%, obesity at 35%, and central obesity at 55%. When age-standardized, the rates of overweight and obesity were 34% and 41%, respectively. Another cross-sectional survey conducted in the UAE in 2000 revealed an overall obesity rate of 34%, with a breakdown of 26% for men and 40% for women [26].

According to data from a cross-sectional study, the prevalence of obesity and overweight in adult expatriates in the UAE was found to be 32.2% and 43%, respectively, taking into consideration ethnicity-specific BMI, gender, waist circumference, and waist-to-hip ratio [11].

In Arab Gulf countries, the prevalence of obesity varies among adult genders, with rates ranging from 2% to 55% in females and 1% to 30% in males. For children and adolescents, the prevalence ranges from 5% to 14% in males and 3% to 18% in females [14]. According to WHO estimates for 2016, the obesity rates among adults were 37% in Kuwait, 35% in Saudi Arabia, and 34% in Qatar. The prevalence was notably higher among adult females, particularly in Kuwait (44%), Qatar (42%), and Saudi Arabia (41%) [15].

A recent cross-sectional study examined the occurrence of obesity in adolescents aged 13–19 years attending both public and private schools. The study utilized various measures, including BMI above the 85th percentile for age, abdominal obesity, and body fat percentage, to determine overweight and obesity. The findings indicated that 37.4% of participants were overweight or obese, 40.6% had a high body fat percentage, and abdominal obesity was observed in 47.3%, 22.7%, and 27.1% of participants based on waist circumference, waist-to-hip ratio, and waist-to-height ratio, respectively. Interestingly, students from public schools exhibited a significantly higher prevalence of overweight and obesity compared to students from private schools (37.8% vs. 31.1%). The predictors of abdominal obesity included being male, studying at a public school, being Emirati, being physically inactive, and consuming less than five servings of fruits and vegetables [16].

Compared to students attending private schools, some studies in other countries showed that students attending public schools were found to have less physical activity and exercise, and a lower intake of fruits, vegetables, water, fiber, vitamins, and minerals [19]; however, some studies showed the opposite trend, which could be explained by the type of diet, school environment, socioeconomic status, and factors pertaining to infancy [16].

According to cross-sectional studies, there is evidence indicating higher rates of obesity among youth aged 13–15 years residing in various cities in the UAE. The reported prevalence of obesity varied between 18.9% in Abu Dhabi and 35% in Dubai [17, 18].

The prevalence of obesity and overweight in youth aligns with studies conducted in different Arab countries. The reported rates of obesity and overweight are as follows: Lebanon (32.2%), Egypt (35%), Saudi Arabia (39%), and Kuwait (44.3%), while studies from European countries showed lower rates of obesity and overweight among adolescents, ranging from 22% to 25%, and the United States showed a rate of 30% for overweight and obesity among adolescents [16].

19.4 Children's Obesity

Children's obesity is linked to an increased risk of adult obesity, premature death, and disability. An obese child may experience breathing difficulties, sleep apnea, asthma, fractures, high blood pressure, insulin resistance, early markers of cardiovascular disease, and psychological manifestations [12, 13]. In 2020, the WHO estimated that 39 million children (0–5 years) were overweight or obese, and 340 million children and adolescents (5–19 years) were overweight or obese. The prevalence of overweight and obesity in children and adolescents has risen dramatically from just 4% in 1975 to over 18% in 2016, occurring at similar rates among both boys and girls [13].

A study on the lifetime direct medical costs of childhood obesity estimated that the incremental cost of an obese child, relative to a normal-weight child who maintains a normal weight in adulthood, is $19,000 per child. This number does not take into account the indirect costs of childhood obesity [27].

According to the WHO's global school-based student health survey, the rate of physical inactivity among children and adolescents was estimated at 72% in the UAE and 85% in Qatar [15]. This is an incredibly concerning statistic.

The significant socioeconomic changes in the UAE necessitate careful monitoring of obesity in the pediatric population, as it has become an alarming epidemic. Studies estimate that each year, an additional 0.5–1% of children gain excess body fat, with approximately 32% of these individuals becoming overweight and 8% becoming obese [12].

In a large cohort study conducted in Ras Al-Khaimah governmental schools, the prevalence of obesity was examined in 44,942 students using different BMI interpretation methods, including those by the Centers for Disease Control and Prevention (CDC), the World Health Organization (WHO), and the International Obesity Task Force (IOTF). The study revealed a linear increase in obesity rates from ages 3 to 12, with an additional 2.3% of students becoming obese each year. The rate of extreme obesity was 9.6 times higher among boys than girls. Among students aged 15–18, 10.3% of boys and 3% of girls were classified as extremely obese [12].

Table 19.2 from the study shows that the IOTF method underestimated obesity and extreme obesity, while the WHO method overestimated them in all age groups. The CDC values fell between those of the IOTF and WHO methods. The prevalence of overweight, obesity, and extreme obesity for different age groups and genders in 2014–2015 ($n = 27{,}113$) is shown using the IOTF, WHO, and CDC methods [12].

The prevalence of obesity is on the rise among children and adolescents aged 3–18 years, compared to previous reports. This increase begins in toddlers and

Table 19.2 Prevalence of overweight, obesity and extreme obesity for age and gender (2014–2015, $n = 27,113$ citizens) using the IOTF, WHO and CDC methods

IOTF

Age, Y	Overweight, obesity and extreme obesity (BMI =25 kg/m² equivalent)			Obesity and extreme obesity (BMI =30 kg/m² equivalent)			Extreme obesity (BMI =35 kg/m² equivalent)		
	All	Girls	Boys	All	Girls	Boys	All	Girls	Boys
3–6 ($n = 6,731$)	11.5	12.7	10.4	5.2	5.8	4.7	2.9	3.4	2.5
7–10 ($n = 9,058$)	27.6	28.9	26.2	12.4	12.7	12.1	4.1	4.4	3.9
11–14⁽?⁾ ($n = 7,437$)	41.2	38.3	43.1	18.9	17.3	20.7	6.4	5.6	7.1
15–18⁽?⁾ ($n = 3,852$)	38.0	35.6	42.4	19.3	17.2	22.6	8.1	7.2	9.6

WHO

Age, Y	Overweight, obesity and extreme obesity (BMI for age =85th percentile)			Obesity and extreme obesity (BMI for age =95th percentile)			Extreme obesity (BMI for age =99th percentile)		
	All	Girls	Boys	All	Girls	Boys	All	Girls	Boys
3–6 ($n = 6,731$)	14.0	15.1	13.0	11.2	11.9	10.6	–	–	–
7–10 ($n = 9,058$)	31.2	32.3	30.2	27.0	28.2	25.9	–	–	–
11–14⁽?⁾ ($n = 7,437$)	43.1	42.6	43.8	37.5	37.0	38.2	–	–	–
15–18⁽?⁾ ($n = 3,852$)	38.4	36.0	41.6	33.8	31.2	37.4	–	–	–

CDC

Age, Y	Overweight, obesity and extreme obesity (BMI for age =85th percentile)			Obesity and extreme obesity (BMI for age =95th percentile)			Extreme obesity (BMI for age =99th percentile)		
	All	Girls	Boys	All	Girls	Boys	All	Girls	Boys
3–6 ($n = 6,731$)	14.2	15.2⁽¶⁾	13.3	7.4	7.7⁽#⁾	7.1	3.3	3.1⁽#⁾	3.5
7–10 ($n = 9,058$)	29.0	28.6⁽#⁾	29.3	16.7	15.7⁽¶⁾	17.6	3.8	3.6⁽#⁾	4.0
11–14⁽?⁾ ($n = 7,437$)	41.2	38.7	39.5	24.3	21.6	27.5	5.7	4.4	7.1
15–18⁽?⁾ ($n = 3,852$)	37.2	33.8	41.3	22.2	18.3	27.2	8.8	3.0	10.3

Prevalence values are percent.
P-value between girls and boys is >0.05.
¶ *P*-value between girls and boys is <0.01.
? *P*-value between girls and boys is <0.001 in all BMI categories.
Source: https://www.ncbi.nlm.nih.gov/pmc/articles/PMC5074293/

Table 19.3 Prevalence of overweight, obesity, and extreme obesity for age (2014–2015, $n = 2332$ residents) using the CDC method [12]

Age, Y	Overweight, obesity, and extreme obesity (BMI for age ≥85th percentile)	Obesity and extreme obesity (BMI for age ≥95th percentile)	Extreme obesity (BMI for age ≥99th percentile)
3–6 ($n = 289$)	$n = 37$ (12.8%)	$n = 19$ (6.6%)	$n = 7$ (2.4%)
7–10 ($n = 516$)	$n = 146$ (28.3%)	$n = 74$ (14.3%)	$n = 11$ (2.1%)
11–14 ($n = 867$)	$n = 323$ (37.3%)	$n = 187$ (21.6%)	$n = 41$ (4.7%)
15–18 ($n = 660$)	$n = 242$ (36.7%)	$n = 138$ (20.1%)	$n = 25$ (3.8%)

Source: https://www.ncbi.nlm.nih.gov/pmc/articles/PMC5074293/

continues to escalate linearly with age. It is noteworthy that obesity is more prevalent among boys. In fact, approximately 25% of children aged 11–14 are classified as either obese or extremely obese [12]. Table 19.3 shows the prevalence of overweight, obesity, and extreme obesity for age using the CDC method.

This rise in obesity is believed to be associated with several factors. One contributing factor is the substitution of healthy foods with energy-dense products that are high in fat and sugar but lack essential nutrients. Additionally, sedentary lifestyles, characterized by excessive screen time and engagement in video games, have become increasingly common among children and adolescents. These lifestyle factors, including poor dietary choices and sedentary behaviors, are believed to play a significant role in the increasing prevalence of obesity in this age group [12].

19.5 Social Determinants of Health

Social determinants of health include the conditions in which we live, learn, work, and play. It is hard to establish healthy food choices and engage in enough physical activity if health is not supported by these conditions [10]. Differences in social determinants of health can affect the outcomes of chronic illnesses and risks, including obesity, among different racial and socioeconomic groups, different geographies, and people with different physical abilities [10]. Eating patterns and physical activities are affected in childcare centers and schools by the food and drinks offered and the opportunities for exercising in the communities. The prevalence of obesity is shaped by various factors, including the affordability of healthy food choices, the presence of peer and social support networks, marketing and promotional practices, and community policies that dictate the design of the built environment [10].

19.6 Health Systems and Prevention

Both the federal government and individual Emirates are involved in the regulation of the healthcare system in the UAE, and numerous government health insurance programs are in place to support healthcare provision (such as "Thiqa" in Abu Dhabi, "Saada" in Dubai, and the Department of Health Insurance in Sharjah) [43];

these programs provide medical insurance to Emirati nationals to cover health insurance in the private sector, government-funded insurance is also provided for all Emirati nationals in governmental hospitals. Expatriates usually use private health insurance to cover their medical necessities [20]. Significant efforts have been made by the government to prevent obesity in the community, which include prohibiting students from bringing unhealthy foods to school and applying a tax on sugary drinks [20].

The "Weqaya" is a screening program in Abu Dhabi that is designed to prevent obesity and overweight in the community. It operates under the umbrella of the Department of Health (DOH) in Abu Dhabi and provides informative resources on multiple prevention programs that cover aspects of tobacco control, diet, nutrition, obesity, and diabetes [24]. Additionally, the healthcare system in the UAE promotes the practice of booking appointments at the nearest healthcare facilities that offer "Weqaya" screening programs. This initiative aims to encourage individuals to proactively engage in preventive health measures by undergoing regular screenings and check-ups. Moreover, efforts are made to assist community members in locating restaurants that offer "Weqaya"-labeled food. This labeling system helps individuals identify food establishments that adhere to healthy guidelines and offer nutritious options, thereby supporting their overall well-being [20, 24].

In December 2018, the DOH issued a new service requirement standard for the comprehensive periodic screening program for adults. Acknowledging that obesity serves as a prevalent risk factor for various chronic diseases, including cancer, and emphasizing the importance of a unified, comprehensive approach to early detection, the updated standard included a modification of the Weqaya cardiovascular risk factors screening program to include screening for breast cancer, colorectal cancer, cervical cancer, and lung cancer, in addition to mental health, dental health, and special screenings for senior citizens such as hearing and visual acuity and abdominal aortic dilatation [28]. This program, currently called IFHAS (the Arabic word for test or check), is led by the Abu Dhabi Public Health Center (ADPHC). It began its pilot implementation phase in 2020 and launched an extensive accompanying educational campaign to encourage people to take age-appropriate screenings and pursue care for the identified risk factors, including obesity [29].

The DoH has established service requirements for weight management in overweight and obese children. These requirements encompass clinical care and outline the scope of practice for children aged 2–18 years. The aim is to provide comprehensive and effective interventions to address weight-related concerns in this specific age group. The guidelines highlight weight management interventions for general practitioners, family doctors, general pediatricians, pediatric sub-specialists, nurses, and dietitians, focusing on a multi-disciplinary approach and making it a family-centered program to basically include different component lifestyle recommendations that need the empowerment and awareness of parents. The guidelines also include pharmacological and surgical interventions when required [22, 23].

In addition to this standard, the DOH has issued several other important standards and initiatives to prevent and fight obesity by improving the nutrition of children and adults, improving early detection and screening for risk factors and obesity-related diseases, and enhancing the quality of care and management received by patients with obesity, as part of the cross-sectoral, multistakeholder Abu Dhabi government strategy, Ending Childhood Obesity Strategy: A Call to Action, launched in 2016. The Department of Health in Abu Dhabi has introduced various measures to address obesity and weight management. These include the publication of the "Standard for Obesity and Weight Diagnosis, Pharmacological, and Surgical Management Interventions" in 2018 [30]. Additionally, the DoH has set service requirements for the provision of the periodic comprehensive screening program (PCSP) for adults since 2018. Furthermore, school canteen guidelines have been established for schools in the Emirate of Abu Dhabi, focusing on food establishments. The Abu Dhabi nutrition labeling program, known as Weqaya, has been implemented to promote nutritional awareness. The Department of Health has also issued guidelines for implementing sugar reduction in food entities within the Emirate of Abu Dhabi. Furthermore, specific guidelines have been introduced for declaring calories on menus by manufacturers and food suppliers of ready-to-eat foods in Abu Dhabi. These measures collectively demonstrate the department's commitment to combating obesity and promoting healthier practices within the Emirate of Abu Dhabi [31].

At the national level, the UAE has implemented various strategies and plans aimed at preventing and detecting overweight and obesity. Notably, the publication of the National Plan for Prevention and Response for Non-communicable Diseases 2017–2021 in 2017 signifies the country's commitment to addressing this issue. Additionally, the UAE has developed the National Nutrition Plan, which aims to enhance the nutritional status of the population across all stages of life and reduce the health risks associated with diet-related factors contributing to NCDs. It is also worth mentioning that the National Agenda 2021 targeted reducing childhood obesity and established monitoring the prevalence of obesity among children as a priority [21, 33].

The UAE strategic plans for wellbeing for 2031 and 2071 include physical activity and dietary interventions as key points to be provided in the "quality of life for individuals" initiative [34]. There are also multiple national and emirate-based initiatives and programs worth mentioning that target improving governance and engaging stakeholders, such as the establishment of a national committee to combat obesity, the launch of the National Nutrition Strategy 2017–2021, the establishment of the Abu Dhabi Childhood Obesity Combat Committee 2014–2016, the Abu Dhabi Childhood Obesity Taskforce by the Abu Dhabi Public Health Center in 2019, and the Abu Dhabi Childhood Obesity Research Committee in 2019.

Other initiatives targeting the strengthening the regulations include imposing taxes of 50% on carbonated drinks and 100% on energy drinks in 2017, followed by the inclusion of all sweetened beverages in the 50% taxation in 2019 [34]; additionally, the national labeling of prepacked food products was introduced in 2018, along with the front-of-pack labeling policy implemented in 2022. Regarding the national school canteen guidelines, the Emirate of Abu Dhabi has developed specific guidelines for school canteens, targeting both caterers and schools. These guidelines provide clear instructions and recommendations for promoting healthy food choices and creating a nutritious environment within school canteens [35]. The Council of

Ministers Resolution No. 21 of 2018 was enacted to regulate the marketing of products specifically related to infant and young child nutrition. This resolution aims to ensure that marketing practices surrounding such products adhere to established guidelines and standards, with a focus on safeguarding the health and well-being of infants and young children [36].

Initiatives focusing on improving surveillance include the chronic disease registries in Abu Dhabi, which also incorporate the obesity register. The "Mutabah" system is an online surveillance system implemented at the federal level by the Ministry of Health and Prevention (MOHAP) to gather data on obesity among school students. It is an integral component of the Basic School Screening Program in schools across the UAE [36]. Initiatives and programs enabling the public to practice a healthy lifestyle and improve their nutrition and physical activity include the urban planning guidelines for health encouraging cities in Abu Dhabi, the Abu Dhabi nutrition-labelling program Weqaya (a voluntary menu labelling program for adults and kids, the Abu Dhabi Guideline for voluntary implementation of declaring calories on menus for manufacturers and food suppliers of ready-to-eat foods in the Emirate of Abu Dhabi, which encourages and provides guidance for manufacturers and food suppliers to voluntarily include calorie information on menus [37], the supermarket of the future program in Abu Dhabi where healthy food is clearly labelled and easy for customers to choose, and all Weqaya nutrition programs in Abu Dhabi, which have recently been reviewed, revamped, and launched under the umbrella of the "SEHHI," the Arabic word for healthy) nutrition program.

In the UAE, there are several programs with a specific emphasis on early detection, such as screening programs designed to identify cardiovascular disease risk factors and detect cancer at an early stage. These programs are implemented to proactively assess individuals for potential health risks, enabling timely interventions and treatment (e.g., Etminan, IFHAS). In addition, multiple large-scale public education campaigns have been launched, including "Mane and Takhtookh," a mass media campaign that aims to increase awareness around childhood obesity; the Ma'kom program [38], aimed at healthy diet, healthier environments at work, in schools and universities, and an active lifestyle in general; the "lose to win" program; move it UAE; it all adds up; rethink your drink; eat right and get active; health champions game [39]; and National Sports Day, held annually on March 7.

It is worth noting that in the Emirate of Abu Dhabi, all obesity-related efforts and their leading factors, i.e., prevention, early detection, and health education programs, are under the care and custody of the Abu Dhabi Public Health Center (ADPHC), which is a newly established government entity, created under Law No. 14 of 2019. ADPHC, operating under the Department of Health Abu Dhabi, is an autonomous organization with complete legal authority to carry out its functions. Its primary objective is to safeguard the well-being of Abu Dhabi's residents and ensure the protection of all individuals working within the Emirate. By upholding the principles of public and preventative health, the center strives for excellence in promoting a healthy and secure society. Its mission is to enhance the overall health of Abu Dhabi's population and ensure the safety of its workforce through the implementation of a comprehensive public health management system that adheres to the highest standards of innovation, excellence, and creativity [40].

19.7 Opportunities for Improvement

There are many achievements to be celebrated in the UAE when it comes to combating obesity efforts, especially in the fields of regulation, prevention, early detection, education, and management. Yet, there are still many opportunities for improvement. In terms of managing identified overweight and obese patients, there are multiple standards, guidelines, and recommendations, some of which were mentioned above in the Emirate of Abu Dhabi. Additionally, there is a set of "Clinical Practice Recommendations for the Management of Obesity in the United Arab Emirates," which was published in 2018. It was developed by a team of experts consisting of international and regional professionals from various disciplines who specialize in the treatment of patients with obesity and overweight conditions [41].

Furthermore, the report titled "Regional Recommendations for the Treatment and Management of Adult Obesity in the Gulf and Lebanon" also received contributions from numerous clinical experts in the UAE. This report provides specific recommendations for obesity management tailored to the Middle Eastern region, taking into account the unique health systems and cultural aspects of the community [42].

But we still do not have a nationally unified obesity management guideline that is officially recognized by all the relevant health authorities across the different Emirates. We also need a comprehensive, nationwide, integrated care model of obesity management in primary health care (PHC) through lifestyle clinics and weight management clinics. Additionally, we need to review our insurance coverage of obesity treatment modalities (including lifestyle interventions, counselling, medication, and surgery) and reach a consensus that ensures access to the appropriate level of care for the right patients in a cost-effective and sustainable model.

Strong, widespread, and sustainable work and education wellness programs are also very important to face the globally rising levels of obesity, especially after the COVID-19 pandemic and some of the necessary precautionary measures that were implemented during the pandemic response period.

We also recognize the need for national-level regulations on the marketing and advertising of unhealthy food, including on social media platforms, especially for children. Given that obesity is multifactorial, we cannot overemphasize the importance of research to identify modifiable and non-modifiable factors and test the effectiveness of current preventative and curative practices. One very promising example is the "UAE Healthy Future"study, which aims to enroll over 20,000 UAE nationals in order to identify risk factors among adults and determine the need for interventions [15, 25]. This study will provide valuable evidence on the lifestyle and genetic factors associated with common chronic diseases among the Emirati population. However, more research specifically focused on obesity and innovative approaches to its prevention and management is still needed.

19.8 Conclusion

Obesity is considered a global epidemic caused by a wide range of factors, such as genetic, epigenetic, physiological, iatrogenic, environmental, and sociocultural influences. Obesity has been acknowledged as a significant risk factor for various medical conditions within the UAE.

The rapid urbanization of the UAE has led to the adoption of modern, fast-paced, and technology-driven lifestyles, resulting in a significant decline in physical activity. This, coupled with the increased consumption of unhealthy diets lacking essential nutritional value, has contributed to the growing prevalence of obesity and overweight among youth in the country. These findings align with studies conducted in various Arab countries across the Middle East, indicating a similar trend. The significant socioeconomic changes in the UAE require close monitoring of obesity in the pediatric population, where current rates are very alarming. Eating patterns and physical activities are influenced by schools through the food and drinks offered and the opportunities for physical activity in the communities; obesity is influenced by the affordability of options. Health systems in the UAE have established guidelines to highlight weight management interventions for healthcare providers, focusing on a multidisciplinary approach that requires empowerment and awareness. The guidelines include pharmacological and surgical interventions when required. More research focusing on obesity and innovative approaches to prevent and manage it is needed.

Conflicts of Interest The authors have no conflicts of interest to declare.

References

1. Bray GA, Kim KK, Wilding JPH. World obesity FederTL: Bitte den zweiten Punkt löschen. Ation. Obesity: a chronic relapsing progressive disease process. A position statement of the world obesity federation. Obes Rev. 2017;18(7):715–23. https://doi.org/10.1111/obr.12551.
2. Ferri F. Ferri's clinical advisor 2019. 21st ed, 2018
3. Olshansky SJ, Passaro DJ, Hershow RC, Layden J, Carnes BA, Brody J, et al. A potential decline in life expectancy in the United States in the 21st century. N Engl J Med. 2005 Mar 17;352(11):1138–45.
4. Ul-Haq Z, Mackay DF, Fenwick E, Pell JP. Meta-analysis of the association between body mass index and health-related quality of life among adults, assessed by the SF-36. Obesity. 2013;21(3):E322–7.
5. Nawar R, Ibrahim E, Abusnana S, Al Awadi F, Al Hammadi FH, Farghaly M, Fiad TM, Aly H, Aly Mohamed Y, Ben Serghin Z. Understanding the gaps in obesity management in the UAE: perceptions, barriers, and attitudes. Dubai Diabetes Endocrinol J. 2021;27:37–49. https://doi.org/10.1159/000514359.
6. Radwan H, Ballout RA, Hasan H, Lessan N, Karavetian M, Rizk R. The epidemiology and economic burden of obesity and related cardiometabolic disorders in The United Arab Emirates: a systematic review and qualitative synthesis. J Obes. 2018;2018:2185942.
7. InternMoHAPet M. MoHAP ramps up efforts to improve results of national indicator on prevalence of obesity. [online] Ministry of Health and Prevention – UAE; 2022. Available at:

https://mohap.gov.ae/en/media-center/news/4/3/2022/mohap-ramps-up-efforts-to-improve-results-of-national-indicator-on-prevalence-of-obesity. Accessed 31 May 2022.
8. WHO W. 2018. [online] Cdn.who.int. Available at: https://cdn.who.int/media/docs/default-source/ncds/ncd-surveillance/data-reporting/united-arab-emirates/uae-national-health-survey-report-2017-2018.pdf?sfvrsn=86b8b1d9_1&download=true. Accessed 31 May 2022.
9. CDC C. n.d. Defining adult overweight & obesity. [online] Available at: https://www.cdc.gov/obesity/basics/adult-defining.html. Accessed 4 June 2022.
10. CDC C. n.d. Causes of obesity. [online] Available at: https://www.cdc.gov/obesity/basics/causes.html. Accessed 4 June 2022.
11. Sulaiman N, Elbadawi S, Hussein A, Abusnana S, Madani A, Mairghani M, Alawadi F, Sulaiman A, Zimmet P, Huse O, Shaw J, Peeters A. Prevalence of overweight and obesity in United Arab Emirates Expatriates: the UAE National Diabetes and Lifestyle Study; 2017. [online] Available at: https://pubmed.ncbi.nlm.nih.gov/29118852/. Accessed 4 June 2022.
12. AlBlooshi A, Shaban S, AlTunaiji M, Fares N, AlShehhi L, AlShehhi H, AlMazrouei A, Souid A. Increasing obesity rates in school children in United Arab Emirates; 2016. [online] Available at: https://www.ncbi.nlm.nih.gov/pmc/articles/PMC5074293/. Accessed 4 June 2022.
13. WHO W. Obesity and overweight; 2021. [online] Who.int. Available at: https://www.who.int/news-room/fact-sheets/detail/obesity-and-overweight. Accessed 4 June 2022.
14. Alnohair S. Obesity in gulf countries; 2014. [online] Available at: https://pubmed.ncbi.nlm.nih.gov/24899882/. Accessed 5 June 2022.
15. AlAbdulKader A, Tuwairqi K, Rao G. Obesity and cardiovascular risk in the Arab Gulf States; 2020. [online] Available at: https://link.springer.com/article/10.1007/s12170-020-00642-8. Accessed 5 June 2022.
16. Baniissa W, Radwan H, Rossiter R, et al. Prevalence and determinants of overweight/obesity among school-aged adolescents in The United Arab Emirates: a crosssectional study of private and public schools. BMJ Open. 2020;10:e038667. https://doi.org/10.1136/bmjopen-2020-038667.
17. Al Junaibi A, Abdulle A, Sabri S, et al. The prevalence and potential determinants of obesity among school children and adolescents in Abu Dhabi, United Arab Emirates. Int J Obes. 2013;37:68–74. https://pubmed.ncbi.nlm.nih.gov/22890490/
18. Bin Zaal AA, Musaiger AO, D'Souza R. Dietary habits associated with obesity among adolescents in Dubai, United Arab Emirates. Nutr Hosp. 2009;24:437–44.
19. Provenzano S, Santangelo OE, Catalano R, et al. Determinants associated with obesity and physical activity in the public and private schools of the city of Palermo. Acta Med Mediterr. 2018;34:443–8.
20. Global Obesity Observatory. Health systems; 2020. [online] Available at: https://data.worldobesity.org/country/united-arab-emirates-225/#data_health-systems. Accessed 8 June 2022.
21. National Nutrition Strategy 2017–2021. [online] Available at: https://u.ae/en/about-the-uae/strategies-initiatives-and-awards/federal-governments-strategies-and-plans/national-nutrition-strategy-2017-2021. Accessed 9 June 2022.
22. Doh.gov.ae. DOH service requirements for the weight management program for overweight and obese children; 2018. [online] Available at: https://www.doh.gov.ae/-/media/007172E5F6 7B48ECB4F15B0FC8E81BD3.ashx. Accessed 10 June 2022.
23. Doh.gov.ae. Department of health—Abu Dhabi calls for participation in its new program for weight management and obesity in children – News – Department of health; 2019. [online] Available at: https://www.doh.gov.ae/en/news/doh-abu-dhabi-calls-for-participation-in-its-new-program. Accessed 10 June 2022.
24. Weqaya.doh.gov.ae. n.d. Weqaya. [online] Available at: https://weqaya.doh.gov.ae/en-us/home.aspx. Accessed 10 June 2022.
25. Abdulle A, Alnaeemi A, Aljunaibi A, Al Ali A, Al Saedi K, Al Zaabi E, Oumeziane N, Al Bastaki M, Al-Houqani M, Al Maskari F, Al Dhaheri A, Shah S, Loney T, El-Sadig M, Oulhaj A, Wareth L, Al Mahmeed W, Alsafar H, Hirsch B, Al Anouti F, Yaaqoub J, Inman C, Al Hamiz A, Al Hosani A, Haji M, Alsharid T, Al Zaabi T, Al Maisary F, Galani D, Sprosen T, El Shahawy O, Ahn J, Kirchhoff T, Ramasamy R, Schmidt A, Hayes R, Sherman S, Ali R. The UAE healthy future study: a pilot for a prospective cohort study of 20,000 United Arab

Emirates nationals; 2018. [online] Available at: https://bmcpublichealth.biomedcentral.com/articles/10.1186/s12889-017-5012-2. Accessed 12 June 2022.
26. Hajat C, Harrison O, Al Siksek Z, Weqaya: a whole population cardiovascular screening programme in Abu Dhabi, United Arab Emirates; 2012. [online] Available at: https://ajph.aphapublications.org/doi/full/10.2105/AJPH.2011.300290. Accessed 12 June 2022.
27. Finkelstein, E et al. Lifetime direct medical costs of childhood obesity. Pediatrics. 2014;133, 5. Available online at: Lifetime direct medical costs of childhood obesity – PubMed (nih.gov). Accessed 20 July 2022.
28. DOH Program Service Requirements for the Provision of Cardiovascular Risk Factors Screening and Follow-up, PH/PH/NCD/SR/1.2, published Dec 2018. Available on line at: https://www.doh.gov.ae//media/4CEA97DEE7F64DCAA5202AC376C4D0A4.ashx. Accessed 20 July 2022.
29. The Periodic comprehensive periodic screening program (IFHAS), available on line at: https://www.adphc.gov.ae/Public-Health-Programs/Comprehensive-screening-Program%2D%2DIFHAS. Accessed on 20 July 2022.
30. Standard for Obesity and Weight Diagnosis, Pharmacological and Surgical Management Intervention, Available online at: https://www.doh.gov.ae/en/news/doh-abu-dhabi-calls-for-participation-in-its-new-program. Accessed on 20 July 2022.
31. Abu Dhabi Guideline for Implementing the Declaring of Calories on the Menus for Manufacturers and Food Suppliers for Ready-to-Eat foods in the Emirate of Abu Dhabi. Available on line at: https://qcc.gov.ae/-/media/Project/QCC/QCC/Documents/Quality-Infrastructure-Documents/Abu-Dhabi-Specification/Abu-Dhabi-Guideline/ADG-26%2D%2D-Abu-Dhabi-Guideline-for-Implementing-the-Declaring-of-Calories-on-the-Menus-for-Manufactu.pdf. Accessed on 20 July 2022.
32. The UAE National Agenda 2021. Available online at: https://www.vision2021.ae/en/national-agenda-2021. Accessed on line 20th of July 2022.
33. The National Strategy for Wellbeing 2031 for UAE. Available on line at: https://u.ae/en/about-the-uae/strategies-initiatives-and-awards/federal-governments-strategies-and-plans/national-strategy-for-wellbeing-2031
34. UAE: Definition of sugar sweetened beverages for Excise Tax purposes – what to do next?, PWC report Aug 2019 available on line at: https://www.pwc.com/m1/en/services/tax/me-tax-legal-news/2019/uae-definition-sugar-sweetened-beverages-excise-tax-purposes-what-do-next.html. Accessed on 23rd July 2022.
35. WHO Policy – School Canteen Guidelines of the Emirate of Abu Dhabi, Available on line at: https://extranet.who.int/nutrition/gina/en/node/63350. Accessed on 23 July 2022.
36. MOHAP M. 2018. Mohap, cabinet resolution. Available at: https://mohap.gov.ae/documents/20117/1421791/PHP-LAW-EN-77.pdf/e9b4190b-f9a7-bbff-0834-6255af3b17c8?t=1739453134704 (Accessed: 02 June 2025).
37. Health of vulnerable groups, Available on line at the UAE Government portal: https://u.ae/en/information-and-services/health-and-fitness/health-of-vulnerable-groups. Accessed on 23 July 2022.
38. Declaring of Calories on the Menus for Manufacturers and Food Suppliers for Ready-to-Eat foods in the Emirate of Abu Dhabi, Available on line at: https://qcc.gov.ae/-/media/Project/QCC/QCC/Documents/Quality-Infrastructure-Documents/Abu-Dhabi-Specification/Abu-Dhabi-Guideline/ADG-26%2D%2D-Abu Dhabi Guideline-for-Implementing-the-Declaring-of-Calories-on-the-Menus-for-Manufactu.pdf. Accessed on 23 July 2022.
39. Ma'kom program, MOHAP. Available on line at: https://makom-fcsa.hub.arcgis.com/ Accessed on 24 July 2022.
40. In Collaboration with ADEK and In Partnership with SHF Department of Health kicks off 'Healthy Champions' an innovative educational experience for School Students in Abu Dhabi, Available on DOH website at: https://www.doh.gov.ae/en/news/in-collaboration-with-adek-and-in-partnership-with-shf. Accessed on 24 July 2022.
41. Abu Dhabi Public Health Center. Available on line at ADPHC website: https://www.adphc.gov.ae/en. Accessed on 24 July 2022.

42. Abusnana S, Fargaly M, Alfardan SH, Al Hammadi FH, Bashier A, Kaddaha G, McGowan B, Nawar R, Sadiya A. Clinical practice recommendations for the management of obesity in The United Arab Emirates. Obes Facts. 2018;11(5):413–28.
43. The World Obesity Federation The "Regional Recommendations for the Treatment and Management of Adult Obesity in the Gulf & Lebanon" report. Available on line at: https://www.worldobesity.org/resources/resource-library/gulf-lebanon-regional-recommendations. Accessed on 24 July 2022.
44. https://u.ae/en/information-and-services/health-and-fitness/health-insurance. n.d. Health insurance. [online] Available at: https://u.ae/en/information-and-services/health-and-fitness/health-insurance. Accessed 4 Aug 2022.

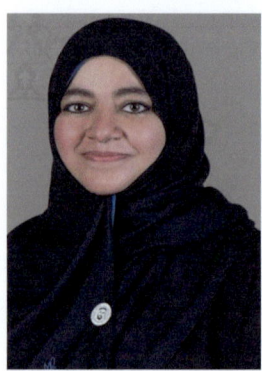

H.E. Dr. Omniyat Mohammed Al Hajeri is a consultant in diabetes, endocrinology, and metabolic diseases and the Executive Director for community health at the Abu Dhabi Public Health Center. She graduated from the Royal College of Surgeons in Ireland (1999) and has been a member of the Royal College of Physicians since 2001. She earned her MPH and DrPH in Public Health and Leadership from the Bloomberg School of Public Health at Johns Hopkins University in 2011 and 2020, respectively.

In addition to her clinical practice, Dr. Omniyat has worked at the first Health Authority established in Abu Dhabi and continued to help shape the health sector and its major reforms from 2001 until today. She has served in the Department of Health as the Director of Public Health and Research since 2011 and was a founding member of the AD Public Health Center in 2019, where she is currently working. She and her team have initiated and implemented many public health initiatives and programs that are still serving the Abu Dhabi community, including initiatives that systematically target combating obesity on multiple levels, including advocacy, policy and guidelines, surveillance and early detection, disease management, and secondary and tertiary prevention, in addition to education and empowerment targeting the involved stakeholders, the public, and industry.

She is a board member of the Abu Dhabi Sports Council and the vice chairwoman of the Sheikha Fatima Bint Mubarak Ladies Sports Academy. She also previously served as an assistant professor of internal medicine at the University of Medicine and Health Sciences.

Dr. Omniyat was awarded the "Chairman of The Executive Council Medal" in the Executive Directors category in 2013, in addition to more than 25 academic awards and medals and 10 other recognition awards during her professional career. She was elected a member of the Delta Omega Honor Society in May 2011 and was re-elected in 2020 for lifelong membership in the U.S. national honor society.

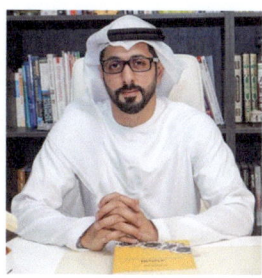

Omar Al Hammadi is a consultant in internal medicine. He graduated from the Royal College of Surgeons, Ireland, in 2009, then completed an internal medicine residency at Sheikh Khalifa Medical City in Abu Dhabi, UAE, accredited by the Accreditation Council for Graduate Medical Education (ACGME-I) in 2014. He has been an Arab Board examiner since 2022. He was a TEDx Inspiring figure for young Emirati students at the UAE University Faculty of Medicine in 2014. He holds a Master's degree in Leadership in Health Professions Education from both the Royal College of Surgeons in Dubai and the University of Sharjah (2017). He holds a Diploma in Obesity and Weight Management from the University of South Wales (2020). He has been the Vice President of the Emirates Internal Medicine Society since 2019. He established a weight management clinic and chaired the Continuous Medical Education Committee at Al Rahba Hospital (2018). He was chosen to be the UAE government's official spokesperson for COVID-19 media briefings between 2020 and 2021. He was the head of medical affairs at Al Rahba Hospital in 2022–2023. Currently, he is Vice President of Medical Services at ADNOC Group and a consultant in internal medicine at Al Dhannah Hospital.

Open Access This chapter is licensed under the terms of the Creative Commons Attribution 4.0 International License (http://creativecommons.org/licenses/by/4.0/), which permits use, sharing, adaptation, distribution and reproduction in any medium or format, as long as you give appropriate credit to the original author(s) and the source, provide a link to the Creative Commons license and indicate if changes were made.

The images or other third party material in this chapter are included in the chapter's Creative Commons license, unless indicated otherwise in a credit line to the material. If material is not included in the chapter's Creative Commons license and your intended use is not permitted by statutory regulation or exceeds the permitted use, you will need to obtain permission directly from the copyright holder.

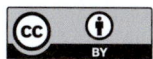

Burden and Characteristics of Diabetes and the Outcome of Care in the UAE

20

Khaled M. Al Dahmani, Mohamed Suliman, Khadija Hafidh, and Salem A. Beshyah

20.1 Introduction

Diabetes is a complex metabolic disorder with increased mortality and morbidity. Based on the most recent International Diabetes Federation (IDF) data from 2021, diabetes mellitus (DM) affects 537 million and is projected to reach 783 million people by 2040. [1] In the Middle East and North Africa (MENA) region, diabetes affects 1 in 6 adults, and this number is predicted to increase to 136 million by 2045.

The Arab Gulf countries, including the United Arab Emirates (UAE), have an increased prevalence of type 2 diabetes (T2D). These countries have similar populations and cultural and socioeconomic characteristics (lifestyle, diet, income, language, and religion). The rates of diabetes, primarily T2D, range from 8 to 22%, according to the latest IDF report. Several risk factors contribute to the increased

---

K. M. Al Dahmani (✉)
Division of Endocrinology, Tawam Hospital, Al Ain, United Arab Emirates

Department of Medicine, UAE University, Al Ain, United Arab Emirates
e-mail: kmdahmani@seha.ae

M. Suliman
Imperial College London Diabetes Center, Al Ain, United Arab Emirates
e-mail: msuliman@icldc.ae

K. Hafidh
Department of Diabetes and Endocrinology, Rashid Hospital, Dubai, United Arab Emirates

Department of Medicine, College of Medicine and Health Sciences, Khalifa University, Abu Dhabi, United Arab Emirates

S. A. Beshyah
Department of Medicine, College of Medicine and Health Sciences, Khalifa University, Abu Dhabi, United Arab Emirates

Department of Medicine, Dubai Medical College for Girls, Dubai, United Arab Emirates

The Endocrine Clinic, Bareen International Hospital, Abu Dhabi, United Arab Emirates

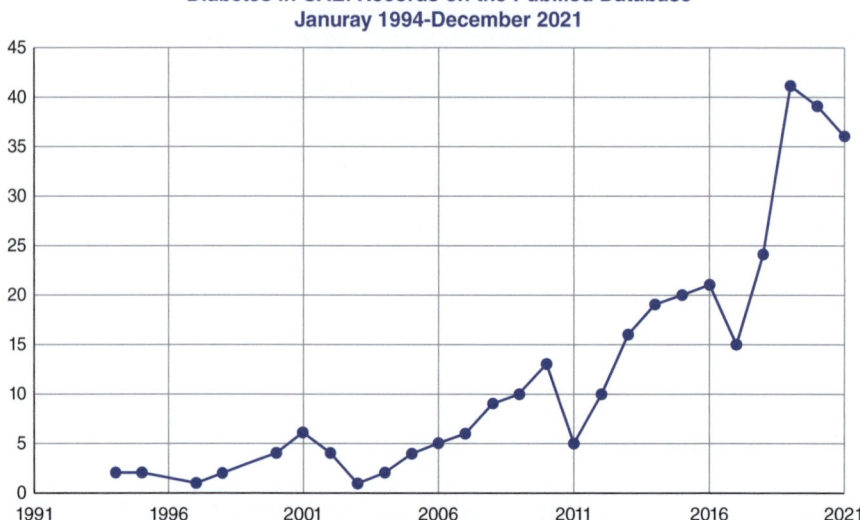

Fig. 20.1 The increasing scientific research on diabetes in the UAE is reflected in the increasing number of articles identified by the search term (Diabetes and Emirates) in the abstract or title fields of the PubMed database up to 31.12.2021. Retrieved on 21.7.2022

prevalence of diabetes in this region, particularly obesity and an unhealthy lifestyle. As a result of increased wealth and prosperity, Gulf countries now experience higher healthcare expenditures and life expectancies. However, genetic susceptibility and the incidence of T2D among children and young people are also rising. Diabetes has severe implications for individuals, families, and society.

A good body of scholarly work on diabetes in the UAE has been published over the last three decades (Fig. 20.1). Diabetes prevalence in the UAE is estimated at 12.3% for the 20–79 age group (age-adjusted prevalence: 16.4%) [1]. Given its importance for public health, this chapter reviews the literature on the epidemiology, types, clinical characteristics, complications, and quality of care, including the role of technology in diabetes care. We also explore the challenges of diabetes management and future directions in clinical practice and research.

20.2 Epidemiology

20.2.1 Prevalence

Several studies have evaluated the epidemiology of diabetes in the UAE. The majority focused on T2D and reported on the prevalence of the disease. However, only a few studies provided data representing the entire country (Table 20.1). Malik M. et al. studied the diabetes prevalence in 5,844 adults (>20 years) between October 1999 and June 2000 [2]. Diabetes diagnosis was based on fasting blood glucose

Table 20.1 Summary of the T2DM prevalence studies in the UAE

Authors, year [ref]	Patient population/setting	Prevalence	Comments
Malik M et al. 2005 [2]	5844 adults (>20 years) between Oct 1999 and June 2000	Crude 20% Age-adjusted: UAE: 25% Expats: 16–21%	40% of UAE citizens of the cohort DM Dx: FBG >7 mmol/l and or BG >11.1 mmol/l post 2 h OGTT Of interest, 41% of those with diabetes were undiagnosed prior to the survey IFG/IGT prevalence: 5%/21% in women, 7%/16% in men
Saadi H et al. et al. 2007 [3]	Survey of 2455 adults in 452 houses in Al Ain (Dec 2005 – Nov 2006)	29% (among 373 people who underwent testing; 30–64 years)	Microvascular complications were present in 35–52% of patients with diabetes, while peripheral vascular disease and coronary heart disease were present in 11.1% and 10.5%, respectively PreDM prevalence: 20.2%
Hajat C et al. 2012 [4]	50,138 self-enrolled adults at primary care clinics for weqaya screening in Abu Dhabi (2009–2010)	Age-standardized 24.6%	DM Dx: HbA1c > 6.5%, RBG >11.1 mmol/l or history of DM on medications Limitations: Selection bias due to self-enrollment of participants, data from Abu Dhabi emirate only, and type of DM not defined PreDM prevalence: 29.5%
Suliman N et al. 2018 [7]	2724 migrants in UAE	19.1%	Results were derived from the UAEDIAB study. The cohort was derived from individuals coming to medical centers for visa renewal. The majority were males, Asians, non-Arabs, and 40 years or younger. Data from all emirates except Abu Dhabi
Suliman N et al., 2018 [6]	872 adult UAE nationals living in the Northern Emirates	Crude: 25.1%	Results were derived from the UAEDIAB study Diabetes Dx based on HbA1c of >6.5% Undiagnosed diabetes was reported in 14.8% of the participants Data from all emirates except Abu Dhabi
Hamoudi R et al. 2019 [5]	3203 individuals	UAE nationals (M: 21%/ F: 23%) Asian non-Arabs (M: 23%/ F: 20%).	Results were derived from the UAEDIAB study. DM Dx: HbA1c > 6.5%, FBG > 7 mmol/l. 25% of UAE nationals in this cohort. Nationals with DM had the highest rate of positive family history of diabetes (64%) compared to other ethnicities. Data from all emirates except Abu Dhabi
Alawadi F et al. [8]	2245 adults from the Dubai household survey	UAE nationals: 19.3%; expats: 12.4%	The results are similar to the data from the DHHS 2014/17, with the reported prevalence of 19% for UAE nationals and 14.7% for expats (9)

Abbreviations: *UAEDIAB* UAE National Diabetes and Lifestyle Study

(FBG) and/or 2-h post-oral glucose tolerance test (OGTT) criteria. The overall crude diabetes prevalence was 20%. The age-adjusted prevalence was higher among UAE nationals (25%) compared with expatriates (16–21%). However, expatriates in the UAE had a higher risk of diabetes and prediabetes compared with populations in their respective home countries. Of interest, 41% of those with diabetes were unrecognized before the survey. The prevalence of impaired fasting glucose (IFG) was 5% in women and 7% in men. Saadi H. et al. surveyed 2455 adults in 452 houses in Al Ain between December 2005 and November 2006 [3]. Of those, 10.2% reported having diabetes. Among the 373 non-pregnant women and men who underwent testing, the age-standardized rate for diabetes was 29% among the 30–64 age group. Microvascular complications were present in 35–52% of patients with diabetes, while coronary heart disease and peripheral vascular disease were present in 10.5 and 11.1%, respectively. The reported prevalence of prediabetes was 20.2% in this study. Hajat et al. evaluated cardiovascular risk factors among 50,138 self-enrolled adults (>18 years) presenting to 25 primary care clinics. This was part of the screening program in the Emirate of Abu Dhabi (*Weqaya; Arabic for prevention*) between April 2009 and June 2010 [4]. In this study, the age-standardized prevalence rates of diabetes were 24.6 and 29.5% for prediabetes. A cross-sectional study by Hamoudi et al. evaluated the diabetes prevalence among UAE nationals and expatriates residing for at least 4 years in Sharjah, Dubai, and the rest of the Northern Emirates [5]. A total of 3,202 individuals (25% UAE nationals) were included. The reported adjusted diabetes rates were highest among UAE nationals (males 21% and females 23%) and non-Arab Asians (males 23% and females 20%). Suliman N. et al. reported a crude diabetes prevalence of 25.1% in a sample of 872 adult UAE nationals from the five Northern Emirates [6]. The results were derived from the UAE National Diabetes and Lifestyle Study, collected in 2013. The diagnosis of diabetes was based on HbA1c values >6.5%. Previously undiagnosed diabetes was reported in 14.8% of the participants. The same group reported an age-adjusted diabetes prevalence of 19.1% among 2724 migrants in the UAE [7]. This cohort was derived from individuals coming to medical centers for visa renewal. The majority were males (81%), Asian non-Arabs (71%), and younger than 40 years (65%) [7]. Furthermore, Alawadi F. et al. recently reported on 2245 adults from the Dubai household survey, indicating an overall diabetes prevalence. The prevalence was significantly higher among UAE nationals than among expats (19.3 vs. 12.4) [8]. The findings are similar to the DHHS 2014/17 data, with a reported prevalence of 19% for UAE nationals and 14.7% for expats [9].

20.2.2 Incidence

There is limited information on the incidence of diabetes in the UAE. A small study by Sreedharan J. et al. evaluated the incidence of diabetes in Emiratis in the Emirate of Ajman in 2010 [10]. The study included 101 patients with a new diagnosis of T2D (aged 23–78 years, 65% were female). The overall incidence was calculated as 4.8/1000 person-years (PY). The incidence was higher in females than in males, with the highest incidence observed in the 55–59-year age group [10].

20.2.3 Special Population

20.2.3.1 Latent Autoimmune Diabetes in Adults (LADA)
Autoimmune diabetes, defined as diabetes-associated autoantibodies without ketoacidosis or not requiring insulin for at least 6 months following the date of diagnosis, was assessed in a study from a large center in Abu Dhabi [11]. Among 17,062 patients with diabetes aged between 30 and 70 years, the prevalence of LADA was 2.6% in this setting.

20.2.3.2 Neonatal Diabetes Mellitus (NDM)
The characteristics of NDM in patients across pediatric diabetes clinics in Abu Dhabi were studied. Twenty-five cases were identified, and the incidence of NDM was approximately 1:29,000 live births. Of those, 23 had permanent NDM, while 2 had transient NDM [12]. Genetic alterations were detected in 21 cases (9 EIF2AK3 mutations, 6 INS mutations, 2 PTF1A enhancer deletions, 1 KCNJ11 mutation, 1 ABCC8 variant, and four without mutations). For the transient NDM, the genetic abnormalities were a homozygous INS c-331C > G mutation and a 6q24 methylation defect [12].

20.2.3.3 Sex and Diabetes
A couple of studies provided UAE sex-based diabetes data. The prevalence of prediabetes and diabetes was evaluated among 555 young female college students in a cross-sectional study in 2021 in Al Ain. Diagnosis in Emirati girls was based on HbA1c and fasting plasma glucose (FPG) [13]. The age range was 17–25 years. Based on HbA1c values, the prevalence of diabetes and prediabetes was 8.6 and 24.0%, respectively. Remarkably lower corresponding estimates were detected using FPG at 9.2% and 0.5%, respectively. Abnormal glycemic status was significantly associated with abnormal lipids and increased inflammatory markers. However, using FPG to evaluate glycemic control underestimated the size of the problem of unrecognized diabetes, which could have serious implications for public health and clinical practice. Furthermore, Meo SA et al. estimated the prevalence of T2D among males in the Middle East (including the UAE) from a review of 74 studies [14]. From 17 studies included the prevalence of T2D among males in the UAE was 25.8%. The prevalence in the Gulf in general correlated directly with the gross domestic product of these states ($p = 0.0005$).

20.2.3.4 Adolescents
A large nationwide cross-sectional study investigated the prevalence of diabetes and risk factors among adolescents attending schools in the UAE in 2021 [15]. A stratified random sample survey of public and private schools (number = 151) across the seven UAE emirates involved 6365 students (12–22 years). Overall, diabetes was reported in 0.9% of students. This was significantly more evident in males than in females (1.5% vs. 0.5%, respectively). Diabetes status was positively associated with some characteristics of adolescents, such as parental marital status, male sex, smoking, and illegal drug use. The increased frequency of smoking and/or illegal

drug use suggests a need for mental health and behavioral interventions and better parental support and involvement.

20.2.3.5 Diabetes During Pregnancy

Emirati women, similar to other Arab women, have been identified as carrying a high risk of gestational diabetes and diabetes during pregnancy on several counts. A comprehensive discussion of this aspect is beyond the scope of the current chapter. Nonetheless, contributing factors include obesity, ethnicity, and high fertility with pregnancies continuing to the third and fourth decades of life. The earlier research was mainly conducted by obstetricians from the UAE, mostly in clinic-based surveys, and addressed overall frequency and the contribution of diabetes to the general outcome of pregnancy and some specific complications, such as macrosomia and shoulder dystocia. Also, several studies particularly from Al Ain, investigated the validity and utility of various strategies for the screening and diagnosis of gestational diabetes in this high-risk, multiethnic population. However, more recent studies are larger and include epidemiology of diabetes in pregnancy in the UAE, applicability of several diagnostic guidelines, and the impact of lifestyle management. The Mutaba'ah study is the largest multi-center mother and child cohort study in the UAE, with an 18-year follow-up. The findings indicate discrepancies among the diagnostic criteria in identifying GDM cases. This emphasizes the need to unify GDM diagnostic criteria in this population to provide accurate and reliable incidence estimates for healthcare planning, especially because the agreement with the recommended criteria was not optimal.

20.3 Evaluation and Management

20.3.1 The Need for International and National Diabetes Guidelines

Diabetes requires continuous medical care, consisting of multi-factorial risk modification strategies, not merely glycemic control. Diabetes care is constantly changing with new evidence, therapies, and technologies that may improve the well-being and outcomes of people with diabetes. Consequently, most international bodies concerned with diabetes (e.g., the ADA, EASD, IDF) produce and regularly update guidelines that cover all aspects of diabetes care based on the interpretation of the latest available evidence [16, 17]. These international guidelines targeted mainly the needs of the West. In 2020, the Emirates Diabetes Society (EDS) revised its national consensus guidelines for managing T2D [18, 19]. The guidelines considered the screening, diagnosis, and management of T2D in adults and also for those individuals with prediabetes and obesity (i.e., those at risk for developing the disease). These guidelines have been adapted for national use to enhance the level of care for people with diabetes by increasing knowledge among healthcare providers practicing in the country.

20.3.2 Goals of Treatment and Organization of Diabetes Care

Diabetes management aims to reduce the risk of complications and maintain a good quality of life [16–20]. To achieve this, hyperglycemia and cardiovascular risk factors should be controlled, which necessitates regular follow-up. A patient-centered approach should be adopted to increase patients' engagement in self-care activities. Individualized treatment goals and strategies should be informed by carefully considering patient factors and preferences. Patients with diabetes benefit from the services of coordinated multidisciplinary teams. Such teams include physicians experienced in diabetes management, diabetes educators, dietitians, and podiatrists. Other healthcare professions, such as pharmacists, ophthalmologists, cardiologists, nephrologists, and vascular surgeons, contribute their relevant expertise [20].

20.3.3 Glycemic Targets

Glycemic control is usually assessed by HbA1c, since it reflects the average glycemic status over the previous 3 months. Real-time assessments involve self-monitoring of capillary blood glucose (SMBG) and continuous glucose monitoring (CGM) [21]. For most patients with diabetes, a target HbA1c lower than 7% should be the goal. This target corresponds to SMBG fasting glucose values of 80–130 mg/dL and postprandial levels of <180 mg/dL [21]. However, individualized targets should be based on age, hypoglycemic risk, diabetes duration, patient motivation, and comorbidities, especially cardiovascular disease.

20.3.3.1 Strategies for Glycemic Management
To achieve the glycemic targets stated above, a comprehensive diabetes care program is required. This program consists of diabetes self-management education (DSME), lifestyle modification through diet and physical activity, glucose monitoring, and appropriately selected pharmacotherapeutic agents [19–22].

20.3.3.2 Structured Education
DSME in a structured manner should be accessed by all patients with diabetes and/or their family members appropriately. DSME and support should be patient-centered and may be offered in group or individual settings. DSME aims to empower patients and families with the necessary knowledge, skills, and capabilities needed for confident self-management of diabetes, and to provide activities necessary to sustain the lifestyle modifications required to manage the condition in the long term [19, 22].

20.3.3.3 Nutrition
All patients with diabetes should have access to a qualified dietitian at diagnosis and as needed later (at times of intensification, suboptimal responses, problems with hypoglycemia, weight gain, etc.,). The aim is to provide patients with personalized nutritional recommendations. These recommendations should consider specific

needs and goals based on personal and cultural preferences, and provide practical tools to adopt healthy eating patterns. As most patients with T2D are either overweight or obese, nutritional plans should aim for a weight loss of 5% or more to achieve favorable outcomes in the optimal control of blood glucose, plasma lipids, and arterial blood pressure [19, 22].

There is not enough evidence to advocate for the ideal percentage of calories derived from carbohydrates, fat, and protein for all people with diabetes. Hence, the distribution of macronutrients should be based on an individualized evaluation of metabolic goals, personal eating patterns, and patient preferences. In general, nutritional advice emphasizes the use of non-starchy vegetables, minimizes refined grains and added sugars, and gives preference to whole foods over highly processed foods [22].

Dietary plans for UAE patients need to consider the local custom of eating dates [18]. For instance, dates are a popular food item incorporated into staple food and as a dessert. Dates are rich in calories; any meal plan should account for this. Dates have been shown to have a high fiber content and to be a source of antioxidants and minerals [23]. A local UAE study showed that dates have a low glycemic index and may not result in significant postprandial glycemic excursions [24]. Nonetheless, excessive intake of dates is not uncommon, especially in the summer, and has a negative impact on diabetes control, albeit transiently for many patients.

20.3.3.4 Physical Activity
Regular physical activity improves the control of blood glucose levels, contributes to weight reduction efforts, lowers cardiovascular risk, and enhances overall well-being and self-esteem [22]. Consequently, international and national guidelines recommend that patients with T2D undertake moderate aerobic exercise for more than 150 min, together with 2–3 sessions of resistance exercise per week [19, 21]. Of particular concern is that a local study found that 3% of patients with T2D in the UAE perform physical activity levels that meet the recommendations above. Therefore, much effort is needed to encourage patients with diabetes to exercise and to identify and address barriers preventing them from doing so [25].

20.3.3.5 Antihyperglycemic Pharmacotherapy

20.3.3.5.1 Initial Treatment
Because of the progressive nature of T2D, most patients experience relentless deterioration of beta-cell function and rising hyperglycemia. Therefore, lifestyle changes alone will not be enough to maintain target blood glucose levels. For this reason, the increasing pharmacotherapy will be needed in most patients [16, 19, 26]. Traditionally, first-line therapy starts with metformin combined with comprehensive lifestyle modification.

20.3.3.5.2 Intensification of Therapy
After metformin, other drugs can be added as required. Choices include sulphonylureas, DPP-4 inhibitors, GLP-1 receptor agonists, SGLT2 inhibitors, pioglitazone, and insulin [16, 17, 19, 26]. Over the last decade, several cardiovascular outcomes

trials (CVOTs) have provided evidence that two classes of anti-diabetic medications (the GLP-1RAs and the SGLT2 inhibitors) have resulted in cardiovascular and renal benefits beyond their glycemic efficacy. These findings have significantly influenced the latest guidelines on the choice of anti-diabetic medications [16, 17, 19, 26].

The national UAE diabetes guidelines have classified patients with T2D into four risk groups: very high, high, moderate, or low, depending on several factors, including CVD or target organ damage, age, diabetes duration, and cardiovascular risk [19]. The guidelines suggested that drugs with proven cardiovascular and renal benefits (i.e., GLP-1RAs and SGLT2 inhibitors) should be offered to patients in the very high-risk category and should be considered for those in the high-risk category regardless of the level of glycemic control. For those at moderate and low risk, the choice of drugs will depend on other factors, such as hypoglycemia risk, impact on weight, and cost [19].

20.3.3.5.3 Insulin Therapy for T2D

Many patients with T2D eventually require insulin therapy. Patients should be made aware of the progressive nature of T2D, and the use of insulin should be viewed as a phase in the natural progression of the disease, and not as a sign of the patient's personal failure. With careful patient education and an explanation of the efficacy of insulin in maintaining glycemic control, patients' reluctance to use insulin can be overcome [26]. Healthcare professionals should avoid clinical inertia, and should not delay recommending treatment intensification for patients who are not meeting treatment goals. Patients' resistance can be overcome with appropriate education and support [26].

20.3.4 Cardiovascular Disease and Risk Management

20.3.4.1 The Overall Approach

Atherosclerotic cardiovascular disease (ASCVD) encompasses all diseases presumed to be of atherosclerotic origin, such as coronary heart disease (CAD), peripheral arterial disease (PAD), and cerebrovascular disease (CeVD). These are the leading causes of morbidity and mortality in patients with diabetes [16, 17, 27]. Established risk factors for ASCVD, such as hypertension and dyslipidemia, are commonly associated with diabetes. Other risk factors for ASCVD include smoking, obesity, albuminuria, chronic kidney disease, and a family history of premature CAD. All modifiable risk factors should be eagerly identified and adequately treated. In addition to CAD, heart failure has been more recently recognized as a critical cardiovascular complication in patients with diabetes. There is clear and undisputed evidence that controlling these risk factors prevents or slows the progression of ASCVD in patients with diabetes. For this reason, control of these ASCVD risk factors is vital in the management of patients with diabetes [17, 27].

CVD risk factors need to be addressed more aggressively in patients with cardiovascular disease in the Middle East, as their risk is higher than that of their counterparts in

Western countries. It has been shown that patients who present with acute coronary attacks in the Middle East are 10–12 years younger than those in Western countries [28]. Furthermore, patients from the UAE with T2D were found to have a high prevalence of comorbidities, such as hypertension, dyslipidemia, and obesity [29].

20.3.4.2 Blood Pressure Targets

Hypertension is a major risk factor for both ASCVD and microvascular complications, and the current targets agreed upon by most international guidelines are a BP of <140/90 mmHg in patients with low risk for CVD, while a target of <130/80 should be aimed for in those with high CV-risk [17, 27]. Specific anti-hypertensive drug classes that have been shown to decrease cardiovascular events and should be used in patients with diabetes include ACE inhibitors, ARBs, dihydropyridine calcium channel blockers, and thiazide-like diuretics. Therefore, there is a compelling indication for patients with diabetes to receive ACE inhibitors or ARBs as their first-line medications, especially in the presence of CAD or albuminuria in patients [17, 27].

20.3.4.3 Lipid Targets

LDL-cholesterol has been shown to correlate linearly with the risk of IHD; therefore, it is considered the primary lipid parameter to be addressed. Together with lifestyle modification, statins are the drugs of choice for treating dyslipidemia in patients with diabetes. Patients should be prescribed high-intensity or moderate-intensity statins to achieve the appropriate lipid targets [17, 27]. Patients with a previous ASCVD event are considered very high risk, whereas those with multiple risk factors are at high risk. The target LDL-c for those at very high risk for ASCVD is <55 mg/dL, for high risk <70 mg/dL, and for moderate risk <100 mg/dL. For patients who do not achieve targets on the maximum tolerated dose of a statin, consideration should be given to adding ezetimibe or a PCSK9 inhibitor [17, 27].

20.3.4.4 Use of Antiplatelet Therapy

Aspirin is recommended for all patients with diabetes who have had a previous ASCVD event (i.e., for secondary prevention). However, aspirin is generally not recommended for patients with no prior evidence of ASCVD (i.e., for primary prevention), as, for most patients, the risk of bleeding outweighs any ASCVD reduction benefits [17, 27].

20.4 Diabetes and Technology

20.4.1 Diabetes Technology in Context

In general, technology has transformed healthcare; patients with diabetes have the potential to benefit most from the integration of technology with management paradigms. Technology has revolutionized insulin delivery systems, blood glucose monitoring, and screening for diabetes-related complications through artificial intelligence and remote consultation (telemedicine) applications. Digital tools, like platforms, apps, and devices for managing diabetes are increasingly utilized. They can facilitate treatment delivery and monitoring to personalize diabetes care depending on each patient's individual needs. Introducing communication tools easily connects patients with health professionals remotely.

In the context of diabetes, technology denotes all hardware, software, and devices that people with diabetes utilize to assist in their management of the condition [30]. Practically, diabetes technology encompasses two main categories: insulin delivery tools and blood glucose monitoring technology.

Currently, insulin can be administered by different types of pen devices for multiple-dose injection regimens or via pumps for continuous subcutaneous insulin infusion [CSII]. The adequacy of blood glucose control is assessed by self-monitoring of blood glucose (SMBG), continuous glucose monitoring (CGM), and intermittent (flash) glucose monitoring (FGM). However, advanced diabetes technology includes hybrid devices that can monitor glucose and deliver insulin simultaneously. Some of these devices function automatically. The software also provides support for diabetes self-management. Various forms of diabetes technology, patients' education, and professional close follow-up obviously enhance the health and well-being of people with diabetes and reduce the anxiety of families and caregivers. However, the rapidly changing and increasingly complex diabetes technology landscape can potentially hinder patient's and healthcare providers' abilities to implement it.

Mobile health ("mHealth") is defined as "medical and public health practice supported by various mobile devices." These devices include all monitoring devices, mobile phones, personal digital assistants, and other wireless devices [31]. Generally, digital health apps may be considered under three categories depending on the purpose of their use, such as for tracking wellness, for stand-alone medical devices, or for display, download, and/or use of data from medical devices that diagnose, monitor, treat, or prevent a given medical condition [32]. These devices enhance quality of life and health outcomes by coaching patients, supporting their healthy behavior, maintaining lifestyle modification, guiding dosing, encouraging glucose monitoring, even remotely, assisting with interpreting results, and reducing complications [33].

Several studies have confirmed that self-care behaviors specific to glucose monitoring are essential to managing glycemic levels. Incorporating technology into diabetes management can augment and facilitate self-management. Indeed, CGM systems have fully revolutionized the management of diabetes [34–36].

20.4.2 Benefits of CGM

Recent abilities to continuously measure interstitial glucose allow the detection of time in range (TIR), glucose variability, and hypoglycemic events [37]. In 2017, an international consensus on continuous glucose monitoring standardized the use of CGM technology [38]. TIR is a novel concept based on the time between near-normal glucose levels. TIR is usually 70–180 mg/dL for most patients but can vary individually. The use of CGM helps promote therapy adjustments in T1D and T2D, especially for patients with frequent hypoglycemia [38]. Based on current evidence, a TIR of >70% is recommended for most individuals. Other metrics derived from CGM technology include mean glucose, glucose variability, and the glucose management indicator (formerly called estimated HbA1c), in addition to time below range (TBR) and time above range (TAR). All metrics should be examined in every patient-physician encounter and appraised against the recommendations.

20.4.3 Summary of Technology-Related Studies in the UAE

The UAE has been an early adopter of CGM technologies. Glucose monitoring devices are available to most patients with diabetes in both public and private healthcare facilities. Several groups have published their CGM experiences in different patient populations and clinical settings (Table 20.2) [39–44].

Two prospective studies from the same tertiary care center in the UAE employed Freestyle-Libre continuous glucose monitoring (FSL-CGM) in two high-risk groups (e.g., CAD and CKD) who were observing Ramadan fasting in 2016 [39, 40]. Firstly, a prospective interventional study included 25 patients with T2D with stage 3 CKD [39]. FSL-CGM data showed significantly longer duration and more frequent hypoglycemic episodes during Ramadan than during non-Ramadan. The mean blood glucose was significantly lower during Ramadan than in the non-fasting period. There was no significant change in renal function during fasting. Secondly, the other study aimed to determine the safety of fasting in 21 diabetic patients with CHD who insisted on fasting [40]. Similarly, FSL-CGM data showed a higher frequency of hypoglycemia during Ramadan. However, no adverse cardiovascular effects were observed due to fasting in patients with stable CHD. These studies demonstrated higher rates of FSL-CGM-detected hypoglycemia, but there were no renal or cardiac adverse effects during Ramadan.

In a different patient population, Afandi et al. studied hypoglycemia in 21 adolescents (mean age 16 years) with T1D while fasting during Ramadan [41]. They were monitored using the FSL-CGM system. Glucose profiles are determined by the eating pattern and the times of the day and night. Hypoglycemia typically occurs in the early evening, immediately before iftar. This suggests that reducing basal insulin may be needed to reduce hypoglycemia [41].

Ehtisham and Adhami compared the sensor-estimated HbA1c and the measured HbA1c. Twenty-four children with T1D used glucose sensors (20 FSL-CGM and 4 Dexcom G5). [42] The estimated HbA1c tended to be lower than the measured HbA1c, but the mean difference was negligible (measured HbA1c: 7.9% vs. predicted HbA1c: 7.7%). There was no relation between lower sensor wear time and estimated HbA1c. With increasing sensor accuracy, three-monthly HbA1c blood tests may eventually be replaced with the estimated HbA1c.

Farooqi HM et al. evaluated the impact of telemonitoring (TM) on glycemic control and compliance in 38 patients with T2D who were lost to follow-up in an interventional single-center study in Dubai [43]. Patients were given home-based

Table 20.2 Summary of the studies on CGM and telemonitoring conducted in the UAE

Authors, year [ref]	Patient population (N)	Clinical setting	Technology used	Summary of findings
Alawadi F et al., 2019 [39]	High-risk patients with DM and chronic kidney disease stage 3 (CKD 3) $N = 25$	Ramadan fasting (RF)	Freestyle libre flash glucose monitoring system	RF under close supervision and optimal diabetes care was not associated with worsening of HbA1c and renal function. More frequent and prolonged hypoglycemic episodes occurred during RF
Hassanein M et al. 2019 [40]	Patients with T2DM with stable known CHD $N = 21$	During and after RF	Freestyle libre monitoring device (FSL-CGM)	No associated adverse cardiovascular effects with RF in patients with stable CHD under optimal diabetes care. A higher frequency of hypoglycemia occurred during RF
Afandi B et al., 2018 [41]	Children with type 1 DM ($N = 24$)		Freestyle libre or Dexcom G5	Hypoglycemia is typically encountered during the hours preceding *Iftar*, indicating an over-effect of basal insulin; hence, basal insulin reduction is necessary to minimize hypoglycemia risk
Ashraf, T et al. 2021 [42]	T2DM adults $N = 21$	COVID lockdown	FreeStyle libre flash glucose monitoring (FGM)	Despite reduced exercise and the psychological stress of the COVID-related lockdown period, FGM-derived markers of glycemic control were improved
Farooqi H M, et al. 2022 [43]	Lost-to-follow-up T2DM patients. $N = 38$	Routine follow-up	Home-based Telemonitoring (TM) devices	TM significantly improved overall DM outcomes (glycemic control and body weight), indicating its effectiveness in a challenging population previously lost to follow-up
Ehtisham & Adhami 2019 [44]	Children with T1DM	Routine follow-up	Comparison of FL-CGM-derived estimated HbA1c (eHbA1c) with measured HbA1c (mHbA1c)	eHbA1c tended to be lower than the mHbA1c, with no relationship between sensor wear time and HbA1c. eHbA1c was within 0.75% of the mHbA1c 79.2% of the time

RF Ramadan Fasting

TM devices at the initial visit, and they were evaluated 3 months later. The mean HbA1c decreased significantly to 7.4% at 3 months of follow-up from 10.3% at baseline. This suggests that TM significantly improved overall diabetes outcomes, demonstrating its effectiveness in this challenging population of T2D patients who were lost to follow-up [43]. Another group from Abu Dhabi described their experience with TM [44]. They described data on 21 individuals using FSL-CGM who were remotely connected to the diabetes clinic. Glycemic control improved during the COVID-19 lockdown compared to the preceding weeks. Therefore, despite the reduced exercise and the lockdown-associated psychological stress, FGM-CGM-derived markers of glycemic control improved [44].

These few studies in our region show how integrating technology into diabetes management can improve diabetes care, particularly on ethnically relevant issues such as Ramadan fasting. As the technology continues to be refined and upgraded, healthcare providers will have access to tools that can monitor patients more accurately and provide real-time management recommendations. Improvements in monitoring have the potential to translate into a better quality of life with fewer diabetes-related complications. The UAE has been at the forefront of embracing these advances.

Insulin delivery systems are valuable tools for diabetes management. However, not every patient with diabetes may be eligible for pump use. Identifying candidates is the first step. The ADA recommends a list of questions to be answered when choosing a given approach for insulin therapy (i.e., pump versus multiple-dose injections) [26]. These questions need to be addressed under regional circumstances to get the best possible approach for the individual patient within his or her skills, financial means, and access to professional support.

20.5 Professional and Patient Perspectives

In 2007, DM prevalence in the UAE ranked as the second highest in the world, according to the IDF's annual report. Since then, there has been a significant public, governmental, and professional interest in the challenges of diabetes [45]. Several epidemiological studies have documented the increased prevalence of diabetes in both the native population and expatriates. Centers of excellence for diabetes care were established as stand-alone centers (such as the Rashid Center of Diabetes and Research (RCDR), Imperial College London Diabetes Center, and Dubai Diabetes Center (ICLDC)) or within the major health facilities (Sheikh Khalifa Medical City, Dubai Hospital, and Tawam Hospital). Diabetes care received appropriate prominence in all public and private healthcare facilities, with high-caliber physicians recruited from all over the world. An increasing volume of research has been published (Fig. 20.1). Several annual and occasional conferences on diabetes have been conducted by the Emirates Diabetes Society and the Gulf Chapter of the American Association of Clinical Endocrinologists (now the Gulf Association of Endocrinology and Diabetes (GAED)) to improve the understanding and management of diabetes. The UAE recently became a focal point for health-related Ramadan fasting research, including diabetes. To support physicians' knowledge and expertise, several international universities providing postgraduate education in diabetes, particularly from the UK (Cardiff, Warwick, and Leicester), have extended their presence in the UAE. A national university (University of Sharjah) recently provided an MSc degree in diabetes care. In addition, an endocrinology fellowship program was established in Abu Dhabi as a collaboration between ICLDC and SEHA hospitals (3 years of training: one in the UAE and two in the UK). Another endocrinology fellowship program started at Dubai Hospital in 2022. Two medical journals specializing in diabetes and endocrinology are in the UAE (*Dubai Diabetes and Metabolism Journal* by Dubai Health Authority and *Journal of Diabetes and Endocrine Practice* by GAED). This may encourage more locally conducted research to find its way to publication. In addition, the Arab Society of Pediatric Endocrinology and Diabetes (ASPED) has its headquarters in the UAE and runs many of its activities locally.

The UAE pioneered early access to the latest types and therapies, including modern pharmacological classes, shortly after their approvals in their manufacturing countries. Also, health insurance schemes widely support the adoption of high technology, such as CGM and insulin pump therapy, as discussed above. Trained and qualified diabetes educators increasingly support patients. There is a single lay patient society named Friends for Diabetes Association, based in Sharjah, which plays a vital patient advocacy role and conducts regular activities.

20.6 Conclusions, Challenges, and Future Directions

20.6.1 Conclusions

This chapter reviewed the available knowledge on the burden and challenges and solutions for the problem of diabetes in the UAE. Diabetes in the UAE considerably burdens the healthcare system. A concerted effort is needed to adopt uniform diabetes care nationwide, use standardized methods to document the national burden, explore possible differences in various epidemiological phenomena, improve access to healthcare, assess the impact on outcomes, and evaluate the cost-effectiveness of care using different models.

20.6.2 Highlights from Local Data

Among Emirati female college students, the prevalence of prediabetes and diabetes, based on HbA1c, was 9.2% and 24%, respectively [13]. The incidence of T2D among overweight or obese Emiratis was 16.3 per 1,000 person-years. Age over 44 years and obesity in women, and prediabetes in men, predicted the development of diabetes [45]. The prevalence of metabolic syndrome among adults in the UAE is about 37%. Age, sex, BMI, ethnicity, marital status, and educational level were positively associated with metabolic syndrome [46]. Microalbuminuria is highly prevalent (61%) among patients with diabetes in the UAE, with higher rates in men, individuals with elevated BMI, and in the presence of other diabetes-related microvascular complications [47]. Non-optimal glycemic control may account for more than one in three deaths among adult UAE nationals with diabetes [48].

20.6.3 Limitations and Future Directions

A remarkable body of literature has been produced over the last two decades on diabetes and diabetes care in the UAE. However, there are notable limitations in the available literature. Several studies are based on a single city or locality rather than on a more comprehensive national basis. In addition, some outcome studies rely on data collected from different healthcare systems with differing levels of coverage and access to conventional and advanced resources. These may introduce methodological and conceptual confounders that prevent the generalization of conclusions on a national level or direct comparisons due to the different methods employed in various settings. Many studies are limited to observational methodology rather than to reflections on quality improvement exercises. There are limited data on the incidence of diabetes in the UAE, particularly T1DM and monogenic form of diabetes. In addition, the different models of healthcare provision (national health services, independent sector, and employer-associated provision) and financing (national, insurance-based, and out-of-pocket) add further complexity.

A concerted effort is needed to evaluate diabetes nationwide using a unified methodology. Specifically, documenting the nationwide burden, exploring possible differences in various epidemiological phenomena, and assessing healthcare are crucial. These efforts should ascertain the impact on outcomes and evaluate the cost-effectiveness of care using different models.

Authors' Contributions Equal.

Conflicts of Interest The authors have no conflicts of interest to declare.

Funding and Sponsorship None.

Compliance with Ethical Principles Not applicable.

References

1. International diabetes federation. IDF diabetes atlas, 10th edn 2021. Accessed 2022 July 27. Available from: https://www.diabetes-atlas.org/en/resources
2. Malik M, Bakir A, Saab BA, Roglic G, King H. Glucose intolerance and associated factors in the multi-ethnic population of The United Arab Emirates: results of a national survey. Diabetes Res Clin Pract. 2005;69(2):188–95.
3. Saadi H, Carruthers SG, Nagelkerke N, Al-Maskari F, Afandi B, Reed R, Lukic M, Nicholls M, Kazam E, Algawi K, Al-Kaabi J, Leduc C, Sabri S, El-Sadig M, Elkhumaidi S, Agarwal M, Benedict S. Prevalence of diabetes mellitus and its complications in a population-based sample in Al Ain, United Arab Emirates. Diabetes Res Clin Pract. 2007 Dec;78(3):369–77.

4. Hajat C, Harrison O, Al Siksek Z. Weqaya: a population-wide cardiovascular screening program in Abu Dhabi, United Arab Emirates. Am J Public Health. 2012;102(5):909–14.
5. Sulaiman N, Mahmoud I, Hussein A, El-badawi S, Abusnana S, Zimmet P, et al. Diabetes risk score in The United Arab Emirates: a screening tool for the early detection of type 2 diabetes mellitus. BMJ Open Diabetes Res Care. 2018;6(1):e000489.
6. Sulaiman N, Albadawi S, Abusnana S, Mairghani M, Hussein A, Al Awadi F, et al. High prevalence of diabetes among migrants in The United Arab Emirates using a cross-sectional survey. Sci Rep. 2018;8(1):6862.
7. Hamoudi R, Sharif-Askari NS, Sharif-Askari FS, Abusnana S, Aljaibeji H, Taneera J, Sulaiman N. Prediabetes and diabetes prevalence and risk factors comparison between ethnic groups in the United Arab Emirates. Sci Rep. 2019 Nov;25(1):17437.
8. Alawadi F, Hassanein M, Sulaiman E, Hussain HY, Mamdouh H, Ibrahim G, et al. The prevalence of diabetes and prediabetes among the population: finding from Dubai household survey 2014 and 2017. Dubai Diabetes Endocrinol J. 2020;26(2):1–7.
9. Al Awadi F, Hassanein M, Hussain HY, Mohammed H, Ibrahim G, Khater A, Suliman A. Prevalence of diabetes and associated health risk factors among adults in Dubai, United Arab Emirates: results from Dubai household survey 2019. Dubai Diabetes Endocrinol J. 2020;26:164–73.
10. Sreedharan J, Muttappallymyalil J, Al Sharbatti S, Hassoun S, Safadi R, Abdirahman I, Hameed WA, Ibrahim AM, Takana MT, Fouda AM. Incidence of type 2 diabetes mellitus among Emirati residents in Ajman, United Arab Emirates. Korean J Fam Med. 2015;36:253–7.
11. Maddaloni E, Lessan N, Al Tikriti A, Buzzetti R, Pozzilli P, Barakat MT. Latent autoimmune diabetes in adults in The United Arab Emirates: clinical features and factors related to insulin-requirement. PLoS One. 2015 Aug 7;10(8):e0131837.
12. Deeb A, Habib A, Kaplan W, Attia S, Hadi S, Osman A, Al-Jubeh J, Flanagan S, DeFranco E, Ellard S. Genetic characteristics, clinical spectrum, and incidence of neonatal diabetes in the emirate of Abu Dhabi, United Arab Emirates. Am J Med Genet A. 2016 Mar;170(3):602–9.
13. Mohamad MN, Ismail LC, Stojanovska L, Apostolopoulos V, Feehan J, Jarrar AH, Al Dhaheri AS. The prevalence of diabetes amongst young Emirati female adults in The United Arab Emirates: a cross-sectional study. PLoS One. 2021 June 17;16(6):e0252884. https://doi.org/10.1371/journal.pone.0252884.
14. Meo SA, Sheikh SA, Sattar K, Akram A, Hassan A, Meo AS, Usmani AM, Qalbani E, Ullah A. Prevalence of type 2 diabetes mellitus among men in the Middle East: a retrospective study. Am J Mens Health. 2019 May-Jun;13(3):1557988319848577. https://doi.org/10.1177/1557988319848577.
15. Barakat C, Yousufzai SJ, Booth A, Benova L. Prevalence of and risk factors for diabetes mellitus in the school-attending adolescent population of The United Arab Emirates: a large cross-sectional study. BMJ Open. 2021 Sep 15;11(9):e046956. https://doi.org/10.1136/bmjopen-2020-046956.
16. Buse J, Wexler D, Tapas A, et al. 2019 update to management of hyperglycemia in type 2 diabetes, 2018. A consensus report by the American Diabetes Association (ADA) and the European Association for the Study of Diabetes (EASD). Diabetes Care. 2020;43(2):487–93.
17. Cosentino F, Grant P, Aboyans V, et al. 2019 ESC guidelines on diabetes, prediabetes, and cardiovascular disease developed in collaboration with the EASD. Eur Heart J. 2020;41:255–323.
18. UAE National Diabetes Committee. National diabetes guidelines: United Arab Emirates 2009. Abu Dhabi: The UAE National Diabetes Committee; 2009.
19. Alawadi F, Abusnana S, Afandi B, et al. Emirates diabetes society consensus guidelines for the Management of Type 2 diabetes mellitus. Dubai Diabetes Endocrinol J. 2020;26:1. https://doi.org/10.1159/000506508.
20. American Diabetes Association. 4 comprehensive medical evaluation and assessment for comorbidities: standards of medical care in diabetes-2022. Diabetes Care. 2022;45(Suppl. 1):S46–59.
21. American Diabetes Association. 6 glycemic targets: standards of medical care in diabetes-2022. Diabetes Care. 2022;45(Suppl. 1):S83–96.

22. American Diabetes Association. 5 facilitating behavior change and well-being to improve health outcomes: standards of medical care in diabetes-2022. Diabetes Care. 2022;45(Suppl. 1):S60–82.
23. Al-Farsi M, Yong LC. Nutritional and functional properties of dates: a review. Crit Rev Food Sci Nutr. 2008;48:877–87.
24. Alkaabi J, Al-Dabbagh B, Ahmad S, et al. Glycemic indices of five varieties of dates in healthy and diabetic subjects. Nutr J. 2011;10:59.
25. Al-Kaabi J, Al-Maskari F, Saadi H, et al. Physical activity and reported barriers to activity among type 2 diabetic patients in The United Arab Emirates. Rev Diabet Stud. 2009;6:271–8.
26. American Diabetes Association. 9 pharmacologic approaches to glycemic treatment: standards of medical Care in Diabetes-2022. Diabetes Care. 2022;45(Suppl. 1):S125–43.
27. American Diabetes Association. 10 cardiovascular disease and risk management: standards of medical Care in Diabetes-2022. Diabetes Care. 2022;45(Suppl. 1):S144–74.
28. Gehani A, Al Hinai A, Zubaid M, et al. Association of risk factors with acute myocardial infarction in middle eastern countries: the INTERHEART Middle East study. Eur J Prev Cardiol. 2014;21(4):400–10.
29. Alzaabi A, Al-Kaabi J, Al-Maskari F, et al. Prevalence of diabetes and cardio-metabolic risk factors in young men in The United Arab Emirates: a cross-sectional national survey. Endocrinol Diabetes Metab J. 2019;2:e00081.
30. American Diabetes Association. 7. Diabetes technology: standards of medical care in diabetes-2022. Diabetes Care. 2022;45(Suppl. 1):S97–S112. https://doi.org/10.2337/dc22-S007.
31. WHO. mHealth: new horizons for health through mobile technologies. Based on the findings of the second global survey on eHealth. Global observatory for eHealth series – volume 3. Geneva: WHO; 2011. Available from www.who.int/goe/publications/goe_mhealth_web.pdf. Accessed 17 Sep 2018.
32. Elenko E, Speier A, Zohar D. A regulatory framework emerges for digital medicine. Nat Biotechnol. 2015;33(7):697–702. https://doi.org/10.1038/nbt.3284.
33. American Association of Diabetes Educators. AADE7 self-care behaviors. Diabetes Educ. 2008;34:445–4.
34. Dungan K, Verma N, Reddy N. Monitoring technologies–continuous glucose monitoring, mobile technology, biomarkers of glycemic control. South Dartmouth: Endotext; 2015.
35. Mcgarraugh G, Bragg R, Weinstein R. Free style navigator continuous glucose monitoring system with TRUstart algorithm, a 1-hour warm-up time. J Diabetes Sci Technol. 2011;5:99.
36. Welsh JB, Gao P, Derdzinski M, Puhr S, Johnson TK, Walker TC, Graham C. Diabetes Technol Ther. 2019;21:128.
37. Wright LA, Hirsch IB. Metrics beyond hemoglobin A1C in diabetes management: time in range, hypoglycemia, and other parameters. Diab Technol Ther. 2017;19:S16–26.
38. Danne T, Nimri R, Battelino T, Bergenstal RM, Close K, DeVries H, et al. International consensus on the use of continuous glucose monitoring. Diab Care. 2017;40:1631–40.
39. Alawadi F, Rashid F, Bashier A, Abdelgadir E, Al Saeed M, Abuelkheir S, et al. Free Style Libre Continues Glucose Monitoring (FSL-CGM) to monitor the impact of Ramadan fasting on glycemic changes and kidney function in high-risk patients with diabetes and chronic kidney disease stage 3 under optimal diabetes care. Diabetes Res Clin Pract. 2019;151:305–12.
40. Hassanein M, Rashid F, Elsayed M, Bashir A, Al Saeed M, Abdelgadir E, et al. Assessment of risk of fasting during Ramadan under optimal diabetes care in high-risk patients with diabetes and coronary heart disease through FreeStyle Libre flash continuous glucose monitor (FSL-GCMS). Diabetes Res Clin Pract. 2019;150:308–14.
41. Afandi B, Kaplan W, Majd L, Roubi S. Rate, timing, and severity of hypoglycemia in adolescents with type 1 diabetes during Ramadan fasting: a study with freestyle libre flash glucose monitoring system. Ibnosina J Med Biomed Sci. 2018;10:9–11.
42. Ehtisham S, Adhami S. Accuracy of glucose sensor estimate of HbA1c in children with type 1 diabetes. ESPE Abstracts. 2019;92(RFC7):1.
43. Farooqi HM, Abdelmannan DK, Al Buflasa MM, Abbas H, Moataz A, Xavier M, et al. The impact of Telemonitoring on improving glycemic and metabolic control in previ-

ously lost-to-follow-up patients with type 2 diabetes mellitus: a single-center interventional study in The United Arab Emirates. Int J Clin Pract. 2022;2022:6286574. https://doi.org/10.1155/2022/6286574.
44. Ashraf T, Helal R, Majeed M, Lessan N. An analysis of flash glucose monitoring (FGM) data on insulin-treated patients with diabetes: effects of COVID-19 lockdown. Endocr Abstr. 2021;73:AEP161.
45. Regmi D, Al-Shamsi S, Govender RD, Alkaabi J. Incidence and risk factors of type 2 diabetes mellitus in an overweight and obese population: a long-term retrospective cohort study from a gulf state. BMJ Open. 2020;10:e035813.
46. Mahmoud I, Suliman N. Prevalence of metabolic syndrome and associated risk factors in The United Arab Emirates: a cross-sectional population-based study. Front Public Health. 2021;9:811006.
47. Al-Maskari F, El-Sadig M, Obineche E. Prevalence and determinants of microalbuminuria among diabetic patients in The United Arab Emirates. BMC Nephrol. 2008;9(1)
48. Al-Shamsi S, Govender RD, Soteriades ES. Mortality and potential years of life lost attributable to non-optimal glycaemic control in men and women with diabetes in The United Arab Emirates: a population-based retrospective cohort study. BMJ Open. 2019;9:e032654.

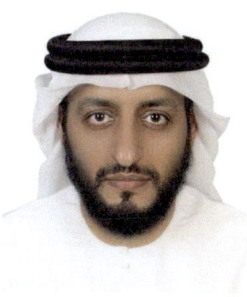

Dr. Khaled M. Al Dahmani obtained his medical degree from UAE University in 2006 and then completed his internal medicine residency training at the University of British Columbia in Canada (2011). He completed subspecialty training in endocrinology and metabolism at Dalhousie University in 2013, followed by a 1-year combined clinical and research fellowship training in pituitary disorders and thyroid cancer at the same university. He is board-certified in internal medicine and endocrinology in the USA and Canada.

Dr. Aldahmani is the scientific committee chairperson of the Emirates Diabetes and Endocrinology Society (EDES) and the Past President of the Gulf Association of Endocrinology and Diabetes (GAED).

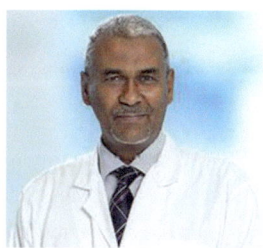

Dr. Mohamed Suliman worked as a consultant endocrinologist in the United Kingdom before moving to the UAE in 2013. He is interested in education, training, and obesity management and has been the lead doctor for clinical guidelines at the ICLDC.

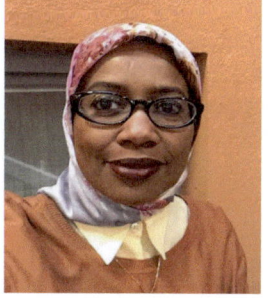

Dr. Khadija Hafidh has over 20 years of experience in internal medicine, diabetes, obesity, metabolism, and medical education. Currently, she heads the Diabetes Unit at Rashid Hospital, Dubai Health Authority. She is a Fellow of the Royal College of Physicians of Edinburgh and a member of the American College of Physicians. She is an associate professor and clinical tutor at Dubai Medical College, UAE. She is a steering committee member for the UAE National Diabetes Guidelines and an Editorial Board Member of the *Dubai Diabetes and Endocrine Journal*. Her research interests include the cardiovascular complications of diabetes and obesity.

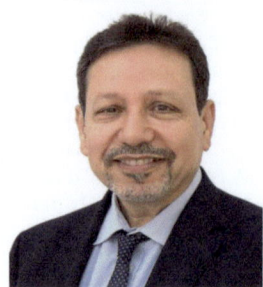

Dr. Salem A. Beshyah graduated from the Medical School of Tripoli in 1981. After receiving basic clinical training in Tripoli and Glasgow (1982–1986) and passing the MRCP in 1987, he trained as a clinical registrar in Leicester and Bedford (1987–1989), where he developed an interest in diabetes care. Following this, he undertook a 4-year clinical research fellowship and training in clinical endocrinology at Imperial College London. He has been a consultant general physician interested in diabetes and endocrinology for the past 25 years in Harlow, Essex, UK, and Abu Dhabi, UAE. He is particularly interested in cultural aspects of medicine, education, and culturally relevant clinical research. He has been involved in local and regional educational and research activities and maintained a vast network of local, regional, and international collaborations.

Open Access This chapter is licensed under the terms of the Creative Commons Attribution 4.0 International License (http://creativecommons.org/licenses/by/4.0/), which permits use, sharing, adaptation, distribution and reproduction in any medium or format, as long as you give appropriate credit to the original author(s) and the source, provide a link to the Creative Commons license and indicate if changes were made.

The images or other third party material in this chapter are included in the chapter's Creative Commons license, unless indicated otherwise in a credit line to the material. If material is not included in the chapter's Creative Commons license and your intended use is not permitted by statutory regulation or exceeds the permitted use, you will need to obtain permission directly from the copyright holder.

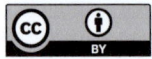

Cardiovascular Healthcare in the UAE

21

Yosef Manla ⓘ, Laszlo Göbölös, Sultan Abdulali, Azan Salem Binbrek, Arif Al Nooryani, Srinath Kidambi, and Wael Almahmeed ⓘ

21.1 The UAE Demographics

The United Arab Emirates (UAE), a country in Western Asia, is formed from a federation of seven emirates, consisting of Abu Dhabi (the capital), Ajman, Dubai (the most populous), Fujairah, Ras Al Khaimah, Sharjah, and Umm Al Quwain. In 2021, the UAE population was estimated to be 9.4 million, with an estimated life expectancy of 77.2 years (for males) and 80.9 years (for females) [1, 2]. Birth and death rates were estimated to be 10.3% and 1.9%, respectively [2]. Current health expenditure per capita in the UAE measured $ 2191.8, representing 5.67% of the gross domestic product in 2020 [3, 4]. With the establishment of highly specialized centers, international healthcare partnerships, and the initiation of training programs to train the next generation of UAE physicians, the healthcare sector in the UAE has undergone massive development in the last two decades.

Y. Manla · W. Almahmeed (✉)
Department of Cardiology, Heart, Vascular and Thoracic Institute, Cleveland Clinic Abu Dhabi, Abu Dhabi, United Arab Emirates

L. Göbölös
Department of Cardiac Surgery, Heart, Vascular and Thoracic Institute, Cleveland Clinic Abu Dhabi, Abu Dhabi, United Arab Emirates

S. Abdulali
Department of Cardiology, Sheikh Khalifa Medical City, Abu Dhabi, United Arab Emirates

A. S. Binbrek
Department of Cardiology, Rashid Hospital, Dubai Health Authority, Dubai, United Arab Emirates

A. Al Nooryani
Cardiac Center, Al Qassimi Hospital, Al Sharjah, United Arab Emirates

S. Kidambi
Division of Cardiology, Sheikh Shakhbout Medical City, Abu Dhabi, United Arab Emirates

© The Author(s) 2025
H. O. Al-Shamsi (ed.), *Healthcare in the United Arab Emirates*, https://doi.org/10.1007/978-981-96-0523-1_21

21.2 The Burden of Cardiovascular Disease and Its Associated Risk Factors in the UAE

21.2.1 Cardiovascular Disease Prevalence in the UAE

According to estimations of the 2021 Global Burden of Disease (GBD) Study [5], there were 729,852 (95% uncertainty interval (UI) [674,007.3 – 791,870.8]) prevalent cases of cardiovascular disease (CVD) in the UAE, corresponding to an increase of 85% in the rate of prevalent cases (4,105 to 7,578 cases per 100,000) and a rise of 2% (10,842 to 11,067 cases per 100,000) in the age-standardized rate of prevalent cases between 1990 and 2021. Figure 21.1a shows temporal trends in age-standardized rates of CVD prevalence in the UAE between 1990 and 2021, which exceed global rates [6]. In the year 2021, ischemic heart disease contributed the most to the number of prevalent CVD cases in the UAE (52.7%), followed by stroke (15.6%), other cardiovascular and circulatory diseases (14.2%), rheumatic heart disease (11.9%), lower extremity peripheral arterial disease (6.7%), atrial fibrillation and flutter (1.8%), and hypertensive heart disease (1.6%) Table 21.1 [5]. Furthermore, data from the GBD 2021 study estimated that 45,606.15 (95% UI [37,436–54,719.2]) cases lived with HF in the UAE in 2021, with the age-standardized prevalence increasing by 8% (795.6 to 861.3, cases per 100,000) between the years 1990 and 2021 [5,7].

Notably, the UAE population features an early presentation of CVD; this is clearly evident in the GBD 2021 study as the rate of CVD prevalence in the UAE

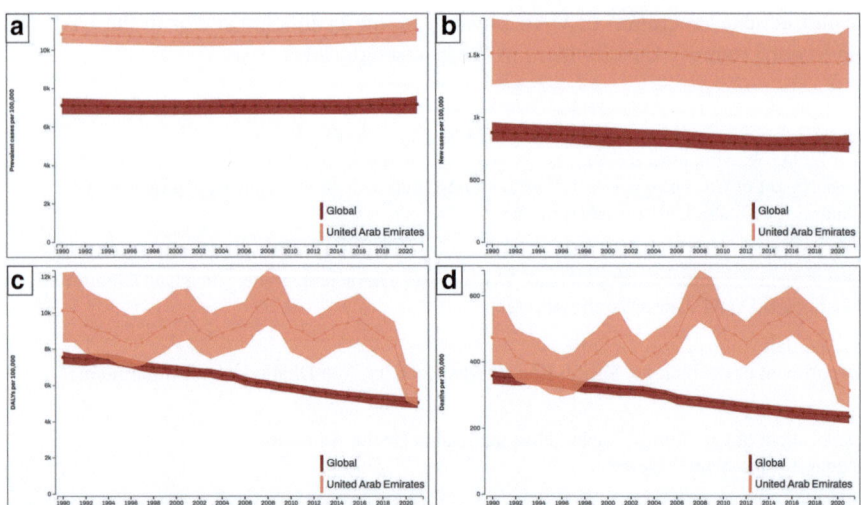

Fig. 21.1 Trends in the age-standardized rates of cardiovascular disease globally and in the UAE from 1990 to 2021. (**a**)Prevalence. (**b**)Incidence. (**c**) Disability-adjusted life years Disability-adjusted life years (DALYs). (**d**) Mortality. Source: Institute for Health Metrics and Evaluation. Used with permission. All rights reserved [6]

Table 21.1 Estimates on the incidence, prevalence, and mortality of various cardiovascular conditions in the UAE in 2021 [5]

Cardiovascular diseases	Incidence	Prevalence	Mortality
All	85,873.1 [69,396.2–104,217.3]	729,852 [674,007.3–791,870.8]	5,122.7 [4,113.3–6,191.9]
Ischemic heart disease	62,589.1 [45,589.4–80,890.7]	384,627.5 [344,256.3–428,314.1]	2,885.1 [2,296.3–3,515.4]
Stroke	10,210.1 [8,910.5–11,682.8]	113,378.9 [108,776.8–117,974.6]	1,243.5 [970.5–1,518.7]
Rheumatic heart disease	3,039 [2,358.2–3,863.8]	86,912.6 [67,764–109,241.4]	72.5 [52.2–120.2]
Lower extremity peripheral artery disease	5,687.8 [4,693.3–6,983.2]	48,988.4 [40,585.6–58,286.3]	19.4 [14.7-25.5]
Hypertensive heart disease	–	12,043.3 [9,192.8–16,089.8]	451.15 [334.4–595.8]
Atrial fibrillation and flutter	1,662 [1,236–2,172.9]	13,474.7 [9,821–18,266.3]	30.1 [23.5–37.4]
Non-rheumatic valvular heart disease	844.2 [709.2–1,008.7]	7,281.7 [6,076.7–8,738]	68.3 [53.3–85.6]
Other cardiovascular and circulatory diseases	–	103,822.7 [71,576.3–141,227.9]	95.2 [64.5–123.5]
Cardiomyopathy and myocarditis	1,106.4 [794.5–1,486.4]	8,429.3 [6,654.3–10,606]	175.1 [134.1–225.7]
Endocarditis	688.8 [523.9–891.7]	341.1 [276.6–428.2]	29.4 [20–44.2]

Values were represented as estimates, 95% uncertainty interval for the age group (20–54 years) exceeded the global rate (6,464.4 vs. 3,910 cases per 100,000) in 2021 [5]. This aligns with prior reports from the Emirates [8, 9]. Results from a 3-year prospective registry of acute coronary syndrome in the UAE (UAE-ACS Registry) featured young patients with high-risk profiles [9]. Another prospective study of patients hospitalized with heart failure in Dubai featured younger patients and a higher prevalence of diabetes compared to developed countries [8].

21.2.2 Cardiovascular Disease Incidence in the UAE

According to estimates of the 2021 GBD Study [5], there were 85,873.1 (95% UI [69,396.2–104,217.3]) incident cases of CVD in the UAE in 2021, corresponding to an increase of 89% in the rate of incident cases (470.7 to 891.6 cases per 100,000) and a deccrease of 3% (1,516.4 to 1,464.5 cases per 100,000) in the age-standardized rate of incident cases between 1990 and 2021. Figure 21.1b shows temporal trends in age-standardized rates of CVD incidence in the UAE, which exceed global rates [6]. In the year 2021, ischemic heart disease contributed the most to the number of incident CVD cases in the UAE (72.9%), followed by stroke (11.9%), lower extremity peripheral arterial disease (6.6%), rheumatic heart disease (3.5%), and atrial fibrillation and flutter (1.9%) (Table 21.1) [5]. These estimates align with a study by Al-Shamsi et al., which was conducted on 977 subjects with a median follow-up of 9 years and reported an incidence rate of 12.7 per 1000 person-years (95% confidence interval [CI] 10.4–15.4) in the UAE [10]. Al-Shamsi et al. reported that systolic blood pressure, estimated glomerular filtration rate, and serum glycosylated hemoglobin A1c level were strong predictors of major CVD events in both sexes [10]. Another recent study has shown a rate of recurrent CVD events of 92.1 per 1000 person-years among patients with a history of CVD; in addition, older age, female sex, and diabetes mellitus were reported as significant predictors of these events [11].

21.2.3 Disability-Adjusted Life Years Due to Cardiovascular Diseases in the UAE

In 2021, the number of disability-adjusted life years [(DALY), defined as the sum of years of life lost and years lived with disability of years of life lost] due to CVD was 190,482.8 years, corresponding to a decrease of 33% in the rate of DALYs (2,942.7 to 1,977.8 years per 100,000) between 1990 and 2021. The age-standardized rate of DALYs decreased significantly (a decrease of 43%, from 10,135.3 to 5,758.5 years per 100,000) between 1990 and 2021 [5]. Figure 21.1c shows the temporal trends in age-standardized rates of DALYs due to CVD in the UAE [6].

21.2.4 Mortality Rates Due to Cardiovascular Diseases and Their Attributable Risk Factors in the UAE

In 2021, CVD was the leading cause of death overall in the UAE, accounting for an estimated 5,122.7 deaths. This represented around 25.5% of all-cause deaths and corresponded to a decrease of 38% in the death rate (86 to 53.2 deaths per 100,000) between 1990 and 2021. Additionally, the age-standardized rate of deaths decreased by 34% (from 473.2 to 314.1 per 100,000) between 1990 and 2021 [5]. Figure 21.1d shows the temporal trends in age-standardized rates of CVD deaths in the UAE [6].

In 2021, ischemic heart disease contributed the most to the number of deaths due to CVD (56.3%), followed by stroke (24.3%), hypertensive heart disease (8.8%), and cardiomyopathy and myocarditis (3.4%) (Table 21.1) [5].

The 2021 GBD study identified major attributable risk factors for the age-standardized CVD death rate; the top four risk factors were high systolic blood pressure, followed by particular matter pollution, high LDL cholesterol, and high fasting plasma glucose [5]. Comparing these risk factors to the year 1990, CVD mortality attributable to high body mass index ranked higher in 2021, while smoking ranked lower (Fig. 21.2) [6].

Results of the UAE STEPS 2017–2018 survey [12], a survey of 8214 participants with an 87% response rate, funded by the Ministry of Health and Prevention and conducted in collaboration between local entities and the World Health Organization Eastern Mediterranean Region Office, demonstrated that 2.7% [1.7–3.7%] of the participants aged 40–69 had a 10-year CVD risk of =30 or an existing CVD with a male to female predominance of 2:1. In terms of CVD risk factors (current daily smokers, less than five servings of fruits and vegetables per day, insufficient physical activity, BMI = 25 kg/m^2, raised blood pressure (BP) [systolic BP = 140 and/or diastolic BP = 90 mmHg or currently on medication for raised BP]), the results of

1990 rank	2021 rank
1 High blood pressure	1 High blood pressure
2 Particulate matter	2 Particulate matter
3 High LDL	3 High LDL
4 High fasting plasma glucose	4 High fasting plasma glucose
5 Kidney dysfunction	5 High body-mass index
6 High body-mass index	6 Kidney dysfunction
7 Low whole grains	7 High temperature
8 Low temperature	8 Low whole grains
9 Smoking	9 Low temperature
10 High temperature	10 Smoking
11 Lead	11 Lead
12 Secondhand smoke	12 Secondhand smoke

Fig. 21.2 Changes in the rank of risk factors attributable to age-standardized cardiovascular death rates in the UAE from 1990 to 2021. Source: Institute for Health Metrics and Evaluation. Used with permission. All rights reserved

the survey showed that 49.5% [47.1–51.9], 61.7% [58.0–65.5], and 52.5% [50.5–54.6] of the age groups 18–44, 45–69, and 18–69, respectively, had three or more of the above risk factors. While only 1.5% [0.9–2.0] had no risk factors. One of the landmark CVD screening programs in Abu Dhabi was the "Weqaya" (Arabic for "protection") Population-wide Screening Program that commenced in April 2008, using self-reported indicators, anthropometric measures, and blood tests [13, 14]. In a Weqaya analysis of 50,138 adults aged 18 years or older taking part in the screening program, the rates of prevalence of CVD risk factors were 35%, 18%, 44%, and 23.1% for obesity, diabetes, dyslipidemia, and hypertension, respectively [13, 14]. Furthermore, within its first 2 years, Weqaya has delivered a Framingham Risk Score for almost every adult Emirati, predicting approximately 8,800 CVD events during a 10-year period, with most of these events occurring in the age group (>35 years) for males and (>45 years) for females [13, 14].

According to a recent cross-sectional study in Al Ain City, this high burden of cardiometabolic risk factors was also evident in Emirati school-aged children with excess body weight compared to those with normal weight [15]. In addition to the high prevalence of these risk factors, data from the UAE Health Future Study, an ongoing population-based prospective cohort study that aims to explore risk factors for non-communicable disease, have shown a high association between these risk factors, such that dyslipidemia and obesity co-existed with other cardiometabolic risk factors more than 70% and 50% of the time, and 40% of the population accumulated more than two risk factors. Therefore, creating a heavy burden of risk factors and forecasting an increase in the burden of CVD in the UAE [16, 17]. Currently, there is a substantial focus in the UAE on adopting novel models of care for patients with cardiometabolic syndrome through multidisciplinary cardiometabolic clinics, a form of collaboration between multiple specialties to achieve optimal management [18].

21.3 Milestones in the Development of the UAE Cardiovascular Healthcare System

21.3.1 Historical Overview

A half-century ago, with the union of the seven Emirates, the Trucial Sheikhdoms transformed from a traditional society to a modern one. This change has notably affected all segments of everyday life, including human medicine. The initial essential care level hospitals could not provide a sufficient answer for complex patient care demands; many needed to travel abroad to receive specialized treatment, including cardiosurgical procedures. Since the region features a high burden of CVD and its cardiometabolic risk factors, as well as a growing burden of heart failure (HF), traveling abroad for medical treatment by itself does not provide a sufficient response for the everyday needs of the entire society, especially in emergencies [19–22]. The initial medical expansion steps included the local establishment of smaller, specialized hospitals with locum surgeon coverage, but reliable, constant patient care required complex medical units, including but not limited to Mafraq

Hospital and Sheikh Khalifa Medical City, Abu Dhabi; Dubai and Rashid Hospitals, Dubai; and Al Qassimi Hospital, Sharjah. These hospitals have covered a good generic cardiovascular (CV) spectrum with established, well-cooperative teams. However, subspecialty fields and complex approaches were unavailable or just temporarily supported by external guest surgeons or teams.

21.3.2 Healthcare Sectors in the UAE

The private sector is playing an increasingly prominent role in healthcare across the U.A.E., supported by the government's strategies to promote public-private partnerships and attract private investment. Still, public institutions and government-linked entities continue to play a comparatively large role in healthcare provision [23]:

- Public sector institutions:1-Dubai Health : an integrated academic health system comprised of 6 hospitals, 26 ambulatory health centers, including facilities previously operated by the Dubai Health Authority. Its flagship facilities encompass Dubai Hospital, Rashid Hospital, Latifa Women and Children Hospital, Hatta Hospital, Jebel Ali Hospital, and Al Jalila Children's Hospital. 2- Emirates Health Services (EHS): It consists of all hospitals, primary care facilities, and public healthPublic health services previously provided under the Ministry of Health and Prevention (MOHAP)Ministry of Health and Prevention (MOHAP) umbrella, including at least 17 hospitals and nearly 100 clinics throughout the UAE, especially in the northern emirates [23].
- Major government-linked entities: including M42 and PureHealth. M42 is a partnership between Mubadala Investment Company, a major Abu Dhabi government investment vehicle, and G42 Healthcare. Its subsidiaries include Cleveland Clinic Abu Dhabi, Imperial College London Diabetes Center, National Reference Laboratory, Danat Al Emarat, Healthpoint, and Malaffi. In 2022, the Abu Dhabi Health Services Company (SEHA), previously operating all public hospitals and clinics in Abu Dhabi, became part of PureHealth-a subsidiary of an Abu Dhabi-based holding company—forming the largest integrated healthcare network in the U.A.E. with 25 hospitals, 100 clinics, and 160 laboratories [23].

21.3.3 Milestones in Cardiovascular Care in Abu Dhabi

Central Hospital opened its doors in 1968 with 50 beds and expanded progressively; a coronary care unit was established there 10 years later, and the hospital had a cardiac catheterization lab under the radiology department to treat valvular heart diseases [24, 25]. In 1978, a 320-bed hospital, Al-Jazeera, was built adjacent to Central Hospital, and both hospitals were working together as a composite unit. In the same year, Mafraq Hospital was built, 35 kilometers away from the populated island. The hospital gradually developed to encompass a dedicated accident and emergency unit and a surgical department specializing in cardiac, neuro, thoracic, pediatric, and plastic surgery, as well as kidney transplantation. Dr. Amin Fikree, a pioneer in cardiovascular care in the UAE, established Mafraq Hospital's state-of-the-art cardiology department, staffed by physicians who worked at Central Hospital, and some equipment was also moved from there [24, 25]. The establishment of a cardiac catheterization lab and cardiac surgery department at Mafraq Hospital in 1985 was an important milestone, with percutaneous coronary intervention being conducted in the year 1990; until then, less than 100 cases were performed annually [26]. Despite having a single operation theater and only six cardiac surgery intensive care unit beds, the number of heart surgeries increased and reached 300–320 open-heart surgical procedures per year. These surgeries included mitral and aortic valve replacements. In addition, the hospital also encompassed the only neonatal cardiac surgery unit in the country, with Prof. Gerald Brom performing the first ASD closure. The pediatric cardiac surgery program performed complex surgeries with very good results, including in neonates. Many cases were referred from neighboring countries, including Oman, Yemen, and Bahrain. On average, 100 pediatric cases were done annually from 1990 until 2007, when Sheikh Khalifa Medical Center (SKMC) started the pediatric program. From 1989 until 2003, Mafraq Hospital was the major Cardiac Surgery Centre for the whole of the UAE.

SKMC opened in 2000 as a tertiary referral center with a particular interest in cardiac sciences. Al-Jazeera, Central, and SKMC hospitals were all "amalgamated" in 2005 to form the new Sheikh Khalifa Medical City (maintaining the same acronym). In 2003, Shaikh Khalifa Medical City started Cardiac Services. In 2005, a 24/7 primary PCI center was established under the leadership of Prof. Wael Al Mahmeed, considered to be the first in the Middle East Region. Following that, the cardiology department at SKMC became the most comprehensive cardiac department in the UAE, providing all the necessary services, from electrophysiology and adult congenital heart disease to rehabilitation. The department was accredited by the Society of Chest Pain Centers, the European Association of Echocardiography, and the American College of Cardiology (ACC) as an International Centre of Excellence (ICOE) Program in 2009, 2012, and 2015 respectively. The first extracorporeal membrane oxygenation (ECMO) device in a child was implanted at SKMC in 2008, followed by the first BiVentricular Assist Device (Berlin Heart Excor) in 2009. In 2011, SKMC also performed its first ECMO implantation in an adult. Although, to some extent, pediatric cardiosurgical procedures were performed in Mafraq Hospital, the complete institutional framework was missing and was eventually fulfilled by the pediatric cardiosurgical program that started at SKMC in April 2007 (Dr. Laszlo Királby). This dedicated, high-performing team saved nearly 5000 little lives until March 2021, setting a milestone in regional pediatric cardiosurgical care with outstanding outcomes comparable with the European Association for Cardio-Thoracic Surgery standards (EACTS).

The opening of Cleveland Clinic Abu Dhabi (CCAD) in 2015 reshaped the CV care landscape in the country, with century-old medical expertise delivered by one of the largest and most impactful healthcare systems in the United States, offering patients an integrated, multidisciplinary care, from prevention to acute care through rehabilitation [27]. The facility offers cutting-edge diagnostic cardiovascular imaging techniques to detect heart valve disease. CCAD currently performs more than two-thirds of all structural heart disease cases in the UAE. Transcatheter aortic valve replacement (TAVR) procedures are performed in a transfemoral or non-transfemoral (trans-axillary, trans-carotid) approach by the team at CCAD. Drs. A. Edris and E. Tuzcu et al. described five-year outcomes of the CCAD TAVR program, which showed favorable outcomes compared with TAVR procedures performed at hospitals with the lowest quartile of procedural volumes in the United States [28]. In addition, these outcomes were comparable to surgical aortic valve replacement in terms of ventricular and functional recovery [29]. Physicians at CCAD performed the UAE's first tricuspid clip heart procedure in 2021 [30], and first cases of Tricvalve system implantation (Drs. Mahmoud Traina and Emad Hakemi) in 2023. In addition, cases of mitral valve repair with MitraClip®, valve-in-valve transcatheter mitral valve replacement, TAVR-in-TAVR, and pulmonary vein stenting were performed at CCAD. In 2025, CCAD was recognized as an ICOE by the ACC.

As a result of the high level of quality and efficiency in delivering both conventional and minimal invasive mitral and aortic valve surgeries, coronary artery bypass graft surgeries for complex cases, and the application of novel aortic surgical techniques [31–33], CCAD was designated a center of excellence for adult cardiac surgery in 2023 by the Department of Health—Abu Dhabi [34].

Furthermore, endoscopic coronary artery bypass and robotic mitral valve repair were undertaken at CCAD. Besides the above activities, mitral valve replacement, tricuspid valve repair, atrial septal defect closure, unroofing of a coronary myocardial bridge, and permanent epicardial pacemaker placement for ventricular re-synchronization therapy were performed in a robotic fashion at CCAD.

At CCAD, a total of 15,563 cardiac rehabilitation sessions were attended between 2015 and 2022, with 1774 patients attending at least one session. The most common referral diagnoses were coronary artery bypass grafting, valve surgery, and percutaneous coronary intervention [35].

Regarding the care of HF patients, significant progress has been made at CCAD under the leadership of Prof. Feras Bader. Important highlights include the establishment of the country's first multidisciplinary HF program, including physicians, nurses, pharmacists, social workers, physical therapists, dieticians, patient educators, and administrators. The program housed several specialized outpatient clinics, including the region-first pharmacist-led HF medication optimization clinic, cardiomyopathy clinic, and advanced HF clinic specifically dedicated to patients with ventricular assist devices and heart transplantation [36–41]. The program also established the first dedicated multidisciplinary inpatient service for HF patients in the region [39] and eventually implemented for the first time in the UAE, in a systemic, multidisciplinary fashion, the use of ventricular assist devices both as a bridge to transplantation and also as a destination therapy [42, 43, 44]. In May 2017, successful implantation of such device took place. Later that year, the UAE's first successful heart transplant was done in December 2017 [44, 45]. Dozens of abstracts and papers were published to reflect the structure, operations, and outcomes of the program since its inception in 2015 [36–44, 46, 47]. Additionally, this program formed the nucleus of what gradually became the largest HF conference in the Middle East Region, also chaired by Prof. Feras Bader.

21.3.4 Milestones in Cardiovascular Care in Dubai

Rashid Hospital was built in 1973 and is Dubai's second-oldest hospital. At that time, the cardiology department was an integral part of the medical department. Rashid Hospital had only four CCU beds, and the rest of the cardiac patients were admitted to the general medical department. It had only 12 lead ECG machines, and an exercise ECG was carried out on wooden steps. In 1980, proper treadmill exercises with ECG monitoring, echocardiography, and Holter monitoring were introduced to Rashid Hospital. Patients with acute myocardial infarction were admitted to the CCU, which had a cardiac trolley with a defibrillator, and the only treatment was oxygen and morphine (the typical treatment worldwide at that time). In 1976, a temporary pacemaker was implanted in a patient with a complete heart block. A year later, a permanent pacemaker with VVI pacemakers was performed at Rashid Hospital. The pioneer Professor Joseph Muscat Baron arrived in Dubai in 1977 and, alongside Dr. James Harries, was responsible for running the medical unit at Rashid Hospital. In 1988, he became the founding professor of Dubai Medical College for Girls and was later appointed Dean in 2002. As chair of the Medical Education Committee, he played a key role in developing the internship and residency programs at the Department of Health and Medical Services.

Dubai Hospital was the second-biggest hospital in Dubai and opened in 1982. In 1983, diagnostic coronary angiography was carried out at Dubai Hospital with staff from both Dubai and Rashid Hospitals. Patients who required intervention were only offered coronary artery bypass surgery, which was available at Dubai Hospital [48]. The doctors in Rashid Hospital worked together with the doctors in Dubai Hospital for 2 days to perform coronary angiography. In 1984, cardiologists at Rashid Hospital performed angiography and shared the X-ray suite with the radiography department. By 1986, dedicated state-of-the-art angiographic X-ray equipment had been installed in Rashid Hospital. Patients who required bypass surgery were sent to Dubai Hospital, where a cardiac surgery program was established in 1992. The published outcomes of the first 522 consecutive patients undergoing coronary artery bypass graft surgery in Dubai Hospital suggested that despite high rates of multiple CVD risk factors, the surgery was well tolerated [48]. Since the 1990s, Rashid Hospital under Dr. Azan Binbrek participated in Multi Center interventional trials. The first balloon valvuloplasty was carried out at both Rashid Hospital and Dubai Hospital in early 2000. In November 2003, percutaneous coronary intervention (PCI) was started in Dubai Hospital, and a year later, it was also done in Rashid Hospital. In 2015, The Adult Congenital Heart Disease Department was established at Rashid Hospital. More recently, in 2021, a fully-fledged electrophysiology department was set up and carried out SVT and AF ablations with good results. Currently, the Dubai Health Authority is planning to build a state-of-the-art cardiac center in Dubai to be included in the Rashid Medical Complex, which will house state-of-the-art equipment, 250 wards, and 1000 outpatient clinics [23, 49].

21.3.5 Milestones in Cardiovascular Care in the Northern Emirates

Al Qassimi Hospital is the largest tertiary hospital under MOHAP in the Northern Emirates; it was founded in May 1991, and has a capacity of 362 beds, including 10 critical care beds. Early on, the cardiology department was integrated with the medical department. Over time and in light of the expansion of cardiac services, the cardiac catheterization laboratory was inaugurated in 2003 to provide a multidisciplinary model for preventing, treating, and eradicating heart diseases [50].

Since then, it has witnessed continuous development and innovations in terms of adding renowned international cadres and novel technology that keep the standards of provided services up to date with implementing international recommendations and state-of-the-art cardiology practice. The laboratory is currently one of the busiest interventional catheterization laboratories and a regional resource center for cardiac emergency care in Sharjah and the Northern Emirates of the UAE [34]. The lab covers 11 government hospitals and referrals from private hospitals in Sharjah and the Northern Emirates, and primary coronary interventions are performed 24/7 for patients from these regions. Until 2011, 9000 cases were completed. The "Cath Lab" undertakes primary and secondary interventions and emergency pacemaker implantations. The diagnostic and therapeutic services offered by the facility include coronary angiography, peripheral angiography, pediatric cardiac catheterization, renal angiography, electrophysiology studies, radiofrequency ablations, and the usage of intra-aortic balloon pumps and Impella devices, among others. Interventional procedures, such as coronary angioplasty, robotic guided coronary intervention, peripheral angioplasty, and pediatric interventions, include atrial septal defect and ventricular septal defect device closure, patent ductus arteriosus device and coil closure, cerebral embolization and carotid angioplasty, valvuloplasty, permanent pacemaker implantation, alcohol septal ablation, and left atrial appendage closure device. Trans-catheter aortic valve implantation is regularly performed. The unit also treats cardiogenic shock cases [50].

21.4 Cardiovascular Fellowship Training in the UAE

The UAE's first cardiology fellowship program was established at SKMC in 2013; the program is currently running under Sheikh Shakhbout Medical City (SSMC), with fellows rotating between SKMC and SSMC. Each year, two fellows are accepted for a 3-year, dedicated cardiology training program. The program is accredited by the Arab Board, the Accreditation Council for Graduate Medical Education-International (ACGME-I), the Jordanian Board, and the Emirati Board [51]. In September 2022, another cardiology fellowship program was established at CCAD with a capacity of three fellows in an effort to train the next generation of UAE cardiologists. As of 2025, there are five cardiology fellowship programs in the UAE, with a total of 36 fellows in training.

21.5 The Emirates Cardiac Society

The Emirates Cardiac Society (ECS) is a non-profit organization established in 1999 under the Emirates Medical Association [36]. ECS is striving to promote CV health in the UAE through education, research, and high-quality, evidence-based practice. The society currently encompasses nine working groups inlcuding the intervention, imaging, congenital and genetic heart disease, heart failure, prevention, surgical, electrophysiologic studies, hypertension, and fellows in training working groups. The society conducts annual scientific meetings, in addition to regular seminars and educational gatherings, through its working groups. Furthermore, it hosts local and international conferences affiliated with the Gulf Heart Association, Asian Pacific Society of Cardiology, World Heart Federation, European Society of Cardiology, and American Heart Association. In August 2018, the ECS was officially recognized as an affiliated cardiac society with the European Society of Cardiology. Through annual health campaigns, ECS also helps people understand the importance of healthy lifestyle choices [52].

21.6 Cardiovascular Research Highlights from the UAE

Since the 1990s, small studies have been carried out in Abu Dhabi and Dubai hospitals and published in local and regional journals. Also, the UAE hospitals participated in multicenter international studies such as the Continuous Infusion versus Double-Bolus Administration of Alteplase (COBALT) study, the Assessment of the Safety of a New Thrombolytic (ASSENT) I, II, and III studies, and the Telmisartan Randomized Assessment Study in ACE-Intolerant Subjects with Cardiovascular Disease (TRANSCEND) studies, which were published in high-quality journals [53–56]. The Emirates participated as well in regional multicenter studies such as the Gulf Registry of Acute Coronary Events (Gulf RACE), Gulf RACE-2, Gulf Survey of Atrial Fibrillation Events (Gulf SAFE), Gulf Acute Heart Failure Registry (Gulf CARE), Gulf COAST, Gulf Familial Hypercholesterolemia (Gulf FH), and the Gulf Left Main registries [57–63].

Results of a bibliometric study by the UAE Ministry of Health and Prevention and Monash University Australia for the years 2014–2018 revealed that 350 (7.8%) out of a total of 4504 medicine research outputs in the UAE were related to CVD. The top three institutions in terms of CV research output were the UAE University, Dubai Hospital, and SKMC. Interestingly, 15.1% of these CV research outputs were among the world's top 10% cited publications, according to SciVal® (by September 20th, 2019) [64]. Moreover, the UAE hosted 115 clinical trials over the reference period; approximately one-third of these trials were focused on CVD ($n = 18$) and its major risk factors, diabetes and obesity ($n = 23$) [64].

A recent study by Ghader et al. aiming to identify clinically relevant research priorities for the treatment and prevention of CVD in the UAE 65. The study included 37 delegates from MOHP, the DOH, SEHA, DHA, Abu Dhabi Police, Dubai Corporation for Ambulance Services, ECS, National Ambulance, the

American Heart Association, the University of Sharjah, and the American University of Sharjah. The delegates identified five research priorities to tackle CVD mortalities in the UAE for the upcoming 5 years, including the development of evidence-based CVD algorithms; the availability, accessibility, and affordability of CVD treatment and rehabilitation; identifying relationships between CVD, lifestyle, and mental health; the efficacy and constraints in the management of cardiac emergencies; and finally epidemiological studies that trace CVD in the UAE [65].

21.7 Challenges and Future Directions

Public awareness and behaviors toward CVD and its associated risk factors pose a major challenge in tackling the burden of CVD in the UAE. Data from a survey on the public's awareness of CVD in Dubai in 2021 has shown that more than half of the participants had high knowledge and attitudes toward CVD, but their behaviors were not satisfactory. Highlighting the need for more effective educational interventions to promote positive health behaviors [66]. Promising outcomes from the city of Al Ain were reported on implementing behavioral and educational tools to improve patient adherence to CV medications [67]. In another study of Emirati women, participants were generally unaware of the atypical symptoms commonly experienced by women, and major barriers to seeking treatment were identified, including, among others, a lack of awareness of disease severity and symptoms, sociocultural influences, and distrust in the healthcare system. Therefore, there is a substantial need for culturally relevant, gender-specific, and age-focused CVD awareness campaigns in the UAE [68]. One of the major experiences of such campaigns in the Emirates was the Dubai Shopping for Cardiovascular Risk Study (DISCOVERY), which included comprehensive screening for CVD risk factors in four shopping malls, nine healthcare facilities, and three labor camps in five cities in the United Arab Emirates, with the majority of the subjects (85%) having at least one CVD risk factor. At 1-month post-screening follow-up, three in five participants reported positive lifestyle changes; however, only one-third consulted a doctor after the screening [69]. Another initiative incorporating a pharmacy screening intervention has proven its efficacy and feasibility in identifying and referring patients with CVD [70, 71].

In light of the evolving field of CV medicine, it is essential to adhere to recent guidelines for diagnosing and managing CVD. Data from the UAE on adherence to guideline therapies for various CV conditions revealed good, satisfactory, or poor compliance with guidelines [72–74]. Increasing adherence to the recent guidelines can be achieved by the following: addressing knowledge gaps of physicians and conducting regular seminars and scientific workshops; eliminating obstacles in the process of care that limit the adoption of these guidelines; and adapting the multidisciplinary models of care, which have proven their efficiency in improving patients' outcomes and overall adherence to the recent guidelines. Finally, the UAE's successful experiences in partnering with world-renowned health institutions brought an unparalleled level of CV care to the UAE and the wider Gulf region; such experiences can help local institutions to establish international collaborations to improve outcomes of CVD in the UAE [23].

21.8 Conclusion

The CV healthcare sector in the UAE has undergone massive development through the years; while CVD still imposes a significant burden on both patients and healthcare systems, efforts should be made to increase public awareness of CVD and positive health practices, in addition to increasing providers' adherence to recent guidelines, in order to improve screening, diagnosis, and management of CVD in the Emirates.

Conflicts of Interest The authors declare no conflicts of interest.

References

1. https://www.worldometers.info/world-population/united-arab-emirates-population/. United Arab Emirates Population, 2022. Accessed 1 Nov 2023.
2. https://www.worlddata.info/life-expectancy.php#by-population. Life expectancy. Accessed 1 Nov 2023.
3. World Bank. Current health expenditure per capita [Internet]. Available from: https://data.worldbank.org/indicator/SH.XPD.CHEX.PC.CD. Accessed 1 Nov 2023.
4. World Bank. Current health expenditure (% of GDP). Available from https://data.worldbank.org/indicator/SH.XPD.CHEX.GD.ZS. Accessed 1 Nov 2023.
5. Institute for Health Metrics and Evaluation (IHME). GBD Results. Seattle, WA: IHME, University of Washington, 2024. Available from https://vizhub.healthdata.org/gbd-results/. Accessed 5 May 2025.
6. Institute for Health Metrics and Evaluation (IHME). GBD Compare Data Visualization. Seattle, WA: IHME, University of Washington, 2024. Available from http://vizhub.healthdata.org/gbd-compare. Accessed 5 May 2025.
7. Ferrari AJ, Santomauro DF, Aali A, Abate YH, Abbafati C, Abbastabar H, Abd ElHafeez S, Abdelmasseh M, Abd-Elsalam S, Abdollahi A, Abdullahi A. Global incidence, prevalence, years lived with disability (YLDs), disability-adjusted life-years (DALYs), and healthy life expectancy (HALE) for 371 diseases and injuries in 204 countries and territories and 811 subnational locations, 1990–2021: a systematic analysis for the Global Burden of Disease Study 2021. The Lancet. 2024;403(10440):2133-61.
8. Saheb Sharif-Askari N, Syed Sulaiman SA, Saheb Sharif-Askari F, Al Sayed Hussain A, Tabatabai S, Abdullatif A-MA. Hospitalized heart failure patients with preserved vs. reduced ejection fraction in Dubai, United Arab Emirates: a prospective study. Eur J Heart Fail. 2014;16(4):454–60.
9. Yusufali AM, AlMahmeed W, Tabatabai S, Rao K, Binbrek A. Acute coronary syndrome registry from four large centres in United Arab Emirates (UAE-ACS Registry). Heart Asia [Internet]. 2010;2(1):118. Available from: http://heartasia.bmj.com/content/2/1/118.abstract.
10. Al-Shamsi S, Regmi D, Govender RD. Incidence of cardiovascular disease and its associated risk factors in at-risk men and women in The United Arab Emirates: a 9-year retrospective cohort study. BMC Cardiovasc Disord. 2019;19(1):148.

11. Govender RD, Al-Shamsi S, Soteriades ES, Regmi D. Incidence and risk factors for recurrent cardiovascular disease in middle-eastern adults: a retrospective study. BMC Cardiovasc Disord. 2019;19(1):253.
12. Mujahed M, Harbi A, Madi H, Belaila DRBA Bin, Jaber M. WHO-STEPS non-communicable disease risk factor survey.
13. Hajat C, Harrison O, Al SZ. Weqaya: a population-wide cardiovascular screening program in Abu Dhabi, United Arab Emirates. Am J Public Health. 2012;102(5):909–14.
14. Hajat C, Harrison O. The Abu Dhabi cardiovascular program: the continuation of Framingham. Prog Cardiovasc Dis. 2010;53(1):28–38.
15. Bhagavathula AS, Al-Hamad S, Yasin J, Aburawi EH. Distribution of Cardiometabolic risk factors in school-aged children with excess body weight in the Al Ain City, United Arab Emirates: a cross-sectional study. Children. 2021;8(10):884.
16. Mezhal F, Oulhaj A, Abdulle A, AlJunaibi A, Alnaeemi A, Ahmad A, et al. The interrelationship and accumulation of cardiometabolic risk factors amongst young adults in The United Arab Emirates: the UAE healthy future study. Diabetol Metab Syndr. 2021;13(1):140.
17. Abdulle A, Alnaeemi A, Aljunaibi A, Al Ali A, Al Saedi K, Al Zaabi E, et al. The UAE healthy future study: a pilot for a prospective cohort study of 20,000 United Arab Emirates nationals. BMC Public Health. 2018;18(1):1–9.
18. Manla Y, Almahmeed W. Cardiometabolic clinics: is there a need for a multidisciplinary clinic? Front Clin Diab Healthcare [Internet]. 2022;3. Available from: https://www.frontiersin.org/articles/10.3389/fcdhc.2022.880468.
19. Malekpour MR, Abbasi-Kangevari M, Ghamari SH, Khanali J, Heidari-Foroozan M, Moghaddam SS, et al. The burden of metabolic risk factors in North Africa and the Middle East, 1990–2019: findings from the Global Burden of Disease Study. EClinicalMedicine. 2023;60:102022.
20. Manla Y, Almahmeed W. The pandemic of coronary heart disease in the Middle East and North Africa: what clinicians need to know. Curr Atheroscler Rep [Internet]. 2023;25(9):543–57. https://doi.org/10.1007/s11883-023-01126-x.
21. Mansouri A, Khosravi A, Mehrabani-Zeinabad K, Kopec JA, Adawi KII, Lui M, et al. Trends in the burden and determinants of hypertensive heart disease in the Eastern Mediterranean region, 1990–2019: an analysis of the Global Burden of Disease Study 2019. EClinicalMedicine. 2023;60:102034.
22. Manla Y, Bader F. Heart failure burden in asia: the full picture. JACC Asia. 2024;4(7):569.
23. The U.S.-U.A.E. Business Council. 2025 Healthcare Report [Internet]. [cited 2025 May 4]. Available from: https://usuaebusiness.org/wp-content/uploads/2024/01/Final-Report-23-January.pdf.
24. Beshyah S, Beshyah A. Central hospital of Abu Dhabi: forty years of service to the community (1968-2008). Ibnosina J Med Biomed Sci. 2013;5(02):99–108.
25. Kazi N. Early days of health service in Abu Dhabi, United Arab Emirates: a personal perspective. Ibnosina J Med Biomed Sci. 2013;5(02):109–13.
26. Sheikh Shakhbout Medical City. Annual Reports | Sheikh Shakhbout Medical City Abu Dhabi [Internet]. 2020 [cited 2023 Jul 19]. Available from: https://ssmc.ae/assets/uploads/2023/02/SSMC_Annual_Report_English_2020.pdf.
27. Best Heart, Vascular & Thoracic Institute in Abu Dhabi, UAE [Internet]. [cited 2023 Nov 4]. Available from: https://www.clevelandclinicabudhabi.ae/en/institutes-and-specialties/heart-vascular-and-thoracic-institute.
28. Edris A, Manla Y, Al Badarin F, Hasan K, Hashmani S, Traina M, et al. Outcomes of Transcatheter aortic valve replacement in The United Arab Emirates: real-world, single-Centre experience from an emerging programme. Interv Cardiol Rev Res Resour. 2023;18:e08.
29. Manla Y, Khalouf A, Edris A, Hasan K, Hashmani S, El Zouhbi A, et al. Left ventricular remodelling and changes in functional measurements in patients undergoing transcatheter vs surgical aortic valve replacement: a head-to-head comparison. Asia Interv. 2022;8(2):153–5.

30. https://www.clevelandclinicabudhabi.ae/en/media-center/news/pages/cleveland-clinic-abu-dhabi-performs-uaes-first-tricuspid-clip-heart-procedure.aspx [Internet]. Cleveland Clinic Abu Dhabi performs UAE'S first tricuspid clip heart procedure.
31. Aljabery Y, Manla Y, Gobolos L, Bhatnagar G, Traina M. Abstract 17147: multidisciplinary-team management of a severely-ill pregnant Covid-19 patient with a newly diagnosed severe mitral stenosis. Circulation. 2021:144(Suppl_2):A17147–A17147.
32. Manla Y, Bhatnagar G, Gobolos L, Aljabery Y. The impact of initiating quality of care improvement protocols on intensive care unit length of stay in patients undergoing coronary artery bypass grafting: an insight from a nascent program. Eur Heart J Acute Cardiovasc Care. 2022;11(Supplement_1):zuac041-163.
33. Manla Y, Bhatnagar G, Khan N, Al Badarin F, AlJabery Y, Kakar V, et al. Management of acute aortic services during the COVID-19 pandemic: a retrospective cohort study from the Middle East. Ann Med Surg. 2023;85(7):3279–83.
34. Cleveland Clinic Abu Dhabi. Department of Health—Abu Dhabi announces Cleveland Clinic Abu Dhabi as a Centre of Excellence for Adult Cardiac Surgery. 2023 [cited 2023 Oct 23]; Available from: https://www.clevelandclinicabudhabi.ae/en/media-center/news/cleveland-clinic-abu-dhabi-as-a-centre-of-excellence-for-adult-cardiac-surgery.
35. Thrush AH. Cardiac rehabilitation in Abu Dhabi: a retrospective investigation of program delivery, participants, and factors associated with program completion utilizing a hospital registry. J Saudi Heart Assoc. 2023;35(3):235.
36. Alsindi F, Manla Y, Bader F. Patient characteristics of heart failure with improved ejection fraction (HFimpEF) following treatment with Sacubitril/Valsartan: a real-world experience from the Middle East. J Card Fail [Internet]. 2022;28(5, Supplement):S85. Available from: https://www.sciencedirect.com/science/article/pii/S1071916422003177.
37. Manla Y, Vest AR, Anderson L, Ducharme A, Gomez-Mesa JE, Jadhav UM, et al. Global innovations in the care of patients with heart failure. Int J Heart Fail. 2025;7(2):47–57. https://doi.org/10.36628/ijhf.2024.0062.
38. Atallah B, Sadik ZG, Osoble AA, Ghalib H, Hamour I, AlTakruri M, et al. Establishing the first pharmacist-led heart failure medication optimization clinic in the Middle East Gulf region. J Am Coll Clin Pharm. 2020;3(5):877–84.
39. Manla Y, Ghalib HH, Al BF, Ferrer R, Lee-St. John T, Abdalla K, et al. Implementation of a multidisciplinary inpatient heart failure service and its association with hospitalized patient outcomes: first experience from the Middle East and North Africa region. Heart Lung. 2023;61:92–7.
40. Manla Y, Kholoki O, Bader F, Kanwar O, Abidi E, El Nekidy WS, et al. The prevalence of cardiorenal anemia syndrome among patients with heart failure and its association with all-cause hospitalizations: a retrospective single-center study from the Middle East. Front Cardiovasc Med. 2023;10:1244305.
41. Alaryani J, Manla Y, Hisham M, Abidi E, Salti Y, Attallah N, et al. Screening and prevalence of iron deficiency in an outpatient heart failure clinic in the Middle East Gulf region. J Card Fail [Internet]. 2023 [cited 2023 Apr 14];29(4):592–3. Available from: http://www.onlinejcf.com/article/S107191642200848X/fulltext.
42. Gabra G, Manla Y, Al Badarin F, Ghalib H, Kakar V, Ghisulal P, et al. Survival to discharge among cardiogenic shock patients supported by VA-ECMO: an insight from the largest VA-ECMO experience in the middle east-gulf region. J Card Fail. 2024;30(1):170-1.
43. Gabra G, Hamour I, Soliman M, El Tahlawy W, Manla Y, Al Badarin F, et al. Association of Multidisciplinary Heart Failure Team with outcomes in patients requiring extracorporeal membrane oxygenation. J Heart Lung Transplant. 2021;40(4):S416.
44. Bader F, Manla Y, Ghalib H, Al Matrooshi N, Khaliel F, Skouri H. Advanced heart failure therapies in the Eastern Mediterranean Region: current status, challenges, and future directions. Curr Probl Cardiol. 2024;49(7):102564.
45. Bader F, Atallah B, Rizk J, AlHabeeb W. Heart transplantation in the Middle East Gulf region. Transplantation. 2018;102(7):1023.

46. Alsindi F, Manla Y, Soliman M, Hamour IM, Ghalib H, Bader F. Heart failure clinic no-show rates and effect on heart failure hospitalizations: a real-world experience from the Middle East. J Card Fail [Internet]. 2022;28(5, Supplement):S115–6. Available from: https://www.sciencedirect.com/science/article/pii/S1071916422003992.
47. Hamour IM, Ferrer R, AbuBaker S, ElBanna M, ElHajj S, Bajwa G, et al. Beyond borders: our Middle Eastern experience of international collaboration to run a successful heart transplantation program. J Card Fail. 2018;24(8):S127.
48. Sadanandam R, Al Khaja N, Aziz MA, Turner MA. Profile of coronary artery bypass surgery in United Arab Emirates: Dubai Hospital experience. http://dx.doi.org/101177/021849239800600210 [Internet]. 2016 [cited 2023 Feb 8];6(2):118–24. Available from: https://journals.sagepub.com/doi/abs/10.1177/021849239800600210?journalCode=aana.
49. Gulf News. https://gulfnews.com/business/new-dubai-hospital-to-be-built-on-public-private-model-1.60940790. New Dubai hospital to be built on public-private model.
50. http://hmaward.org.ae/profile.php?id=176 [Internet]. Cardiac Cath Lab Department - Al Qassimi Hospital, Sharjah.
51. Sheikh Shakhbout Medical City Abu Dhabi. Available from: https://ssmc.ae/cardiology-fellowship-program/. Cardiology Fellowship Program.
52. Emirates Cardiac Society. Available from: https://ecsociety.com/about-us/. About Us.
53. of the Safety TA. Efficacy and safety of tenecteplase in combination with enoxaparin, abciximab, or unfractionated heparin: the ASSENT-3 randomised trial in acute myocardial infarction. Lancet. 2001;358(9282):605–13.
54. Fu Y, Goodman S, Chang WC, Van de Werf F, Granger CB, Armstrong PW. Time to treatment influences the impact of ST-segment resolution on one-year prognosis: insights from the assessment of the safety and efficacy of a new thrombolytic (ASSENT-2) trial. Circulation. 2001;104(22):2653–9.
55. Investigators CI versus DBA of A (COBALT). A comparison of continuous infusion of alteplase with double-bolus administration for acute myocardial infarction. N Engl J Med. 1997;337(16):1124–30.
56. Investigators TRAS in ACE iNtolerant subjects with cardiovascular D (TRANSCEND). Effects of the angiotensin-receptor blocker telmisartan on cardiovascular events in high-risk patients intolerant to angiotensin-converting enzyme inhibitors: a randomised controlled trial. Lancet. 2008;372(9644):1174–83.
57. Daoulah A, Elfarnawany A, Al Garni T, Hersi AS, Alshehri M, Almahmeed W, et al. Outcomes of myocardial revascularization in diabetic patients with left main coronary artery disease: a multicenter observational study from three gulf countries. Cardiovasc Revasc Med. 2023;46:52–61.
58. Alhabib KF, Al-Rasadi K, Almigbal TH, Batais MA, Al-Zakwani I, Al-Allaf FA, et al. Familial hypercholesterolemia in the Arabian Gulf region: clinical results of the gulf fh registry. PLoS One. 2021;16(6):e0251560.
59. AlHabib KF, Sulaiman K, Al-Motarreb A, Almahmeed W, Asaad N, Amin H, et al. Baseline characteristics, management practices, and long-term outcomes of Middle Eastern patients in the Second Gulf Registry of Acute Coronary Events (Gulf RACE-2). Ann Saudi Med [Internet]. 2012 [cited 2023 Mar 12];32(1):9–18. Available from: https://www.annsaudimed.net/doi/10.5144/0256-4947.2012.9.
60. Zubaid M, Rashed W, Alsheikh-Ali AA, Garadah T, Alrawahi N, Ridha M, et al. Disparity in ST-segment elevation myocardial infarction practices and outcomes in Arabian Gulf countries (Gulf COAST registry). Heart Views. 2017;18(2):41.
61. Sulaiman KJ, Panduranga P, Al-Zakwani I, Alsheikh-Ali A, Al-Habib K, Al-Suwaidi J, et al. Rationale, design, methodology and hospital characteristics of the first Gulf Acute Heart Failure Registry (Gulf CARE). Heart Views. 2014;15(1):6.
62. Zubaid M, Rashed WA, Alsheikh-Ali AA, AlMahmeed W, Shehab A, Sulaiman K, et al. Gulf survey of atrial fibrillation events (Gulf SAFE) design and baseline characteristics of

patients with atrial fibrillation in the Arab middle East. Circ Cardiovasc Qual Outcomes. 2011;4(4):477–82.
63. Zubaid M, Rashed WA, Al-Khaja N, Almahmeed W, Al-Lawati J, Sulaiman K, et al. Clinical presentation and outcomes of acute coronary syndromes in the gulf registry of acute coronary events (Gulf RACE). Saudi Med J. 2008;29(2):251.
64. MOHAP Open Data | Open Data | Ministry of Health and Prevention - UAE. https://mohap.gov.ae/en/open-data/mohap-open-data. The state of Health Research in the United Arab Emirates.
65. Ghader N, Al-Yateem N, Dalibalta S, Razzak HA, Rahman SA, Al Matrooshi F, et al. Cardiovascular health research priorities in The United Arab Emirates. Front Public Health. 2023;11:1130716.
66. Kazim MN, AbouMoussa TH, Al-Hammadi FA, Al Ali A, Abedini FM, Ahmad FSM, et al. Population awareness of cardiovascular disease risk factors and health care seeking behavior in the UAE. Am J Prev Cardiol. 2021;8:100255.
67. Shehab A, Elnour AA, Al SS, Bhagavathula AS, Hamad F, Shehab O, et al. Evaluation and implementation of behavioral and educational tools that improves the patients' intentional and unintentional non-adherence to cardiovascular medications in family medicine clinics. Saudi Pharm J. 2016;24(2):182–8.
68. Khan S, Ali SA. Exploratory study into awareness of heart disease and health care seeking behavior among Emirati women (UAE)-cross sectional descriptive study. BMC Womens Health. 2017;17(1):1–10.
69. Yusufali A, Bazargani N, Muhammed K, Gabroun A, AlMazrooei A, Agrawal A, et al. Opportunistic screening for CVD risk factors: the Dubai shopping for cardiovascular risk study (DISCOVERY). Glob Heart. 2015;10(4):265.
70. Alzubaidi H, Hasan S, Saidawi W, Mc Namara K, Chandir S, Krass I. Outcomes of a novel pharmacy screening intervention to address the burden of type 2 diabetes and cardiovascular disease in an Arabic-speaking country. Diabet Med. 2021;38(8):e14598.
71. Alzubaidi HT, Chandir S, Hasan S, McNamara K, Cox R, Krass I. Diabetes and cardiovascular disease risk screening model in community pharmacies in a developing primary healthcare system: a feasibility study. BMJ Open. 2019;9(11):e031246.
72. AlAhmad M, AbuRuz S, Beiram R. Application of the American College of Cardiology(ACC/AHA) 2017 guideline for the management of hypertension in adults and comparison with the2014 eighth joint National Committee Guideline. J Saudi Heart Assoc. 2021;33(1):16–25.
73. Saheb Sharif-Askari N, Sulaiman SAS, Saheb Sharif-Askari F, Hussain AAS, Al-Mulla AA. Assessment of guideline adherence in hospitalised heart failure patients with systolic dysfunction in Dubai, United Arab Emirates. Int J Cardiol. 2014;172(3):e491–3.
74. Alliabi FJA, Jaber AAS, Jallo MKI, Baig MR. Adherence of physicians to evidence-based management guidelines for treating type 2 diabetes and atherosclerotic cardiovascular disease in Ajman, United Arab Emirates. BMC Prim Care. 2022;23(1):70.

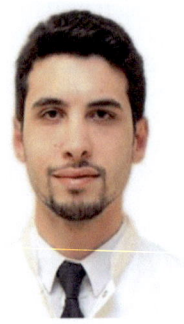

Yosef Manla earned his MD from the University of Aleppo, Syria in 2020. He then worked as a Research Scholar at the Heart, Vascular, and Thoracic Institute at Cleveland Clinic Abu Dhabi. Afterwards, he completed a postdoctoral research fellowship in heart transplantation at the Smidt Heart Institute, Cedars-Sinai Medical Center in Los Angeles, California. He has been academically active, with several publications in high-impact journals and presentations at the foremost cardiovascular and transplantation conferences. He received multiple research recognitions and awards from major American and European cardiac societies, including the American Heart Association, American College of Cardiology, and the European Society of Cardiology .

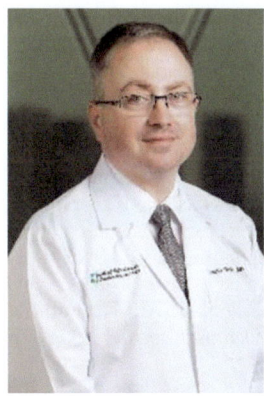

Laszlo Göbölös MD, PhD, is serving as a cardiac surgeon at the Heart, Vascular, and Thoracic Institute, Cleveland Clinic Abu Dhabi. In his current position, besides the daily clinical routine, he is active in education and clinical research. Prior to joining CCAD, he served at the Department of Cardiothoracic Surgery, Southampton University Hospital Trust, UK, and was a certified Educational Supervisor of Wessex Deanery (PGMDE). He graduated from the University of Pécs (est. 1367), Hungary, and defended the MD thesis "Functional and biochemical changes following coronary occlusion and reperfusion in an experimental canine model." In addition, his PhD thesis, "New techniques and principles in acute aortic pathologies requiring emergency surgical interventions," achieved an outstanding rating in the accreditation process. He was appointed as an Assistant Professor at the University of Pécs in 2007 and as a Clinical Associate Professor in 2019 at the Cleveland Clinic Lerner College of Medicine, Case Western Reserve University, USA. Recently, he was promoted to Clinical Professor of Surgery at CCLCM, CWRU. Dr. Göbölös is a Fellow of the ACS, ESC, ACC, and GHA, a member of the ESC Cardiovascular Surgery Working Group, and an ASCVTS. He possesses an excellent track record of both basic scientific investigation and clinical research and is the author and co-author of a number of book chapters .

Sultan Abdulali is a former consultant interventional cardiologist at Mafraq and Sheikh Khalifa Medical City Hospitals (1984–2018). Since 2009, he has been appointed Director of the Presidential Medical Wing in Abu Dhabi. After finishing his medical school training (1967–1971) at Makerere University, Uganda, he worked in various hospitals in Portsmouth and London, UK. He obtained his MRCP (UK) in 1977, then did his cardiology training in Leeds, UK, between 1980 and 1984.

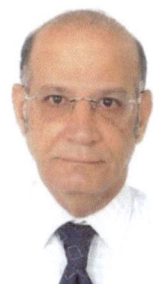

Dr. Azan Salem Binbrek is a consultant cardiologist at Rashid Hospital in Dubai, United Arab Emirates. Dr. Binbrek was educated in the UK. He received his MBChB from the University of Glasgow in 1971. He obtained various qualifications subsequently in the UK: DCH, Glasgow in 1973; MRCP, UK in 1975; FRCP, Edinburgh in 1986; and FRCP, London in 1988.

Dr. Binbrek returned to Dubai in 1976 and worked as a specialist in Medicine. In 1978, he returned to London and was a research fellow in Cardiology until 1980. He settled in Dubai afterward and became a consultant cardiologist in 1984. Dr. Binbreak is actively involved in clinical trials. He was the principal investigator for the Continuous Infusion versus Double-Bolus Administration of Alteplase (COBALT) study and the Assessment of the Safety of a New Thrombolytic (ASSENT) I, II, and III studies. He has also published articles on various clinical studies, meta-analyses, and registry studies conducted in the UAE and the Middle East and has presented abstracts at international congresses. Dr. Binbrek was honored with the Hamdan Medical Award for his research work .

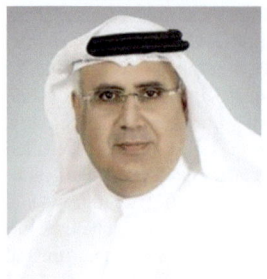

Arif Al Nooryani has been the CEO of Al Qassimi Hospital Sharjah, UAE (Since 2009) and Head of Cardiac Centre and Cardiac Cath Lab at Al Qassimi Hospital in Sharjah. He is also the Associate Professor of Cardiology at the University of Sharjah (since September 2018) and has completed PhD studies in Cardiovascular Medicine at the Medical Faculty of the University of Belgrade, Serbia (since 2018). He holds the German Board of Internal Medicine and Cardiology. Dr. Al Nooryani is an expert in interventional cardiology with high-level experience in coronary stents, peripheral artery intervention, and management of structural heart disease, including TAVI, aortic valve implantation, and mitral valve repair through catheterization. Dr. Arif is an official reviewer for international journals such as *Catheterization and Cardiovascular Interventions*.

Srinath Kidambi is a consultant cardiologist at Sheikh Shakhbout Medical City. In addition, he is a Clinical Associate Professor of Cardiology at Khalifa University, Abu Dhabi, UAE, and Gulf Medical University, Ajman, UAE. He earned his MBBS (1977) and MD (General Medicine, 1981) from Osmania University in India and his DM (Cardiology, 1986) from Sri Chithra Thirunal Institute of Medical Sciences and Technology. He worked at Sheikh Khalifa Medical City, Abu Dhabi, from 2015 to 2020, and served as acting Head of the Department of Medicine at Al Rahba Hospital, Abu Dhabi, between April 2012 and January 2015. In addition, he is involved in various educational and research activities at his current institution.

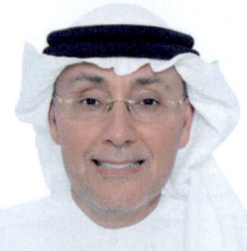

Wael Almahmeed has been a staff physician in the Heart, Vascular, and Thoracic Institute at Cleveland Clinic Abu Dhabi since 2014. Before joining Cleveland Clinic Abu Dhabi, Dr. Almahmeed served as Head of Cardiology from 2007 to 2014 and the Deputy Chief Medical Officer from 2007 to 2012 at Sheikh Khalifa Medical City (SKMC), Abu Dhabi, and as a Clinical Associate Professor, Faculty of Medicine and Health Sciences, UAEU, from 2007 to 2016. Dr. Almahmeed received his medical degree from the University of Southampton, England, in 1988. He completed his residency in Internal Medicine and his fellowship in Cardiology and Echocardiography at the University of British Columbia, Vancouver, Canada. He has been practicing for more than 25 years. Echocardiography is his specialty, and prevention is his focus, as he is eager to contribute to better heart awareness and disease outcomes.

Dr. Wael Almahmeed received the first Mohammed bin Rashid Award for Investing in Scientific Research in recognition of his efforts to support research and the scientific community in the UAE. In addition, Dr. Wael Almahmeed has been awarded the Hamdan Award for Honoring Individuals Working in the Field of Medicine and Health for the 2021–2022 term.

Open Access This chapter is licensed under the terms of the Creative Commons Attribution 4.0 International License (http://creativecommons.org/licenses/by/4.0/), which permits use, sharing, adaptation, distribution and reproduction in any medium or format, as long as you give appropriate credit to the original author(s) and the source, provide a link to the Creative Commons license and indicate if changes were made.

The images or other third party material in this chapter are included in the chapter's Creative Commons license, unless indicated otherwise in a credit line to the material. If material is not included in the chapter's Creative Commons license and your intended use is not permitted by statutory regulation or exceeds the permitted use, you will need to obtain permission directly from the copyright holder.

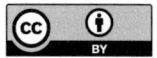

Women's Health in the UAE

22

Cosette Fakih El Khoury, Jennifer Fortin, and Samantha Dumas

22.1 Introduction

Despite being a small country in the Arabian Gulf, the United Arab Emirates (UAE) has shown a commitment to the establishment of a world-class health system, and over the past decade it has seen many changes in the healthcare sector [1]. Given the cultural, religious, and demographic context of the UAE, women's health and quality of life have also undergone changes. Women are holding more leadership roles both in politics and in the public sector and now have more access to education, which has led to a generation of more qualified and competent women [2].

In May 2018, the UAE announced that married couples and unmarried women would be given the option to freeze their embryos and eggs, marking a major milestone in providing women with more choices and empowering them to take charge of their reproductive health [3].

The UAE has been described as a pro-natal society because of the cultural importance of having children [4], and women's health plays a major role in sexual and reproductive health, but it should extend beyond this to cover all physical and mental health concerns and conditions among women [5].

The UAE population is varied, with over 200 different nationalities residing in the country, with a majority being expatriates. Women make up 31% of the population (3.15 million), and the largest group consists of females aged 25 to 54 (1.76

C. F. El Khoury (✉)
Nabta Health Clinics LLC, Dubai, United Arab Emirates

Nutrition and Public Health, INSPECT-LB, Beirut, Lebanon
e-mail: cosette.fakihelkhoury@inspect-lb.org

J. Fortin
Public Health Intern at Nabta Health Clinics LLC, Dubai, United Arab Emirates

S. Dumas
Nabta Health FZE, Dubai, United Arab Emirates

© The Author(s) 2025
H. O. Al-Shamsi (ed.), *Healthcare in the United Arab Emirates*,
https://doi.org/10.1007/978-981-96-0523-1_22

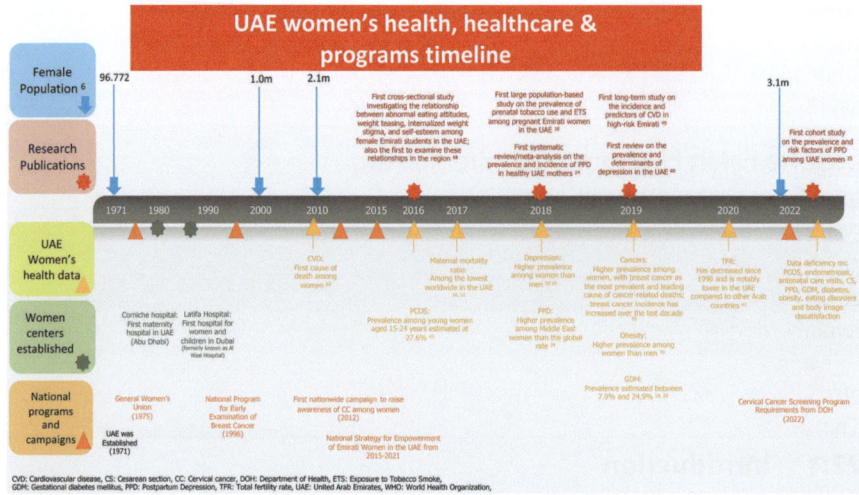

Fig. 22.1 UAE women's health, healthcare, and program timeline

million), followed by young girls under the age of 14 (0.75 million) [6]. Given the demographic and age distribution, women of childbearing age represent the largest segment of the female population. This chapter aims to describe the status of women's health in the UAE across the different life stages that women experience. The following timeline, depicted in Fig. 22.1, provides an overview of this chapter, along with additional information regarding research, national programs, and healthcare facilities.

22.2 Women's Health in the UAE Across the Lifecycle

22.2.1 Menstrual Health

In Arab culture, a woman who experiences menarche is considered to have become a woman. Although menarche is celebrated among Arabs, it may be accompanied by social restrictions on her and may impact her interactions with men [7].

There are many beliefs around menstruation across the world. In Arab culture, for instance, some women believe that showering during menstruation is not preferred, that herbal teas should be primarily used to alleviate menstrual pain, and that pads should be the sole menstrual product used by young girls, given the cultural value of virginity in this region [7].

Although menstruation is a normal part of a woman's life, there are times when the symptoms that accompany it may disturb a woman's quality of life by impacting relationships, emotional well-being, and work productivity [8]. Premenstrual syndrome (PMS) is a condition that most menstruating women experience to a certain extent. It is characterized by feelings of bloating, changes in appetite, weight gain, breast tenderness, aches and pains, poor concentration, sleep disturbances, and psychological discomfort [9]. The prevalence of PMS in the UAE is notable; a study among school-aged girls reported a PMS prevalence of 16.5%. It also reported that having UAE nationality, a sister with PMS, and dysmenorrhea increased the likelihood of PMS. This indicates the need for further studies exploring PMS among Emirati women. The same study also reported that the quality of life of girls suffering from PMS was adversely affected. Regrettably, almost 60% of the girls with PMS recounted that during encounters with their family physicians or specialists, the symptoms experienced around menstruation were not addressed [8]. This suggests that the detection and management of PMS among young girls in the UAE remain neglected.

Menstrual health and its role in women's overall health, well-being, and quality of life (QoL) are under-researched in the UAE, particularly among local women. The available data indicate the need for school, adolescent, and women's health services to address young girls' needs. The aim should be to educate girls and women on menstruation and to promote better detection and management of menstruation-related symptoms and conditions such as PMS. School programs and national campaigns are warranted. For better adoption, such programs should be designed and delivered by women so that cultural norms around the privacy of menarche and menstruation are respected [10]. This is particularly relevant in Arab culture, where menstruation is rarely discussed around men and is considered a "women's issue" only [7].

22.2.2 Fertility

Fertility is estimated at 1.5 crude births per woman, according to the latest data reported by the World Bank in 2020. The total fertility rate (TFR) in the UAE is relatively lower compared to other Arab countries such as Syria, Saudi Arabia, and Lebanon, which have fertility rates of 2.8, 2.5, and 2.1 births per woman, respectively, in the same year. This number is alarmingly low, especially when compared to data from 1990 to 2000, when the UAE had a fertility rate of 4.5 births per woman [11]. It is important, however, to understand how such data are computed and to keep in mind that the UAE population is made up of 200 different nationalities, with an average length of stay of 4.4 years for expatriate residents. Additionally, the total fertility rate (TFR) is computed using data from household surveys based on age-specific fertility rates. Careful interpretation and further investigation are needed in this regard, particularly given that a decrease in fertility at the national level is usually accompanied by an increase in the use of contraceptives, which is not the case in the UAE. The percentage of married women using contraception remains low (28%), especially compared to other Arab countries, where about 50% of married women use contraception [11].

22.2.3 Pregnancy

Pregnancy is a dynamic process in which anatomic and physiological changes occur from fertilization to parturition. In the UAE, data on maternal health reported by UNICEF indicate remarkable maternal outcomes. For instance, 99% of births in the UAE are attended by skilled health personnel (2018). The maternal mortality ratio in the UAE is 3 per 100,000 live births based on data from 2017 [10]; this ratio is among the lowest globally. For instance, the maternal mortality ratios for Sweden, the United Kingdom, and Saudi Arabia were 4, 7, and 17, respectively, for the same year [12].

Although available data are scarce and indicators such as antenatal care visits and cesarean section (CS) rates are not officially available for the UAE, it seems that CS rates are increasing. Based on data from the Mutaba'ah[1*] study, pregnant women aged 18–24 years reported either having or preferring CS [13]. The World Health Organization (WHO) recommends limiting population-based cesarean section (CS) rates to 10–15% as higher rates may not reduce maternal, neonatal, and infant mortality [14]. The same study reported that 78.4% of pregnant Emirati women did not have adequate knowledge of delivery modes [13].

One of the determinants of conception and pregnancy outcomes is women's knowledge. However, it seems that knowledge about antenatal care and related outcomes are rather low. For example, a study that aimed to determine knowledge and attitudes toward pregnancy in the UAE found that 31.7% of women were not sure or did not know the importance of an ultrasound examination during pregnancy [15]. The majority of women in this study also thought that the fetus had a better chance of survival at 7 months of gestation than at 8 months (75%) and believed that intercourse during pregnancy was harmful to the fetus (56.6%) [15]. Alternatively, women in the UAE perceived herbal supplements as safe during pregnancy (42.9%), while most women (94.2%) agreed that not all over-the-counter medications (OTC) are safe to consume during pregnancy [16]. The perception of safety regarding the use of herbal supplements during pregnancy is worrying, as such products are uncontrolled; however, attitudes toward medications in general are also poor. Another study [17] reported that pregnant women in the UAE tend to be more skeptical of drugs and tend not to use medications unless a serious health condition is present. Women's beliefs and knowledge about medicines can affect their decisions regarding herbal, drug, and prescription intake during pregnancy. More national awareness campaigns are warranted to improve maternal knowledge and empower women to participate in informed decision-making during pregnancy.

Exposure to tobacco smoking (ETS) is yet another determinant of pregnancy outcomes, as it increases the risk of premature birth, congenital defects, smaller head circumference, and shorter baby length [18]. Although the use of tobacco among pregnant women in the UAE is low (0.7%), secondhand smoke from the

---

[1*] The Mutaba'ah Mother and Child Health Study is an ongoing prospective cohort study in Al Ain, UAE. It includes pregnant women from the Emirati population who are 18 years and above, and are residents of Al Ain.

parental side is significant. A study [18] revealed that more than a third (34.8%) of Emirati pregnant women were exposed to tobacco smoking at home.

A few studies have reported that conditions such as gestational diabetes and hypertension during pregnancy require special consideration. In the UAE, gestational diabetes mellitus (GDM) prevalence is estimated to be between 7.9% and 24.9% [19, 20], while the frequency of hypertension is reported to be around 3.1% during pregnancy [21]. Given the importance of lifestyle management in conditions such as GDM and hypertension, clinical encounters with a dietitian among women with GDM were investigated, and 22% of women with GDM never had an appointment with a dietitian for counseling, while 65% visited a dietitian once or twice during pregnancy. The same study also reported low nutrition knowledge among women with GDM [22].

22.2.4 Postpartum Depression

Depressive and anxiety disorders are common during the antenatal and postpartum periods, and they can persist for up to 1 year after giving birth. Postpartum depression (PPD) can be defined as the onset of symptoms during the first 4 weeks after delivery. Symptoms such as depressed mood, lack of pleasure or interest, sleep disturbances, and agitation, among others, are usually used to identify PPD [23].

According to a 2018 systematic review [24], the Middle East has a prevalence rate of 26% for PPD, which is higher than the global rate of 17%. PPD among women in the UAE is understudied. Prevalence rates vary from 12% to 33% and may be explained by the rapid growth of the country and its cultural diversity [25]. Moreover, a study published in 2022 [25] reported that 35% of mothers in the UAE experienced depressive symptoms during the first 6 months postpartum.

Factors that may increase the likelihood of developing postpartum depression symptoms include young age, being of the Muslim faith, part-time employment, low socioeconomic status, difficulty managing family income, and maternity leave that exceeds 3 months. Protective factors, on the other hand, include breastfeeding, living in one's own house, partner support, paternal employment status, and the perception of a healthy infant [25]. Such studies highlight the importance of developing interventions to identify and address maternal mental health.

22.2.5 Breastfeeding

The World Health Organization (WHO) and the United Nations' Children's Fund (UNICEF) recommend the initiation of breastfeeding within the first hour of birth, for a period of at least 6 months exclusively (meaning no other foods or liquids are provided, including water), and continued breastfeeding up to 2 years or beyond thereafter [26].

Data on breastfeeding in the UAE is promising, and most women living in the Emirates (Emirati and expatriate women) initiate breastfeeding during their hospital stay, with about 70% doing so within an hour of delivery. At 6 months, 81.5% of women were still breastfeeding, of whom about 27% were exclusively breastfeeding. The study reported that older women who initiated breastfeeding within 1 hour of giving birth were more likely to still be breastfeeding by the age of 6 months [27]. Similarly, a study from Abu Dhabi reported that 60% of women initiate breastfeeding within an hour of delivery, and about 44% of women breastfeed exclusively until 6 months of age [28].

22.2.6 Menopausal Health

A natural biological transition in every woman's life, and an area attracting increased research attention worldwide, is the link between understanding of, and attitudes toward, menopause and the strength of reported symptoms.

Increased life expectancy among Emirati women [29] means more women in the UAE are reaching menopause; according to data from the World Bank, 91% of women survive to the age of 65 in the UAE [11].

Numerous global studies [30] show that culture influences the way women's health and menopause are approached. Culture also has a powerful effect on how women experience emotional and physical perimenopausal symptoms. The word for menopause in Arabic translates as "Age of Despair," a clear signal of the social stigma linked with the peri- and postmenopausal decline in fertility, and the eventual end of reproductive life. Recognizing the powerful role of language in communicating universal experiences, the UAE-based hybrid healthcare platform, Nabta Health, is working to change this perception by challenging the existing Arabic terminology for menopause and seeking to celebrate menopause as a time of regeneration and renewal, an "Age of Hope" [31].

A 2019 Quality of Life (QoL) study [32] among menopausal Emirati women aged 40 to 64 years found that the most common menopausal symptoms reported as a result of the decline in reproductive hormones were physical, with 78.6% reporting muscle and joint aches and 75.7% reporting backaches. This contrasts with the reported experiences of menopausal Western and European women, whose most common symptoms reported are hot flashes [29].

A study researching knowledge and understanding of menopausal hormone therapy (MHT) [29] among Emirati women in the UAE found that participating women had fairly low levels of understanding about menopause, the physical and mental changes that occur in a woman's body, and the health risks linked with the natural decline in reproductive hormones. 95.6% of the Emirati women surveyed had not used MHT and had not received advice on the benefits and risks of hormonal treatment. The same study discussed a potential link between educational level, employment status, and understanding the pros and cons of MHT.

Another study [33] from the UAE aimed to determine the knowledge and use of hormonal treatment to manage menopausal symptoms among Arabic- and English-speaking women in Sharjah and Abu Dhabi. The authors found that 48% were using MHT, 45% felt positive about MHT, and 25% felt negative about it.

22.3 Nutrition and Lifestyle Considerations

A balanced, nutritious diet is essential for health and development; it prevents malnutrition in all its forms and contributes to the prevention and progression of non-communicable diseases such as diabetes, heart disease, stroke, and cancer. Eating a healthy food diet is also linked to better mental health and has been associated with happiness and a higher self-perception of health [34].

Despite the UAE government's education-based interventions on the importance of eating healthy [35], diet-related health conditions remain prevalent in the UAE, with the younger population following poor eating habits and relying too heavily on junk foods as well as foods high in fat and sugar [35]. Remarkably, women in the UAE have higher nutritional knowledge than men, which contributes to an improved overall diet [35]. However, Arab women find it difficult to balance eating a healthy, nutritious diet with family and work responsibilities and with traditional gender role expectations [36].

Dietary patterns are particularly important among pregnant women, and maintaining a high dietary diversity has been shown to be associated with higher diet quality. The Mother-Infant Study Cohort (MISC), a two-year prospective cohort study of pregnant women living in the United Arab Emirates, identified two distinct dietary patterns. The authors showed that adherence to a dietary pattern rich in fruits, vegetables, mixed dishes, meat, dairy products, legumes, nuts, and oils reduced the risk of insufficient gestational weight gain. Conversely, higher consumption of the "Western" pattern (more sweets and sweetened beverages, added-fats and processed foods sugar, and fast food) increased the risk of excessive gestational weight gain [20].

Based on data from the Ministry of Health and Prevention, about 40% of women are advised by a healthcare provider to reduce salt intake in their diet; about 47% are advised to increase their daily fruit and vegetable intakes; and 49% are advised to reduce their fat intakes [37].

Physical activity also plays an important role in the prevention of non-communicable diseases. A 2021 survey of young adults in the UAE found a lack of awareness of the importance of physical exercise, with both females and males spending up to 80% of their waking hours engaged in sedentary behavior. The same study reported that 76.6% of women were identified as "low-active" according to step counts [38].

A survey performed in 2010 by the Dubai Health Authority [39] found that nearly 58% of the UAE adult population is physically inactive, and while men do less physical activity than women, only 25% of women get sufficient exercise for good health. The same survey found that women from the Philippines were the most physically active women residing in the UAE, at 41%, compared with the average of 25% among UAE Nationals. Physical activity rates drop drastically among women in the UAE as they age, with just 5% of Emiratis over the age of 60 consistently performing enough regular exercise for good health.

22.4 Non-communicable Diseases

22.4.1 Obesity

Obesity is a chronic condition associated with non-communicable diseases (NCDs), including conditions that are specific to women, such as polycystic ovarian syndrome (PCOS). NCDs, such as cardiovascular disease, diabetes, cancer, and chronic respiratory disease, are responsible for about 77% of all deaths in the UAE [40].

The prevalence of adult obesity (defined as BMI $\geq 30 Kg/m^2$) in the UAE is higher among women, particularly Arab women (40%), while the prevalence of overweight (defined as $25 \leq$ BMI ≥ 30 Kg/m^2) was about 35% among women and higher among men (48%). Previous data had shown that older Emirati women are more likely than younger women to struggle with weight and obesity; however, in this study, this was not the case [41].

Obesity among women is particularly relevant during the preconception period, as pregnancy initiated with a healthy BMI is associated with better outcomes. Results from the MISC study showed that almost 60% of women were either overweight or obese before pregnancy, and 57.4% experienced excessive weight gain during pregnancy [20].

22.4.2 Polycystic Ovarian Syndrome (PCOS) and Endometriosis

Polycystic ovarian syndrome (PCOS) is a metabolic disorder characterized by hormonal imbalance, irregular menstrual cycles, and reduced fertility. As an emerging global public health concern, it is increasingly being recognized as a public health concern in the UAE as well [42]. The prevalence of PCOS in the UAE is estimated at 27.6% among young women aged 15–24 years [43]. Currently, there is no official data reporting PCOS prevalence in the UAE.

While local research has been limited, a study published in 2020 [42] assessing reproductive health knowledge and awareness among Emirati students found that only 38% of students had heard of PCOS. Additionally, students were not aware that unhealthy lifestyle choices could affect their reproductive health. Although most surveyed students (91%) considered it important to be educated about PCOS, 62% said they would prefer to learn about PCOS from a trusted medical professional. The study highlighted the importance of early detection and management of PCOS and of healthy lifestyle education.

Endometriosis is another chronic female reproductive disorder associated with inflammation. Endometriosis mainly presents as pelvic pain and infertility; however, the clinical manifestations of endometriosis are varied [44]. Accurate prevalence data for endometriosis in the UAE are not available; however, a study of self-reported endometriosis estimated the prevalence to be 1.5%, with the highest rates among young women aged between 20 and 29 years, women with period irregularities, and long menses [45].

Endometriosis and PCOS can both affect women's quality of life [46, 47]. Arab women have reported a negative impact of endometriosis on all aspects of their lives and a negative outcome from the associated psychological impact of delayed diagnosis and potential infertility [47].

22.4.3 Cardiovascular Diseases

In 2010, cardiovascular diseases were the principal cause of death among women in the UAE. Women's incidence of major cardiovascular diseases (CVDs) is 9.0 per 1,000 person-years [48].

Gender differences in cardiovascular diseases include presentation and delays in diagnosis among women. Data retrieved from the Gulf Registry in 2007 indicated a higher mortality rate among women in the UAE following heart conditions (4.6%) compared to men (1.2%) [49, 50]; in the same study, women were also reported to be treated less aggressively [50].

Women have many risk factors for heart diseases, and they are more likely to experience atypical symptoms of CVD [49]. An independent predictor of major CVD events among women is the ratio of total cholesterol to high-density lipoprotein cholesterol (TC/HDL-C), with an estimated 44% increase in risk per unit increase in the ratio. The TC/HDL-C ratio is a modifiable risk factor [48] that can be improved with lifestyle changes and medications.

Although heart diseases are among the leading causes of death among women, the perception of risk is low (only 10.5% of women perceived themselves as susceptible to heart disease), and only 17.7% believed they were not well informed about heart diseases [49]. Alarmingly, awareness of symptoms is particularly low, especially regarding atypical symptoms. Only a minority of women identified atypical symptoms of heart diseases, including anxiety (12%), pain in the back (8.4%), vomiting (6.1%), pain in the jaw (5.5%), pain in the stomach (4.1%), and elbow pain (2.4%) [49].

Although the data reported in this section may not be a comprehensive or accurate representation of the current situation in the UAE, gender differences should be further investigated regarding CVD.

22.4.4 Diabetes

According to the Ministry of Health's National Health Survey, 30.7% of Emirati women and 16% of non-Emirati women reported having impaired glycemia or diabetes [51]. Among women diagnosed with diabetes, 15.7% tended to consult traditional healers for diabetes management, and 11% reported using herbal treatment [37]. Based on a meta-analysis published in 2019, the prevalence of pre-diabetes among women is 14.4% (pooled prevalence), while the prevalence of type 2 diabetes is 7.7% (pooled prevalence) [52].

Impaired glycemia among women of childbearing age may influence the uterine environment, modulating the pathogenesis of diabetes in the offspring. Accordingly, identifying and treating women to prevent elevated glucose levels in the pregestation, gestation, and postpartum stages can decrease the intergenerational risk of diabetes [52, 53].

22.4.5 Cancer

The UAE Ministry of Health and Prevention published an annual cancer report (2023) [54] reporting that 60.1% of cancer cases in the UAE were among women (compared with 39.9% in men). The most frequent cancers among women were breast (36.6%), thyroid (14.4%), colorectal (5.7%), uterus (5.4%), and cervix uteri (3.7%). In addition to being the most common cancer among women, breast cancer is ranked second in mortality in 2023 [54]. Some data [55, 56] suggest that the average age of diagnosis of breast cancer in the UAE and other Arab countries is a decade earlier than in Western countries (49 years vs. 60 years in developed countries). Most available studies investigating cancer in the UAE highlight the importance of increasing screening and awareness among women. For more information on cancer in the UAE, refer to Chap. 26.

22.5 Mental Health

Mental disorders are a significant public health and socioeconomic burden on individual women, their families, and the community. Under the National Agenda, the UAE government set a goal to be ranked among the happiest nations; policies, programs, and tools have been established to support happiness-related initiatives [57]. This was an important step in emphasizing mental health at the national level. However, mental health in general, and depression in particular, remain the leading causes of disability worldwide. Gender disparities are especially remarkable when it comes to mental health, and women are more affected by depression compared with men (5.1% women, 3.6% men globally) [58].

In the UAE, a systematic review [59] reported a prevalence of depression ranging from 12.5% to 28.6%. The review also identified important risk factors such as female gender, indicating that women are more likely to suffer from depression in the UAE (consistent with global data). Other risk factors identified include financial difficulties, stressful life events, a lack of social support, and the presence of chronic illnesses [59]. All of this creates even greater gender inequalities, particularly among women from vulnerable populations, such as women from low-income households, women with disabilities, and women with chronic illnesses.

Irrespective of a mental health diagnosis, prolonged exposure to stress is associated with negative outcomes for health, including physical and mental health disorders [60]. Women can experience high levels of stress by juggling multiple roles, such as domestic work, childbearing, and professional work. Nonworking women, or housewives, seem to experience even more stress than working women [61]. A study [62] from the UAE reported higher salivary cortisol among nonworking women compared with working women, indicating that they exhibit higher levels of stress and highlighting the urgent need to support nonworking women with policies and coping mechanisms.

Studies among female Emirati students [63] and young Muslim women [64] in the UAE suggest that self-stigma and societal stigma about mental health disorders are significant barriers to help-seeking. Among female Emirati students, 36.5% identified social stigma as the main barrier to seeking treatment, and 19.8% identified self-stigma as a barrier. Another 13.5% of female students reported misconceptions about the role of psychologists, available treatments, and mental health services as a barrier.

Eating disorders and body image dissatisfaction greatly impact mental health and wellbeing among women, and in the UAE, as in other countries, body image dissatisfaction and disturbed eating behaviors are also common [65]. Although there does not seem to be solid data on this topic from the UAE, some studies among young women [65] and Emirati university students [66] suggest that women may have high levels of body dissatisfaction. These studies reported that 74–78% of young women were dissatisfied with their body image. Additionally, 20–30% of the women had at least one symptom of an eating disorder [65–67]. Risk factors that are associated with higher levels of eating disorders and related symptoms include depressive symptoms [65], internalized weight stigma, negative body image [66], and being bothered by teasing from family or friends [67]. Accordingly, eating disorders and body dissatisfaction are additional mental health conditions that affect a large number of women in the UAE and require public health programs to improve the health and wellbeing of young women.

22.6 Conclusion

The women's health sector in the UAE has seen many changes and improvements in the past decades; however, gender disparities in the diagnosis and treatment of women still exist.

While policies aimed at preventing, identifying, and treating physical and mental health conditions among women are warranted, programs aimed at educating and empowering women to take charge of their own health and that of their families are also needed. National programs, starting with school education, should be initiated and continued across the spectrum of a woman's life cycle. After all, a well-known African proverb states, "If you educate a woman, you educate a nation."

Conflicts of Interest The authors have no conflicts of interest to declare.

References

1. Koornneef E, Robben P, Blair I. Progress and outcomes of health systems reform in The United Arab Emirates: a systematic review. BMC Health Serv Res. 2017;17(1):1–13.
2. Kemp LJ, Madsen SR, El-Saidi M. The current state of female leadership in The United Arab Emirates. J Glob Respons. 2013;4:99.
3. Council U-UB. The UAE Healthcare Sector-Sector Updates. United Arab Emirates 2021.
4. Khayata G, Rizk D, Hasan M, Ghazal-Aswad S, Asaad M. Factors influencing the quality of life of infertile women in United Arab Emirates. Int J Gynecol Obstet. 2003;80(2):183–8.
5. World Health Organization. Women's health 2023. Available from: https://www.who.int/health-topics/women-s-health.
6. Global Media Insights. United Arab Emirates population statistics 2023, 2023.
7. Kridli SA-O. Health beliefs and practices among Arab women. MCN Am J Matern Child Nurs. 2002;27(3):178–82.
8. Rizk DE, Mosallam M, Alyan S, Nagelkerke N. Prevalence and impact of premenstrual syndrome in adolescent schoolgirls in The United Arab Emirates. Acta Obstet Gynecol Scand. 2006;85(5):589–98.
9. Steiner M, Macdougall M, Brown E. The premenstrual symptoms screening tool (PSST) for clinicians. Arch Womens Ment Health. 2003;6(3):203–9.
10. UNICEF. United Arab Emirates Key Demographic Indicators 2023. Available from: https://data.unicef.org/country/are/.
11. World Bank. Fertility rate, total (births per woman) - United Arab Emirates 2020. Available from: https://data.worldbank.org/indicator/SP.DYN.TFRT.IN?locations=AE.
12. UNICEF. UNICEF Data Warehouse. Available from: https://data.unicef.org/resources/data_explorer/unicef_f/?ag=UNICEF&df=GLOBAL_DATAFLOW&ver=1.0&dq=ARE+LBN+SAU+GBR+USA+FRA+SWE.MNCH_MMR+MNCH_MATERNAL_DEATHS..&startPeriod=2016&endPeriod=2022.
13. Al-Rifai RH, Elbarazi I, Ali N, Loney T, Oulhaj A, Ahmed LA. Knowledge and preference towards mode of delivery among pregnant women in The United Arab Emirates: the Mutaba'ah study. Int J Environ Res Public Health. 2020;18(1):36.
14. Betran AP, Torloni MR, Zhang J, Ye J, Mikolajczyk R, Deneux-Tharaux C, et al. What is the optimal rate of caesarean section at population level? A systematic review of ecologic studies. Reprod Health. 2015;12(1):1–10.
15. Alkaabi MS, Alsenaidi LK, Mirghani H. Women's knowledge and attitude towards pregnancy in a high-income developing country. J Perinat Med. 2015;43(4):445–8.
16. Abduelkarem AR, Mustafa H. Use of over-the-counter medication among pregnant women in Sharjah, United Arab Emirates. J Pregnancy. 2017;2017:4503793.
17. Mohamed Ibrahim OH, Ibrahim RM, Al-Tameemi NK, Bahy Mohammed Ebaed S, AlMazrouei N, Riley K. Evaluation of the use and attitudes of pregnant and postpartum women towards medicine utilisation during pregnancy in The United Arab Emirates: a national cross-sectional study. Int J Clin Pract. 2021;75(9):e14344.
18. Taha MN, Al-Ghumgham Z, Ali N, Al-Rifai RH, Elbarazi I, Al-Maskari F, et al. Tobacco use and exposure to environmental tobacco smoke amongst pregnant women in The United Arab Emirates: the Mutaba'ah study. Int J Environ Res Public Health. 2022;19(12):7498.
19. Bashir MM, Ahmed LA, Alshamsi MR, Almahrooqi S, Alyammahi T, Alshehhi SA, et al. Gestational diabetes Mellitus: a cross-sectional survey of Its knowledge and associated factors among United Arab Emirates University students. Int J Environ Res Public Health. 2022;19(14):8381.
20. Itani L, Radwan H, Hashim M, Hasan H, Obaid RS, Ghazal HA, et al. Dietary patterns and their associations with gestational weight gain in The United Arab Emirates: results from the MISC cohort. Nutr J. 2020;19(1):1–12.
21. Jijiwa H, Sabitu A, Danbello Z, Jumba F, Haruna H, Al SS. Hypertension among pregnant women attending GMC Hospital, Ajman, UAE. Gulf Med Univ Proc. 2015;2015(4–5 Poster):47–54.

22. Ali HI, Jarrar AH, El Sadig M, K BY. Diet and carbohydrate food knowledge of multi-ethnic women: a comparative analysis of pregnant women with and without Gestational Diabetes Mellitus. PLoS One. 2013;8(9):e73486.
23. Sharma V, Sharma P. Postpartum depression: diagnostic and treatment issues. J Obstet Gynaecol Can. 2012;34(5):436–42.
24. Shorey S, Chee CYI, Ng ED, Chan YH, Tam WWS, Chong YS. Prevalence and incidence of postpartum depression among healthy mothers: a systematic review and meta-analysis. J Psychiatr Res. 2018;104:235–48.
25. Hanach N, Radwan H, Fakhry R, Dennis CL, Issa WB, Faris ME, et al. Prevalence and risk factors of postpartum depression among women living in The United Arab Emirates. Soc Psychiatry Psychiatr Epidemiol. 2022;58:395.
26. World Health Organization. Breastfeeding 2023. Available from: https://www.who.int/health-topics/breastfeeding#tab=tab_2.
27. Radwan H, Fakhry R, Metheny N, Baniissa W, Faris MAIE, Obaid RS, et al. Prevalence and multivariable predictors of breastfeeding outcomes in The United Arab Emirates: a prospective cohort study. Int Breastfeed J. 2021;16(1):1–13.
28. Taha Z, Garemo M, Nanda J. Patterns of breastfeeding practices among infants and young children in Abu Dhabi, United Arab Emirates. Int Breastfeed J. 2018;13(1):1–10.
29. Shahzad D, Thakur AA, Kidwai S, Shaikh HO, AlSuwaidi AO, AlOtaibi AF, et al. Women's knowledge and awareness on menopause symptoms and its treatment options remains inadequate: a report from The United Arab Emirates. Menopause. 2021;28(8):918–27.
30. Avis N, Crawford S. Cultural differences in symptoms and attitudes toward menopause. Menopause Manag. 2008;17:8–13.
31. Kimani M. Did you know that 'menopause' translates to 'Age of Despair' in Arabic? That label stops now with Nabta. Dubai, UAE: Nabta Health FZE; 2022. Available from: https://nabtahealth.com/articles/nabta-health-celebrates-women-during-their-age-of-hope/.
32. Smail L, Jassim G, Shakil A. Menopause-specific quality of life among Emirati women. Int J Environ Res Public Health. 2020;17(1):40.
33. Mohamed Ibrahim O, Hussein R. Knowledge, attitude, and prevalence of use of hormone replacement therapy among women in United Arab Emirates. Asian J Pharm Clin Res. 2016;9:115–8.
34. Badri MA, Alkhaili M, Aldhaheri H, Alnahyan H, Yang G, Albahar M, et al. Understanding the interactions of happiness, self-rated health, mental feelings, habit of eating healthy and sport/activities: a path model for Abu Dhabi. Nutrients. 2022;14(1):55.
35. AlBlooshi S, Khalid A, Hijazi R. The Barriers to Sustainable Nutrition for Sustainable Health among Zayed University Students in the UAE. Nutrients. 2022;14(19):4175.
36. Al-Thani MA, Khaled SM. "Toxic pleasures": a study of eating out behavior in Arab female university students and its associations with psychological distress and disordered eating. Eat Behav. 2018;31:125–30.
37. Ministry of Health and Prevention UAE. Non-Communicable Disease Risk Factor Survey (STEPS). Data Book for UAE 2017–2018, 2017–2018.
38. Dalibalta S, Majdalawieh A, Yousef S, Gusbi M, Wilson JJ, Tully MA, et al. Objectively quantified physical activity and sedentary behaviour in a young UAE population. BMJ Open Sport Exerc Med. 2021;7(1):e000957.
39. Authority DH. Dubai Household Health Survey 2009, 2010.
40. Fadhil I, Belaila B, Razzak H. National accountability and response for noncommunicable diseases in The United Arab Emirates. Int J Noncommun Dis. 2019;4(1):4–9.
41. Sulaiman N, Elbadawi S, Hussein A, Abusnana S, Madani A, Mairghani M, et al. Prevalence of overweight and obesity in United Arab Emirates Expatriates: the UAE National Diabetes and Lifestyle Study. Diabetol Metab Syndr. 2017;9(1):88.
42. Pramodh S. Exploration of lifestyle choices, reproductive health knowledge, and Polycystic Ovary Syndrome (PCOS) awareness among female Emirati university students. Int J Women's Health. 2020;12:927–38.

43. Saidunnisa B, Atiqulla S, Ayman G, Mohammad B, Housam R, Khaled N. Prevalence of polycystic ovarian syndrome among students of rak medical and health sciences University United Arab Emirates. Int J Med Pharm Sci. 2016;6:109–18.
44. Lee S-Y, Koo Y-J, Lee D-H. Classification of endometriosis. Yeungnam Univ J Med. 2021;38(1):10–8.
45. Al-Jefout M, Alawar S, Balayah Z, Al-Hareb A, Al-Ameri F, Alhosani M. Self-reported prevalence of endometriosis and its symptoms in The United Arab Emirates (UAE). Biomed Pharm J. 2018;11(1):265–75.
46. Zaitoun B, Al Kubaisi A, AlQattan N, Alassouli Y, Mohamed A, Alameeri H, et al. Polycystic ovarian syndrome awareness among females in the UAE: a cross-sectional study. BMC Womens Health. 2022;23(1):181.
47. Mousa M, Al-Jefout M, Alsafar H, Becker CM, Zondervan KT, Rahmioglu N. Impact of endometriosis in women of Arab ancestry on: health-related quality of life, work productivity, and diagnostic delay. Front Glob Womens Health. 2021;2:708410.
48. Al-Shamsi S, Regmi D, Govender RD. Incidence of cardiovascular disease and its associated risk factors in at-risk men and women in The United Arab Emirates: a 9-year retrospective cohort study. BMC Cardiovasc Disord. 2019;19(1):148.
49. Khan S, Ali SA. Exploratory study into awareness of heart disease and health care seeking behavior among Emirati women (UAE) - Cross sectional descriptive study. BMC Womens Health. 2017;17(1):88.
50. Shehab A, Yasin J, Hashim MJ, Al-Dabbagh B, Mahmeed WA, Bustani N, et al. Gender differences in acute coronary syndrome in Arab Emirati women—implications for clinical management. Angiology. 2013;64(1):9–14.
51. Ministry of Health and Prevention UAE. UAE National Health Survey report 2017–2018, 2017–2018.
52. Al-Rifai RH, Majeed M, Qambar MA, Ibrahim A, AlYammahi KM, Aziz F. Type 2 diabetes and pre-diabetes mellitus: a systematic review and meta-analysis of prevalence studies in women of childbearing age in the Middle East and North Africa, 2000–2018. Syst Rev. 2019;8(1):1–32.
53. Clausen TD, Mathiesen ER, Hansen T, Pedersen O, Jensen DM, Lauenborg J, et al. High prevalence of type 2 diabetes and pre-diabetes in adult offspring of women with gestational diabetes mellitus or type 1 diabetes: the role of intrauterine hyperglycemia. Diabetes Care. 2008;31(2):340–6.
54. Cancer Incidence in United Arab Emirates Annual Report of the UAE-National Cancer Registry-2023.pdf.
55. Najjar H, Easson A. Age at diagnosis of breast cancer in Arab nations. Int J Surg. 2010;8(6):448–52.
56. Bendardaf R, Saheb Sharif-Askari F, Saheb Sharif-Askari N, Yousuf Guraya S, Abusnana S. Incidence and clinicopathological features of breast cancer in the Northern Emirates: experience from Sharjah breast care center. Int J Women's Health. 2020;12:893–9.
57. UAE Government. Happiness 2016. Available from: https://u.ae/en/about-the-uae/the-uae-government/government-of-future/happiness.
58. WHO. Global Health Estimates; Depression and other common mental disorders, 2017.
59. Razzak HA, Harbi A, Ahli S. Depression: prevalence and associated risk factors in the United Arab Emirates. Oman Med J. 2019;34(4):274–82.
60. Yaribeygi H, Panahi Y, Sahraei H, Johnston TP, Sahebkar A. The impact of stress on body function: a review. EXCLI J. 2017;16:1057–72.
61. Durak M, Senol-Durak E, Karakose S. Psychological distress and anxiety among housewives: the mediational role of perceived stress, loneliness, and housewife burnout. Curr Psychol. 2022;42:14517.
62. Bani-Issa W, Radwan H, Al Shujairi A, Hijazi H, Al Abdi RM, Al Awar S, et al. Salivary cortisol, perceived stress and coping strategies: a comparative study of working and nonworking women. J Nurs Manag. 2022;30:3553.

63. Al-Darmaki F, Thomas J, Yaaqeib S. Mental health beliefs amongst Emirati female college students. Community Ment Health J. 2016;52(2):233–8.
64. Vally Z, Cody BL, Albloshi MA, Alsheraifi SNM. Public stigma and attitudes toward psychological help-seeking in The United Arab Emirates: the mediational role of self-stigma. Perspect Psychiatr Care. 2018;54(4):571–9.
65. Schulte SJ, Thomas J. Relationship between eating pathology, body dissatisfaction and depressive symptoms among male and female adolescents in The United Arab Emirates. Eat Behav. 2013;14(2):157–60.
66. Thomas J, Khan S, Abdulrahman AA. Eating attitudes and body image concerns among female university students in The United Arab Emirates. Appetite. 2010;54(3):595–8.
67. O'Hara L, Tahboub-Schulte S, Thomas J. Weight-related teasing and internalized weight stigma predict abnormal eating attitudes and behaviours in Emirati female university students. Appetite. 2016;102:44–50.

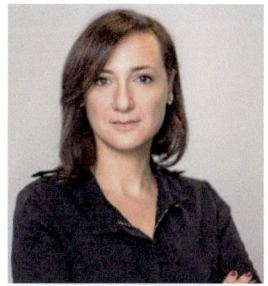

Cosette Fakih El Khoury is a clinician, researcher, and nutrition and public health consultant with a BS and MS in Nutrition and Dietetics from the American University of Beirut and a PhD in Health Services Research from Maastricht University. She has worked in academia and as a nutrition and public health consultant to international organizations and UN agencies in multiple countries in the Eastern Mediterranean Region. She is also the former general manager of Nabta Health Clinic, a women's health startup in the United Arab Emirates. Dr. El Khoury is passionate about the prevention and management of noncommunicable diseases and is a strong supporter of gender equality in health .

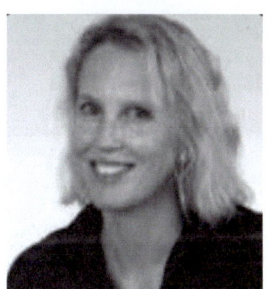

Jennifer Fortin is a passionate *public* health specialist currently focused on women's health and mental health in the GCC region. She specializes in raising awareness, advocacy, and education initiatives related to these areas. Prior to her work in the Gulf, Jennifer contributed to a range of public health initiatives across Canada. She collaborated on projects addressing housing insecurity, developed strategies for early STBBI detection, and conducted analyses of chronic disease trends among Canadian First Nations. Her policy work is research-driven, responsive to community needs, and focused on long-term impact. Holding a Master of Public Health and a Bachelor's in Psychology from the University of Montreal, Jennifer is guided by a strong commitment to social justice. Her early involvement with marginalized children, isolated seniors, and justice-involved individuals continues to shape her inclusive and equity-centered approach to public health.

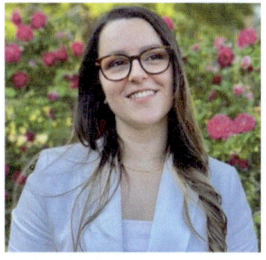

Samantha Dumas is a *content* and strategic communications specialist with 25 years of writing and advisory experience across organizations, sectors, and markets. Her focus is on developing content for disruptors, start-ups, and individuals working to make the world a better, fairer, greener place for all, with an emphasis on improving outcomes for girls and women.

Open Access This chapter is licensed under the terms of the Creative Commons Attribution 4.0 International License (http://creativecommons.org/licenses/by/4.0/), which permits use, sharing, adaptation, distribution and reproduction in any medium or format, as long as you give appropriate credit to the original author(s) and the source, provide a link to the Creative Commons license and indicate if changes were made.

The images or other third party material in this chapter are included in the chapter's Creative Commons license, unless indicated otherwise in a credit line to the material. If material is not included in the chapter's Creative Commons license and your intended use is not permitted by statutory regulation or exceeds the permitted use, you will need to obtain permission directly from the copyright holder.

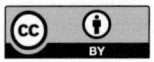

Midwifery Care in the UAE

23

Saloua El Azzabi and Etab Omar Salem

23.1 Introduction

In 2021, the United Arab Emirates (UAE) formulated a strategy for the nursing/midwifery development plan vision through 2071, in which it draws the framework for a 5-year plan as a roadmap to strengthening the nursing and midwifery professions, as they are considered crucial contributing elements to reducing neonatal, infant, and maternal mortality rates in the UAE [1].

The midwifery profession stands as a cornerstone within the healthcare system, playing a pivotal role in ensuring comprehensive and high-quality maternal and newborn care. Midwives, equipped with specialized knowledge and skills, contribute significantly to the well-being of expectant mothers and their infants.

In recent years, the UAE has recognized the importance of midwifery and has taken significant strides to enhance the profession. This chapter focuses on the evolving landscape of midwifery in the UAE, exploring the importance of midwives in providing high-quality maternal healthcare and the efforts being made to empower and elevate this noble profession.

23.2 International Midwifery Definition

"A Midwife is a person who has successfully completed a midwifery education program based on the ICM Essential Competencies for Midwifery Practice and the framework of the ICM Global Standards for Midwifery Education, recognized in the country where it is located; who has acquired the requisite

S. El Azzabi (✉)
Danat Al Emarat Hospital for Women and Children, Abu Dhabi, United Arab Emirates

E. O. Salem
Burjeel Specialty Hospital, Sharjah, Sharjah, United Arab Emirates

qualifications to be registered and/or legally licensed to practice midwifery and use the title 'Midwife'; and who demonstrates competency in the practice of midwifery" [2].

23.3 Licensing and Certification

In order to practice as a Midwife in the UAE, individuals must be licensed by the Dubai Health Authority (DHA), the Ministry of Health and Prevention (MOHAP), or the Department of Health Abu Dhabi (DOH). These licensing bodies ensure that midwives meet the specific requirements and qualifications imposed by government authorities to demonstrate the necessary knowledge, skills, and competence to perform duties safely and effectively [1].

23.4 Scope of Midwifery Practice

Midwifery is recognized as an autonomous and independent profession. Midwives work in partnership with women to provide the necessary support, care, and advice during pregnancy, labor, and the postpartum period, and to conduct vaginal births under the midwife's own responsibility, in addition to newborn care. This care includes preventive measures, the promotion of normal birth, the detection of complications in the mother and infant, and facilitating access to medical care or other appropriate assistance, including carrying out emergency measures [2].

The Midwife has an important role in health counseling and education, not only for the women and gender-diverse people they serve but also within the family and the community.

This work includes antenatal education and preparation for parenthood and may extend to sexual and reproductive healthcare, as well as care for infants and young children.

A Midwife may practice in any setting, including the home, community, hospitals, clinics, or health units.

23.5 Scope of Practice of Midwives in the UAE

Midwives in the UAE have a wide scope of practice, which includes providing antenatal care, assisting in childbirth, providing postnatal care, and offering counseling and education to women and their families. They also play a crucial role in promoting and supporting breastfeeding. Due to specific regulations, the practices and requirements of midwifery might vary from one emirate or healthcare facility in the UAE to the next [3].

23.6 Role of Midwifery in Maternal Healthcare

Midwives in the UAE work closely with obstetric physicians and other healthcare providers to deliver comprehensive care to pregnant women and their newborns. They monitor the progress of pregnancy, conduct regular check-ups, and provide guidance on nutrition, exercise, and overall well-being. Midwives also play a critical role in supporting women's health throughout the entire childbirth process. Their role is crucial during antenatal care, labor and delivery, and the postpartum period. They possess unique qualities and skills, such as providing emotional support, promoting breastfeeding, and ensuring the well-being of both mother and child [4].

23.7 Midwifery and Cultural Sensitivity

Midwives in the UAE prioritize cultural sensitivity when providing their care. During induction and orientation, they undergo comprehensive training to align their practices with the diverse cultural and religious beliefs of the community they serve. This includes respecting privacy, dignity, and traditions while ensuring the safety of both mother and baby. UAE facilities actively incorporate these cultural considerations into their training for midwives, reflecting a commitment to providing patient-centered and culturally competent care.

Midwives are integrated within the cultural variation of the UAE. This includes education on religious customs, traditional birthing practices, and the importance of family involvement. By fostering cultural competence, midwives can establish trust and rapport with the women in their care, creating a supportive and inclusive environment [2, 5].

23.8 Challenges and Recommendations

Like in other countries worldwide, midwives in the UAE face challenges with regard to the growth of their profession on the one hand, and enjoy great opportunities on the other. From a national midwifery perspective, there is significant opportunity to develop midwifery services and to curb a culture of medicalized childbirth, especially in private hospitals. On average, 35,566 births occurred in 2021 across the culturally diverse healthcare system in Abu Dhabi.

Midwives' practice varies from one facility to the next. Some midwives practice within the full scope of midwifery, providing antenatal, intrapartum, and postnatal care for women and their infants, which includes vaginal birth, suturing, and other necessary care. In other facilities, the midwife's role is limited to providing support for women during labor and assisting obstetricians in conducting vaginal and instrumental births (unless in the case of a precipitous delivery), which is known as a physician-led model of care. This model is currently the dominant model in many healthcare facilities. Several challenges can be identified in midwifery practice, including the following [6, 7]:

- *Patient preference* or lack of knowledge about the midwifery profession and the role of midwives.
- *Political issues:* Midwifery practices in the UAE vary, with some hospitals leaning toward a more medical approach rather than being evidence-based. The shared care model relies on strong support, and the key to success lies in the crucial collaboration and cooperation between obstetricians and midwives.
- *Legal factors:* Compensation for midwifery services and adoption of the most recent scope of practice outlined by the UAE Nursing and Midwifery Council.
- *Economic factors:* This model should be both economical and proficient. Each facility has varying salary structures, and there is a shortage of midwives in certain regions.
- *Social factors:* Certain regions are extremely remote and pose challenges in attracting midwives. There is a need to enlist midwives who are fluent in Arabic.
- *Technical factors:* Providing additional skills to midwives comes with financial and human resource considerations. Maintaining proficiency in smaller obstetric services poses challenges. Strengthening the midwifery network is essential.
- *Environmental factors:* Ensuring the sustainability of the infrastructure is crucial. The model should be backed by ongoing education and professional growth. Sustaining the midwifery program is essential.

Here are some recommendations to enhance midwifery practice in the UAE:

- Enlist the support of Chief Medical Officers and Chief Midwifery and Nursing Officers in each facility to introduce midwifery.
- Continue to work with the midwifery and nursing council to identify gaps and challenges in midwifery practice.
- Explore partnerships with local colleges to develop an education strategy.
- Develop a sustainable and economically viable model to support midwifery growth.
- Create a competency framework based on evidence, led by the midwifery and nursing council.
- Expand the midwifery workforce to align with current demand.
- Create a conducive environment for midwives to practice to their fullest extent, enabling greater autonomy in their scope of practice and promoting an increase in midwife-attended births.
- Establish distinct pathways for low-risk women to access midwifery services. Health plans could adopt midwifery as the primary model for low-risk pregnancy care, reserving referrals to obstetricians or maternal-fetal medicine specialists for more complex pregnancies requiring higher level care.
- Allocate additional focus and public investment in midwifery education, emphasizing the recruitment of a diverse workforce.

23.9 Midwifery Profession's Future in the UAE

The future of midwifery practice in the UAE holds great promise. To ensure continued success, it is crucial to invest in the continuous professional development of midwives, expand training programs, and integrate technological advancements. Community engagement and education efforts can raise awareness about the benefits of midwifery-led care, while research initiatives contribute to evidence-based practices and help identify the potential areas for improvement, such as increasing public awareness and understanding of midwifery. Advocacy for supportive policies, cultural competence training, and fostering public-private partnerships are key components in further strengthening midwifery services. By implementing these recommendations, the UAE can shape a future where midwives play a pivotal role in delivering high-quality, culturally sensitive maternal and neonatal care, emphasizing the importance of ongoing support, mentorship, and professional development opportunities for midwives [1, 7].

23.10 Continuous Professional Development

Midwives in the UAE are encouraged to engage in ongoing professional development to maintain up-to-date, evidence-based practices and stay informed about advancements in the field, which enables them to ensure the delivery of optimal care to women and their families.

1. Professional Development: Ensure that midwives in the UAE engage in continuous professional development programs to stay abreast of evolving evidence-based practices, technological advancements, and emerging trends in maternal healthcare.
2. Training Program Expansion: Expand and diversify midwifery training programs to meet the increasing demand for skilled professionals, in collaboration with educational institutions to offer comprehensive and accessible training opportunities.

23.11 Initiatives and Programs Promoting Midwifery in the UAE

The UAE government, healthcare institutions, and professional associations persist in extensive efforts to acknowledge and enhance the midwifery specialty in the region through establishing training programs, formulating regulations and standards, and seamlessly integrating midwives into the healthcare system. The integration of midwives into the healthcare system is another pivotal aspect of these initiatives. By recognizing and incorporating midwives into the broader healthcare landscape, the UAE aims to optimize the delivery of maternal and newborn care. This integration involves collaboration with other healthcare professionals, fostering a multidisciplinary approach to address the diverse needs of expectant mothers. Additionally, there is an emphasis on highlighting success stories and notable accomplishments in advancing the practice of midwifery [1].

23.12 Empowering Midwives in the UAE

Midwives collaborate with women, their partners, and families as needed, and engage with other healthcare professionals when necessary. They are well-positioned to anticipate and identify changes that may lead to various care needs, encompassing physical, psychological, social, cultural, or spiritual aspects, including situations like perinatal loss and end-of-life care. When such situations arise, midwives take responsibility for immediate response, management, and escalation, collaborating with interdisciplinary colleagues. They ensure continuity and coordination of care, acting as advocates to prioritize the woman's needs, views, preferences, and decisions, as well as those of her newborn [7].

The medicalization of childbirth is prevalent in many countries, with economic growth often paralleled by increased interventions like cesarean sections (CSs). Concerns arise regarding the impact on mortality, morbidity rates, and healthcare costs. To address this, a midwife-led care unit strategy is gaining traction in high-income countries. This approach emphasizes normality, continuity of care, and the presence of a trusted, licensed, and skilled Midwife during labor and childbirth. The focus is on the natural ability of women to experience birth with minimal intervention. Midwife-led units, often located in or near hospitals, exhibit higher rates of spontaneous vaginal births, lower intervention rates, and similarly positive infant outcomes [8].

23.12.1 Midwifery-Led Care

Midwifery-led care is a model of maternity services that places midwives at the forefront of supporting and guiding expectant mothers throughout pregnancy, childbirth, and the postpartum period. This approach is based on the belief that pregnancy and childbirth are natural processes, and midwives play a central role in providing holistic, woman-centered care [9, 10].

23.12.2 Advantages of Midwifery-Led Care

This model offers numerous advantages that contribute to maternity health services, as it facilitates the establishment of a strong and trusting relationship between the Midwife and the expectant mother, which fosters open communication. This approach allows for a more profound comprehension of the woman's individual needs, preferences, and concerns, further enhancing continuity of care.

Midwifery-led care in the UAE context emphasizes this model as having a positive impact on maternal health outcomes, such as reducing maternal and infant mortality rates, increasing breastfeeding rates, and improving overall patient satisfaction levels.

23.13 Successful Personal Stories of Midwife Home Visits That Showcase the Transformative Impact of Midwifery Care

One of the leading UAE facilities in Dubai introduced Midwife home visits in 2023. The project had several benefits with a positive outcome.

1. Comfort and convenience: Midwife postnatal home visits allow new couples to benefit from necessary care in the comfort of their own homes, fostering a personalized and familiar environment. This reduces the need for frequent clinic or hospital visits, saving time and decreasing stress. It also provides a relaxed environment for the couple, which can contribute to a positive and healthy postnatal recovery.
2. Personalized care: Midwife postnatal home visits offer individualized attention and care to couples. The Midwife takes time to build a relationship with the couples, understanding their unique needs, concerns, and preferences. This personalized approach ensures that the care provided is tailored to each couple's specific situation.
3. Emotional support: Midwives provide emotional support and encouragement to mothers and fathers during the first days and weeks of postnatal recovery. They play a crucial role in listening, answering questions, and addressing concerns, fostering empowerment and confidence in parents' ability to care for their newborns.

This support is necessary during the first days and weeks of postnatal transition; it has an incredible impact on identifying postnatal blues and depression in postpartum mothers and enables early detection and referral of high-risk cases that require medical interventions or treatment.

23.14 National Strategy for Nursing and Midwifery-2026 in the UAE

The UAE National Strategy for Nursing and Midwifery-2026 outlines a comprehensive plan for the advancement and enhancement of nursing and midwifery services in the UAE. The strategy includes key objectives, policies, and initiatives aimed at promoting the growth, development, and effectiveness of nursing and midwifery practices within the country. It focuses on areas such as education, professional development, recruitment, and the overall elevation of the nursing and midwifery workforce to meet the evolving healthcare needs of the UAE [1].

The National Strategy for Nursing and Midwifery-2026 aims to enhance the scope of the profession through professional organizational policies and practices to:

- Guarantee the sustainability of the profession and its active contribution to achieving the Sustainable Development Goals.
- Ensure the effective planning of the nursing and midwifery workforce, focusing on recruitment and retention in alignment with evolving needs and priorities.
- Guarantee that nursing personnel fulfill their responsibilities in accordance with their qualifications and experience, delivering high-quality nursing care services.
- The strategy also aims to qualify nursing and midwifery staff to participate in evidence-based research and practice, address national health priorities, and contribute to the development of professional policies and practices.

The strategy was launched with the objectives to:

- Encourage increased participation of citizens in the nursing and midwifery professions
- Promote both public and specialized nursing academic programs
- Elevate the quality of nursing care and midwifery services within the country

The key pillars of the strategy likely include the following:

- Governance and leadership
- Effective legislation
- A comprehensive labor administration system designed for the nursing and midwifery professions
- High-quality health and nursing services
- Enhancing excellence and creativity in education and professional growth, as well as advancing scientific research and evidence-based practices

The strategy incorporates the following promptly executable strategic solutions:

- Creating a structured career advancement system within the human resources trajectory
- Incorporating the nursing profession into the curricula from the first to twelfth grades to cultivate a fresh perception of the profession within society
- Implementing a nationwide accreditation program to uphold excellence in nursing care and midwifery
- Allocating resources to enhance the leadership skills of nursing cadres, with a particular focus on leadership during crises and emergencies

23.15 Conclusion

In conclusion, midwifery in the UAE plays a crucial role in providing healthcare services to women during pregnancy, childbirth, and the postpartum period. The profession has seen significant growth and development over the years, with increased recognition of the importance of midwives in promoting safe and positive birth experiences.

The UAE government has taken steps to improve midwifery services by implementing regulations and guidelines that ensure the competency and qualifications of midwives. This includes the requirement for midwives to be registered and licensed by the relevant authorities and the initiation of educational programs.

Overall, midwifery in the UAE is an essential component of the healthcare system, contributing to the well-being of women and their families. The profession continues to evolve and improve, with ongoing efforts to enhance the quality of midwifery services and further integrate midwives into the healthcare system.

Conflicts of Interest The authors have no conflicts of interest to declare.

References

1. National Strategy for Nursing and Midwifery - Roadmap for 2026 | The Official Portal of the UAE Government [Internet 2022]. Available from: https://u.ae/en/about-the-uae/strategies-initiatives-and-awards/strategies-plans-and-visions/health/national-strategy-for-nursing-and-midwifery#:~:text=The%20National%20Strategy%20for%20Nursing,midwifery%20services%20in%20the%20country.
2. Icm. ICM Definitions. ICM, n.d.. https://www.internationalMidwives.org/our-work/policy-and-practice/icm-definitions.html.
3. NURSING AND MIDWIFERY SCOPE OF PRACTICE USERGUIDE [Internet]. UAE Nursing and Midwifery Council. 2015. Available from: http://www.uaenmc.gov.ae/Data/Files/2016June/User%20Guide%20SOP.pdf.
4. Role of nurse in midwifery and obstetrical care [Internet]. Rawat Nursing. Available from: https://www.rawatnursingcollege.com/blog/role-of-nurse-in-midwifery-and-obstetrical-care.
5. Mantula F, Chamisa JA, Nunu WN, Nyanhongo PS. Women's perspectives on cultural sensitivity of midwives during intrapartum care at a maternity ward in a national referral hospital in Zimbabwe. SAGE Open Nurs [Internet]. 2023;9:237796082311604. https://doi.org/10.1177/23779608231160476.
6. Safari K, McKenna L, Davis J. Midwifery in Middle Eastern and North African countries: a scoping review. Women Birth [Internet]. 2021;34(6):503–13. https://doi.org/10.1016/j.wombi.2020.11.002.
7. Grace F, Philidah S. Empowering midwives in The United Arab Emirates. Worldwide Matern Serv [Internet]. 2016;26:387–90. Available from: https://ecommons.aku.edu/cgi/viewcontent.cgi?article=1086&context=eastafrica_fhs_sonam.
8. Johanson R, Newburn M, Macfarlane A. Has the medicalisation of childbirth gone too far? BMJ [Internet]. 2002;324(7342):892–5. Available from: https://doi.org/10.1136/bmj.324.7342.892.
9. Ricchi A, Rossi F, Borgognoni P, Bassi MC, Artioli G, Foà C, et al. The midwifery-led care model: a continuity of care model in the birth path. PubMed [Internet]. 2019;90(6–S):41–52. Available from: https://pubmed.ncbi.nlm.nih.gov/31292414.

10. Symon A, Pringle J, Cheyne H, Downe S, Hundley V, Lee EC, et al. Midwifery-led antenatal care models: mapping a systematic review to an evidence-based quality framework to identify key components and characteristics of care. BMC Pregnan Childbirth [Internet]. 2016;16(1). https://doi.org/10.1186/s12884-016-0944-6.

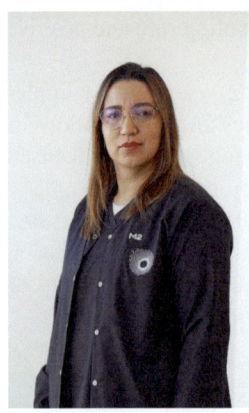

Saloua El Azzabi is an experienced healthcare professional with a passion for midwifery and nursing. She has dedicated her career to providing exceptional care to patients and leading teams to deliver high-quality services. She began her journey in healthcare by completing her Bachelor of Science in Midwifery from the Ministry of Health in Morocco in 2009. During her studies, she developed a keen interest in women's health and decided to move to the UAE and expand her specialization in midwifery. After obtaining her license as a Registered Midwife in 2014 from the Department of Health in Abu Dhabi, Saloua started working in a busy labor and delivery unit at a renowned hospital. Her dedication to providing compassionate and evidence-based care quickly earned her recognition among her colleagues and patients. Saloua's ability to handle complex cases and her strong leadership qualities led to her promotion as a unit manager within a few years. She went on to pursue a Master's degree in Healthcare at Swiss Business School University in 2023, further expanding her knowledge and skills in this field. Saloua's commitment to her profession extends beyond her workplace. She actively participates in professional organizations and conferences, where she shares her expertise and contributes to the advancement of midwifery and nursing.

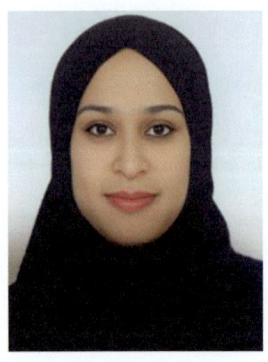

Etab Omar Salem is a compassionate Registered Midwife who is dedicated to supporting the journey of mothers and their newborns. She graduated from Jordan University in 2009 with a Bachelor's degree in Nursing Science and began her professional career in 2012 as a registered nurse in the labor and delivery unit. Over the years, she developed a strong interest in obstetrics and gynecology, which motivated her to advance her education. In 2023, she successfully earned a Master's degree in Midwifery from Ras Al Khaimah Medical and Health Science University in the United Arab Emirates. This academic achievement, part of her continuous professional development, underscores her commitment to enhancing her skills and making meaningful contributions to the field of women's health.

Open Access This chapter is licensed under the terms of the Creative Commons Attribution 4.0 International License (http://creativecommons.org/licenses/by/4.0/), which permits use, sharing, adaptation, distribution and reproduction in any medium or format, as long as you give appropriate credit to the original author(s) and the source, provide a link to the Creative Commons license and indicate if changes were made.

The images or other third party material in this chapter are included in the chapter's Creative Commons license, unless indicated otherwise in a credit line to the material. If material is not included in the chapter's Creative Commons license and your intended use is not permitted by statutory regulation or exceeds the permitted use, you will need to obtain permission directly from the copyright holder.

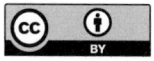

24. The Children's Health Service in the UAE: The Past, Present, and Future

Ahmed Elghoudi, Sara Awad, and Rana Ahmad Bitar

24.1 History

At the beginning of the twentieth century, the medical service in the Gulf region was mainly based on traditional medicine, which used specific remedies from plants and seeds and procedures such as cautery, cupping, and casting limbs.

In the 1960s, there were missionary groups of Americans and Canadians touring the Gulf region, particularly in the nearby parts of Bahrain and Oman. Among these groups were doctors who used to provide healthcare services within their charitable mission. The late Sheikh Zayed Bin Sultan Al Nahyan, the UAE's founder, had an intelligent instinct and knew the quality of modern medicine after experiencing it firsthand. He did not hesitate to request that doctors provide medical services to his local community. It was not long before Dr. Burwell Kennedy and his wife, Dr. Marian Kennedy, landed in the Al Ain region in March 1960 and established work in a converted guest house, later given the name of the Oasis Hospital [1].

Therefore, in 1960, the first-ever facility for providing modern medical healthcare services in the Al Ain region and the United Arab Emirates was founded by the American couple, Dr. Purwell and Dr. Marian Kennedy.

A. Elghoudi (✉)
Sheikh Khalifa Medical City, Abu Dhabi, United Arab Emirates

UAE University, Al Ain, United Arab Emirates

S. Awad
Cleveland Clinic, Lerner Research Institute, Cleveland, OH, USA

R. A. Bitar
Sheikh Khalifa Medical City, Abu Dhabi, United Arab Emirates

Khalifa University, Abu Dhabi, United Arab Emirates
e-mail: rahmed@seha.ae

Sheikh Zayed Bin Sultan Al Nahyan, the area governor, welcomed and supported Dr. Burwell and Dr. Marian. The service was mainly focused on maternity and infant care, as the prenatal and neonatal morbidity and mortality figures were very high compared to similar international statistics. It was estimated that one in two newborn babies and one in three mothers died due to a lack of proper prenatal healthcare [2].

It did not take long for the local community to realize and appreciate the quality of the services provided by the Kennedys. They gained the trust of the locals, and they became a popular destination, with hundreds of locals seeking medical care. The number of children born at the Oasis jumped from 2 to 67 in 1 year, many of them being members of the royal family, the most notable being HH Sheikh Mohammad Bin Zayed Al Nahyan in 1961, the ruler of the United Arab Emirates. After that, the hospital relocated twice to an elementary building before settling in a concrete building with 20 rooms in the Al Muwaiji area of Al Ain [3].

Drs. Pat and Marian Kennedy did exceptionally well by establishing a modern hospital that served the local community in the Al Ain area and its district. The couple's hard work, supported by the late Sheikh Zayed, the site's governor at the time, set the stage for further expansion and growth, from a small palm hut to a sophisticated hospital serving over 500,000 patients per year [4].

The state of Kuwait played a significant role in the development of the health sector and health-related services in areas of the United Arab Emirates from 1960 until the founding of the United Arab Emirates in 1971 by building several hospitals, such as the Kuwait hospitals in Al Baraha and Ras Al-Khaimah, in addition to primary care centers in Khorfakan and Al Fujairah. These hospitals and centers remained under Kuwaiti supervision until the establishment of the United Arab Emirates in 1971 [5].

Since the foundation of the United Arab Emirates in 1971, the economy has improved significantly, and special attention has been paid to providing the best available healthcare services to the residents of the country and particularly to children. This dramatic improvement is reflected in the remarkable drop in neonatal and maternal deaths to figures that are even superior to those in developed countries such as the USA, with the infant mortality rate being 5.6 per 1000 live births in the UAE and 5.8 per 1000 live births in the USA [6].

24.2　Current Status

The rapid economic growth coincided with an increase in healthcare facilities specializing in pediatric and child health, whether in the governmental or private sectors. It was not only the economy that drove child healthcare forward but also the ambition of the leaders of the UAE one of the best countries in the world in terms of public service, happiness, and quality of life [7].

Since the early 2000s, the UAE has been actively working to find the best health system that matches the unique demographic structure of its residents, the aim of which is to improve fitness and health. These reforms have focused on introducing health insurance and a boom in private health provisions against a speedy population increase and a rising prevalence of chronic conditions such as diabetes and obesity [8].

The current status of child health services in the UAE is continuously improving, encouraged by many initiatives driven by decision-makers in both the public and private sectors. In addition, the national vaccination program ensured the eradication and control of various infectious diseases in childhood, such as measles, mumps, rubella, diphtheria, tetanus, hepatitis, and rotavirus.

Primary care clinics are of paramount importance and have been recognized by the Department of Health for providing an array of interventions to the community, ranging from routine screening to specialty-focused clinics like child psychiatry and pediatric dentistry, among others. They are also the centers offering a unique program aimed at screening couples willing to get married to check for communicable, familial, and hereditary diseases that could impact the health of the partner or their offspring. The screening includes tests for determining blood type, hemoglobin level, inherited hemoglobinopathies, blood sugar level, hepatitis B virus, acquired immunodeficiency syndrome (AIDS).

Detecting disease early and delivering timely treatment is of essential. The Maternal and Child Health Department of the Ministry of Health is offering newborn screening services across the country to ensure early detection of specific diseases in early life. These diseases, if detected early and early treatment is initiated, will have a significant impact on the future health and well-being of these children. The treatment for these conditions is accessible and readily available in the UAE. The newborn screening program includes but is not limited to testing for phenylketonuria, congenital hypothyroidism, congenital adrenal hyperplasia, sickle cell disease, and thalassemia.

To offer specialized-level healthcare services, the UAE developed healthcare cities. The cities are complexes containing clinics of diverse specialties that house consultant physicians from around the world with expertise in all medical fields, including pediatrics and pediatric subspecialties. Currently, there are three such cities in the UAE: Abu Dhabi, Dubai, and Sharjah. In 2008, the first standalone pediatric tertiary hospital was established in Dubai, Al Jalila Hospital. It is home to the first pediatric organ transplant center. It also houses the first pediatric clinical genomics center, where complex genetic testing takes place as well as family counselling for genetic diseases (Fig. 24.1). Another children's hospital has been proposed to be established within Sheikh Khalifa Medical City in Abu Dhabi. It will be home to advanced medical treatments and procedures such as bone marrow and organ transplants.

The UAE has become a platform of excellence in pediatric and child health throughout the region, with world-class neonatal units provided with the most advanced techniques and modalities of invasive/noninvasive ventilation, pediatric emergency departments that are easily accessible across the country, acute pediatric wards, and specialized outpatient clinics.

Transferring patients across the Emirates and the world for specialized services is facilitated to enable access to the best available service regardless of the child's residence within the UAE.

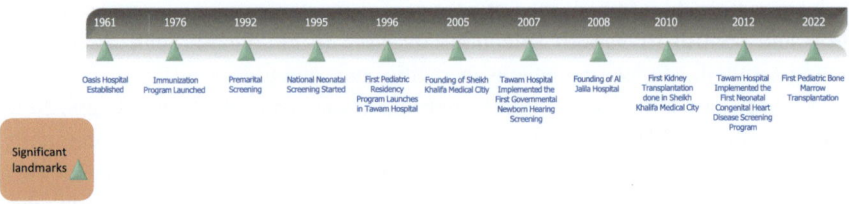

Fig. 24.1 Pediatrics service in the UAE timeline

There are international collaborations with world-renowned children's hospitals in Europe and the USA, such as Cincinnati Children's Hospital and Children's Hospital of Philadelphia. UAE pediatricians will continue regular collaboration between these centers to ensure patients are appropriately managed upon their return to the UAE.

The UAE also opened its doors to medical students across the country to further support medical education and train future competent physicians. In addition to this, several pediatric residency programs and fellowships have been established in the Emirates of Abu Dhabi, Dubai, Sharjah, Ajman. Moreover, the incorporation of medical technology into everyday practice has transformed the quality of services provided; therefore, it was no surprise that in 2021, the UAE ranked 20th globally in the World Index of Healthcare Innovation [9].

In 2016, a federal law known as Wadeema's Law was passed, which protects children from all forms of abuse. With the establishment of the "Child Protection Unit" initiative, the public and childcare specialists can easily report abuse to protect children and ensure their medical, social and emotional wellbeing. It stresses that all children have the right to access healthcare regardless of social, religious, or ethnic backgrounds [10].

24.3 Challenges and Opportunities

Over the last decades, a clear and dramatic improvement in child healthcare within the UAE has been evident. Nonetheless, medical care for children and young adults continues to face challenges globally. Pediatric medical care within the UAE is no exception; these challenges must be addressed and overcome. Expanding the current success of preventing childhood disease is a challenge. Building on current pediatric services to establish super-specialized medical centers is another challenge; providing high-quality pediatric health accessible to all children within the United Arab Emirates closer to their homes remains a challenge.

Chronic diseases in childhood such as obesity and it's complications is a significant challenge for children healthcare providers. Modern life eating attitudes, lack of physical exercise and relying more on electronic gaming has contribute to the global issue of obesity. It has been seem to decrease direct engagement with family members and friends. Although obesity may not endanger a child's health immediately, it would have a major impact on adult life if measures were not put in place to control it. Obese children may develop diseases early in their lives, such as diabetes, hypertension, respiratory diseases, and cardiovascular diseases. Ischemic heart disease, stroke, and diabetes remain the leading causes of death and disability in the UAE [11]. Therefore, even more emphasis needs to be placed on current initiatives tackling obesity, healthy nutrition, and exercise to enhance children's health further and tackle disease prevention early on. Moreover, the consumption of sugary foods and drinks is associated with an increased incidence of dental caries. SEHA conducted a mass screening for school hygiene among 26,000 schoolchildren in Abu Dhabi, Al Ain, and Al Gharbia. It showed that almost 60% of the screened children have dental decay [12].

The screening programs for pre-married couples and newborn babies need to be extended to tackle developmental delays with early intervention and support services, mental and brain health support programs, smoking cessation, and injury prevention.

Healthcare provision for children in the UAE has developed tremendously, with centers of excellence evolving in the public and private sectors. However, one challenge that needs to be overcome is establishing super-specialized services such as pediatric liver, heart, lung, pancreas, and bowel transplantation. Pediatric bone marrow transplantation is in its initial stages within the UAE but additional efforts need to be put into place to develop this initiative to the highest standards. With this in mind, there is a need to recruit specialized medical teams such as physicians, nurses, and support teams to establish these specialized services.

As children with chronic and lifelong conditions grow, we need to transition them smoothly to adult care providers when they hit their late teens and effort to ensure effective transition and to anticipate any interruption of the medical care provided; therefore, the need for adolescent medicine practice is on the rise as an unrecognized field of medicine that caters to the pre-adult subset of patients.

Multiple factors can influence the ease with which children access different private and public healthcare facilities. Some of these factors include where a child lives and the type of medical insurance they have. Most specialized pediatric services are present in Abu Dhabi, Dubai, and Sharjah. Children from remote areas have less access to pediatric subspecialty services. The ideal model of pediatric medical care should allow the delivery of high-quality pediatric care to all children, regardless of insurance or geographic location. To complement this, another challenge arises: the development of a connected electronic medical records system for all medical facilities within the UAE.

Challenges come with continuously upgrading pediatric and child health services. The pediatric specialty is more costly with less revenue when compared to other surgical and intervention specialties. However, it remains a primary responsibility to keep the service running and to ensure new technologies are introduced in diagnostic and therapeutic patient care.

Investment in research, innovation and incorporating artificial intelligence in pediatric health services will enhance the quality of care for the patient suh as by identifiying risk groups, support clincal trials, remote robotic surgeries and consultations. This is crucial to improving child health within society and allowing the UAE to become a pediatric health leader worldwide.

24.4 The Future

The UAE leadership look forward to seeing the country as one of the best in the world, and several key performance indicators (KPIs) are now targeted to develop healthcare to the highest level. Examples of such KPIs include increasing life longevity, working on the framework of the current health system, and increasing public awareness of high-risk hazards such as air pollution and global warming.

The future of the pediatric health service is bright and very promising. As our-population grows, there is a need to expand pediatric training programs to train and recruit high quality pediatricians to cater to the increased number of children and adolescents seeking expert medical care. The future may see more senior and qualified general pediatricians in primary care to reduce the pressure on tertiary care centers.

The COVID-19 pandemic resulted in the wide use of virtual clinical care on a vast scale. The experience was excellent, and we believe such practices are here to stay. Across Abu Dhabi Health Services, over 400,000 teleconsultations were successfully conducted from April 2020 to April 2021 [13].

Adolescent medicine is a specialty that still needs to grow and expand. Similar to neonatology and child health, adolescents demonstrate unique physical and emotional challenges requiring specialized knowledge and expertise. If we do not recognize their needs, adolescent medical care will be lost between the general pediatricians, the internists, the gynecologists, and other specialties [14].

We can only conclude the future of pediatric and child health in the UAE by addressing the impact Artificial Intelligence (AI) would have on the service. Software programs would be able to pick up on those children at risk of developing certain diseases, and they would be targeted and acted upon by the preventive medicine teams, thus reducing morbidity and cost and ensuring good health and harmony among them [15].

Promising research in gene therapy and genomic medicine is currently underway to transfer the concept of treatments from a thesis to realistic day-to-day practice, therefore protecting affected children from devastating and life-threatening conditions.

The UAE is a hub and a favorable destination for elites from different medical and non-medical backgrounds. We will continue to see an influx of experts from around the globe, and at the same time, we will witness a higher number of Emirati men and women with world-class qualifications and experience guiding the march towards establishing one of the best health services worldwide.

The commitment of the Department of Health to build a concrete network of family phsyicians would act as the backbone of the health system, by providing comprehensive and continuous care that addresses both acute and chronic conditions. They foster trust through longterm patient relationships, enabling early detection and prevention of health issues. The holistic approach of family medicine reduces healthcare costs by mimimizing unecessary specialist referrals and hospitalization.

24.5 Conclusion

The UAE's vision is to provide cutting-edge and state of the art pediatric medical services aimed at children and adolescents for it's nationals and residents. The government understands that the children are the men and women of the future who will continue the mission of Sheikh Zayed Bin Sultan Al Nahyan, the founder of the nation. The continuous growth of the service growth in all the aspects affecting children's health and well-being. Challenges such as obesity, genetic diseases, allergic diseases, climate change and their impact on children's health are top tasks to tackle in order to provide a high quality standard of medical care to the children of the UAE.

Conflicts of Interest The authors have no conflicts of interest to declare.

References

1. Dyck G. The oasis. Al Ain: Motivate Publishing Limited; 2000.
2. Bell J. Modern UAE health care: from a mud hut to skyscraper hospitals, the national. The National. 2021. Available at: https://www.thenationalnews.com/uae/health/modern-uae-health-care-from-a-mud-hut-to-skyscraper-hospitals-1.300036. Accessed 21 Nov 2022.
3. Samihah Zaman SR. Kanad Hospital: the story of the Al Ain hospital where Sheikh Mohamed was born, year of the 50th – Gulf News. Gulf News. 2021. Available at: https://gulfnews.com/uae/year-of-the-50th/kanad-hospital-the-story-of-the-al-ain-hospital-where-sheikh-mohamed-was-born-1.79714052. Accessed 21 Nov 2022.
4. Uaemodern. Case study: Oasis hospital in Al-Ain, uaemodern. 2014. Available at: https://uae-modern.com/post/88682388043/case-study-oasis-hospital-in-al-ain. Accessed 21 Nov 2022.
5. Muheisen E. Health services in the Emirates, from traditional medicine to the international one, EmaratAlyoum, 22 March; 2015.
6. World Health Organization. World Health Statistics 2015. Geneva: World Health Organization; 2015 [cited 2016 Aug 11]. Available at: http://apps.who.int/iris/bitstream/10665/170250/1/9789240694439_eng.pdf. Accessed 21 Nov 2022.
7. BBC News [Internet]. United Kingdom: BBC; 2016. UAE creates ministers for happiness and tolerance; 2016 [cited 2016 Aug 11]. Available at: http://www.bbc.com/news/world-middle-east-35531174. Accessed 21 Nov 2022.
8. Koornneef EJ, Robben PBM, Al Seiari MB, et al. Health system reform in the emirate of Abu Dhabi. Health Policy. 2012;108(2–3):115–21. https://doi.org/10.1016/j.healthpol.2012.08.026.
9. Roy A. United Arab Emirates: #20 in the 2021 world index of healthcare innovation, Freopp. 2021. Available at: https://freopp.org/united-arab-emirates-freopp-world-index-of-healthcare-innovation-5ccc1512303f. Accessed 21 Nov 2022.
10. Abu Dhabi HA. Abu Dhabi newborn screening program healthcare professional's manual first edition 2009. Abu Dhabi: Health Authority; 2019.

11. GBD 2019 Diseases and Injuries Collaborators. Global burden of 369 diseases and injuries in 204 countries and territories, 1990–2019: a systematic analysis for the Global Burden of Disease Study 2019. Lancet. 2020;396(10258):1204–22. https://doi.org/10.1016/S0140-6736(20)30925-9. Erratum in: Lancet. 2020 Nov 14;396(10262):1562. PMID: 33069326; PMCID: PMC7567026.
12. Khda News. KHDA. 2011. Available at: https://web.khda.gov.ae/en/About-Us/News/2011/Survey-of-school-pupils-reveals-widespread-health. Accessed 21 Nov 2022.
13. Virtual Consultations Charting a New Roadmap for UAE Healthcare. 2021. Seha.ae. Available at: https://www.seha.ae/virtual-consultations-charting-a-new-roadmap-for-uae-healthcare/. Accessed 21 Nov 2022.
14. Lee L, Upadhya KK, Matson PA, Adger H, Trent ME. The status of adolescent medicine: building a global adolescent workforce. Int J Adolesc Med Health. 2016;28(3):233–43. https://doi.org/10.1515/ijamh-2016-5003. PMID: 26167974; PMCID: PMC5039240.
15. Li YW, Liu F, Zhang TN, Xu F, Gao YC, Wu T. Artificial intelligence in pediatrics. Chin Med J. 2020;133(3):358–60. https://doi.org/10.1097/CM9.0000000000000563. PMID: 31929357; PMCID: PMC7004621.

Further Reading

Convention on the rights of the child text UNICEF. Available at: https://www.unicef.org/child-rights-convention/convention-text. Accessed 21 Nov 2022.

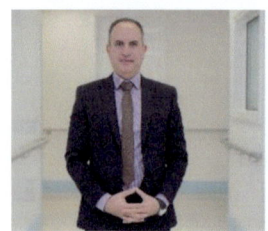

Ahmed Elghoudi is a consultant in general paediatrics and allergy at Sheikh Khalifa Medical City in Abu Dhabi, United Arab Emirates, and an adjunct assistant clinical professor at the College of Medicine and Health Sciences, UAE University. He graduated in Libya and completed his pediatric and allergy training in the UK, holding a certificate of completion of pediatric training and an MSc in allergy from the University of Southampton. With over 20 years of experience across Libya, the Republic of Ireland, and the UK, he is skilled in managing a range of pediatric conditions, including food allergy, asthma, and eczema. Dr. Elghoudi is a recognised speaker in pediatric allergy, a peer reviewer for international journals, and actively involved in several professional organisations. He is passionate about medical education and engages in volunteer work.

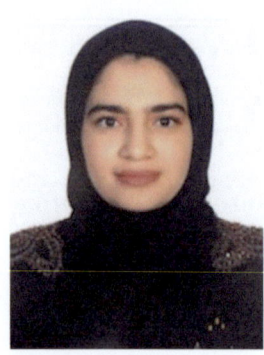

Sara Awad Hailing from the UAE, my journey began with a childhood in its vibrant embrace. Dedicated to pediatric medicine, I completed my training locally, refining skills that now converge in the specialized realm of pediatric hematology oncology. The intricate world of healing young lives fuels my professional path, where each day is a step toward making a profound impact. Rooted in the rich tapestry of my upbringing, I am driven by a deep-seated commitment to fostering health and hope in the realm of pediatric care.

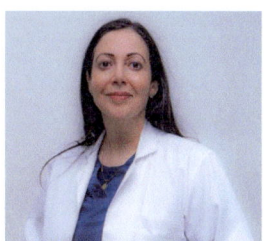

Dr. Rana Ahmad Bitar underwent postgraduate training in pediatric gastroenterology, hepatology, and nutrition in the United Kingdom. She was the head of pediatric hepatology in the North of England and led pediatric nutrition and pediatric endoscopy training. Dr. Rana has been a pediatric gastroenterology consultant at Sheikh Khalifa Medical City since 2016 and an assistant professor at Khalifa University since 2021. She is a clinical director at the Special Olympics UAE. She is a member of the Royal College of Paediatrics and the British Society of Paediatric Gastroenterology Hepatology and Nutrition (BSPGHAN).

Open Access This chapter is licensed under the terms of the Creative Commons Attribution 4.0 International License (http://creativecommons.org/licenses/by/4.0/), which permits use, sharing, adaptation, distribution and reproduction in any medium or format, as long as you give appropriate credit to the original author(s) and the source, provide a link to the Creative Commons license and indicate if changes were made.

The images or other third party material in this chapter are included in the chapter's Creative Commons license, unless indicated otherwise in a credit line to the material. If material is not included in the chapter's Creative Commons license and your intended use is not permitted by statutory regulation or exceeds the permitted use, you will need to obtain permission directly from the copyright holder.

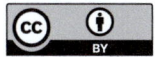

Geriatric Medicine in the UAE

25

Salwa Alsuwaidi and Abdulla Al Ali

25.1 Geriatric Population Demographics

Since the foundation of the United Arab Emirates (UAE), the country has undergone a major transformation, from a region with scarce resources and underdeveloped infrastructure in many aspects of life to a contemporary nation that is considered among the top countries worldwide in terms of quality of life and other standards.

The healthcare system has made great progress over the last few decades. Federal and local governmental health strategies' main focus has been the welfare of UAE citizens, who are considered the nation's greatest asset and the main target of many national initiatives to meet the needs of diverse members of the UAE community.

The estimated UAE population was 69,588 in 1950, which significantly increased to 9.68 million in 2019, with further increases expected by 2050, reaching 13,163,548 [1].

As a result of the above-mentioned positive progress in healthcare standards, life expectancy has increased over the last few decades. Life expectancy before 1971 was 53 years, rising significantly to 79.9 years in 2018, which is considered the highest life expectancy in the Middle East. Furthermore, life expectancy was 80.4 years for females and 79.4 years for males in 2018 [1].

In 2017, the Ministry of Community Development estimated that the percentage of the total elderly population over the age of 60 years was 6%, expected to increase to 11% by 2032 and 19% by 2050 [1].

A recent observational study showed an increase in the prevalence of noncommunicable diseases among the elderly in the UAE. In this study, the average number

---

S. Alsuwaidi
Dubai Academic Health Corporation (DAHC), Dubai, United Arab Emirates
e-mail: saalsuwaidi@dha.gov.ae

A. Al Ali (✉)
Zayed Military Hospital, Abu Dhabi, United Arab Emirates

© The Author(s) 2025
H. O. Al-Shamsi (ed.), *Healthcare in the United Arab Emirates*,
https://doi.org/10.1007/978-981-96-0523-1_25

of chronic diseases per elderly person was found to be at least four. Hypertension and diabetes are the most common chronic illnesses. The prevalence of depression was 38.3% [2]. On the other hand, data regarding the prevalence of geriatric syndromes remain scarce.

Regarding mortality data, based on a systematic review published in 2013, the top four causes of death are cardiovascular diseases, injuries, cancer, and respiratory diseases [3]. However, there is no data on the most common causes of death among individuals aged 65 or older.

Elderly people enjoy high regard in the UAE community. Most of them live with their families, and their care is provided through informal caregivers. A very small proportion reside in nursing homes under certain conditions, mainly those without first-degree relatives.

Emirati society, over generations, has valued the care and appreciation of the elderly as part of its religious, cultural, and social obligations. The extended family, in which several generations of members of family members live in one house or in close proximity, is still maintained to some extent. This structure has a positive impact on the ability to provide care for elderly family members with one or several geriatric syndromes, especially dementia, by other family members, particularly female offspring [4].

25.2 Geriatric Services

25.2.1 Home Care Services

The Dubai Health Authority (DHA) has taken the lead in terms of implementing geriatric medicine services. These services include home care targeting both UAE citizens and expatriates through the implementation of a comprehensive geriatric assessment, skilled nursing care, home safety assessment and modification, rehabilitation, nutritional evaluation, psychological assessment, and support by multidisciplinary teams.

In addition, mobile healthcare services were added to the home care services, offering several health-related investigations, especially blood tests, with immediate results provided within 10 minutes. During the COVID-19 pandemic, Telehealth was also added [5].

The Ministry of Health and Prevention (MOHAP) has launched the "Mobile Healthcare Initiative," targeting senior citizens in remote areas. This initiative provides a variety of diagnostic, therapeutic, rehabilitative, and preventive services free of charge. In 2021, the services of this initiative had reached 3000 beneficiaries [6].

Abu Dhabi Health Services Company (SEHA) has launched several home care services, which include regular home visits targeting home-bound senior citizens, provided by multiple multidisciplinary teams offering a range of diagnostic, therapeutic, rehabilitative, and preventive services. In addition, mental health home care services have been established [7].

The Ministry of Community Development also launched several services, which include primary healthcare, social, psychological, and physical therapy for senior citizens aged 60 years and older, delivered through a home care program at elderly care centers [8].

The private healthcare sector has expanded its home healthcare services, covering elderly patients throughout the UAE. These services include skilled nursing care and rehabilitative services, as well as diagnostic and therapeutic services.

25.2.2 Residential Long-Term Services

It is expected that the number of elderly individuals with frailty, multiple geriatric syndromes, and multiple morbid conditions leading to cognitive, functional, mobility, and psychological impairments will increase, necessitating both formal and informal care. The aim is to provide the required care to an elderly person with the above-mentioned limitations at home, supported by available community services. Nevertheless, the development of long-term residential care services is equally important, both in terms of the number of long-term facilities and the quality of care provided. The reason for this expected shift in long-term care for the elderly may be partly explained by a change in social patterns, from extended families, which are the primary source of informal care, to smaller family units [9].

25.2.2.1 The Seniors' Happiness Center in Dubai
- It was established in October 1993. It belongs to the Dubai Health Authority (DHA), and it is considered a long-term care facility that provides inpatient care for elderly individuals with first-degree relatives, and a daycare program for seniors who do not live in the facility. In addition, it provides respite care services for caregivers and end-of-life care services for terminal cases. Seniors residing in the facility and the community receive medical, rehabilitative, clinical dietary, and social services delivered by a multidisciplinary team led by a geriatrician. The inpatient service consists of 20 beds, and the outpatient service served more than 700 seniors in 2021.
- Seniors' Happiness Centre achieved JCI accreditation against the standards of LTC, becoming the first standalone governmental entity in the GCC, MENA, and Asia to do so in 2021.
- Seniors' Happiness Centre in 2013 established the "Alzheimer's Support Group." The aim of this initiative is to raise awareness about Alzheimer's dementia among members of the community and to provide an opportunity for caregivers to share their experiences and exchange information about caring for relatives with dementia. Several meetings have been held with a series of educational lectures provided by multidisciplinary team members to improve caregivers' knowledge and skills. These activities were attended by more than 100 caregivers over the last few years [1].

In addition, several other long-term facilities are available in governmental and private healthcare settings, where elderly residents can receive medical, psychological, rehabilitative, skilled nursing, and social services.

25.2.3 Outpatient Services and Programs

There are several outpatient services and programs that have been established and developed to address the complexity of geriatric patients. In the primary healthcare department in Dubai, several specialty clinics have been established, including a geriatric clinic, where elderly patients receive comprehensive geriatric care, in addition to an osteoporosis clinic and a memory clinic.

In addition, a caregiver education program was launched, focusing on training caregivers in various aspects of daily personal care, nursing care, home safety, handling home medical equipment, and managing caregiver burden.

Moreover, smart clinics have been established to provide telemedicine services for elderly patients. Over the last few years, several specialized clinics and services have been established in other governmental and private sectors, helping to improve diagnostic, therapeutic, rehabilitative, and preventive care for elderly patients [5].

25.3 Policies

- On October 21, 2018, the UAE government approved a national policy for the elderly, aligned with the UAE Vision 2021 and the UAE Centennial Strategy 2071. The policy, titled "The National Policy for Senior Emiratis," is based on an integrated care system to ensure that seniors remain active and have access to government services.
- The UAE government also decided to replace the term "elderly Emiratis" with "Senior Emiratis." "They are senior in experience, in service to this country, and the highest in our eyes and hearts," His Highness Sheikh Mohammed Bin Rashid, the Prime Minister and Ruler of Dubai, stated on Twitter.
- According to national policy, senior Emiratis will have access to special health insurance.
- Senior Citizens will have access to discounts. In addition, protection programs have been developed to safeguard them from violence and abuse. The policy focuses on seven main domains:
  - Healthcare
  - Community involvement and active life
  - Effective civic participation
  - Infrastructure and transportation
  - Financial stability
  - Safety and security
  - Quality of future life [10].

- "In January 2017, His Highness Sheikh Dr. Sultan bin Mohamed Al Qasimi, Supreme Council Member and Ruler of Sharjah, issued an administrative decree (No. 2 of 2017) formally heralding the Emirate's decision to join the Global Network for Age-Friendly Cities and Communities. The administrative decree emphasizes the importance of the environment in promoting healthy aging and encourages the creation of an age-friendly environment in the Emirate. It aims to create a physical, healthy, social, economic, and culturally sustainable environment in Sharjah, making the Emirate an ideal place for the elderly to live and enjoy a high quality life." Forty strategic initiatives have been launched according to the WHO's eight age-friendly domains, which include: "external spaces and buildings; transportation; housing; community participation; respect and social inclusion; civil participation and employment; communications and information; community support; and health services" [11].
- Federal Law No. 9 of 2019 on the Rights of Senior Emiratis was announced in December 2019 and signed by the previous president of the UAE, His Highness Sheikh Khalifa Bin Zayed Al Nahyan. In this law senior Emiratis were defined as UAE nationals over the age of 60. In addition, the following rights are guaranteed for senior citizens:
  - The right to independence and privacy
  - The right to protection from violence and abuse
  - The right to an enabling environment, housing, education, and work
  - The right to social care includes the provision of elderly community centers and social clubs
  - The right to medical care includes preventive health services, medical insurance, mobile nursing units, and supportive medical devices
  - The right to confidentiality of information pertaining to them
  - The right to preferential treatment with respect to government transactions, facilities, social aid, and medical services
- This law specifies various punishments for circumstances in which senior citizens are abused or neglected [10].

25.4 Challenges and Recommendations

Populations around the world are rapidly aging. Aging presents both challenges and opportunities. It is expected to increase demand for primary healthcare and long-term care, require a larger and better-trained workforce, and heighten the need for environments to be more age-friendly. Aging is a global phenomenon that is occurring rapidly in developing countries. People worldwide are living longer. Today, for the first time in history, most people can expect to live into their 60s and beyond.

The main challenges in the UAE with regard to aging are the following:

- Geriatric medicine experience was introduced as a core requirement in certain residency programs a few years ago, and a geriatric residency or fellowship pro-

grams was established by AHS in 2024. In addition, the availability of a well-established undergraduate geriatric medicine curriculum is still lacking.
- Research related to elderly demographics, health-related issues, and geriatric syndromes remains limited.
- The high number of beds occupied by senior patients at the main acute hospitals reduces the bed capacity for acute cases in need.
- The UAE has no national dementia care strategy, and epidemiological data on dementia in the country remain scarce [12].
- Lack of geriatric rehabilitation center facilities in the UAE limits the facilitation of early discharge from acute hospitals and the restoration of pre-hospitalization status. Currently, post-acute care is provided by several rehabilitation centers not specifically designed for elderly patients, and these centers are mainly available in the private sector.
- In spite of progress in the development of healthcare services provided in the community for elderly persons, there are still no well-established programs and services in hospitals to prevent hospital-related hazards, reduce hospital length of stay, and avoid further functional decline.
- There is a lack of a database, proper statistics, and studies regarding seniors' issues, as well as a lack of family or caregiver awareness about the consequences of the aging process, mental illnesses, and medication complications.
- The growth of the elderly population does not align with the planned future services.
- Most of the current senior citizens have a low educational level which makes engagement with smart applications and new technological solutions difficult.
- Ensure equal, and high-quality healthcare for every older person worldwide.
- Expand the geriatrics knowledge base through regular practical training.
- Increase the number of healthcare professionals who apply the principles of geriatric medicine in caring for older people.
- Recruit physicians and other healthcare professionals into careers in geriatric medicine, and unite professional and lay groups in efforts to influence public policy to continually improve the health and healthcare of seniors.
- Educate and train seniors on how to use technology and smart applications [13].
- Create intermediate care or step-down facilities to facilitate early discharge from acute hospitals and provide proper rehabilitation.
- Collaborate with insurance companies to define and approve standards of home nursing, enabling families to care for their seniors at home.
- Introduce a geriatric medicine curriculum in medical schools.
- Implement pre-retirement courses and training to help seniors plan for their future more effectively.

Collaboration with the government, organizations, agencies, foundations, and other partners is essential to achieve these goals in response to the needs of the growing elderly population. Over the last 10 years, a few conferences and workshops in the field of elderly healthcare have taken place for physicians and healthcare providers in different Emirates, but the UAE, like many other Arab countries, still lacks specialist physicians and nurses in elderly care (geriatricians) and geriatric academic training programs.

25.5 Conclusion

In summary, the United Arab Emirates has made tremendous progress in establishing multiple high-standard healthcare services, which have helped to improve the care of the elderly population. Despite current challenges, geriatric medicine is a promising and evolving specialty in the UAE, with expected growth in education, research, and services.

Conflicts of Interest The authors have no conflicts of interest to declare.

References

1. Abyad A, Farmosa F. Population aging in Middle East & North Africa: research and policy implications; 2021. p. 55–63.
2. AlShaali A, Al Jaziri A. Health profile of elderly patients registered in the elderly home based primary care, Dubai, United Arab Emirates. Middle East J Age Aging. 2015;12(1):13–9.
3. Loney, et al. An analysis of the health status of The United Arab Emirates: the 'big 4' public health issues. Glob Health Action. 2013;6:20100.
4. Ostler GJ, Tadro. Behavioral and psychlogical symtoms in dementia. Arab J Psychiatr. 2011:164–9.
5. Dubai Academic Health Corporation. Primary health care elderly services in Dubai. Dubai; n.d.
6. Mobile Healthcare initiative enaya. Ministry of Health and Prevention – UAE. https://mohap.gov.ae/en/about-us/projects-and-initiatives/mobile-healthcare-initiative-enaya.
7. Seha.ae. n.d. https://www.seha.ae/media-detail/48.
8. Ministry of Community Development. 2019. Retrieved from https://www.mocd.gov.ae/en/home.aspx.
9. Woo J. Geriatrics in the rest of the world. In: Brocklehurst's textbook of geriatric medicine and gerontology, vol. 2010; 2010. p. 1010–5.
10. The National Policy for Senior emiratis | The Official Portal of the... n.d. https://u.ae/en/about-the-uae/strategies-initiatives-and-awards/policies/social-affairs/the-national-policy-for-senior-emiratis.
11. Sharjah age-friendly initiative: 52% implementation of 2017–20 strategic plan. https://www.sgmb.ae/en/media-centre/news/28/1/2019/sharjah-age-friendly-initiative-52-implementation-of-2017-20-strategic-plan.aspx#page=148.
12. Ahmed AI, Suwaidi SA, Ali AA. Dementia care international perspectives/UAE. Oxford: Oxford University; 2019.
13. Malik WA. The universal challenges and the future of geriatric medicine discpline. J Gerontol Geriatr Res. 2017;67.

Dr. Salwa Alsuwaidi is a consultant in internal medicine and geriatrics. She is the Director of the Seniors' Happiness Center at Dubai Academic Health Corporation (DAHC).

Dr. Salwa is a graduate of the UAE Faculty of Medicine and Health Sciences. She holds MRCP UK (Glasgow), MRCP SCE Geriatrics, PhD Arab Board Internal Medicine, Post Graduate Diploma of Gerontology & Geriatrics, Clinical Leadership Diploma from RCSI, and a Professional Diploma in Medicine for the older person from the Royal College of Physicians of Ireland. Dr. Salwa was the first Emirati geriatrician. She was the founder and first chairperson of the Emirates Seniors' Friends Association. She is a board member of the Middle East Academy for the Medicine of Ageing (MEAMA) and a board member of the IAGG (AFMEE) program.

Dr. Abdulla Al Ali is an American board certified in geriatric medicine. He works as a consultant in geriatric medicine at Zayed Military Hospital, Abu Dhabi, United Arab Emirates. Abu Dhabi Ambulatory health services geriatric fellowship program director

Open Access This chapter is licensed under the terms of the Creative Commons Attribution 4.0 International License (http://creativecommons.org/licenses/by/4.0/), which permits use, sharing, adaptation, distribution and reproduction in any medium or format, as long as you give appropriate credit to the original author(s) and the source, provide a link to the Creative Commons license and indicate if changes were made.

The images or other third party material in this chapter are included in the chapter's Creative Commons license, unless indicated otherwise in a credit line to the material. If material is not included in the chapter's Creative Commons license and your intended use is not permitted by statutory regulation or exceeds the permitted use, you will need to obtain permission directly from the copyright holder.

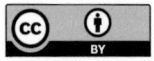

Cancer Care in the UAE

26

Humaid O. Al-Shamsi ⓘ and Faryal Iqbal ⓘ

26.1 Introduction

Cancer represents a significant health concern in the United Arab Emirates (UAE), resulting in considerable morbidity and mortality. It contributes to 12.4% of all fatalities in the UAE, positioning it as the third most prevalent cause of death in 2023 [1]. The UAE is committed to achieving an almost 18% reduction in cancer-related deaths by the year 2025. Decreasing the mortality rate associated with cancer stands as a significant benchmark within the UAE's national agenda, aligning with its aspiration to be recognized as a leader in providing world-class healthcare [2].

H. O. Al-Shamsi (✉)
Burjeel Cancer Institute, Burjeel Medical City, Abu Dhabi, United Arab Emirates

Department of Medical Oncology, Dana-Farber Cancer Institute, Harvard Medical School, Boston, MA, United States

Harvard Medical School, Harvard University, Boston, MA, United States

College of Medicine, Ras Al Khaimah Medical and Health Sciences University, Al Juwais, Al Qusaidat, Ras Al Khaimah, United Arab Emirates

Gulf Medical University, Ajman, United Arab Emirates

Gulf Cancer Society, Alsafa, Kuwait

Emirates Oncology Society, Dubai, United Arab Emirates

College of Medicine, University of Sharjah, Sharjah, United Arab Emirates
e-mail: humaid.al-shamsi@medportal.ca

F. Iqbal
Burjeel Cancer Institute, Burjeel Medical City, Abu Dhabi, United Arab Emirates
e-mail: Faryal.iqbal@burjeelmedicalcity.com

© The Author(s) 2025
H. O. Al-Shamsi (ed.), *Healthcare in the United Arab Emirates*,
https://doi.org/10.1007/978-981-96-0523-1_26

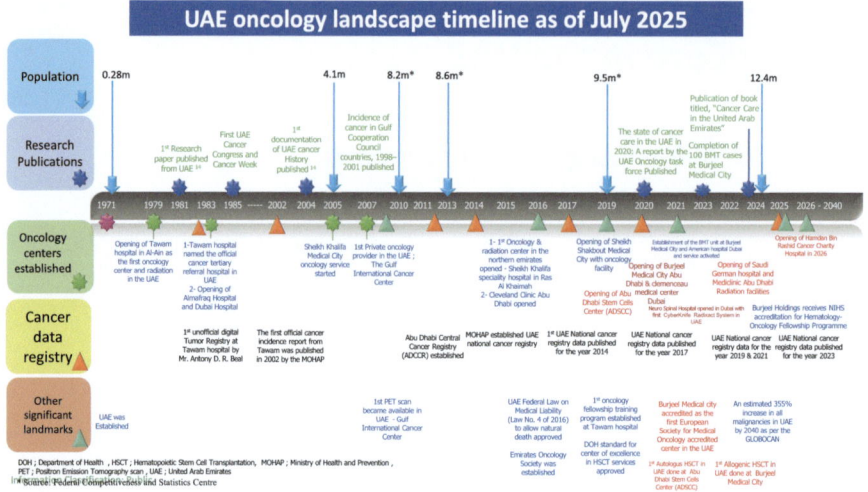

Fig. 26.1 Timeline of UAE oncology care in the UAE

26.2 History of Cancer Care in the UAE

The origin of cancer treatment in the UAE dates back to 1979 when Tawam Hospital was inaugurated in Al Ain [2]. Notable developments in the UAE over recent years include the introduction of cyberknife radiation technology and the commencement of hematopoietic stem cell transplantation (HSCT) [3, 4]. Additionally, more cancer centers have been established. Figure 26.1 provides an overview of the oncology landscape in the UAE.

26.3 Cancer Epidemiology in the UAE

From January 1 to December 31, 2023, the UAE National Cancer Registry (UAE-NCR) recorded a total of 7487 newly identified cases of cancer, including both malignant and in situ diagnoses [1]. Of these cases, 7098 (equivalent to 94.8%) were identified as malignant, and 389 (comprising 5.2%) were categorized as in situ cases. Cancer occurred more frequently in females than in males, affecting 4200 (56.1%) of the female population and 3287 (43.9%) of the male population. Among individuals who were citizens of the UAE, there were 1736 newly diagnosed cases of cancer, with 1648 (94.9%) being malignant and 88 (5.1%) being in situ cases. Similarly, among non-UAE citizens, there were 5751 newly diagnosed cancer cases, with 5450 (94.8%) being malignant and 301 (representing 5.2%) being in situ cases. This data translates to an overall crude incidence rate of 66.5 cases per 100,000 people for both genders [1]. The crude incidence rate was higher in females, standing at 102.9 cases per 100,000 people, compared to males, who had a rate of 46.1

cases per 100,000. The overall age-standardized incidence rate (ASR) for both genders was 105.4 per 100,000. Breast, thyroid, colorectal, skin (carcinoma) and prostate were the most prevalent types of cancer among all newly diagnosed cases in both males and females. For males, the leading cancers were colorectal, prostate, thyroid, leukemia, and skin (carcinoma). Among females, the top-ranked cancer types were breast, thyroid, colorectal, uterus, and cervix uteri [1].

In 2023, there were 237 new cancer diagnoses among children aged 0–14 in the UAE. Among these cases, 40.1% were females, and 59.9% were males. This accounted for approximately 3.3% of all malignant cases that were registered. The most frequently occurring types of cancer among both boys and girls in this age group were leukemia, brain and central nervous system (CNS) cancers, non-Hodgkin's lymphoma, bone and articular cartilage, and kidney and renal pelvis [1].

Cancer was identified as the third leading cause of mortality in the UAE. The total number of deaths attributed to cancer was 1432, with 738 occurring in males and 693 in females. This accounted for approximately 12.4% of all deaths, irrespective of nationality, cancer type, or gender, as indicated in Table 3. This translates to an estimated age-standardized mortality rate of 30.37 per 100,000 for both genders. Colorectal cancer emerged as the primary cause of cancer-related deaths in 2023, accounting for an estimated average of 10.6% of all cancer-related deaths annually. Breast cancer ranked as the second most prevalent cause of cancer-related deaths, while lung cancer held the position of the third most common cause of cancer-related deaths [1].

26.3.1 Evolving Patterns in Cancer Burden

Figure 26.2 sheds light on the cancer incidence trend from 2015 till the most recent published report 2023 [1].

Thyroid (+33.4%) and prostate (+29%) cancers saw the biggest increases. Breast cancer remains the most common, with a 27.8% rise [1]. Lung cancer cases slightly declined (−0.43%), reflecting the impact of the UAE's strong anti-smoking measures, such as smoke-free public spaces, advertising bans, and stricter age limits for tobacco sales [5]. Colorectal cancer (+10.5%), leukemia (+6.57%), and non-Hodgkin lymphoma (+0.6%) showed modest increases [1] (Table 26.1).

The most significant trend from the report was observed in the clear shift toward middle-aged and older adults over time, particularly in the 40–49 age groups. From 2015 to 2023, the percentages in these age brackets steadily increased. Conversely, younger age groups (0–14 years) show a consistent decline [1], might indicating an aging population or a demographic shift toward middle and older age groups (Fig. 26.3).

In Fig. 26.4, a comparison of cancer incidence between Emirati and non-Emirati populations suggests a continued predominance of cases among non-Emiratis, consistent with their larger demographic share. However, the gap between Emirati and non-Emirati rates is narrowing, suggesting more equitable healthcare access.

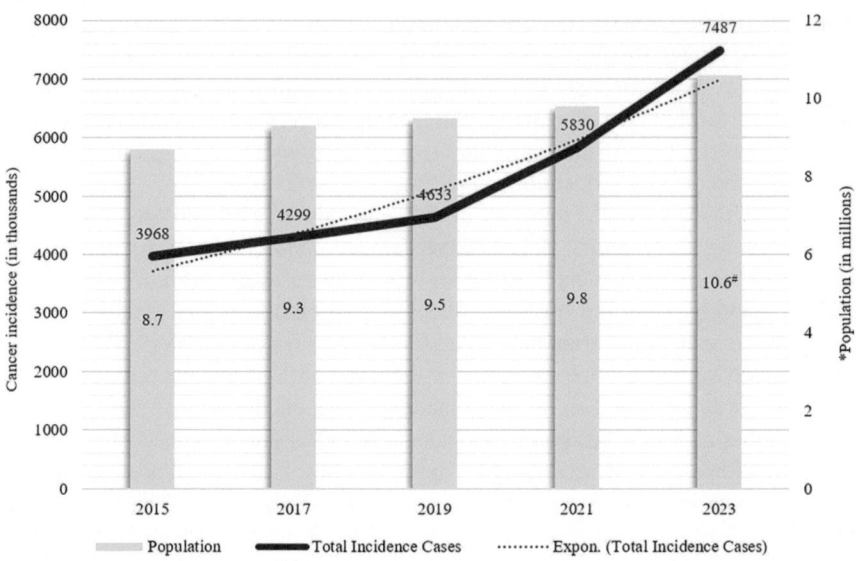

*Source: Federal Competitiveness and Statistics Centre

#Note: Preliminary data

Fig. 26.2 Cancer incidence in the UAE over the years. (Source: Ministry of Health and Prevention, Statistics and Research Center, National Disease Registry—UAE National Cancer Registry Report, 2015–2023. *Source: Federal Competitiveness and Statistics Centre. #Note: Preliminary data)

Table 26.1 A comparison of top malignant primary sites among all UAE population in between the years 2021 and 2023

Cancer type	2021 Cases	2023 Cases	% Change
Breast	1139	1456	+27.8
Thyroid	595	794	+33.4
Colorectal	532	588	+10.5
Skin (carcinoma)	273	333	+21.97
Prostate	251	324	+29
Non-Hodgkin lymphoma	228	324	+0.62
Leukemia	304	324	+6.57
Bronchus and lung	231	230	- 0.43
Uterus	173	215	+24.27
Lip, oral cavity, and pharynx	154	197	+27.9

Source: Ministry of Health and Prevention, Statistics and Research Center, National Disease Registry—UAE National Cancer Registry Report, 2021–2023

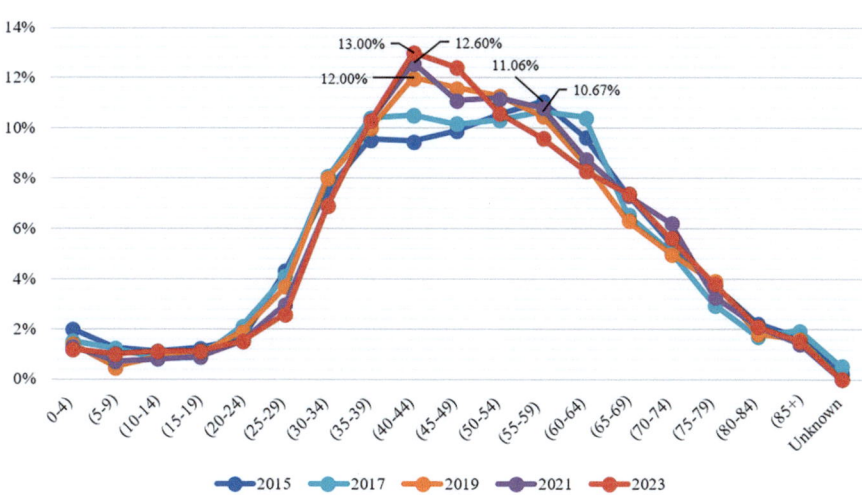

Fig. 26.3 Age group comparison of malignant cases in the UAE across all genders (2015–2023). (Source: Ministry of Health and Prevention, Statistics and Research Center, National Disease Registry—UAE National Cancer Registry Report, 2015–2023)

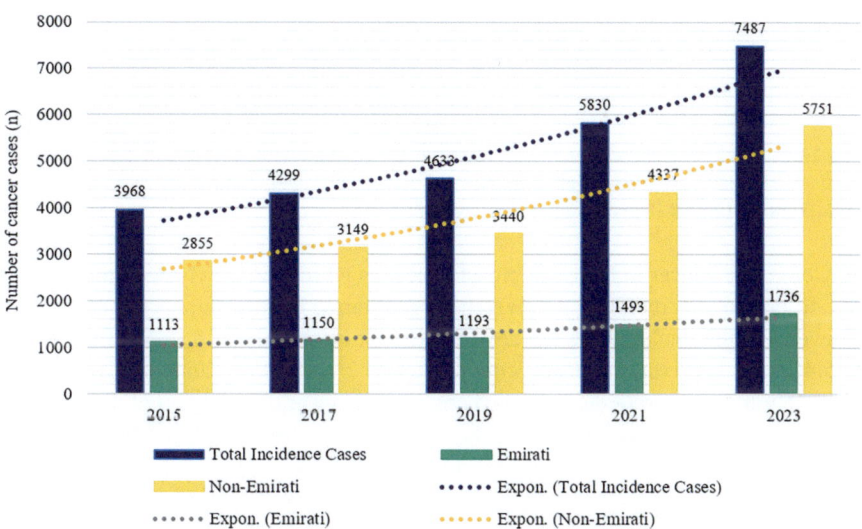

Fig. 26.4 A comparison of Emirati and non-Emirati cancer cases over the years. (Source: Ministry of Health and Prevention, Statistics and Research Center, National Disease Registry—UAE National Cancer Registry Report, 2015–2023)

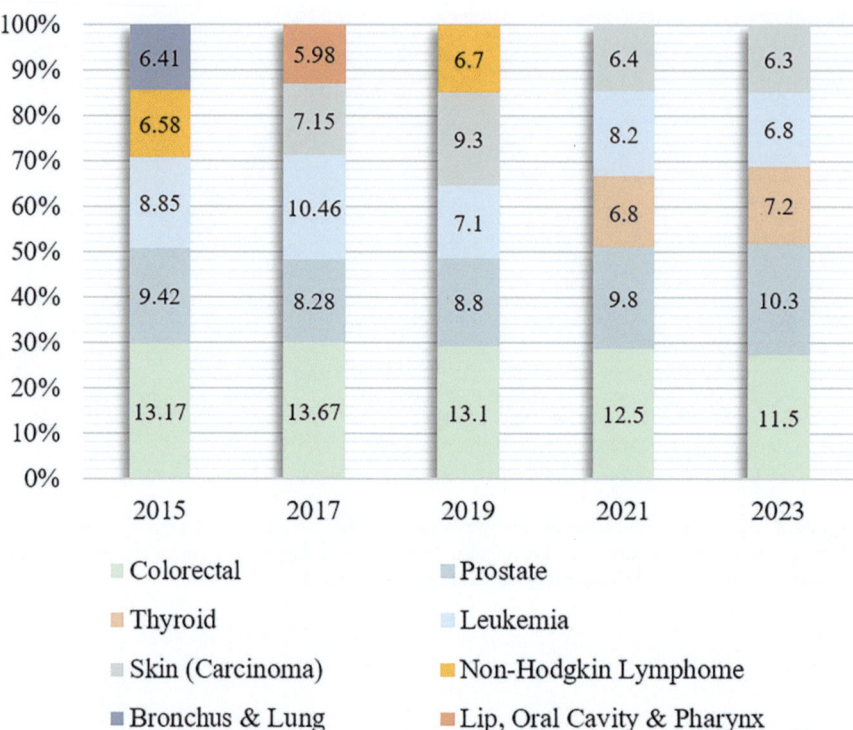

Fig. 26.5 The five most commonly diagnosed cancers in males in the UAE, 2015–2023. (Source: Ministry of Health and Prevention, Statistics and Research Center, National Disease Registry—UAE National Cancer Registry Report, 2015–2023)

Colorectal cancer in men and breast cancer in women is slowly declining, likely due to effective screening and awareness programs. Uterus and cervix uteri rates showed a slight decline between 2021 and 2023; uterus cancer dropped from 5.7% to 5.4%, and cervix uteri cancer from 4.6% to 3.7% [1] (Figs. 26.5 and 26.6). This positive trend likely reflects improved preventive care and the impact of the national HPV vaccination program. The UAE was the first in the Eastern Mediterranean region to introduce the vaccine for schoolgirls aged 13–14 in 2018, and in 2023, the program expanded to include boys of the same age, enhancing community-wide protection [6]. In contrast, a concerning rise in prostate cancer highlights the need for targeted interventions.

Figure 26.7 indicates a sharp decline in leukemia cases, with a 12.1% decrease in occurrence in 2023. Brain and CNS cancers also show a slight declining trend of 1.4% in the pediatric population in the same year [1].

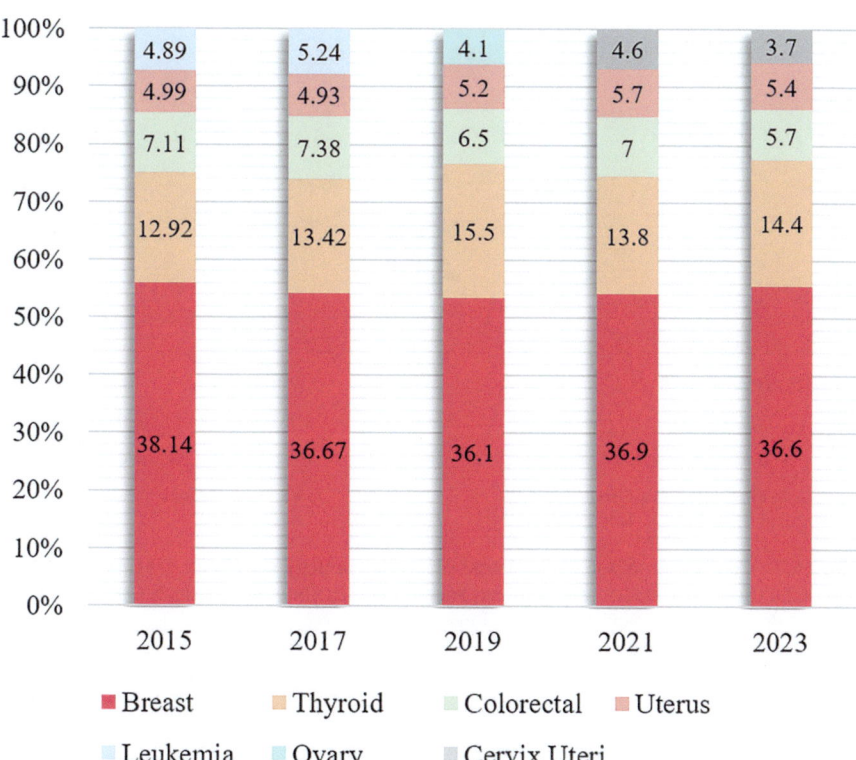

Fig. 26.6 The five most commonly diagnosed cancers in females in the UAE, 2015–2023. (Source: Ministry of Health and Prevention, Statistics and Research Center, National Disease Registry—UAE National Cancer Registry Report, 2015–2023)

Figure 26.8 presents an age group comparison, highlighting a significant decline in two female age brackets (0–4 and 5–9 years) from 2021 to 2023. Additionally, the 0–4 age group in the male population exhibits a gradual 5% decline over the same period [1].

A comparative analysis of total cancer incidence versus mortality over recent years highlights important insights into healthcare outcomes. A growing divergence between rising incidence and relatively stable mortality rates suggests improvements in early detection, treatment access, and patient survival, underscoring the progress made in the UAE's cancer care infrastructure (Fig. 26.9).

A key observation in the trend is that females consistently exhibit a higher age standardized mortality rate than males, suggesting potential gender-based differences in mortality risks. The increase in mortality cases from 975 in 2021 to 1432 in 2023 [1] could be influenced by factors such as population growth, healthcare advancements, or emerging health challenges (Table 26.2).

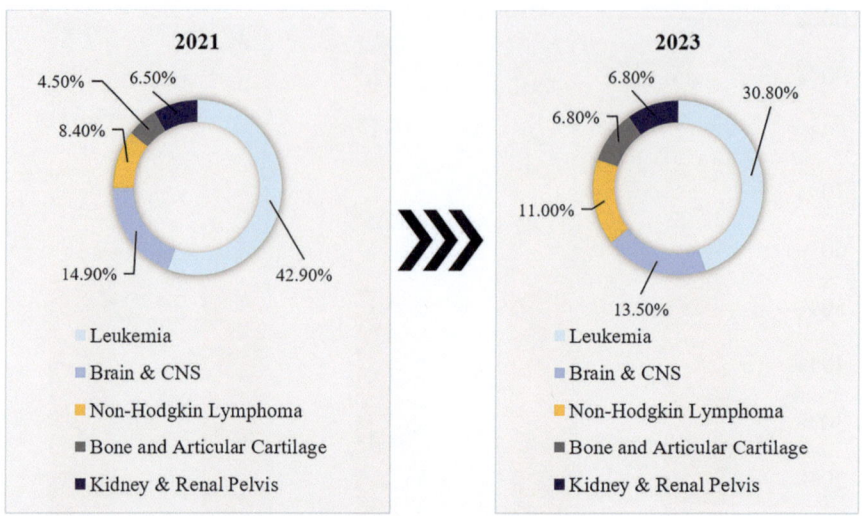

Fig. 26.7. Comparison of top five pediatric cancers by primary sites in the UAE between 2021 and 2023. (Source: Ministry of Health and Prevention, Statistics and Research Center, National Disease Registry—UAE National Cancer Registry Report, 2021–2023)

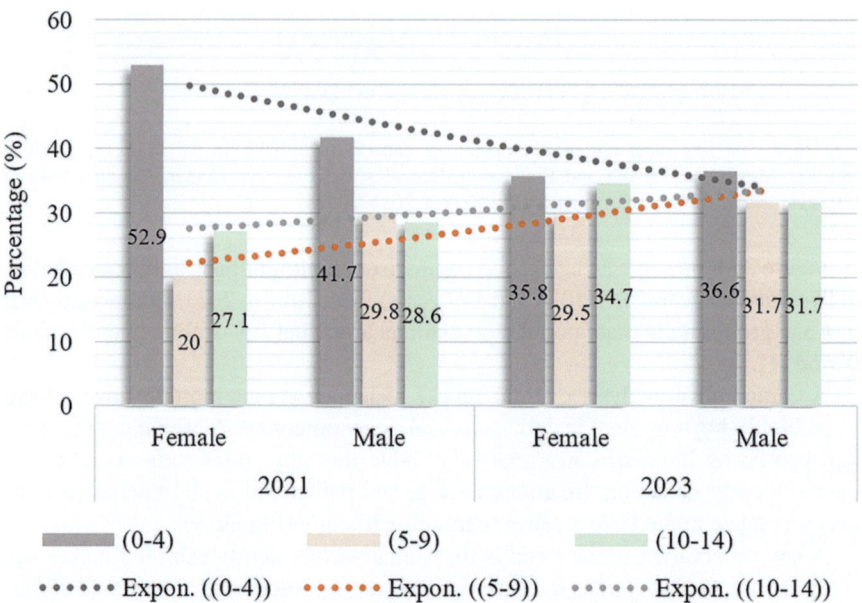

Fig. 26.8 Age group comparison of pediatric cancers among both genders in the UAE. (Source: Ministry of Health and Prevention, Statistics and Research Center, National Disease Registry—UAE National Cancer Registry Report, 2021–2023)

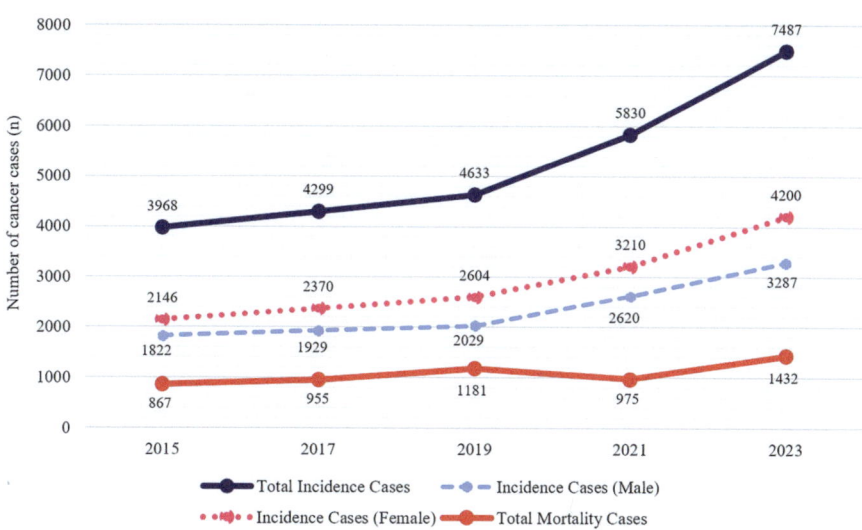

Fig. 26.9 A comparison of total cancer incidence and mortality cases over the years. (Source: Ministry of Health and Prevention, Statistics and Research Center, National Disease Registry—UAE National Cancer Registry Report, 2015–2023)

Table 26.2 Trends in total mortality cases and age-standardized mortality rates by gender (2015–2023)

Year	Total number of mortality cases (n)	Age standardized mortality rate[a] (both genders)	Age standardized mortality rate[a] (male)	Age standardized mortality rate[a] (female)
2023	1432	30.37	28.6	34.8
2021	975	29.6	29.3	33.4
2019	1181	33.3	–	–
2017	955	26.4	26	31
2015	867	–	–	–

Source: Ministry of Health and Prevention, Statistics and Research Center, National Disease Registry—UAE National Cancer Registry Report, 2015–2023
[a]Per 100,000 population

26.4 Cancer Screening Programs

While the UAE has made notable progress in developing cancer screening initiatives, it has not yet implemented a comprehensive nationwide screening program. Instead, there are multiple localized screening programs serving specific regions. The programs are detailed below [7–13]:

- Simply Check, introduced in September 2014 in the Emirate of Abu Dhabi, covered breast, colorectal, cervical, and lung cancer screenings. It has now been integrated into the IFHAS program.

- ITMENAN, which translates to "Contentment" in Arabic, was launched in November 2016 in the Northern Emirates, focusing on breast, colorectal, and cervical cancer screenings. This program is currently ongoing.
- WEQAYA, which translates to "Prevention" in Arabic, was launched in January 2021 in the Emirate of Abu Dhabi, targeting breast, colorectal, and cervical cancers. This initiative has now been integrated into the IFHAS program.
- IFHAS, meaning "Check" in Arabic, was introduced in June 2022 in the Emirate of Abu Dhabi, covering breast, colorectal, cervical, and lung cancer screenings. This program is currently active.
- The Cancer Screening Program by the Dubai Health Authority was established in November 2017 in the Emirate of Dubai to focus on breast, colorectal, and cervical cancer screenings. This initiative remains actively ongoing.
- The Cancer Patient Support Program, known as BASMAH, which translates to "Smile" in Arabic, was launched in November 2020 in the Emirate of Dubai, targeting breast, colorectal, and cervical cancers. This program is currently active.

Despite efforts to enhance cancer screening and early detection in the UAE, the number of deaths continues to rise. In the largest survey to date in the UAE distributed via social media, it was found that most respondents were comfortable discussing cancer and understood the importance of early detection, yet the willingness to undergo screening was suboptimal, with 75.2% reporting, they were unwilling to undergo cancer screening. The study highlights the need for increased cancer awareness and calls for updated screening guidelines. It also suggests that hospitals, cancer charities, educational institutions, and media should target the general population and specific groups to boost cancer awareness [14].

26.5 Modifiable Cancer Risk Factors in the UAE

The occurrence of cancer has been linked to various risk factors that have the potential to be altered on a broad, national level [15]. Reducing the prevalence of five modifiable cancer risk factors, including obesity, fast food consumption, smoking, and the presence of human papillomavirus (HPV) and hepatitis B virus (HBV), can lead to a decrease in cancer cases.

The high occurrence of obesity and overweight among young people in the UAE is similar to that observed in other Middle Eastern Arab nations, primarily due to the widespread consumption of unhealthy diets lacking in nutritional value [16].

In our previous publications, we have discussed the UAE government's proactive approach towards managing cancer risk factors, particularly focusing on obesity and all forms of smoking. The government has undertaken numerous initiatives to address these issues [2]. Furthermore, we suggest the implementation of calorie information on fast-food menus and the prohibition of advertising for fast-food establishments, as such promotions are increasingly prevalent on the internet and throughout the streets of the UAE [17].

The government had previously declared its intention to impose excise taxes on a few items. Starting in December 2019, these taxes were applied to carbonated beverages, tobacco products, energy drinks, electronic smoking devices, liquids used in such devices, and any product containing added sugar or alternative sweeteners. Furthermore, a minimum excise tax per individual cigarette, per gram of waterpipe tobacco, ready-to-use tobacco, or similar products was also introduced in December 2019 [18]. Additional preventive measures are currently in place, which include the provision of counseling services and programs as well as the promotion and adoption of healthy lifestyles in the UAE [15].

Nationwide smoking cessation programs have been implemented [15]. On February 5, 2006, the United Arab Emirates became a party to the WHO Framework Convention on Tobacco Control and has since implemented several key policies, which include the following [19]:

- Prohibition of smoking in specific enclosed public spaces and public transportation. While some places and transport options may designate smoking areas, healthcare, educational facilities, sports facilities, and places of worship do not allow smoking. Moreover, outdoor areas adjacent to educational, health, sports, places of worship, and industrial facilities are also designated as smoke-free zones.
- Banning tobacco advertising in all forms of print and electronic media, including at points of sale.
- Mandating health warnings on tobacco product packaging that are both pictorial and textual, covering at least 50% of the primary display areas on the packaging (e.g., front and back).
- Regulating the specified contents of cigarettes, including restrictions on the use of certain herbs, spices, and flavorings.
- Prohibiting the sale of tobacco products near schools, places of worship, and through vending machines and online platforms. Additionally, there are regional restrictions on the sale of specific smokeless tobacco products. Selling tobacco products to individuals under the age of 18 is strictly forbidden.
- Allowing the sale of e-cigarettes with specific restrictions on flavors, ingredients, nicotine concentration, and product quality standards. E-cigarette packaging must feature text-only health warnings that cover 50% of both the front and back of the packaging.

Cervical cancer ranks as the fifth most frequently occurring cancer among women in the UAE [1]. The UAE took the lead in the MENA region by introducing the HPV vaccine. In 2008, the Department of Health (DOH) in Abu Dhabi initiated the HPV vaccination program for all eligible schoolgirls, whether in public or private schools. Then, in 2013, the DOH extended the HPV vaccination initiative to encompass all females aged 15–26, irrespective of their nationality. Additionally, the Dubai Health Authority (DHA) advised the commencement of HPV vaccination for all girls aged 11–12 years [2]. On February 29, 2024, the Ministry of Health and Prevention (MoHAP) announced that it has expanded the scope of HPV vaccine to include males in the National Immunisation Programme, making the UAE as one of the first countries in the MENA region to implement a gender-neutral HPV vaccine approach [20].

The Hepatitis B vaccine was implemented and made obligatory in the UAE in 1991 [21]. Starting in 2006, all new expatriates relocating to the UAE for employment are required to undergo testing for hepatitis B and C infections. If an individual is found to be nonimmune to HBV, it is compulsory for them to receive the Hepatitis B vaccination [2].

26.6 Cancer Prevention and Awareness Programs

Numerous organizations in the UAE are actively involved in community engagement initiatives aimed at raising awareness about cancer among the local population.

26.6.1 Friends of Cancer Patients

Friends of Cancer Patients is a notable nongovernmental organization (NGO) dedicated to promoting cancer awareness throughout the UAE. They have various programs and activities to achieve this goal, including the following [22].

26.6.1.1 Pink Caravan

The Pink Caravan is a breast cancer initiative that covers the entire UAE and operates as part of the "Kashf" program under the umbrella of Friends of Cancer Patients. Established in 2011 with the support of His Royal Highness Sheikh Dr. Sultan bin Mohammed Al Qasimi, a member of the Supreme Council and the Ruler of Sharjah, and Her Highness Sheikha Jawaher Bint Mohammed Al Qasimi, the wife of the Ruler of Sharjah and the Founder and Patron of Friends of Cancer Patients, the Pink Caravan has the following objectives [23]:

- Raising awareness and promoting cancer prevention
- Early detection of breast cancer

A. *Pink Caravan Medical Mobile Clinic Services*

The Pink Caravan Medical Mobile Clinic is a healthcare facility that roams throughout the UAE, delivering on-site education and screening services for breast and cervical cancer, thereby enhancing the prospects of detecting these conditions early and improving survival rates. Pink Caravan medical mobile clinic services include the following [23]:

- Clinical Breast Examination (CBE): A CBE, which stands for Clinical Breast Examination, is a medical assessment carried out by a healthcare expert. It entails a thorough examination and manual inspection of all breast tissue, including the examination of lymph node areas.

- Mammogram Screening: Mammogram screenings are performed on asymptomatic women aged 40 and above, utilizing the advanced HOLOGIC Tomosynthesis 3Dimensions Mammography System.
- Ultrasound Screening: Additional imaging evaluation is conducted to acquire a conclusive and prompt diagnosis for any potential abnormalities identified during CBE or mammogram screening.
- Pap Test: The Papanicolaou test, commonly known as the Pap test, is the established method for cervical cancer screening. It is available to all sexually active women between the ages of 25 and 65, regardless of their marital status (married, divorced, or widowed), as long as they are free of symptoms.

B. *Pink Ride*

Every year, the Pink Caravan conducts the Pink Caravan Ride, spanning all seven emirates and extending its reach to remote regions. Annually, more than 150 skilled equestrians come together, uniting various sectors and enlisting the backing of schools, universities, businesses, Pink Caravan advocates, and members of royalty. Up to this point, the Pink Caravan Ride has covered a distance exceeding 2100 kilometers throughout the seven emirates, involving over 9754 riders, more than 1250 volunteers, and conducting more than 1300 medical clinics for early breast cancer detection examinations for a total of 93,201 individuals [23].

C. *Pink October*

The Pink Caravan by FOCP has been journeying through the UAE since 2011, with a mission to increase awareness regarding early detection and breast cancer, offering complimentary screenings and professional medical support, advocating for healthy lifestyles, and empowering both citizens and residents to safeguard themselves from the threat of this disease [24].

In preparation for the annual International Breast Cancer Awareness Month in October, the Pink Caravan invites private sector companies nationwide to participate in their "Corporate Wellness Day" initiative. This program aims to educate employees about the importance of early detection and treatment of breast cancer [24].

26.6.1.2 Shanab

Shanab is a men's health campaign operating under the "Kashf" initiative of Friends of Cancer Patients. It focuses on the early detection of cancer, specifically targeting prostate and testicular cancer. Introduced in November 2014, Shanab, which means "moustache" in English, primarily emphasizes the significance of early detection while working to dispel any associated stigmas related to these two forms of cancer [25].

Shanab aims to form partnerships with diverse entities, such as government bodies, private companies, sports associations, and similar organizations, with the goal of expanding the reach of awareness efforts and encouraging a culture where prioritizing health takes precedence over other concerns. Shanab's objectives include the following [25]:

- Increasing awareness among its target audience about the significant health challenges that men encounter
- Encouraging men to share their health issues with their peers

26.6.1.3 Ana

Ana is a childhood cancer campaign that operates within the "Kashf" initiative of Friends of Cancer Patients, focusing on the early detection of cancer in children. This initiative was established in November 2014, following the guidance of Her Highness Sheikha Jawaher Bint Mohammed Al Qasimi, the wife of the Ruler of Sharjah, Founder and Patron of the Friends of Cancer Patients organization. The name "Ana," which translates to "I" in English, was deliberately chosen to inspire children with cancer to embrace their individuality regardless of their physical appearance. Ana's goals include the following [26]:

- Improving the well-being of children with cancer and their families
- Promoting awareness regarding the seven typical indicators of childhood cancer and emphasizing the significance of early detection

A. *Ana-vation*

As part of the Ana initiative, Ana-vation, a unique program merging "Ana" and "innovation," stands out by promoting awareness through enjoyable and educational activities. These activities include innovative do-it-yourself robotic kits, app development, and more. Ana-vation underscores the significance of early detection in childhood cancer by incorporating essential S.T.E.A.M. (Science, Technology, Engineering, Arts, and Mathematics) principles and coding, aiming to inspire future developers, researchers, doctors, and engineers [26].

The third Ana-vation competition, organized by FOCP, empowers 150 students in an app development program aimed at tackling childhood cancer. This initiative not only enhances students' app development capabilities but also educates them on creating innovative solutions for contemporary challenges. Additionally, it fosters awareness about childhood cancer among both the participating students and their families. The app's objective is to address a genuine and practical requirement that benefits cancer patients in real-world settings [26].

B. *Ana-Nutrition*

Ana-Nutrition is an initiative that places significant emphasis on promoting a healthy lifestyle. It achieves this by organizing small workshops, where children learn to prepare delicious and nutritious snacks. Simultaneously, it encourages discussions with parents about recognizing early signs and symptoms of childhood cancer and the significance of proper nutrition. Ana-nutrition's goal is to educate children on the importance of maintaining a healthy lifestyle and adopting good nutritional practices [26].

26.6.1.4 Relay for Life

The inaugural Relay For Life event in the region was introduced in 2017, following the guidance of Sheikha Jawaher Bint Mohammed Al Qasimi, who is the wife of the

Ruler of Sharjah and the Founder and Patron of the Friends of Cancer Patients organization. Relay For Life stands as one of the globe's largest community engagement events aimed at raising awareness and collecting funds. Relay for Life UAE has the following objectives [27]:

- Relay For Life endeavors to provide support to individuals in their cancer journey by fostering empowerment and building a supportive network for them and their families.
- It is geared towards raising awareness and generating funds to combat cancer.

26.6.2 Brest Friends

Brest Friends was founded in 2005 by Dr. Houriya Kazim. The support group brings together patients and survivors on a monthly basis to exchange knowledge, share their journeys, and provides essential moral and emotional support. This support network has proven to play a vital role in the healing process for women affected by breast cancer. Al Jalila Foundation, in collaboration with Brest Friends, is a leader in advocating for the significance of early breast cancer detection, enhancing patient assistance through medical care, and making substantial investments in local breast cancer research [28].

26.6.3 Emirates Oncology Society

Emirates Oncology Society has led numerous events for raising awareness of various cancers. Some of them are [29]:

26.6.3.1 Breast Cancer Awareness Event
The Emirates Breast Cancer Working Group within EOS, with Dr. Aydah Al Awadhi as its president and Dr. Nahla Al Mansoori and Dr. Mona Al Ayyan as board members, organized its inaugural event for breast cancer patients. The event was remarkable, offering valuable education, insightful information, and the exchange of stories with inspiring and resilient breast cancer survivors, as well as experts in the field [29]. The recent breast cancer awareness event was organized in October 2024, with a theme "Stronger Together". This day was dedicated to supporting and empowering those navigating a breast cancer diagnosis and recovery [30].

26.6.3.2 Cancer Survivor Graduation Day
To commemorate Cancer Survivor Month, the Emirates Oncology Society organized an informative panel discussion on June 18, 2023, at the Museum of the Future in Dubai. The event was graced by the presence of H.E. Obaid Khalfan Al Ghoul Al Salami and EOS President Prof. Humaid Al-Shamsi. Its purpose was to promote awareness and honor the unwavering courage and resilience of our cancer patients. After the panel discussion, a Graduation Ceremony for Cancer Survivors

took place. It was a touching event that brought together survivors, their families, and kind-hearted members of our community who wanted to offer their steadfast support [29]. The second Graduation Day was held on June 7, 2024, and is planned to be an annual event.

26.6.3.3 World Cancer Day

To mark World Cancer Day, the Emirates Oncology Society organized a Panel Discussion on February 4 at the Museum of the Future in Dubai. The event featured the presence of notable individuals including H.E. Dr. Hussain Al Rand (Assistant Undersecretary for health centers and clinics, Ministry of Health and Prevention), H.E. Sawsan Jafar (Chairperson & President of the Board of Directors, Friends of Cancer Patients, UAE), Dr. Mouza Al-Sharhan (President of the Emirates Medical Association), and esteemed members of EOS along with President Prof. Humaid Al-Shamsi. Subsequent to the panel discussion, there was a tree-planting event at the Museum of the Future, where Ghaf Tree Seeds were sown. This act symbolized resilience and vitality, serving as an inspiration for all cancer patients to confront challenges and remain steadfast and resilient [29].

26.6.3.4 Liver Cancer

EOS paid tribute to a month dedicated to raising awareness about liver cancer by illuminating the world's tallest observation wheel in Dubai with a "Liver Stronger" art installation, generously sponsored by AstraZeneca [31].

These are very few instances illustrating the various initiatives undertaken by different institutions in the UAE to promote cancer awareness among people of all age groups, addressing various types of cancer.

26.7 Established Comprehensive Cancer Centers

A Comprehensive Cancer Center (CCC) should serve as a single destination for all cancer care requirements. From our perspective, a CCC must offer the following services to qualify: medical oncology, hematology, bone marrow transplant services for both adults and children, surgical oncology, radiation oncology, nuclear medicine, and palliative care [32].

At present, there are four centers that meet the criteria for being classified as CCCs. However, other prominent cancer centers do not fulfill our CCC criteria [13].

The Hamdan Bin Rashid Cancer Hospital, part of Dubai Health, will be Dubai's first integrated and comprehensive cancer hospital, bringing a groundbreaking model of advanced and accessible cancer care to the region [33].

26.8 Treatment

26.8.1 Oncology Manpower

As of January 2024, it is estimated that there are approximately 100 medical oncologists, radiation oncologists, and specialists in malignant hematology practicing in the United Arab Emirates (UAE). The majority of these oncologists are concentrated in the emirates of Abu Dhabi and Dubai. These healthcare professionals hail from diverse national backgrounds, with a significant portion originating from the United Kingdom, the United States, and Arab nations like Lebanon, Syria, and Jordan. Many of them have chosen to relocate to the UAE, attracted by better remuneration and the high quality of life offered in the country. These oncologists have received their training from various educational backgrounds, including a substantial number who hold board certifications from American and UK institutions. Additionally, there are numerous oncologists with training from neighboring countries such as Lebanon, Jordan, and Syria. Among these oncologists, approximately 10–12 individuals (comprising about 10% of all oncologists in the UAE) are local UAE residents. Most of the locally trained UAE oncologists have received their education and advanced fellowships from prestigious institutions like MD Anderson Cancer Centers. It is imperative to promote oncology as a career choice among UAE physicians, and this can be achieved by raising awareness about this specialty among medical students and early-career physicians [13].

26.8.2 Surgical Oncology/Robotic Surgery

Surgical oncology has a long history in the UAE, but a significant number of surgeons in this field lack formal training. However, there has been a recent influx of formally trained surgical oncologists to the UAE in recent years. Research indicates that a surgeon's training significantly influences the outcomes of cancer patients [13].

Out of the 27 studies that investigated the outcomes of surgeons in relation to their training and specialization, a majority of 25 studies discovered that specialized surgeons achieved superior results in cancer surgery when compared to their non-specialized counterparts [34]. The UAE has expanded the availability of robotic surgery, although only a limited number of cancer centers offer this technology [13].

A significant hurdle in the field of surgical oncology in the UAE is the quality of surgeries conducted for cancer patients. Regrettably, many surgeons lacking formal training in surgical oncology do not refer their patients to specialized surgical oncologists for procedures. This reluctance is often driven by financial conflicts of interest and competition, as most of these surgeons operate within private practices. Surgeries performed by non-specialized surgeons typically do not involve consultations with a multidisciplinary team (MDT), resulting in inadequate surgical management, particularly in cases of breast and rectal cancers. These patients may undergo surgery when they actually require neoadjuvant therapy for improved treatment outcomes [13].

To tackle this problem, it is crucial for regulatory authorities to take action by mandating that a multidisciplinary team (MDT) reviews every cancer case before granting insurance approval for cancer surgeries. This mandate should apply in all cases, except for emergency surgeries, and there should also be oversight in the form of audits for surgeons who perform a significant number of emergency cancer surgeries. Moreover, the utilization of robotic surgery should be limited to surgeons who have received accredited surgical training [35], as some surgeons attend short courses and promote themselves as robotic surgeons, which can influence the choices made by cancer patients regarding their surgical treatment [13].

26.8.3 Anticancer Therapies in the UAE

Healthcare authorities in the UAE have streamlined the process to ensure patients have sufficient access to all authorized medications, including innovative and recently developed drugs for cancer treatment. These medications are typically provided to patients after undergoing rigorous evaluation and receiving approval from the Food and Drug Administration (FDA). In the UAE, stringent packaging and storage regulations are enforced to guarantee the safety of these medications. Additionally, best practices are upheld to ensure the secure transportation of these drugs. Typically, hospitals directly request specific medications from pharmaceutical companies that supply them, and the expenses for these drugs are covered when they are deemed necessary. As recommended by the EOS consensus group, an approach to lowering the cost of these drugs involves the government making bulk orders for medications instead of hospitals procuring them directly [2]. Recently, Rafed was established, which aims to ensure the availability and quality of essential goods and services for Abu Dhabi's healthcare sector. Rafed is the first Group Purchasing Organization in the region that is primarily focused on healthcare procurement [36].

26.8.4 Radiation Therapy

Presently, there are a minimum of ten facilities offering radiation therapy services in the UAE. Among these, four are situated in Abu Dhabi and Al Ain, five in Dubai, and one in Ras Al-Khaimah, which serves as the sole radiation center in the Northern Emirates. These centers are equipped with a total of seven linear accelerators (LINACs), a tomotherapy unit, and two brachytherapy units in the Abu Dhabi/Al Ain area. At the moment, Ras Al-Khaimah has two linear accelerators and a ViewRay MR Linac in operation. In contrast, Dubai has four linear accelerators, a tomotherapy unit, a Cyberknife machine, and two brachytherapy units actively in use. The majority of linear accelerators (LINACs) in the UAE are of the latest generation and have a new status, with Elekta Versa HD™ and Varian—TrueBeam® being the most commonly utilized models in the country.

All of these facilities utilize sophisticated techniques such as complex intensity-modulated radiation therapy (IMRT), RAPID-ARC, and volumetric modulated arc therapy (VMAT), in conjunction with advanced image-guided radiation therapy (IGRT) [13]. The Neurospinal Hospital in Dubai incorporated CyberKnife radiosurgery in its services in 2022 [3]. In 2022, Burjeel Medical City introduced a complete Novalis system equipped with BrainLab and Elements software, which is a technology used for providing precision radiotherapy and stereotactic radiosurgery (SRS) in the UAE [37]. Lastly, in Ras Al-Khaimah, you can find the sole ViewRay—MRIdian system in the Middle East. This system, the first FDA-cleared MRI-Guided Radiation Therapy cancer treatment system in the Middle East, blends magnetic resonance imaging with adaptive radiotherapy [13, 38].

The Emirates Medical Association (EMA) has approved the establishment of a radiation oncology working group under the Emirates Oncology Society (EOS) umbrella. It was launched in September 2023. Dr. Ibrahim Abu-Gheida has been named the Chairman of the radiation oncology working group. The group conducted the first radiation oncology conference in UAE history, the BEST of ASTRO Gulf, in April 2024 (Fig. 26.11) [39, 40].

26.9 HSCT in the UAE

Hematopoietic stem cell transplantation (HSCT) has evolved into a firmly established therapeutic approach that offers a potential cure or life-saving treatment for a wide range of noncancerous and cancerous hematologic conditions, immune disorders, and solid tumors. During the years 2016 to 2018, a total of 164 pediatric patients and 161 adult patients, who were citizens of the UAE, received hematopoietic stem cell transplantation (HSCT) abroad [4].

Each year, an estimated 200 patients in the UAE, both citizens and non-citizens, require hematopoietic stem cell transplantation (HSCT) [13]. The UAE's first hematopoietic stem cell transplantation (HSCT) service was introduced in 2019 by the Abu Dhabi Stem Cell Center. In October 2021, Burjeel Medical City established a comprehensive HSCT unit for both adults and pediatric patients, introducing cryopreservation HSCT to the UAE [13]. Over 100 patients who underwent HSCT from the initiation of the transplant program in 2021 at BMC to May 2024 were included in the adult and pediatric categories. Out of 120 patients, most underwent autologous transplantation; others underwent allogeneic transplantation during this period. Patients who underwent allogeneic transplants were haploidentical, fully matched, and related stem cell transplants. The most common malignancies for which patients underwent HSCT at our center were multiple myeloma, followed by Hodgkin's lymphoma, non-Hodgkin lymphoma, amyloidosis, thalassemia, germ cell tumors, chronic myeloid leukemia, acute myeloid leukemia, myelodysplastic syndrome, neuroblastoma, and premature immunodeficiency. Transplants for solid tumors have also been completed for germ cell tumors, neuroblastoma, and gestational trophoblastic disease (GTD). The majority of patients who underwent stem cell transplants were in complete remission at the time of the transplant. Acute graft-versus-host disease (GvHD) was rarely observed in our patients. Over 90% of the patients survived post-transplant (unpublished data on file).

26.10 Gynecologic Oncology in the UAE

In 2023, gynecologic cancers affecting women ranked as one of the most prevalent categories of cancers in the UAE. This category included 215 cases of uterus cancer, 146 cases of cervix uteri, and 125 cases of ovarian cancer, bringing the total of 486 cases of women's cancers. These cases accounted for 6.84% of all malignancies recorded in the UAE in 2023 [1]. At present, the UAE lacks specialized gynecologic oncology units. Furthermore, the number of adequately trained gynecologic oncology surgeons is exceedingly scarce, with an estimated count of fewer than ten throughout the entire UAE. Our recommendation is to create specialized gynecologic oncology facilities, enforce mandatory referrals to these units throughout the UAE, and restrict general surgeons from conducting surgeries related to gynecologic oncology. Additionally, it's important to tackle the low uptake of cervical cancer screening and conduct research to identify the obstacles hindering screening. As mentioned earlier, the HPV vaccine is integrated in the UAE's nationwide vaccination initiative for girls, and this implementation has been effective. Lastly, there is currently no availability of gynecologic oncology fellowship training programs in the UAE, and we strongly advocate for the establishment of such programs [13].

26.11 Pediatric Oncology in the UAE

According to the UAE-National Cancer Registry, in 2023, there were 237 new invasive cancer cases diagnosed among children aged 0–14 in the UAE. These cases represented approximately 3.3% of all documented malignant cases, with females making up 40.1% and males accounting for 59.9%. The data reveals that the highest occurrence of pediatric cancer cases was in the 0–4 age group, comprising 86 cases or 36.3% of the total, followed by the 10–14 age group with 78 cases, accounting for 32.9%. It's worth noting that a smaller number of cancer cases in the pediatric population were identified in the 5–9 age group, totaling 73 cases or 30.8%. The data shows that the most frequently diagnosed cancer type was leukemia, accounting for 73 cases (30.8%). This was followed by brain and central nervous system (CNS) cancers at 32 cases (13.5%), non-Hodgkin lymphoma at 26 cases (11.0%), bone and articular cartilage cancers at 16 cases (6.8%), and kidney & renal pelvis at 16 cases (6.8%) [1].

Seven hospitals offer services in pediatric hematology-oncology, staffed by approximately 28 to 30 physicians specialized in this field. Among these, Tawam Hospital, Sheikh Khalifa Medical City, and Dubai Hospital are the public healthcare facilities that provide these services and experience the highest patient volume. It's worth mentioning that there are no pediatric hematology-oncology services available in the Northern Emirates (Table 26.3) [13].

Table 26.3 Hospitals providing pediatric oncology in the UAE [13]

Hospital	Emirate	Facility type
American Hospital Dubai	Dubai	Private
Burjeel Medical City	Abu Dhabi	Private
Dubai Hospital	Dubai	Public
NMC Hospital Abu Dhabi	Abu Dhabi	Private
Mediclinic City Hospital	Dubai	Private
Sheikh Khalifa Medical City	Abu Dhabi	Public
Tawam Hospital	Al Ain	Public

Burjeel Medical City was the first hospital in the UAE to start a pediatric bone marrow transplant (BMT) service. In a notable achievement, this facility carried out the first-ever five successful allogeneic BMTs in the UAE, commencing with the inaugural procedure in April 2022 [41]. Pediatric hematology-oncology services are distributed across multiple providers, serving a relatively small patient population. Our suggestion is to consolidate pediatric hematology-oncology services in the UAE to enhance treatment outcomes [42].

The pediatric HSCT service at BMC is the first and only pediatric HSCT service in the UAE. The service started in March 2022. The median day of engraftment at the pediatric HSCT service at BMC for thalassemia is 29 days, and the median day of engraftment for sickle cell anemia is also 29 days. Severe combined immunodeficiency had an 11-day engraftment. Primary immunodeficiency (PID) had 32 days for engraftment (unpublished data on file).

26.12 Palliative and Supportive Care

Over the past 4 years, since the release of the earlier report titled "Palliative care in the UAE, A desperate need" in 2018 [43], there has been significant progress in palliative and supportive care within the UAE. The availability of palliative care services has expanded from two centers to four centers across the UAE. The palliative care department at Tawam Hospital was established in 2007 to cater to oncology patients at that hospital. It's important to note that this is the sole government-supported palliative care initiative in the UAE. In addition, the American Hospital in Dubai initiated its palliative care service in December 2014 [43].

Mediclinic Hospital Dubai initiated this service in 2019. Burjeel Medical City (BMC) in Abu Dhabi introduced its palliative and supportive care service in March 2020, marking the first provider of such services in Abu Dhabi. In May 2022, a significant milestone was achieved, as the UAE obtained its first representative in the World Health Organization's (WHO) palliative care network. Dr. Neil A. Nijhawan, the Director of Palliative Care Services at Burjeel Medical City in Abu Dhabi, was appointed by WHO as an expert member of the EMRO Expert Network on Palliative Care [13].

The Emirates Medical Association (EMA) has granted approval for the creation of a palliative and supportive care working group, which falls under the Emirates Oncology Society (EOS). This working group was officially launched in September 2023 [44]. This development represents a significant move towards increasing public awareness of palliative care and advocating for its availability in the UAE. The working group will also have a crucial role in advocating for this specialized field with relevant stakeholders and regulatory bodies in the UAE. Additionally, education and training will be a central focus of the group's mission [13].

Dr. Neil Arun Nijhawan was named the chairman of the EOS palliative and supportive care working group [39].

Enhancing the delivery of palliative care in the UAE demands a thoughtful and well-structured strategy, rather than a direct adoption of Western palliative care methods. Our earlier publication outlined recommendations for enhancing palliative care in the UAE, and these have been further developed as detailed below [45]:

- The establishment of a comprehensive palliative and supportive care strategy at the national level as an integral component of the UAE's cancer control initiative
- Ensuring that vital pain relief and palliative medications are accessible across all healthcare settings, including the provision of injectable opioids or morphine pumps for patients receiving end-of-life care in their own homes
- Fundamental palliative care education for nonspecialists, emphasizing pain management, along with the integration of palliative care into the curricula of undergraduate medical schools and nursing programs
- Provisions for additional key roles within the multidisciplinary team that necessitate training and support (governance), such as clinical nurse specialists, imams, and chaplains
- Enhancing and expanding the 2016 Allow Natural Death (AND) policy to incorporate advance care planning and treatment-de-escalation plans

26.13 Emirates Oncology Society

The Emirates Oncology Society (EOS) is committed to advancing and nurturing comprehensive cancer patient care in the United Arab Emirates. This mission is achieved by uniting cancer specialists from various fields who are actively practicing in the country [39]. The primary objective of EOS is to furnish its members with the latest information to turn this objective into a quantifiable achievement for the benefit of all patients. EOS working groups were established in September 2023 (Figs. 26.10 and 26.11) [39].

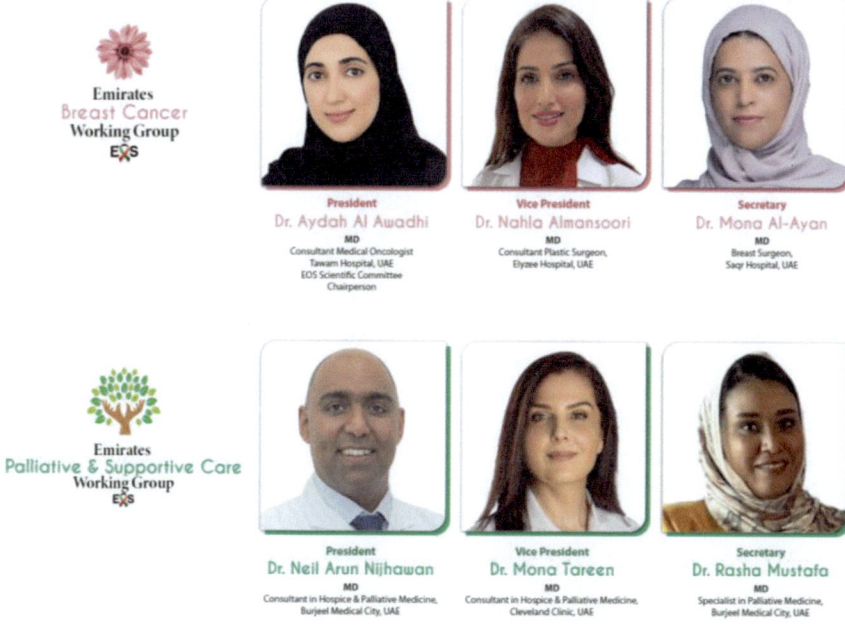

Fig. 26.10 EOS' breast cancer and palliative and supportive care working group members [39]

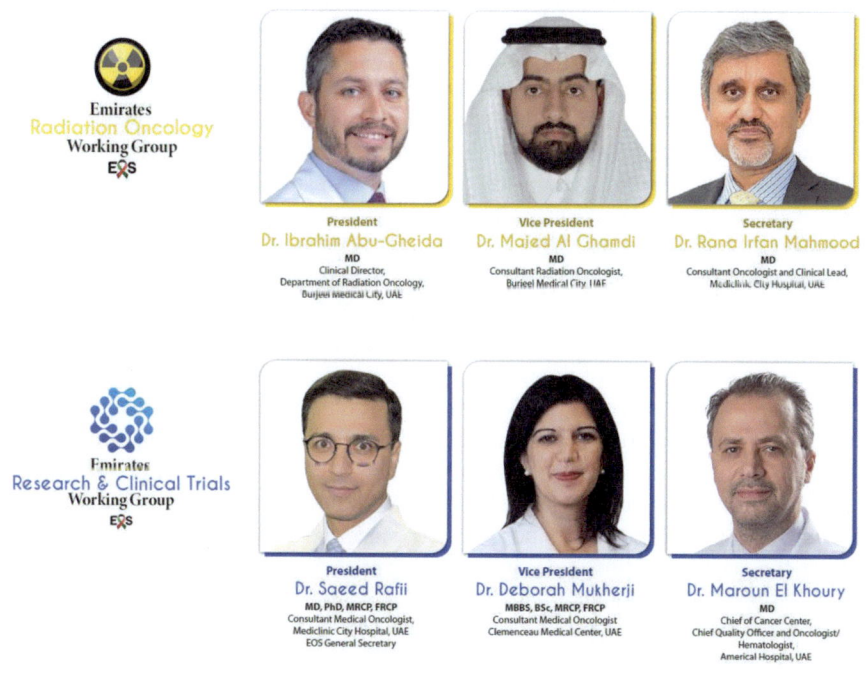

Fig. 26.11 EOS' radiation oncology, and research and clinical trials working group members [39]

26.14 Research and Education

26.14.1 Research

In general, the productivity of cancer research is changing over time, but there are still some gaps in the available evidence. The opportunities for both basic and translational research are growing within the country, thanks to the increasing number of academic institutions and research programs focused on molecular and cellular research. Until now, most observational studies have primarily concentrated on screening and fundamental epidemiological aspects. However, moving forward, it is essential to emphasize the growth of national registries and the continuous collection of clinically significant data over time. This will provide a more comprehensive understanding of the clinical and molecular characteristics of breast cancer within the country and, notably, improve the assessment of survival metrics for guiding effective management strategies. Finally, a noticeable shortage of therapeutic clinical trials exists, a challenge that extends to neighboring areas. Presently, there are several ongoing initiatives aimed at establishing collaborations with sponsors of clinical trials to facilitate the hosting of interventional studies in the country. This is due to the advanced and flexible regulatory and resource infrastructures, which are adaptable to international standards and criteria. Similarly, there needs to be an equivalent focus on comprehending lifestyle factors that can be changed to reduce the risk of cancer, such as smoking, obesity, dietary choices, and lack of physical activity. These factors are believed to have suboptimal status in the UAE, although the precise prevalence rates among Emiratis compared to expatriates and their connections to cancer incidence are still not well-established [46]. There are many barriers to conducting oncology clinical trials in the UAE (Fig. 26.12) [47].

It is essential for all stakeholders to come together and collaborate in addressing significant challenges associated with conducting oncology clinical trials in the UAE. Due to the ongoing expansion of academic institutions and research initiatives dedicated to cellular and molecular studies, the opportunities for basic and translational research in the UAE are generally on the rise. However, when it comes to clinical research as a whole and, more specifically, clinical trials, there is considerable room for improvement, both in terms of quantity and focus. There is a pressing requirement for a call to action from both local and global communities to enhance the involvement of the UAE in global clinical trials. Additionally, it is crucial to establish local funding opportunities for domestic studies to ensure that the effectiveness and safety of drugs are assessed within the local population, rather than "assumed" from data from Western countries [47]. In September 2023, the Emirates Oncology Society established the "Emirates Research and Clinical Trials Working Group" to promote and enhance cancer research in the UAE [44]. To ensure the success of this endeavor, it is essential for all stakeholders to provide mutual support and collaborate in improving cancer care in the UAE [47].

In September 2024, a book publication titled *Cancer Care in the United Arab Emirates*, edited by Prof. Humaid O. Al-Shamsi, was launched. This groundbreaking book marks the nation's first specialized scientific work on cancer. It

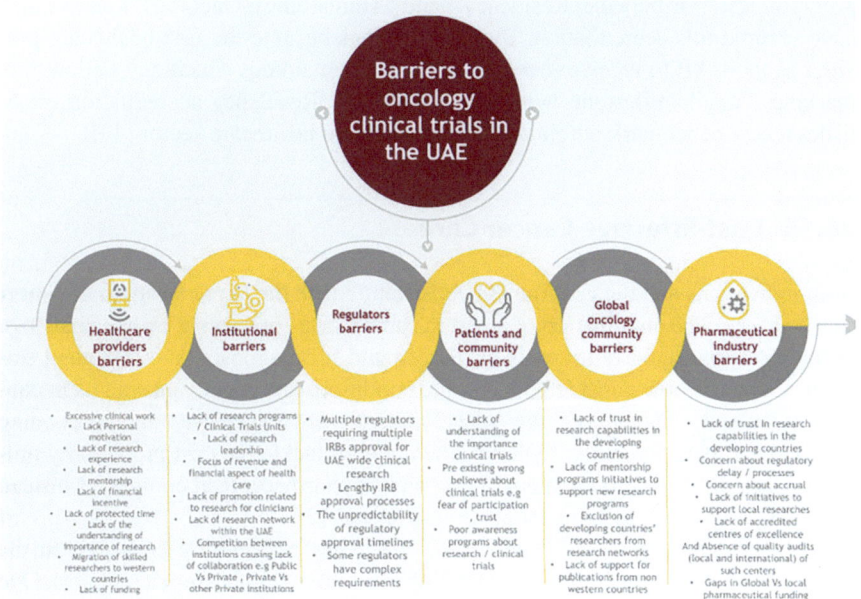

Fig. 26.12 Barriers to oncology-clinical trials in the UAE

comprehensively covers all aspects related to cancer, including statistics, extensive data, and in-depth research on various types of cancer within the country. Furthermore, the book sheds light on the continuous state-led initiatives aimed at advancing this crucial sector [48].

26.14.2 Education

The UAE has boosted the availability of specialized oncology training programs within the country. Tawam Hospital inaugurated its inaugural medical oncology fellowship program in November 2019, and several other public and private hospitals in the country also offer a limited number of oncology training programs. With the expanding realm of medical practice, the UAE has devised strategies to implement more advanced training programs. These programs aim to enable medical professionals from the region to receive training and engage in medical practice within the UAE [2]. It is crucial to recruit a competent workforce, enhance their abilities through training and ongoing education, and closely assess their performance. Obtaining international accreditations from reputable global organizations is also essential for maintaining a continuous path of improvement [46]. On February 15, 2025, Burjeel Holdings achieved a significant milestone in healthcare education by receiving accreditation from the National Institute for Health Specialties (NIHS), a prestigious accreditation program in the UAE. The two specialized medical training programmes, "Orthopedic Residency" and "Hematology-Oncology Fellowship", have secured this accreditation. Burjeel Holdings became the first healthcare provider in the UAE to receive recognition for its Hematology-Oncology Fellowship, marking a major milestone, while the Orthopedic Residency accreditation establishes a new benchmark within Abu Dhabi's private healthcare sector [49].

26.15 Cost-Effective Cancer Care

Both individuals and the government consistently face the financial strain of cancer care services. The anticipation of a rise in cancer cases presents a unique challenge in the UAE, particularly in terms of the demand for diagnostic and treatment services. Cancer is now considered a chronic condition, driving advancements in cancer treatment, including the development of expensive therapies like immunotherapies. Recently, EOS has attempted to tackle the cost problem by proposing the collective procurement of drugs from pharmaceutical companies instead of individual purchases by hospitals or institutions [2].

An alternative approach to enhancing efficiency and cutting costs within the healthcare system would involve embracing innovative reimbursement models. One such example is shifting from a "per-fraction" radiation model to a "per-site" model [15, 50]. This results in more cost-effective cancer therapy, leading to a decrease in the number of treatments required. Consequently, patients and their caregivers, who frequently accompany them to the radiotherapy centers, may experience fewer days of potential work or other commitments missed [15].

Protocols concerning the utilization of advanced imaging techniques, such as Positron Emission Tomography (PET/CT) scans have been implemented, resulting in reduced follow-up costs that are typically incurred by oncology patients. Moreover, unnecessary X-rays or CT scans have been regulated to avoid subjecting patients to scans that are not essential and could pose potential risks [51].

Last, but certainly not least, screening and early identification of prevalent cancers play a vital role. The UAE health authorities have introduced nationwide cancer screening initiatives. Nevertheless, these screening programs still face a challenge in terms of low participation rates. Despite this obstacle, the proportion of patients diagnosed with advanced stage IV breast cancer has notably dropped from 20% to 6% [15].

26.16 Challenges and Advantages

26.16.1 Medical Tourism

The UAE government has provided financial assistance to a substantial number of individuals who are seeking cancer treatment in foreign countries [52]. Each case is evaluated on an individual basis, and a decision to offer medical treatment in another country is made. Several sponsoring agencies in the UAE, including the official health authorities, Armed Forces, Presidential Affairs, Police, and charitable organizations, participate in this process. Additionally, patients have the option to cover their expenses directly through self-payment. UAE citizens predominantly engage in medical tourism for oncology and orthopedic surgery, with cancer treatment accounting for the largest number of trips and associated costs (Salim et al. in 2008). The United States, South Korea, Germany, Singapore, and Thailand are among the countries that cancer patients consider as treatment destinations [53, 15].

Conversely, there has been a recent trend of medical tourism in the opposite direction. In this case, patients from foreign countries are coming to the UAE to access medical assistance. This can be largely attributed to the contemporary healthcare facilities established and backed by the government, as well as prominent private healthcare providers, which have been successful in attracting international professionals to work in the UAE [15].

26.16.2 Future Outlook for Cancer Care in the UAE

As the UAE progresses towards enhancing cancer care services, the collaboration between the public and private sectors has resulted in the formation of entities like the Emirates Oncology Society (EOS), aimed at standardizing oncology healthcare in the UAE [2]. While the UAE possesses a comprehensive range of cancer treatment options and therapies, the government maintains its commitment to assisting individuals who require and opt for treatment abroad. Within the UAE, cancer patients receive ongoing support from the government [15].

The UAE has revealed several new cancer-care tertiary centers, both in the public and private sectors. These hospitals often engage in partnerships with renowned international oncology-care institutions, such as the collaboration between the Mayo Clinic and Sheikh Shakhbout Medical City, or the affiliation between Johns Hopkins Hospital and Tawam Hospital, along with Burjeel Medical City, which earned its 2021 European Society of Medical Oncology (ESMO) accreditation, among other initiatives. The growing presence of exceptionally skilled doctors in the UAE can be attributed to these collaborative endeavors, which provide both intricate and all-encompassing cancer treatment services [15].

With the UAE's economy and population on the rise, the incidence of cancer patients is also increasing, despite the relatively small population. This suggests that there will be a higher number of cancer patients who can achieve improved clinical outcomes when treated in specialized cancer care facilities [54]. EOS has proposed an optimal solution, which involves outfitting cancer care facilities with several satellite centers to establish a centralized cancer care system with conveniently located clinics throughout the country [2].

Another valuable suggestion put forward by EOS is the implementation of a cancer—electronic-health-record system throughout the entire country [2]. Oncologists have the option to access all the genetic workup platforms provided on the website (www.eos.ae). These platforms can be integrated into unified treatment protocols involving different institutions, and there is a plan to establish a national ordering system for chemotherapy/immunotherapy with the goal of enhancing resource allocation in the UAE in the future [15].

A comprehensive approach to cancer care involving a centralized virtual multidisciplinary tumor board that encompasses various healthcare facilities across the UAE can be a valuable resource for advancing cancer care by providing guidance on the diagnosis and treatment of newly diagnosed cancer cases in the UAE [15].

26.17 Conclusion

Despite having a relatively younger population, the United Arab Emirates boasts one of the world's top healthcare systems. A number of public and private healthcare institutions offer comprehensive cancer care services. Strategic initiatives are being devised to position the UAE as a prominent destination for medical tourism in the near future. The quality of complex cancer care in the UAE has been enhanced thanks to highly skilled healthcare professionals and robust governmental backing and logistical support. Further progress is needed to strengthen cooperation with cancer centers, both within the country and on a global scale, including those situated in the Arab region. Clinical trials and cancer research represent key areas for further development and enhancement to support advancements in UAE cancer care.

Conflicts of Interest The authors have no conflicts of interest to declare.

References

1. Ministry of Health and Prevention, Statistics and Research Center, National Disease Registry—UAE National Cancer Registry Report, 2015–2023.
2. Al-Shamsi H, Darr H, Abu-Gheida I, Ansari J, McManus MC, Jaafar H, Tirmazy SH, Elkhoury M, Azribi F, Jelovac D, et al. The state of cancer care in The United Arab Emirates in 2020: challenges and recommendations, a report by The United Arab Emirates oncology task force. Gulf J Oncol. 2020;1:71–87.
3. Shanbhag NM, Antypas C, Msaddi AK, Murphy SC, Singhet TT. Meningioma treated with hypofractionated stereotactic radiotherapy using CyberKnife®: first in The United Arab Emirates. Cureus. 2022;14:e21821. [CrossRef] [PubMed].
4. Al-Shamsi HO, Abyad A, Kaloyannidis P, El-Saddik A, Alrustamani A, Abu Gheida I, Ziade A, Dreier NW, Ul-Haq U, Joshua TLA, et al. Establishment of the first comprehensive adult and pediatric hematopoietic stem cell transplant unit in The United Arab Emirates: rising to the challenge. Clin Pract. 2022;12:84–90. [CrossRef] [PubMed].
5. https://uaelegislation.gov.ae/en/legislations/1206/download#:~:text=It%20is%20prohibited%20to%20smoke,Executive%20Regulations%20of%20this%20Law. (Accessed on 14 Jul 2025).
6. https://www.wam.ae/en/article/bj0bze7-uae-vaccinate-90-girls-aged-13%E2%80%9314-against-hpv. Accessed on 14 Jul 2025.
7. Available online: https://www.doh.gov.ae/en/news/Early-Cancer-Diagnosis-Saves-Lives. Accessed 30 Dec 2023.
8. Available online: https://mohap.gov.ae/en/about-us/projects-and-initiatives/itmenan. Accessed 30 Dec 2023.

9. Available online: https://www.khaleejtimes.com/health/uae-new-screening-facility-launched-for-early-detection-of-diseases. Accessed 30 Dec 2023.
10. Cancer Patient Support Program (BASMAH). Available online: https://www.isahd.ae/content/docs/PD%20PSP%20Program_Basmah%20Guidelines_24-11-2020.pdf. Accessed 30 Dec 2023.
11. Available online: https://www.adphc.gov.ae/en/Public-Health-Programs/Comprehensive-screening-Program%2D%2DIFHAS. Accessed 30 Dec 2023.
12. Available online: https://dha.gov.ae/uploads/112022/National%20Periodic%20Health%20Screening%20Manual%20final20221111119.pdf. Accessed 30 Dec 2023.
13. Al-Shamsi HO. The state of cancer care in the united arab emirates in 2022. Clin Pract. 2022;12(6):955–85. https://doi.org/10.3390/clinpract12060101. PMID: 36547109; PMCID: PMC9777273.
14. Humaid Al-Shamsi S, Humaid Al-Shamsi A, Humaid Al-Shamsi M, Sajwani A, Alzaabi MS, Al Hammadi O, Iqbal F, Al-Shamsi HO. The perception and awareness of the public about cancer and cancer screening in The United Arab Emirates, a population-based survey. Clin Pract. 2023;13:701–14. https://doi.org/10.3390/clinpract13030064.
15. Abu-Gheida IH, Nijhawan N, Al-Awadhi A, Al-Shamsi, HO. General oncology care in the UAE. In: Al-Shamsi HO, Abu-Gheida IH, Iqbal F, Al-Awadhi A. (eds) Cancer in the Arab World. Springer; Singapore. https://doi.org/10.1007/978-981-16-7945-2_19.
16. Radwan H, Ballout RA. The epidemiology and economic burden of obesity and related cardiometabolic disorders in The United Arab Emirates: a systematic review and qualitative synthesis. J Obes. 2018;2018:2185942.
17. Alkharfy KM. Food advertisements: to ban or not to ban? Ann Saudi Med. 2011;31:567–8.
18. https://gulfnews.com/uae/from-december-payextra-for-sweetened-drinks-juices-1.1575109321210. Accessed 2 Jan 2024.
19. https://www.tobaccocontrollaws.org/legislation/united-arab-emirates/summary. Accessed 2 Jan 2024.
20. https://gulfnews.com/uae/mohaps-new-vaccination-policy-for-school-boys-what-uae-parents-need-to-know-1.101890417.
21. Al Awaidy ST, Ezzikouri S. Moving towards hepatitis B elimination in Gulf Health Council states: from commitment to action. J Infect Public Health. 2020;13:221–7.
22. https://www.focp.ae/program-category/community-engagement/.
23. https://www.focp.ae/our-programs/womens-health/.
24. https://www.focp.ae/pink-ocotber/.
25. https://www.focp.ae/our-programs/mens-health/.
26. https://www.focp.ae/our-programs/child-health/.
27. https://www.focp.ae/our-programs/relay-for-life/.
28. https://www.aljalilafoundation.ae/what-we-do/partnerships/brest-friends/.
29. https://eos-uae.com/events/.
30. https://eos-uae.com/breast-cancer-awareness-event-2024/. Accessed on 11 Jul 2025.
31. https://eos-uae.com/liver-cancer/.
32. Grosso D, Aljurf M, Gergis U. Building a comprehensive cancer center: overall structure. In: The comprehensive cancer center: development, integration, and implementation. Cham: Springer International Publishing; 2022. p. 3–13.
33. https://aljalilafoundation.ae/en/our-program/care/hamdan-bin-rashid-cancer-hospital/.
34. Bilimoria KY, Phillips JD, Rock CE, Hayman A, Prystowsky JB, Bentrem DJ. Effect of surgeon training, specialization, and experience on outcomes for cancer surgery: a systematic review of the literature. Ann Surg Oncol. 2009;16:1799–808.
35. Chen IA, Alan H, Ghazi A, Sridhar A, Stoyanov D, Slack M, Kelly JD, Collins JW. Evolving robotic surgery training and improving patient safety, with the integration of novel technologies. World J Urol. 2021;39:2883–93.
36. https://purehealth.ae/rafed/.
37. Available online: https://gulfnews.com/uae/health/burjeel-medical-city-introduces-4d-radiation-radiosurgery-to-treat-cancer-1.88281497. Accessed 4 Jan 2024.

38. Available online: https://viewray.com/find-mridian-mri-guided-radiation-therapy/. Accessed 8 Aug 2022.
39. https://eos-uae.com/.
40. https://eos-uae.com/best-of-astro-gulf/.
41. Available online: https://www.wam.ae/en/details/1395303041032. Accessed 9 Aug 2022.
42. Available online: https://www.cancer.org/cancer/cancer-in-children/how-are-childhood-cancers-treated.html. Accessed 9 Aug 2022.
43. Al-Shamsi HO, Tareen M. Palliative care in The United Arab Emirates, a desperate need. Palliat Med Care. 2018;5:1–4.
44. Emirates Oncology Society. https://eos-uae.com/. Accessed 4 Jan 2024.
45. Nijhawan NA. An update on the state of palliative care development in The United Arab Emirates. Palliat Med Hosp Care Open J. 2022;8:27–9.
46. Al-Shamsi HO, Abyad AM, Rafii S. A proposal for a National Cancer Control Plan for the UAE: 2022–2026. Clin Pract. 2022;12:118–32. https://doi.org/10.3390/clinpract12010016.
47. Al-Shamsi HO. Barriers and facilitators to conducting oncology clinical trials in the UAE. Clin Pract. 2022;12:885–96. https://doi.org/10.3390/clinpract12060093.
48. https://link.springer.com/book/10.1007/978-981-99-6794-0. Accessed on 11 Jul 2025.
49. https://www.wam.ae/en/article/15f6bdn-burjeel-holdings-receives-nihs-accreditation-for. Accessed on 14 Jul 2025.
50. Proposed radiation oncology (RO) model. https://www.cms.gov/newsroom/fact-sheets/proposed-radiation-oncology-ro-model. Accessed 5 Jan 2024.
51. Martinuk SD. The use of positron emission tomography (PET) for cancer care across Canada, Time for a National Strategy. 2011. https://www.triumf.ca/sites/default/files/TRIUMF-AAPS-Martinuk-PET-Across-Canada-REPORT.pdf. Accessed 1 July 2020.
52. 600 million UAE Dirhams spent on cancer care medical tourism. 16 June 2014. http://www.alittihad.ae/details.php?id=90507&y=2014.
53. Sahoo S. Rising numbers in outbound medical tourism. http://www.thenational.ae/business/industry-insights/tourism/risingnumbers-in-outbound-medical-tourism.
54. Pfister DG, Rubin DM, Elkin EB, Neill US, Duck E, Radzyner M, Bach PB. Risk adjusting survival outcomes in hospitals that treat patients with cancer without information on cancer stage. JAMA Oncol. 2015;1(9):1303–10.

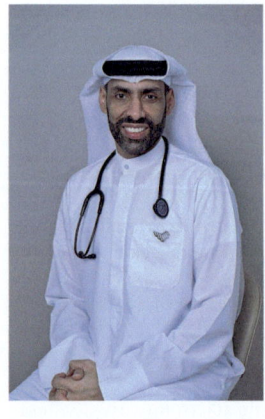

Professor Humaid Obaid Al-Shamsi is the Chief Executive Officer of Burjeel Cancer Institute in Abu Dhabi, UAE; President of the Emirates Oncology Society; Visiting Professor at Harvard Medical School at Harvard University; Visiting Scientist at Dana-Farber Cancer Center, Harvard Medical School, Boston, USA; Full Professor of Oncology at Ras Al Khaimah Medical and Health Sciences University; Ras Al Khaimah, UAE; an Adjunct Professor of Oncology at the College of Medicine, University of Sharjah; and Clinical Professor at Gulf University, Ajman, UAE. He is the first Emirati to be promoted as a professor in oncology in UAE history. He is also the Chairman for Colorectal Cancer in the MENA region, appointed by the prestigious National Comprehensive Cancer Network® in the USA. He is also the only member of the Lung Cancer Policy Network in the MENA region, which aims to advance lung cancer research and screening globally. He is the Chairman of the Oncology and Hematology Fellowship Training Program for the National Institute for Health Specialties in the United Arab Emirates. He is also the only member in the GCC in the WIN Consortium, which comprises organizations representing all stakeholders in personalized cancer medicine globally.

He is board-certified in both internal medicine and oncology from the UK, the USA (ABIM), the National Board of Physicians and Surgeons in the USA, and Canada (FRCPC). He has also been awarded the FRCP (Canada) in 2012, FRCP (London) in 2023, FRCP (Glasgow) in 2024, and FRCP (Edinburgh) in 2025. He is the only physician in the UAE with a subspecialty fellowship certification and training in gastrointestinal oncology and the first Emirati to complete a clinical post-doctoral fellowship in palliative care. He was an Assistant Professor at the University of Texas MD Anderson Cancer Center between 2014 and 2017. He has published more than 170 peer-reviewed articles in *JAMA Oncology, Lancet Oncology, Journal of Clinical Oncology, The Oncologist, BMC Cancer,* and many others. His area of expertise includes precision oncology and cancer care in the UAE. In 2016, he published with his group from MD Anderson in the *Journal of Clinical Oncology* a study describing a new distinct subgroup of colorectal cancer, NON-V600 BRAF-mutated colorectal cancer. In 2022, he published the first book about cancer research in the UAE and also the first book about cancer in the Arab world, both of which were launched at Dubai Expo 2020. *Cancer in the Arab World* has been downloaded more than 500,000 times in its first 2 years of publication and is the ultimate source of cancer data in the Arab region. He also published the first comprehensive book, *Cancer Care in the United Arab Emirates,* which is the first book in UAE history to document cancer care in the UAE, with many topics addressed for the first time. The book was also another success with over 100,000 downloads in the first 2 months of publication.

He is passionate about advancing cancer care in the UAE and the GCC and has made significant contributions to cancer awareness and early detection for the public using social media platforms. He engages actively with the public through awareness campaigns and serves on numerous national health committees, including with the UAE Ministry of Health and the Department of Health, Abu Dhabi.

He is considered the most followed oncologist in the world, with over half a million followers across his social media platforms (Instagram, Twitter, LinkedIn, and TikTok). In 2022, he was awarded the prestigious Feigenbaum Leadership Excellence Award from Sheikh Hamdan Smart University for his exceptional leadership and research, and he was also awarded the Sharjah Award for Volunteering. He was also named the Researcher of the Year in the UAE in 2020 and 2021 by the Emirates Oncology Society.

In May 2024, HH Sheikh Mansour bin Zayed Al Nahyan, Vice President of the United Arab Emirates, awarded him first place in the Emirati Talent Competitiveness Council (NAFIS) program for outstanding leadership in the private sector across all business and medical disciplines. In February 2025, he was awarded the *Sheikha Fatima bint Mubarak Family Award* for being a successful role model in UAE society.

As CEO of Burjeel Cancer Institute, he is leading the largest cancer network in the UAE with over 30 oncologists and hematologists and built the first pediatric bone marrow transplant program in the UAE. He secured the UAE's first European Society for

Medical Oncology (ESMO) accreditation for a cancer center in the UAE at Burjeel Cancer Institute.

Besides his clinical and administrative duties, he is engaged in education and various levels of research training for medical trainees to enhance their clinical and research skills. He established the UAE's first hematology and oncology fellowship training program accredited by the UAE National Institute for Health Specialties at Burjeel Cancer Institute.

His mission is to advance cancer care in the UAE and the MENA region and make cancer care accessible to everyone in need around the globe.

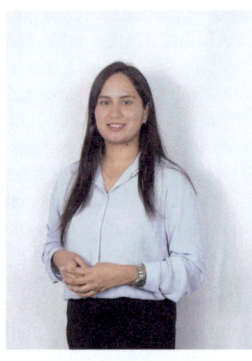

Faryal Iqbal is the Research Manager at Burjeel Cancer Institute, Burjeel Medical City in Abu Dhabi, UAE. She earned her undergraduate degree in Molecular Biology & Biotechnology, followed by a postgraduate qualification in Molecular Genetics in Pakistan, where her thesis explored the association between XRCC1 gene polymorphism and radiation exposure in healthcare workers. At Burjeel Cancer Institute, she is deeply involved in shaping the institute's research landscape. Her role extends beyond managing data and coordinating clinical studies; she mentors medical interns, supports scientific writing, and contributes significantly to the academic and editorial aspects of cancer research.

She is the co-editor of *Cancer in the Arab World*, the first comprehensive book covering cancer care across all Arab countries. The book has resonated widely across the region and beyond, gathering over half a million downloads within just two years. She has authored numerous peer-reviewed publications and contributed to at least ten book chapters, with her research interests rooted in oncology, hematology, and genetics.

In recognition of her growing contributions to the field, she was honored with the "EOS Research Award" by the Emirates Oncology Society in September 2023, an accolade that reflects both her professional excellence and her passion for advancing cancer research in the region.

Open Access This chapter is licensed under the terms of the Creative Commons Attribution 4.0 International License (http://creativecommons.org/licenses/by/4.0/), which permits use, sharing, adaptation, distribution and reproduction in any medium or format, as long as you give appropriate credit to the original author(s) and the source, provide a link to the Creative Commons license and indicate if changes were made.

The images or other third party material in this chapter are included in the chapter's Creative Commons license, unless indicated otherwise in a credit line to the material. If material is not included in the chapter's Creative Commons license and your intended use is not permitted by statutory regulation or exceeds the permitted use, you will need to obtain permission directly from the copyright holder.

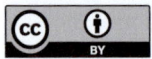

Palliative and Hospice Medicine in the UAE

27

Neil A. Nijhawan, Humaid O. Al-Shamsi, and Halah Ibrahim

27.1 Introduction to Palliative Care

Palliative care (PC) is a comprehensive approach to the care of people who experience severe health-related suffering due to serious illnesses, particularly those approaching the end of life. Its primary objective is to enhance the quality of life for patients, their families, and their caregivers. The fundamental principles and goals

---

N. A. Nijhawan (✉)
Khalifa University College of Medicine and Health Sciences, Abu Dhabi, United Arab Emirates

Burjeel Cancer Institute, Burjeel Medical City, Abu Dhabi, United Arab Emirates

Emirates Oncology Society, Emirates Medical Association, Dubai, United Arab Emirates

Gulf Medical University, Ajman, United Arab Emirates

H. O. Al-Shamsi
Burjeel Cancer Institute, Burjeel Medical City, Abu Dhabi, United Arab Emirates

Department of Medical Oncology, Dana-Farber Cancer Institute, Harvard Medical School, Boston, MA, United States

Harvard Medical School, Harvard University, Boston, MA, United States

College of Medicine, Ras Al Khaimah Medical and Health Sciences University, Al Juwais, Al Qusaidat, Ras Al Khaimah, United Arab Emirates

Gulf Medical University, Ajman, United Arab Emirates

Gulf Cancer Society, Alsafa, Kuwait

Emirates Oncology Society, Dubai, United Arab Emirates

College of Medicine, University of Sharjah, Sharjah, United Arab Emirates
e-mail: humaid.al-shamsi@medportal.ca

© The Author(s) 2025
H. O. Al-Shamsi (ed.), *Healthcare in the United Arab Emirates*,
https://doi.org/10.1007/978-981-96-0523-1_27

- Includes prevention, early identification, comprehensive assessment, and management of physical issues, including pain and other distressing symptoms, psychological distress, spiritual distress, and social needs. Whenever possible, these interventions must be evidence-based.
- Provides support to help patients live as fully as possible until death by facilitating effective communication, helping them and their families determine goals of care.
- Is applicable throughout the course of an illness, according to the patient's needs.
- Is provided in conjunction with disease-modifying therapies whenever needed.
- May positively influence the course of an illness.
- Intends neither to hasten nor postpone death, affirms life, and recognizes dying as a natural process.
- Provides support to the family and the caregivers during the patient's illness and in their own bereavement.
- Is delivered by recognizing and respecting the cultural values and beliefs of the patient and the family.
- Is applicable throughout all health care settings (places of residence and institutions) and at all levels (primary to tertiary).
- Can be provided by professionals with basic palliative care training.
- Requires specialist palliative care with a multiprofessional team for the referral of complex cases.

Fig. 27.1 Principles and aims of palliative care [1]

of palliative care, as defined by the World Health Organization (WHO) [1] (Fig. 27.1), form the basis for this specialized field.

Although the roots of palliative care can be traced back to the post-Second World War period, palliative care gained UK medical specialty status in 1987 and in the U.S. in 2006. In 1967, Dr. Cicely Saunders established the first hospice, St. Christopher's Hospice, in Southeast London. A pivotal moment occurred in 1973 when Dr. Balfour Mount, inspired by his visit to St. Christopher's Hospice, helped establish the first palliative care ward at Montreal's Royal Victoria Hospital in Canada. The term "palliative care" is widely attributed to Dr. Mount.

Essentially, palliative care embodies a multidisciplinary approach to care that one would desire for oneself or a loved one facing a life-limiting illness. It is driven by patient need rather than solely focusing on the diagnosis and is appropriate at any point in a patient's illness, from the point of diagnosis to the end-of-life phase and beyond (Fig. 27.2) [2]. Traditionally, palliative care has been associated with end-of-life care, predominantly based on the experiences of adult patients in advanced stages of cancer. However, an expanding body of literature supports the integration of palliative care with disease-modifying treatments for both nonmalignant conditions [3] and cancer [4].

A groundbreaking study by Jennifer Temel in 2010 [4] demonstrated the benefits of early palliative care involvement from the time of diagnosis for patients with advanced metastatic lung cancer. Patients reported significant improvements in both quality of life and mood. Notably, despite receiving less aggressive end-of-life care compared to the control group, patients receiving early palliative care had a longer median survival of 11.6 months, compared to 8.9 months ($P = 0.02$).

The progression of palliative care from a philosophy of care for the dying to an interprofessional discipline focusing on enhancing the quality of life for patients

H. Ibrahim
Khalifa University College of Medicine and Health Sciences,
Abu Dhabi, United Arab Emirates
e-mail: halah.ibrahim@ku.ac.ae

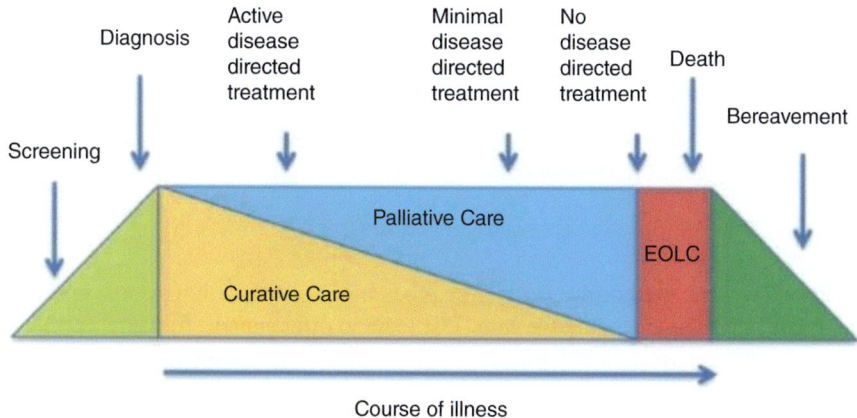

Fig. 27.2 The continuum of palliative and end-of-life care [2]

and their families throughout the disease trajectory is evident. This transformation is evident by the expanded concept of supportive care, particularly in the field of oncology [5]. The benefits of palliative care for patients with noncancer, life-limiting illnesses cannot be overstated. With a globally aging population and the concurrent rise in multimorbidity, the demand for palliative care services will continue to increase [6], including in the United Arab Emirates (UAE).

27.2 Palliative Care Provision in the UAE

Palliative care is a relatively recent addition to the healthcare landscape in the UAE (Fig. 27.3). The first public health palliative care service was established in 2007 at Tawam Hospital in Al Ain, Abu Dhabi, initially as a consultative service for its oncology service. This then evolved into a distinct division within the oncology department, providing outpatient clinics, an inpatient consult service, dedicated inpatient beds, and a palliative care nurse outreach service. Currently, the Tawam palliative care team is the sole provider of palliative care services within the public health service. Since 2015, the number of palliative care services has grown within the private healthcare sector. The American Hospital in Dubai offers outpatient clinics, inpatient consult services, and inpatient palliative care beds, with the majority of their referrals coming from patients with cancer diagnoses.

In September 2019, Mediclinic City Hospital in Dubai launched its palliative care service, which currently includes outpatient clinics, inpatient reviews, and a consult service. A consult service was also initiated at Parkview Hospital, a sister facility, in 2020. Most recently, a new palliative and supportive care service at Burjeel Medical City (BMC) in Abu Dhabi was established in March 2020. Similar to Tawam Hospital, BMC offers a comprehensive palliative care service, integrating outpatient clinics with pain medicine, physical medicine, and rehabilitation clinics. They provide dedicated palliative care inpatient beds and a palliative care nurse

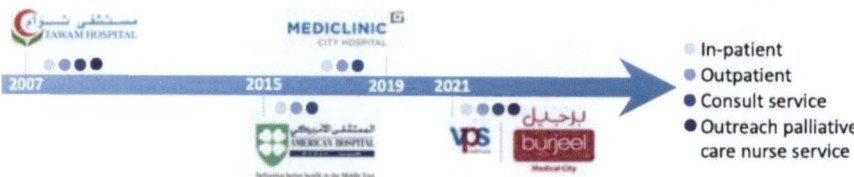

Fig. 27.3 The UAE Palliative Care landscape timeline [7]

outreach service. Within the Burjeel healthcare ecosystem, a homecare service is available, enabling the palliative care (PC) team to offer support for patients requiring palliative care and end-of-life care in the comfort of their own homes.

27.3 Factors Influencing Palliative Care Provision in the UAE

27.3.1 Philosophy and Culture

While the focus in Western medical ethics is on the autonomy of the individual patient, in contrast, in Middle Eastern cultures, the extended family is the central social institution and the main decision-maker. Middle Eastern patients typically rely heavily on their personal support network during a crisis or illness; this contrasts with Western ideals of individual autonomy and maintaining personal independence. Within the UAE, such support networks, particularly the extended family support network, are not always available, particularly for expatriate workers, who comprise almost 90% of the population [8].

Islam in the Middle East is a way of life, with particular beliefs that inform attitudes towards health and illness. Common themes include the beliefs that [9]:

- Each person's fate is sealed the moment their soul is created. Even though fate is predetermined, a person cannot know their fate, so it is wise to strive for God's favor through obedience.
- Illness is sent from God as a punishment.
- Everything is in accordance with God's master plan.

These beliefs are reflected in the almost fatalistic attitude of acceptance of death and disease. This attitude is tempered by the belief that Islam views it as a duty to preserve life until God decides that it will slip away. Such a dichotomy results in healthcare providers being faced with the common scenario where a patient with an advanced progressive illness is rapidly deteriorating and not expected to survive, but the family will often insist that "everything must be tried." Discussions focused on maintaining the quality of life for the patient by not subjecting them to medically futile interventions are often poorly received and viewed in a negative light, with the perception being that the doctors are giving up hope. Because only God knows how poor a prognosis is, hope should never wane, and to give up hope would mean forfeiting God's help. Even if hope is futile by Western medical standards, the belief remains that hope helps a patient cope with their illness. Taking this hope away from the patient by communicating openly is considered both tactless and unforgivable [10]. These beliefs usually underlie the differences in opinion that are apparent when doctors talk about the need to be open and honest with patients about their illness and contribute to the high levels of expectation that the population has about what medical interventions are able to provide. Hope is not a static phenomenon; there is evidence that what patients hope for changes over time [11]. It is also well documented that patients will often wait for family members to leave the room before asking the doctor to be honest with them and confirm their suspicions about their illness, this is a global phenomenon [11, 12].

While it is important to be open and honest in conversations with the patient and their family, it is important to acknowledge that not all patients wish to know all the details of their condition. PC consultations will often begin with a question about how much information the patient wants to have. Are they the sort of person who likes having all the details, or are they satisfied with knowing just enough. It is useful to have this conversation in the presence of family members in order to reassure them that there is no hidden agenda to the consultation and that it will be done according to the patient's or family's preference and at their pace.

27.3.2 Workforce Capacity and Training

The availability of a skilled and trained workforce is crucial for palliative care service provision. Palliative care requires a multidisciplinary approach involving physicians, nurses, social workers, psychologists, and other healthcare professionals. In the UAE, there is a need for increased palliative care clinical capacity across various healthcare disciplines to ensure a competent workforce capable of addressing the complex needs of patients and their families.

Almost all publications that focus on the barriers to PC provision comment on the attitudes of healthcare providers. The stigma attached to PC teams is present globally, including here in the UAE, with the prevailing impression that palliative care is just about pain management and end-of-life care [13].

The WHO notes that improving palliative care services in a country requires the incorporation of palliative medicine education into the country's medical schools and health professional training programs [14, 15]. Teaching palliative and end-of-life care is increasingly recognized as an important component of medical education [15]. There is a large body of literature, however, that reveals that palliative medicine education is limited and inconsistent in undergraduate and postgraduate medical curricula worldwide, leaving students and residents ill-prepared to manage seriously ill patients.

A recent publication confirmed that palliative medicine is not prioritized in the country's medical schools and postgraduate programs. A survey of medical school graduates revealed that over half of the respondents did not receive any formal PC education in medical school [16]. Only 13% of respondents participated in clinical PC rotations, with only 25% reporting any assessment of PC knowledge or skills during medical school. Approximately 75% of the students admitted that they never or rarely witnessed patient-physician communication regarding a terminal prognosis. The vast majority described a lack of comfort in providing care for dying patients and their families.

A study of UAE medical schools highlighted the gaps in PC education [17]. Only one medical school offered a dedicated palliative medicine course within the curriculum, and none of the schools required a palliative care rotation to be a core requirement. Typically, PC topics were most often incorporated into other topics. The number of hours allocated to PC content differed widely between the schools, as did the concepts covered. The most frequently taught topics were pain management, end-of-life communication skills, and the ethics of terminal care. None of the universities had academic faculty positions for PC specialists. Clinical and bedside teaching in PC was limited and primarily led by faculty who lacked prior PC training or expertise. Other professions, including nurses, social workers, and faith-based leaders, were not routinely involved in PC teaching. Although the UAE medical school deans all recognized the importance of inculcating palliative and end-of-life care into the undergraduate curriculum, they reported several barriers, including limited clinical PC training facilities, a lack of specialized faculty, and cultural barriers to PC education.

Residency programs in the UAE also face similar challenges. In a qualitative study of all internal medicine residency program directors in the UAE, the program directors agreed that PC knowledge and skills were an essential component of postgraduate training but had mixed results in implementing its components [17]. The program directors cited the lack of specialized PC faculty, cultural resistance to PC services, and the lack of formal end-of-life hospital policies as the main barriers to teaching PC. Only one residency program offered a structured PC curriculum, and only one program mandated a dedicated PC clinical rotation, but the allotted time was two weeks, and exposure was limited to patients with cancer diagnoses. PC training was most often embedded into other rotations, namely oncology, intensive care, general internal medicine, and geriatrics. The most common topics covered included the core principles of PC, pain management, and end-of-life communication. Symptom management at the end of life was rarely taught.

As education is a central measure of PC status worldwide, the lack of standardized PC education in the country's medical schools and residency programs can impede the advancement of PC services in the UAE. However, curricular changes are currently underway. Many medical schools and residency programs are working to develop and implement PC curricula. In addition, several academic medical centers in the UAE have planned the expansion of their oncology centers with dedicated PC units and anticipate the recruitment of trained PC specialists. This will increase clinical training opportunities for medical students and residents. With these reforms, the UAE medical education system will better prepare a future generation of health professionals to provide quality PC services to UAE patients and their families.

While social workers and psychologists do exist within some UAE hospitals, many of them may not have received specific training in palliative care. This highlights the need for additional training and education in palliative care for these professionals to ensure comprehensive and holistic care for patients and their families.

Spiritual care is an essential component of palliative care, as it addresses the spiritual needs and concerns of patients and their families. While most palliative care clinicians have some training in assessing patients' spiritual care needs, the role of a chaplain is important in providing specialized support in this area. Chaplains are trained to offer a nonjudgmental listening presence to patients and their families, regardless of their religious or spiritual beliefs. However, the role of hospital chaplains is not yet established in the UAE, despite the country's diverse population comprising expatriates from different cultural and religious backgrounds. Being able to provide culturally sensitive spiritual care for patients approaching the end of life is crucial.

27.3.3 Access to Essential Palliative Care Medications

The impression that PC is primarily about pain management is understandable, given that pain is the single most prevalent symptom for patients receiving PC [18]. Pain control at the end of life is the right of the patient and the duty of the healthcare provider. The World Health Organization's position is clear: patients have a right to have their pain treated and controlled adequately based on clear guidelines and recommendations [19]. We know from experience that uncontrolled pain affects all aspects of a person's life. When pain is better controlled, there is a sense of well-being, and therefore an improved quality of life. It is important, however, to highlight the fact that the availability of analgesics has not eliminated the problem of ineffective pain control, with the WHO estimating that there are approximately 5 billion people living in countries with little or no access to pain medicines, including 5.5 million terminal cancer patients [20], 80% of whom are estimated to experience moderate to severe pain due to inequitable access to medicines.

In PC, pain relief is a priority. When pain is better controlled, there is improved overall comfort, which makes it easier for patients to talk openly about their hopes, fears, and dreams. Although we utilize the full range of interventions to help alleviate pain, including nonpharmacological techniques and radiation therapy in the case of certain cancers, opioids remain essential for the management of moderate to severe pain.

Severe cancer-related pain is poorly managed by nonspecialists. The WHO guidelines for cancer pain in adults [21] recommend the three-step analgesic ladder (Fig. 27.4), although there is no pharmacological need for Step 2, and compared to

Fig. 27.4 The World Health Organization three-step analgesic ladder [21]

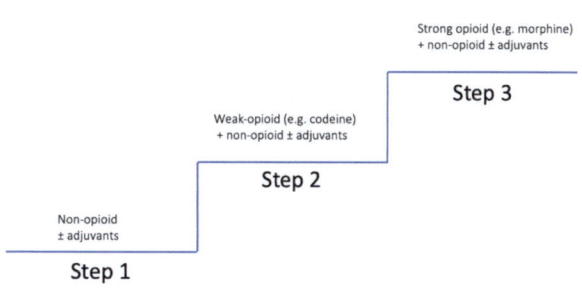

weak Step 2 opioids, the benefit from low-dose morphine (20–30 mg/24 h PO) is greater and more rapid [22]. Step 2 opioids exist because in many countries, accessing strong (Step 3) opioids is difficult and sometimes impossible, despite the fact that morphine is relatively cheap and is the most widely available and best-characterized opioid analgesic.

According to the *Atlas of Palliative Care in the Eastern Mediterranean region*, the median consumption of opioids (excluding Methadone) within the UAE is 3.03% as compared to the regional median of 3.27% [23]. International Narcotic Control Board (INCB) data demonstrate that overall opioid consumption within the UAE is lower than expected, with an defined daily dose for statistical purposes SDDD-defined daily dose for statistical purposes per million inhabitants per day of 162, where <200 is categorized as inadequate and <100 as very inadequate usage [24].

Severe cancer-related pain can be difficult to manage without opioids. This may be exacerbated by a physician's discomfort with treating pain with strong opioids, especially in cases of severe complex pain. This fear of opioid abuse or misuse by the patient may actually be a barrier to effective pain management.

In actual fact, within the UAE, we have access to the majority of the essential PC medicines as recommended by the International Association of Hospice and Palliative Care (IAHPC)—Table 27.1 [25]. One exception is the oral preparation of Levomepromazine, an antipsychotic medication that is commonly used in PC for delirium, nausea, vomiting, and terminal restlessness. Oral Methadone 5 mg tablets are available, as are both oral (immediate and sustained release) and injectable forms of Hydromorphone.

27.3.3.1 Barriers to Opioid Prescribing

The two main barriers to opioid prescribing are (1) the general perception that taking a strong opioid will invariably lead to addiction, and (2) restrictions on accessing and prescribing strong opioids and other commonly used medications. Opioid-phobia is made worse by increased public awareness of the issue of illicit substance abuse within the region. A 2015 study [26] examined the use of illicit substances among 250 male patients recruited from the National Rehabilitation Centre in Abu Dhabi and illustrated that opioids and alcohol were the most common substances used. In the younger age group (<30 years), Tramadol was the most commonly used, with Heroin preferred among the older age group (=30 years). Other drugs of abuse among younger patients included Pregabalin, Procyclidine, and Carisoprodol.

The implementation, in 2019, of a national online prescribing platform [27] that requires the insertion of the patient's national identity card (Emirates ID) into a specialized card reader has meant that it is easier to track and monitor the prescription and dispensing of controlled and narcotic medications (including opioids). This has provided a degree of safety for the prescriber and reduced the risk of misuse of opioid medications. Additionally, the platform helps reduce inefficiencies caused by the loss of paper prescriptions, in addition to ensuring accurate tracking of prescriptions and dispensing of drugs.

Table 27.1 The IAHPC list of essential medications for palliative care [25]

Medication	Formulation	Indication	UAE availability
Amitriptyline	50 mg tablets	Depression Neuropathic pain	Yes
Bisacodyl	10 mg tablets 10 mg rectal suppositories	Constipation	Yes Yes
Carbamazepine	100–200 mg tablets	Neuropathic pain	Yes
Citalopram	10–20 mg tablets	Depression	Yes
Codeine	30 mg tablets	Pain: mild to moderate Diarrhea	Yes
Dexamethasone	0.5–4 mg tablets 4 mg/ml injection	Anorexia Nausea & vomiting Neuropathic pain	Yes
Diazepam	2.5–10 mg tablets 5 mg/ml injection 10 mg rectal suppository	Anxiety Muscle relaxant	Yes Yes Yes
Diclofenac	25–50 mg tablets 50–75 mg/3 ml injection	Inflammatory pain	Yes
Diphenhydramine	25 mg tablets 50 mg/ml injection	Antihistamine Motion sickness	
Fentanyl transdermal patch	12.5–100 micrograms/hour	Pain: moderate to severe	Yes
Gabapentin	300–400 mg tablets	Neuropathic pain	Yes
Haloperidol	0.5–5 mg tablets 0.5–5 mg/ml injection	Delirium Nausea & vomiting Terminal restlessness	Yes
Hyoscine butylbromide	10 mg tablets 10 mg/ml injection	Visceral pain Nausea & vomiting Terminal respiratory congestion	Yes
Ibuprofen	200–400 mg tablets	Inflammatory pain	Yes
Levomepromazine	5–50 mg tablets 25 mg/ml injection	Delirium Terminal restlessness	No No
Loperamide	2 mg tablets	Diarrhea	Yes
Lorazepam	0.5–2 mg tablets 2–4 mg/ml injection	Anxiety	Yes Yes
Megestrol acetate	160 mg tablets 40 mg/ml solution	Anorexia	Yes Yes
Methadone	5 mg tablets	Pain: moderate to severe Neuropathic pain	Yes
Metoclopramide	10 mg tablets 5 mg/ml injection	Nausea & vomiting	Yes
Midazolam	1–5 mg/ml injection	Anxiety Terminal restlessness	Yes
Fleet® Mineral oil enema			Yes

(continued)

Table 27.1 (continued)

Medication	Formulation	Indication	UAE availability
Mirtazapine	15–30 mg tablets	Depression Anorexia	Yes
Morphine	Immediate release 10–60 mg tablets Immediate release 10 mg/5 ml solution Immediate release 10 mg/ml injection Sustained release 10 mg tablets Sustained release 30 mg tablets	Pain: moderate to severe Dyspnea	Yes Yes Yes Yes Yes
Octreotide	100micrograms/ml injection	Diarrhea Vomiting	Yes
Oral rehydration salts		Diarrhea	Yes
Oxycodone	5 mg tablets	Pain: moderate to severe	Yes
Paracetamol	100–500 mg tablets 500 mg rectal suppositories	Pain: mild to moderate	Yes
Prednisolone (dexamethasone alt)	5 mg tablets	Anorexia	Yes
Senna	8.6 mg tablets	Constipation	Yes
Tramadol	50 mg immediate release tablets/capsules 50 mg/ml injection	Pain: mild to moderate	Yes
Trazodone	25–75 mg tablets	Insomnia	Yes
Zolpidem	5–10 mg tablets	Insomnia	Yes

More pertinent is the restrictive regulation of prescribing controlled medications. More specifically:

- Only consultant physicians can prescribe a 30-day supply of controlled medications, all other physicians are permitted to prescribe only a 7- to 14- day supply.
- Current regulations do not permit the prescription of injectable controlled medicines (including opioids and other centrally acting medicines) for patients outside the hospital. We are therefore unable to initiate an intravenous or subcutaneous infusion for patients at home who are approaching the end of life and who require injectable medications for symptom control.

27.3.4 Legal and Regulatory Framework

Legal and regulatory frameworks play a crucial role in shaping palliative care services. In the UAE, there is currently no palliative care-specific legislation or regulatory framework. This lack of clear guidelines and policies can create challenges in the provision of palliative care, including issues related to medication access, controlled substances, and advance care planning. However, efforts are underway to address these gaps and develop appropriate regulations for palliative care.

27.3.5 Public Awareness and Perception

Public awareness and perception of palliative care can influence its acceptance and utilization. Lack of awareness about the benefits of palliative care, misconceptions, and cultural beliefs and attitudes towards pain and pain management, including opioids, can contribute to its underutilization or delayed access to palliative care services. Public education campaigns and initiatives are essential for raising awareness, dispelling myths, and promoting a better understanding of palliative care among the population. Although there have been recent newspaper articles in the UAE highlighting the need for palliative care [28], there remains a significant mismatch between patient and family expectations and the reality of what modern medicine is able to achieve [29].

27.3.6 Financing Palliative Care Services

Remuneration for healthcare services, whether delivered within the government health service or the private sector, is either part of a health insurance ecosystem or self-paid by the patient. Within the UAE, each emirate has different laws for medical insurance, with Abu Dhabi and Dubai mandating that employers are legally obligated to provide medical cover for employees and their dependents. The current reimbursement system has added complexity to being able to offer PC input to patients. Traditionally, medical insurance companies did not cover palliative care input for their policy holders, although this has now changed with the adoption of specific diagnosis-related group (DRG) codes for palliative care, covering both inpatient and outpatient consultations. Although the financial justifications for PC have been clearly established, there is no UAE-specific data available at present.

Addressing these factors requires a comprehensive and collaborative approach involving government authorities, healthcare institutions, healthcare professionals, educators, and the community. By addressing these challenges, the UAE can further enhance the provision of palliative care and thus improve the quality of life for patients with serious life-limiting illnesses.

27.3.7 Advanced Care Planning (ACP)

ACP is an important aspect of palliative care, particularly for patients with progressive, life-limiting illnesses. ACP involves making decisions about the care a person would like to receive in case they are unable to communicate their preferences. While advance directives, which outline specific healthcare wishes, are not legally recognized in the UAE, discussions about a patient's preferences with their relatives are considered standard of care. Cultural attitudes towards serious illness in the UAE often emphasize reliance on faith and continuing with all medical treatments, even if they are deemed futile. This may lead to moral distress among healthcare workers who feel compelled to prolong patients' suffering in pursuit of curative treatments.

Allowing natural death and Do Not Attempt Cardio-Pulmonary Resuscitation (DNACPR) decisions are important considerations in end-of-life care. CPR is an invasive medical treatment intended for patients with reversible conditions and is not appropriate for those who are dying from irreversible illnesses. The UAE Federal Law No. 4 on Medical Liability [30] of 2016 permits healthcare professionals to refrain from performing CPR on terminally ill or dying patients who have exhausted treatment options and when resuscitation is deemed medically useless. However, if a patient explicitly requests CPR, it cannot be prevented, even if it is considered futile. The frequency of utilizing the allow natural death policy or patient requests for full CPR in terminally ill patients in the UAE is not currently available through national-level statistics, although data from the Burjeel palliative care service demonstrate that 90% of patients receiving end-of-life care on the ward agreed to a do not resuscitate status [29]. Currently, the majority of patients receive end-of-life care in hospitals in the UAE [29]. Patients who desire home-based end-of-life care are highly unlikely to have this preference honored due to the lack of (1) formalized community PC teams or community palliative care units (Hospices), and (2) the inability to prescribe injectable medicines (e.g., opioids) outside the hospital environment.

27.4 Conclusion

PC provision remains significantly lacking within the UAE. As the world's population ages and the prevalence of cancer and other life-limiting illnesses increases, so too will the need for more comprehensive palliative care services. Given the worldwide shortage of PC-trained nurses and doctors, improving PC within the UAE will not simply be a matter of recruiting more healthcare professionals. Our recommendations for improving palliative care in the UAE were highlighted in a previous publication [31], and these have been refined further and illustrated diagrammatically [29] in Fig. 27.5.

These recommendations take into account the specific challenges and cultural context of the UAE. It is important to address issues related to the availability and training of healthcare professionals, including all members of the interdisciplinary team. Providing specialized palliative-care training for these professionals is essential to ensuring the delivery of high-quality, holistic care.

In conclusion, improving palliative care in the UAE requires a comprehensive and multidisciplinary approach that addresses the availability and training of

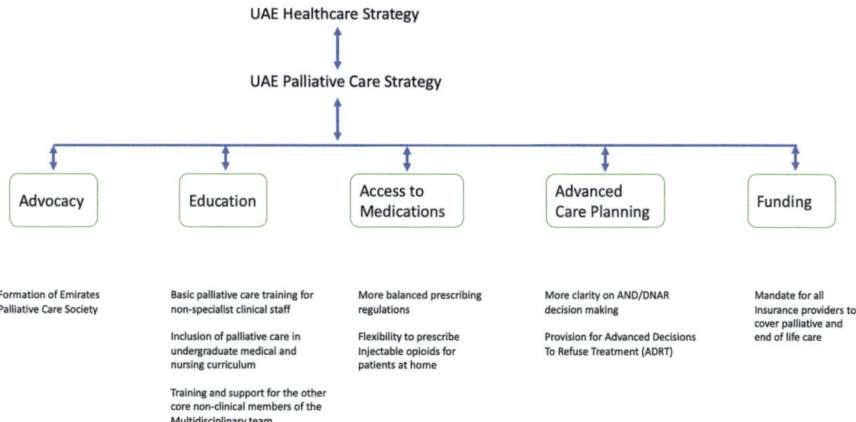

Fig. 27.5 Recommendations for palliative care in the UAE

healthcare professionals, recognizes the importance of spiritual care, involves physiotherapists and occupational therapists, promotes advanced care planning, and ensures appropriate financial support. By implementing these recommendations, the UAE can enhance its palliative care services and provide compassionate and comprehensive care to patients and their families facing life-limiting illnesses.

Conflicts of Interest The authors have no conflicts of interest to declare.

References

1. https://www.who.int/cancer/palliative/definition/en/.
2. Myatra SN, Salins N, Iyer S, Macaden SC, Divatia JV, Muckaden M, et al. End-of-life care policy: an integrated care plan for the dying: a Joint Position Statement of the Indian Society of Critical Care Medicine (ISCCM) and the Indian Association of Palliative Care (IAPC). Indian J Crit Care Med. 2014;18;615–35. https://doi.org/10.4103/0972-5229.140155.
3. Kingston AEH, Kirkland J, Hadjimichalis A. Palliative care in non-malignant disease. Medicine. 2020;48(1):37–2. https://doi.org/10.1016/j.mpmed.2019.10.010.
4. Temel 2010 paper. https://doi.org/10.1056/NEJMoa1000678.
5. https://www.esmo.org/guidelines/supportive-and-palliative-care?page=2.
6. Etkind, et al. How many people will need palliative care in 2040? Past trends, future projections and implications for services. BMC Med. 2017;15:102. https://doi.org/10.1186/s12916-017-0860-2.
7. Nijhawan NA. An update on the state of palliative care development in the United Arab Emirates. Palliat Med Hosp Care Open J. 2022;8(2):27–9. https://doi.org/10.17140/PMHCOJ-8-149.
8. https://www.statista.com/statistics/984373/uae-expat-population-by-country-of-origin/.
9. Lipson JG, Meleis AI. Issues in health care of Middle Eastern patients. West J Med. 1983;139(6):854–61. PMID: 6364575.
10. Meleis AI, Jonsen AR. Ethical crises and cultural differences. West J Med. 1983;138:889–93. PMID: 6613119.
11. Daneault S. Ultimate journey of the terminally ill, ways and pathways of hope. Can Fam Physician. 2016;62(8):648–56. PMID: 27521394.

12. Srivastava guardian article. https://www.theguardian.com/commentisfree/2018/apr/04/should-a-doctor-always-disclose-a-terminal-diagnosis.
13. Al-Alfi N. Palliative care in the United Arab Emirates: a nurse's perspectives. J Palliat Care Med. 2015;S5:S5–005. https://doi.org/10.4172/2165-7386.1000S5006.
14. World Health Organization. Worldwide hospice palliative care alliance. Global atlas of palliative care. 2nd ed. Geneva; 2020.
15. Mason S, Paal P, Elsner F, et al. Palliative care for all: an international health education challenge. Palliat Support Care. 2020;18(6):760–2. https://doi.org/10.1017/S1478951520000188.
16. Ibrahim H, Lootah S, Satish KP, Harhara T. Medical student experiences and perceptions of palliative care in a middle eastern country. BMC Med Educ. 2022;22(1):371.
17. Harhara T, Ibrahim H. Undergraduate palliative care education in the United Arab Emirates: a nationwide assessment of medical school deans. BMC Med Educ. 2021;21:526.
18. https://doi.org/10.1191/0269216303pm760oa.
19. Carlson CL. Effectiveness of the World Health Organisation cancer pain relief guidelines: an integrative review. J Pain Res. 2016;2016(9):515–34. https://doi.org/10.2147/JPR.S97759.
20. Global Alliance to Pain Relief Initiative (GAPRI). Access to essential pain medicines brief. 2010. Available from: http://www.gapri.org/understand-problem.
21. https://www.who.int/cancer/palliative/painladder/en/.
22. Twycross RG, et al. Palliative care formulary. 6th ed; 2019. p. 295–6. ISBN 9780857113481.
23. Osman H, Rihan A, Garralda E, Rhee JY, Pons JJ, de Lima L, Tfayli A, Centeno C. Atlas of palliative care in the eastern Mediterranean region. Houston: IAHPC Press; 2017.
24. INCB. Narcotic drugs estimated world requirements for 2020. 2019. ISBN: 978-92-1-148309-3.
25. IAHPC list of essential medications. https://hospicecare.com/what-we-do/projects/palliative-care-essentials/iahpc-essential-medicines-for-palliative-care/.
26. Alblooshi H, et al. The pattern of substance use disorder in the United Arab Emirates in 2015: results of a National Rehabilitation Centre Cohort Study. Subst Abuse Treat Prev Policy. 2016;11:19. https://doi.org/10.1186/s13011-016-0062-5.
27. https://doh.gov.ae/en/news/Department-of-Health-adopts-Unified-Electronic-Platform-for-narcotic-drugs-and-controlled-medicines.
28. https://www.khaleejtimes.com/lifestyle/health/caring-for-the-terminally-ill-in-uae-how-palliative-care-providers-help-patients-families.
29. Nijhawan NA, Al-Shamsi HO. Experiences and challenges of a new palliative care service in the United Arab Emirates. Palliat Med Hosp Care Open J. 2022;8(2):30–4. https://doi.org/10.17140/PMHCOJ-8-150.
30. https://www.dha.gov.ae/Asset%20Library/MarketingAssets/20180611/(E)%20Federal%20Decree%20no.%204%20of%202016.pdf.
31. https://doi.org/10.1007/978-3-319-74365-3_102-1.

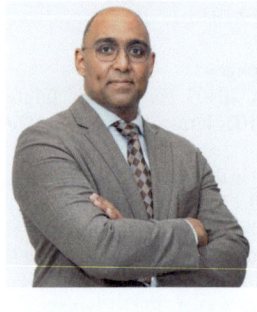

Dr. Neil A. Nijhawan is a UK-trained consultant in Palliative Medicine at Burjeel Cancer Institute, Burjeel Medical City. After medical school at King's College London, he pursued specialty training in Palliative Medicine in London, with rotations in acute general hospitals, domiciliary visits, community hospices, and tertiary oncology centres. Before completing his palliative medicine training, Neil returned to his childhood home, Trinidad in the West Indies, to help set up and commission the new Caura Hospital Palliative Care Unit, where he was the Medical Director. This unit was opened in 2014 and provides a comprehensive palliative care service, including a 12-bed inpatient unit, weekly outpatient clinics, and a palliative care consult service at the local university hospital. After completing his specialty training, Neil worked as a consultant in palliative medicine at the Imperial College Healthcare NHS Trust in London, where he was the clinical lead for palliative medicine. His clinical area of interest is symptom control (including pain, nausea, breathlessness, and fatigue) and assistance with complex treatment decision-making at the end of life, and he is often called on to provide an independent second opinion. He is active in palliative care education and palliative care advocacy and is currently the UAE representative to the WHO Eastern Mediterranean Region Palliative Care Expert Network. Neil holds adjunct faculty positions with both Khalifa University and Gulf Medical University, where he is Clinical Associate Professor in Hospice & Palliative Medicine.

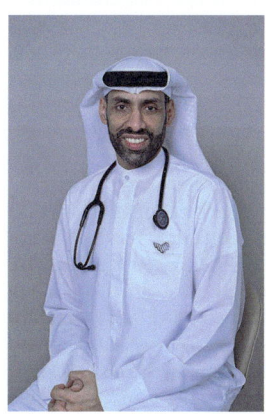

Professor Humaid Obaid Al-Shamsi is the Chief Executive Officer of Burjeel Cancer Institute in Abu Dhabi, UAE; President of the Emirates Oncology Society; Visiting Professor at Harvard Medical School at Harvard University; Visiting Scientist at Dana-Farber Cancer Center, Harvard Medical School, Boston, USA; Full Professor of Oncology at Ras Al Khaimah Medical and Health Sciences University; Ras Al Khaimah, UAE; an Adjunct Professor of Oncology at the College of Medicine, University of Sharjah; and Clinical Professor at Gulf University, Ajman, UAE. He is the first Emirati to be promoted as a professor in oncology in UAE history. He is also the Chairman for Colorectal Cancer in the MENA region, appointed by the prestigious National Comprehensive Cancer Network® in the USA. He is also the only member of the Lung Cancer Policy Network in the MENA region, which aims to advance lung cancer research and screening globally. He is the Chairman of the Oncology and Hematology Fellowship Training Program for the National Institute for Health Specialties in the United Arab Emirates. He is also the only member in the GCC in the WIN Consortium, which comprises organizations representing all stakeholders in personalized cancer medicine globally.

He is board-certified in both internal medicine and oncology from the UK, the USA (ABIM), the National Board of Physicians and Surgeons in the USA, and Canada (FRCPC). He has also been awarded the FRCP (Canada) in 2012, FRCP (London) in 2023, FRCP (Glasgow) in 2024, and FRCP (Edinburgh) in 2025. He is the only physician in the UAE with a subspecialty fellowship certification and training in gastrointestinal oncology and the first Emirati to complete a clinical post-doctoral fellowship in palliative care. He was an Assistant Professor at the University of Texas MD Anderson Cancer Center between 2014 and 2017. He has published more than 170 peer-reviewed articles in *JAMA Oncology, Lancet Oncology, Journal of Clinical Oncology, The Oncologist, BMC Cancer,* and many others. His area of expertise includes precision oncology and cancer care in the UAE. In 2016, he published with his group from MD Anderson in the *Journal of Clinical Oncology* a study describing a new distinct subgroup of colorectal cancer, NON-V600 BRAF-mutated colorectal cancer. In 2022, he published the first book about cancer research in the UAE and also the first book about cancer in the Arab world, both of which were launched at Dubai Expo 2020. *Cancer in the Arab World* has been downloaded more than 500,000 times in its first 2 years of publication and is the ultimate source of cancer data in the Arab region.

He also published the first comprehensive book, *Cancer Care in the United Arab Emirates*, which is the first book in UAE history to document cancer care in the UAE, with many topics addressed for the first time. The book was also another success with over 100,000 downloads in the first 2 months of publication.

He is passionate about advancing cancer care in the UAE and the GCC and has made significant contributions to cancer awareness and early detection for the public using social media platforms. He engages actively with the public through awareness campaigns and serves on numerous national health committees, including with the UAE Ministry of Health and the Department of Health, Abu Dhabi.

He is considered the most followed oncologist in the world, with over half a million followers across his social media platforms (Instagram, Twitter, LinkedIn, and TikTok). In 2022, he was awarded the prestigious Feigenbaum Leadership Excellence Award from Sheikh Hamdan Smart University for his exceptional leadership and research, and he was also awarded the Sharjah Award for Volunteering. He was also named the Researcher of the Year in the UAE in 2020 and 2021 by the Emirates Oncology Society.

In May 2024, HH Sheikh Mansour bin Zayed Al Nahyan, Vice President of the United Arab Emirates, awarded him first place in the Emirati Talent Competitiveness Council (NAFIS) program for outstanding leadership in the private sector across all business and medical disciplines. In February 2025, he was awarded the *Sheikha Fatima bint Mubarak Family Award* for being a successful role model in UAE society.

As CEO of Burjeel Cancer Institute, he is leading the largest cancer network in the UAE with over 30 oncologists and hematologists and built the first pediatric bone marrow transplant program in the UAE. He secured the UAE's first European Society for Medical Oncology (ESMO) accreditation for a cancer center in the UAE at Burjeel Cancer Institute.

Besides his clinical and administrative duties, he is engaged in education and various levels of research training for medical trainees to enhance their clinical and research skills. He established the UAE's first hematology and oncology fellowship training program accredited by the UAE National Institute for Health Specialties at Burjeel Cancer Institute.

His mission is to advance cancer care in the UAE and the MENA region and make cancer care accessible to everyone in need around the globe.

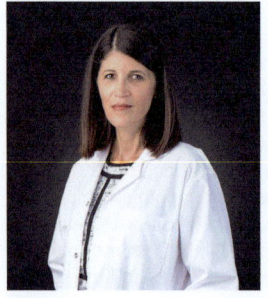

Halah Ibrahim, MD, MEHP is an internist and clinician-educator with over 25 years of experience in undergraduate and postgraduate medical education in the United States and United Arab Emirates. Her research interests include international medical education reform and end-of-life education and communication. Dr. Ibrahim is a graduate of the Mount Sinai School of Medicine and completed her internship and residency at The New York Hospital - Cornell Medical Center (currently New York Presbyterian University Hospital of Columbia and Cornell). She holds a master's degree in health professions education from Johns Hopkins University.

Open Access This chapter is licensed under the terms of the Creative Commons Attribution 4.0 International License (http://creativecommons.org/licenses/by/4.0/), which permits use, sharing, adaptation, distribution and reproduction in any medium or format, as long as you give appropriate credit to the original author(s) and the source, provide a link to the Creative Commons license and indicate if changes were made.

The images or other third party material in this chapter are included in the chapter's Creative Commons license, unless indicated otherwise in a credit line to the material. If material is not included in the chapter's Creative Commons license and your intended use is not permitted by statutory regulation or exceeds the permitted use, you will need to obtain permission directly from the copyright holder.

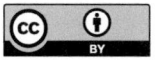

Pathology and Laboratory Medicine in the UAE

28

Laila Osama AbdelWareth and Annisah Binti Abdullah

28.1 The Birth of Pathology and Laboratory Medicine (PLM) in the UAE

Laboratory medicine was first founded as a department under the preventive medicine division in the Ministry of Health (MOH) back in 1972. The MOH at that time was tasked with operating all healthcare facilities in the United Arab Emirates (UAE), including hospital laboratories and later blood donor centers. In the 1970s, there were only seven hospitals in the entire UAE and one main laboratory at that time, called "The Central Laboratory," which was located at Central Hospital in Abu Dhabi. The Central Laboratory had the only anatomic pathology laboratory for the MOH hospitals at that time.

28.2 Regulatory Landscape

Pathology and laboratory medicine are branches of medicine that are heavily regulated. Quality control processes and standards are deeply embedded in this profession.

L. O. AbdelWareth (✉)
National Reference Laboratory, Abu Dhabi, United Arab Emirates

Clinical Pathology, Cleveland Clinic, Abu Dhabi, United Arab Emirates

Department of Pathology, College of Medicine & Health Sciences, Khalifa University, Abu Dhabi, United Arab Emirates

Global Patient Care, M42, Abu Dhabi, United Arab Emirates
e-mail: WarethL@nrl.ae

A. B. Abdullah
National Reference Laboratory, Abu Dhabi, United Arab Emirates

© The Author(s) 2025
H. O. Al-Shamsi (ed.), *Healthcare in the United Arab Emirates*,
https://doi.org/10.1007/978-981-96-0523-1_28

At its onset, the MOH had limited regulatory standards to govern the profession and practice, as its focus was mainly on the provision and expansion of services.

The UAE used to import blood and blood products from abroad for transfusion services but felt the pressure to secure its own blood products with the emergence of the AIDS pandemic. In 1986, the Dubai Blood Donor Center was founded, and with that came the initial regulatory framework and requirements. The MOH subsequently opened and operated four donor centers throughout the country, and until 1994, donors were paid for their blood donations.

In 1994, the National Blood Services Act was published, mandating that blood donations be voluntary.

Realizing that there was a potential conflict if the provider of health services was also the regulator, the Emirate of Abu Dhabi created the General Authority for Health Services (GAHS) in 2005, which subsequently split into the Health Authority for Abu Dhabi (HAAD), now known as the Department of Health (DoH), and SEHA. HAAD took on the regulatory function for health services in the Emirate of Abu Dhabi, while SEHA looked after the provision of government health services. The Dubai Health Authority (DHA) was also formed with a similar mission in 2007 to regulate health services in the Emirate of Dubai and participate in the provision of healthcare services.

In 2010, HAAD created the first hospital regulatory standards, which included a chapter on medical laboratory standards [1]. With the introduction of the Professional Qualification Requirement (PQR) [2] and primary source verification, licensing of medical professionals became more rigorous. HAAD then started auditing various hospitals and laboratories according to these standards, an action that helped tremendously in improving laboratory services in Abu Dhabi and the UAE. Licenses for medical laboratories as well as hospitals were provided based on passing the HAAD or DHA audits. HAAD as well as DHA also encouraged laboratories to pursue other laboratory accreditations to add an extra layer of rigor to the regulation of the practice and the provision of laboratory services according to high levels of international quality standards. In 2015, a movement to obtain ISO 15189 accreditation, as well as accreditation by the College of American Pathologists and the American Association of Blood Banks, was heavily encouraged and later mandated for reimbursement. This was coupled with the introduction of Joint Commission International Accreditation (JCIA) for hospitals and healthcare facilities and the creation of the Emirates International Accreditation Center (EIAC) [3].

28.3 Technology Evolution

In the 1970s and early 1980s, technology in clinical chemistry laboratories was limited to spectrophotometers, radioimmunoassays (RIA), and manual procedures in both clinical pathology and anatomic pathology. Central Hospital hosted the reference clinical pathology laboratory at that time, where most hormone analysis were performed using radioimmunoassays (RIA), which was the standard method back then for hormone testing. Analysis and testing were classically performed in batch fashion, with various tests run on certain days of the week, and the turnaround time was typically 1–2 weeks for most routine hormonal investigations.

Clinical chemistry tests like liver function tests (LFTs), lipid tests, etc. were performed manually using prepared reagents pipetted into secondary tubes. Most of the end-point reactions were conducted by this method, and enzymes assays were carried out by taking readings after specified times. The readings were taken on manual spectrophotometers, and the results were manually calculated using graphs.

With these spectrometers, laboratory scientists had to use water baths, managing temperatures with mercury or alcohol thermometers for most enzyme analysis. Periodically, these water baths had to be cleaned to prevent fungal growth. These were time-consuming, tedious, and manpower-intensive processes. Analysis was limited in throughput to 20–100 tests per hour, and the turnaround time for those tests was 1–2 days after all the manual calculations and transcription of the results were completed.

The 1990s witnessed rapid growth in technology as fully automated random-access analyzers were introduced in clinical chemistry laboratories. The introduction of the modular design allowed for the integration of electrolytes, enzymes, and hormone analyses on the same platform and from the same test tube. The first total laboratory automation (TLA) system was installed at Sheikh Khalifa Medical City Laboratory in 2009, where each laboratory workstation was coupled to a track or conveyor belt so that samples could be moved from one workstation to another. The TLA allowed the processing of a large number of samples in a very short time, with a throughput of up to 2,000 tests per hour.

Near-patient, or point-of-care testing (POCT), adoption also developed in the 1990s with the introduction of blood gas analysis in intensive care units. Placing these instruments outside the laboratory and near patients certainly helped save time and effort in transporting samples to the laboratory for analysis and returning the reports manually via porters.

The United Arab Emirates (UAE) has a universal neonatal screening program that started in January 1995 with limited screening for phenylketonuria (PKU), followed by the introduction of congenital hypothyroidism (CH) and wide-scale screening in January 1998, and has continued to grow and expand ever since [4]. This program was initiated in Mafraq and Al Qassemi hospitals under the MOH.

From 2000 to the present, we have witnessed the rapid growth of molecular diagnostics, chromosomal analysis, and the introduction of genomic testing and precision medicine. Technologies such as next-generation sequencing and real-time polymerase chain reaction (PCR) became available in several laboratories throughout the UAE. Most of these tests were sent outside the country to reference laboratories in Europe and the USA for analysis. Many sophisticated technologies were also introduced in this era, including flow cytometry, electrophoresis, high-performance liquid chromatography (HPLC), LC-MS/MS, MALDI-TOF, and ICP-MS, among others.

28.4　Test Requisition and Pre-Analytics Evolution

In the early days of the establishment of hospital laboratories, all processes were manual. Request forms were manually written and sent with the patient or kept in the ward for the nurse. The request forms were on duplicate pages with carbon copies.

Samples were received from the phlebotomist through dedicated windows in the lab, and they were then checked against the request forms that accompanied them. Samples were collected in trays with the patients' names written in marker or pen. The only identification methods were the name and the hospital file number. Samples were then manually sorted according to the manual request forms.

After sorting, they were labeled with numbers starting from 0001 every morning. This was the only way to track the number of samples or requests received each day.

The labels were printed every morning by the clerical staff using manual handheld devices.

Samples are then labeled to match their corresponding request forms. For the forms, the labels were placed on the top copy as well as the duplicate, which was retained in the lab for records.

The request forms were then handed over to the clerical staff, who manually registered them in the lab registration book with the date, lab number, name of the patient, and the tests requested.

This was a very cumbersome and manual process, and technicians had to remember to pass the samples to the next bench with the request form.

With the introduction of the physician order entry modules in 2000, most of these manual request forms and registrations were eliminated.

In the mid-1990s, vacutainers were introduced in the MOH, which improved the safety of blood collection and reduced needle prick injuries. The gel separation also helped prevent pre-analytical errors such as fibrin threads and clots and improved the integrity of serum and plasma samples.

28.5 Reporting and Information Technology Evolution

Up until the late 1970s, the management of laboratory samples and the associated analysis and reporting were time-consuming manual processes, often riddled with transcription errors.

Reporting results in a timely manner was challenging in the early days because of multi-step processes.

The request forms with the results were returned to the clerical station, and the results were then registered in the logbook where the forms were initially logged.

The top copy was then placed on dedicated pigeonhole shelves for the corresponding wards where the request was initially sent.

The carbon copy was retained in the lab, again in a pigeonhole shelf, for about one month. The pigeonhole shelf had about 30 slots.

The retrieval of reports was only possible by searching through the logbook according to the dates. These logbooks were kept in the lab for about six months. Urgent results were often relayed by phone to the wards or the doctors.

The results in the pigeonholes were periodically retrieved by the assistants from the wards.

Samples of the manual reports used then are depicted in Fig. 28.1.

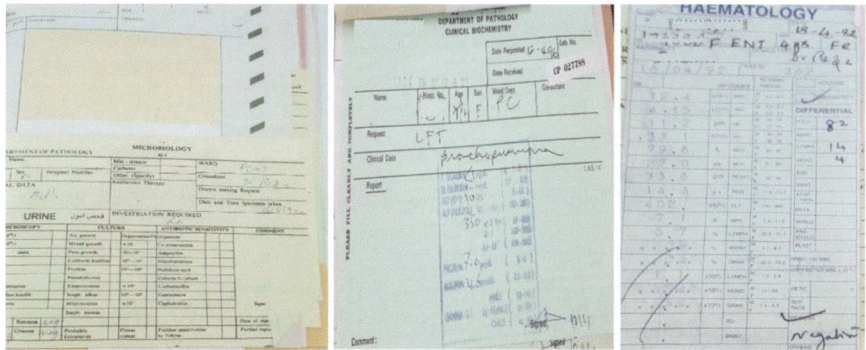

Fig. 28.1 Samples of manual reports in microbiology, chemistry, and hematology (1980s & 1990s)

In 1982, the first generation of the Laboratory Information Management System (LIMS) was introduced in the form of a centralized minicomputer that offered automated reporting tools.

By 1988, the second generation was developed, using relational databases to expand LIMS into more application-specific territory. By 1990, a third generation of LIMS was available, which took advantage of a client-server architecture and allowed laboratories to implement better data processing and exchange.

The first Laboratory Information System (LIS) was introduced in the 1990s in a few hospitals throughout the UAE, with another wave in 2001 that included more hospitals at that time. The LIS was used only within the laboratory. Requests had to be entered into the system, and then the samples were processed after barcodes were assigned.

Results were returned to the LIS and stored. This eliminated the manual entries in the large sample register. Results were, however, still printed and sent physically to the wards or clinics.

In 2006, SEHA contracted with Cerner Middle East and embarked on a major project linking all its hospitals and laboratories through Cerner HIS and LIS. The project went live with a big bang in 2011, and it was very successful in linking all hospitals, primary healthcare centers, and laboratories under SEHA at that time.

From 2011 onward, more sophisticated LISs were introduced, with a bidirectional interface to physician order entry modules, analyzers, and direct reporting into the hospital information system or electronic medical records.

The LIS introduction eliminated many clerical errors, saved considerable time, and improved efficiency, patient safety, confidentiality, and clinical care.

In 2018, the DoH embarked on a very impressive project to integrate medical records from all the hospitals in Abu Dhabi. The project was named "Malaffi", a health information exchange in the Emirate of Abu Dhabi [5]. The project went live in 2019, with 85% of hospitals connected by 2020 and reaching 100% by September 2021. Malaffi enabled the Emirate to harness its response during the COVID-19 pandemic in 2020 and exchange critical information between healthcare facilities. It also prevented duplication of testing in various healthcare facilities.

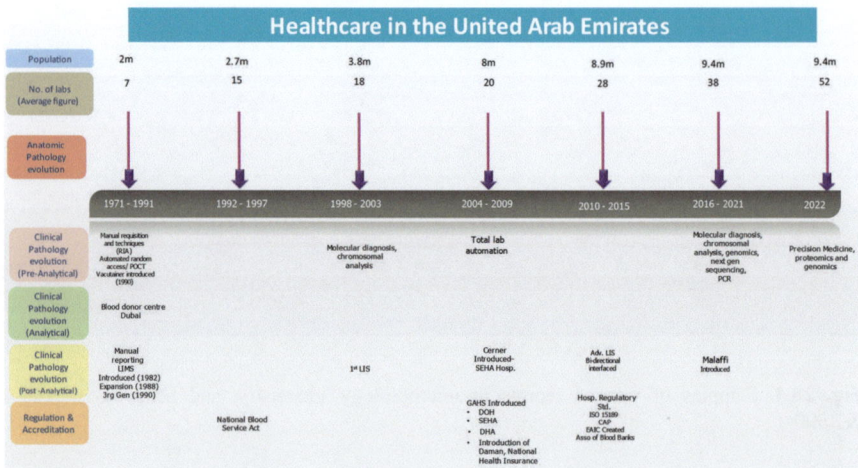

Fig. 28.2 Summary of the major milestones in pathology and laboratory medicine in the UAE

Nowadays, patients can access their laboratory results through a secure patient portal in real time and discuss those results with their physicians online.

28.6 Current Laboratory Landscape in the UAE

Over 50 private laboratories are available throughout the UAE. The majority of the private laboratories are situated in the Emirate of Dubai. There is a movement towards the privatization of laboratories previously owned by the public sector, such as MOHAP and SEHA, and the wide-scale introduction of precision medicine and advanced genetic testing in the UAE.

Major milestones and developments in pathology and laboratory medicine in the UAE are summarized in Fig. 28.2.

28.7 Conclusion

Pathology and laboratory medicine have developed very rapidly over the span of 20 years in the United Arab Emirates. Major developments that contributed to this development include total laboratory automation, advances in genomics and molecular testing, laboratory information systems, and information technology.

Conflicts of Interest The authors have no conflicts of interest to declare.

References

1. HAAD Clinical Laboratory Standards. https://Standards | Department of Health Abu Dhabi (doh.gov.ae).
2. Introduction to Professional Qualification Requirement (PQR). https://www.doh.gov.ae.

3. The Emirates International Accreditation Centre (EIAC). https://eiac.gov.ae/.
4. Al Hosani H, Salah M, Osman HM, Farag HM, El-Assiouty L, Saade D, Hertecant J. Expanding the comprehensive national neonatal screening programme in the United Arab Emirates from 1995 to 2011. East Mediterr Health J. 2014;20(1):17–23.
5. Malaffi to highlight Abu Dhabi's regional leadership in digital transformation in healthcare at HIMSS23 in Chicago USA. https://Malaffi.ae.

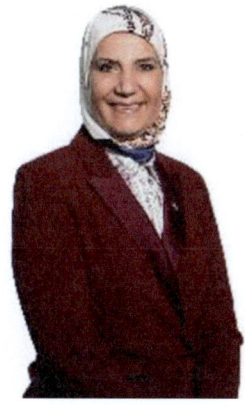

Dr. Laila Osama AbdelWareth is the Executive Director at the National Reference Laboratory and the Diagnostic Cluster at M42, and the President of the Emirates Clinical Chemistry Society.

Prior to joining the National Reference Laboratory, Dr. AbdelWareth served as the Chair of Clinical Pathology at Cleveland Clinic Abu Dhabi Pathology & Laboratory Medicine Institute, Chief Medical Officer of SEHA Pathology and Laboratory Medicine Services and Chair of the Pathology and Laboratory Medicine Institute at Sheikh Khalifa Medical City.

Previous appointments included British Columbia Children's & Women's Hospital in Vancouver, Canada, and Mafraq Hospital, Abu Dhabi, UAE.

Dr. AbdelWareth earned her medical degree from Ain Shams University Cairo, Egypt, and completed her postgraduate training at the University of British Columbia.

She obtained Canadian and American Board certification in Medical Biochemistry and Clinical Pathology and is a fellow of the Royal College of Physicians and Surgeons in Canada as well as the College of American Pathologists. She also obtained an Executive master's degree in healthcare administration from Zayed University, UAE. She is an active member of various scientific societies and has several publications to her credit in the field of laboratory medicine.

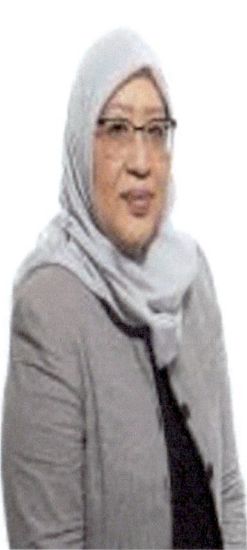

Annisah Binti Abdullah is the retired technical director of Imperial College Laboratories NRL under Mubadala Health Care, with four decades of experience in medical technology and research. She began her career at Fatima Hospital and the Ipoh Specialist Centre in Ipoh W. Malaysia. She then joined Mafraq Hospital in 1983, where she played a key role in establishing the medical laboratory and its research sector.

Subsequently, Annisah assumed leadership roles in three Imperial College London Diabetes Centre laboratories, situated in Al Ain and Abu Dhabi. She liaised with researchers from Imperial College London to help establish the RIA Research Lab. Her tenure continued until her retirement in December 2021.

Even after retirement, Annisah's commitment to laboratory medicine remains undiminished. She is currently registered as a freelance ISO Technical Assessor with the local accreditation body, ENAS.

She earned a BSc in Chemistry and an MSc in Biochemistry from Madras University. She holds the Chartered Biomedical Scientist certification from IBMS UK and a license from the University of New York, USA.

Open Access This chapter is licensed under the terms of the Creative Commons Attribution 4.0 International License (http://creativecommons.org/licenses/by/4.0/), which permits use, sharing, adaptation, distribution and reproduction in any medium or format, as long as you give appropriate credit to the original author(s) and the source, provide a link to the Creative Commons license and indicate if changes were made.

The images or other third party material in this chapter are included in the chapter's Creative Commons license, unless indicated otherwise in a credit line to the material. If material is not included in the chapter's Creative Commons license and your intended use is not permitted by statutory regulation or exceeds the permitted use, you will need to obtain permission directly from the copyright holder.

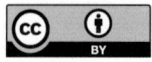

Emergency Medicine in the UAE

29

Saleh Fares Al-Ali , Rasha Buhumaid, Khalifa Alqaydi, Muna Aljallaf, and Hind Aldhaheri

29.1 Emergency Medicine Journey in the UAE

Although emergency care has been provided in several hospitals for years, "emergency medicine" (EM) is considered a new specialty in the United Arab Emirates (UAE). This is not unlike many other countries, given the milestones in the field. Since the establishment of the country in 1971, the "accident units" within hospitals have been mainly run by general practitioners with no formal training in EM. It was even a place where "low-performing" physicians could occasionally be placed as a form of "punishment". This gradually changed when board-certified emergency physicians (EPs) started working in certain areas across the country. During the early 2000s, Sheikh Khalifa Medical City was one of the first hospitals to hire qualified American and Canadian emergency physicians through

---

S. F. Al-Ali (✉)
Emergency Medicine, EMS and Disaster Medicine, International Federation for Emergency Medicine, Abu Dhabi, United Arab Emirates

Emirates Society of Emergency Medicine, Dubai, United Arab Emirates

R. Buhumaid
Emirates Society of Emergency Medicine, Dubai, United Arab Emirates

Mohammed Bin Rashid University of Medicine and Health Sciences, Dubai, United Arab Emirates

K. Alqaydi
Emergency Department, Zayed Military Hospital, Ministry of Defense, Abu Dhabi, United Arab Emirates

M. Aljallaf
Dubai Academic Health Corporation (DAHC), Dubai, United Arab Emirates
e-mail: MuKAlQubaisi@dha.gov.ae

H. Aldhaheri
Adult Division and EM Residency Program, Tawam Hospital, Al Ain, United Arab Emirates
e-mail: hidhaheri@seha.ae

© The Author(s) 2025
H. O. Al-Shamsi (ed.), *Healthcare in the United Arab Emirates*,
https://doi.org/10.1007/978-981-96-0523-1_29

a staffing company called InterHealth Canada. It was an important milestone in transforming the UAE's "accident units" into true "emergency departments." With the subsequent increase in job opportunities, the UAE started attracting more qualified emergency physicians (EPs), which helped improve awareness of the specialty and highlighted the importance of encouraging Emirati junior physicians to pursue it as a career. The first Emirati board-certified emergency physician graduated from McGill University in 2007. This was followed by an increasing number of Emirati EM-certified graduates from Canada, the United States, France, and UAE-based Arab Board programs.

With the increasing numbers in the EM community, there was a pressing need for a professional organization to represent the EM specialty in the country, similar to those in other developed countries. Therefore, a group of EPs (including EM residents) gathered on August 28, 2012, and founded the first EM society in the country, naming it the Emirates Society of Emergency Medicine (ESEM), under the Emirates Medical Association. The first elected ESEM board included Dr. Saleh Fares, Dr. Ayesha Al Memari, Dr. Mahmoud Ghaniam, Dr. Moin Fikri, and Dr. Abdel Noureldin. The society launched several educational outreach activities targeted toward physicians in rural hospitals, with a focus on life-saving skills.

The society launched the first meeting of the annual ESEM Scientific Conference in December 2014 in Dubai, which was attended by over 500 delegates; it is now considered the largest EM conference in the Middle East, with over 1,500 delegates annually. During the ESEM Conference in 2014, ESEM proposed the idea of founding the "Gulf Federation of Emergency Medicine (GFEM)," and a task force was formed to take the idea forward. The federation was officially launched during the ESEM Conference in 2017, with Dr. Ghada Qassim from Bahrain as the first General Secretary. The federation's aim is to standardize emergency care across the Gulf Cooperation Council (GCC) countries.

ESEM continued to build its international presence and was able to win a historic bid to host the main conference of the 2021 International Federation for Emergency Medicine (IFEM). The International Conference on Emergency Medicine (ICEM21) was held in June 2021 for the first time in the Middle East and North Africa (MENA) region, with over 2,500 delegates. At an official level, ESEM is currently a respected representative of EM in the UAE and is steadily gaining recognition. In September 2020, a major achievement of ESEM was a joint effort with the Ministry of Health to pass a law equivalent to the "Good Samaritan Law" in other countries, which is considered the first law of its kind in an Arab country [1]. The UAE Emergency Medicine landscape timeline is summarized in Fig. 29.1.

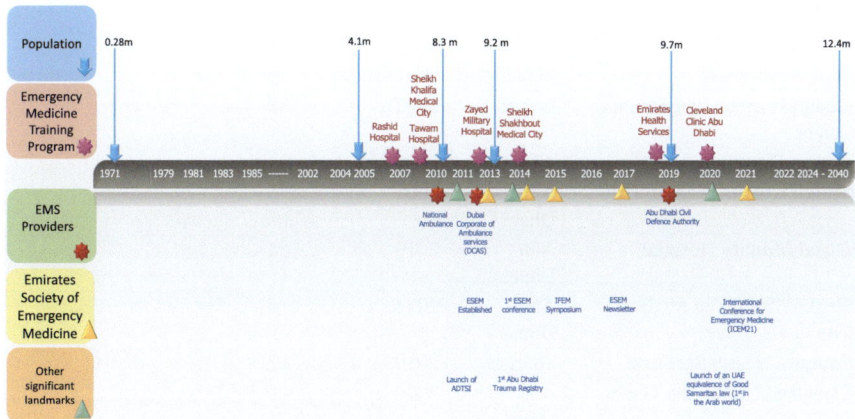

Fig. 29.1 UAE emergency medicine landscape timeline

29.2 Research and Education

Exposing medical students to EM early in their careers is essential to attracting them to the specialty; this is best accomplished by having a mandatory EM internship in the undergraduate medical curriculum [2]. There are eight medical schools in the UAE, which collectively graduate around 450 students annually [3]. Most of the undergraduate programs have dedicated time in their curriculum for an EM internship during the clinical years [4–8], although some only offer it as an elective rotation [9, 10]. The UAE has seven EM residency training programs. The first batch of locally trained EPs graduated in 2012 [11]. Over the past 15 years, six more training programs have been started (Table 29.1).

Two-thirds of the programs are in Abu Dhabi. All programs are 4 years long, and their curricula are based on the North American EM residency program training model. More than half of the programs are accredited by the Accreditation Council for Graduate Medical Education–International [12]. Graduates from the programs are eligible to obtain the Arab Board of Health Specializations (ABHS) in EM or the Jordanian Board of EM. The main limitation of these board certifications is that they lack international recognition compared to other EM board certificates. To address this limitation, the National Institute for Health Specialties (NIHS) was established in 2014 to organize specialty training and enhance the quality of training in the UAE. The NIHS began accrediting EM programs in 2022 and offer the graduates of its accredited programs eligibility for the Emirati board of EM [13]. The annual capacity of EM training posts in the UAE increased from 20 seats per year in 2010 to

Table 29.1 Emergency medicine residency training programs in the UAE

Training program	Location	Year established	Number of training posts per year
Rashid Hospital and Trauma Center	Dubai	2007	8
Tawam Hospital	Al Ain	2009	10
Sheikh Khalifa Medical City	Abu Dhabi	2009	6
Zayed Military Hospital	Abu Dhabi	2013	4
Sheikh Shakhbout Medical City	Abu Dhabi	2014	4
Emirates Health Services	Sharjah	2019	3
Cleveland Clinic Abu Dhabi	Abu Dhabi	2020	4

40 seats per year in 2020 [14, 15]. The doubling of EM training posts both reflects the popularity of the programs and responds to the local demand for the specialty. Fifteen years after the first EM residency program was established, the first EM subspecialty fellowship training program was launched in the field of pediatric EM [14].

With the establishment of ESEM in 2012, the UAE became a hub for high-caliber scientific conferences and courses in EM, such as the annual ESEM Scientific Conference, the International Conference for Emergency Medicine, the Asian Society for Emergency Medicine Conference, the WINFOCUS World Congress, and the Middle East and North Africa Clinical Toxicology Association Conference [16–20]. These conferences attract local, regional, and international experts who discuss evidence-based updates and advancements in EM.

However, EM research in the UAE, the Gulf, and the MENA region is underdeveloped [21]. According to the latest review of global EM literature in 2018, the MENA region is one of the lowest producers of EM research across the various study types [22–24]. To enhance the culture of research in EM in the UAE, the Emirati board will include a mandatory research rotation in the EM residency program curriculum. In addition, ESEM is launching the EM Researcher Award to encourage EPs to participate in research and enhance the field.

29.3 Emergency Medicine Model of Care

Common emergency care practices like trauma response, medical emergencies, and disaster medicine differ across the country. This variation can be explained by differences in EM practitioners' backgrounds (North American, European, Asian, etc.). It is of utmost importance to have a systematic approach to designing an integrated system to improve emergency care delivery [25, 26].

When it comes to medical emergencies, the WHO prioritizes an integrated approach to early recognition and resuscitation. This high-impact and cost-effective approach significantly reduces morbidity and mortality. Primary prevention and outbreak response are best managed with effective disease surveillance in acute care settings [25].

Another attempt to propose an integrated model of care was presented by the Emergency Management Integrated Roadmap Aimed Toward Every Healthcare System, (the EMIRATES Framework), which outlines a simplified approach to integrating the different emergency services in healthcare, complementing the WHO approach. The EMIRATES Framework organizes the emergency medical management system into four key components: governance, pre-hospital, hospital, and public health.

The governance component emphasizes the importance of having "an owner of EM" or a "lead agency" within the government. This helps in setting related strategies, standards, and policies to ensure an efficient emergency medical management system. The pre-hospital component highlights the importance of integrating the Emergency Medical Services (EMS) with other field services, including search and rescue efforts, disaster medical assistance teams, mass fatality management, and casualty care in hazardous material incidents. The hospital component highlights the need for full-time emergency managers within hospitals to coordinate the hospital-based emergency management program according to international standards. The public health component aims to create emergency services with a system-wide scope that integrates with the other components to provide an effective response during day-to-day emergencies or disaster situations (e.g., poison control centers, blood banks, and strategic stockpiles). The framework argues that all four of these components need a well-orchestrated operations management model (in the form of operations centers) to align the different components and ensure a seamless response [26]. The EMIRATES Framework is currently considered a foundation for establishing an Abu Dhabi Healthcare Emergency Management "Ecosystem."

29.4 Specialized EM Programs

Thus, the targeted integrated model of care aims to coordinate and deliver the right care for critical emergencies in the right place, using the right expertise, and at the right time without interruption. Building on that, developing specialized programs becomes a natural path for growth in the emergency system to provide proper care for common emergencies like trauma, burns, ST-elevation myocardial infarction (STEMI), and stroke, thereby improving outcomes.

29.4.1 Trauma Care

An advanced trauma system is being developed in Abu Dhabi and Dubai, with plans to extend this program to the whole UAE. The system is based on key components outlined by the Committee on Trauma of the American College of Surgeons [27]. This system is being developed to deliver trauma care on a "continuum of care" principle, which means it spans the whole spectrum of care, extending back to prevention and continuing through injury care and then rehabilitation. Several milestones have been successfully reached to date, including the successful introduction of numerous injury prevention programs across the UAE; the launch of the trauma registry in Abu Dhabi and Dubai; the establishment of specialized regional trauma centers (Sheikh Shakhbout Medical City in Abu Dhabi and the Rashid Hospital Trauma Center in Dubai); and the establishment of specialized burn units associated with the regional trauma centers.

29.4.2 STEMI Care

Cardiovascular diseases are the leading cause of mortality worldwide, especially acute coronary syndromes (ACS) [28]. Almost half of ACS-related deaths in the Middle East occur in a prehospital setting [29]. To improve the outcomes of STEMI patients, a task force has been created to provide a comprehensive pathway to ensure a smooth transfer of STEMI patients to the designated center. This has resulted in reducing the door-to-balloon time to well below the 90-minute target for the majority of cases in several cities [30].

29.4.3 Stroke Care

With the rapid development of the healthcare sector in the UAE, multiple stroke centers have been established (e.g., Cleveland Clinic Abu Dhabi and Rashid Hospital in Dubai). These centers provide comprehensive diagnostic and treatment options for stroke patients, and they are working closely with a special stroke task force to streamline initial emergency stroke care and implement telemedicine even before transferring the patient to the specialized center.

29.4.4 Toxicology Care

Toxicology care is currently developing in the UAE. Specialized hospital-based toxicology services have been established in both Abu Dhabi and Dubai. Sheikh Khalifa Medical City (SKMC) opened its specialized toxicology unit in late 2021, marking an important milestone in providing comprehensive care for toxicology patients. The emergency department of Rashid Hospital established its own toxicology consultation service as well, to cover the Dubai region. In February 2023, the Department of Health (DOH) established an Abu Dhabi-wide Poison Center; which is closing a critical gap in the system. The center provides 24/7 service to healthcare providers across Abu Dhabi, and occasionally from other emirates. It will be be accessible to the public in the near future.

29.4.5 Pediatric Emergency Care

Pediatric patients represent a special challenge for emergency care providers because of their unique needs. Pediatric patients receiving care in general emergency departments are less likely to receive proper, evidence-based care than when treated in pediatric emergency departments [31–34]. Awareness of this data prompted the establishment of dedicated pediatric emergency departments and tertiary centers like Sheikh Khalifa Medical City in Abu Dhabi and the Al Jalila Hospital in Dubai. An organized, system-wide provision for pediatric emergency care is still under development.

29.5 Prehospital Care

Prehospital care in the UAE has gone through several stages. Initially, it started as a hospital-based ambulance service, with very limited care provided en route. In the late 1990s and early 2000s, the Ministry of Interior took the lead in managing EMS. There were no Emirati paramedics at the beginning, but over the years, they have started graduating and taking leadership positions across the country. In Abu Dhabi, EMS was initially provided by the police service until 2020, when it was moved to a newly established entity named the Abu Dhabi Civil Defense Authority.

In Dubai, it started as a police-run service until 2010, when the Dubai Government decided to transfer the service to a new independent entity called the Dubai Corporation for Ambulance Services (DCAS), which reports to the Dubai Executive Council. In the other Northern Emirates, the service was initially scattered between hospital-based and police-run services. In 2010, the Ministry of Interior signed a joint venture with a private provider to establish a government-owned company named "National Ambulance." National Ambulance started providing EMS services to several government entities, including Abu Dhabi airports and military units. In 2014, National Ambulance was tasked with fully managing EMS in the Northern Emirates. Formal Helicopter EMS (or HEMS) is still in the development stage, as it is currently provided by several non-health entities that supply medical teams when needed. This is expected to change as the EMS system matures further over the next few years.

With such positive changes in the EMS system, the care provided has dramatically improved over the years. Around the same time, several private EMS providers entered the market, focusing on interfacility transportation. These prehospital clinical providers range from paramedics with basic skills to highly qualified critical care paramedics from different parts of the world. The provider's levels follow the national Professional Qualifications Requirements (PQR), which has evolved over the years [35]. The levels were originally based on the American system (Basic EMT, Intermediate EMT, and Paramedic). In the summer of 2023, the levels were unified and simplified across different providers to ensure alignment with international best practices. The new levels include Emergency Medical Technician (EMT), Paramedic, Advanced Care Paramedic (ACP), and Critical Care Paramedic (CCP).

The educational programs for paramedics are still going through unsynchronized development, mainly due to the lack of a national EMS regulatory body. Promising efforts to provide paramedicine programs have started at several academic institutions, such as the Higher Colleges of Technology, Sheikha Fatima College, and the University of Sharjah.

Efforts are currently underway to fill key gaps in the EMS system, including establishing clear standards and policies, improving medical direction, developing evidence-based clinical practice guidelines, and defining a clear scope of practice. Standardizing services across the country will be a major goal in the upcoming years.

29.6 Disaster Medicine

Following several devastating mass casualty incidents [36, 37], the UAE government realized the importance of establishing an entity dedicated to coordinating and managing emergency management efforts among different emirates. This resulted in the establishment of the National Emergency Crisis and Disasters Management Authority in 2007. Following that, the practice of emergency management matured dramatically, and this has slowly been reflected in the healthcare sector. The Ministry of Health and Prevention is the official lead ministry for preparing the healthcare system for any emergency. This preparation occurs in close collaboration with the local health regulatory bodies in each emirate. In 2008, a review of Abu Dhabi government hospitals' disaster plans highlighted several challenges in preparing for future incidents [38]. These included the lack of an all-hazards approach, the absence of a standardized incident management system, the fact that plans were not data-driven, limited coordination and collaboration between hospitals, a primitive information-sharing mechanism across the system that caused frequent miscommunication, and, most importantly, a lack of structured emergency management programs.

Following the recommendations of that review, the hospitals involved adopted the Hospital Incident Command System framework for managing emergencies. Similarly, plans are shifting more toward an all-hazards approach with an annual hazard vulnerability analysis. Zayed Military Hospital was the first hospital in the UAE to introduce a full-time emergency manager in 2014 to run the emergency management program within the facility. Such practices continue to differ from hospital to hospital, although there are efforts to standardize them. The Department of Health in Abu Dhabi launched a hospital preparedness program that unifies the process to manage emergencies within hospitals and evaluates hospitals' compliance with the requirements.

Like many other countries, the COVID-19 pandemic was another test for the UAE to evaluate the response of the different entities in supporting the healthcare sector. Fortunately, the many years of hard work paid off on several levels, and the various emergency response systems were able to position the UAE as one of the most successful countries in terms of the COVID-19 response. Despite the expected areas for improvement, the healthcare sector was able to ensure full alignment with other sectors and managed to record several global successes, including the highest COVID-19 vaccination rate in the world, one of the lowest mortality rates, status as the first country to receive monoclonal antibodies, and, last but not least, no significant shortage of personal protective equipment (PPE) [39].

The growing successes of the UAE's healthcare emergency management continue to boost confidence in the country's ability to adopt a well-integrated model to deal with health-related emergencies.

29.7 Injury Prevention Programs

Injury prevention requires cohesive and comprehensive programs to address community needs. Trauma, ischemic cardiac disease, and occupation-related events are some notable causes of injury in the UAE.

As previously mentioned, one of the more remarkable programs was the Abu Dhabi Trauma System Initiative, established in 2010, which implemented an advanced trauma approach and, in turn, managed to establish the Abu Dhabi Trauma Registry in 2014. The registry currently offers insight into trauma epidemiology and helps to support further research and program refinements [40]. Analyzing the trauma registries should enable policymakers to address trauma as a public health problem, thus tailoring specific preventative interventions to decrease mortality and morbidity and eventually improve trauma care outcomes in the Emirate [41].

Additionally, we expect to improve the outcomes of out-of-hospital cardiac arrest by encouraging community involvement in such incidents, as awareness of the UAE equivalent of the Good Samaritan Law increases. Bystanders are being encouraged to intervene in emergency situations until adequate help arrives. Similarly, the government has launched several initiatives to enforce safe workplace environments, including heat precautions during the summer, ensuring workers wear safety gear, and requiring the availability of first aid providers. In general, the injury prevention field is growing and can be enriched with many programs to counter the high number of possible injuries and to leverage the different registries that are available [1, 42].

29.8 Challenges and Advantages

Emergency medicine in the UAE continues to face some critical challenges that affect this enthusiastic growth. The lack of a clear governing body overseeing emergency medical issues in certain emirates creates confusion in handling key issues related to the specialty. Another important challenge is the shortage of trained emergency medical providers across the country. This shortage is not limited to emergency physicians but also includes emergency nurses and paramedics. The focus on attracting talent to local education programs is expected to address part of that shortage. On the other hand, the lack of structured primary care places unnecessary pressure on the emergency medical system [43]. Emergency research is also facing significant challenges, which will hopefully be overcome through increased government grants and greater involvement from residency programs.

Despite the challenges, the UAE has several advantages that can help boost the emergency medicine specialty. The country is an attractive destination for talented emergency providers, making it a hub for a wide range of experiences from around the world. Other advantages include the government's ambitious vision of becoming one of the most developed countries in the region, which has facilitated strong support and funding for the development of emergency medical infrastructure. The country's robust information technology (IT) infrastructure enables the implementation of cutting-edge solutions such as telehealth and artificial intelligence to enhance emergency care.

ESEM is an active society in the region and is participating in the rapid growth of the specialty of emergency medicine through numerous educational activities and internationally recognized conferences. Such activities make it feasible to stay up to date on the latest EM developments.

29.9 The Future of EM in the UAE

Emergency medicine in the UAE is heading toward a promising future as the government continues to reach a series of milestones to support its development and success. There is a clear emphasis on the importance of providing a high level of emergency care across the country. This support is well invested in establishing key projects that are expected to improve patient outcomes. These projects include establishing a national poison center; special programs like trauma, STEMI, and stroke; building an integrated model of care; and, most importantly, investing in research and education. With the establishment of accredited specialty training programs, many EM board-certified physicians are overseeing and coordinating emergency care efforts. This process will continue to flourish. There is a growing need for accredited fellowship programs to address the increasing demand for robust emergency services. Following the pediatric EM fellowships, other fellowships in areas like ultrasound, toxicology, disaster medicine, and trauma will surely follow soon.

The ESEM is similarly heading in the right direction. Following its numerous outstanding achievements, it is well-positioned to be recognized as an international society through its collaboration with WHO, IFEM, GFEM, and many others. This will continue to position EM prominently on the world map [2, 11, 42, 44, 45].

29.10 Conclusion

Emergency medicine in the UAE has gone through different phases of development over the years. The country is focusing on developing a full "EM Ecosystem" model of care to integrate policymakers with prehospital providers, hospital-based emergency care, and strategic system-wide projects. To support that goal, EM education is rapidly growing, feeding the system with qualified practitioners who will take the specialty forward for years to come.

Conflicts of Interest The authors have no conflicts of interest to declare.

References

1. Federal Decree (No. 31), Criminal law, Article 55. 2020, September. Retrieved Aug 20, 2022, from: https://laws.uaecabinet.ae/ar/materials/law/1529.
2. Cevik AA, Cakal ED, Shaban S, El Zubeir M, Abu-Zidan FM. A mandatory emergency medicine clerkship influences students' career choices in a developing system. Afr J Emerg Med. 2021;11(1):70–3. https://doi.org/10.1016/j.afjem.2020.08.003.
3. World Federation for Medical Education. World Directory of Medical Schools. 2016, June 1. Retrieved July 13, 2022, from https://www.wdoms.org/.
4. Dubai Medical College. n.d. Retrieved July 13, 2022, from https://www.dmcg.edu/.
5. Gulf Medical University. Doctor of Medicine MD program. 2022, July 13. Retrieved July 13, 2022, from https://gmu.ac.ae/college-medicine/bachelor-of-medicine-and-bachelor-of-surgery-mbbs/#structure.
6. Mohammed Bin Rashid University of Medicine and Health Sciences. Bachelor of Medicine and Bachelor of Surgery (MBBS). n.d. Retrieved July 13, 2022, from https://www.mbru.ac.ae/programs/bachelor-of-medicine-and-bachelor-of-surgery-mbbs-program-mbru/.
7. RAK Medical & Health Sciences University. MBBS study plan. 2022, July 4. Retrieved July 13, 2022, from https://www.rakmhsu.ac.ae/rakcoms-study-plan.
8. United Arab Emirates University. Undergraduate programs: doctor of medicine. 2022, July 4. Retrieved July 13, 2022, from https://cmhs.uaeu.ac.ae//en/programs/undergraduate/doctor-of-medicine.shtml.
9. Khalifa University. College of Medicine and Health Sciences. n.d. Retrieved July 13, 2022, from https://www.ku.ac.ae/academics/college-of-medicine-and-health-sciences.
10. University of Sharjah. Bachelor of Medicine and Bachelor of Surgery (MBBS). n.d. Retrieved July 13, 2022, from https://www.sharjah.ac.ae/en/academics/Colleges/Medicine/Pages/Bachelor-of-Medicine-and-Bachelor-of-Surgery.aspx.
11. Fares S, Irfan FB, Corder RF, Al Marzouqi MA, Al Zaabi AH, Idrees MM, Abbo M. Emergency medicine in the United Arab Emirates. Int J Emerg Med. 2014;7(1):4. Retrieved July 13, 2022, from https://doi.org/10.1186/1865-1380-7-4.
12. ACGME-I, Accreditation Council for Graduate Medical Education–International. Where we are. n.d. Retrieved July 13, 2022, from https://www.acgme-i.org/about-us/where-we-are/.
13. United Arab Emirates University. NIHS establishment. 2022, June 27. Retrieved July 13, 2022, from https://nihs.uaeu.ac.ae/en/index.shtml.
14. Department of Health Abu Dhabi. Residency and fellowship application 2022. 2022, July 13. Retrieved July 13, 2022, from https://www.doh.gov.ae/en/Announcements/Residency-and-fellowship-application-process-2022.
15. Dubai Health Authority. Dubai residency training program. 2022, July 13. Retrieved July 13, 2022, from https://www.dha.gov.ae/en/MedicalEducationandResearch/DubaiResidencyTrainingProgram.
16. Emirates Society of Emergency Medicine. Emirates Society of Emergency Medicine conference. n.d. Retrieved July 13, 2022, from https://esemconference.ae/.
17. International Federation for Emergency Medicine. International Federation for Emergency Medicine: about. n.d. Retrieved July 13, 2022, from https://www.ifem.cc/about_icem.
18. Asian Society for Emergency Medicine. ASEM academic meeting. n.d. Retrieved July 13, 2022, from https://www.asiansem.org/events-and-sponsorship.
19. Middle East & North Africa Clinical Toxicology Association. n.d. Retrieved July 13, 2022, from https://www.menatox.org/.
20. World Interactive Network Focused on Critical Ultrasound. 15th World Interactive Network Focused on Critical Ultrasound (WINFOCUS) World Congress on ultrasound in emergency & critical care: post event report 2019. 2020. Retrieved July 13, 2022, from https://www.winfocus.org/wp-content/uploads/2020/04/WINFOCUS-WC-Report-2019.pdf.
21. Abuzeyad FH, Shujaa AS, Dawood Al-Balushi AS, Farooq M, Alqasem L, Al-Awadhi A, Bashmi L, Aljawder SS, Hsu S. The journey of emergency medicine in the Arabian Gulf States. Saudi J Emerg Med. 2021;2(3):205–17. https://doi.org/10.24911/SJEMed/72-1628743646.

22. Hansoti B, Aluisio AR, Barry MA, Davey K, Lentz BA, Modi P, Newberry JA, Patel MH, Smith TA, Vinograd AM, Levine AC, on behalf of the Global Emergency Medicine Think Tank Clinical Research Working Group. Global health and emergency care: defining clinical research priorities. Acad Emerg Med. 2017;24(6):742–53. https://doi.org/10.1111/acem.13158.
23. Trehan I, Kivlehan SM, Pousson AY, Quao NSA, Rybarczyk MM, Selvam A, Bonney J, Bhaskar N, Becker TK, on behalf of the Global Emergency Medicine Literature Review (GEMLR) Group. Global emergency medicine: a review of the literature from 2019. Acad Emerg Med. 2019;28(1):117–28. https://doi.org/10.1111/acem.14107.
24. Partridge R, Abbo M, Virk A. Emergency medicine in Dubai, UAE. Int J Emerg Med. 2009;2(3):135–9.
25. WHO Emergency Care. World Health Organization. 2019, September 24. Retrieved July 24, 2022, from https://www.who.int/health-topics/emergency-care#tab=tab_2.
26. Fares S. The EMIRATES framework: Emergency management integrated roadmap aimed towards every healthcare system a conceptual framework. Saudi J Emerg Med. 2021;2(1):3–3.
27. American College of Surgeons. Resources for the optimal care of the injured patient. Chicago: ACS; 2006.
28. World Health Organization. Cardiovascular diseases. NMH Fact Sheet. World Health Organization; 2014. p. 1–2.2.
29. Fares S, Zubaid M, Al-Mahmeed W, Ciottone G, Sayah A, Al Suwaidi J, et al. Utilization of emergency medical services by patients with acute coronary syndromes in the Arab Gulf States. J Emerg Med. 2011;41:310–6.
30. Batt A, Al-Hajeri A, Delport S, Jenkins S, Norman S, Cummins F. Implementation of a STEMI bypass protocol in the northern United Arab Emirates. Heart Views. 2019;19:121–7. https://doi.org/10.4103/HEARTVIEWS.HEARTVIEWS_81_17.
31. Horner KB, Jones A, Wang L, Winger DG, Marin JR. Variation in advanced imaging for pediatric patients with abdominal pain discharged from the ED. Am J Emerg Med. 2016;34(12):2320–5.
32. Michelson KA, Hudgins JD, Monuteaux MC, Bachur RG, Finkelstein JA. Cardiac arrest survival in pediatric and general emergency departments. Pediatrics. 2018;141(2):e20172741.
33. Bekmezian A, Hersh AL, Maselli JH, Cabana MD. Pediatric emergency departments are more likely than general emergency departments to treat asthma exacerbation with systemic corticosteroids. J Asthma. 2011;48(1):69–74.
34. Strauss KJ, Somasundaram E, Sengupta D, Marin JR, Brady SL. Radiation dose for pediatric CT: comparison of pediatric versus adult imaging facilities. Radiology. 2019;291(1):158–67.
35. Professional Qualification Requirement. Department of Health. Retrieved July 26, 2022, from: https://www.doh.gov.ae/en/pqr.
36. Absal R, Scott K. Horrific accident on Abu Dhabi-Dubai highway near Ghantoot. 2008, March. Cited 24 Mar 2019.
37. Ahmed SA, Jarsh MB, Al-Abdooli S, Al-Radhi MK, Galadari A. Forecasting tropical storms in the eastern region of the United Arab Emirates: lessons learnt from gonu. In: Causes, impacts and solutions to global warming. New York: Springer; 2013. p. 183–94.
38. Fares S, Femino M, Sayah A, Weiner DL, Yim ES, Douthwright S, et al. Health care system hazard vulnerability analysis: an assessment of all public hospitals in Abu Dhabi. Disasters. 2014;38(2):420–33.
39. Al Hosany F, Ganesan S, Al Memari S, Al Mazrouei S, Ahamed F, Koshy A, Zaher W. Response to COVID-19 pandemic in the UAE: a public health perspective. J Glob Health. 2021;11:03050.
40. Hafizur RM, Allen KA, Hyder AA. Descriptive epidemiology of injury cases: findings from a pilot injury surveillance system in Abu Dhabi. Int J Inj Control Saf Promot. 2014:1–10. https://doi.org/10.1080/17457300.2014.908225.
41. Al-Ali SF. Establishing a trauma registry in the Emirate of Abu Dhabi. Doctoral dissertation. Johns Hopkins University; 2021.
42. Fares S. Together for emergency medicine in the United Arab Emirates! Mediterr J Emerg Med Acute Care. 2019;1(1).

43. DaCruz DJ. Unnecessary emergency visits: Middle East has an answer. BMJ: Br Med J. 2008;336(7655):1206.
44. Emirates Society of Emergency Medicine (ESEM). https://esem.ae/about-esem/.
45. Alper CA, Cakal ED, Alao D, Margret E, Sami S, Abu-Zidan F. Self-efficacy beliefs and expectations during an emergency medicine clerkship. Int J Emerg Med (Online). 2022;15(1):4.

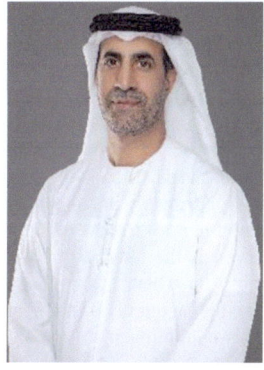

Dr. Saleh Fares Al-Ali is the first Canadian and American board-certified emergency physician from the United Arab Emirates. He completed the Royal College Emergency Medicine Residency Program at McGill University in Montreal, Canada (2002–2007). In 2008, he completed a fellowship in EMS at the University of Toronto in Canada, followed by a Disaster Medicine Fellowship at BIDMC in Boston, a teaching hospital of Harvard Medical School, as Harvard's first Disaster Medicine fellow and co-founder of the program (2009). In May 2011, he obtained his MPH from Johns Hopkins University and his DrPH in Health Care Management and Leadership from the same school (May 2021).

Dr. Fares Al-Ali is the former head of the ED and the former program director at Zayed Military Hospital. He is the founder and former chairman of the Trauma System Initiative of the Emirate of Abu Dhabi, and he is also the founder and past president of the Emirates Society of Emergency Medicine (ESEM). Dr. Fares Al-Ali was able to establish several key initiatives, including the first official trauma registry in the Emirate of Abu Dhabi, the Abu Dhabi STEMI network involving different stakeholders, and the approval of the UAE "Good Samaritan Law," which is considered the first law of its kind in an Arab country. He led the ESEM Conference to be the largest emergency conference in the MENA region and successfully hosted ICEM21 for the first time in the MENA region, with over 2500 delegates. He was appointed as the Executive Director of the Center of Emergency Preparedness and Response (CEPAR) at the Department of Health—Abu Dhabi from April 2021 to July 2024, during which he was able to introduce a new concept of Health Emergency Management in Abu Dhabi. Dr. Saleh Fares Al-Ali has contributed to several international textbooks and peer-reviewed articles in the fields of EM, EMS, and disaster medicine and has presented at several conferences regionally and internationally.

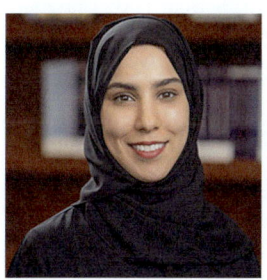

Rasha Buhumaid is a Consultant Emergency Physician and Assistant Professor at Mohammed Bin Rashid University of Medicine and Health Sciences (MBRU). She is the Past President of the Emirates Society of Emergency Medicine (ESEM) and currently serves as President-Elect of the Asian Society for Emergency Medicine (ASEM), reflecting her growing influence in regional and international emergency medicine leadership.

She completed her Emergency Medicine residency at George Washington University in Washington, D.C., and a fellowship in Emergency Ultrasound at Massachusetts General Hospital, Boston. She is also pursuing a Master's in Medical Education at the University of Dundee.

Dr. Buhumaid is a recognized authority in point-of-care ultrasound (POCUS) education and has led numerous regional and international workshops. Her work continues to shape emergency medicine education and practice across the Middle East and Asia.

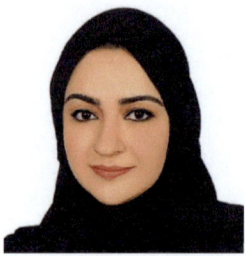

Khalifa Saeed Alqaydi is a Consultant Emergency Physician and a prominent leader in military and academic emergency medicine in the UAE. He serves as Head of the Emergency Department and Director of the Emergency Medicine Residency Program at Zayed Military Hospital in Abu Dhabi, under the Ministry of Defense.

Dr. Alqaydi earned his medical degree from the University of Manchester (UK) and completed his Emergency Medicine residency at McGill University (Canada), followed by fellowships in Trauma Team Leadership and Resuscitation Leadership.

His professional interests lie in caring for critically ill patients in the Emergency Department and contributing to trauma system improvement. Notably, Dr. Alqaydi serves as the Co-chair of the Education Sub-Task Force within the Abu Dhabi Emergency Medicine Task Force, focusing on enhancing the quality of medical education in the emirate. This reflects his commitment to shaping the education and training of healthcare professionals in Abu Dhabi. Overall, Dr. Khalifa Saeed Alqaydi plays a multifaceted role, combining clinical expertise, leadership in emergency medicine, and a commitment to advancing medical education in Abu Dhabi.

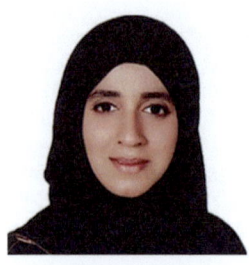

Muna Al Jallaf is an Emergency Medicine Specialist at Rashid Hospital, one of the UAE's leading trauma and emergency care centers. As the General Secretary of the Emirates Society of Emergency Medicine (ESEM), she actively contributes to the development of emergency care practices and professional education in the UAE. Dr. Al Jallaf is committed to clinical excellence and continuous improvement in emergency services.

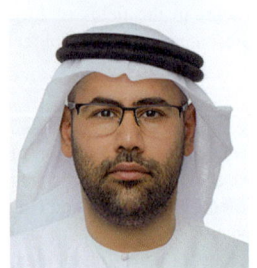

Hind Al Dhaheri is a Consultant Emergency Physician and a senior academic leader at Tawam Hospital, where she serves as Deputy and Associate Program Director of the Emergency Medicine Residency Program. She holds an MBBS from UAE University (2009), the Jordanian Board of Emergency Medicine (2015), and an Executive Master's in Healthcare Administration from Zayed University (2017).

Dr. Al Dhaheri is the Vice-President of the Emirates Society of Emergency Medicine (ESEM), contributing to national initiatives in emergency care education and policy. She also plays a key role in hospital administration, serving on multiple strategic committees including the Blood Utilization Committee, Hospital-wide Morbidity and Mortality Committee, and the Graduate Medical Education Committee.

She is also a member of the Emergency Medicine Specialty Committee at the UAE National Institute for Health Specialties, supporting the advancement of emergency medicine standards nationwide.

Open Access This chapter is licensed under the terms of the Creative Commons Attribution 4.0 International License (http://creativecommons.org/licenses/by/4.0/), which permits use, sharing, adaptation, distribution and reproduction in any medium or format, as long as you give appropriate credit to the original author(s) and the source, provide a link to the Creative Commons license and indicate if changes were made.

The images or other third party material in this chapter are included in the chapter's Creative Commons license, unless indicated otherwise in a credit line to the material. If material is not included in the chapter's Creative Commons license and your intended use is not permitted by statutory regulation or exceeds the permitted use, you will need to obtain permission directly from the copyright holder.

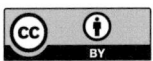

Intensive Care in the UAE

30

Ayesha Almemari, Saif Mohammed Alkaabi, Abdullah AlNaqbi, and Fayez Alshamsi

30.1 History of Intensive Care

Intensive care medicine can be traced back to the nineteenth century, specifically to the Crimean War (1850s), when Florence Nightingale (the founder of the modern nursing profession) and her team moved the sick and wounded soldiers to a specific area close to the nursing station so that they could be observed closely [1]. The modern intensive care medicine practice likely started in the mid-twentieth century with the invention of positive pressure ventilation (PPV) [2]. The first intensive care unit (ICU) in Europe was established by Bjorn Ibsen, an anesthetist, who suggested treating polio patients with PPV, and he is considered the father of intensive care in Europe [3]. In North America, the first ICU is believed to have been at the University of South California Medical Center, established by Max Harry Weil, who is credited with being the father of the ICU in the USA; at the same time, the University of Pittsburgh started their first ICU [3, 4].

In the United Arab Emirates (UAE), ICUs are usually staffed by trained intensivists of diverse backgrounds. The number of intensive care beds varies widely between countries. The economic status of the country is the main determinant of the number of ICU beds available to the population. ICU care is one of the most expensive services in any health system [5, 6]. Published data from 2012 reported that public hospitals in the Emirate of Abu Dhabi had 18 ICU units across 7 secondary

---

A. Almemari
Sheikh Shakhbout Medical City (SSMC), Abu Dhabi, United Arab Emirates
e-mail: amemari@ssmc.ae

S. M. Alkaabi · A. AlNaqbi
Zayed Military Hospital, Abu Dhabi, United Arab Emirates

F. Alshamsi (✉)
College of Medicine and Health Sciences, United Arab Emirates University, Al Ain, United Arab Emirates
e-mail: f_ebrahim@uaeu.ac.ae

and tertiary care hospitals, with a total bed capacity of 287, distributed among 10 adult ICUs, 5 neonatal ICUs, and 3 pediatric ICUs, excluding coronary care units (CCUs) [7]. The number of hospital beds in the UAE had almost doubled from 8,000 beds in 2010 to 14,000 beds in 2017, and the number of ICU beds was rising too [8, 9]. There is no consensus on the number of beds per 100,000 people worldwide. In Asian countries, the number of ICUs per 100,000 population varies; in high-income countries, it ranges between 8.1 and 20.8, with a median of 12.3. In the neighboring country, Oman, there are 14.6 ICU beds per 100,000 population, and in Saudi Arabia, there are 22.8 ICU beds per 100,000 population [10]. In 2017, data from the Department of Health (DoH) in Abu Dhabi showed that Abu Dhabi (population 3,000,000) had a total of 848 ICU beds (approximately 28 ICU/CCU beds per 100,000 population), of which 81 were pediatric, 263 neonatal, and 504 adult ICU beds in both private and government hospitals [11]. Data from the Dubai Health Authority (DHA) in 2018 showed that Dubai's population was 3.1 million, and critical care beds totaled 902 beds (29 ICU beds per 100,000 population), comprising 526 adult, 299 neonatal, and 77 PICU beds in both private and government hospitals. The remaining cities in the UAE are under the authority of the Ministry of Health and Prevention (MOHAP), where no data about ICU beds could be found; however, they are expected to be similar to Dubai and Abu Dhabi [12]. The UAE population in 2020 was 9.28 million. The total number of hospital beds was 18,005 in the same year in both private and government hospitals [11]. The COVID-19 pandemic changed global health services dramatically; at some stages, almost all ICU beds worldwide were full. The supply-demand estimation for the need for actual ICU beds was not accurate, as the magnitude of the pandemic was not expected. The pandemic was a disaster situation, straining hospitals' capacity to accommodate critically ill patients. Expansion of ICU services during the pandemic to accommodate the high number of ventilated patients was the only solution. Many areas in the hospitals were utilized for critically ill patients, such as the Post Anesthesia Recovery Unit (PACU), High Dependency Unit (HDU), and Emergency Department (ED). The ratio of ICU beds to normal hospital beds changed, and many ICU beds were added to the system; some were temporary in field hospitals, and others became operational on a daily basis, in addition to the standby surge-ready ICU beds [13, 14]. This experience will affect the future design and disaster preparedness of any hospital [15]. In the UAE, there was no official data available at the time of writing this chapter about the actual current capacity of ICU beds since the beginning of the pandemic or regarding manpower; this is an area for future research.

30.2　Epidemiology of Critically Ill Patients in the UAE

The UAE is known for its diverse population in terms of gender, age, and culture. The UAE population reached 10.08 million in March 2022. Males comprise the majority of the population at 68.7% (6.9 million), while females are at 31.2% (3.1 million). Age-wise, the majority of the population is young working class (age 25–54) (6.5 million), and, when coupled with a developed healthcare system, this results in a long life expectancy [16]. Emiratis are only 11% of the population, while 89% are expatriates, which poses a unique health challenge, as the pathologies that present to the ICU are diverse (both communicable and non-communicable diseases), reflecting the population [17]. Mortality due to injuries accounted for 21% of the 2008 data, followed by cardiovascular disease (16%) and oncology (12%) [17]. Up until the update of UAE medical liability law in 2016, which allowed natural death "Do Not Resuscitate" orders in futile medical conditions, all patients were dying in the ICU, and almost all received cardiopulmonary (CPR) at the time of death, even when death was expected [18, 19]. During wave one of the COVID-19 pandemic, one of the major ICUs dedicated to COVID-19 patients reported combined ICU and hospital mortality due to COVID-19 pneumonia of 20%. This was lower than the reported mortality in other countries, such as Italy, where it reached 50%, a difference that reflects multiple factors, one of which may be the young age of the UAE population [20]. Another study from Dubai reported COVID-19 pneumonia overall mortality of 30%, with ICU mortality being 50%, noting that ICU patients were older and 85% of them required mechanical ventilation [21].

30.3 Intensive Care Delivery

Intensive care (IC) delivery may differ between institutions based on the ICU operating model, staffing, intensivist-to-patient ratios, care delivered by non-physician providers, and unit specialization. IC operating models are described as either "open" or "closed." In open models, the care of the patient is delivered by multiple clinicians, which may or may not include an intensivist, as opposed to a single intensivist in a closed model [22]. In the UAE, no published data exists on which model is more common; however, the authors' experience is that both models are utilized, with open units being more common in smaller private and community hospitals. Staffing also differs with intensivists' availability around the clock inside the unit, usually through shift work, versus being on-call and summoned as needed, with a specific expected time of arrival. In 2017, a systematic review by the American Thoracic Society, focusing on patient-important outcomes of mortality and length of stay in the ICU, concluded that limited observational evidence suggests around-the-clock intensivist availability was not linked to better outcomes [23]. The authors' experience in the UAE is that most units have around-the-clock in-house intensivist coverage, backed up by a senior intensivist on call, depending on the institution. Another aspect of staffing that impacts patient care is the intensivist-to-patient ratio. For closed units, the Society of Critical Care Medicine found a negative impact on patient care and staff wellbeing when the ratio was less than 1:14 [24]. Data from the DoH of the Emirate of Abu Dhabi Master Plan showed that in 2017, there were a total of 120 licensed intensivists and 767 ICU beds [11, 25]. However, calculating an accurate ratio from raw data is difficult.

Care of critically ill patients is complex and is best delivered by interprofessional collaboration among caregivers with different expertise, such as ICU nurses, respiratory therapists, clinical pharmacists, dieticians, rehabilitation therapists, social workers, and spiritual care providers [26]. This model has been recommended by an expert panel, as it has been shown to improve outcomes [27]. Delivering care in a mixed general ICU versus a specialized ICU varies between institutions and is determined by several factors, including the level of care of the hospital and expertise, such as cardiac surgical care and neurocritical care [28]. Admissions to neurocritical care units for patients with acute ischemic strokes and intracerebral hemorrhages were associated with better outcomes compared with patients with these conditions admitted to a mixed general ICU [28, 29]. Granular data on the distribution of unit specializations in the UAE is not available. However, in the author's experience, tertiary centers of excellence often have specialized critical care units. Finally, critical care delivery in crises is integral to the planning and preparedness of healthcare systems, as seen recently with the COVID-19 pandemic and the challenges it imposed, as well as its implications for the future of critical care delivery [15]. The UAE's response focused on emergency response with regulatory documents, surge capacity, risk communication and public engagement, case and contact tracing, surveillance, and robust containment public health measures [13].

30.4 Community Perception of Intensive Care

Family needs in ICU are similar around the world, with slight differences related to cultural, social, and economic factors. A better understanding of these needs improves the overall experience of families, enhances interaction with healthcare workers, and probably leads to better satisfaction while decreasing anxiety and uncertainty. There are two main elements to be considered. First is the ICU patient's family perception of their needs, and second is the healthcare worker's perception of family needs. Information and assurance appear to be the greatest universal needs of ICU patient families. Families want timely, clear, and understandable information about their relatives' medical conditions without leaving room for unrealistic hope. In most literature, healthcare staff ranked the need for information and assurance as the top two important needs; yet, despite this, both needs were the most frequently cited by family members as being unmet by healthcare staff. Overall, the ICU patient family is highly satisfied with the care their relative receives, especially regarding aspects of care such as the skill and competence of staff and the respect given to the patient. Families were less satisfied with emotional support, the provision of understandable, consistent information, and the coordination of care. Families felt more satisfied when clear, honest information was delivered to them in understandable language, as this enabled them to actively participate in the decision-making process. Some family members are prone to being impacted by the critical illness of their loved one. Risk factors associated with an increase in symptoms of anxiety include female gender, being a spouse, unplanned ICU admission, lower educational status, poor sleep patterns, fatigue, a lack of regular meetings with medical staff, and failing to meet family needs [30].

In Saudi Arabia, where the society has similar values to the UAE, the most important need identified by family members was the need for assurance, followed by information, proximity, comfort, and support. A higher level of education was significantly associated with a higher level of need for assurance, information, and proximity [31]. A study looking specifically at the family needs of Muslim patients found that family members and healthcare providers ranked assurance, information, and cultural and spiritual needs as the most important, and support and proximity as the least important. A significant finding not identified in other studies was the extreme importance of postmortem care, ranked first by family members but fifth by healthcare providers [32].

30.5 Intensive Care Training

In the eighteenth and nineteenth centuries, medical school graduates used to start practicing immediately after graduation from medical school. Only elite doctors pursued further education and sought a PhD, which, back then, was mainly attained in Europe; afterward, they returned to their home country to practice and pioneer their field. After the First World War and the Industrial Revolution, people moved to cities; hence, more hospitals were established, and the demand to staff the hospitals with physicians in various specialties increased, which in turn increased the training opportunities. Physicians in training historically used to *live in the hospital*, and that is how they got the term resident physicians [33]. Michael Pinsky defined an intensivist as "The physician providing the most efficient primary care for the critically ill, bringing some aspects of all specialties to the bedside and allowing titration of resources in a patient-specific fashion; a primary generalist" [34]. There are four major IC training models known internationally (Fig. 30.1) [35]. The first model is the multiple sub-specialty model, where IC training is "owned" by multiple parent specialties, and access to training is limited to trainees within the respective parent discipline. Multidisciplinary access can begin during or after base training, and each specialty has its own national IC curriculum. At the end, physicians can choose to have dual certification, or base specialty certification, which includes IC [34]. The second model is the single sub-specialty model, where IC training is "owned" by one parent specialty, and access is limited to trainees within this specialty, either during or after base training; trainees from other disciplines are not accepted. Toward the end of the training, trainees can have dual certification or base specialty certification, which includes IC. This model is the classic combination of anesthesia

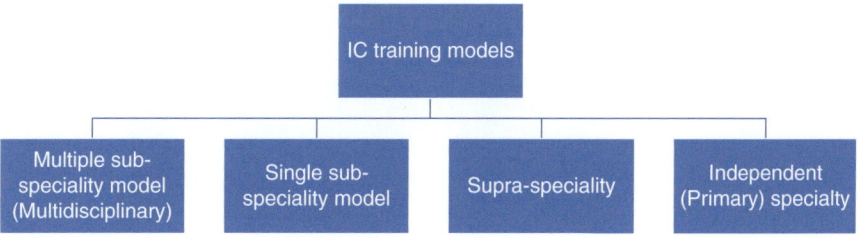

Fig. 30.1 Intensive care (IC) training models

and critical care that dominated most European countries, specifically Scandinavian countries, until the 1990s, when, on average, about 30% (6–9 months) of the training period (5 years) was dedicated to IC and 70% to anesthesia. The third model is where IC is considered a supra-specialty, and physicians need to complete base specialty training and certification before entering IC as a subspeciality; this is the main model in North America. The basic specialty training that physicians can completed before specializing in IC includes internal medicine, general surgery, emergency medicine, and anesthesia. In this model, all graduates of various disciplines join the same IC training program. The fourth model is IC training as an independent (primary) specialty, a model that was started in Spain in 1978 with the goal of having intensivists dedicated to ICU care to reduce mortality. Switzerland and Germany adopted this model in the 1980s, the UK in the 1990s, and Saudi Arabia in 2015. In this model, trainees join a 5-year IC program directly after medical school, and their certificate is only in IC [34, 35]. Figure 30.2 outlines the IC training models in various countries worldwide. Data from Spain comparing ICU outcomes to those of other European countries did not show any difference. However, perhaps the measured outcome was not the correct reflection of the IC training model as an advantage. Having a closed ICU design instead might have been the factor that influenced the ICU outcome more than the IC training model [36]. Outcomes that need to be measured to assess if IC as a primary specialty training model performs better than other models are patient and family satisfaction, nurse perception, and physician turnover and satisfaction [37]. The clinical care that is required of ICU physicians is by nature stressful, fast-paced, and potentially chaotic, which may lead to burnout. A study on burnout among intensivists demonstrated that the timing of work, rather than the volume of work, is associated with burnout. On the other hand, having professional activities outside of bedside care, such as involvement in a work group or research team, may be protective against burnout. In addition,

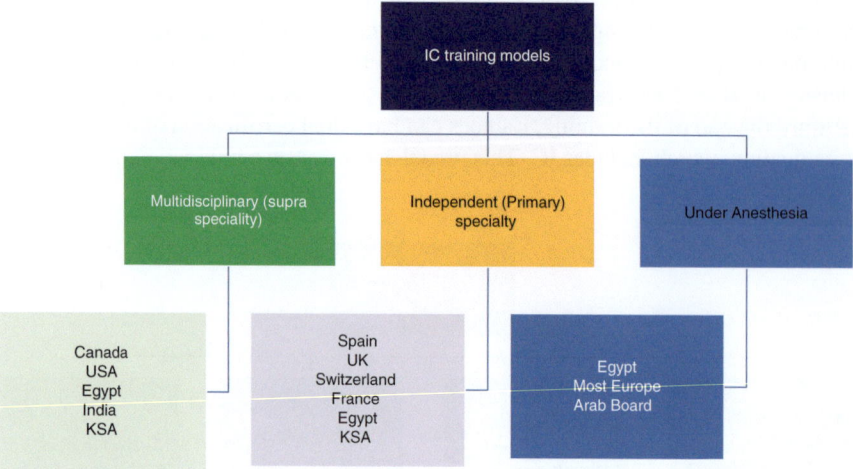

Fig. 30.2 Intensive care training models in different countries worldwide

changing intensivist rotations from 14 consecutive days to either 7 consecutive days or giving the weekend off in the middle is associated with reduced burnout symptoms. Moreover, having a dual specialty allows for flexibility in scheduling and less ICU direct clinical care, an advantage that is not available for physicians with IC training as their primary specialty [38]. In the UAE, the IC training model adopted is a multidisciplinary, supra-specialty training one in which trainees from various disciplines apply to one fellowship and complete training with dual specialization in their base specialty and IC. The fellowship training programs are accredited by the National Institute for Health Specialties (NIHS), and the first program was accredited in 2024 [39].

30.6 Conclusion

After discussing intensive care in the United Arab Emirates, including historical background, epidemiology of critically ill patients, intensive care delivery, community perceptions and needs, and intensive care training, we conclude this chapter with IC outcomes and a future outlook in the UAE.

Published data on IC outcomes preceding the COVID-19 pandemic are scarce, as evident from a PubMed search combining the MeSH terms "United Arab Emirates" and "critical care outcomes." The country's response and COVID-19 outcomes have been reported previously [13, 20, 40–42]. Mass screening, contact tracing, vaccination, and early recognition and management of patients led to outcomes that were comparable to and sometimes better than those reported in the literature, owing to factors such as an overall younger population, among others.

With a growing population, unique demographics, increased life expectancy, a rising prevalence of cardiovascular diseases and their complications (such as dialysis), and emerging infectious threats such as the monkeypox virus, the healthcare system in the UAE is faced with several challenges [43–45]. With increasing life expectancy, the average age of referrals to intensive care will inevitable rise, as already observed in some countries where the median age of the ICU population is above 65 years old [46, 47]. Caring for such a population is challenging due to the frequent coexistence of chronic illnesses and altered physiology that affects functional recovery, often resulting in prolonged critical care and hospital stays, as well as increased mortality [46, 47]. Addressing these challenges should be a priority for research and healthcare planning [47].

In 2016, death by neurological criteria (DNC) was adopted as a legal definition, with the first case of deceased multiorgan donation happening on July 15, 2017. Since then, donation activity has steadily increased, with 109 donors recorded as of this writing [48]. Globally, donors after DNC accounted for 77% of all in 2020, understanding the critical role of intensive care in identifying, referring, and managing donors after DNC to ensure successful donation and transplant outcomes [49].

Innovative solutions such as tele-intensive care (Tele-ICU) can improve several aspects of critical care delivery both before or during an ICU stay. They also help mitigate staff shortages and expand access to expertise, particularly during disasters

[50, 51]. Artificial intelligence has also gained traction, especially during the COVID-19 pandemic; however, its impact on improving intensive care outcomes remains an area of active research [15, 52].

MOHAP, DoH, and DHA, the primary healthcare regulatory entities in the UAE, continue to update their future outlooks and capacity plans to address the aforementioned needs [11, 12, 25, 43].

Conflicts of Interest The authors have no conflicts of interest to declare.

References

1. Wallace DJ, Kahn JM. Florence nightingale and the conundrum of counting ICU beds. Crit Care Med. 2015;43(11):2517–8. https://doi.org/10.1097/CCM.0000000000001290.
2. Slutsky AS. History of mechanical ventilation. From Vesalius to ventilator-induced lung injury. Am J Respir Crit Care Med. 2015;191(10):1106–15. https://doi.org/10.1164/rccm.201503-0421PP.
3. Kelly FE, Fong K, Hirsch N, Nolan JP. Intensive care medicine is 60 years old: the history and future of the intensive care unit. Clin Med (Lond). 2014;14(4):376–9. https://doi.org/10.7861/clinmedicine.14-4-376.
4. History of Critical Care | NEJM Resident 360. https://resident360.nejm.org/content_items/277. Accessed 04 July 2022.
5. Rhodes A, Ferdinande P, Flaatten H, Guidet B, Metnitz PG, Moreno RP. The variability of critical care bed numbers in Europe. Intensive Care Med. 2012;38(10):1647–53. https://doi.org/10.1007/s00134-012-2627-8.
6. Murthy S, Wunsch H. Clinical review: international comparisons in critical care – lessons learned. Crit Care. 2012;16(2):218. https://doi.org/10.1186/cc11140.
7. Latif A, et al. Implementing a multifaceted intervention to decrease central line–associated bloodstream infections in SEHA (Abu Dhabi Health Services Company) intensive care units: the Abu dhabi Experience. Infect Control Hosp Epidemiol. 2015;36:1–7. https://doi.org/10.1017/ice.2015.70.
8. UAE needs 1,000 ICU beds to meet patient demands. Arabian Business. 16 May 2017. https://www.arabianbusiness.com/gcc/uae-needs-1-000-icu-beds-meet-patient-demands-674000. Accessed 04 July 2022.
9. UAE: number of hospitals beds 2017. Statista. https://www.statista.com/statistics/822693/uae-number-of-hospitals-beds/. Accessed 04 July 2022.
10. Phua J, et al. Critical care bed capacity in Asian countries and regions. Crit Care Med. 2020;48(5):654–62. https://doi.org/10.1097/CCM.0000000000004222.
11. Department of Health Abu Dhabi. Abu Dhabi health statistics 2017. 2017. [Online]. Available: https://www.doh.gov.ae/-/media/Feature/Resources/AbuDhabiHealthStatistics.ashx. Accessed 18 Aug 2022.
12. Dubai Health Authority. Dubai clinical services capacity plan 2018–2030. 2018. [Online]. Available: https://www.dha.gov.ae/uploads/122021/e9b6b25d-1339-4f2e-8fbf-2b8ea3217315.pdf.
13. Al Hosany F, et al. Response to COVID-19 pandemic in the UAE: a public health perspective. J Glob Health. 2021;11:03050. https://doi.org/10.7189/jogh.11.03050.
14. Digital T. Al Rahba Hospital opens new Urgent Care Center for COVID-19 medical services. Department of Health Abu Dhabi. 2022. [Online]. Available: https://www.doh.gov.ae/en/news/Al-Rahba-Hospital-opens-new-Urgent-Care-Center-for-COVID-19-medical-services. Accessed 04 July 2022.

15. Arabi YM, et al. How the COVID-19 pandemic will change the future of critical care. Intensive Care Med. 2021;47(3):282–91. https://doi.org/10.1007/s00134-021-06352-y.
16. United Arab Emirates (UAE) Population Statistics 2022 | GMI. Official GMI Blog. https://www.globalmediainsight.com/blog/uae-population-statistics/. Accessed 04 July 2022.
17. Blair I, Sharif AA. Population structure and the burden of disease in The United Arab Emirates. J Epidemiol Glob Health. 2012;2(2):61–71. https://doi.org/10.1016/j.jegh.2012.04.002.
18. Masood UR, Said A, Faris C, Al Mussady M, Al Jundi A. Limiting intensive care therapy in dying critically ill patients: experience from a tertiary care center in United Arab Emirates. Int J Crit Illn Inj Sci. 2013;3(3):200–5. https://doi.org/10.4103/2229-5151.119201.
19. The-UAE-new-law-on-medical-liability. https://ach-legal.com/blog/The-UAE-New-Law-on-Medical-Liability. Accessed 04 July 2022.
20. Ismail K, et al. Characteristics and outcome of critically ill patients with coronavirus disease-2019 (COVID-19) pneumonia admitted to a tertiary care center in The United Arab Emirates during the first wave of the SARS-CoV-2 pandemic. A retrospective analysis. PLoS One. 2021;16(10):e0251687. https://doi.org/10.1371/journal.pone.0251687.
21. Nadeem R, et al. Clinical profile of mortality and treatment profile of survival in patients with COVID-19 pneumonia admitted to Dubai hospital. Dubai Med J. 2021;4(3):256–62. https://doi.org/10.1159/000516591.
22. Garland A, Gershengorn HB. Staffing in ICUs: physicians and alternative staffing models. Chest. 2013;143(1):214–21. https://doi.org/10.1378/chest.12-1531.
23. Kerlin MP, et al. An official American Thoracic Society systematic review: the effect of nighttime intensivist staffing on mortality and length of stay among intensive care unit patients. Am J Respir Crit Care Med. 2017;195(3):383–93. https://doi.org/10.1164/rccm.201611-2250ST.
24. Ward NS, et al. Intensivist/patient ratios in closed ICUs: a statement from the Society of Critical Care Medicine Taskforce on ICU Staffing. Crit Care Med. 2013;41(2):638–45. https://doi.org/10.1097/CCM.0b013e3182741478.
25. Department of Health Abu Dhabi. Healthcare capacity master plan. 2020. [Online]. Available: https://www.doh.gov.ae/-/media/Files/Capacity-Masterplan.ashx.
26. Donovan AL, et al. Interprofessional care and teamwork in the ICU. Crit Care Med. 2018;46(6):980–90. https://doi.org/10.1097/CCM.0000000000003067.
27. Michalsen A, et al. Interprofessional shared decision-making in the ICU: a systematic review and recommendations from an expert panel. Crit Care Med. 2019;47(9):1258–66. https://doi.org/10.1097/CCM.0000000000003870.
28. Lott JP, Iwashyna TJ, Christie JD, Asch DA, Kramer AA, Kahn JM. Critical illness outcomes in specialty versus general intensive care units. Am J Respir Crit Care Med. 2009;179(8):676–83. https://doi.org/10.1164/rccm.200808-1281OC.
29. Chang CWJ, Provencio JJ, Shah S. Neurological critical care: the evolution of cerebrovascular critical care. Crit Care Med. 2021;49(6):881–900. https://doi.org/10.1097/CCM.0000000000004933.
30. Scott P, Thomson P, Shepherd A. Families of patients in ICU: a scoping review of their needs and satisfaction with care. Nurs Open. 2019;6(3):698–712. https://doi.org/10.1002/nop2.287.
31. Alsharari AF. The needs of family members of patients admitted to the intensive care unit. Patient Prefer Adherence. 2019;13:465–73. https://doi.org/10.2147/PPA.S197769.
32. Al-Mutair AS, Plummer V, Clerehan R, O'Brien AT. Families' needs of critical care Muslim patients in Saudi Arabia: a quantitative study. Nurs Crit Care. 2014;19(4):185–95. https://doi.org/10.1111/nicc.12039.
33. Why do we have residency training? The Health Care Blog. https://thehealthcareblog.com/blog/2020/01/16/why-do-we-have-residency-training/. Accessed 04 July 2022.
34. Bion J, Rothen HU. Models for intensive care training. A European perspective. Am J Respir Crit Care Med. 2014;189(3):256–62. https://doi.org/10.1164/rccm.201311-2058CP.
35. Barrett H, Bion JF. An international survey of training in adult intensive care medicine. Intensive Care Med. 2005;31(4):553–61. https://doi.org/10.1007/s00134-005-2583-7.

36. van der Sluis FJ, Slagt C, Liebman B, Beute J, Mulder JW, Engel AF. The impact of open versus closed format ICU admission practices on the outcome of high risk surgical patients: a cohort analysis. BMC Surg. 2011;11(1):18. https://doi.org/10.1186/1471-2482-11-18.
37. Burnout and Joy in the profession of critical care medicine | critical care | full text. https://ccforum.biomedcentral.com/articles/10.1186/s13054-020-2784-z. Accessed 05 July 2022.
38. Mikkelsen ME, Anderson BJ, Bellini L, Schweickert WD, Fuchs BD, Kerlin MP. Burnout, and fulfillment, in the profession of critical care medicine. Am J Respir Crit Care Med. 2019;200(7):931–3. https://doi.org/10.1164/rccm.201903-0662LE.
39. https://nihs.uaeu.ac.ae/en/accr_program.shtml. Accessed 20 Sep 2025.
40. Al Harbi M, et al. Clinical and laboratory characteristics of patients hospitalised with COVID-19: clinical outcomes in Abu Dhabi, United Arab Emirates. BMC Infect Dis. 2022;22(1):136. https://doi.org/10.1186/s12879-022-07059-1.
41. Hannawi S, et al. Clinical and laboratory profile of hospitalized symptomatic COVID-19 patients: case series study from the first COVID-19 center in the UAE. Front Cell Infect Microbiol. 2021;11:632965. https://doi.org/10.3389/fcimb.2021.632965.
42. Nadeem A, Hamed F, Saleh K, Abduljawad B, Mallat J. ICU outcomes of COVID-19 critically ill patients: an international comparative study. Anaesth Crit Care Pain Med. 2020;39(4):487–9. https://doi.org/10.1016/j.accpm.2020.07.001.
43. Ministry of Health and Prevention. UAE statistical annual report 2019. 2019. [Online]. Available: https://mohap.gov.ae/assets/download/7758bf4d/UAE%20Statistical%20Annual%20Report%202019.pdf.aspx. Accessed 18 Aug 2022.
44. Richards N, et al. Epidemiology and referral patterns of patients with chronic kidney disease in the Emirate of Abu Dhabi. Saudi J Kidney Dis Transpl. 2015;26(5):1028–34. https://doi.org/10.4103/1319-2442.164600.
45. Alakunle EF, Okeke MI. Monkeypox virus: a neglected zoonotic pathogen spreads globally. Nat Rev Microbiol. 2022;20(9):9. https://doi.org/10.1038/s41579-022-00776-z.
46. Pugh R, Subbe C, Thorpe C, Szakmany T. The Baby Boom and later life: is critical care fit for the future? Anaesthesiol Intensive Ther. 2019;49(5). [Online]. Available: https://www.termedia.pl/The-Baby-Boom-and-later-life-is-critical-care-fit-for-the-future-,118,38117,1,1.html. Accessed 23 Aug 2022.
47. Flaatten H, et al. The status of intensive care medicine research and a future agenda for very old patients in the ICU. Intensive Care Med. 2017;43(9):1319–28. https://doi.org/10.1007/s00134-017-4718-z.
48. Kumar S, Sankari BR, Miller CM, Obaidli AAKA, Suri RM. Establishment of solid organ transplantation in the United Arab Emirates. Transplantation. 2020;104(4):659–63. https://doi.org/10.1097/TP.0000000000003030.
49. 2020 International Activities report. GODT. http://www.transplant-observatory.org/2020-international-activities-report/. Accessed 24 Aug 2022.
50. Subramanian S, et al. Tele-critical care: an update from the Society of Critical Care Medicine Tele-ICU Committee. Crit Care Med. 2020;48(4):553–61. https://doi.org/10.1097/CCM.0000000000004190.
51. Lilly CM, et al. Critical care telemedicine: evolution and state of the art. Crit Care Med. 2014;42(11):2429–36. https://doi.org/10.1097/CCM.0000000000000539.
52. Mamdani M, Slutsky AS. Artificial intelligence in intensive care medicine. Intensive Care Med. 2021;47(2):147–9. https://doi.org/10.1007/s00134-020-06203-2.

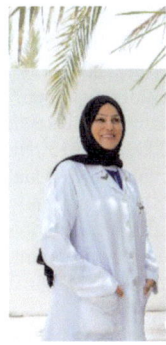

Dr. Ayesha Almemari is a consultant in emergency medicine and critical care in Abu Dhabi, UAE. She is a Canadian board-certified in emergency medicine as well as critical care medicine. She did her Master's in Quality and Safety in Health Care Management at RCSI in Dubai in 2014. Also, she earned a Master's in International Tissue and Organ Transplant and Donation from the University of Barcelona, Spain, in 2017. She holds an executive Master's in Business Administration from Hult University in Dubai in 2019. Dr. Ayesha has research interests in physician wellbeing and burnout; emergency medicine quality improvement; medical liability; and community health and well-being regulation.

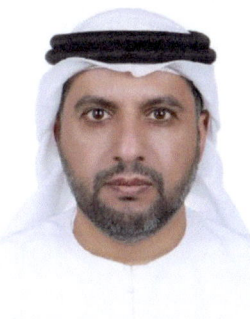

Dr. Saif Mohammed Alkaabi is an Emirati physician who earned his MBBS degree from the UAE University School of Medicine in 1998. He furthered his medical education by completing postgraduate studies at McMaster University in Hamilton, Canada. Between 2002 and 2007, Dr. Alkaabi received specialized training in internal medicine and critical care. He holds fellowships from the Royal College of Physicians of Canada and the American Board of Internal Medicine in Critical Care Medicine. In 2022, he achieved certification as a diplomate of the American Board of Internal Medicine in Neurocritical Care.

Dr. Alkaabi has been a dedicated ICU physician at Zayed Military Hospital in Abu Dhabi, UAE, since 2007 and has served as the head of the department since 2009. Additionally, he is actively involved in teaching within the Arab Board Internal Medicine Residency Program at Zayed Military Hospital, imparting his expertise in Advanced Cardiac Life Support (ACLS). Furthermore, he leads the hospital's Code Blue Committee.

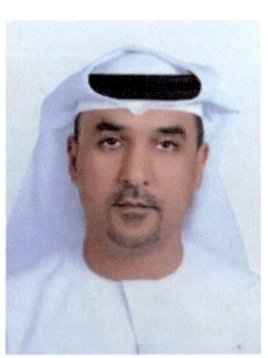

Abdullah AlNaqbi works as a medical director and head of the ICU at Zayed Military Hospital-Batayeh. His journey in medicine started after graduation from the College of Medicine and Health Science, UAE University. He pursued further education and training, completing a residency in Canada at the University of Toronto from 2005 to 2010, specializing in both internal medicine and critical care. Additionally, he holds a Master's degree in Health Care Management from RCSI, the Royal College of Surgeons in Ireland. Dr. AlNaqbi is also a member of the Supreme Medical Liability Committee in the UAE.

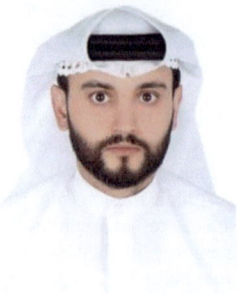

Fayez Alshamsi is an assistant professor of internal medicine at the College of Medicine and Health Sciences, United Arab Emirates University (UAEU). After earning his medical degree from UAEU in 2007, he underwent postgraduate training in internal medicine, critical care medicine, and neurocritical care at McMaster University, Ontario, Canada, from 2009 to 2015. He provides clinical services as a consultant in internal medicine and critical care medicine at Tawam Hospital, Al Ain. He is currently enrolled in the International Master in Donation and Transplantation of Organs, Tissues and Cells at the University of Barcelona, Spain, and is due to graduate in June 2019. He also serves on the National Transplant Committee in the UAE as Deputy Chairman.

Open Access This chapter is licensed under the terms of the Creative Commons Attribution 4.0 International License (http://creativecommons.org/licenses/by/4.0/), which permits use, sharing, adaptation, distribution and reproduction in any medium or format, as long as you give appropriate credit to the original author(s) and the source, provide a link to the Creative Commons license and indicate if changes were made.

The images or other third party material in this chapter are included in the chapter's Creative Commons license, unless indicated otherwise in a credit line to the material. If material is not included in the chapter's Creative Commons license and your intended use is not permitted by statutory regulation or exceeds the permitted use, you will need to obtain permission directly from the copyright holder.

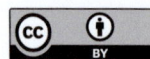

Road Traffic Collisions in the UAE

31

Hani O. Eid, Yasin J. Yasin, and Fikri M. Abu-Zidan

31.1 Introduction

The burden of road traffic collisions (RTCs) is global. According to the World Health Organization, around 1.35 million deaths annually worldwide are attributed to RTCs [1]. RTC death rates generally decrease when income increases. This is not true for high-income countries (HIC) in the Eastern Mediterranean Region, where RTC death rates increase when income increases [1]. This is particularly relevant to the United Arab Emirates (UAE), which is a rich country with rapid economic growth. It has modern, high-speed roads with a large number of cars [1, 2]. During 2016, around 3.39 million vehicles were registered in the UAE, of which 1.6% were motorized two- and three-wheelers [1]. The economic growth attracted foreign workers, who make up 87% of the population [3]. Many of them have low salaries and use walking, cycling, and motorized two- and three-wheelers as affordable transportation methods [2, 4–7]. Accordingly, a policy was adopted to build up a sustainable environment for all road users [8].

H. O. Eid
Rescue and Air Ambulance, Abu Dhabi Police Aviation, Abu Dhabi, United Arab Emirates

Y. J. Yasin
Institute of Public Health, College of Medicine and Health Sciences, United Arab Emirates University, Al-Ain, United Arab Emirates

Department of Environmental Health and Behavioral Sciences, School of Public Health, College of Health Sciences, Mekelle University, Mekelle, Ethiopia
e-mail: 201990037@uaue.ac.ae

F. M. Abu-Zidan (✉)
Department of Surgery, College of Medicine and Health Sciences, United Arab Emirates University, Al-Ain, United Arab Emirates

In the UAE, RTCs are ranked as the seventh cause of death and the fifth cause of disability-adjusted life years (DALYs), with death and DALY rates higher than those in other HICs [1, 9, 10]. During 2016, approximately 31% of all road deaths in the UAE were among vulnerable road users, with 24.3%, 1.5%, and 5.5% among pedestrians, cyclists, and motorized two- and three-wheelers, respectively, compared with 54.5% among vehicle occupants [1]. RTC injuries in the UAE cost 0.263% of its total GDP, with an average per capita cost of around 1900 USD [11]. This cost is nearly 2.5 times higher than the cost of other HICs [11]. Despite that, the RTC death and DALY rates have decreased. Road death rates and DALY rates per 100,000 population dropped by 44% and 42%, respectively, during the period 2000–2019 [9, 10]. This is attributed to improvements in road safety, injury prevention (e.g., installation of speed cameras, signaled pedestrian crossings, enforcement of safety regulations, use of safety devices), the emergency medical system (EMS), prehospital care, in-hospital care, trauma registries, trauma education, and trauma research [12–14]. In this chapter, we describe the nature of RTCs in the UAE and efforts made to reduce them, as documented by the published research of the Trauma Group of the College of Medicine and Health Sciences, United Arab Emirates University, which was conducted during the last two decades.

31.2 Biomechanisms of RTC

Clinicians need to understand the biomechanics of RTCs, which helps them diagnose patients' injuries, recognize their severity, and define their workup [15, 16]. A proper history of the crash should always be recorded. With knowledge, understanding, imagination, and critical thinking, trauma biomechanics becomes very useful for clinicians [15]. When two objects collide, each has a certain amount of energy. The energy can be calculated from the formula: Energy = ½ mass × V^2, where V is velocity. The relationship between energy and mass is linear, while the relationship between energy and velocity is exponential. That is why the relationship between velocity and mortality from RTCs is exponential. During a collision, energy transfers from one object to another; this depends on the object's direction, speed, position, and the characteristics of the injured tissues. Elderly pedestrians with osteoporosis easily sustain cervical spine injuries, while children with soft, elastic tissues may have significant tissue injuries without fractures [15, 16].

Motor vehicle collisions can be front impact, rear impact, side impact, or combined; the vehicle may roll over or the occupants may be ejected from it. The energy transfer and its direction determine the outcome of a collision [17]. The severity of injuries in RTCs in the UAE increases in the following sequence: rear impact, front impact, side impact, rollover, and finally, ejection. Those who are ejected have injuries that are five times more severe than those with a rear impact. Those involved in a front impact have injury severity twice that of those involved in a rear impact. The injury severity of ejected vehicle occupants was double that of those with a lateral impact or rollover [16].

A front impact is a deceleration injury. The force of the initial frontal collision is usually transmitted through the lower limbs. It may result in an ankle injury, a stress fracture of the femur, or a hip dislocation, depending on the collision's severity and the position of the lower limbs. Passengers without seatbelts may hinge at the hip and lean forward, leading to chest compression against the steering wheel or hitting the head against the windscreen [15]. The greater the severity of injury sustained by an occupant's lower limb in a frontal-impact collision, the less severe their head injuries [18, 19].

Rear impact is associated with acceleration of the vehicle, which pushes the back of the passengers against the seat, leading to minor injuries. Restrained vehicle occupants will sustain whiplash injuries, which are higher among front-seat occupants, but head restraints help reduce the injury's severity [15]. Side impacts are associated with more severe brain and thoracic injuries and higher mortality compared with other types of crashes [15]. In rollover collisions, the vehicle roof can be compressed, leading to occupants' head and spinal cord injuries. If occupants are unrestrained, more serious injuries occur as they move freely. Furthermore, injury severity triples with ejection, leading to higher mortality. Unprotected ejected victims are more susceptible to being run over by another moving vehicle [15].

31.3 Effects of Safety Devices

RTCs are predictable and preventable. Seatbelts are the most important safety innovation in injury prevention. They limit the movement of car occupants to prevent them from hitting the interior parts of the car or being ejected during a crash [20, 21]. Seatbelt usage reduces the severity of injuries, hospital admission rates, duration of hospital stays, and the number of operations [22]. It reduces the risk of death, serious injuries, and minor injuries among front-seat occupants by up to 50%, 45%, and 25%, respectively, and among rear-seat occupants by 25%, 25%, and 20%, respectively [23]. In the UAE, the implementation of seatbelt legislation began in January 1999 [24]. As of 2017, it became mandatory for all car passengers [25]. Despite this, seatbelt non-compliance remains a major challenge in the UAE, mainly among young adults [22, 26, 27], and is a major contributor to injuries and deaths [26, 28, 29] (Fig. 31.1).

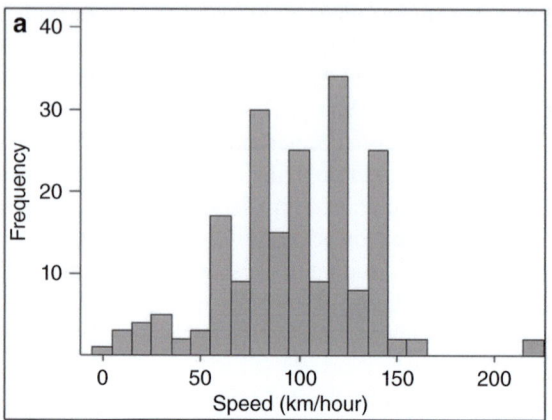
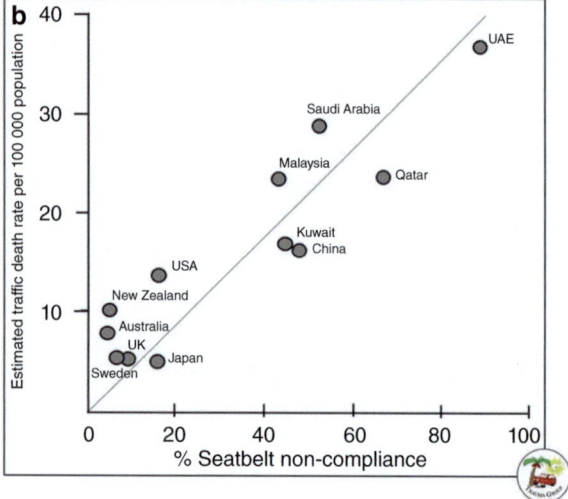

Fig. 31.1 The two most important factors that contributed to the high rate of RTC mortality in the United Arab Emirates 15 years ago (2007) were (1) over-speeding and (2) the low rate of seatbelt compliance. Figure (**a**) shows the distribution of speed of the cars involved in road traffic collisions ($n = 196$); 42% were higher than the legal speed limit of 100 km/hr at that time, while Figure (**b**) shows the RTC death rate in the United Arab Emirates compared with other selected countries. The United Arab Emirates had the highest morality and non-compliance with seatbelt usage. (Figure (**a**) is reproduced from Grivna et al. [65] which is distributed under the terms of the Creative Commons Attribution 4.0 International License)

A recent study from the UAE showed that nearly half of the drivers involved in vehicle crashes were not wearing seatbelts [26]. This is similar to other Gulf Cooperation Council (GCC) countries but not to other HICs [28]. Factors affecting seatbelt usage include law enforcement, road user characteristics (such as age, gender, and educational level), occupant type (driver versus passenger), position in the car (front-seat versus rear-seat), and vehicle type [27, 28, 30, 31]. Seatbelt usage, although useful in reducing mortality, is associated with specific spinal, pelvic, and abdominal injuries [32]. The presence of a combined seatbelt sign on the abdominal wall and a fractured spine increases the probability of bowel injury [33] (Fig. 31.2).

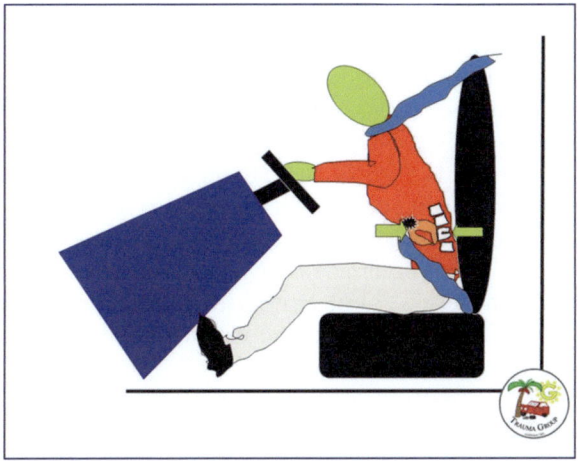

Fig. 31.2 Seatbelt syndrome is defined as a seatbelt sign associated with lumbar spine fracture and bowel perforation. (This figure was reproduced from Abbas et al. [32] which is distributed under the terms of the Creative Commons Attribution 4.0 International License. Illustrated by Professor Fikri Abu-Zidan, College of Medicine and Health Sciences, United Arab Emirates University, Al-Ain, UAE)

31.4 Risk Factors for RTCs

Distraction while driving is a serious road safety issue that causes preventable deaths [34, 35]. It is responsible for about 80% of collisions and 65% of near-collisions [36]. Distraction takes the driver's attention away from driving, either visually by taking their eyes off the road, manually by taking their hands off the wheel, or cognitively by taking the mind off the driving task. The eyes need to be on the road, the hands on the wheel, and the mind on the driving task to avoid distraction. A prospective study on distraction-related RTC injuries in the UAE showed that distraction by alert drivers accounted for 13% of road traffic collisions, the majority of which were middle-aged males [37]. Distraction occurred due to using mobile phones, deep thinking, talking to others, manipulating objects inside the vehicle, and using entertainment systems [37]. Using mobile phones without headsets, smoking, and eating or drinking while driving are illegal and banned by UAE traffic law.

Driving while drunk is deadly for all age groups. However, this risk is greater among young drivers, regardless of their blood alcohol concentration. A prospective study in the UAE showed a low incidence (2.1%) of self-reported alcohol-related RTCs, with injuries mainly to the head and face (94%) [38]. The alcohol group was much younger (median age 35 years) compared with international figures and stayed in the hospital twice as long as the non-alcohol group [38]. Patients with traumatic brain injury (TBI) need comprehensive medical care and have high mortality rates [38, 39]. Management of patients with alcohol intoxication and severe TBI is usually delayed by more than two hours compared with non-alcohol patients

[40]. This is attributed to the assumption that the low level of consciousness was induced by alcohol use and not by the TBI. The absence of routine blood alcohol concentration testing upon admission to hospitals has led to an underestimation of the contribution of alcohol to fatal TBI [41]. This problem is aggravated by the absence of national guidelines on blood alcohol testing.

Sleepiness contributes to 3.9% of all RTCs in Western countries [42]. A study from the UAE showed that it accounts for 5% of all collisions [43]. Most drivers (79%) who slept while driving and had a collision drove at 100 km/h or more. Sleepiness-related collisions occurred mainly during the month of Ramadan (42%) and while driving on highways (83%). Drivers in our community should be advised to stop driving when feeling sleepy, especially during Ramadan and on highways.

31.5 Injuries to Vehicle Occupants

Unintentional injuries cause 11.5% of all deaths in the UAE [44]. Injuries cause 17% of all deaths in the Abu Dhabi Emirate, 77% of which are unintentional. Sixty-two percent of unintentional injuries are caused by RTCs [45]. Vehicle occupants are the most injured road users and the majority are drivers [39]. Head injury is the main cause of hospitalization and mortality in victims of RTCs, especially in unrestrained vehicle occupants. Unrestrained rear vehicle occupants are frequently injured, with the same severity of injury as front-seat occupants [39]. The risk of death for restrained front vehicle occupants increases fivefold if the rear vehicle occupants are unbuckled because they act as flying objects within the vehicle, hitting front-seat passengers. Wearing seatbelts by rear vehicle occupants reduces their risk of death by 60% [46, 47]. It was a very lengthy battle to make seatbelt usage mandatory for all vehicle occupants in the UAE, which became law only in 2017.

Prompt diagnosis of life-threatening vascular injuries is essential for a favorable outcome. The incidence, mechanism, and anatomical distribution of vascular injuries following RTCs are not well studied in the Middle East [48]. In the UAE, the incidence of hospitalized vascular injury due to RTCs is 1.87 cases per 100,000 inhabitants. The most serious of these is thoracic aortic injury, which results from severe acceleration-deceleration impacts [48]. The most frequent cause of genitourinary (GU) injuries in severely injured patients in the UAE is RTCs, constituting 1.8% of hospitalized RTC patients [49]. Vehicle occupants make up the majority (78%), and renal injuries account for 74% of all injuries [49]. GU organs have a well-protected location; therefore, a high-energy impact is required to injure these retroperitoneal and intrapelvic organs [49].

31.6 Motorcycle Injuries

Motorized two- and three-wheelers account for 1.6% of all registered vehicles in the UAE [1], with a recent increasing trend [1]. They are used for transportation, delivery, sporting, and recreational activities [5]. Their riders are vulnerable road users because of their high speeds and exposed bodies [5]. Their risk of death from a crash is 30 times greater than that of a car occupant [50]. In 2016, motorized two- and three-wheeler deaths accounted for approximately 5.5% of all road deaths in the UAE [1]. However, the incidence of motorized two- and three-wheeler injuries decreased by about 40% over the period 2003–2017 [5]. This was attributed to improvements in injury prevention measures, such as the use of safety devices (like helmets), enforcement of safety regulations (e.g., speed and helmet law enforcement), installation of road safety cameras, penalties for speed violations, and educational programs [5, 7, 51]. Motorcycle injuries have recently increased in homes, workplaces, and public areas in the UAE [5]. This indicates the increasing use of motorized two- and three-wheelers, such as scooters, e-bikes, and motorcycles, as affordable means of transportation.

On the other hand, there was a sharp increase in motorized two- and three-wheeler deaths in the UAE, from 2.6% in 2013 to 5.5% in 2016 [1, 21]. This rise cannot be explained by the recent minimal increase in motorized two- and three-wheelers [5]. Instead, other factors contributing to crashes and increasing deaths include a high percentage of younger motorcycle license holders combined with risky driving behaviors such as speeding, drug and alcohol abuse, not using helmets, and violations of traffic laws [51]. In contrast, the mortality of hospitalized motorcycle-related injured patients reduced from 6% to 0% in the last 15 years (2003–2017) [5]. This indicates a significant improvement in the trauma care system, mainly in pre-hospital and in-hospital care. This reduction also highlights that most motorized two- and three-wheeler deaths occur on the roads rather than in hospitals. Overall, the UAE achieved the United Nations (UN) target of reducing road user deaths by half in 2020 [52], which was not achieved globally [53].

31.7 Pedestrian Injuries

Walking is a common, low-cost mode of transport method that has health, physical, and environmental benefits, but it is unsafe when walking on roads that lack pedestrian infrastructure, especially when combined with an increased number of vehicles [54, 55]. Despite the hot weather in the UAE, low-income workers walk as a low-cost transport option [6], making pedestrians the most vulnerable road users [6, 29], with remarkably higher rates of severe injuries compared with other road users [1, 21]. Approximately a quarter of people killed on UAE roads are pedestrians, which is higher than in other high-income countries and above the global average [1, 54]. Head injuries are the main cause of death among injured pedestrians [6]. Most of these injuries occur during work shift changes and on the last working day [6].

Risk factors contributing to pedestrian injuries in the UAE include low visibility due to walking at night, being younger and male [6], and engaging in improper pedestrian behavior, such as illegal crossings outside designated pedestrian lines, using a mobile phone while walking, inattention, and distraction [31, 56]. About 20% of the pedestrians in the UAE cross outside designated pedestrian areas, and

8% cross while using their mobile phones [56]. Those who cross outside the designated area are more likely to use their mobile phones compared with those walking within the area [56]. Improving road user behavior is a challenge [31]. Pedestrians who are involved in RTCs have a higher risk of death compared with vehicle occupants [29]. There was a reduction in the global pedestrian death rate by 28% during the period 2007–2016, mainly in HICs [55]. This was attributed to the high gross national income per capita, vehicle-per-person ratio, safety improvements over time, legislation, and effective law enforcement [55, 57].

31.8 Bicycle Injuries

Cycling is a common mode of urban transportation all over the world. It is cheap, environmentally friendly, increases physical fitness, and promotes health, yet it also has its hazards. Cycling is the preferred mode of transportation method for low-income foreign workers. Currently, electric bicycles are common on city roads. There are no separate bicycle paths on UAE roads; however, there are efforts to build separate bicycle lanes for sports and recreational activities, but not as an essential component of transportation safety [2, 7].

In comparison with the protected body of the car occupant, cyclists are more prone to serious RTC injuries because of their exposed bodies, which leads to hospitalization mainly for head injuries. Riding a bicycle without a helmet and collisions with motor vehicles are important risk factors for bicycle-related injuries [58]. Safety measures while cycling include wearing helmets, using front and rear lights, wearing reflective vests at night, and using cycle paths. These measures are not all mandatory by law in most of the UAE. Wearing a helmet protects against brain injury by 65% and severe brain injury by 74% [59]. Although the UAE Traffic Law requires that all bicyclists use helmets, helmet use in our community is alarmingly low, ranging between 0.5% and 2% [2, 7, 60]. This has not changed over the last 15 years.

Most of the hospitalized injured bicyclists in the UAE are expatriate adult males. The majority were injured during the evening, on main roads, through collisions with moving vehicles. Head injuries caused by a collision with a motor vehicle were the main cause of hospital admissions [2, 7, 60].

31.9 Environmental Effects on RTCs

RTCs are caused by complex, interlinked environmental, vehicle, and human risk factors. Many of these have been well studied. Nevertheless, the impact of the COVID-19 pandemic on RTCs was less studied, both globally and locally. We have shown in a recent review that the most important factors affecting RTCs during the COVID-19 pandemic include reduced traffic volume, empty lanes, over-speeding, less law enforcement, alcohol and drug abuse, and not wearing seatbelts [61], Fig. 31.3a. The impact of the COVID-19 pandemic in the UAE is attributed to

Fig. 31.3 The impact of the COVID-19 pandemic on road traffic collisions both globally (**a**) and in the United Arab Emirates (**b**). (**a**) Overall impact of the COVID-19 pandemic on traffic volume, traffic lanes, vehicle speed, number of road traffic collisions, injury severity, hospitalization, and RTC deaths. (**b**) Monthly number of hospitalized road traffic collision trauma patients in Al-Ain City, United Arab Emirates, during the pre-COVID-19 pandemic period (March 2019–February 2020, yellow bars) and during the COVID-19 pandemic period (March 2020–February 2021, red bars). (Figure (**a**) is reproduced from Yasin et al. [61]. Figure (**b**) is reproduced from Yasin et al. [62]. Both figures are distributed under the terms of the Creative Commons Attribution 4.0 International License)

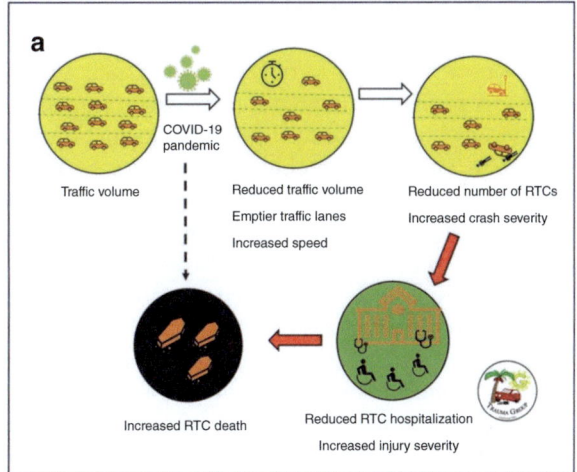

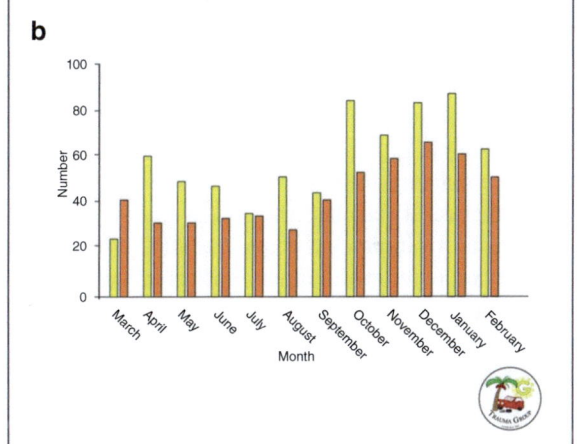

various national measures implemented by the government to reduce the spread of the virus, including physical distancing, stay-at-home orders, closure of schools, working from home, quarantine, restrictions on travel and mass gatherings, and complete lockdown [61, 62]. These measures reduced traffic movements and changed traffic characteristics and driving behaviors, which in turn decreased the number of RTCs and their injuries during the pandemic [61, 62]. There was a reduction in the number of hospitalized RTC-injured patients by 33.5% during the pandemic in Al-Ain City, UAE [62], Fig. 31.3b. This was mainly due to the reduction in motor vehicle, bicycle, and pedestrian injuries, while motorcycle injuries increased [62]. In contrast, injury severity and mortality significantly increased among hospitalized RTC-injured patients during the pandemic in Al Ain City [62].

31.10 RTCs of Special Groups

RTCs are a major cause of injury and death among children and youth in the UAE. These injuries impose a tremendous burden on the affected children, their families, and healthcare facilities. Risk factors for RTCs vary across different settings [63]. The ability of children to make safe decisions on the roads is not fully developed, especially during their cognitive development process. Young children may unintentionally take risks because they lack appropriate skills. On the other hand, older children and adolescents may actively seek out risk [63].

Studies from the UAE revealed the most frequent mechanisms of injury among children and youth that necessitate hospitalization. These were rollovers of vehicles and auto-pedestrian crashes, with head injury as the primary cause of admission [63–65]. Young UAE-national males are at higher risk of being injured on the roads. Rollover crashes have a high risk of ejection, increasing the proportion of head injuries. Pedestrian injuries are a major cause of morbidity and mortality. The bodies of pedestrians are not protected when hit by a vehicle. The pattern of injuries is affected by the size of both the vehicle and the victim. Serious head injuries can occur if the vehicle hits the child pedestrian's head [60].

Trauma in women, which has a major impact on families, is not well studied in our region. Injuries to the vertebrae and pelvis in women may cause urinary incontinence, pelvic organ prolapse, dyspareunia, infertility, and an increased risk of operative delivery [66]. A study from the registry of a trauma center in the UAE shows that most females involved in trauma were 20–34 years old. The primary mechanism for injury and death was RTC. More cervical injuries were observed in females compared with lumbar injuries in males [66].

31.11 Effects of the Trauma System and Trauma Registries

Injury is a global burden that requires effective measures for prevention and treatment. To address this issue, countries establish trauma systems, which are pre-planned, comprehensive, organized, and coordinated injury control efforts to be implemented [67]. It has been more than two decades since the UAE started to establish this system to tackle the burden of trauma [12]. The United Arab Emirates University has actively participated in these efforts by establishing the Trauma Group in 2001, which has the mission of improving trauma research and education to high international standards to improve care for trauma patients. The Trauma Group established the Al-Ain Hospital Trauma Registry on March 15, 2003, followed by the Tawam Hospital Trauma Registry in April 2006 [13, 14]. These registries were useful clinical and epidemiological databases that prospectively documented patient information collected by full-time trained trauma fellows. These data can be used for quality improvement, planning, policy, and trauma research [14, 68]. These data were used by the Trauma Group to produce numerous high-quality publications on injury prevention [5, 12, 13], which brought the burden of trauma, including RTCs, into the public domain. This was used to advocate injury

Table 31.1 Demography and severity of injury of hospitalized patients during the period 2003–2006 ($n = 2573$) and 10 years later ($n = 3519$) during the period 2014–2017, Al-Ain Hospital, Al-Ain, United Arab Emirates

Variable	Years 2003–2006	Years 2014–2017	p value
Age group			<0.0001
<18 years	419 (16.3%)	610 (17.3%)	
18–60 years	2059 (80.5%)	2646 (75.2%)	
>60 years	79 (3.1%)	263 (7.5%)	
Sex			<0.0001
Male	2228 (86.6%)	2901 (82.4%)	
Female	345 (13.4%)	618 (17.6%)	
UAE nationals	461 (17.9%)	745 (21.2%)	0.002
ISS[a]	4 (1–43), 5.61 (6)	4 (1–75), 6.48 (6.21)	<0.0001
ICU admission	202 (7.9%)	559 (6.3%)	0.02
Hospital stay (days)	9.2 (12.6)	5.9 (7.5)	<0.0001
Death	58 (2.3%)	35 (1%)	<0.0001

This table was reproduced and modified from the study of Alao et al. [12] which is distributed under the terms of the Creative Commons Attribution 4.0 International License

[a]Data are presented as mean (SD), median (range) or number (%) as appropriate. Ordinal data are occasionally presented in addition as mean (SD) if the median is the same. ISS = injury severity score. p = Pearson Chi square or Fisher's Exact test as appropriate for categorical data and Mann-Whitney U test for ordinal or continuous data

prevention strategies that improved road, work-related, and home safety. Additionally, the registries were used to evaluate trauma clinical management as part of the trauma system [5, 12]. Numerous injury prevention interventions were introduced, which included the installation of speed cameras, signaled pedestrian crossings, the use of safety devices (like helmets), the enforcement of road safety regulations (e.g., helmet and speed law enforcement), and educational and awareness programs [25, 31]. The reduction of trauma incidence by 38% and the reduction of the incidence of motorcycle-related injuries by 37% over the past 15 years reflect improvements in injury prevention [5, 12].

Another significant improvement was in the trauma educational activities run by the Trauma Group. These included the establishment of the Advanced Trauma Life Support program (ATLS) [69], and Point-of-Care Ultrasound (POCUS) courses [70], which became an integral part of the clinical practice [71]. Improvements also occurred in prehospital care, emergency medical services (EMS), and in-hospital care, an increased number of health care providers and EMS-trained staff [72], mandatory ATLS training [69], use of POCUS, 24-h angioembolization and interventional radiology, damage control surgery, and adherence to trauma management updates, including hypotensive resuscitation [71, 73, 74]. The reduction of mortality in hospitalized trauma patients by 56% and the reduction of mortality in hospitalized motorcycle-related patients to 0% over the last 15 years indicate improved trauma care within the hospital [12]. Table 31.1 shows the changes in trauma patterns and management outcomes in Al-Ain City, UAE, over time. Trauma among women, UAE nationals, and geriatric patients increased significantly. Despite the increased severity of injury in the admitted patients, ICU admissions, length of hospital stay, and trauma deaths decreased significantly.

31.12 Conclusions

The heavy burden of RTCs requires genuine efforts to find solutions for both injury prevention and treatment. Our experiences over the last two decades as part of the Trauma Group at the United Arab Emirates University have taught us that a multidisciplinary approach that builds bridges with all stakeholders in a *trauma system* is the most effective strategy to reduce the toll of injury. This should include injury prevention, trauma education, prehospital care, in-hospital trauma management, patient transportation between hospitals, trauma registries for data collection, trauma research, quality improvement programs, and disaster management plans. We are proud and honored to be part of this collective effort, which has borne fruit after 20 years of hard work.

Conflicts of Interest The authors have no conflicts of interest to declare.

References

1. World Health Organization. The Global status report on road safety, vol. 2. Geneva; 2018. Available at: https://www.who.int/violence_injury_prevention/road_safety_status/2018/en/. Accessed 21 Oct 2021.
2. Grivna M, AlKatheen A, AlAhbabi M, AlKaabi S, Alyafei M, Abu-Zidan FM. Risks for bicycle-related injuries in Al Ain city, United Arab Emirates. Medicine (Baltimore). 2021;100:1–7.
3. Gulf Labour Market and Migration. Percentage of nationals and non-nationals in Gulf population (2020), 2020. Available at: https://gulfmigration.grc.net/media/graphs/Figure1percentageofnationalsnon-nationals2020v2.pdf. Accessed 5 Aug 2022.
4. Fargues P, Shah NM, Brouwer I. Working and living conditions of low-income migrant workers in the hospitality and construction sectors in the United Arab Emirates. 2019;(2/2019):1–77. Available at: https://cadmus.eui.eu/bitstream/handle/1814/65986/Report_GLMM02.pdf?sequence=1&isAllowed=y. Accessed 5 Aug 2022.
5. Yasin YJ, Eid HO, Alao DO, Grivna M, Abu-Zidan FM. Reduction of motorcycle-related deaths over 15 years in a developing country. World J Emerg Surg. 2022;17:1–7.
6. Hefny AF, Eid HO, Abu-Zidan FM. Pedestrian injuries in The United Arab Emirates. Int J Inj Control Saf Promot. 2015;22:203–8.
7. Hefny AF, Eid HO, Grivna M, Abu-Zidan FM. Bicycle-related injuries requiring hospitalization in The United Arab Emirates. Injury. 2012;43:1547–50.
8. Abu Dhabi Urban Planning Council. Abu Dhabi urban street design manual, 2013. Available at: https://bicycleinfrastructuremanuals.com/manuals4/Abu-Dhabi-StreetDesignManual.pdf. Accessed 5 Aug 2022.
9. World Health Organization, Global Health estimates 2019: deaths by cause, age, sex, by country and by region, 2000–2019. Geneva; 2020. Available at: https://www.who.int/data/gho/data/themes/mortality-and-global-health-estimates/ghe-leading-causes-of-death. Accessed 25 July 2021
10. World Health Organization. Global health estimates: disease burden by cause, age, sex, by country and by region, 2000–2019. Geneva; 2020. Available at: https://www.who.int/data/gho/

data/themes/mortality-and-global-health-estimates/global-health-estimates-leading-causes-of-dalys. Accessed 25 July 2021
11. Chen S, Kuhn M, Prettner K, Bloom DE. The global macroeconomic burden of road injuries: estimates and projections for 166 countries. Lancet Planet Heal. 2019;3:e390–8.
12. Alao DO, Cevik AA, Eid HO, Jummani Z, Abu-Zidan FM. Trauma system developments reduce mortality in hospitalized trauma patients in Al-Ain City, United Arab Emirates, despite increased severity of injury. World J Emerg Surg. 2020;15:1–6.
13. Shaban S, Ashour M, Bashir M, El-Ashaal Y, Branicki F, Abu-Zidan FM. The long term effects of early analysis of a trauma registry. World J Emerg Surg. 2009;4:1–4.
14. Shaban S, Eid HO, Barka E, Abu-Zidan FM. Towards a national trauma registry for The United Arab Emirates. BMC Res Notes. 2010;3:187.
15. Eid HO, Abu-Zidan FM. Biomechanics of road traffic collision injuries: a clinician's perspective. Singapore Med J. 2007;48:693–700.
16. Abu-Zidan FM, Eid HO. Factors affecting injury. Severity of vehicle occupants following road traffic collisions. Injury. 2015;46:136–41.
17. American College of Surgeons. ATLS advanced trauma life support program for doctors. 7th ed. Chicago; 2004. p. 315–35.
18. Ammori MB, Abu-Zidan FM. The biomechanics of lower limb injuries in frontal-impact road traffic collisions. Afr Health Sci. 2018;18:321–32.
19. Ammori MB, Eid HO, Abu-Zidan FM. Lower limb and associated injuries in frontal-impact road traffic collisions. Afr Health Sci. 2016;16:306–10.
20. Lee J, Conroy C, Coimbra R, Tominaga GT, Hoyt DB. Injury patterns in frontal crashes: the association between knee-thigh-hip (KTH) and serious intra-abdominal injury. Accid Anal Prev. 2010;42:50–5.
21. World Health Organization. Global status report on road safety, vol. 15. Geneva; 2015. Available at: https://www.afro.who.int/sites/default/files/2017-06/9789241565066_eng.pdf. Accessed 21 Oct 2021.
22. Abu-Zidan FM, Abbas AK, Hefny AF, Eid HO, Grivna M. Effects of seat belt usage on injury pattern and outcome of vehicle occupants after road traffic collisions: prospective study. World J Surg. 2012;36:255–9.
23. Elvik R, Høye A, Vaa T, Sørensen M. The handbook of road safety measures. 2nd ed; 2009. Available at: https://silo.pub/qdownload/handbook-of-road-safety-measures-second-edition.html. Accessed 21 Oct 2021.
24. El-Sadig M, Sarfraz Alam M, Carter AO, Fares K, Al-Taneuiji HOS, Romilly P, et al. Evaluation of effectiveness of safety seatbelt legislation in The United Arab Emirates. Accid Anal Prev. 2004;36:399–404.
25. United Arab Emirates Government Portal. Road safety, 2022. Available at: https://u.ae/en/information-and-services/justice-safety-and-the-law/road-safety. 2 Aug 2022.
26. Alketbi LMB, Grivna M, Al DS. Risky driving behaviour in Abu Dhabi, United Arab Emirates: a cross-sectional, survey-based study. BMC Public Health. 2020;20:1–11.
27. Bendak S, Alnaqbi SS. Rear seat belt use in The United Arab Emirates. Policy Pract Heal Saf. 2019;17:3–13.
28. Abbas AK, Hefny AF, Abu-Zidan FM. Seatbelt compliance and mortality in the Gulf Cooperation Council countries in comparison with other high-income countries. Ann Saudi Med. 2011;31:347–50.
29. AlKheder S, AlRukaibi F, Aiash A. Analysis of risk factors affecting traffic accident injury in United Arab Emirates (UAE). Eur J Trauma Emerg Surg. 2022;48:4823–35.
30. Forjuoh SN. Are successful safety devices being used universally? Int J Inj Control Saf Promot. 2019;26:127–8.
31. Grivna M, Aw TC, El-Sadig M, Loney T, Sharif AA, Thomsen J, et al. The legal framework and initiatives for promoting safety in The United Arab Emirates. Int J Inj Control Saf Promot. 2012;19:278–89.
32. Abbas AK, Hefny AF, Abu-Zidan FM. Seatbelts and road traffic collision injuries. World J Emerg Surg. 2011;6:18.

33. Hefny AF, Al-Ashaal YI, Bani-Hashem AM, Abu-Zidan FM. Seatbelt syndrome associated with an isolated rectal injury: case report. World J Emerg Surg. 2010;5:2–7.
34. World Health Organization. Global status report on road safety: supporting a decade of action, vol. 19. Geneva; 2013. Available at: http://www.who.int/violence_injury_prevention/road_safety_status/2013/en/%5Cn. http://www.who.int/violence_injury_prevention/road_safety_status/2015/en/. Accessed 21 Oct 2021.
35. Lee VK, Champagne CR, Francescutti LH. Fatal distraction: cell phone use while driving. Can Fam Physician. 2013;59:723–5.
36. Virginia Tech Transportation Institute. 100-car naturalistic study fact sheet. Virginia Tech Transportation: Blacksburg; 2005. Available at: https://vtx.vt.edu/articles/2005/06/2005-834.html. Accessed 6 Jan 2014.
37. Eid HO, Abu-Zidan FM. Distraction-related road traffic collisions. Afr Health Sci. 2017;17:491–9.
38. Osman OT, Abbas AK, Eid HO, Salem MO, Abu-Zidan FM. Alcohol-related road traffic injuries in Al-Ain City, United Arab Emirates. Traffic Inj Prev. 2015;16:1–4.
39. Eid HO, Barss P, Adam SH, Torab FC, Lunsjo K, Grivna M, et al. Factors affecting anatomical region of injury, severity, and mortality for road trauma in a high-income developing country: lessons for prevention. Injury. 2009;40:703–7.
40. Golan JD, Marcoux J, Golan E, Schapiro R, Johnston KM, Maleki M, et al. Traumatic brain injury in intoxicated patients. J Trauma. 2007;63:365–9.
41. O'Toole O, Mahon C, Lynch K, Brett FM. Is the contribution of alcohol to fatal traumatic brain injuries being underestimated in the acute hospital setting? Ir Med J. 2009;102:207–9.
42. Sagberg F. Road accidents caused by drivers falling asleep. Accid Anal Prev. 1999;31:639–49.
43. Al-Houqani M, Eid HO, Abu-Zidan FM. Sleep-related collisions in United Arab Emirates. Accid Anal Prev. 2013;50:1052–5.
44. United Arab Emirates Ministry of Health and Prevention. Distribution of deaths by cause, sex and nationality, UAE. Int J Nurs Stud. 2019; Available at: https://mohap.gov.ae/en/open-data/mohap-open-data. Accessed 13 Aug 2022.
45. Department of Health. Abu Dhabi Health Statistics 2017, 2018. Available at: https://www.doh.gov.ae/-/media/Feature/Resources/AbuDhabiHealthStatistics.ashx. Accessed 13 Aug 2022.
46. Ichikawa M, Nakahara S, Wakai S. Mortality of front-seat occupants attributable to unbelted rear-seat passengers in car crashes. Lancet. 2002;359:43–4.
47. Zhu M, Cummings P, Chu H, Cook LJ. Association of rear seat safety belt use with death in a traffic crash: a matched cohort study. Inj Prev. 2007;13:183–5.
48. Jawas A, Hammad F, Eid HO, Abu-Zidan FM. Vascular injuries following road traffic collisions in a high-income developing country: a prospective cohort study. World J Emerg Surg. 2010;5:1–5.
49. Hammad F, Eid H, Jawas A, Abu-Zidan F. Genitourinary injuries following road traffic collisions: a population-based study from the Middle East. Ulus Travma Acil Cerrahi Derg. 2010;16:449–52.
50. Lin MR, Kraus JF. A review of risk factors and patterns of motorcycle injuries. Accid Anal Prev. 2009;41:710–22.
51. Abbas AK, Hefny AF, Abu-Zidan FM. Does wearing helmets reduce motorcycle-related death? A global evaluation. Accid Anal Prev. 2012;49:249–52.
52. United Nations. Global plan for the decade of action for road safety 2011–2020. Geneva: WHO; 2010. p. 25. Available at: http://scholar.google.com/scholar?hl=en&btnG=Search&q=intitle:Global+Plan+for+the+Decade+of+Action+for+Road+Safety+2011-2020#0. Accessed 21 Oct 2021.
53. Yasin YJ, Grivna M, Abu-Zidan FM. Motorized 2–3 wheelers death rates over a decade: a global study. World J Emerg Surg. 2022;17:1–8.
54. World Health Organization. Pedestrian safety: a road safety manual for decision-makers and practitioners. World Health Organization, 2013. Available at: https://apps.who.int/iris/bitstream/handle/10665/79753/9789241505352_eng.pdf;jsessionid=94498E0501AADE66F373ED7101AD298F?sequence=1. Accessed 21 Oct 2021.

55. Yasin YJ, Grivna M, Abu-Zidan FM. Reduction of pedestrian death rates: a missed global target. World J Emerg Surg. 2020;15:1–6.
56. Bendak S, Alnaqbi AM, Alzarooni MY, Aljanaahi SM, Alsuwaidi SJ. Factors affecting pedestrian behaviors at signalized crosswalks: an empirical study. J Saf Res. 2021;76:269–75.
57. Eid HO, Abu-Zidan FM. Pedestrian injuries-related deaths: a global evaluation. World J Surg. 2015;39:776–81.
58. Thompson MJ, Rivara FP. Bicycle-related injuries. Am Fam Physician. 2001;63:2007–14.
59. Lee AJ, Mann NP. Cycle helmets. Arch Dis Child. 2003;88:465–6.
60. Eid HO, Bashir MM, Muhammed OQ, Abu-Zidan FM. Bicycle-related injuries: a prospective study of 200 patients. Singapore Med J. 2007;48:884–6.
61. Yasin YJ, Grivna M, Abu-Zidan FM. Global impact of COVID-19 pandemic on road traffic collisions. World J Emerg Surg. 2021;16:1–14.
62. Yasin YJ, Alao DO, Grivna M, Abu-Zidan FM. Impact of the COVID-19 pandemic on road traffic collision injury patterns and severity in Al-Ain City, United Arab Emirates. World J Emerg Surg. 2021;16:1–7.
63. Grivna M, Eid HO, Abu-Zidan FM. Pediatric and youth traffic-collision injuries in Al Ain, United Arab Emirates: a prospective study. PLoS One. 2013;8:1–8.
64. Grivna M, Barss P, Stanculescu C, Eid HO, Abu-Zidan FM. Child and youth traffic-related injuries: use of a trauma registry to identify priorities for prevention in The United Arab Emirates. Traffic Inj Prev. 2013;14:274–82.
65. Grivna M, Eid HO, Abu-Zidan FM. Youth traffic-related injuries: a prospective study. World J Emerg Surg. 2017;12:1–7.
66. Abbas AK, Mirghani H, Eid HO, Abu-Zidan FM. Trauma in women of child-bearing age in a high-income developing country. Ulus Travma ve Acil Cerrahi Derg. 2012;18:239–42.
67. Tien CH. The Canadian forces trauma care system. Can J Surg. 2011;54:s112–7.
68. Moore L, Clark DE. The value of trauma registries. Injury. 2008;39:686–95.
69. Abu-Zidan FM, Mohammad A, Jamal A, Chetty D, Gautam SC, Van Dyke M, et al. Factors affecting success rate of advanced trauma life support (ATLS) courses. World J Surg. 2014;38:1405–10.
70. Abu-Zidan FM, Dittrich K, Czechowski JJ, Kazzam EE. Establishment of a course for focused assessment sonography for trauma. Saudi Med J. 2005;26:806–11.
71. Abu-Zidan FM. Optimizing the value of measuring inferior vena cava diameter in shocked patients. World J Crit Care Med. 2016;5:7.
72. Fares S, Irfan FB, Corder RF, Al Marzouqi MA, Al Zaabi AH, Idrees MM, et al. Emergency medicine in The United Arab Emirates. Int J Emerg Med. 2014;7:1–8.
73. Bashir MM, Abu-Zidan FM. Damage control surgery for abdominal trauma. Eur J Surg Suppl. 2003;588:8–13.
74. Saleh A, Potemkowski A, Abu-Zidan FM. Endovascular aortic stent graft repair for blunt traumatic thoracic aortic transection. Singapore Med J. 2008;49:847–8.

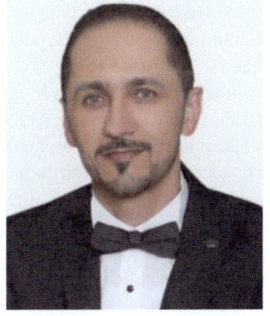

Hani O. Eid is a general practitioner who obtained his MBBS degree from the University of Gezira, Sudan, in 2002. He has been working for Abu Dhabi Police Aviation-Air Ambulance since December 2021. Before that, he worked in the emergency departments of different governmental and private-sector hospitals in the United Arab Emirates. He has also worked in a prehospital setting, including ground ambulance service, helicopter emergency medical service (HEMS), flying physicians, and motor sports events such as Formula 1. He has a deep interest in medical research, trauma registries, and medical informatics. His efforts and IT skills were pivotal for the establishment of two leading major trauma registries in the United Arab Emirates under the direct training of Professor Fikri Abu-Zidan, one of the leading trauma surgeons in the Middle East. He worked as a full-time research fellow (2003–2007) and as a senior research fellow (2013–2014) in the Department of Surgery, College of Medicine and Health Sciences, United Arab Emirates University. He has co-authored more than 50 publications in refereed international journals and has been invited by international journals to review articles and join their editorial boards .

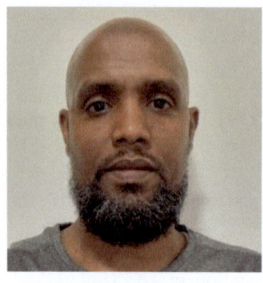

Yasin J Yasin has a BSc degree in Environmental Health from Haramaya University, Ethiopia; a Master's Degree in Public Health (MPH) from Addis Ababa University, Ethiopia; an MSc in Environmental Sciences from King Fahd University of Petroleum and Minerals (KFUPM), Saudi Arabia; and a Certificate in Clinical Research from Harvard Medical School, Harvard University, USA. He is a faculty member at the School of Public Health, College of Health Sciences, Mekelle University, Ethiopia. He has more than 15 years of teaching and research experience at several public universities in Ethiopia. He has successfully defended his PhD, which is titled "Factors affecting changes in road traffic collision related injuries and death over time: The global and the United Arab Emirates perspectives" in April 2023, at the Institute of Public Health, College of Medicine and Health Sciences, United Arab Emirates University, UAE. He was working under the supervision of Prof. Michal Grivna and Prof. Fikri Abu-Zidan. His research interests include pedestrian injuries, motorized two- and three-wheeler injuries, road traffic injuries, road safety, school safety, global health, GIS and spatial epidemiology, environmental epidemiology, environmental health, one health, and public health. He has published 14 manuscripts in highly ranked international medical journals .

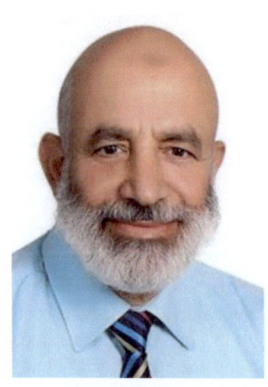

Fikri M Abu-Zidan is an international expert in statistics, research methodology, acute care surgery, disaster medicine, and point-of-care ultrasound. He graduated (MD) from Aleppo University (Syria) in 1981; gained the FRCS in Glasgow, Scotland, in 1987; achieved his PhD in Trauma and Disaster Medicine from Linkoping University (Sweden) in 1995; and obtained his Postgraduate Diploma of Applied Statistics from Massey University (New Zealand) in 1999. His clinical experience includes treating war-injured patients during the Gulf War (1990). He has been promoting the use of point-of-care ultrasound for more than 35 years, in which he is a world leader. Furthermore, he is an international translational medicine consultant developing novel clinically relevant animal models. He has made major contributions to trauma management, education, and research in Kuwait, Sweden, New Zealand, Australia, and the United Arab Emirates. He has authored more than 520 publications, presented more than 800 invited lectures and abstracts, and received more than 40 national and international awards. He is recognized as the most active researcher on road traffic collisions in the Gulf Region. He is serving as the statistics editor of the *World Journal of Emergency Surgery* and the *European Journal of Trauma and Emergency Surgery*. He has chaired the organization committees of seven highly successful international conferences on trauma management, critical care and prevention, and disaster medicine.

Open Access This chapter is licensed under the terms of the Creative Commons Attribution 4.0 International License (http://creativecommons.org/licenses/by/4.0/), which permits use, sharing, adaptation, distribution and reproduction in any medium or format, as long as you give appropriate credit to the original author(s) and the source, provide a link to the Creative Commons license and indicate if changes were made.

The images or other third party material in this chapter are included in the chapter's Creative Commons license, unless indicated otherwise in a credit line to the material. If material is not included in the chapter's Creative Commons license and your intended use is not permitted by statutory regulation or exceeds the permitted use, you will need to obtain permission directly from the copyright holder.

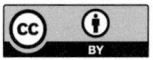

32. Mental Health in the UAE: Current Landscape and Future Directions

Ammar Albanna, Meshal A. Sultan, Faisal A. Nawaz, Hanan Derby, Mehnaz Zafar Ali, Nusrat Khan, Nahida N. Ahmed, and Omer El Rufaei

32.1 Introduction

In its constitution, the World Health Organization (WHO) defines health as "… a state of complete physical, mental and social well-being …" placing mental health at the core of health. Mental disorders are among the leading causes of disease burden globally and constitute a significant challenge to healthcare systems worldwide. Further, the burden of mental disorders is rising, as reflected in the increased global rate of disability-adjusted life years (DALYs), from 80.3 million in 1990 to 125.3 million in 2019 [1]. Surprisingly, despite the importance and burden of mental disorders, only a small fraction of health budgets is allocated to mental health [2]. Therefore, the lack of adequate services continues to be an essential barrier to providing accessible mental health services [3]. Furthermore, the Coronavirus Disease 2019 (COVID-19) pandemic triggered a significant increase in mental health needs

---

A. Albanna (✉)
Al Amal Psychiatric Hospital, Emirates Health Services, Dubai, United Arab Emirates

Mohamed Bin Rashid University of Medicine and Health Sciences, Dubai Health, Dubai, United Arab Emirates
e-mail: Ammar.Albanna@ehs.gov.ae

M. A. Sultan · N. Khan
Mohamed Bin Rashid University of Medicine and Health Sciences, Dubai Health, Dubai, United Arab Emirates
e-mail: meshal.sultan@ehs.gov.ae; Nusrat.Khan@dubaihealth.ae

F. A. Nawaz · M. Zafar Ali
Al Amal Psychiatric Hospital, Emirates Health Services, Dubai, United Arab Emirates
e-mail: faisal.nawaz@ehs.gov.ae; mehnaz.ali@ehs.gov.ae

H. Derby
Al Jalila Children's Hospital, Dubai Health, Dubai, United Arab Emirates
e-mail: hanan.derby@dubaihealth.ae

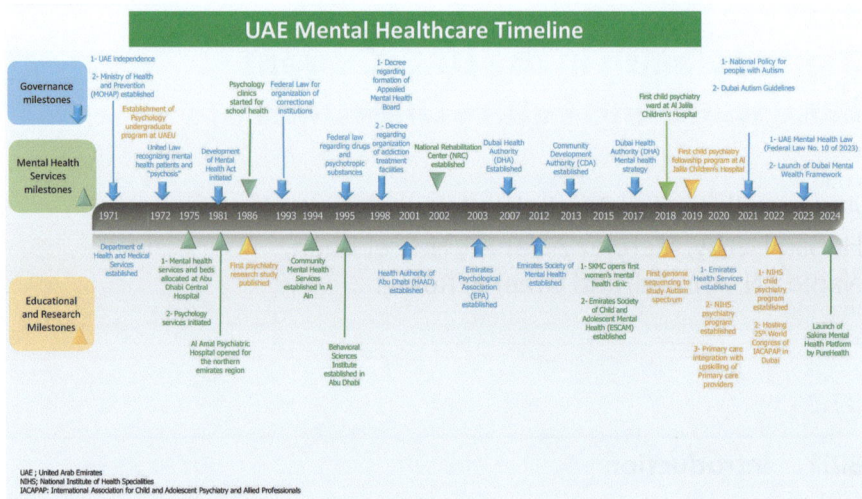

Fig. 32.1 Timeline of mental healthcare in the UAE

across different countries in the context of pandemic measures and other factors [4]. This acute upsurge in mental health demands served as a wake-up call for governments to urgently step up and address the mental health needs of their populations.

The United Arab Emirates (UAE) has been unswervingly attentive to its population's mental health and well-being over the past several decades, beginning in 1971. This was expressed through various steps and achievements, including but not limited to establishing state-of-the-art mental health services, developing laws and policies related to mental health, and announcing a national strategy for happiness and well-being. This is also reflected in the UAE government's vision and national agenda [5]. There are ongoing challenges, and the recent pandemic further underscores the importance of investing in effective mental health systems.

This chapter provides a brief overview of mental health in the UAE, including clinical services, research, education, policy, and workforce development. The chapter also highlights the critical challenges, potential solutions, and opportunities for the region's future direction in mental health (Fig. 32.1).

N. N. Ahmed
SEHA Mental Health Services, Abu Dhabi, United Arab Emirates

College of Medicine and Health Sciences (CMHS) of the United Arab Emirates University,
Al Ain, United Arab Emirates
e-mail: nnahmed@seha.ae

O. El Rufaei
College of Medicine, Mohamed Bin Rashid University of Medicine and Health Sciences,
Dubai Health, Dubai, United Arab Emirates
e-mail: omer.elrufaie@dubaihealth.ae

32.2 Mental Health Landscape of the UAE

The UAE has an estimated population of 9.2 million, comprising over 200 nationalities that shape a culturally diverse community [6]. The local Emirati population makes up 11.5% of the total population, with the significant expatriate population composed of Indians (27.5%), Pakistanis (12.7%), Bangladeshis (7.4%), and Filipinos (5.56%). Males significantly outnumber the female population (6.4 million males to 2.8 million females), and over one-quarter of the population is under 25 years old [7]. These vital statistics have important implications, especially given that most mental disorders have their onset during childhood.

32.3 Mental Health Statistics in the UAE

Mental disorders affect 1 in 8 people globally (970 million people), with anxiety (301 million people) and depression (280 million people) being the most common [8, 9]. The prevalence of mental disorders among the general population in the UAE is 14%, similar to the global prevalence of 13%. Mental health disorders in the UAE account for 9% of DALYs, compared with 5% globally [10]. Studies indicate that the COVID-19 pandemic has increased rates by 26% for anxiety and 28% for depression [8].

It has been reported that the UAE has witnessed a recent surge in mental illness, drug use disorders, and self-harm among the top 10 causes of the total number of deaths in 2019 [11, 12]. When considering mortality and disability combined, drug use disorders and depressive disorders ranked among the top 10 causes in the UAE [12]. Approximately 20% of the UAE's disease burden is attributable to neuropsychiatric disorders [13]. The prevalence and epidemiological data for mental health disorders in the UAE are limited; this challenge also applies to common mental health conditions such as depression [14]. Prevalence rates for depression range from 12.5% to 28.6% in the UAE [10, 14]. Suicide rates were 6.5 (per 100,000 population) in 2019, 8.0 (per 100,000) for males, and 3.0 for females. It has been noted that the rate of suicide in the expatriate population was seven times that of the national population [15]. It is also important to note that the rates of mental disorders in the UAE may be exacerbated due to the young population (23.9% of children in the UAE are reported to have mental health problems) and the increasing burden of noncommunicable diseases [16, 17]. The prevalence of mental disorders among a primary healthcare sample was estimated at around 28% (30% among females, 20% among males), with depression being the most prevalent [18]. A study exploring the mental health of migrant workers in the UAE showed that around one quarter met the threshold for depression, and 2.5% had suicidal ideations [19]. Such studies emphasize the importance of investigating mental health among subpopulations in the UAE, as this may inform service planning.

In terms of mental disorders among children, an earlier study by Eapen et al. estimated the prevalence of psychiatric disorders among children in the UAE at around 10%, with mood disorders, anxiety disorders, and oppositional defiant disorders being the most prevalent [16]. This study identified adverse family factors as

Table 32.1 Global age-standardized prevalence estimates per 100,000 (95% UI) applied to the UAE population estimate of 9.2 million

	Age-standardized prevalence estimates per 100,000 (95% UI)	Applied to UAE population (9.2 million)
Mental disorders	12,262·0 (11,382·9–13,213·3)	1,127,920
Anxiety disorders	3779·5 (3181·1–4473·3)	347,368
Depressive disorders	3440·1 (3097·0–3817·6)	316,480
ADHD	1131·9 (831·7–1494·5)	104,052
Bipolar disorder	489·8 (407·5–580·6)	44,988
ASD	369·4 (305·9–441·2)	33,948
Schizophrenia	287·4 (246·2–330·9)	26,404
Eating disorders	174·0 (130·1–222·1)	16,008

The same study estimated age-standardized DALY rates per 100,000 at 1712.2 (95% uncertainty intervals (age-standardized rates) 1256·7–2253·0) and total DALYs in 1000 s at 192·4 (140·0–253·3) [1]

the most important correlates of childhood mental disorders. Subsequent research exploring child psychiatric disorders in primary healthcare centers found that more than 40% of referred children met the criteria for a psychiatric disorder, and only 1% were referred for appropriate services, highlighting the need to enhance awareness and screening for mental disorders [20]. The prevalence of mental disorders among children has been studied in specific populations, such as conduct disorder among juvenile delinquents, which was estimated at around 25% and was correlated with psychosocial factors such as living with a single parent [21]. One study estimated the prevalence of anorexia nervosa among adolescent girls in the UAE at around 2%, while about 25% had subthreshold symptoms of disordered eating [22]. This study also showed that family and social factors were associated with disordered eating. Studies exploring neurodevelopmental disorders in the UAE estimated the prevalence of attention deficit/hyperactivity disorder (ADHD) and autism spectrum disorder (ASD) at 4% and 0.3%, respectively [23, 24].

A significant recent study attempted to estimate the prevalence and burden of mental disorders worldwide across 204 countries, including the UAE [1]. This study's prevalence rates of common mental disorders were applied to the UAE population of 9.2 million; see Table 32.1.

In summary, the above studies demonstrate that mental disorders are prevalent in the UAE and are associated with significant healthcare and societal burdens.

32.4 Mental Health Systems in the UAE

Mental health systems in the UAE are rapidly progressing toward a sustainable and scalable model of mental healthcare, employing innovation, an integrated approach, and international evidence-based best practices. The UAE National Agenda aims to achieve a world-class healthcare system, and significant attention is given to mental and behavioral disorders at the national level [5]. This section provides a brief overview of different aspects pertaining to mental health systems in the UAE, including legislation, governance, services, and other aspects.

32.4.1 Mental Health Legislations and Policies

UAE federal laws pertaining to mental health have existed since the country was united in 1971. These laws cover different mental health domains, including protecting the rights of people with mental disabilities, protecting child rights, and numerous constitutional guarantees for the promotion of human rights [25]. Law No. (5) of 2019 was passed for addiction treatment and rehabilitation facilities for UAE residents and Emiratis, with emphasis on providing a safe environment, the right to privacy, and freedom to seek treatment [26]. Legal reforms were introduced in the UAE, including decriminalizing suicide and attempted suicide in Federal Decree Law No. 15 of 2020 [27]. Members of the Federal National Council passed the mental health draft law in 2021, which aims to provide the necessary healthcare for these patients according to the best standards, protect their rights and dignity, reduce the negative effects of mental disorders on the lives of individuals, families, and society, and promote the integration of the psychiatric patients into the community [28].

The Ministry of Health and Prevention developed "The National Policy for the Promotion of Mental Health in the United Arab Emirates," issued by the UAE Cabinet in 2017, with a human rights-based approach in line with the National Health Strategy, the UAE Vision 2021, the UAE Centennial 2071, and the Next 50-year Plan. Its strategic objectives align with mental health awareness, prevention, service provision, multi-sectoral collaboration, and the development of research.

Dubai Health Authority (DHA) formulated the first comprehensive mental health strategy, titled "Happy Lives, Healthy Communities," 2017–2021, to assess mental health gaps and articulate guiding principles for a responsive, culturally appropriate mental health system [11]. The "National Strategy for Wellbeing 2031" also aims to promote good mental health and adopt positive thinking as a strategic objective [29]. As a component of its health Sector strategy, the Department of Health (DOH) Abu Dhabi has put forth an extensive Mental Health plan built upon a capacity and demand assessment, gap analysis, and benchmarking effort in the mental healthcare field. The resulting strategy represents a comprehensive and holistic framework encompassing numerous initiatives organized into three overarching categories: "Staying Healthy," "Getting Better," and "Sustaining Health." A multitude of government entities have joined forces to implement this holistic model, emphasizing prevention and recovery rather than solely access to healthcare services.

The UAE Government has taken strategic steps to ensure the integration of people with disabilities (PWD) within society at large and improve access to services. This includes adopting "People of Determination" (POD) as an official label to recognize their efforts and achievements [30]. Adopting strategies and policies pertaining to POD is quite relevant to mental health, given that the concept of disability overlaps with some mental disorders, and many disabilities have a significant impact on mental well-being. Policies include the UAE National Policy for Empowering People of Determination [31], the Abu Dhabi Comprehensive Strategy for People of Determination, and the Dubai Inclusive Education Framework announced by the Dubai Knowledge and Human Development Authority (KHDA) [32]. With regard to ASD, the Ministry of Community Development (MOCD) announced a UAE National Policy aiming to empower individuals with ASD across the lifespan [33]. To improve the standards of services provided for children with ASD and enhance the system of care, the Dubai Health Authority announced the first edition of the Dubai Autism Guidelines in 2021, following consultation with parents and stakeholders [34, 66, 67]. In summary, policies play a fundamental role in mental health, and the UAE has taken significant strides in developing its mental health guidelines.

32.4.2 Mental Health Governance

Mental health service provision is governed by different regulatory authorities in the UAE, including the federal health authority, which comprises the Ministry of Health and Prevention (MOHAP), responsible for providing healthcare services, and Emirates Health Services (EHS), which works to enhance the efficiency of the federal health sector by implementing strategic health-related policies and standards and preventive care. The Department of Health (DoH), Dubai Health Authority (DHA), Dubai Health Care Authority (DHCA) in Dubai, and Sharjah Health Authority carry out similar responsibilities [35]. In 2021, a decree was issued by the ruler of Dubai declaring the establishment of the Dubai Academic Health Corporation (DAHC) [65]. At the time of writing this chapter, the healthcare system of Dubai is undergoing a transformation under this decree towards an integrated academic system.

The Emirates Society of Mental Health (ESMH) is a scientific society under the umbrella of the Emirates Medical Association (EMA), composed of psychiatrists and healthcare specialists proactively promoting mental health awareness in the Middle Eastern region through its various activities. The Emirates Psychological Association (EPA) was established in 2003 in Dubai by the Ministry of Social Affairs. It is the only officially recognized professional association for psychologists in the UAE. In 2015, the Emirates Society for Child and Adolescent Mental Health (ESCAM) was established under EMA, focusing on enhancing mental healthcare, research, and awareness in the UAE. Notably, ESCAM hosted the 25th World Congress of the International Association of Child and Adolescent Psychiatrists and Allied Professionals (IACAPAP) in December 2022, which was held for the first time in an Arab city since the congress commenced in 1937 and was attended by delegates from more than 80 countries [36].

32.4.3 Mental Health Services

Psychiatric services are delivered primarily through the public and private sectors as outpatient clinics. Under the umbrella of Emirates Health Services, Al Amal Psychiatric Hospital serves as the leading tertiary care facility in the UAE, offering acute and specialized inpatient care, a 24/7 emergency department, community home care services, and outreach services catering to Dubai and the Northern

Emirates. The Rashid Hospital Psychiatry Unit, currently under Dubai Health, provides psychiatry outpatient, inpatient, community, and liaison services.

Recent years have witnessed the development of specialized services, such as Clinical Academic Groups under Al Amal Psychiatric Hospital, in partnership with Maudsley Health, that includes specialized forensic psychiatry, addictions psychiatry, old-age psychiatry, Intellectual disabilities, children and adolescents' mental health, and community mental health. Al Amal Psychiatric Hospital, operating under the umbrella of Emirates Health Services, functions within a comprehensive healthcare system that integrates preventive care, clinical services, research, innovation, and education to deliver world-class mental health services to the population. Innovative approaches currently being explored include the integration of generative artificial intelligence to support the mental well-being of older adults, exemplified by the 'Synthetic Memories' project. In parallel, AI-driven tools such as remote eye-tracking and deep typing technologies are being employed to facilitate the early detection of autism within home environments. These and other forward-looking initiatives reflect a broader commitment to harnessing emerging technologies in order to advance population mental health at scale. One of the milestones in child and adolescent mental health in the UAE is the establishment of the Mental Health Center of Excellence at Al Jalila Children's Hospital (AJCH) in Dubai, which aims to provide state-of-the-art clinical services, as well as research and education [37]. Specialized mental healthcare at AJCH is delivered through comprehensive outpatient and inpatient services for individuals up to 18 years of age. Treatment and rehabilitation for substance misuse disorders are provided at specialized facilities like the National Rehabilitation Center in Abu Dhabi and Erada in Dubai. Police and prison services are integral to substance misuse programs, where treatment is offered on a voluntary basis, and mental health cases [38]. Satellite clinics in primary healthcare (PHC) centers were launched to improve access to mental healthcare through psychiatry consultations for patients visiting the PHCs. The UAE offers a mixed health insurance system, with public and private insurance. Public insurance grants access to government-funded hospitals and clinics.

Abu Dhabi Health Services Company (SEHA), part of the PureHealth network, has restructured its mental health services into a unified, tiered model of care. In May 2024, it launched Sakina, now the largest integrated mental health network in Abu Dhabi, as a cornerstone of the emirate's mental health strategy. Sakina offers holistic, accessible, and stigma-free services across outpatient hubs, neurodiversity centers, and inpatient units. Built on the pillars of Awareness & Prevention, Clinical Excellence, and Rehabilitation & Reintegration, it aims to embed mental health within general healthcare, reduce barriers, and meet the needs of vulnerable populations through community-based and tertiary care [39].

32.4.4 Mental Health Workforce

According to the WHO, the number of mental health workers employed in the UAE increased sevenfold between 2017 and 2020. These include psychiatrists, mental health nurses, psychologists, social workers, and other specialized staff members, such as occupational therapists. The total number of mental health professionals employed in 2020 was 4914, including 3777 mental health nurses, 414 psychiatrists, and 282 psychologists [13].

32.4.5 Mental Healthcare Initiatives in the UAE

The government of the UAE is continuously advocating for mental health through active participation in "World Mental Health Day" and making efforts to improve access to care and reduce stigma by launching community mental health activities, digital mental health initiatives, school mental health programs, awareness talks, and extensive media campaigns. In 2010, the UAE mental health plan was reviewed, focusing on the wider accessibility of mental health services in the government's facilities across the region and their incorporation into primary care [40].

The Ministry of Health and Prevention (MOHAP) launched its innovation strategy (2019–2021) for the future of healthcare under the theme "Innovate for Health", aiming to make the UAE a leading international destination for a sustainable future in smart healthcare through technological integration into diagnostic and therapeutic methods [41]. The Mental Health Innovation Lab 2021 brought together leaders and experts to collaborate and achieve a common goal of supporting mental health and wellness sustainably by integrating care and promoting intersectoral action and collaboration in mental health to establish evidence-based standards [42].

A free mental health support network was built in Abu Dhabi under the theme of "Darkness into Light UAE" to raise awareness about mental health issues. To raise awareness of mental health challenges, reduce stigma, and end discrimination against those with mental illness within the UAE, the Al Jalila Foundation awarded three Emirati journalists the "Mental Health Journalism Fellowship" [43]. The Emirates Health Services (EHS) launched the "Theqa" program in 2021 to provide moral and psychological support for healthcare providers (HCPs) who have been traumatized due to their involvement in an unanticipated adverse patient event. The Community Psychiatry Department at Al Amal Psychiatric Hospital also launched "Nadamukum" in 2022, which is a caregiver forum and support group for families and loved ones of patients with severe and chronic mental illnesses.

In 2022, the Department of Health (DOH) Abu Dhabi launched a primary care upskilling program to increase the scope of primary care providers to screen, intervene, and treat individuals suffering from mental health issues early in the illness [68]. The program had two components: psychopharmacology training designed for primary care physicians, and psychotherapy training designed for primary care physicians and nurses. The Department of Community Medicine launched a helpline for the psychological support of the community [69]. The Family Care Authority (FCA) was launched in 2023 as an affiliate under Abu Dhabi's Department of Community Development (DCD), tasked with advancing the psychosocial quality of life for families in Abu Dhabi [70].

32.4.6 Initiatives During the COVID-19 Pandemic

The government made tremendous efforts to offer uninterrupted mental health services during the COVID-19 pandemic by developing effective smart systems that offered innovative therapeutic, preventive, and mental health rehabilitation services while ensuring safety and privacy across the community.

1. Mental healthcare was delivered by tele-psychiatry and tele-mental health services, including the psychological counseling helpline service "Talk, We Do Hear You," and the launch of relevant virtual clinics. These included virtual psychiatric and psychological clinics for outpatient clinic patients, virtual pharmacy services, remote guidance for psychiatric drugs, psychosocial rehabilitation programs for patients with addiction, and medication home delivery services.
2. The Health Ministry formed multidisciplinary teams to provide 24/7 psychiatric emergency services to COVID-19-affected patients in accordance with the best international standards and practices.
3. Community mental health services provided continuity of care through the designation of home care and support teams for chronic cases, and the activation of a virtual visit program for inpatients to enable them to meet their families [44].
4. The National Program for Happiness and Wellbeing launched the Mental Support Line (800 HOPE) to provide safe and confidential mental support to individuals impacted by COVID-19, and an online national campaign titled "The National Campaign for Mental Support" to help the community overcome the psychological impact of the pandemic. This campaign was promoted with the hashtag #DontWorry.
5. The "Employees Assistance Program," named "Hayat," was introduced as a psychological and moral support program to help federal government employees deal with the circumstances and anxiety associated with COVID-19 [45].
6. Awareness campaigns during the COVID-19 period were of high caliber, and many programs, such as "Rest Assured," were launched by the Ministry of Community Development [46].
7. From 2020–2022, SEHA operated the "Ma'akum" (With you) helpline for close to 20,000 healthcare staff members in its network to provide psychological support during the pandemic

32.5 Mental Health Research and Education in the UAE

32.5.1 Research

The Arab world produces approximately 1% of the world's publications in peer-reviewed journals on mental health [47]. In the context of this relatively low research output, the United Arab Emirates has been emphasizing research education. For instance, major medical schools have introduced research into their curriculum, and conducting research has become a requirement in undergraduate medical education.

Furthermore, leading and conducting a research project has been a training requirement in postgraduate psychiatry programs [48]. Research on mental health in the United Arab Emirates is being conducted in multiple areas. The main areas of research include epidemiological studies, diagnosis and classification of disorders, translation, development, and validation of psychiatric instruments, personality and psychosocial aspects of physical illness, biological and genetic research, and transcultural psychiatry [38]. The DOH, Abu Dhabi, has issued grants up to 500,000 AED for research ideas exploring innovations for dementia care.

More recently, and since the COVID-19 pandemic, multiple studies have been published exploring its psychological impact on the UAE population. These studies targeted the general population as well as vulnerable groups, including healthcare professionals, pregnant women, children, and their families [49–54]. The number of publications in the mental health field in the UAE has been increasing gradually. A total of 43 PubMed-indexed publications were reported from 1987 to 2002 [55]. This number increased by about threefold, reaching 132 during the period from 2003 to 2019 [43].

32.5.2 Education and Training

The introduction of psychiatry training in undergraduate medical education in the UAE started in 1990 with the establishment of the Academic Department of Psychiatry at the Faculty of Medicine and Health Sciences, in the form of a clinical clerkship lasting 3 to 8 weeks. This has been incorporated into the curriculum in all major universities that have established colleges of medicine in the country. With the graduation of medical students, various general psychiatry residency programs have also been established. Psychiatry specialty programs offer four-year clinical training under the supervision of qualified professionals. Efforts have been made to ensure that training meets the highest international standards [38]. Al Amal Psychiatric Hospital under Emirates Health Services, offer an accredited psychiatry residency program by the UAE National Institute of Health Specialities, as well as providing mental health training experiences for approximately 1000 trainees annually.

Postgraduate training expanded to sub-specialized fields with the establishment of a Child and Adolescent Psychiatry two-year fellowship program in 2019 [48]. The field of psychology started in the UAE in the 1970s with the launch of the undergraduate psychology program at UAE University [40]. Education and training for allied mental health services have advanced since then and are provided in several institutions. Current programs include a Bachelor of Science in Psychology, a Master of Science in Clinical Psychology, and a Master of Science in Mental Health Nursing [56, 57]. Moreover, education and international collaborative opportunities have been ongoing through the hosting of world-class scientific conferences. Prominent conferences in the UAE include the "Systems of Care for Autism Spectrum Disorder" held in 2017, the International Association for Child and Adolescent Psychiatry and Allied Professions (IACAPAP) World Congress 2022

[36, 58], the annual Emirates Health Services Mental Health Conference, and the annual Abu Dhabi Integrated Mental Health Conference.

The SEHA network supports two psychiatry residency programs accredited by the Accreditation Council for Graduate Medical Education-International (ACGMEI) in the Emirate of Abu Dhabi, affiliated with the esteemed UAE University in the city of Al Ain and Khalifa University in Abu Dhabi city. These programs have received endorsement from the Royal College of Psychiatrists. The government of the UAE has invested in sending medical graduates to prestigious psychiatric programs in the USA, Canada, the UK, and Germany for residency and fellowship training.

32.6 Current Challenges and Future Directions

The UAE's mental health system is founded upon values and principles that support mental healthcare. As discussed in this chapter, the UAE strongly supports mental health at the highest levels.

32.6.1 Mental Health Law

In recent years, the UAE has made significant strides in strengthening its legal and policy frameworks for mental health. A key milestone was the enactment of Federal Law No. 10 of 2023 on Mental Health, signed by the President of the United Arab Emirates. This law represents a landmark development in the country's efforts to modernize mental health governance and align with international standards. Currently in the implementation phase, the legislation lays the groundwork for a rights-based approach to mental healthcare, emphasizing patient autonomy, dignity, and access to care. The introduction of this law opens new opportunities to further enhance access to quality mental health services, including for children and adolescents. Its successful implementation will not only clarify the roles and responsibilities of mental health professionals, but also promote equity, reduce stigma, and ensure early and appropriate care across the lifespan. As the UAE continues to advance its mental health strategy and implementation, Federal Law No. 10 of 2023 serves as a foundational pillar for building a modern, inclusive, and patient-centered mental health system [59].

32.6.2 Universal Mental Health Coverage

One of the crucial challenges impacting the accessibility of mental healthcare in the UAE is related to insurance coverage. Although insurance companies are increasing their coverage for various mental disorders, there is still no universal coverage. This is especially the case with less-urgent, longer-term psychosocial interventions that are required [60]. Concerning research and education, the UAE has undoubtedly taken significant steps toward academic advancement. However, there is a need to expand existing training programs in order to match the population's needs. Furthermore, there is a need to develop additional specialty programs for allied mental health professionals and subspecialties.

32.6.3 Accessibility of Mental Health Services

The future direction of mental healthcare in the UAE can be strategized by evaluating existing challenges and promoting innovative tools for preventing, detecting, and treating mental illnesses. One of the critical challenges that the COVID-19 outbreak emphasized is the lack of sufficient mental health resources, resulting in difficulties accessing mental healthcare globally. Even when mental health services are available, many individuals may be unable to afford them. Addressing the accessibility of services systemically and sustainably is essential to improving mental healthcare in the UAE. This may be achieved through different initiatives, including primary care integration, robust screening programs, training professionals across schools and non-mental health disciplines, revamping mental healthcare systems, shifting to functional recovery-based community services, and using technology and the latest advancements [66].

With regard to training, a national approach to the needs of mental health professionals will be of great importance, as will adopting strategies to fulfill these needs sustainably. This includes developing advanced psychology training programs, providing more training opportunities, and supporting trained psychologists in finding and maintaining careers in mental health. This aforementioned step is especially important in the UAE context, given the presence of undergraduate psychology programs and, on the other hand, the limited post-graduate and training opportunities for undergraduate alumni. Indeed, countries with high per-capita mental health professionals continue to struggle with access to services. Training non-mental health professionals in basic mental health skills may significantly help bridge this gap.

Furthermore, moving toward community mental health is an essential step. A stepped approach to care is currently being adopted by many mental healthcare systems globally, with significant resources being invested in prevention and primary care. This enables early screening of mental disorders in diverse settings within primary care systems. Increased funding for community mental health services can take this one step further by allowing care to be integrated within homes. This, in turn, reduces the burden on healthcare settings, where underdiagnosis, polypharmacy, and unnecessary referrals can be avoided due to direct access to personalized mental healthcare.

Another aspect of enhanced care is adopting digital health technologies in the community. Using chatbots as a mental health triage system can be an effective method of risk stratification among larger patient populations [61]. Mental health apps are another example of screening tools used for remote mental health assessments [62]. Integrating such tools into the healthcare system allows direct access pathways for the workforce to manage existing patients and monitor their long-term prognosis. Data integration across mental health facilities can facilitate the creation of a unified mental health assessment and care system across different facilities. Artificial intelligence-based models can then be utilized to analyze such data and predict trends in psychiatric illnesses within vulnerable populations. This could guide public health entities in planning nationwide targeted mental health awareness initiatives. Increased funding is warranted for digital infrastructure unique to the UAE population's needs to establish remote mental health support using telepsychiatry platforms. While technology can play a positive role in advancing mental healthcare, the adverse effects of technology on the population also require further research, particularly in the context of social media's implications on the mental health of youth in the UAE and the impact of cyberbullying on this population [63, 64].

32.7 Conclusion

To conclude, the UAE has taken significant strides in improving its population's mental health. This has been reflected, since the establishment of the UAE, in the necessary steps of adopting national policies and country-wide plans. Furthermore, the UAE has pioneered advancements in mental healthcare, research, and education. Expanding mental health capacity, increasing accessibility of services, and adopting innovative mental healthcare systems while endorsing innovation will further pave the way toward achieving the UAE's vision for accessible mental healthcare.

Conflicts of Interest The authors have no conflicts of interest to declare.

References

1. GBD 2019 Mental Disorders Collaborators. Global, regional, and national burden of 12 mental disorders in 204 countries and territories, 1990–2019: a systematic analysis for the Global Burden of Disease Study 2019. Lancet Psychiatry. 2022;9(2):137–50.
2. Vigo DV, Kestel D, Pendakur K, Thornicroft G, Atun R. Disease burden and government spending on mental, neurological, and substance use disorders, and self-harm: cross-sectional, ecological study of health system response in the Americas. Lancet Public Health. 2019;4(2):e89–96.
3. World Health Organization. Mental health investment case: a guidance note, 2021.
4. Santomauro DF, Herrera AMM, Shadid J, Zheng P, Ashbaugh C, Pigott DM, et al. Global prevalence and burden of depressive and anxiety disorders in 204 countries and territories in 2020 due to the COVID-19 pandemic. Lancet. 2021;398(10312):1700–12.
5. UAE Vision 2021 [Internet]. Available from: https://www.vision2021.ae/en.
6. Federal Competitiveness and Statistics Center [Internet]. Available from: https://u.ae/en/about-the-uae/fact-sheet.
7. UAE Population Statistics [Internet]. Available from: https://www.globalmediainsight.com/blog/uae-population-statistics/.
8. Mental Disorders [Internet]. Available from: https://www.who.int/news-room/fact-sheets/detail/mental-disorders.

9. Global Health Data Exchange [Internet]. Available from: https://vizhub.healthdata.org/gbd-results/.
10. Global Burden of Disease [Internet]. Available from: https://www.healthdata.org/gbd/2019.
11. DHA mental strategy [Internet]. Available from: https://www.dha.gov.ae/ar/uploads/062022/Dubai_Health_Strategy_2016-2021_En2022649600.pdf.
12. Health Data UAE [Internet]. Available from: https://www.healthdata.org/united-arab-emirates.
13. Mental Health Atlas 2020 Country Profile: United Arab Emirates [Internet]. Available from: https://www.who.int/publications/m/item/mental-health-atlas-are-2020-country-profile.
14. Razzak HA, Harbi A, Ahli S. Depression: prevalence and associated risk factors in The United Arab Emirates. Oman Med J. 2019;34(4):274.
15. Dervic K, Amiri L, Niederkrotenthaler T, Yousef S, Salem MO, Voracek M, et al. Suicide rates in the national and expatriate population in Dubai, United Arab Emirates. Int J Soc Psychiatry. 2012;58(6):652–6.
16. Eapen V, Al-Gazali L, Bin-Othman S, Abou-Saleh M. Mental health problems among schoolchildren in United Arab Emirates: prevalence and risk factors. J Am Acad Child Adolesc Psychiatry. 1998;37(8):880–6.
17. Cohen A. Addressing comorbidity between mental disorders and major noncommunicable diseases: background technical report to support implementation of the WHO European Mental Health Action Plan 2013–2020 and the WHO European Action Plan for the Prevention and Control of Noncommunicable Diseases 2016–2025. 2017.
18. El-Rufaie OE, Absood GH. Minor psychiatric morbidity in primary health care: prevalence, nature and severity. Int J Soc Psychiatry. 1993;39(3):159–66.
19. Al-Maskari F, Shah S, Al-Sharhan R, Al-Haj E, Al-Kaabi K, Khonji D, et al. Prevalence of depression and suicidal behaviors among male migrant workers in United Arab Emirates. J Immigr Minor Health. 2011;13(6):1027–32.
20. Eapen V, Ai-Sabosy M, Saeed M, Sabri S. Child psychiatric disorders in a primary care Arab population. Int J Psychiatry Med. 2004;34(1):51–60.
21. Al Banna A, Al Bedwawi S, Al Saadi A, Al Maskari F, Eapen V. Prevalence and correlates of conduct disorder among inmates of juvenile detention centres, United Arab Emirates. EMHJ-East Mediterr Health J. 2008;14(5):1054–9.
22. Eapen V, Mabrouk AA, Bin-Othman S. Disordered eating attitudes and symptomatology among adolescent girls in The United Arab Emirates. Eat Behav. 2006;7(1):53–60.
23. Eapen V, Mabrouk AA, Zoubeidi T, Sabri S, Yousef S, Al-Ketbi J, et al. Epidemiological study of attention deficit hyperactivity disorder among school children in The United Arab Emirates. Hamdan Med J. 2009;2(3):119–27.
24. Eapen V, Mabrouk AA, Zoubeidi T, Yunis F. Prevalence of pervasive developmental disorders in preschool children in the UAE. J Trop Pediatr. 2007;53(3):202–5.
25. Alhassani G, Osman OT. Mental health law profile: The United Arab Emirates. BJPsych Int. 2015;12(3):70–2.
26. Mohammed Bin Rashid issues new law to tackle rehabilitation of substance and alcohol abuse in Dubai. Available from: https://gulfnews.com/uae/mohammed-bin-rashid-issues-new-law-to-tackle-rehabilitation-of-substance-and-alcohol-abuse-in-dubai-1.66478449.
27. Latest Legislations and Laws [Internet]. Available from: https://www.moj.gov.ae/en/laws-and-legislation/latest-legislations-and-laws.aspx#page=1.
28. UAE passes mental health care draft law. Available from: https://gulfnews.com/uae/health/uae-passes-mental-health-care-draft-law-1.79769430.
29. National Strategy for Wellbeing 2031 [Internet]. Available from: https://u.ae/en/about-the-uae/strategies-initiatives-and-awards/federal-governments-strategies-and-plans/national-strategy-for-wellbeing-2031.
30. People of determination [Internet]. Available from: https://u.ae/en/information-and-services/social-affairs/people-of-determination.
31. The National Policy for empowering people of determination [Internet]. Available from: https://u.ae/en/about-the-uae/strategies-initiatives-and-awards/federal-governments-strategies-and-plans/the-national-policy-for-empowering-people-with-special-needs.

32. Dubai Inclusive Education Policy Framework [Internet]. Available from: https://web.khda.gov.ae/getattachment/About-Us/Legislation/Private-Schools-Regulations/Dubai-inclusive-education-policy-framework/Education_Policy_En.pdf.aspx?lang=en-GB.
33. The National Policy for autism [Internet]. Available from: https://www.mocd.gov.ae/en/about-mocd/autism/the-national-policy-for-autism.aspx.
34. Dubai clinical practice guidelines for autism spectrum disorder (ASD) in children and adolescents [Internet]. Available from: https://www.dha.gov.ae/uploads/112021/f5d3aa75-37c3-4237-ba9a-d9e4fba52531.pdf.
35. Health regulatory authorities [Internet]. Available from: https://u.ae/en/information-and-services/health-and-fitness/health-authorities.
36. IACAPAP 2022 [Internet]. Available from: https://www.iacapap2022.com, https://iacapap.org/events/world-congresses.html.
37. Child and Adolescent Mental Health Centre of Excellence, Al Jalila Children's Hospital [Internet]. Available from: https://aljalilachildrens.ae/centers-services/child-and-adolescent-mental-health.
38. Eapen V, El-Rufaie O. United Arab Emirates (UAE). Int Psychiatry Bull Board Int Aff R Coll Psychiatr. 2008;5(2):38–40.
39. PureHealth 2024. PureHealth launches Sakina, the region's largest mental health platform. Abu Dhabi Media Office.
40. Psychology and mental health services in the United Arab Emirates [Internet]. Available from: https://www.apa.org/international/pi/2015/06/psychology-arab.
41. Innovation Health Strategy [Internet]. Available from: https://mohap.gov.ae/en/about-us/innovation-health-strategy.
42. MoHAP and EHS hold Mental Health Innovation Lab [Internet]. Available from: https://mohap.gov.ae/en/media-center/news/1/11/2021/mohap-and-ehs-hold-mental-health-innovation-lab.
43. Mental health [Internet]. Available from: https://u.ae/en/information-and-services/health-and-fitness/mental-health.
44. MoHAP highlights its mental health services provided during COVID-19. Available from: https://www.wam.ae/en/details/1395302875919.
45. Maintaining mental health in times of COVID-19 [Internet]. Available from: https://u.ae/en/information-and-services/justice-safety-and-the-law/handling-the-covid-19-outbreak/maintaining-mental-health-in-times-of-covid19.
46. "Rest Assured" Social Mental Health Initiative During COVID-19 Current Wave Achieves Broad Social Interaction [Internet]. Available from: https://www.mocd.gov.ae/en/media-centre/news/23/2/2022/23022022.aspx.
47. Maalouf FT, Alamiri B, Atweh S, Becker AE, Cheour M, Darwish H, et al. Mental health research in the Arab region: challenges and call for action. Lancet Psychiatry. 2019;6(11):961–6.
48. The curriculum of the fellowship child and adolescent psychiatry training, Al Jalila Children's Speciality Hospital [Internet]. Available from: https://aljalilachildrens.ae/fellowship/curriculum/Educational%20Activities.
49. Thomas J, Barbato M, Verlinden M, Gaspar C, Moussa M, Ghorayeb J, et al. Psychosocial correlates of depression and anxiety in The United Arab Emirates during the COVID-19 pandemic. Front Psych. 2020;11:564172.
50. Cheikh Ismail L, Mohamad MN, Bataineh MF, Ajab A, Al-Marzouqi AM, Jarrar AH, et al. Impact of the coronavirus pandemic (COVID-19) lockdown on mental health and well-being in The United Arab Emirates. Front Psych. 2021;12:633230.
51. AlGhufli F, AlMulla R, Alyedi O, Zain AlAbdin S, Nakhal MM. Investigating the impact of COVID-19 pandemic on mental health status and factors influencing negative mental health among health-care workers in Dubai. United Arab Emirates Dubai Med J. 2021;4(4):301–9.
52. Hashim M, Coussa A, Al Dhaheri AS, Al Marzouqi A, Cheaib S, Salame A, et al. Impact of coronavirus 2019 on mental health and lifestyle adaptations of pregnant women in The United Arab Emirates: a cross-sectional study. BMC Pregnancy Childbirth. 2021;21(1):515.

53. Saddik B, Hussein A, Albanna A, Elbarazi I, Al-Shujairi A, Temsah MH, et al. The psychological impact of the COVID-19 pandemic on adults and children in The United Arab Emirates: a nationwide cross-sectional study. BMC Psychiatry. 2021;21(1):224.
54. Ghader NA, Mheiri NA, Fikri A, AbdulRazzak H, Saleheen H, Saddik B, et al. Prevalence and factors associated with mental illness symptoms among school students post lockdown of the COVID-19 pandemic in The United Arab Emirates: a cross-sectional national study [Internet]. Psychiat Clin Psychol. 2022; [cited 2022 Nov 13]. Available from: http://medrxiv.org/lookup/doi/10.1101/2022.07.20.22277866
55. Afifi M. Mental health publications from the Arab world cited in PubMed, 1987-2002. EMHJ-East Mediterr Health J. 2005;11(3):319–28.
56. RAK College of Nursing [Internet]. Available from: https://www.rakmhsu.ac.ae/rakcon-programs-offered.
57. Bachelor of Science in Psychology, Zayed University [Internet]. Available from: https://www.zu.ac.ae/main/en/colleges/colleges/__college_of_natural_and_health_sciences/_course_descriptions/bachelor-of-Science-in-Psychology.aspx.
58. Systems of care for autism spectrum disorder [Internet]. Available from: https://ghd-dubai.hms.harvard.edu/files/ghd_dubai/files/autism_digital.pdf.
59. United Arab Emirates 2023. Federal Law No. (10) of 2023 on Mental Health. https://uaelegislation.gov.ae/en/legislations/2166/download.
60. DHA EBP Plans [Internet]. Available from: https://www.sukoon.com/individuals/health-insurance/plans/dha-ebp-plans.
61. Almalki M, Azeez F. Health Chatbots for fighting COVID-19: a scoping review. Acta Inform Medica. 2020;28(4):241.
62. Klein A, Clucas J, Krishnakumar A, Ghosh SS, Van Auken W, Thonet B, et al. Remote digital psychiatry for mobile mental health assessment and therapy: MindLogger platform development study. J Med Internet Res. 2021;23(11):e22369.
63. Keles B, McCrae N, Grealish A. A systematic review: the influence of social media on depression, anxiety and psychological distress in adolescents. Int J Adolesc Youth. 2020;25(1):79–93.
64. Abaido GM. Cyberbullying on social media platforms among university students in The United Arab Emirates. Int J Adolesc Youth. 2020;25(1):407–20.
65. Law No. (13) of 2021 Establishing the Dubai Academic Health Institution (no date). Available at: https://dlp.dubai.gov.ae/Legislation%20Reference/2021/Law%20No.%20(13)%20of%202021%20Establishing%20the%20Dubai%20Academic%20Health%20Institution.html#_ftn1.
66. Albanna A, Soubra K, Alhashmi D, Alloub Z, AlOlama F, Hammerness P, et al. Effectiveness of collaborative tele-mental health care for children with attention deficit hyperactivity disorder in primary care centres: randomized controlled trial in Dubai. East Mediterr Health J. 29:742. https://doi.org/10.26719/emhj.23.076.
67. Suha A, Karina S, Deena A, Fathumo M, Sarah M, Saeeda A, Zeinab A, Sandra W, Ammar A. Parental perceptions of autism spectrum disorder (ASD) services in the UAE. New Emirates Med J. 2024;5:e180823220001. https://doi.org/10.2174/0250688205666230818113555.
68. Reporter, S. Z. S. How Abu Dhabi is reforming mental health treatment and access for all. Gulf News: Latest UAE news, Dubai news, Business, travel news, Dubai Gold rate, prayer time, cinema, 2023, Jan 21. https://gulfnews.com/uae/health/how-abu-dhabi-is-reforming-mental-health-treatment-and-access-for-all-1.93353881.
69. DCD and DOH Collaborate to enhance individuals mental health through Istijaba Hotline. Home, n.d. https://addcd.gov.ae/Media-Center/News/DCD-and-DOH-Collaborate-to-Enhance-Individuals-Mental-Health-Through-Istijaba-Hotline.
70. FCA. Home, n.d. https://www.addcd.gov.ae/en/FCA.

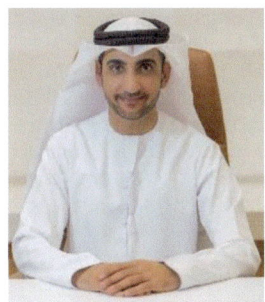

Ammar Albanna is a consultant child and adolescent psychiatrist trained in Canada and is currently the director of Al Amal Psychiatric Hospital, the premier psychiatric facility in the UAE under Emirates Health Services. Graduating from McGill University, Canada, Dr. Albanna completed his psychiatry residency and pursued child and adolescent psychiatry training. He furthered his expertise with a fellowship in pediatric neuropsychiatry at the Toronto Hospital for Sick Children. In addition to being a Fellow of the Royal College of Physicians and Surgeons of Canada, he's also an international fellow of the American Psychiatric Association. Dr. Albanna holds a Master's in Healthcare Leadership from McGill University. He is distinguished as the founding head of the Child and Adolescent Mental Health Center of Excellence at Al Jalila Children's Specialty Hospital in Dubai. Under the Emirates Medical Association, he initiated the Emirates Society for Child and Adolescent Mental Health, representing the field nationally. He is presently on the executive board of the Emirates Medical Association. Internationally, he currently serves as Vice President of the International Association of Child and Adolescent Psychiatrists and Allied Professionals (IACAPAP). He is an Adjunct Associate Professor in psychiatry at the Mohammed Bin Rashid University of Medicine and Health Sciences in Dubai (MBRU) and Sharjah University. Dr. Albanna's research, primarily centered on neuropsychiatric disorders in the UAE and innovative healthcare models, has earned him acclaim. He is the co-principal investigator for a study funded by SWARD exploring machine intelligence's role in autism spectrum disorders. His endeavors have garnered numerous research grants, including the Dubai Harvard Center for Global Healthcare Delivery Research Award, the Al Jalila Foundation grant and the Dubai Future foundation Grant for Autism Innnovation. He has championed significant initiatives, like the Dubai Declaration for Autism in 2017 and the 2021 Dubai Autism Guidelines. Recognized for his contributions, Dr. Albanna has received numerous accolades for his clinical, research, and educational pursuits. A regular speaker at local and international scientific forums, Dr. Albanna has also chaired pivotal global conferences, including the Autism Congress in 2017 and the 25th Congress of the International Association of Child and Adolescent Psychiatrists and Allied Professionals (IACAPAP) in 2022. He provides peer reviews for esteemed medical journals, is a member of MBRU's Institutional Review Board (2017–2024), and has served on jury committees for prominent awards, such as the Fatima Bint Mubarak Award for Motherhood and Childhood. He is the chair of the Research and Innovation Committee at Al Amal Psychiatric Hospital.

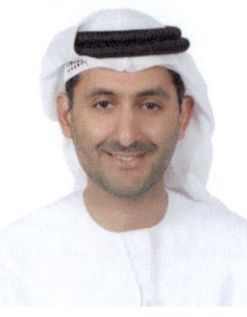

Meshal A. Sultan is a Consultant Child and Adolescent Psychiatrist at Al Amal Psychiatric Hospital, Emirates Health Services. He chairs the Committee of Academic and Professional Advancement at Al Amal Psychiatric Hospital. He is also an adjunct associate professor of psychiatry at the Mohammed Bin Rashid University of Medicine and Health Sciences (MBRU), Dubai, UAE. He is the inaugural chair of the Scientific Committee for the Specialty of Child and Adolescent Psychiatry at the National Institute for Health Specialties (NIHS), United Arab Emirates.

Dr. Sultan obtained his medical degree from UAE University in 2007. He completed his psychiatry residency training as well as a child and adolescent psychiatry subspecialty fellowship at the University of Ottawa. He has obtained certification from the Royal College of Physicians and Surgeons of Canada in psychiatry as well as in child and adolescent Psychiatry. He is an International Fellow of the American Psychiatric Association and a Fellow of the Royal College of Physicians of Canada. He served as a consultant child and adolescent psychiatrist at Al Jalila Children's Specialty Hospital in Dubai from 2017 to 2023. Dr. Sultan has more than 22 publications in peer-reviewed journals. He presented at international conferences on several topics, including attention-deficit/ hyperactivity disorder (ADHD), collaborative care, and mindfulness. He was the Chair of the Local Organizing Committee of the 25th World Congress of the International Association for Child and Adolescent Psychiatry and Allied Professions (IACAPAP), held in Dubai from December 5 to 9, 2022.

Dr. Sultan has been actively involved in leadership and academic roles. He served as the General Secretary of the Emirates Society for Child and Adolescent Mental Health after being elected in 2018. He was then elected for the position of vice president of the society in 2021. He was appointed as the Deputy Director of Academic Affairs at Al Jalila Children's from 2019 to 2022. He has actively participated in establishing the first Child and Adolescent Psychiatry Fellowship Program in the UAE, which started in 2019. He served as the Deputy Director of the Fellowship Program from 2018 to 2023.

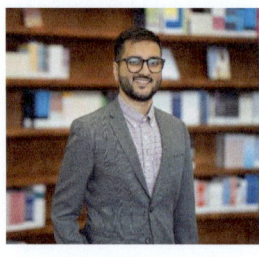

Faisal A. Nawaz is a psychiatry resident doctor at Al Amal Psychiatric Hospital in Dubai, United Arab Emirates. As a graduate of the Mohammed Bin Rashid University of Medicine and Health Sciences, Dr. Nawaz completed 6 years of medical training and was awarded the "Alumni Excellence Award" upon completion of the Bachelor of Medicine and Bachelor of Surgery program. Dr. Nawaz later pursued his interest in joining as a psychiatry resident as part of the 4-year Arab Board of Psychiatry Residency program at Emirates Health Services, UAE. During his undergraduate training years in the UAE, Dr. Nawaz also shared the privilege of exploring diverse health systems in countries including the USA, Jordan, and India. With an unwavering commitment to advancing the field of mental health, he has authored over 60 peer-reviewed research publications and delivered presentations at international and local conferences. Dr. Nawaz's research expertise extends across diverse domains, including mental health, global health, digital health, and medical education. Dr. Nawaz's efforts in scaling interdisciplinary collaborations have created an impactful presence in the social media community, which has led to further research developments in the field of social media research. Beyond his clinical and academic pursuits, Dr. Nawaz serves as the Chief Operating Officer and is a co-founder of the Global Remote Research Scholars Program. This innovative training program exemplifies his dedication to providing mentorship and guidance to the global healthcare community, fostering the development of future leaders in medical research. Additionally, Dr. Nawaz's leadership extends to the United Kingdom, where he serves as the strategy lead for the Clinician Engineer Hub. In this role, he plays a pivotal role in bridging the collaboration gap between physicians and engineers on a global scale. By fostering new areas for growth in mental health innovations, Dr. Nawaz aims to strengthen the digital infrastructure and knowledge base for technology-enhanced care in psychiatric services worldwide.

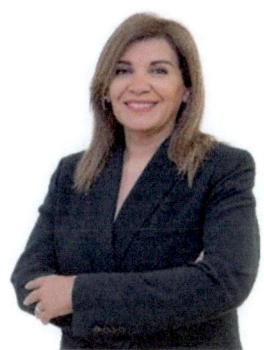

Hanan Derby is a child and adolescent psychiatry consultant at Al Jalila Children's. She is also the program director of the child and adolescent psychiatry fellowship program and adjunct professor at Mohammed Bin Rashid University Medical College.

Dr. Derby is a Fellow of the Royal College of Psychiatrists, UK, and has been a member of the Royal College of Paediatrics and Child Health, UK, the Royal College of Physicians of London, UK, and the Association of Child and Adolescent Mental Health, UK.

Prior to joining Al Jalila Children's, Dr. Derby was a senior consultant in child and adolescent psychiatry and the director and head of the Child and Adolescent Mental Health Service (CAMHS) at Hamad Medical Corporation (HMC). She also served as an assistant professor in psychiatry at Weill Cornell Medical College in Doha, Qatar.

Dr. Derby started her medical career as a pediatrician in the UK, attaining MRCP in Pediatrics. She then trained in psychiatry, accomplishing MRCPsych and achieving her Higher Specialist Training degree (the CCT) in Child and Adolescent Psychiatry. She has special interests in neurodevelopmental disorders, family-based therapy, infant mental health, mood and eating disorders, and medical education. In the UK, she established and led the CAMH subspecialty service for learning disabilities in Derbyshire, UK. In addition to her clinical role, Dr. Derby has always been active in medical training and teaching.

She is experienced in medical management, has led several psychiatrist services, and has sat on numerous departmental committees, including the Child Psychiatry Fellowship Training Committee, Academic Affair Committee, Institutional Training Committee, MBRU, JCI Academic Committee, Psychiatry Education, Clinical Competency, and Pharmacy and Therapeutic Committees. She was also an author member of the Autism Action Plan for Dubai. She has also served on the Children's Work Stream Governance Committee at Hamad Medical Corporation and the Qatar Strategic Health Committee of the Supreme Council of Health.

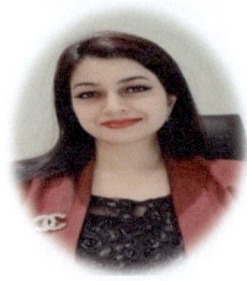

Dr. Mehnaz Zafar Ali is a Consultant Psychiatrist and the clinical lead for Community Psychiatry Services at Al Amal hospital, under Emirates Health Services (EHS). She also serves as Associate professor of Psychiatry at University of Sharjah and Sheikh Mohammad Bin Rashid University. She has accomplished her MD in Psychiatry, MRCPsych from UK and American Board Certification in Community Psychiatry. Her extensive contributions to global mental health advocacy are reflected in her international roles as Director at Large at the World Federation of Mental Health and middle eastern representative for the World Health Organization. Dr. Zafar has been elected as Co-Chair of Women Mental Health section at World Psychiatry Association (WPA) and Board member of Rehabilitation Psychiatry at the Royal College of Psychiatrists, UK. Her dedication to the field of medical education and research is demonstrated through her role on the International Advisory Board of the Journal of Psychiatry and Clinical Neurosciences and as the accreditation surveyor for the fellowship programs at National Institute for Health specialties, UAE. In addition, she leads the Behavioral health information system at EHS, spearheading the development of digital mental health solutions by integrating cutting-edge technologies with evidence-based practices.

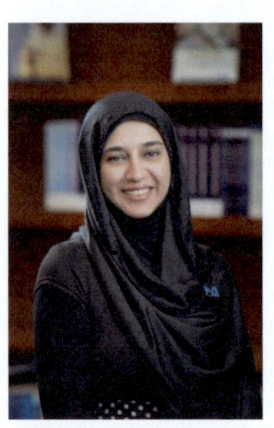

Nusrat Khan earned her Bachelor of Medicine and Bachelor Surgery (MBChB) from the University of Leicester (UK) and passed her membership examinations, becoming a Member of the Royal College of Psychiatrists in 2004. She received her Certificate of Completion of Training (CCT) in General Adult Psychiatry in 2007 and became a Fellow of the Royal College of Psychiatrists (UK) in 2020. Dr. Nusrat Khan gained her legal qualification of Master of Laws with commendation in Medical Law from Northumbria University School of Law, UK. She has also completed a Masters in Medical Education from the University of Dundee and is a Fellow of the Academy of Medical Educators. Dr. Nusrat Khan is an associate professor of psychiatry, teaching undergraduate medical students and postgraduate students. Clinically, she works in the private sector in Dubai and is a judicial member working as a medical member of the First-tier Tribunal, Health, Education, and Social Care Chamber (Mental Health) in the UK.

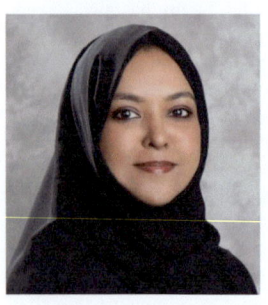

Dr. Nahida Nayaz Ahmed is an American Board-Certified Consultant Psychiatrist and Chief Medical Officer at SAKINA. She has held several senior leadership roles in the UAE government health sector and is a leading figure in mental health reform. Dr. Ahmed completed her psychiatry residency at Tufts University and a Consultation-Liaison Fellowship at Harvard University. She is a Certified Physician Executive (CPE), Adjunct Associate Professor at UAE University, and Associate Lecturer at Khalifa University.

She led the integration of mental health services across the Primary Health Network in Abu Dhabi and established clinics in tertiary centers under SEHA and Pure Health. Dr. Ahmed has authored numerous publications, guidelines, and policies, contributing significantly to mental health transformation efforts in the UAE.

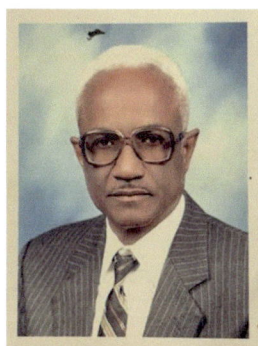

Omer El Rufaei earned his MBBS from the University of Khartoum, followed by training jobs in various specialties. He then joined the Institute of Psychiatry, University of London, and the Maudsley Hospital for higher psychiatric training. This resulted in obtaining the DPM and Membership of the Royal College of Psychiatrists (MRCPsych) in 1974. He became a Fellow of the Royal College of Psychiatrists (FRCPsych) in 1989. Previous university jobs for Professor Omer included Associate Professor at King Faisal University, KSA, for about 8 years, followed by more than a decade as Professor and Chair of the Department of Psychiatry, College of Medicine, United Arab Emirates University (UAEU).

The main research theme for Professor Omer was primary care psychiatry, but he also published in other epidemiological fields, e.g., transcultural psychiatry and somatized mental disorders, among others. Based on his research record at UAEU and other scholarly work, Professor Omer was granted the USA Green Card under the "Exceptional Ability" category. In addition, and by virtue of professional excellence, his name was included in "Who's Who in the World," "Who's Who in Medicine and Healthcare" (A Marquis Who's Who Publication), as well as "2000 Outstanding People of the 20th Century" by the International Biographical Centre, Cambridge, England. Prof El Rufaei was conferred the title of the first Professor Emeritus at MBRU in recognition of his lifetime of excellence and unwavering dedication to advancing mental health care and education in the UAE.

Open Access This chapter is licensed under the terms of the Creative Commons Attribution 4.0 International License (http://creativecommons.org/licenses/by/4.0/), which permits use, sharing, adaptation, distribution and reproduction in any medium or format, as long as you give appropriate credit to the original author(s) and the source, provide a link to the Creative Commons license and indicate if changes were made.

The images or other third party material in this chapter are included in the chapter's Creative Commons license, unless indicated otherwise in a credit line to the material. If material is not included in the chapter's Creative Commons license and your intended use is not permitted by statutory regulation or exceeds the permitted use, you will need to obtain permission directly from the copyright holder.

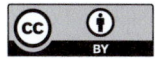

Rheumatic Disease History in the UAE

33

Ahmed Abogamal, Atheer Al-Ansari, and Ghita Harifi

33.1 Demographics

Rheumatic diseases (RD) represent a high percentage of health consultations worldwide. They are estimated to account for around 25% in certain parts of the world [1]. There is no accurate data about the prevalence of rheumatic disorders, other musculoskeletal (MSK) conditions, and bone health diseases in the United Arab Emirates (UAE). Historically, the UAE was originally divided between three health authorities, but in recent years, there has been a strong emphasis on amalgamating services and the data collected from all three regions. The lack of data or registries is prominently due to the two-tier health system between the private and government sectors. Figure 33.1 shows the diseases treated in rheumatology.

A recent study by Al-Salah et al. on the common RD conditions seen by primary care physicians (PHC) in the Dubai region demonstrated that low back pain is the most common presentation in these clinics (33%), followed by knee osteoarthritis (25%) and inflammatory arthritis (3%) [2]{Bulatovic, 2021, Barriers to Medical Tourism Development in the United Arab Emirates (UAE)}. The degenerative and mechanical presentations are both associated with older age groups and high body mass index (BMI) status. Interestingly, within the inflammatory arthritis group, seronegative spondylarthritis was estimated to be threefold higher than rheumatoid arthritis and significantly higher than in the other countries in the COPCORD study, which compared RD prevalence rates among different Middle Eastern countries [3]. For bone health conditions, they found that 3% of the attending cohort had osteoporosis, while 22% had osteopenia.

A. Abogamal (✉)
Rheumatology, Al Zahra Hospital, Dubai, United Arab Emirates

A. Al-Ansari
Mediclinic Airport Road Hospital, Abu Dhabi, United Arab Emirates

G. Harifi
HBG Medical Center, Dubai, United Arab Emirates

© The Author(s) 2025
H. O. Al-Shamsi (ed.), *Healthcare in the United Arab Emirates*,
https://doi.org/10.1007/978-981-96-0523-1_33

Fig. 33.1 Diseases treated under rheumatology [9]

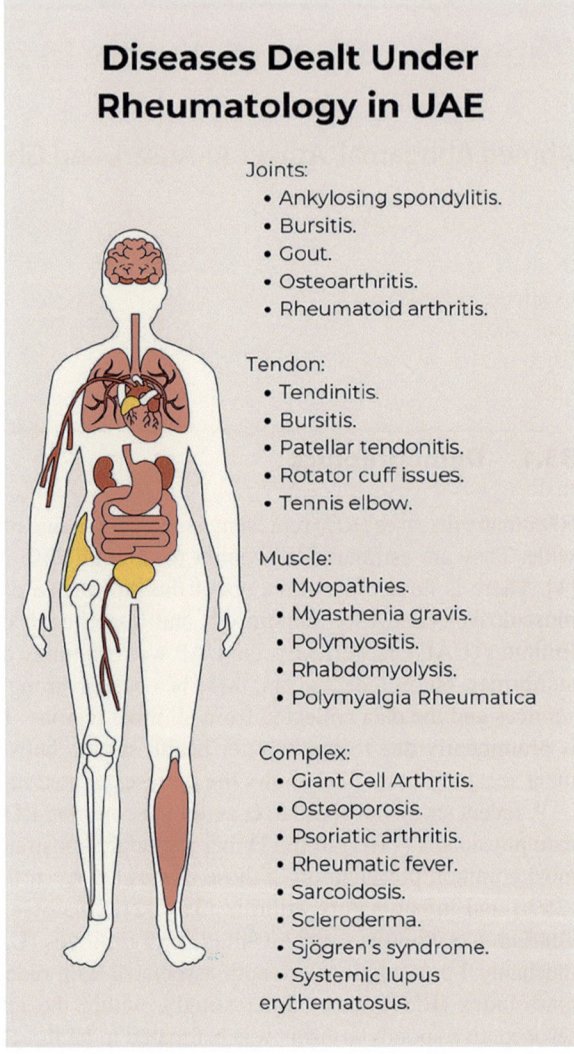

A similar study from the Emirate of Ajman involving 304 patients demonstrated that 17.5% had musculoskeletal manifestation (arthritis), and it is estimated that around 1% of this cohort was suffering from rheumatoid arthritis [4]. The prevalence of rheumatoid arthritis in this center's attendance is comparable to the international prevalence of the disease. However, it is important to note that this cohort was small.

There is no published immunological study conducted in the primary care setting in the Dubai region, but there is a tertiary center observation of patients specifically attending for rheumatoid arthritis (RA) disease by Namas et al. in 2019. They studied patients attending a rheumatology clinic at the Cleveland Hospital in Abu Dhabi over a four-year period via retrospective analysis [5]. This study covered UAE nationals demographically as the main ethnic group (81%), with the rest from other expatriate backgrounds. One of the main findings of the study was that the time to diagnosis is delayed by an average of 6.1 years. This is similar to what was observed in Kuwait, Saudi Arabia, and Iran. This is the first study showing the comparison of inflammatory diseases like RA in the national groups, similar to regional patterns, and could indirectly refer to the similarity of prevalence in the population size compared to other countries in the region.

Almoallem et al. (2021) from KSA studied the regional comparison in terms of the data available, and their main conclusions were that late diagnosis, inadequate treatment, and female preponderance are similar among all Middle Eastern countries, including the UAE [6]. Based on these limited studies, the Emirates Rheumatology Society and affiliated groups are urging the development of a national registry for patients with inflammatory joint diseases across all categories.

Osteoporosis, the leading condition in bone health, also lacks accurate prevalence or incidence data, including for primary osteoporosis and fractures. One of the main sources of data is the Dubai Bone and Joint Centre and the Ministry of Health screening program in 2007 [2]. The problem with the study is that its cohort included only 20% UAE nationals, while 80% were expatriates. In the study, around 25% of the screened population had osteoporosis (T-score less than -2.5), and 35% were in the osteopenia range (between -1.0 and -2.5). Among the 20% nationals, the male-to-female ratio was somewhat equal and did not conform to international ratios [2].

The overall estimation of osteoporosis in individuals over the age of 50 is around 7% in Dubai's studied population. Another cohort assessing the incidence of hip fracture estimated that there are 2.5 hip fractures per 100 individuals. This is alarmingly high compared to the data from the International Osteoporosis Foundation (IOF), which is based on data collected from international centers. They estimated the hip fracture rate to be around 2.25 to 1000 individuals per year [7]. There is no national hip fracture registry data in the UAE; however, recently, in both Abu Dhabi and Dubai, health authorities have established registries that feed the FRAX requirement for data, enabling the inclusion of Dubai and Abu Dhabi in separate FRAX registries.

It is quite prevalent within the UAE population to be serologically deficient in vitamin D, despite the recent confusion regarding the correct level at which deficiency can be defined. Nevertheless, it has been considered one of the risk factors for people with osteoporosis in the UAE, in addition to the sedentary lifestyle common among most patients in the over-50 age group.

Vitamin D deficiency status might not necessarily have musculoskeletal manifestations at the time of the test, but there is greater emphasis on the community-wide deficiency that could eventually lead to musculoskeletal diseases. In one study by Al Anouti et al. (2022), it was concluded that 67% of people subjected to routine screening are serologically vitamin D deficient, i.e., their levels are below 30 ng/mL [8]. In expatriate Arabic females, this is exceptionally high, with up to 80% of them being deficient. It was even lower in the Filipino ethnic group (15%), but there is no clear indication of the percentage of UAE nationals who are vitamin D deficient.

Additionally, true data on osteomalacia or rickets as the pathophysiological sequelae of critically low vitamin D levels are lacking as well.

There are no clear statistics on hyperuricemia or gout, but some specified sources claim that hyperuricemia could affect 70% of the UAE population, mainly attributed to a higher BMI and sedentary lifestyle. The prevalence of true gout monoarthritic is very scarce, but the general observation by the rheumatology community is that it might be intelligible to people with high BMIs as well as workers from East Asia in particular [1].

33.2 Current Healthcare for Rheumatology in the UAE

Being a relatively young society, the Emirates Society of Rheumatology has given considerable attention to teaching and education from the beginning. From a small-scale journal club in 1999 to several renowned educational entities, the journey of rheumatology education in the UAE has been both exciting and fascinating. Let us look at some of the most important milestones in the history of rheumatology education in the country.

33.2.1 From a Rheumatology Club to an Active Rheumatology Society

The first UAE rheumatology club was established by Dr. Ayman Al Mofti in 1999. The club, which gathered a handful of rheumatologists initially, grew gradually and saw its membership build up year after year. Some of the current eminent rheumatologists, such as Dr. Jamal Al Saleh and Dr. Mustafa Al Izzi, have taken the lead of the rheumatology club since then and have organized a couple of scientific events.

In 2008, the Emirates Society of Rheumatology was officially launched and replaced the Rheumatology Journal Club. Dr. Waleed Al Shehhi became the first president of the ESR. In the same year, the Emirates Society of Rheumatology (ESR) joined APLAR at the APLAR Yokohama Congress in Japan. Since then, it has been an active national rheumatology association member along with other APLAR Arab members, including Syria, Iraq, Kuwait, Oman, and Jordan [10].

The ESR now has more than 70 rheumatologist members. The society works tirelessly towards the establishment of local guidelines for the management of rheumatic diseases, in line with international guidelines and recommendations [the European Alliance of Associations for Rheumatology (EULAR) and the American College of Rheumatology (ACR)]. It also collaborates with governmental authorities to facilitate the implementation of best practices in rheumatology [9].

The society has published guidelines for rheumatoid arthritis, which have been included in the standard of care in Dubai for RA [11]. More recently, it published consensus statements on psoriatic arthritis in the United Arab Emirates [12].

ESR holds regular, high-quality educational monthly and annual meetings, bringing together international, regional, and local speakers and delegates to exchange knowledge and expertise.

The ESR has also collaborated with some of the highly esteemed regional societies to organize important conferences, such as the Pan-Arab Rheumatology Congress in 2014, which witnessed the emergence of ARLAR (Arab League Against Rheumatism). Another major collaboration took place in 2017 with APLAR (Asia Pacific League of Rheumatology Associations), when Dubai was elected to host the annual APLAR conference in partnership with the ESR [13].

It is noteworthy that the ESR is very well represented in a couple of APLAR Special Interest Groups (SIGs), such as the Imaging SIG, the spondyloarthropathies SIG, and the APLAR Young Rheumatologists, where the UAE holds the vice chair position through Dr. Ghita Harifi [13].

33.2.2 Emirates Rheumatology Academy: A New Academic Entity Focused on Education

Founded in 2019, the Emirates Rheumatology Academy (ERA) is a licensed non-profit organization that collaborates with the main global rheumatology organizations, including EULAR, ACR, GRAPPA, ASAS, etc., to bring the most up-to-date, high-quality rheumatology education expertise to UAE rheumatologists. The ERA has given special attention to some forms of arthritis that have not received enough coverage in the past decade, such as psoriatic arthritis and spondyloarthropathies. For three consecutive years, the ERA and GRAPPA (Group for Research and Assessment of Psoriasis and Psoriatic Arthritis) have been collaborating closely to bring the latest updates in the field and the most up-to-date psoriatic arthritis management guidelines [14].

Moreover, ERA has been a pioneer in organizing imaging workshops and courses. A couple of very successful magnetic resonance imaging (MRI) master classes and musculoskeletal courses have been organized by ERA in the last three years. Most of them have been conducted in collaboration with international societies, such as ASAS (the Assessment of SpondyloArthritis International Society), with whom an MRI Master class was organized in 2020, ISEMIR (International Society for Musculoskeletal Imaging in Rheumatology), and EULAR (European Alliance of Associations for Rheumatology). The partnership with EULAR has led to the organization of prestigious and widely popular EULAR-endorsed courses in MSK ultrasonography, under the leadership of Prof. Ahmed Abogamal, Dr. Waleed Al Shihhi, and Dr. Ghita Harifi. Basic and intermediate-level courses have been extremely successful and have attracted participants from the UAE, the Middle East, Asia, and Europe [14].

Finally, ERA has partnered with EULAR and ACR to bring their famous "Post-Conference" highlights annually to Dubai.

33.2.3 Abu Dhabi Advanced Rheumatology Review Course (ADARRC)

An annual rheumatology course was created by Dr. Mustafa Al Maini in 2011. This course is known for its high-quality lectures and workshops covering all aspects of rheumatology. Throughout the years, ADARRC has become a very popular course in the region and has loyal attendees [15].

33.2.4 The GCC Association of Immunology and Rheumatology Conference

The first edition took place in December 2021. This conference aims to provide comprehensive and intensive scientific sessions and enhance rheumatology knowledge across other specialties [16].

33.3 Patients' Education in Rheumatology Within the UAE

33.3.1 The Middle East Arthritis Foundation

Founded in 2006 by Dr. Humeira Badsha, the Middle East Arthritis Foundation (MEAF, formerly Emirates Arthritis Foundation) is a non-profit organization that strives to raise awareness about arthritis and breathe life into leading ideas on health, hope, and happiness among patients living with arthritis. Its goal is to improve the quality of life for people with arthritis through leadership, training in the prevention, control, and cure of the disease. The foundation has grown to support more than 2000 patients today across the UAE. MEAF conducts an extensive range of events and programs to support arthritis patients, share inspirational stories, and promote the support network for better accessibility. Every year, on World Arthritis Day, the foundation organizes a popular annual event that gathers more than 200 patients on average, with a diverse and engaging program including circles of care, talks on well-being, diet, mental health, yoga, Tai chi, and live dance sessions [17].

33.3.2 Friends of Arthritis Patients Association

The Friends of Arthritis Patients Association, chaired by Her Excellency Waheeda Abdul Aziz, was established under the umbrella of the Health Promotion Department at the Supreme Council for Family Affairs in Sharjah in 2008.

In conjunction with the vision of Her Highness Sheikha Jawaher Bint Mohammed Al Qasimi, Wife of His Highness the Ruler of Sharjah and Chairperson of the Supreme Council for Family Affairs, the association aims to support arthritis patients, assist the needy and those who are unable to bear treatment expenses, raise public awareness about arthritis, and encourage members of society to participate in supporting patients and their families.

The association has launched several community initiatives and activities, including an annual charity run for arthritis and an annual health forum, where screening for osteoporosis and other health tests is offered to the participants [18].

33.4 Diagnosis and Management of Rheumatic Diseases

33.4.1 Diagnostic Processes

The UAE stands as a global healthcare center, attracting individuals seeking specialized medical care. Remarkably, healthcare centers like HBG Medical Center in Dubai have significantly enhanced the diagnosis and management of rheumatic conditions over the years [19].

33.4.1.1 Rheumatoid Arthritis (RA)
Early diagnosis, as supported by research, plays a pivotal role in minimizing pain and disability associated with arthritis, potentially improving the prognosis. The adoption of the new ACR/EULAR criteria in local and regional guidelines by rheumatological associations has shown promising results [20].

33.4.1.2 SpondyloArthritis
Diagnosis of SpA has been a challenge in Middle Eastern countries. Previously, owing to restricted access to magnetic resonance imaging and anti-TNF agents, the delay in diagnosis was a crucial problem, requiring urgent attention [21, 22].

However, with evolution, the UAE has paid considerable attention to the problem. Currently, imaging studies, a cornerstone in diagnostics, are extensively utilized in UAE medical centers for precise diagnoses and monitoring of disease progression [19, 23].

33.4.1.3 Osteoporosis and Gout
Specialized bone scans and testing for elevated uric acid levels, along with synovial fluid aspiration, when necessary, contribute to accurate diagnoses. UAE medical centers boast advanced diagnostic facilities for both conditions.

33.4.2 Management Approaches

33.4.2.1 Rheumatoid Arthritis
In combating rising RA cases, the "Dubai Arthritis Task Force," "General Assembly of Dubai Rheumatologists," and "Dubai Standard of Care—Rheumatology" have formulated comprehensive guidelines, emphasizing the utilization of analgesics, physical activity, patient education, weight management, surgical interventions, and corticosteroids as part of the management protocol [11]. Moreover, a study by

Zaffar et al. found that diagnosis and initiation of therapy in RA have significantly improved in the UAE over the past five years, owing to increased public awareness and support groups [24].

Since 2006, efforts to improve public awareness regarding RA have been carried out continuously. This is being done via awareness campaigns, charity drives, and patient support group establishments such as the Emirates Arthritis Foundation (EAF) and the Women's Initiative for Rheumatoid Arthritis (WIRA) [25]. Medical societies, private companies, and the UAE Rheumatology Club are supporting these campaigns. In 2007, the WIRA launched an awareness campaign in conjunction with the Dubai Electricity and Water Authority and the Emirates National Oil Company. Results from a 2010 study demonstrated that the lag to diagnosis of RA in the UAE is now aligned with other high-GDP nations, with the lag time from symptom onset to diagnosis being reduced to 7.8 (T12.1) months [26]. Most importantly, an improvement of 34.9% from 2006 has been recorded in prescribing disease-modifying antirheumatic drugs (DMARDs) [27].

33.4.2.2 Vitamin D Deficiency

Efforts by the UAE Ministry of Health and Prevention (MOHAP), notably through the "e-Etmnan" program launched in 2019, have heightened awareness and screening for various non-communicable diseases, including vitamin D deficiency. Screening initiatives not only aid in prevention but also demonstrate the cost-saving potential in treatment [28].

33.4.2.3 Osteoporosis

As a growing global problem, the Ministry of Health and Prevention, MOHAP, reinforces its services for osteoporosis patients via innovative health services as part of its strategy aimed at delivering comprehensive and innovative healthcare services, as well as building quality systems and therapeutic, health, and pharmaceutical safety in accordance with international standards [28].

MoHAP offers specialized clinics, well-qualified medical staff, and medications to osteoporosis patients, along with diagnostic checkups and osteoporosis-related medical consultations for those visiting outpatient clinics, which are fully equipped with the latest medical equipment and an advanced bone densitometer (bone-density scan).

However, the MENA Geriatric Summit, launched in 2017 by the Dubai Health Authority (DHA) in partnership with the Swiss Business Council, Dubai, and the Northern Emirates, presented facts that, as healthcare delivery improves, mortality numbers are dropping and there is an increasingly aging population that healthcare professionals must take care of. The conference's scientific program showcases new developments and share international views on different topics in elderly care, which cover healthy aging, nutrition for aging, sensory and neurological disorders of aging, anti-aging medicine, and chronic disease, to name a few [29].

33.5 Advancements and Future Prospects

The UAE has established accredited rheumatology fellowship programs in Abu Dhabi and Dubai. There are currently two rheumatology fellowship programs: one in Sheikh Shakhbout Medical City (SSMC) in Abu Dhabi and another in Dubai [30]. Notably, Sheikh Shakhbout Medical City (SSMC) in Abu Dhabi has gained Accreditation Council for Graduate Medical Education (ACGME) accreditation and is in the process of obtaining National Institute for Health Specialties (NIHS) accreditation. Moreover, in early 2023, the Dubai Academic Health Corporation's rheumatology program was also accredited by the Saudi Central Board for Accreditation of Healthcare Institutions (CBAHI) [31]. The future fellowship proposal can be categorized into two classes, as discussed in the following.

33.5.1 Pediatric Rheumatology Fellowship

With the rising cases of rheumatological disorders in childhood, consideration is being given to developing a separate fellowship program for this demographic, focusing solely on disorders encircling early life.

33.5.2 Adult Rheumatology Fellowship

In a meeting in December 2022, an adult rheumatology fellowship curriculum was devised. The key points for development were inspired by ACGME's proposed guidelines.

33.6 Conclusion

The landscape of rheumatology care in the UAE reflects dynamic growth marked by the evolution of societies like the ESR, academia such as the Emirates Rheumatology Academy, and influential educational initiatives like ADARRC. Despite advancements in diagnostic processes and disease management, challenges persist in comprehensive data gathering, especially in areas like osteoporosis, gout, and vitamin D deficiency. Efforts by governmental bodies and healthcare institutions to create guidelines and establish specialized clinics demonstrate a commitment to enhancing patient care. The accreditation of fellowship programs and discussions around pediatric rheumatology training highlight a concerted effort to address the scarcity of specialists. Moving forward, fostering collaboration, expanding educational endeavors, and bolstering research efforts are imperative to bridge existing gaps and elevate rheumatology care in the UAE to international standards.

Conflicts of Interest The authors have no conflicts of interest to declare.

References

1. Rheumatic Diseases and Pain. https://www.cdc.gov/arthritis/communications/features/rheumatic-diseases-and-pain.html. Accessed 19 Nov 2023.
2. Al Saleh J, Sayed ME, Monsef N, Darwish E. The prevalence and the determinants of musculoskeletal diseases in Emiratis attending primary health care clinics in Dubai, (in eng). Oman Med J. 2016;31(2):117–23. https://doi.org/10.5001/omj.2016.23.
3. Chaaya M, et al. High burden of rheumatic diseases in Lebanon: a COPCORD study, (in eng). Int J Rheum Dis. 2012;15(2):136–43. https://doi.org/10.1111/j.1756-185X.2011.01682.x.
4. Abdullah A, et al. Arthritis among patients attending GMC hospital, Ajman, UAE: a cross sectional survey [Online] Available: https://pesquisa.bvsalud.org/portal/resource/pt/emr-178222
5. Namas R, Joshi A, Ali Z, Al Saleh J, Abuzakouk M. Demographic and clinical patterns of rheumatoid arthritis in an Emirati cohort from United Arab Emirates, (in eng). Int J Rheumatol. 2019;2019:3057578. https://doi.org/10.1155/2019/3057578.
6. Almoallem AM, et al. Top ethical issues concerning healthcare providers working in Saudi Arabia, (in eng). J Epidemiol Glob Health. 2020;10(2):143–52. https://doi.org/10.2991/jegh.k.191211.001.
7. Al Anouti F, Taha Z, Shamim S, Khalaf K, Al Kaabi L, Alsafarb H. An insight into the paradigms of osteoporosis: from genetics to biomechanics. Bone Rep. 2019;11:100216.
8. Anouti FA, et al. Vitamin D deficiency and its associated factors among female migrants in The United Arab Emirates, (in eng). Nutrients. 2022;14(5) https://doi.org/10.3390/nu14051074.
9. Emirates Society for Rheumatology. https://esr.ae/. Accessed.
10. Prakash P, Shankar S. Voice of aplarheumatology, FirstAnniversary special, 2017.
11. Al Yousuf H. Dubai standards of care-rheumatoid arthritis, 2017.
12. Alnaqbi KA, Hannawi S, Namas R, Alshehhi W, Badsha H, Al-Saleh J. Consensus statements for evaluation and nonpharmacological Management of Psoriatic Arthritis in UAE, (in eng). Int J Rheum Dis. 2022;25(7):725–32. https://doi.org/10.1111/1756-185X.14357.
13. Asia Pacific League of Associations for Rheumatology (APLAR). aplar.org. Accessed.
14. Emirates Rheumatology Academy. https://era-rheumatology.org/. Accessed.
15. Advanced Academic Rheumatology Review Course. https://www.adarrc.org/. Accessed.
16. GCC Association of Immunology and Rheumatology. https://gccair.org/. Accessed.
17. Middle East Arthritis Foundation. https://arthritis.ae. Accessed.
18. FOAP Marathon. https://foapmarathon.com/404.html. Accessed.
19. H. M. Center. https://www.hbgmc.com/. Accessed.
20. Cross M, et al. The global burden of rheumatoid arthritis: estimates from the global burden of disease 2010 study, (in eng). Ann Rheum Dis. 2014;73(7):1316–22. https://doi.org/10.1136/annrheumdis-2013-204627.
21. El Zorkany B, et al. The treatment journey for patients with axial spondyloarthritis in North Africa and the Middle East: from diagnosis to management (in eng). Int J Rheum Dis. 2020;23(11):1574–80. https://doi.org/10.1111/1756-185X.13961.
22. Hammoudeh M, et al. Challenges of diagnosis and management of axial spondyloarthritis in North Africa and the Middle East: an expert consensus (in eng). J Int Med Res. 2016;44(2):216–30. https://doi.org/10.1177/0300060515611536.
23. Hammoudeh M, Al Rayes H, Alawadhi A, Gado K, Shirazy K, Deodhar A. Clinical assessment and management of Spondyloarthritides in the Middle East: a multinational investigation, (in eng). Int J Rheumatol. 2015;2015:178750. https://doi.org/10.1155/2015/178750.

24. Zafar S, et al. Efforts to increase public awareness may result in more timely diagnosis of rheumatoid arthritis, (in eng). J Clin Rheumatol. 2012;18(6):279–82. https://doi.org/10.1097/RHU.0b013e3182676975.
25. Kuller LH, et al. Rheumatoid arthritis in the Women's Health Initiative: methods and baseline evaluation, (in eng). Am J Epidemiol. 2014;179(7):917–26. https://doi.org/10.1093/aje/kwu003.
26. Aletaha D, Eberl G, Nell VP, Machold KP, Smolen JS. Attitudes to early rheumatoid arthritis: changing patterns. Results of a survey (in eng). Ann Rheum Dis. 2004;63(10):1269–75. https://doi.org/10.1136/ard.2003.015131.
27. Sokka T, et al. QUEST-RA: quantitative clinical assessment of patients with rheumatoid arthritis seen in standard rheumatology care in 15 countries, (in eng). Ann Rheum Dis. 2007;66(11):1491–6. https://doi.org/10.1136/ard.2006.069252.
28. United Arab Emirates Ministry of Health & Prevention. mohap.gov.ae. Accessed 19 Nov 2023.
29. DHA launches the MENA Geriatric Summit 2017. https://www.dha.gov.ae/en/media/news/398. Accessed 19 Nov 2023.
30. Arab World. https://www.arab-board.org/?utm_medium=email&utm_source=transaction. Accessed 19 Nov 2023.
31. Alnaqbi KA, Al Cheikh SA. Shaping the future: the transformative path of the Arab Board of Rheumatology (in eng). Cureus. 2023;15(9):e45624. https://doi.org/10.7759/cureus.45624.

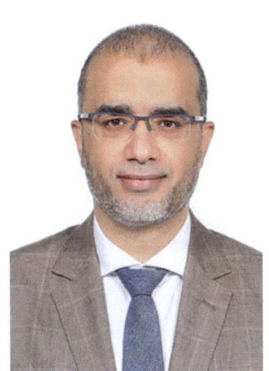

Ahmed Abogamal is a Full Professor of Rheumatology, Consultant Rheumatologist, and Head of the Rheumatology Department at Al Zahra Hospital in Dubai, UAE. He graduated with honors from the Faculty of Medicine at Al-Azhar University, where he went on to earn both his Master's and PhD degrees in Rheumatology, ultimately attaining the rank of Full Professor.

Abogamal completed advanced training with the European Alliance of Associations for Rheumatology (EULAR), becoming one of the first certified musculoskeletal ultrasound (MSUS) teachers and trainers from EULAR. He has played a leading role in initiating and organizing the collaborative EULAR annual training courses with the Emirates Rheumatology Association (ERA) in Dubai, with the goal of advancing ultrasound skills among Arab rheumatologists. In 2019, he co-founded the MSUS interest group under the Arab League of Associations for Rheumatology (ARLAR), where he currently chairs the Scientific Committee.

From 2001 to 2022, Prof. Abogamal served as the Scientific Chair of the Emirates Osteoporosis Society. He has also been appointed as a board member of APLAR 2024. In addition to his clinical and academic responsibilities, he is a certified specialist in Healthcare Organizations and Hospital Management. Prof. Abogamal is an active member of the GRAPPA network and has made significant contributions to the field through numerous research articles published in national and international journals indexed by Web of Science.

Atheer Al-Ansari graduated from the medical college of Baghdad University and completed his career postgraduate and specialty training CCST 2008 in the UK.

He became a consultant rheumatologist and head of department at Hollinswood Rheumatology Unit/ Telford.

He moved to Abu Dhabi in 2013 with the same position at Mediclinic Airport Road Hospital Abu Dhabi. He held many other positions.

He has served as ex-vice president of Emirates Society for Rheumatology (ESR) 2016–2019 and has served as head of scientific committee for Annual Asian and Pacific Rheumatology Conference in (APLAR 2017) Dubai. Currently, he serves as scientific advisor for Emirates Academy for Rheumatology.

He was a member of the National Osteoporosis foundation (NOF) in the UK, and member of Emirates Osteoporosis Society (EOS) in UAE.

He is a peer review panel member for APLAR and ELAR journals. He contributed to various conferences, talks, publications, articles, and committees.

He is a member of International Psoriatic arthritis research group (GRAPPA).

Ghita Harifi is a consultant rheumatologist and a French-certified musculoskeletal ultrasonographer. She is also an adjunct assistant professor at Mohammed Bin Rashid University of Medicine and Health Sciences (MBRU) and a General Civil Aviation Authority (GCAA) Specialist Aeromedical Examiner, since 2018. She has been practicing in Dubai since 2012.

Dr Harifi is a board-certified rheumatologist, a Fellow of the Université de Strasbourg, one of France's best research universities specialized in auto-immune diseases. She completed her Post-Graduate Certificate in Interventional Rheumatology, and her French Certificate in Musculoskeletal Ultrasound from L'Université Pierre et Marie Curie (UPMC), Sorbonne Universités, Paris.

Dr Harifi represents the UAE in the APLAR Young Rheumatologists (AYR) Committee, where she has been nominated as Vice-Chairperson.

In 2022, she has received the Emirates Women Award, a prestigious distinction for women who thrive in the UAE.

Open Access This chapter is licensed under the terms of the Creative Commons Attribution 4.0 International License (http://creativecommons.org/licenses/by/4.0/), which permits use, sharing, adaptation, distribution and reproduction in any medium or format, as long as you give appropriate credit to the original author(s) and the source, provide a link to the Creative Commons license and indicate if changes were made.

The images or other third party material in this chapter are included in the chapter's Creative Commons license, unless indicated otherwise in a credit line to the material. If material is not included in the chapter's Creative Commons license and your intended use is not permitted by statutory regulation or exceeds the permitted use, you will need to obtain permission directly from the copyright holder.

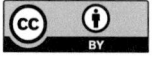

Urology in the UAE

34

Humaid O. Al-Shamsi [iD], Ali Thwaini, Faryal Iqbal [iD],
Omer Darwish, Amrith Rao, Farhad Janahi,
Ahmed Abdul Rahman, Hosam Al-Qudah,
and Thamer Al Kasab

34.1 Introduction

The last century has witnessed a unique evolution of a country. In just over five decades, no other nation has achieved such rapid development. Healthcare in the United Arab Emirates (UAE) has similarly evolved in line with other sectors [1]. This, of course, comes with many challenges; the population of the UAE has dramatically increased over the last few decades, and what is more interesting is the demographic composition of the inhabitants of the UAE [2]. Here are a few

---

H. O. Al-Shamsi
Burjeel Cancer Institute, Burjeel Medical City, Abu Dhabi, United Arab Emirates

Department of Medical Oncology, Dana-Farber Cancer Institute, Harvard Medical School, Boston, MA, United States

Harvard Medical School, Harvard University, Boston, MA, United States

College of Medicine, Ras Al Khaimah Medical and Health Sciences University, Al Juwais, Al Qusaidat, Ras Al Khaimah, United Arab Emirates

Gulf Medical University, Ajman, United Arab Emirates

Gulf Cancer Society, Alsafa, Kuwait

Emirates Oncology Society, Dubai, United Arab Emirates

College of Medicine, University of Sharjah, Sharjah, United Arab Emirates
e-mail: humaid.al-shamsi@medportal.ca

A. Thwaini (✉) · F. Janahi
Mediclinic City Hospital, Dubai, United Arab Emirates
e-mail: farhad.janahi@mediclinic.ze

F. Iqbal
Burjeel Cancer Institute, Burjeel Medical City, Abu Dhabi, United Arab Emirates
e-mail: faryal.iqbal@burjeelmedicalcity.com

O. Darwish · H. Al-Qudah
Fakeeh University Hospital, Dubai, United Arab Emirates
e-mail: omerder@doctors.org.uk

© The Author(s) 2025
H. O. Al-Shamsi (ed.), *Healthcare in the United Arab Emirates*,
https://doi.org/10.1007/978-981-96-0523-1_34

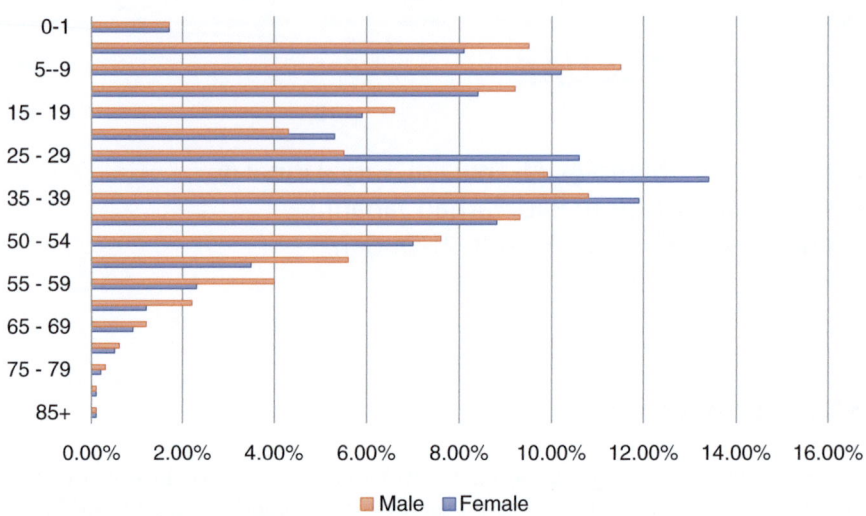

Fig. 34.1 Age-gender distribution of all respondents in surveyed households in the UAE [4]

evidence-based observations that make UAE healthcare stand out, highlighting its advantages and shortcomings.

The indigenous UAE population makes up about 11.5% of the total inhabitants of the country. This percentage has remained relatively constant over the past few decades. Prosperity and easy access to healthcare have led to an increase in the indigenous population. This, along with the vast development of the country at many levels, has necessitated a proportionate increase in expats to help build various aspects of life in the country. Healthcare is no exception [3].

Most of the UAE population is composed of the working class; hence, the majority is a relatively young population, and with the presence of different sociodemographic populations and varied ethnic backgrounds, health-related issues tend to be rather unique to this geographic area [4]. The age distribution in both sexes is shown in Fig. 34.1.

Access to healthcare is generally provided by the public and private sectors. Both sectors provide exceptionally easy access for the public. However, since healthcare

A. Rao
Mediclinic Welcare Hospital, Dubai, United Arab Emirates
e-mail: amrith.rao@mediclinic.ae

A. A. Rahman
NMC Royal Hospital, Sharjah, United Arab Emirates
e-mail: ahmadden@doctors.org.uk

T. Al Kasab
Al Zahra Hospital, Dubai, United Arab Emirates
e-mail: thamer.alkasab@alzahra.ae

providers come from different parts of the world and practices are delivered according to international standards, they may follow different guidelines.

The last two decades have witnessed significant expansion of the healthcare sector with the provision of high-standard treatments.

In line with the above, quality assurance and scrutiny of public and private healthcare providers have developed and gained strong support from the government. This has been translated into the nationwide governance bodies, such as the Dubai Health Authority, the Ministry of Health, the Department of Health, and many others.

Due to the availability of resources, the provision of healthcare has reached levels comparable to other developed healthcare systems in the world. Surgery in general, and urology is no different, have demonstrated a huge leap in their armamentarium; this is reflected clearly by the availability of minimally invasive surgery (including laparoscopic and the latest generation Da Vinci robot), various energy treatments for benign prostatic conditions (such as Holmium LASER, GreenLight LASER, REZUM, and prostatic urethral lift—UroLift).

Stone treatment remains a challenge due to environmental factors that are mainly related to the hot weather and dietary habits (with genetic factors playing another possible role, although complex, considering the genetic mix of this dynamic population). Various medical and endoscopic treatments currently exist, providing a safe and effective way of managing this common condition.

As the trend points toward improving one's image across various aspects of life, humans are no different, especially young adults and adult men and women. This aspiration of improving self-image has driven many men to seek various means of improving their physique, with the resultant increase in the intake of appearance-enhancing drugs in several instances, often without medical supervision. This clearly comes with inherent problems and side effects.

Throughout this chapter, we discuss the development of urology services in the country, go through various urological conditions affecting the population, and discuss the currently available resources and solutions.

34.2 Uro-oncology Services in the UAE

The data from the West clearly suggests that the incidence of urological cancers increases with age. There is more rigorous data collection in the West regarding newly diagnosed cases of cancer from cancer registries that are easily available for analysis. A similar effort has been made in the Gulf Cooperation Council (GCC) countries with the establishment of the Gulf Center for Cancer Registration (GCCR). The contributing countries include the UAE, Saudi Arabia, Bahrain, Kuwait, Qatar, and Oman. The Department of Health in Abu Dhabi established the Central Cancer Registry in 2012. The first publication was released in 2016 and, subsequently, in 2019 [5]. The trend line for genitourinary cancers (2015–2023) is depicted in Fig. 34.2.

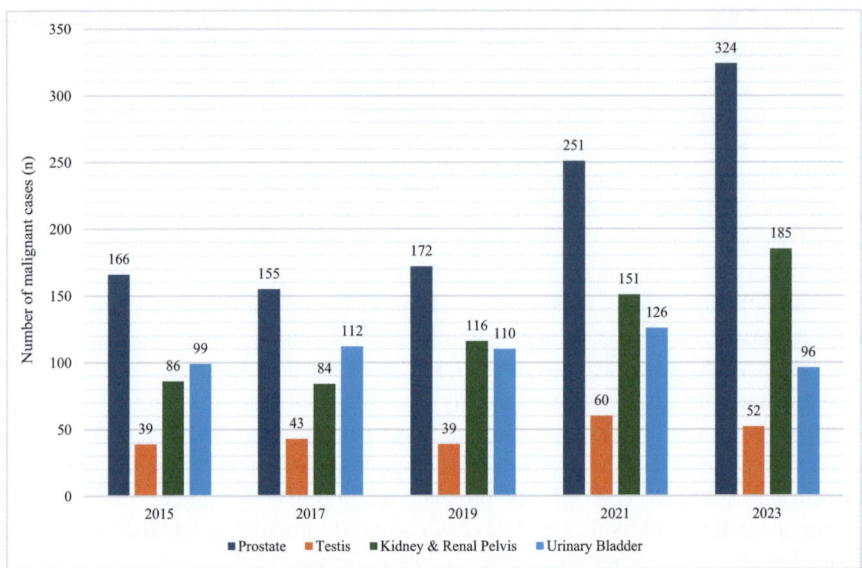

Fig. 34.2 Prevalence of various genitourinary cancers in the UAE from 2015 to 2023 [6]. (Source: Ministry of Health and Prevention, Statistics and Research Center, National Disease Registry—UAE National Cancer Registry Report, 2015–2023)

The current population of the UAE is around 10 million. However, this is expected to increase by nearly 1.47%, with a projection of approximately 12.2 million by 2040. The majority of the population are expatriates who are employed in the UAE. Indeed, the average age in 2020 was 32.6 years. With the introduction of the Golden Visa and its attractiveness in encouraging people to settle down in the country even after retirement, we are expected to see a huge increase in the number of elderly people. This will be reflected by an increase in patients presenting with cancer [1].

Urological cancer care was rudimentary in the past. Local patients would travel to countries like the UK, Germany, or the USA for treatment. Expats would travel to their home countries for further treatment. Therefore, major surgical procedures such as radical nephrectomy, radical cystectomy, and radical prostatectomy were rarely performed. But now the region boasts the latest cutting-edge technology, thus attracting a lot of medical tourism. To provide good cancer care, the government established Tawam Hospital in Al Ain in 1979. By 1983, it had been established as the designated cancer center for the entire nation. Indeed, Tawam Hospital also opened the first radiotherapy center in the UAE [5].

With increasing diagnoses of urological cancers and given the complexity of the cases, the high-volume centers have introduced tumor board discussions for the cases with the involvement of a urologist, medical oncologist, radiation oncologist, radiologist, and pathologist. This ensures the best care is delivered to the patient. Many centers have collaborations with highly specialized centers in the USA or the UK, and second opinions from these centers are also available.

34.2.1 Prostate Cancer

The detection of prostate cancer is increasing due to the acceptance of prostate-specific antigen (PSA) testing by patients. Most established centers are adopting a pre-biopsy multi-parametric diffusion-weighted MRI scan of the prostate. Centers are also offering transrectal prostate needle biopsies. Some centers have started to offer state-of-the-art MR-fusion prostate biopsies. In the past, staging of prostate cancer involved a CECT chest, abdomen, and pelvis scan along with a bone scan. Over the last 3 years, centers of excellence have offered the current "Gold Standard" PSMA PET/CT scan. Therefore, a patient with biopsy-diagnosed prostate cancer has all the investigations available locally and does not need to travel abroad.

Treatment of localized prostate cancer involves radical prostatectomy or radiotherapy. In the past, open radical prostatectomy was rarely performed in this region. Laparoscopic uro-oncological procedures were not routinely offered in the UAE. Patients were referred to specialized centers in Germany, the UK, the USA, or India. With the establishment of laparoscopic services in some centers within the UAE, urologists from overseas would come and perform the procedure. This landscape has changed over the last decade.

External beam radiotherapy (IMRT/IGRT) is offered across many centers in Abu Dhabi, Dubai, and Ras Al Khaimah. Recently, a center in Dubai has also started offering brachytherapy for localized prostate cancer.

Metastatic prostate cancer is usually treated with hormonal treatment with or without chemotherapy. Specialized centers are equipped to provide such services, including the latest medications that have been proven to be effective. Most of these centers follow NCCN guidelines.

However, urologists trained in the West and India began to be invited to the hospitals to perform complex procedures such as a laparoscopic prostatectomy, laparoscopic partial nephrectomy, and radical nephrectomy. With the expansion of medical services and the vision of the leaders of the country, the UAE started to attract talented surgeons from all over the world to settle down in the region and provide their expertise. Highly skilled laparoscopic and robotic surgeons are offering state-of-the-art uro-oncological procedures that benefit patients [7].

Robotic surgery was first introduced in November 2014 at Al Qassimi Hospital, Sharjah (Table 34.1). It was mainly available for gynecological procedures. In August 2015, Cleveland Clinic Abu Dhabi offered advanced uro-oncological procedures such as robotic radical prostatectomy and robotic partial nephrectomy. The American Hospital Dubai was the first private hospital in Dubai to offer robotic urological surgery in 2020. This was subsequently followed by Mediclinic City Hospital (2020), SSMC Abu Dhabi (2020), Clemenceau Medical Center (2021), and Dubai Hospital (2022). Alternative robotic platforms such as CMR (Cambridge Medical Robotics) surgical systems have been established in some centers in Dubai, but data on uro-oncological procedures are lacking.

Table 34.1 History of robotic surgery in the UAE

Center	Installed
Al Qassimi Hospital, Sharjah	November 2014
Cleveland Clinic Abu Dhabi	August 2015
American Hospital Dubai	January 2020
Mediclinic City Hospital, Dubai	June 2020
Sheikh Shakhbout Medical City, Abu Dhabi	August 2020
Clemenceau Medical Center Hospital, Dubai	April 2021
Dubai Hospital, Dubai	May 2022

34.2.2 Bladder Cancer

The evolution of the management of bladder cancer in the UAE has been challenging. Superficial bladder cancers are managed endoscopically, and almost all urological departments in the UAE provide the services. Muscle-invasive bladder cancer requires radical treatment. Due to cultural reasons, the ileal conduit urinary diversion is not readily acceptable. Therefore, bladder-sparing radical treatment in the form of radiotherapy seems to be more preferred than cystectomy. In the past, patients would travel abroad for complex procedures such as radical cystectomy and urinary diversion. However, currently, these procedures are offered within the UAE itself, both openly and minimally invasively, such as through a laparoscopic or robotic approach. Metastatic bladder cancer is managed in specialized centers with chemotherapy. With the advent of immunotherapy, patients have access to the latest medications within the UAE.

34.2.3 Kidney Cancer

In the UAE, the incidence of kidney cancer is increasing due to the rise in cross-sectional imaging. Another reason could also be that surgical treatment options are now available in the UAE. In the past, open procedures were carried out in very few centers. Currently, many centers are offering minimally invasive procedures such as laparoscopic or robotic radical nephrectomy and partial nephrectomy. These procedures were not previously available, and patients used to travel abroad for them. Patients with metastatic disease have access to the latest medications, including immune checkpoint inhibitors. Therefore, the UAE now offers comprehensive kidney cancer management, and this is proving to be attractive not only for residents but also for medical tourism.

34.3 Medical Tourism for Urological Cancer Services

The vision of the leaders of the nation is to establish the UAE as a hub for medical tourism. In 2018, Dubai had 337,011 medical tourists from other countries, and approximately USD 317 million was generated [8]. Complex cancer patients from other GCC countries, as well as other African countries, are choosing the UAE for their medical needs. With the availability of the latest, up-to-date investigations and highly trained surgeons, international patients are receiving the same level of service that they would have in Western countries. The barriers to medical tourism have been well addressed by publications that include high costs for the services, a lack of marketing activities, and a lack of collaboration between medical and tourism service providers [1]. The number of medical tourists doubled in 2021. Dubai received 630,000 international health tourists in 2021, according to a report released by the Dubai Health Authority (DHA) during the ongoing Arab Travel Market in Dubai. Spending by international patients reached nearly AED730 million in the past year despite the global COVID-19 pandemic [9] (Table 34.1).

34.4 Urolithiasis in the UAE

Urolithiasis is defined as the formation of stone concretions in any part of the urinary tract, while nephrolithiasis refers to stone formation in the kidneys, which is often the primary source of the disease. Nephrolithiasis is a highly prevalent disease worldwide, with rates ranging from 7 to 13% in North America, 5 to 9% in Europe, and 1 to 5% in Asia [10]. There is a global increase in the prevalence of nephrolithiasis due to multiple risk factors, including global warming, dietary changes, a lack of physical activity, and the rising trends in some lifestyle diseases [11].

The United Arab Emirates has witnessed outstanding economic development and an increased level of employment, leading to a significant rise in the prevalence of obesity and diabetes.

According to the UAE National Health Survey 2017–2018, 67.8% of the adult population is overweight (BMI $\geq$ 25 Kg/m^2) and 27.8% is obese (BMI $\geq$ 30 Kg/m^2) [13]. The correlation between obesity and nephrolithiasis has been demonstrated by numerous epidemiological studies.

Other studies have shown a strong association between type 2 diabetes mellitus and uric acid stone formation [12, 13].

Moreover, the hot climate in the UAE, especially during the summer, and inadequate compensatory water intake or rehydration can dramatically influence the possibility of disease occurrence, regardless of age or gender. Multiple studies have reported a significant association between higher monthly mean temperatures and the incidence of kidney stone disease-related events [14]. The UAE is considered one of the countries in the stone-forming belt of the world, with a male-to-female ratio of 2:1 [13].

The symptoms of kidney stones are related to their location, whether in the kidney, ureter, or urinary bladder [15]. Initially, stone formation does not cause any symptoms. Later, signs and symptoms of kidney stone disease consist of renal colic (intense cramping pain), flank pain (pain in the lower back), hematuria (bloody urine), obstructive uropathy (urinary tract obstruction), urinary tract infections, blockage of urine flow, and hydronephrosis (dilation of the kidney) [16].

The diagnosis of renal stones is usually made using one of the imaging modalities: an ultrasound scan or a computed tomography (CT) scan. The majority of secondary healthcare facilities in the UAE, both in the public and private sectors, have access to advanced radiology and imaging departments. As a consequence, an increasing number of renal stones are diagnosed incidentally without causing any symptoms. The treatment of these stones depends mainly on their size and composition.

Approximately 80% of all kidney stones are composed of calcium salts, namely calcium oxalate and calcium phosphate [17]. A significant proportion of the remaining stones is composed of uric acid, which accounts for over 10% of all kidney stones [18]. Only pure uric acid kidney stones can be dissolved with medical therapy by urine alkalinization.

Nowadays, healthcare providers in the UAE are investing generously in the equipment for renal and ureteric stone treatment. Fixed and ambulatory extracorporeal shock wave lithotripsy (ESWL) machines are being used to disintegrate kidney stones less than 2 cm in size and ureteric stones less than 1 cm in size. Contrary to what the public believes, this non-invasive procedure does not involve laser energy.

In addition, larger kidney stones can be treated with percutaneous nephrolithotomy using various-sized nephroscopes through a small, less-than-1 cm incision in the back of the patient. Alternatively, retrograde intrarenal minimally invasive approaches have gained momentum following the introduction of miniaturized and flexible uretero-renoscopes. This approach was made possible by using thin and flexible laser fibers delivering holmium lasers to convert renal stones into dust. The open competition among the scope manufacturers has provided a wide range of reusable and single-use digital scopes at an affordable cost.

Patients presenting with ureteric stone obstruction can initially be treated conservatively, provided that there is no compromise of kidney function, infection, or intractable pain. If intervention is needed, the options include a semi-rigid ureteroscope with laser stone fragmentation, or ESWL.

After treating the first episode of renal stone disease, it tends to recur in many patients, as studies have reported recurrence rates of renal stones to be 14% at 1 year, 35% at 5 years, and 52% at 10 years [19]. In addition to their effect on the patient's quality of life, recurrent renal stones increase the risk of a diagnosis of chronic kidney disease [20]. The UAE has recently made a major push to reduce the incidence of chronic diseases by adopting relevant legislation and launching public health campaigns [21]. These measures will help reduce the incidence of renal stone disease in the future.

34.5 Kidney Transplantation in the UAE

Despite the relatively young population in the UAE, chronic medical conditions such as atherosclerosis, diabetes, and hypertension are endemic in the region [22].

This is possibly related to genetic, ethnic, and cultural factors, mainly due to close-related marriages. Added to that is the sedentary lifestyle that comes along with the prosperity-associated disease of metabolic syndrome [23].

This has led to an increase in the number of end-stage kidney disease patients needing dialysis and the subsequent need for organ transplantation.

Despite the advice of healthcare facilities in the UAE, there remains an unmet need for kidney transplantation.

This has inevitably resulted in an increasing exodus of end-stage kidney disease patients across national borders seeking kidney transplantation, utilizing transplant tourism as an alternative source of kidneys, especially for those who are unable to obtain live-related kidneys for donation. However, transplant tourism has always been stigmatized with controversy regarding the source of organs, the donor's care after transplantation, and the recipient's outcomes [24].

The first live-related kidney transplantation occurred in 1985. This was soon followed by two deceased organ donations. The secured organs were donated via Eurotransplant [25].

To address the need for organ donation locally, especially the use of deceased donor kidneys, Mohammed bin Rashid University of Medicine and Health Sciences (MBRU) organized the first UAE Organ Transplant Summit in October 2015 [26]. This was followed by the first UAE Organ Donation Summit in 2016. During these meetings, the Saudi Centre of Organ Transplantation (SCOT) played a significant role in initiating a regional multi-center collaborative network for organ donation between the UAE and Saudi Arabia. Concurrently, a community-based survey was conducted by the university to assess attitudes and knowledge toward organ donation in the UAE. It confirmed the readiness of the public for deceased organ donation [27].

A historical event occurred with the passage of the landmark brain death law in May 2017. This enabled the formal establishment of deceased organ donation.

On June 8, 2016, the first deceased-donor kidney transplant procedure in the history of the UAE took place. A kidney was flown from Saudi Arabia to a female Emirati recipient at Mediclinic City Hospital in Dubai, where the transplantation procedure was performed [28].

The UAE's first multi-organ deceased donation occurred on July 17, 2017, at Al Qassimi Hospital in Sharjah [29].

The launch of the deceased-organ donor program in the UAE eventually paved the way for several firsts, including the first heart, lung, liver, and pancreas transplant surgeries at Cleveland Clinic Abu Dhabi, and the first deceased-donor pediatric kidney transplant at Al Jalila Children's Specialty Hospital in Dubai.

Figure 34.3 demonstrates the total number of deceased kidney transplants that have taken place since.

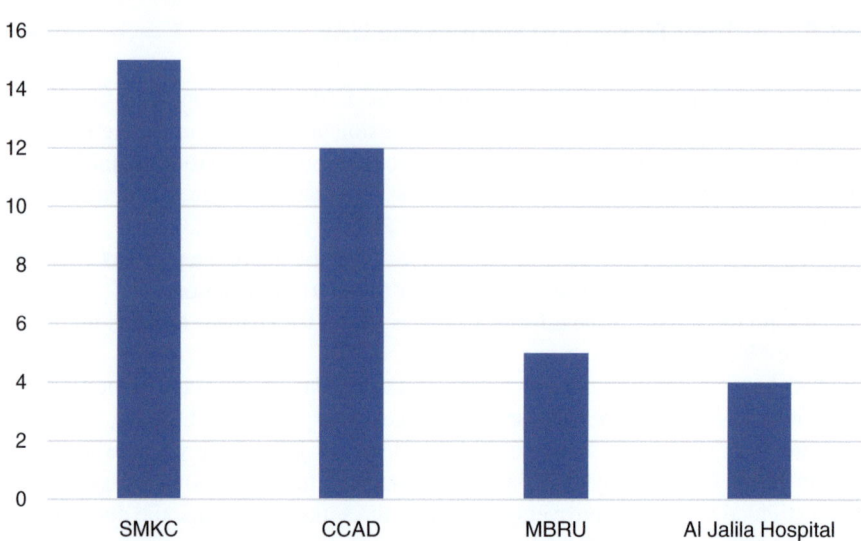

Fig. 34.3 Deceased donor volumes in Abu Dhabi and Dubai for 2017 to date. (SKMC: Sheikh Khalifa Medical City, Abu Dhabi; CCAD: Cleveland Clinic Abu Dhabi; MBRU: Mohammed Bin Rashid University, Dubai)

The kidney transplantation program has recently taken another leap in the transplantation capabilities in the UAE. A three-way swap took place between three families across two different countries [30].

Currently, Cleveland Clinic Abu Dhabi (CCAD) serves as the country's main multi-organ transplant center, along with three other centers performing kidney transplants: Sheikh Khalifa Medical City in Abu Dhabi (adult and pediatric), Mohammed Bin Rashid University at Mediclinic City Hospital (adult) and Al Jalila Children's Specialty Hospital (pediatric), both in the Emirate of Dubai. Organ retrieval in the UAE was valuable in reducing waiting times for organ transplants, not only in the UAE but also in Saudi Arabia and the Gulf region, through coordination with the Saudi Centre for Organ Transplantation. Patients in the UAE suffering from end-stage organ disease can receive life-saving and legally sourced organs in a world-class healthcare system.

34.6 Andrology

It is the urology subspecialty that deals with men's sexual health and fertility. Erectile function is a private matter when it comes to the conservative Middle Eastern man. However, with increasing public knowledge and access to various healthcare and social media platforms, erectile dysfunction (ED) has resurfaced, uncovering an important issue.

Anecdotal reports in the literature have demonstrated an increasing incidence among different age groups, with a further increase in its prevalence due to the increasing life expectancy, leading to a higher incidence of ED in this aging population [31].

ED, though it presents itself as a disease, could potentially be a symptom of a more serious underlying health problem. El-Rufaie et al. investigated ED among men with type II diabetes mellitus (DM) in a controlled study in the UAE, discovering an estimated high prevalence rate of ED among the diabetic group (89.2%). This was significantly greater than in the hypertensive group (43.6%), and the apparently healthy group (16.7%) [32].

This problem has unearthed another important health-related issue. With the increase in public interest in health and body image, there has been an increasing trend toward the use of anabolic steroids (AS), also referred to as appearance-enhancing medications. AS are manufactured testosterone substitutes that last longer than physiological testosterone in the body.

There has been a noticeable increase in AS abuse. This is clearly seen among professionals as well as youths taking part in daily sporting events. Excessive intake of AS is often associated with serious adverse effects. These include the risk of sudden death, chronic liver and kidney damage, and an increased risk of myocardial infarction among young men using them excessively. AS abuse has been associated with psychiatric complications, including violent behavior and suicide [33].

Multivitamin and mineral consumption, which was mostly combined with AS, was significant in the United Arab Emirates (UAE) (44%). A self-administered questionnaire was distributed to all gym users of randomly selected gyms in Al Ain city and showed a very high prevalence of AS misuse (22%) among gym users. This was statistically significantly higher among UAE nationals, bodybuilders, weight-lifters, and commercial club users compared to others [34].

In spite of the general awareness of the potential harm of AS, 7% of non-users were planning future AS use. In addition, abusers perceived more benefits from the use of AS than harms [34].

There has been a recent trend toward the implementation of public programs dedicated to increasing public awareness of the potential harm of AS, with the aim of preventing the propagation of the problem.

Male-factor infertility is another challenging health-related problem. It is defined as the inability to achieve conception after 12 months of unprotected intercourse. A cross-sectional study conducted by the Bourn Hall Fertility Centre, Dubai, in 2017 on 100 men with different nationalities between ages 25 and 56 found that one in five couples in the UAE is affected by this condition [35].

There has been a general global decline in fertility among men, according to the World Health Organization. The UAE is no different. With increasing public awareness, more couples are coming forward to seek treatment, which is a step in the right direction [36].

34.7 Genitourinary Infections in the UAE

Healthcare in the United Arab Emirates has advantages over other healthcare systems in the region due to the outstanding availability of facilities and the ease of access to healthcare services. This is offset by the excessive use of antibiotic treatment for a variety of clinical conditions without strict adherence to national and international guidelines. On many occasions, antibiotics are empirically prescribed in the absence of proven evidence of an infection. This has inevitably resulted in the widespread use of antibiotic-resistant bacterial strains.

In a retrospective review of the microbiology records of just under 500 cases of community-acquired urinary tract infection (UTI) between April 2006 and March 2007, *Escherichia coli* (207 strains) and *Klebsiella* species (90 strains) were identified [37].

Sixty-six percent of gram-negative bacilli were resistant to amoxicillin, 58.5% were resistant to trimethoprim-sulfamethoxazole, and more than 50% were resistant to cephalexin. However, resistance rates to antimicrobials like ciprofloxacin and ceftriaxone remained relatively low at 9.7% and 7.6%, respectively. Interestingly, this old study revealed that quinolone resistance was merely 7% [37].

However, 10 years later, the same author and colleagues researched the prevalence of extended-spectrum β-lactamase (ESBL)-producing bacteria in the UAE, since these bacteria are becoming an evolving and increasingly widespread trend of UTIs around the globe. They studied 399 ESBL-producing *E coli* and *Klebsiella pneumoniae* isolates from UTIs occurring between 2014 and 2016. Astoundingly, the majority of these ESBL-positive isolates were now resistant to quinolones (74%) and trimethoprim-sulphamethoxazole (73%), which are commonly used for treatment of community-acquired urinary tract infections [38].

The above example from the same group of researchers is an illustration of the evolution of microorganisms into resistant strains that were induced by the injudicious use of antimicrobial treatment and is a call to implement better infection control strategies and careful use of antimicrobials, especially in outpatient and community settings [38].

Sexually transmitted infections (STIs) are a challenging and important health issue. Undiagnosed infections in the male population can inevitably result in long-lasting urogenital conditions such as chronic prostatitis, urethritis, urethral stricture disease, ejaculatory duct obstruction, and infertility. Females are more at risk of untreated STIs since most infections are asymptomatic. Untreated women are at risk of long-term pelvic inflammatory diseases, infertility, ectopic pregnancies, dyspareunia, and cervical cancer [39].

With regard to other sexually transmitted infections, a retrospective cross-sectional survey was carried out on 201 female patients aged 16–80 years who were referred to the Obstetrics and Gynecology Department of Iranian Hospital, Dubai, UAE. Cervical swabs were collected from each woman, specifically looking for herpes simplex virus (HSV), *Chlamydia trachomatis* (CT), and *Neisseria gonorrhoeae* (NG). It was found that HSV, CT, and NG were detected in 6.5%, 10.4%, and 5.5% of swab samples, respectively. These rates were lower than expected compared to the literature [40].

With widespread healthcare education among different population groups and readily available access to medical treatment, the level of knowledge of such conditions is a true reflection of an advanced healthcare system. This is demonstrated in a recent study across different population groups in the Middle East. The authors concluded that the level of knowledge of HIV infection in the sampled UAE population of this study group was satisfactory at 70% [41].

34.8 Female Urology

34.8.1 Urinary Incontinence in the UAE

Urinary incontinence (UI) in females is a very common health problem worldwide. It has a severe impact on physical and social activities, as well as interpersonal relationships. More than 40% of women in the UAE suffer from urinary incontinence, which is an embarrassing condition that causes the involuntary leakage of urine. The societies in the Gulf countries are conservative and favor large families, high parity, and short inter-pregnancy intervals. Moreover, there is a high prevalence of gestational diabetes resulting in macrosomic babies [42].

The International Continence Society (ICS) defines urinary incontinence as the complaint of any involuntary leakage of urine. Urine incontinence (UI) is known to affect an individual's health-related quality of life (HRQL). The common types of UI are stress urinary incontinence (SUI), urge urinary incontinence (UUI), and mixed urinary incontinence (MUI). Urinary incontinence can have a negative impact on a person's lifestyle because of the social stigma attached to it. Not only can it affect social and personal relationships, but it can also hinder physical activity, affect a woman's career, and socially isolate her as she is too worried to go out, fearing wetting herself in public [43].

Urinary incontinence is more common in women than men. Older women experience urinary incontinence more often than younger women. This is not always the case, and many younger women can suffer from SUI and UUI, or even a combination of the two. The probable cause of the higher incidence in women can be attributed to pregnancy and childbirth, menopause, and the structure of the female urinary tract [44, 45].

According to a global study published by the Joanna Briggs Institute, an international non-profit research and development center at the University of Adelaide in South Australia, 42.2% of women in the Emirates have urinary incontinence. This compares with 44% in France, 42% in the UK, 30.9% in China, and 23% in Spain. In the Middle East, the overall prevalence of urinary incontinence ranges from 20.3% to 54.8%. In Qatar, it is 20.6%, and in the United Arab Emirates, it is 20.3%. In Saudi Arabia, the prevalence of urinary continence in Jeddah and Riyadh was estimated at 41.4% and 29%, respectively. The reported prevalence in the studies from the Gulf countries appears to be comparable to reports from nearby parts of the world that also studied women from healthcare facilities, such as the one reported by Kilic et al. from Turkey with a prevalence of 37.2% [46].

There are several risk factors associated with urinary incontinence, such as age, obesity, commodities, hysterectomy, and multiparity. Moreover, repeated pregnancies and deliveries may constitute a major risk factor among young and middle-aged women. In addition, increased reporting of urinary incontinence among women is attributed to population aging and increased public awareness that urinary incontinence can be managed and is not an acceptable part of normal aging. Differences in risk factors predisposing women to urinary incontinence were reported in different communities. Hence, the identification of predictors of urinary incontinence for the avoidance of modifiable risk factors is essential in preventing urinary incontinence, which will help to limit the negative impact of incontinence on quality of life and social activities that are common among women with incontinence [47].

Female urinary incontinence is a growing public health concern as it often results in a negative impact on quality of life and affects several aspects of physical activities and emotional relationships. As the majority of the population in the UAE is young, there is a high incidence of stress urinary incontinence following multiple pregnancies. Clearly, this might have a large impact on the community's welfare and healthcare systems. Therefore, primary prevention of urinary incontinence is recommended through necessary health education and awareness programs via mass media about the prevention of urinary incontinence among females by increasing the strength of pelvic floor muscles, particularly after pregnancy. Moreover, having a multidisciplinary team involving female urologists and uro-gynecologists to follow the updated national and international guidelines and, finally, to address the problem and overcome the embarrassment of female patients being seen by male doctors is essential.

34.9 Pediatric Urology

If we look at the statistics of the UAE population, we will clearly see a drift toward a younger population, with a median age of 32.6 years. This is explained by the fact that significant population growth has been witnessed over the past five decades, with most of the growth occurring between 2000 and 2010. Since then, there has been a gradual decline in growth. Following an initial growth of over 5 million people, it has slowed down significantly, reaching 9.89 million people [48].

This decline in growth is in line with the decline in fertility among UAE nationals, to about 1.42 births per woman. Due to the low fertility rate, the UAE government has advocated policies such as offering financial help to young married couples [48].

Another important observation is the rate of closely related marriages and their relationship with the prevalence of congenital malformations among newborns and pediatric patients. Al Gazali et al. studied the rate of congenital malformations among the population of the Al Ain area, which is a large province of the Emirate of Abu Dhabi. Over a two-year period, they found 173 (10.5/1000 births) with major malformations, 90 (52%) with multiple malformations, and 83 (47.97%) with a single systemic malformation. The gastrointestinal, central nervous system, and cardiovascular systems were the most affected. Genitourinary malformations constituted only 42 per 1000 newborns. Expectedly, the consanguinity rate was highest among the syndrome cases, and related parents were more likely to have infants with multiple malformations than with an isolated single system abnormality [49].

One of the most commonly practiced procedures in the pediatric population is ritual circumcision. This is embedded in Muslim culture, which constitutes most of the UAE population. Ritual circumcision is normally practiced at a very early age, preferably in infants. This is normally carried out in a hospital or clinic environment under strict antiseptic conditions. There are different methods of infantile circumcision, which range from the plastic bell to the Gumco clamp and surgical excision. The traditionally applied circumcision using a bone cutter has largely faded due to its globally evident inherent risks of bleeding and, more importantly, penile tip injury [50].

An important and sensitive topic is female genital mutilation (traditionally referred to as female circumcision)-FGM/C. This is defined by the World Health Organization (WHO) as "all procedures involving partial or total removal of the female external genitalia or other injury to the female genital organs for non-medical reasons" [51].

FGM/C is mainly cultural and has no religious background. In fact, the influential Egyptian Muslim institution Dar Al-Ifta Al-Misriyyah recently confirmed in a press statement that FGM/C is religiously forbidden owing to its negative impact on physical and mental well-being [52].

FGM/C has the following types:

Type I—Excision of the prepuce with or without partial or total excision of the clitoris
Type II—Excision of the prepuce and clitoris together with partial or total excision of the labia minora
Type III—Excision of part or all of the external genitalia and stitching or narrowing of the vaginal opening (infibulation)
Type IV—Unclassified: Pricking, piercing, or incision of the clitoris and/or labia [53]

In addition to the lack of any potential medical benefits, FGM/C can immediately cause severe bleeding and urination problems, not to mention subsequent marital, gynecological, and psychological problems. Although there is a high prevalence of FGM/C among older generations of women in the UAE, there is a decrease in its prevalence among younger generations. This clearly reflects a step in the right direction. Clear legislation to criminalize this unfounded practice is an important issue to be addressed, and a national educational and legal program to eradicate this problem should be a priority [52].

34.10 Conclusion

With the increasing population, there is bound to be an increase in the number of urological cancers. With the vision set out by the leaders of the country, the medical services are geared up to meet the demand. There is also an emphasis on making the UAE a hub for medical tourism. The UAE offers patients the same level of expertise as the Western world, from the latest in diagnostics, such as MR Fusion Biopsy, PSMA PET CT scan, and Blue Light Cystoscopy, to minimally invasive approaches such as laparoscopic and robotic surgeries. The latest radiotherapy techniques, including IGRT/IMRT to brachytherapy, are available for patients. The latest medications that are recommended by the NCCN guidelines are available for the benefit of patients.

Conflicts of Interest The authors have no conflicts of interest to declare.

References

1. Bulatovic I, Iankova K. Barriers to medical tourism development in The United Arab Emirates (UAE). Int J Environ Res Public Health. 2021;18(3):1365. https://doi.org/10.3390/ijerph18031365
2. Competitiveness and Statistics Authority, FCSA 2016.
3. https://www.globalmediainsight.com/blog/uae-population-statistics/.
4. UAE National Health Survey 2017-2018. https://cdn.who.int/media/docs/default-source/ncds/ncd-surveillance/data-reporting/united-arab-emirates/uae-national-health-survey-report-2017-2018.pdf?sfvrsn=86b8b1d9_1&download=true.
5. Al-Shamsi et al. Cancer in the Arab World.
6. Cancer incidence in United Arab Emirates, Annual Report of the UAE – National Cancer Registry, 2015–2023. Statistics and research center, ministry of health and prevention. Accessed 09 Sep 2025.
7. About Medical Tourism. Available online: https://www.dha.gov.ae/en/MTC/Pages/About–Medical–Tourism–Council.aspx. Accessed on 20 Oct 2022.
8. https://mediaoffice.ae/en/news/2022/May/09-05/Dubai-receives-630000-health-tourists-in-2021. Accessed on 27/10/2022.
9. Workbook: non-communicable diseases. Cancer Incidence 2016. Department of Health. https://tableau.doh.gov.ae/views/NonCommunicableDiseases/CancerIncidence?%3AisGuest RedirectFromVizportal=y&%3Aembed=y&%3Atoolbar=no. Accessed on 31/10/2022.
10. Sorokin I, Mamoulakis C, Miyazawa K, Rodgers A, Talati J, Lotan Y. Epidemiology of stone disease across the world. World J Urol. 2017;35(9):1301–20. https://doi.org/10.1007/s00345-017-2008-6. Epub 2017 Feb 17. PMID: 28213860.
11. Aldaher HS, Kadhim SZ, Al-Roub NM, Alsadi AH, Salam DA, Tillo EA. Evaluating the understanding about kidney stones among adults in The United Arab Emirates. J Taibah Univ Med Sci. 2021;16(5):788–93. https://doi.org/10.1016/j.jtumed.2021.04.005. PMID: 34690664; PMCID: PMC8498703.
12. Nerli R, Jali M, Guntaka AK, Patne P, Patil S, Hiremath MB. Type 2 diabetes mellitus and renal stones. Adv Biomed Res. 2015;4:180. https://doi.org/10.4103/2277-9175.164012. PMID: 26605219; PMCID: PMC4617153.
13. https://cdn.who.int/media/docs/default-source/ncds/ncd-surveillance/data-reporting/united-arab-emirates/uae-national-health-survey-report-2017-2018.pdf?sfvrsn=86b8b1d9_1&download=true.

14. Alkhayal A, Alfraidi O, Almudlaj T, Nazer A, Albogami N, Alrabeeah K, Alathel A. Seasonal variation in the incidence of acute renal colic. Saudi J Kidney Dis Transpl. 2021;32(2):371–6. https://doi.org/10.4103/1319-2442.335449. PMID: 35017331.
15. Kumar SB, Kumar KG, Srinivasa V, Bilal S. A review on urolithiasis. Int J Univ Pharm Life Sci. 2012;2(2):269–80.
16. Alelign T, Petros B. Kidney stone disease: an update on current concepts. Adv Urol. 2018;2018:3068365. https://doi.org/10.1155/2018/3068365. PMID: 29515627; PMCID: PMC5817324.
17. Worcester EM, Coe FL. Clinical practice. Calcium kidney stones. N Engl J Med. 2010;363(10):954–63. https://doi.org/10.1056/NEJMcp1001011. PMID: 20818905; PMCID: PMC3192488.
18. Prezioso D, Strazzullo P, Lotti T, Bianchi G, Borghi L, Caione P, Carini M, Caudarella R, Ferraro M, Gambaro G, Gelosa M, Guttilla A, Illiano E, Martino M, Meschi T, Messa P, Miano R, Napodano G, Nouvenne A, Rendina D, Rocco F, Rosa M, Sanseverino R, Salerno A, Spatafora S, Tasca A, Ticinesi A, Travaglini F, Trinchieri A, Vespasiani G, Zattoni F, CLU Working Group. Dietary treatment of urinary risk factors for renal stone formation. A review of CLU Working Group. Arch Ital Urol Androl. 2015;87(2):105–20. https://doi.org/10.4081/aiua.2015.2.105. Erratum in: Arch Ital Urol Androl. 2016 Mar;88(1):76. Ferraro, Manuel [added]. PMID: 26150027.
19. Uribarri J, Oh MS, Carroll HJ. The first kidney stone. Ann Intern Med. 1989;111(12):1006–9. https://doi.org/10.7326/0003-4819-111-12-1006. PMID: 2688503.
20. Rule AD, Bergstralh EJ, Melton LJ, Li X, Weaver AL, Lieske JC. Kidney stones and the risk for chronic kidney disease. Clin J Am Soc Nephrol. 2009;4(4):804–11. https://doi.org/10.2215/CJN.05811108. Epub 2009 Apr 1. PMID: 19339425; PMCID: PMC2666438.
21. http://www.usuaebusiness.org/publications/2019-uae-healthcare-sector-report/.
22. Alawadi F, Hassanein M, Suliman E, Hussain HY, Mamdouh H, Ibrahim G, Al Faisal W, Farghaly MN. The prevalence of diabetes and pre-diabetes among the Dubai population: findings from Dubai household health surveys, 2014 and 2017. Dubai Diabetes Endocrinol J. 2020;26:78–84.
23. Shieb M, Koruturk S, et al. Growth of diabetes research in United Arab Emirates: current and future perspectives. Curr Diabetes Rev. 2020;16(4):395–401.
24. Akoh JA. Key issues in transplant tourism. World J Transplant. 2012;2(1):9–18.
25. Masri MA, Shakuntala RV, Dhawan IK, et al. Transplantation in The United Arab Emirates. Transplant Proc. 1993;25:2358.
26. https://www.dhcc.ae/media/news/1st-uae-organ-transplant-summit-concludes-scientific-dialogue.
27. Janahi FK, Al Rais A, Al Rukhaimi M, Khamis AH, Hickey D. Public awareness of knowledge, belief, and attitude regarding organ donation and organ transplantation: A National Survey from The United Arab Emirates. Transplant Proc. 2018;50(10):2932–8.
28. https://gulfnews.com/uae/health/first-successful-kidney-transplant-in-dubai-1.1846518.
29. Kumar S, Sankari BR, Pinna AD, Miller CM, Al Obaidli AAK, Guzman JA, Attallah N, Bajwa G, Bader F, Hamed F, Souilamas R, Kumar A, Abdulbaki A, Siddique H, Kroh MD, El Hajj S, Al Bloooshi A, Suri RM. Establishment of solid organ transplantation in the United Arad Emirates. Transplantation. 2020;104(S3):S281.
30. https://www.shebaonline.org/first-dubai-israel-historic-kidney-donation-and-transplantation/.
31. El-Sakka A. Erectile dysfunction in Arab countries. Part I: prevalence and correlates. Arab J Urol. 2012;10(2):97–103.
32. el-Rufaie OE, Bener A, Abuzeid MS, Ali TA. Sexual dysfunction among type II diabetic men: a controlled study. J Psychosom Res. 1997;43:605–12.
33. Althobiti S, Alqurashi N, Alotaibi A, Alharithi T, Alswat K. Prevalence, attitude, knowledge, and practice of Anabolic Androgenic Steroid (AAS) use among gym participants. Mater Sociomed. 2018;30(1):49–52.

34. Al-Falasi O, Al-Dahmani K, Al-Eisaei K, Al-Ameri S, Al-Maskari F, Nagelkerke N, Schneider J. Knowledge, attitude and practice of anabolic steroids use among gym users in Al-Ain District, United Arab Emirates. Open Sports Med J. 2008;2:75–81.
35. https://gulfnews.com/uae/health/male-infertility-a-reality-in-uae-1.2105864.
36. Kumar N, Singh A. Trends of male factor infertility, an important cause of infertility: A review of literature. J Hum Reprod Sci. 2015;8(4):191–6.
37. Dash N, Al-Zarouni M, Al-Khous N, Al-Shehhi F, Al-Najjar A, Senok A, Panigrahi D. Distribution and resistance trends of community associated urinary tract pathogens in Sharjah, UAE. Microbiol Insights. 2008;2008:41.
38. Dash N, Albataineh M, Alhourani N, Khoudeir M, Ghanim M, Wasim M, Mahmoud I. Community-acquired urinary tract infections due to extended-spectrum β -lactamase-producing organisms in United Arab Emirates. Travel Med Infect Dis. 2018;22:46–50.
39. US Preventive Services Task Force. Screening for chlamydial infection: recommendations and rationale. Am J Prevent Med. 2001;20(3):90–4.
40. Mehrabani D, Behzadi M, Azizi S, Payombarnia H, Vahdani A, Namayandeh M, Ziyaeyan M. Cervical infection with herpes simplex virus, Chlamydia trachomatis, and Neisseria gonorrhoeae among symptomatic women, Dubai, UAE: A molecular approach. Interdisciplin Prespect Infec Dis. 2014;2014:347602.
41. Aldhaleei W, Bhagavathula S. HIV/AIDS-knowledge and attitudes in the Arabian Peninsula: A systematic review and meta-analysis. J Infect Public Health. 2020 Jul;13(7):939–48.
42. Elbis H, Osman N, Hammad F. Social impact and healthcare-seeking behavior among women with urinary incontinence in The United Arab Emirates. Int J Gynaecol Obstet. 2013;122(2):136–9.
43. Abrams P, et al. Fourth International Consultation on Incontinence Recommendations of the International Scientific Committee: evaluation and treatment of urinary incontinence, pelvic organ prolapse, and fecal incontinence, 2010.
44. Milsom MG. The prevalence of urinary incontinence. Climacteric. 2019;22(3):217–22.
45. Minassian VA, Sun H, Yan XS, Clarke DN, Stewart WF. The interaction of stress and urgency urinary incontinence and its effect on quality of life. Int Urogynecol J. 2015;26(2):269–76.
46. Mostafaei H, Bazargani S, Hajebrahimi S, Pourmehr HS, Ghojazadeh M, Onur R, Al MR, Oelke M. Prevalence of female urinary incontinence in the developing world: A systematic review and meta-analysis-A report from the developing World Committee of the International Continence Society and Iranian Research Center for evidence based medicine. Neurourol Urodynamics. 2020;39(4):1063–86.
47. Rizk D, Shaheen H, Thomas L, Dunn E, Hassan M. The prevalence and determinants of health care-seeking behavior for urinary incontinence in United Arab Emirates women. Int Urogynaecol J Pelvic Floor Dysfunc. 1999;10(3):160-5.
48. https://worldpopulationreview.com/countries/united-arab-emirates-population.
49. A-Gazali L, Dawodu A, Sabarinathan K, Varghese M. The profile of major congenital abnormalities in The United Arab Emirates (UAE) population. J Med Genet. 1995;32(1):7–13.
50. Mehmood T, Azam H, Tariq M, Iqbal Z, Mehmood H, Shah S. Plastibell device circumcision versus bone cutter technique in terms of operative outcomes and parent's satisfaction. Pak J Med Sci. 2016;32(2):347–50.
51. Organization WH. Female genital mutilation, 2014.
52. Al AS, Al JM, Osman N, Balayah Z, Al KN, Ucenic T. Prevalence, knowledge, attitude and practices of female genital mutilation and cutting (FGM/C) among United Arab Emirates population. BMC Womens Health. 2020;20:79.
53. Organization WH. A systematic review of the health complications of female genital mutilation including sequelae in childbirth, 2000.

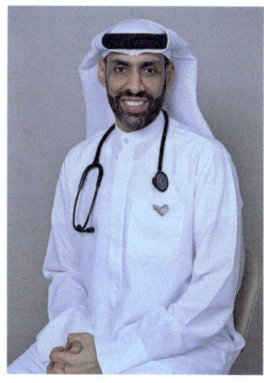

Professor Humaid Obaid Al-Shamsi is the Chief Executive Officer of Burjeel Cancer Institute in Abu Dhabi, UAE; President of the Emirates Oncology Society; Visiting Professor at Harvard Medical School at Harvard University; Visiting Scientist at Dana-Farber Cancer Center, Harvard Medical School, Boston, USA; Full Professor of Oncology at Ras Al Khaimah Medical and Health Sciences University; Ras Al Khaimah, UAE; an Adjunct Professor of Oncology at the College of Medicine, University of Sharjah; and Clinical Professor at Gulf University, Ajman, UAE. He is the first Emirati to be promoted as a professor in oncology in UAE history. He is also the Chairman for Colorectal Cancer in the MENA region, appointed by the prestigious National Comprehensive Cancer Network® in the USA. He is also the only member of the Lung Cancer Policy Network in the MENA region, which aims to advance lung cancer research and screening globally. He is the Chairman of the Oncology and Hematology Fellowship Training Program for the National Institute for Health Specialties in the United Arab Emirates. He is also the only member in the GCC in the WIN Consortium, which comprises organizations representing all stakeholders in personalized cancer medicine globally.

He is board-certified in both internal medicine and oncology from the UK, the USA (ABIM), the National Board of Physicians and Surgeons in the USA, and Canada (FRCPC). He has also been awarded the FRCP (Canada) in 2012, FRCP (London) in 2023, FRCP (Glasgow) in 2024, and FRCP (Edinburgh) in 2025. He is the only physician in the UAE with a subspecialty fellowship certification and training in gastrointestinal oncology and the first Emirati to complete a clinical post-doctoral fellowship in palliative care. He was an Assistant Professor at the University of Texas MD Anderson Cancer Center between 2014 and 2017. He has published more than 170 peer-reviewed articles in *JAMA Oncology, Lancet Oncology, Journal of Clinical Oncology, The Oncologist, BMC Cancer*, and many others. His area of expertise includes precision oncology and cancer care in the UAE. In 2016, he published with his group from MD Anderson in the *Journal of Clinical Oncology* a study describing a new distinct subgroup of colorectal cancer, NON-V600 BRAF-mutated colorectal cancer. In 2022, he published the first book about cancer research in the UAE and also the first book about cancer in the Arab world, both of which were launched at Dubai Expo 2020. *Cancer in the Arab World* has been downloaded more than 500,000 times in its first 2 years of publication and is the ultimate source of cancer data in the Arab region. He also published the first comprehensive book, *Cancer Care in the United Arab Emirates*, which is the first book in UAE history to document cancer care in the UAE, with many topics addressed for the first time. The book was also another success with over 100,000 downloads in the first 2 months of publication.

He is passionate about advancing cancer care in the UAE and the GCC and has made significant contributions to cancer awareness and early detection for the public using social media platforms. He engages actively with the public through awareness campaigns and serves on numerous national health committees, including with the UAE Ministry of Health and the Department of Health, Abu Dhabi.

He is considered the most followed oncologist in the world, with over half a million followers across his social media platforms (Instagram, Twitter, LinkedIn, and TikTok). In 2022, he was awarded the prestigious Feigenbaum Leadership Excellence Award from Sheikh Hamdan Smart University for his exceptional leadership and research, and he was also awarded the Sharjah Award for Volunteering. He was also named the Researcher of the Year in the UAE in 2020 and 2021 by the Emirates Oncology Society.

In May 2024, HH Sheikh Mansour bin Zayed Al Nahyan, Vice President of the United Arab Emirates, awarded him first place in the Emirati Talent Competitiveness Council (NAFIS) program for outstanding leadership in the private sector across all business and medical disciplines. In February 2025, he was awarded the *Sheikha Fatima bint Mubarak Family Award* for being a successful role model in UAE society.

As CEO of Burjeel Cancer Institute, he is leading the largest cancer network in the UAE with over 30 oncologists and hematologists and built the first pediatric bone marrow transplant program in the UAE. He secured the UAE's first European Society for Medical Oncology (ESMO) accreditation for a cancer center in the UAE at Burjeel Cancer Institute.

Besides his clinical and administrative duties, he is engaged in education and various levels of research training for medical trainees to enhance their clinical and research skills. He established the UAE's first hematology and oncology fellowship training program accredited by the UAE National Institute for Health Specialties at Burjeel Cancer Institute.

His mission is to advance cancer care in the UAE and the MENA region and make cancer care accessible to everyone in need around the globe.

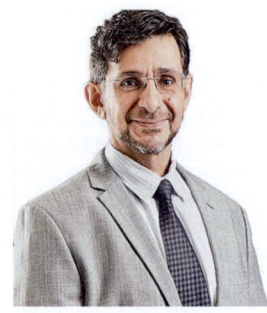

Ali Thwaini is a urologist with a specialist interest in urological cancers, namely renal cancers. He was the lead for renal cancers at the Belfast Health and Social Care Trust (Belfast City Hospital). His main skills are advanced laparoscopy, renal cancer, and renal reconstruction procedures. Dr. Thwaini is also an honorary clinical lecturer at Queens University, Belfast. He is known for his academic contributions throughout his career, with over 40 Medline publications in the field.

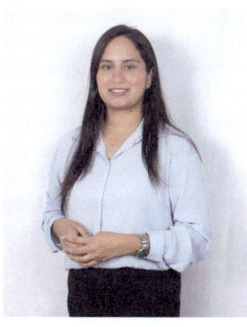

Faryal Iqbal is the Research Manager at Burjeel Cancer Institute, Burjeel Medical City in Abu Dhabi, UAE. She earned her undergraduate degree in Molecular Biology & Biotechnology, followed by a postgraduate qualification in Molecular Genetics in Pakistan, where her thesis explored the association between XRCC1 gene polymorphism and radiation exposure in healthcare workers. At Burjeel Cancer Institute, she is deeply involved in shaping the institute's research landscape. Her role extends beyond managing data and coordinating clinical studies; she mentors medical interns, supports scientific writing, and contributes significantly to the academic and editorial aspects of cancer research.

She is the co-editor of *Cancer in the Arab World*, the first comprehensive book covering cancer care across all Arab countries. The book has resonated widely across the region and beyond, gathering over half a million downloads within just two years. She has authored numerous peer-reviewed publications and contributed to at least ten book chapters, with her research interests rooted in oncology, hematology, and genetics.

In recognition of her growing contributions to the field, she was honored with the "EOS Research Award" by the Emirates Oncology Society in September 2023, an accolade that reflects both her professional excellence and her passion for advancing cancer research in the region.

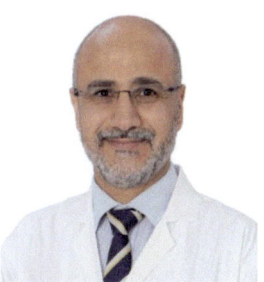

Omer Darwish is a renowned and globally trained consultant urological surgeon. He has trained across the globe in locations like Germany, London, Glasgow, Milan, Barcelona, the UAE, and Eastbourne, to name a few, and has more than 20 years of experience.

He is an expert in all aspects of general and subspecialty urology, including urinary tract stones, urological cancers, bladder dysfunction, and urodynamics, including those related to spinal injuries, female urology, prostatic diseases, sexual dysfunction, and andrology. He can also manage all urological emergencies, such as urinary tract obstructions and injuries. His special interest areas include urological technologies and imaging .

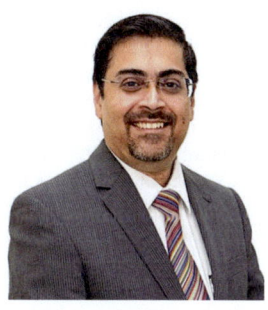

Amrith Rao is a fellowship-trained robotic urologist specializing in urologic cancers. He is a leading uro-oncologist in the region, having performed the maximum number of robotic urological procedures in Dubai. He deals with all aspects of urology and has expertise in prostate, kidney, and bladder disorders. He pays particular attention to men's health disorders and female bladder disorders. Dr. Amrith Rao has presented extensively on urological disorders at international conferences in Europe, the USA, India, and the Middle East. He has published papers in the most prestigious medical journals and is the author of many books .

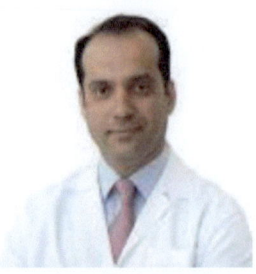

Farhad Janahi is a highly experienced urologist who trained in Ireland and the UK. He is competent in a full range of urological services, such as urology oncological surgery, including radical cystectomies, radical prostatectomies, radical nephrectomies, stone surgeries, and kidney transplantation. He previously worked at Dubai Hospital, where he initiated the process of establishing a renal transplant service in collaboration with the Royal College of Surgeons in Ireland. He currently also works at Mohammad bin Rashid University of Medicine and Health Sciences, where he is an assistant professor .

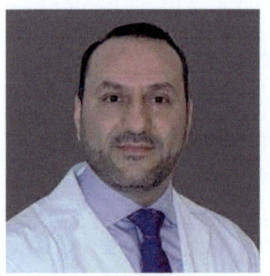

Ahmed Abdul Rahman is one of the leading urologists practicing in Dubai. He has 20 years of experience in his field of specialty, handling cases of general urology, benign urology, and urologic oncology. He has expertise in minimally invasive prostate surgery, female incontinence, prolapse with Erbium YAG laser, Botox, penile implants, erectile dysfunction, andrology, spina bifida, neuropathic bladder, and video-urodynamics .

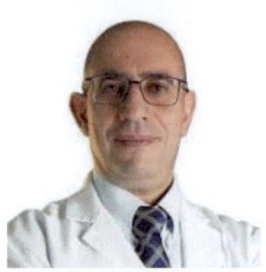

Hosam Al-Qudah is a board-certified consultant urologist. He completed his residency training at Jordan University of Science and Technology and the American University of Beirut; he also had a sub-specialty training in reconstructive urology from Wayne State University and transplant surgery at the University of Maryland. Dr. Al Qudah specializes in minimal invasive urology, stone disease and treatment, including laser therapy, cancer diseases, transplant surgery, female and pediatric urology, male infertility and impotence, urethral strictures, and reconstructive urology .

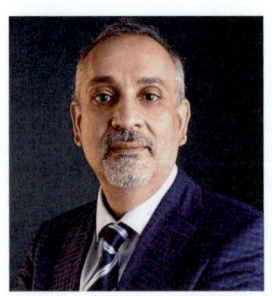

Thamer Al Kasab is a Consultant Urologist with Specialist interest in Renal Cancer he is working in zahra Hospital in Dubai. Dr. Alkasab was the former Medical Director of Alzohoor Private Hospital in Baghdad, Iraq, in 2000. Dr. Alkasab gained his early urology specialty training and residency at Alexandria University, Egypt, from 2004 to 2009, followed by the completion of sub-specialty advanced training in endo-urology and laparoscopy in 2010. Dr. Alkasab started his career and training as a uro-oncologist at the Princess Margaret Cancer Centre, University Health Network, and University of Toronto, Canada, in 2011, and he gained a very comprehensive experience in diagnosing and managing (medically and surgically) prostate cancer, kidney cancer, bladder cancer, and testicular cancer. He has had two fellowships in uro-oncology (clinical and research) throughout his Canadian high-level Training from 2011 to 2016. Dr. Alkasab is a highly trained surgeon on robotic surgery of the prostate and PLND at Princess Margaret Cancer Centre, one of the most famous cancer centers in the world of cancer institutions and of the North American Society of Uro-oncology (SUO). Dr. Alkasab has authored, published, and presented many papers and topics in the field of early diagnosis and treatment of prostate cancer (his main domain of interest) at American and Canadian urological meetings in the last few years.

Open Access This chapter is licensed under the terms of the Creative Commons Attribution 4.0 International License (http://creativecommons.org/licenses/by/4.0/), which permits use, sharing, adaptation, distribution and reproduction in any medium or format, as long as you give appropriate credit to the original author(s) and the source, provide a link to the Creative Commons license and indicate if changes were made.

The images or other third party material in this chapter are included in the chapter's Creative Commons license, unless indicated otherwise in a credit line to the material. If material is not included in the chapter's Creative Commons license and your intended use is not permitted by statutory regulation or exceeds the permitted use, you will need to obtain permission directly from the copyright holder.

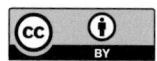

Neurology Care in the UAE

35

U. K. D. Ajith Goonetilleke

35.1 Demographics

The majority of people from the United Arab Emirates (UAE) were traditionally fishermen or had a nomadic life herding sheep and cattle. The discovery of crude oil and natural gas resources in the UAE and subsequent commercial exploitation of these resources in the mid- and late-twentieth centuries has resulted in significant changes in the country. The UAE was formally established in 1971, and is therefore a comparatively young country, and is a member of the Gulf Cooperation Council (GCC). There are seven emirates that comprise the UAE: Abu Dhabi (which is the capital of the UAE), Dubai, Sharjah, Ajman, Ras Al Khaimah, Fujairah, and Umm Al-Quwain. The country has extensive development potential in view of its (i) abundant oil and natural resources; (ii) increasing importance as a trade and financial hub between markets in the Far East and the Indian sub-continent and the West; and (iii) the increasing popularity of the UAE as a shopping and tourism destination. Over the past two decades, the UAE's population has almost tripled, with an estimated current population of around 9.5 million in 2023 [1]. Most of the country's population consists of expatriates, with people from South Asia constituting 58% of expatriates in the UAE [1].

The discovery of oil and natural gas resources transformed the UAE. It is now one of the richest countries in the world, with the UAE population enjoying high standards of living, and access to most modern facilities and technological advancements to pursue a leisurely lifestyle [2].

U. K. D. Ajith Goonetilleke (✉)
Neurology Department, Burjeel Medical City, Abu-Dhabi, United Arab Emirates

Khalifa University College of Medicine & Health Sciences, Abu Dhabi, United Arab Emirates

© The Author(s) 2025
H. O. Al-Shamsi (ed.), *Healthcare in the United Arab Emirates*,
https://doi.org/10.1007/978-981-96-0523-1_35

35.2 Population Health and the Healthcare System in the UAE

The UAE was formed in 1971 as a federation of seven Emirates: Abu Dhabi, Dubai, Sharjah, Ajman, Ras Al Khaimah, Umm Al Quwain, and Fujairah. The UAE's health system is not a single integrated system. The Ministry of Health and Prevention (MOHAP) is the primary federal regulatory health authority for the whole UAE healthcare system. MOHAP works closely with the local regulatory authorities, such as the Department of Health in Abu Dhabi, the Dubai Health Authority, and the Sharjah Health Authority, with MOHAP covering the functions of the other Emirates (i.e., Ajman, Ras Al Khaimah, Umm Al Quwain, and Fujairah) that do not have their own individual regulatory authorities [3].

In 2006, the Abu Dhabi government undertook a number of health system reforms [4]. Previously, a single entity was responsible for both government healthcare provision and regulation, namely the provider itself. As this arrangement was suboptimal, the regulatory functions were assigned to the Health Authority of Abu Dhabi (HAAD) and separated from the health service provider, SEHA (the Abu Dhabi health service company). In 2006, it became mandatory for all residents in the emirate of Abu Dhabi to have health insurance. The local Emirati population was provided with automatic insurance coverage (named Thiqa Insurance) by the government. For the non-UAE population, the onus was on employers to provide healthcare insurance for their employees and, in some cases, their dependents. In 2014, the Dubai government also made private insurance coverage mandatory for non-UAE nationals who are residents of the emirate [4].

The UAE has several factors that can contribute to obesity, including a reliance on motorized vehicles for transport, reduced exercise levels, and poor dietary habits. While the UAE population traditionally ate fish and Arabic bread, such preferences are declining in modern times, with the population now favoring fast foods. Many fast-food franchises have entered the UAE market, resulting in changes in dietary habits toward consuming more fat-rich fast foods and drinking calorie-rich soft drinks. The prevalence of obesity and diabetes is very high in GCC countries, with the UAE being ranked 20th and 23rd highest among all countries regarding the prevalence of obesity and diabetes, respectively [1]. According to a 2017–2018 health survey conducted in the UAE, among 4815 respondents, the prevalence of obesity (i.e., BMI ≥ 30 kg/m^2) was 27.8%, overweight (BMI ≥ 25 kg/m^2) was 67.9%, hypertension was 28.8%, diabetes was 11.8%, and hypercholesterolemia was 43.7% [3]. These are troubling statistics for current and future health issues among the UAE population, suggesting a potential increase in healthcare costs in the future.

In 2020, the reported prevalence of diabetes in the UAE was 16.3%, compared to 9.3% worldwide [5]. Population studies in the UAE show that the prevalence of Diabetes Mellitus (DM) in the Northern Emirates was as high as

25.1% among UAE nationals and 19.1% among expatriates [6, 7]. A cross-sectional household health survey conducted in Dubai in 2019 showed that the prevalence of diabetes among Emiratis (19.3%) was higher than in expatriates (12.4%), with higher rates of DM being strongly correlated with obesity, low levels of physical activity, smoking, and hypertension [8]. According to a World Health Organization (WHO) report, 81.9% of 13–18-year-olds in the UAE have insufficient physical activity, and a high 17.8% rate of tobacco use among 13–15-year-old males [9]. The Gulf countries are ranked among the top 40 countries in the world for high prevalence rates of obesity [10]. The prevalence of overweight and obesity in the UAE appears to have at least doubled between 1989 and 2017 [11], with a UAE obesity prevalence rate of 31.7% in 2016 [10]. These are worrying statistics regarding future health problems in the UAE population. Diabetes and obesity contribute to a number of disorders seen by neurologists, such as cerebrovascular disease (e.g., acute stroke, vascular dementia), peripheral neuropathy, neck and back pain, and benign intracranial hypertension.

To combat these recent worrisome trends, the UAE's commitment to achieving world-class healthcare has been earmarked by the UAE Cabinet as one of six national priorities, as outlined in UAE Vision 2021 [12]. This UAE national strategy includes KPIs (key performance indicators) to achieve specified population health targets (e.g., increasing life expectancy, reducing tobacco consumption), as well as structural and organizational targets (e.g., ensuring that all healthcare facilities are externally accredited). Federal Statistics and Competitive Authority data for 2017 revealed that the governmental health sector provided 45 hospitals (employing 8322 physicians and 20,480 nurses), while the private sector provided 98 hospitals (employing 14,785 physicians and 33,435 nurses) [13]. According to a 2021 report, the percentage of externally accredited healthcare facilities in the UAE had reached 91.27%, with 8.2 physicians and 6.05 nurses per 1000 population [14].

The Legatum Prosperity Index (LPI) ranking is based on 104 variables, analyzing a variety of factors. These include wealth, economic growth, education, health, personal well-being, and quality of life in a country. The UAE set a target of being in the top 20 world rankings for LPI. In 2021, the UAE was ranked 41st out of 149 countries, with national rankings for Denmark first, Germany ninth, the UK 13th, and the USA 20th [15]. For the LPI Health sub-score, the UAE was ranked 36th, with Japan ranked first, Singapore second, Denmark 18th, the UK 31st, Germany 16th, and the USA 68th. The Health Care Index (HCI) was designed to be a more specific indicator of the overall quality of a healthcare system. According to mid-2022 HCI statistics, the UAE was ranked 31st out of 96 countries, with national rankings for Taiwan first, the UK 16th, Germany 23rd, and the USA 33rd [16]. In mid-2022, the UAE had an HCI of 68.02, with only Qatar (73.0) scoring higher in the MENA region (Fig. 35.1).

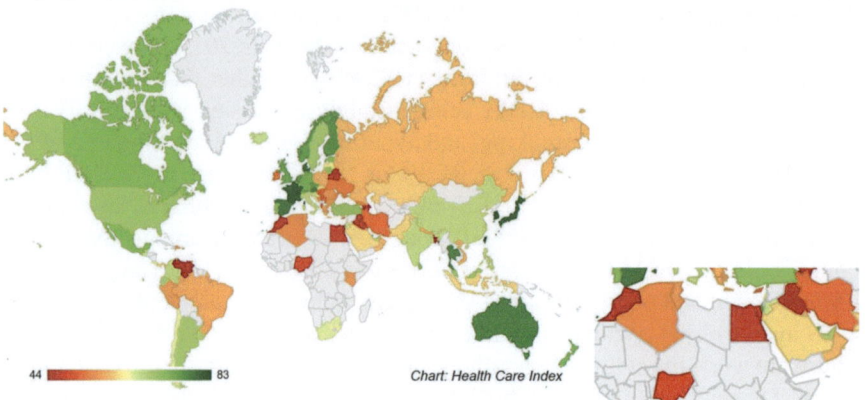

Fig. 35.1 Health Care Index World Map for mid-2022, with insert showing MENA region [16]

35.3 Neurology-Related Statistics in the UAE

There is good availability of neuroimaging and neurophysiology testing in the UAE. The UAE has one of the highest availability rates of CT and MRI scanners in the MENA/Gulf Region (Table 35.1) and compares favorably with the availabilities seen in developed healthcare systems in Western and Eastern European countries, as well as other regions of the world. The waiting time for routine CT or MRI scans, electroencephalograms, evoked potential studies, or nerve conduction studies is approximately 2–4 weeks in the UAE, with the main delays related to waiting for approvals by medical insurance companies.

Cerebral SPECT and PET-CT scanning are useful investigative tools in the diagnostic evaluation of certain neurological disorders [17]. These include dementing disorders (with indications such as use in the early diagnosis and differential diagnosis of Alzheimer's disease and frontotemporal dementia), epilepsy (to identify the epilepsy focus in partial epilepsy and in children to identify the functional deficit zone), movement disorders (in differentiating between Parkinson's disease and atypical parkinsonian syndromes), and neuro-oncology (in assessing the likelihood of malignancy in cerebral space-occupying lesions, for non-invasive grading of malignancies, and for the detection of tumor recurrences). PET scan imaging has been available in the UAE since 2009 (Fig. 35.2). Currently, several centers capable of performing PET-CT scans in the emirates of Abu Dhabi (Burjeel Medical City, Gulf International Cancer Center, and Tawam Molecular Imaging Center), Dubai (Advanced Cancer Oncology Center, American Hospital, City Hospital, Clemenceau Medical Center Hospital, Dubai Hospital, and Neuro-Spinal Hospital), and Ras Al Khaimah (Sheikh Khalifa Specialty Hospital).

Hyperbaric oxygen therapy (HBOT) is currently indicated for, and has been found to have beneficial effects in a number of neurological disorders [20, 21]. These

Table 35.1 The availability of CT and MRI scanners in selected countries around the world in 2019

	Imaging availability, 2019 Scanner density per million population	
	CT	MRI
MENA/Gulf region		
Iran	9.5	3.8
Jordan	5.5	2.1
Kuwait	5.5	5.3
Lebanon	110	41
Libya	13.6	77
Morocco	0.3	0.5
Oman	8.3	1.9
Qatar	9.1	11.2
Saudi Arabia	6.7	3.1
Tunisia	15.7	5.7
UAE	**25.4**	**10.6**
Europe		
Czech Republic	16.4	10.4
Finland	16.3	28.8
France	18.1	15.3
Germany	35.3	34.7
Italy	36.5	30.2
Netherlands	14.9	13.8
Portugal	17.8	10.0
Slovenia	18.2	12.5
Spain	19.2	17.6
Sweden	26.2	16.6
Switzerland	38.7	25.1
UK	8.8	7.4
Other		
Australia	69.8	14.8
Canada	14.6	10.1
Japan	111.5	55.5
New Zealand	15.3	15.4
USA	44.9	40.4

Data obtained from OECD [18, 19]

include idiopathic sudden-onset sensorineural hearing loss, stroke, traumatic brain injury, spinal cord injury, complex regional pain syndrome, elevated intracranial pressure, cluster headaches, refractory migraine, cerebral palsy, multiple sclerosis, intracranial abscess, and fibromyalgia syndrome.

HBOT first became available in the UAE (for non-military personnel) at Al Qassimi Hospital, Sharjah, in 2014 (Fig. 35.2). HBOT is currently available in a limited number of centers in Abu Dhabi (Burjeel Medical City and Gulf Diagnostics) and Dubai (Al Zahra Hospital, Aviv Clinics, and Fakeeh University Hospital).

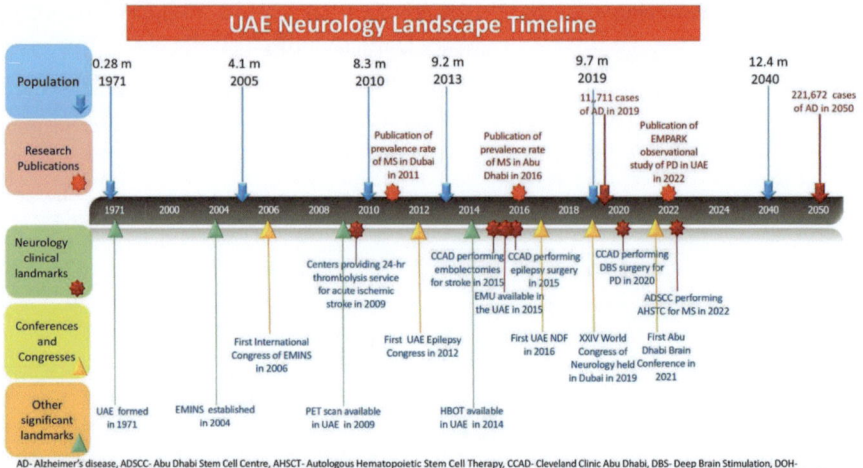

Fig. 35.2 Timeline of UAE neurology-related events

35.4 UAE Neurology Care

35.4.1 Alzheimer's Disease and Other Dementias

Dementia is an umbrella term for a progressive disorder of cognition and is characterized by a decline in information processing abilities, accompanied by changes in personality and behavior. Alzheimer's disease (AD) is the most common cause (50–70%) of dementia, followed by vascular dementia (15–25%), Lewy body dementia (15%), and frontotemporal dementia (5%) [22]. Aggregates of β-amyloid protein peptides (amyloid plaques) and neurofibrillary tangles are thought to be linked with the pathogenesis of AD.

Alzheimer's disease is already the most common neurodegenerative disorder worldwide. Population growth and an increasing proportion of elderly individuals are predicted to further increase the number of people living with dementia globally. In 2019, there were an estimated 57.4 million individuals with dementia globally, with estimates projected to rise to 83.2 million in 2030, 116.0 million in 2040, and 152.8 million in 2050 [20]. The smallest increases were projected in High-Income Asia Pacific (53%) and Western Europe (74%), whereas the largest estimated increases were in the MENA region (367%) and Eastern Sub-Saharan Africa (357%). Qatar is projected to experience the world's largest surge in dementia cases from 2019 to 2050, with a staggering 1926% increase in cases [23], followed by the UAE (1795%), and then Bahrain (1084%).

The Lancet Commission 2020 update on dementia prevention, intervention, and care suggests that up to 40% of cases of dementia may be prevented through targeted interventions on certain risk factors [24]. The evidence to date suggests that there are 12 risk factors for dementia prevention and intervention in a population: low levels of education, poor social contact, traumatic brain injury (TBI), hearing impairment, smoking, excessive alcohol consumption, low levels of physical activity, obesity, depression, hypertension, diabetes, and air pollution [24]. Many of these risk factors are highly prevalent in the UAE and the MENA region.

There have been significant advances in the early diagnosis of AD, including testing for biomarkers in cerebrospinal fluid and blood [25, 26], as well as PET-CT scans, which are now approved as part of the diagnostic algorithm [27, 28].

Treatments for AD were largely limited to symptomatic control (e.g., treatment of depression, agitation, and hallucinations) in the past. The first cholinesterase inhibitor (ChEI) for use in AD was introduced in 1997, with three ChEIs (donepezil, galantamine, and rivastigmine) now available as first-line therapies for mild to moderate AD. Donepezil has also been approved for use in severe AD. Memantine is a non-competitive antagonist of NMDA (N-methyl-D-aspartate) glutamate receptors in the brain and was FDA-approved for use in moderate-to-severe AD in 2003. CHEIs and memantine are available for use by AD patients in the UAE. All these agents may have modest effects on improving or stabilizing some cognitive functions in AD, but they do not have any significant effects on the underlying pathological processes or neuronal loss associated with AD.

In June 2021, the U.S. Food and Drug Administration (FDA) granted conditional accelerated approval for aducanumab for the treatment of mild cognitive impairment and mild dementia in AD. This was the first disease-modifying agent approved by the FDA for use in AD. Aducanumab is a monoclonal antibody that targets soluble (β-amyloid oligomers) and insoluble aggregates of β-amyloid proteins (fibrils and β-amyloid plaques). It is a once-monthly infusion, and side effects include cerebral edema (amyloid-related imaging abnormalities—edema, ARIA-E) and cerebral hemorrhages (amyloid-related imaging abnormalities—hemosiderin deposition, ARIA-H), which encompass microhemorrhages and superficial siderosis. Therefore, close monitoring and repeated brain MRIs are needed to detect these changes. In October 2021, the Ministry of Health and Prevention (MOHAP) in the UAE also approved aducanumab for the treatment of AD, making it the second country in the world to grant approval for the use of this medication. The accumulated evidence to date suggests that aducanumab, when used at higher doses, has a modest impact on the cognitive decline of patients with mild cognitive impairment and at the early stage of AD but does not reverse the prior memory loss associated with AD [29–31].

Lecanemab is a monoclonal antibody that prevents the clumping of amyloid and was shown to reduce markers of amyloid in early AD but resulted in a moderate decline slower than placebo on measures of cognition and function at 18 months [32]. As with aducanumab, adverse events included ARIA-E and ARIA-H. In January 2023, lecanemab became the second disease-modifying agent to obtain FDA approval for use in AD [33].

Neurologists in the UAE have the capability to diagnose and treat AD and other causes of dementia. For difficult-to-diagnose cases of dementia, FDG-SPECT and PET-CT scans are available in certain centers in the UAE, and even the latest disease-modifying agents such as aducanumab have been approved for use in the country. The challenges for the future include adequately screening the UAE population for mild cognitive impairment and dementia as well as having the resources to cope with the expected increases in the prevalence of dementia in the UAE.

35.4.2 Epilepsy

Epilepsy can occur at any age and is the most common of the chronic brain diseases. More than 50 million people worldwide have epilepsy [34]. The estimated prevalence of active epilepsy (i.e., continuing seizures or requiring treatment) worldwide is estimated to be 4–10/1000 [34], with a recent review of 197 prevalence studies suggesting a worldwide point prevalence rate of 6.38/1000 and a lifetime prevalence rate of 7.6/1000 [35]. An early review on epilepsy estimated the prevalence rate to be 2.3/1000 in this region [36], but a more recent review estimated the median prevalence to be 7.5/1000 [37]. This review identified one study from the ELAE (Emirati League Against Epilepsy) from 2014 that suggested a lifetime prevalence rate of 12.9/1000 for epilepsy in the UAE [38].

The high prevalence of epilepsy in the Arabian region may be due to a number of factors. Consanguinity rates are high, with studies showing rates of marriage among first cousins of over 60% [39]. There are increasing rates of consanguinity in Qatar, Yemen, and the UAE [39], with these countries showing higher epilepsy prevalence rates [37]. Although prohibited by Islamic law, alcohol and substance abuse have reached alarming proportions in some Arab countries (e.g., Egypt and Saudi Arabia) [40], where the prevalence of epilepsy is also high. Neurocysticercosis was also considered non-existent in the Arab region, as Islamic law prohibits swine breeding and the consumption of pork. However, the prevalence of neurocysticercosis in this region has been increasing in recent years [41], likely due to the significant increases in the number of migrant workers from Southeast Asia, where neurocysticercosis is common.

For the expatriate epilepsy patient, the choice of anticonvulsant medication is sometimes governed by the level of their medical insurance coverage and the availability of the same medication in their country of origin for use when they return home. Emirati epilepsy patients in the UAE have access to all the anticonvulsant medications approved by the FDA and EMA (European Medicines Agency). In the past, many intractable epilepsy patients would have to go abroad for assessment for possible epilepsy surgery as a treatment option. The UAE developed the capability for prolonged EEG monitoring in an epilepsy monitoring unit in 2016, and SPECT and PET-CT (to identify the epilepsy focus in partial epilepsy and in children to identify the functional deficit zone) as well as the expertise to perform epilepsy surgery in selected centers (e.g., Cleveland Clinic Abu Dhabi) in 2015 (Fig. 35.2).

35.4.3 Headache Disorders

Migraine is a common neurological disorder. The Global Burden of Disease 2016 study suggests a global age-standardized migraine prevalence of 14.3% [42]. Migraine is associated with significant morbidity and reduced quality of life for patients, and results in a significant economic burden in terms of healthcare costs in dealing with the disease, as well as loss of earnings due to absenteeism from work [43, 44]. Migraine is the second-largest cause of disability globally, with women affected more adversely than men [45]. Migraine prevalence rates in the Arab region appear similar to those reported elsewhere, but reported rates vary by country. Migraine prevalence has been reported to be 2.6–5% in Saudi Arabia [46, 47], 7.9% in Qatar [48], 10.1% in Oman [49], and as high as 23% in Kuwait [50].

Headache disorders were found to be the third-highest cause of years lived with disability (YLD) in the Middle East and North Africa in the 2019 Global Burden of Disease study [45]. The common causes of headaches included migraine, tension-type headache, medication-overuse headache, and cervicogenic headache. Neurologists in the UAE have expertise in investigating and treating the spectrum of headache disorders. Treatments that can be provided include the latest oral and injectable medications used in the treatment of migraine and cluster headache, including CGRP (calcitonin gene-related peptide) inhibitors (e.g., erenumab, galcanezumab), gepants (e.g., rimegepant), and ditans (e.g., lasmiditan), as well as botulinum toxin injections and even HBOT for the more chronic headache disorders.

35.4.4 Multiple Sclerosis

Multiple sclerosis (MS) is a demyelinating disorder of the central nervous system. Epidemiological evidence has led to a consensus view that its etiology is multifactorial, with complex interactions between certain susceptibility genes and one or more environmental factors (e.g., sunlight exposure). A longstanding observation has been that MS prevalence is greater at higher latitudes (where sunlight is of lower intensity) than at lower latitudes (Fig. 35.3). Goldberg et al. [51] first reported a link between low levels of sunlight exposure and MS in 1986. A meta-analysis in 2011 confirmed the significant association between latitude and MS prevalence [52]. There is now a body of both epidemiological and experimental evidence suggesting that low vitamin D levels are associated with an increased susceptibility to subsequently developing MS [53–55].

A meta-analysis in 2015 suggested the prevalence of MS in the Middle East was 51.5/100,000 [57], with a reported rate of 54.7/100,000 in a single UAE study based on the population of Dubai [58]. A more recent study conducted in Abu Dhabi [59] showed a prevalence of MS of 64/100,000 (age-standardized), with more than 60% of the patients in the study being native Emiratis. This reported prevalence rate is

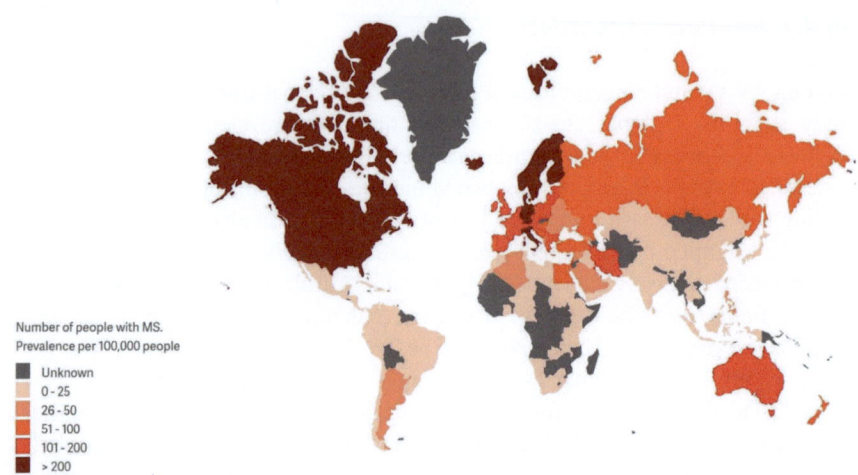

Fig. 35.3 Prevalence of multiple sclerosis. (From Multiple Sclerosis International Federation, Atlas of MS [56])

almost double the global average. Other studies [58, 60] have highlighted an increasing prevalence of MS in the Arab region. Vitamin D deficiency has become epidemic in GCC (Gulf Cooperation Council) countries, with deficiency rates of 81–87.5%, including a vitamin D deficiency rate of 82.5% in the UAE [61]. This may account for increases in the prevalence of MS in the region but requires further investigation.

There have been significant advances in the investigation and treatment of MS in recent decades. In 1993, the FDA approved interferon beta-1b as the first disease-modifying therapy for MS, and since then, there have been significant advances in its treatment of MS. There is now an array of oral, injectable, and infusion therapies that are FDA-approved disease-modifying therapies available for the treatment of MS (Fig. 35.4). Although not FDA-approved, immuno-ablative therapy followed by autologous hematopoietic stem cell therapy has also been shown to be a highly effective treatment for MS and a treatment option that may be considered in patients with aggressive and treatment-refractory MS [62]. All the disease-modifying therapies approved for use in MS are available in the UAE, including the provision for autologous hematopoietic stem cell therapy for MS (Abu Dhabi Stem Cell Centre & Yas Clinic Group) since 2022.

35.4.5 Neuromuscular Disorders

The high DM prevalence rates in the UAE can lead to a number of neurological complications. The recent GulfDiab survey of 1290 diabetic patients in Saudi Arabia, Kuwait, and the UAE found that peripheral neuropathy was the most common diabetes-related complication (present in 34.9% of patients), greater even than

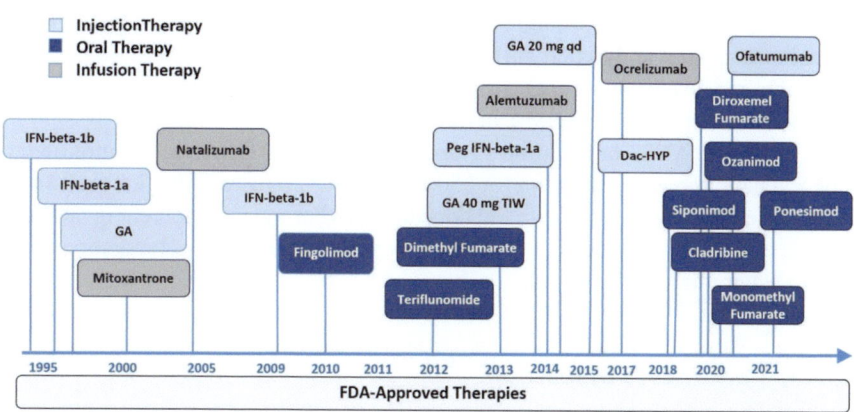

Fig. 35.4 An overview of the timelines of FDA approvals for disease-modifying therapies in multiple sclerosis. DAC HYP Daclizumab High Yield Process, GA Glatiramer Acetate, IFN Interferon. (Based on a figure from De Angelis et al. [63])

background retinopathy (29.9%) and cataract (14.1%) [64]. There was a similar finding in a cross-sectional survey of 513 diabetic patients in Al Ain in 2007, with 39% reporting peripheral neuropathy [65].

Spinal muscular atrophy (SMA) is a genetic disease (mostly autosomal recessive), resulting in the loss of motor neurons in the spinal cord, leading to skeletal muscle wasting and weakness, and possible respiratory failure and subsequent death. SMA patients lack a "survival motor neuron" (SMN) protein, which is a protein that is essential for motor neurons to survive and function. SMA is a leading genetic cause of infantile death. The Centre for Arab Genomic Studies estimates the prevalence of SMA in the GCC to be more than 50 per 100,000 live births, with various studies in the MENA region reporting incidences of SMA ranging from 10 to 193 per 100,000 live births [66]. These rates are much higher than those reported (e.g., 1.2 per 100,000 live births in the United States) in the Western world. The carrier frequency for the SMN1 gene abnormality responsible for the disease is estimated to be 1 in 20 individuals in the MENA region, compared to a global range of 1 in 45 to 1 in 100 [66].

Following studies showing positive results in delaying motor developmental decline and improving mortality [67], in 2016, the FDA approved the use of nusinersen (Spinraza). This was the first disease-modifying therapy approved for use in infantile SMA. Since then, onasemnogene abeparvovec (Zolgensma) and risdiplam (Evrysdi) have also been shown to be effective disease-modifying therapies. However, these agents are highly expensive. Spinraza costs 125,000 USD per injection; after four loading doses administered in the first 2 months (i.e., a total cost of 500,000 USD), it is then administered three times per year (i.e., 375,000 USD per year) for the patient's lifetime. Zolgensma is a one-time treatment, but at a cost of 2.125 million USD, making it the most expensive therapeutic agent in the world. The cost of Evrysdi depends on the infant's weight. The annual cost for an infant under 15 pounds (usually around 2 years of age) is less than 100,000 USD, with an annual cost capped at 340,000 USD (equivalent to an infant weight of 44 pounds). Although expensive, these agents have been made available and are used in the management of infants with SMA in the UAE.

In 2021, the Al Jalila Children's Specialty Hospital's Genomics Centre undertook a genetic screening program for 6500 infants [68]. This was the first such study of this disease in the region, with the hope that newborn genetic screening could be used as a tool for early detection of the disease and that earlier interventions may lead to better clinical outcomes.

35.4.6 Parkinson's Disease

Parkinson's disease (PD) is the second most common of the neurodegenerative disorders, with an increasing prevalence with age. There were estimated to be 6.1 million people with PD globally in 2016, compared to 2.5 million in 1990. The increasing numbers of older people in the population did not entirely account for this increase, as the age-standardized prevalence rate only increased by 21.7%, compared to a 74.3% increase in the crude prevalence rates [69]. The age-adjusted prevalence rates of PD vary around the world, with moderate prevalence rates reported in the MENA region (Fig. 35.5).

Approximately 1 in 10 people in the population aged 45–100 years are at risk of developing PD, with 4% of people diagnosed with PD being younger than 50 years of age (i.e., young-onset PD). Unlike in European and United Kingdom cohorts, Arab families have high rates of consanguineous marriages [39], which may increase the risk of genetic phenotypes (e.g., young-onset PD). Relatively high PD prevalence rates have been reported in North African Arabs [70]. A recent prospective and observational study of 171 UAE patients with PD showed a larger

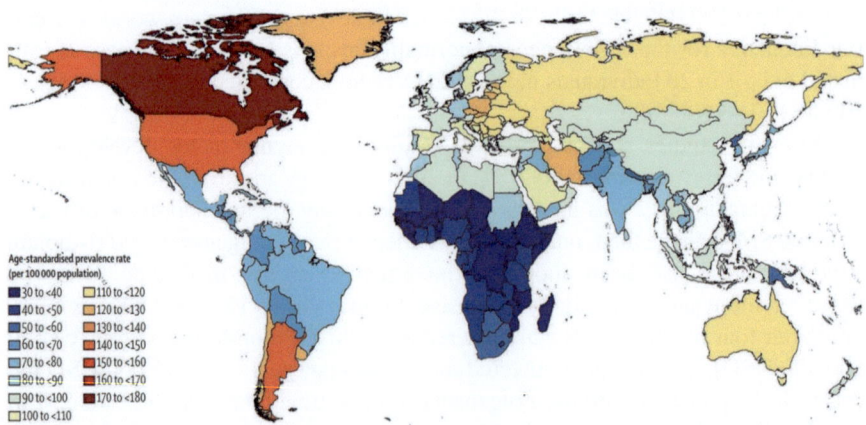

Fig. 35.5 Age-standardized prevalence of Parkinson's disease per 100,000 population by location for both sexes, 2016. (From Fig. 1, GBD 2016 Parkinson's Disease Collaborators [69])

proportion of young-onset PD in the Emirati PD cohort compared to the expatriate PD cohort [71], with a mean age of onset for the Emirati PD patients of 48.5 ± 13.05 years, compared to 64.15 ± 7.7 years for the expat cohort.

In an effort to raise awareness and promote education on PD (and other movement disorders) across the region, the International Parkinson and Movement Disorder Society Task Force for the Middle East was established. The Task Force members conducted a SWOT (strengths, weaknesses, opportunities, and threats) analysis. The consensus statement by the Task Force regarding PD care in the region included the following: greater levels of awareness about PD within the general population and among healthcare professionals; accurate epidemiologic data; enhanced healthcare resources and infrastructure for managing PD; the need for more movement disorders specialists; multidisciplinary care; educational programs; a greater availability of drugs; and the need for an increased availability of more advanced therapy for PD [72].

Neurological expertise is available in the UAE for diagnosing and treating PD. All oral and topical patch medications used in the treatment of PD are available in the UAE. Therapies for more advanced PD (e.g., apomorphine, duo-dopa intestinal gel therapy, and deep brain stimulation surgery) are also now available in the UAE, whereas in the past, PD patients would have had to travel abroad for these treatments.

35.4.7 Stroke

Strokes can be categorized as either ischemic or hemorrhagic (e.g., subarachnoid or intracerebral hemorrhages) in nature, with approximately 85% being ischemic. The Global Burden of Diseases, Injuries, and Risk Factors Study (GBD) in 2017 showed that stroke was the third-leading cause of death and disability combined worldwide and the second-leading cause of death [73, 74].

Recent reviews of stroke publications in the MENA region have highlighted the propensity for hospital-based studies (and a dearth of more informative community- or population-based studies), the lack of age adjustment and prospective designs, and small sample sizes [75, 76]. The Global Stroke Statistics for 2022, published by the World Stroke Organization [77], also highlighted the lack of good-quality data on stroke incidence for the MENA region (Fig. 35.6).

The Global Stroke Statistics for 2022 [77] also showed that the advanced countries in the MENA region (e.g., the UAE) compared favorably to other advanced countries across the world regarding mortality from stroke (Fig. 35.7). This statistic may be the result of a variety of potential contributory factors, including improved socioeconomic conditions, screening programs for risk factors, and quality of care. A recent study also confirmed that the UAE outperformed other countries in the region [78]. The authors speculated that this could possibly be explained by the presence of population-wide screening programs such as "Weqaya" [79], which make risk factor identification possible, and better access to medical care in the UAE, which has a high socio-demographic index [78].

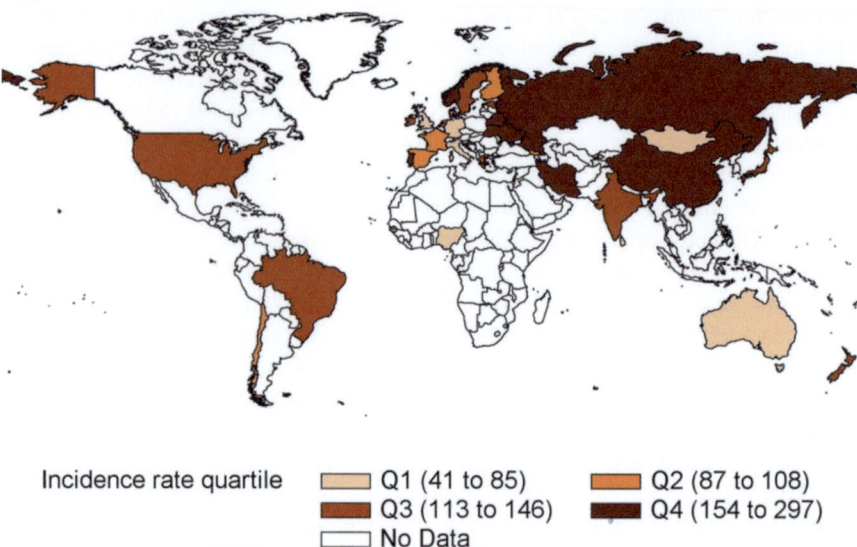

Fig. 35.6 Heat map showing the incidence of stroke adjusted to the world population by quartiles. (From Fig. 2, World Stroke Organization [77])

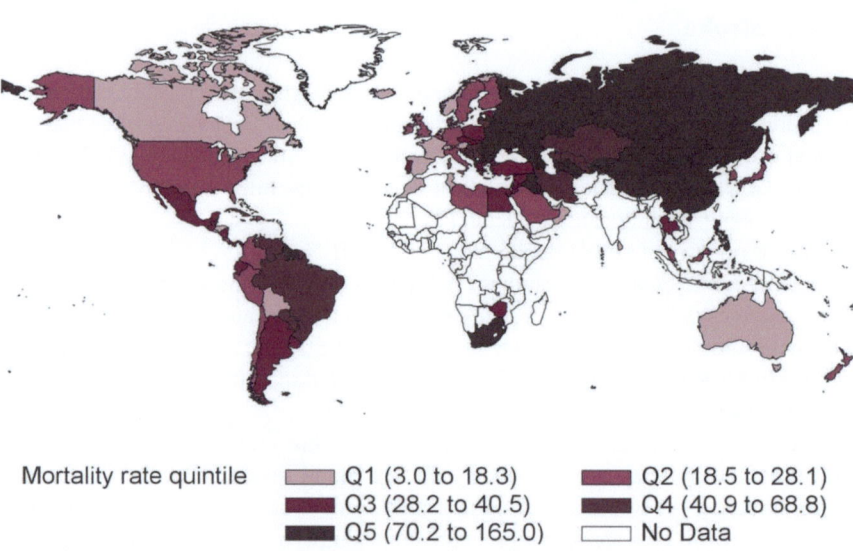

Fig. 35.7 Heat map of mortality (expressed as deaths per 100,000 population) from stroke, displayed as quintiles according to the world population. (From Fig. 10, World Stroke Organization [77])

The data above confirms the existence of relatively well-advanced stroke management in the UAE. In Abu Dhabi and Dubai, there are good availabilities of neurologists, stroke physicians, and healthcare facilities capable of administering intravenous thrombolytics and providing embolectomies for large-vessel occlusions in acute ischemic stroke. The challenge is to provide such care in the remote regions (i.e., the Western region and the Northern Emirates) of the UAE. Future challenges include setting up national registries for stroke and performing community- or population-based studies to ascertain the true incidence and prevalence of stroke in the UAE.

35.5 Challenges and Advantages

35.5.1 Provision of Neurology Care

The provision of care for neurological disorders is not uniform throughout the UAE. Abu Dhabi and Dubai can provide expertise and care comparable to the most advanced healthcare systems in the world, but in other regions of the UAE (e.g., the Western Region and the Northern Emirates), the provision is not as complete. The UAE government and private healthcare facilities are well advanced in the use of electronic medical records, with telemedicine being used extensively and successfully during the recent COVID-19 outbreak. These factors can be harnessed to provide good-quality care throughout the UAE.

National registries are required to document cases of the common neurological disorders encountered in the UAE. This will enhance the accurate ascertainment of the incidence and prevalence of these disorders in the UAE, which in turn will help with healthcare planning. The UAE is a relatively small country, and governmental and private healthcare facilities are employing electronic medical records. Both factors should facilitate the construction of national databases for neurological disorders.

35.5.2 Research

Neurology research in the UAE has been largely limited to attempts at estimating the prevalence and incidence of neurological disorders, descriptions of phenotypes experienced in the UAE population, and local experiences in the management of specific neurological disorders. In order to advance further, there is a requirement for a standardized approach to prevalence and incidence data generated within the UAE. More basic science and clinical research are required, and the former is likely to initially require collaborations with internationally well-established research units. In this regard, the UAE government has already set up initiatives (e.g., the Research and Innovation Centre in Abu Dhabi, the Mohammed Bin Rashid

University of Medicine and Health Science, and the Al Jalila Foundation collaboration to develop biomedical research in Dubai, the Dubai Harvard Foundation for Medical Research) in order to facilitate such collaboration.

35.5.3 Education and Training

UAE physicians wishing to pursue a career in neurology have traditionally traveled to other countries (e.g., the USA, Canada, or Europe) to obtain their required training. After completing their training and obtaining Western certifications, many have returned to the UAE to continue their clinical practice.

In December 2021, Sheikh Shakhbout Medical City in Abu Dhabi announced a neurology residency program, allowing up to two neurology residents to be recruited each year. The certifications achieved upon the successful completion of the training program will be approved by the Arab Board, ACGME-I (Accreditation Council for Graduate Medical Education-International), and the Emirati Board. Further neurology residency programs are likely to be developed in the future, both in governmental and private healthcare facilities.

35.5.4 Medical Tourism in the UAE

Medical tourists are defined as people traveling to other countries in order to seek medical treatments that may be beyond their reach in their own country. The flow of patients has traditionally been from developing countries to developed countries in search of access to advanced medical facilities not available in their home countries. More recently, the trend has changed, with a flow of people from developed countries to developing countries in search of more cost-effective or more immediate medical solutions. Patients travelling overseas for their treatments may do so in order to seek (a) high-quality medical facilities; (b) timely access to healthcare or required interventions, resulting from the significantly long waiting periods in certain countries; and (c) more cost-effective treatments compared to their home country. Indeed, some governmental authorities in Western countries have now started to offer patients the choice of medical tourism in order to gain quicker access and achieve more cost-effective treatments. An increasing number of countries and healthcare facilities have identified the medical tourism industry as a source of income and have started to market themselves as medical tourist destinations. The UAE possesses a number of factors favoring its position as a hub for medical tourism, namely its excellent infrastructure, availability of skilled professionals, excellent tourist attractions and hotel facilities, strong governmental support, and a geographical location that enables easy access to other Gulf countries and European and Asian markets.

Over the last decade, the healthcare industry has been identified as one of the key industrial sectors for UAE economic growth. The UAE medical tourism industry generated $3.29 billion in revenues in 2018, with 350,118 medical tourism visitors to the UAE in 2019 [80]. Government initiatives in Abu Dhabi and Dubai to promote medical tourism include the launch of medical tourism portals (i.e., the Abu Dhabi Medical Tourism Portal and the Dubai Health Experience), which provide medical tourists with the capability to book procedures and access a wide range of tourism services, ranging from direct contact with healthcare providers in the government and private sectors, visa issuance, hotels, and transportation to various recreational activities. In February 2020, the Second Medical Opinion (SMO) program was introduced in the UAE, helping patients make informed decisions about treatment [80]. The program offers a second opinion, provided by a team of multidisciplinary physicians, within 2 working days of the initial request. Patients with neurological disorders were considered one of the sectors to focus on, in addition to other specialties such as cardiology, gynecology, in vitro fertilization (IVF) and other fertility-related treatments, orthopedics, oncology, and urology [80].

The Medical Tourism Index (MTI) ranks the perceptions of people in the United States regarding healthcare across three primary dimensions (destination attractiveness, safety, and quality of care). For 2020–2021, the MTI ranked Dubai sixth and Abu Dhabi ninth among 46 international healthcare destinations [81]. The UAE's medical tourism market was worth $104.68 billion in 2019 and is estimated to rise to $273.72 billion by 2027 [82].

35.6 Conclusion

There have been significant advances in the provision of healthcare since the UAE came into existence as a unified country in 1971. The provision of services for the majority of neurological disorders is similar to that provided by established and advanced healthcare systems elsewhere in the world. Indeed, due to the existence of an extensive network of public and private healthcare providers, there are minimal waiting times for access to both neurological expertise and investigations (e.g., neurophysiology studies, CT scans, and MRI scans) throughout the UAE.

There are major challenges to the continued provision of high-quality neurological care in the UAE. National registries are required for common neurological disorders. The country is also predicted to face an unprecedented increase in cases of Alzheimer's disease and dementia, as well as obesity- and diabetes-related disorders. Fortunately, the UAE government has already prioritized the health of its population, with a commitment to achieving world-class healthcare. The UAE is also currently poised to become one of the preferred destinations in the world for medical tourism.

Conflicts of Interest The author has no conflicts of interest to declare.

References

1. World population review. Available at https://www.worldpopulationreview.com. Accessed 1 Nov 2022.
2. Nydell MK. Understanding Arabs- a guide for westerners. 3rd ed. Maine: Intercultural Press; 2002.
3. United Arab Emirates, Ministry of Health & Prevention: UAE National Health Survey Report 2017–18. p. 92. Available at https://cdn.who.int/media/docs/default-source/ncds/ncd-surveillance/data-reporting/united-arab-emirates/uae-national-health-survey-report-2017-2018.pdf?sfvrsn=86b8b1d9_1&download=true. Accessed 5 Nov 2022.
4. Koornneef EJ, Robben PBM, Al Seiari MB, et al. Health system reform in the emirate of Abu Dhabi. Health Policy. 2012;108(2–3):115–21.
5. International Diabetes Federation. IDF diabetes atlas. 9th ed. Brussels: International Diabetes Federation; 2020. p. 7–44.
6. Sulaiman N, Albadawi S, Abusnana S, et al. High prevalence of diabetes among migrants in The United Arab Emirates using a cross-sectional survey. Sci Rep. 2018;8(1):6862.
7. Sulaiman N, Mahmoud I, Hussein A, et al. Diabetes risk score in The United Arab Emirates: a screening tool for the early detection of type 2 diabetes mellitus. BMJ Open Dib Res Care. 2018;6:e000489.
8. Al Awadia F, Hassaneina M, Hussain HY, et al. Prevalence of diabetes and associated health risk factors among adults in Dubai, United Arab Emirates: results from Dubai household survey 2019. Dubai Diabetes Endocrinol J. 2020;26:164–73.
9. World Health Organization: monitoring health and health system performance in the Eastern Mediterranean Region: core indicators and indicators on the health-related sustainable development goals, 2019. Available at https://applications.emro.who.int/docs/EMHST245E.pdf?ua=1. Accessed 1 Nov 2022.
10. Central Intelligence Agency: The World Fact-Book: Country comparison: obesity – adult prevalence rate, 2016. Available at https://www.cia.gov/library/publications/the-world-factbook/fields/367rank.html. Accessed 1 Nov 2022.
11. Radwan H, Ballout RA, Hasan H, et al. The epidemiology and economic burden of obesity and related cardiometabolic disorders in the United Arab Emirates: a systematic review and qualitative synthesis. J Obes. 2018;2018:2185942. Available at https://doi.org/10.1155/2018/2185942. Accessed 1 Nov 2022.
12. UAE Vision 2021. Available at https://www.vision2021.ae/en. Accessed 4 Nov 2022.
13. Federal Statistics and Competitive Authority. Available at https://fcsa.gov.ae/en-us/pages/home.aspx.
14. UAE National Agenda. Available at https://www.vision2021.ae/en/national-agenda-2021/list/world-class-circle. Accessed 4 Nov 2022.
15. Legatum Institute: The Legatum Prosperity Index: a tool for transformation- overview 2021. Available at https://docs.prosperity.com/3616/3544/3967/the_2021_legatum_prosperity_index_overview_-_web.pdf. Accessed 5 Nov 2022.
16. Numbeo: Health Care Index by Country 2022 Mid-Year. Available at https://www.numbeo.com/health-care/rankings_by_country.jsp?title=2022-mid. Accessed 1 Nov 2022.
17. Varrone A, Asenbaum S, Vander Borght T, et al. EANM procedure guidelines for PET brain imaging using [18F] FDG, version 2. Eur J Nucl Med Mol Imaging. 2009;6(12):2103–10. Available at https://link.springer.com/articale/10.1007/s00259-009-1264-0. Accessed 4 Nov 2022.
18. OECD data: computer tomography (CT) scanners. Available at: Health equipment - Computed tomography (CT) scanners - OECD Data. Accessed 4 Nov 2022.
19. OECD data: magnetic resonance imaging (MRI) units. Available at: Health equipment - Magnetic resonance imaging (MRI) units - OECD Data. Accessed 4 Nov 2022.
20. Al-Waili NS, Butler GJ, Beale J, et al. Hyperbaric oxygen in the treatment of patients with cerebral stroke, brain trauma, and neurologic disease. Adv Ther. 2005;22(6):659–78.

21. Medscape: hyperbaric oxygen therapy: overview, hyperbaric physics and physiology, contraindications. Available at https://emedicine.medscape.com/article/1464149-overview. Accessed 1 Nov 2022.
22. Alzheimer's Association Report. 2020 Alzheimer's disease facts and figures. Alzheimer's Dement. 2020;16:391–460. Available at: https://doi.org/10.1002/alz.12068. Accessed 5 Nov 2022.
23. GBD. Dementia forecasting collaborators: estimation of the global prevalence of dementia in 2019 and forecasted prevalence in 2050: an analysis for the Global Burden of Disease Study 2019. Lancet Public Health. 2019;2022(7):e105–25.
24. Livingston G, Huntley J, Sommerlad A, et al. Dementia prevention, intervention, and care: 2020 report of the Lancet Commission. Lancet. 2020;396:413–46.
25. Barthelemy NR, Horie K, Sato C, et al. Blood plasma phosphorylated-tau isoforms track CNS change in Alzheimer's disease. J Exp Med. 2020;217(11):e20200861. https://doi.org/10.1084/jem.20200861. Accessed 15 Nov 2022.
26. Palmqvist S, Janelidze S, Quiroz YT, et al. Discriminative accuracy of plasma phospho-tau217 for Alzheimer disease vs other neurodegenerative disorders. JAMA. 2020;324(8):772–81. https://doi.org/10.1001/jama.2020.12134. Accessed 15 Nov 2022.
27. Frey KA, Lodge MA, Meltzer CC, et al. ACR-ASNR practice parameter for brain PET/CT imaging dementia. Clin Nucl Med. 2016;41(2):118–25.
28. Nobili F, Bouwman JAF, Drzezga A, et al. European Association of Nuclear Medicine and European Academy of Neurology recommendations for the use of brain 18F-fluorodeoxyglucose positron emission tomography in neurodegenerative cognitive impairment and dementia: Delphi consensus. Eur J Neurol. 2018;25(10):1201–17.
29. Schneider L. A resurrection of aducanumab for Alzheimer's disease. Lancet Neurol. 2020;19(2):111–2.
30. Cummings J, Aisen P, Lemere C, et al. Aducanumab produced a clinically meaningful benefit in association with amyloid lowering. Alzheimers Res Ther. 2021;13(1):10–2.
31. Knopman DS, Jones DT, Greicius MD. Failure to demonstrate efficacy of aducanumab: an analysis of the EMERGE and ENGAGE trials as reported by Biogen, December 2019. Alzheimers Dement. 2021;17(4):696–701.
32. van Dyck CH, Swanson CJ, Aisen P, et al. Lecanemab in early Alzheimer's disease. N Engl J Med. 2023;388:9–21. Available at https://doi.org/10.1056/NEJMoa2212948. Accessed 31 Jan 2023.
33. Reardon S. FDA approved Alzheimer's drug lecanemab amid safety concerns. Nature. 2023;613:227–8. Available at https://doi.org/10.1038/d41586-023-00030-3. Accessed 31 Jan 2023.
34. World Health Organization: Epilepsy. Available at https://www.who.int/news-room/fact-sheets/detail/epilepsy. Accessed 5 Nov 2022.
35. Fiest KM, Sauro KM, Wiebe S, et al. Prevalence and incidence of epilepsy: a systematic review and meta-analysis of international studies. Neurology. 2017;88(3):296–303. Available at https://doi.org/10.1212/WNL.0000000000003509. Accessed 5 Nov 2022.
36. Benamer HTS, Grosset DG. A systematic review of the epidemiology of epilepsy in Arab countries. Epilepsia. 2009;50(10):2301–4.
37. Bhalla D, Lotfalinezhad E, Timalsina U, et al. A comprehensive review of epilepsy in the Arab world. Seizure. 2016;34:54–9.
38. ELAE. Press release congress 2014-experts in the field of neurology to gather at the Third Annual UAE Epilepsy Congress 2014 10 Jan 2015. Available at: http://www.elae.ae/press.html.
39. Tadmouri GO, Nair P, Obeid T, et al. Consanguinity and reproductive health among Arabs. Reprod Health. 2009;6:17.
40. AlMarri TS, Oei TP. Alcohol and substance in the Arabian Gulf region: a review. Int J Psychol. 2009;44(3):222–33.
41. Del Brutto ODH. Neurocysticercosis in the Arabian Peninsula, 2003–2011. Emer Inf Dis. 2013;19(1):172–4.

42. Collaborators GBDH: Global, regional, and national burden of migraine and tension-type headache, 1990–2016: a systematic analysis for the Global Burden of Disease Study 2016. Lancet Neurol 2018;17:954–76. Available at https://doi.org/10.1016/S1474-4422(18)30322-3. Accessed 2 Nov 2022.
43. Agosti R. Migraine burden of disease: from the patient's experience to a socio-economic view. Headache. 2018;58(1):17–32.
44. Foster SA, Chen CC, Ding Y, et al. Economic burden and risk factors of migraine disease progression in the US: a retrospective analysis of a commercial payer database. J Med Econ. 2020;23:1356–64. Available at https://doi.org/10.1080/13696998.2020.1814790. Accessed 2 Nov 2022.
45. Steiner TJ, Stovner LJ, Jensen R, et al. Migraine remains second among the world's causes of disability, and first among young women: findings from GBD2019. J Headache Pain. 2020;21(1):137. Available at https://doi.org/10.1186/s10194-020-01208-0. Accessed 2 Nov 2022.
46. Al Rajeh S, Awada A, Bademosi O, et al. The prevalence of migraine and tension headache in Saudi Arabia; a community-based study. Eur J Neurol. 1997;4:502–6.
47. Jabbar MA, Ogunniyi A. Sociodemographic factors and primary headache syndromes in a Saudi community. Neuroepidemiology. 1997;16:48–52.
48. Bener A. Frequency of headache and migraine in Qatar. Neuroepidemiology. 2006;27:61–6.
49. Deleu D, Khan MA, Al Shehab TA. Prevalence and clinical characteristics of headache in a rural community in Oman. Headache. 2002;42:963–73.
50. Al-Hashel JY, Ahmed SF, Alroughani R. Burden of migraine in a Kuwaiti population: a door-to-door survey. J Headache Pain. 2017;18(1):105. Available at https://doi.org/10.1186/s10194-017-0814-2. Accessed 2 Nov 2022.
51. Goldberg P, Fleming MC, Picard EH. Multiple sclerosis: decreased relapse rate through dietary supplementation with calcium, magnesium and vitamin D. Med Hypotheses. 1986;21(2):193–200. Available at https://doi.org/10.1016/0306-9877(86)90010-1. Accessed 5 Nov 2022.
52. Simpson S Jr, Blizzard L, Otahal P, et al. Latitude is significantly associated with the prevalence of multiple sclerosis: a meta-analysis. J Neurol Neurosurg Psychiatry. 2011;82:1132–41.
53. Holick MF. Vitamin D deficiency. N Engl J Med. 2007;357(3):266–81.
54. Ascherio A, Munger KL, Simon KC. Vitamin D and multiple sclerosis. Lancet Neurol. 2010;9(6):599–612. Available at https://doi.org/10.1016/S1474-4422(10)70086-7. Accessed 5 Nov 2022.
55. Burton JM, Costello FE. Vitamin D in multiple sclerosis and central nervous system demyelinating disease- a review. J Neuroophthalmol. 2015;35(2):194200. Available at https://doi.org/10.1097/WNO.0000000000000256. Accessed 5 Nov 2022.
56. Multiple Sclerosis International Federation, 2023 Atlas of MS, 3rd ed. Available at Number of people with MS | Atlas of MS. Accessed 20 Dec 2023.
57. Heydarpour P, Khoshkish S, Abtahi S, et al. Multiple sclerosis epidemiology in Middle East and North Africa: a systematic review and meta-analysis. Neuroepidemiology. 2015;44:232–44. Available at https://doi.org/10.1159/000431042. Accessed 5 Nov 2022.
58. Inshasi J, Thakre M. Prevalence of multiple sclerosis in Dubai, United Arab Emirates. Int J Neurosci. 2011;121(7):393–8.
59. Schiess N, Huether K, Fatafta T, et al. How global MS prevalence is changing: a retrospective chart review in the United Arab Emirates. Mult Scler Relat Disord. 2016;9:73–9. Available at https://doi.org/10.1016/j.msard.2016.07.005. Accessed 2 Nov 2022.
60. Azami M, Yekta Kooshali MH, Shohani M, et al. Epidemiology of multiple sclerosis in Iran: a systematic review and meta-analysis. PLoS One. 2019;14(4):e0214738.
61. Singh P, Kumar M, Al Khodor S. Vitamin D deficiency in the Gulf Cooperation Council: exploring the triad of genetic predisposition, the gut microbiome and the immune system. Front Immunol. 2019;10:1042.

62. Cuascut FX, Hutton GJ. Stem cell-based therapies for multiple sclerosis: current perspectives. Biomedicines. 2019;7:26. Available at https://www.ncbi.nlm.nih.gov/pmc/articles/pmc6631931/pdf/biomedicines-07-00026.pdf. Accessed 2 Nov 2022.
63. De Angelis F, John NA, Brownlee WJ. Disease-modifying therapies for multiple sclerosis. BMJ. 2018;363:k4674. Available at https://doi.org/10.1136/bmj.k4674. Accessed 6 Dec 2023.
64. Omar MS, Khudada K, Safarini S, et al. DiabCare survey of diabetes management and complications in the Gulf Countries. Indian J Endocrinol Metab. 2016;20(2):219–27. Available at https://doi.org/10.4103/2230-8210.176347. Accessed 10 Nov 2022.
65. Al-Maskari F, El-Sadig M. Prevalence of risk factors for diabetic foot complications. BMC Fam Pract. 2007;8:59. Available at https://doi.org/10.1186/1471-2296-8-59. Accessed 10 Nov 2022.
66. DUPHAT: current treatment and developments for spinal muscular atrophy (SMA) in MENA region. Available at https://duphat.ae/current-treatment-and-development-for-spinal-muscular-atrophy-sma-in-mena-region/. Accessed 10 Nov 2022.
67. Finkel RS, Chiriboga CA, Vajsar J, et al. Treatment of infantile-onset SMA with nusinersen: a phase 2 open-label, dose escalation study. Lancet. 2016;388:3017–26.
68. Omnia Health: first-of-its-kind spinal muscular atrophy study to take place in the UAE. Available at https://insights.omnia-health.com/laboratory-management/first-of-its-kind-spinal-muscular-atrophy-study-take-place-uae. Accessed 10 Nov 2022.
69. GBD 2016 Parkinson's disease collaborators: global, regional, and national burden of Parkinson's disease, 1990–2016: a systematic analysis for the Global Burden of Disease Study 2016. Lancet Neurol 2018;17: 939–53. Available at https://doi.org/10.1016/S1474-4422(18)30295-3. Accessed 12 Nov 2022.
70. Benamer HT, De Silva R. LRRK2 G2019S in the North African population: a review. Eur Neurol. 2010;63:321–5.
71. Metta V, Ibrahim H, Loney T, et al. First two year observational exploratory real life clinical phenotyping, and societal impact study of Parkinson's Disease in Emiratis and expatriate population of United Arab Emirates 2019–2021: The Empark Study. Available at https://doi.org/10.21203/rs.3.rs-1293148/v1. Accessed 10 Nov 2022.
72. Khalil H, Chahine LM, Siddiqui J, et al. Parkinson's disease in the Middle East, North Africa, and South Asia: consensus from the International Parkinson and Movement Disorder Society task force for the Middle East. J Parkinsons Dis. 2020;10:729–41. Available at https://doi.org/10.3233/JPD-191751. Accessed 10 Nov 2022.
73. Kyu HH, Abate D, Abate KH, et al. Global, regional, and national disability-adjusted life-years (DALYs) for 359 diseases and injuries and healthy life expectancy (HALE) for 195 countries and territories, 1990–2017: a systematic analysis for the Global Burden of Disease Study 2017. Lancet. 2018;392:1859–922.
74. Krishnamurthi RV, Ikeda T, Feigin VL. Global, regional and country-specific burden of ischemic stroke, intracerebral hemorrhage and subarachnoid hemorrhage: a systematic analysis of the global burden of disease study 2017. Neuroepidemiology. 2020;54(2):171–9.
75. El-Hajj M, Salameh P, Rachidi S, Hosseini H. The epidemiology of stroke in the Middle East. Eur Stroke J. 2016;1(3):180–98.
76. Streletz LJ, Mushtak A, Gad H, et al. Epidemiology of stroke in the MENA region: a systematic review. Int J Neu Dis. 2017;1(1):10–21.
77. Thayabaranathan T, Kim J, Cadilhac DA, et al. Global stroke statistics 2022. Int J Stroke. 2022;17(9):946–56.
78. Shahbandi A, Shobeiri P, Azadnajafabad S, et al. Burden of stroke in North Africa and Middle East, 1990 to 2019: a systematic analysis for the global burden of disease study 2019. BMC Neurol. 2022;22:279. Available at https://doi.org/10.1186/s12883-022-02793-0. Accessed 11 Nov 2022.
79. Hajat C, Harrison O, Al SZ. Weqaya: a population-wide cardiovascular screening program in Abu Dhabi, United Arab Emirates. Am J Public Health. 2012;102(5):909–14.
80. DUPHAT: The boom of medical tourism in the UAE. Available at https://duphat.ae/the-boom-of-medical-tourism-in-the-uae/. Accessed 5 Nov 2022.

81. Global Healthcare Resources & International Healthcare Resource Centre: Medical Tourism Index 2020–2021. Available at https://www.medicaltourism.com/mti/home. Accessed 4 Nov 2022.
82. Medical Tourism Business. The UAE's medical tourism market size, statjstics, and trends. Available at: The UAE's Medical Tourism Market Size, Statistics, and Trends | Medical Tourism Business. Accessed 27 Nov 2023.

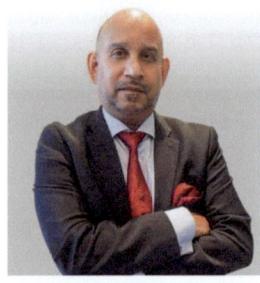

Professor Ajith qualified from St. Thomas's Hospital Medical School in London. He has trained and worked in eminent neurosciences centers, including the Institute of Neurology and the National Hospital for Neurology and Neurosurgery, and Charing Cross and Westminster Hospitals. He was a Consultant and Senior Lecturer in Neurology in Newcastle for 11 years, before moving to Abu Dhabi in the United Arab Emirates in 2009.

At Mafraq Hospital, he was the Chief of Neurology Department from 2009 till 2019, when he became the Chief of Neurology at Sheikh Shakhbout Medical City. In August 2021, he moved to Burjeel Medical City as Head of Department for Neurology. In August 2023, he moved to Clemenceau Medical Centre Hospital in Dubai.

Professor Ajith has published many articles and chapters in international peer-reviewed journals and books, and presented at national and international conferences. In 2016, he organized the first Neurological Disorders Forum, a now popular annual event.

In 2017, the Royal College of Physicians and Birkbeck College (University of London) awarded him a Postgraduate Diploma in Medical Leadership (Merit). He is currently studying for a full-time MBA with the University of Durham, having been awarded the prestigious Durham University Business School Achievement Scholarship.

Open Access This chapter is licensed under the terms of the Creative Commons Attribution 4.0 International License (http://creativecommons.org/licenses/by/4.0/), which permits use, sharing, adaptation, distribution and reproduction in any medium or format, as long as you give appropriate credit to the original author(s) and the source, provide a link to the Creative Commons license and indicate if changes were made.

The images or other third party material in this chapter are included in the chapter's Creative Commons license, unless indicated otherwise in a credit line to the material. If material is not included in the chapter's Creative Commons license and your intended use is not permitted by statutory regulation or exceeds the permitted use, you will need to obtain permission directly from the copyright holder.

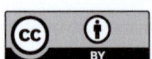

Respirology in the UAE

Bassam Mahboub, Laila Salameh, and Mayank Vats

36.1 Introduction

General Sir T.E. Gordon, a British officer, coined the term "Middle East" in 1900 [1], a phrase that embodies a fluid blend of political and geographic meanings. It typically encompasses a wide expanse, stretching from the Eastern Mediterranean to the western edges of the Indian subcontinent and from the northern borders of Turkey to the southern regions of the Arabian Peninsula. Across time, this region has been a hub for many celebrated civilizations.

The United Arab Emirates (UAE) carries a unique importance in the Middle East, being the fastest and most highly systemized developed country, achieved within a short span of 50 years and with the highest numbers of achievements in all aspects, including infrastructure, education, IT, medicine, health, and almost all fields. The UAE has unique geo-political and social factors contributing to its growth, including high numbers of immigrants, extensive high-rise buildings, a huge degree of construction, and newly established industrial activities with all their possible detrimental health consequences.

The variety of pulmonary diseases found in the UAE likely exceeds that of many other regions worldwide. While traditional lung ailments like pulmonary tuberculosis, chronic obstructive pulmonary diseases due to inhaled tobacco, asthma, lung cancer, and other respiratory conditions remain prevalent, healthcare providers are increasingly facing a rise in "emerging" diseases, notably the unprecedented COVID-19 pandemic. This review is comprehensive but is not intended to cover the full spectrum of these pulmonary health issues.

B. Mahboub (✉) · L. Salameh
Rashid Hospital, Dubai, United Arab Emirates

University of Sharjah, Sharjah, United Arab Emirates

M. Vats
Rashid Hospital, Dubai, United Arab Emirates

36.2 History

It is difficult to chronicle pulmonary pathology in humans throughout antiquity. In addition to historical books, the Middle East—known for its diverse and complex civilizations, such as the Egyptian civilization—has preserved ancient human remains and mummies that show evidence of lung illnesses. Pulmonary TB was a disease that afflicted this area for millennia, but evidence of it has been found in recent research using polymerase chain reaction on Egyptian mummies [2]. According to Zimmerman, *Mycobacterium tuberculosis* potentially evolved from *Mycobacterium bovis* around 5000 years B.C. in the Nile Valley during the process of cattle domestication [3].

The famous "King Tut Curse" or "Mummy's Curse," brought to public attention by the death of Lord Carnarvon after attending the opening of King Tutankhamun's tomb in 1922, might find a potential explanation in recent findings of *Aspergillus niger* and *Aspergillus flavus* in certain ancient mummies. These molds have the capacity to cause allergic bronchopulmonary aspergillosis and pulmonary hemorrhage [4]. However, it remains uncertain whether these mummies were infested by these molds postmortem or before their demise.

The Middle East saw a flourishing Islamic medical renaissance during the Middle Ages. Numerous notable medical professionals made important contributions that still impact contemporary medicine. Ibn-Sina (c. 980–1037), sometimes referred to as Avicenna in Latin and regarded as the founder of modern medicine, is one such person. His many treatises and writings, including "The Canon in Medicine," laid the foundation for risk factor analysis, clinical trials, and experimental medicine. Avicenna instituted quarantine procedures that suggested that microbes exist, and that pulmonary tuberculosis is communicable, and he stressed the significance of cleanliness in inpatient treatment to stop the spread of infectious diseases [5]. Throughout its history, populations in the Middle East have grappled with a range of lung conditions stemming from weather patterns, traditional lifestyles, or genetic predispositions. Contemporary pulmonary diseases persist today due to dietary and lifestyle shifts, human migration, rapid industrialization, and the deliberate use of harmful substances such as uranium during conflicts [5].

36.3 Pulmonary Pathology in the UAE

We emphasize a broad range of lung conditions pertinent to the UAE, classified under several key categories: environmental influences, infections, genetic or idiopathic diseases, sleep-related disorders, lung cancers, pleural ailments, and various other respiratory conditions.

36.3.1 Environmental Influences

A myriad of environmental elements significantly contribute to the expanding array of pulmonary ailments in the UAE. With vast desert-covered areas, the region experiences scorching, highly humid summers and notably cooler temperatures in winter. These fluctuations can exacerbate chronic lung diseases, particularly by making individuals susceptible to conditions such as asthma. Although the detailed prevalence of asthma in this area remains largely undocumented, it is believed to be substantial. A recent study conducted in the United Arab Emirates among children aged 6 to 19 revealed a prevalence of about 13% [6]. Asthma is notorious for its enduring health impact, leading to increased morbidity, school absenteeism, and high treatment costs [7]. In the UAE, numerous sensitizing aeroallergens originating from the desert environment can significantly exacerbate asthma [8, 9]. Contributing factors to the prevalence of asthma in this region include low parental education, low birth weight or prematurity, a family history of asthma, exposure to cigarette smoke, and contact with indoor or outdoor allergens like house dust mites and pollen [10, 11]. Access to adequate asthma care varies across regions and does not always ensure positive health outcomes [12]. Abrupt and heavy exposure to dust and sandstorms may precipitate conditions such as pulmonary alveolar proteinosis and silicosis [13, 14].

36.3.2 Social Factors

In the UAE, the prevalence of tobacco smoking is notably high, correlating with the common occurrence of chronic obstructive pulmonary disease (COPD) [15]. A cross-sectional survey by Al Zaabi A et al., involving a random sample of 520 individuals aged between 40 and 80 in Abu Dhabi, revealed a COPD prevalence of 3.7% [95% CI (2.0–5.3)] [16]. The necessity for preventive education is increasingly urgent [17]. Particular to this region is the practice of smoking through water pipes, known as the hubbly-bubbly or narguile [18]. Globally, water-pipe use is on the rise, particularly in the Eastern Mediterranean region. Misperceptions about safety, health risks, and traditional values often lead to the use of water pipes among women and children [19]. However, water-pipe smoke comprises harmful components, and there is preliminary evidence linking water pipe smoking to various life-threatening conditions, including pulmonary disease, coronary heart disease, and pregnancy-related complications [20].

Another prevalent social habit in the UAE is the burning of incense, which has been documented to trigger asthma attacks upon inhalation of its fumes [21]. A study found that local inhaled exposures, such as water pipe or bakhour use (incense burning) were associated with an increased risk of COPD [16].

36.3.3 Occupational Exposure

The advent of modern industrialization has increased the presence of air pollutants, significantly impacting respiratory health adversely [21]. Factors such as second-hand smoking [22, 23] and exposure to fuel fumes [24] are increasingly prevalent. Numerous agents within the agricultural and industrial sectors significantly contribute to pulmonary diseases in the UAE. These encompass the construction industry, the oil and chemical industries, and the development of various new industries, thereby heightening the likelihood of a rise in respiratory diseases.

36.4 Pulmonary Infections

36.4.1 Tuberculosis

Tuberculosis (TB) poses a significant public health challenge and remains the most commonly occurring infectious disease, with over one-third of the global population harboring latent TB. The World Health Organization (WHO) reported an incidence of TB in the UAE of 3.1% per 100,000 people in 2010. While TB rates in the UAE are relatively low in comparison to other countries, a major concern lies in monitoring the influx of workers arriving from high TB prevalence regions, particularly from Asia and Africa. Statistics from the Health Authority Abu Dhabi (HAAD) indicate that newcomers to the UAE exhibit a 20-fold higher TB rate than UAE nationals, posing a considerable risk to the resident and national populations. There has been a notable increase in the number of potential migrants suffering from TB, paralleling the findings of the WHO on the rise of drug-resistant TB cases in Asia.

As per information from the Dubai Health Authority, supported by findings from HAAD, a significant increase in tuberculosis prevalence has been noted over the last four years among individuals seeking work or residency visas in the UAE. The reported cases in 2008 were 122, increasing in 2009 and notably surging in 2010 to 722 cases. In the initial three months of 2011 alone, there were 606 reported TB cases. In Abu Dhabi in 2010, 450 cases of pulmonary TB and 175 cases of extrapulmonary TB were recorded. Additionally, a study at Al-Qasimi Hospital from 2004 to 2008 revealed a considerable level of resistance to anti-TB medications. Another study conducted in Abu Dhabi between 2001 and 2008 showed high resistance to anti-TB drugs, such as isoniazid and pyrazinamide, reaching as high as 27.7% [25].

A 2010 HAAD study among Abu Dhabi residents underscored the risk of TB, revealing that 14% of the 1558 individuals with TB carried latent forms, which could reactivate at any time. Furthermore, there was a potential risk of TB activation in 9% of the population, which could lead to its spread within the community. The rise of multi-drug resistant (MDR) TB strains is exacerbating this critical health issue [26]. The WHO reports a distressing surge in MDR TB incidence in the Middle East, accounting for 0.9% to 5.4% of new TB cases in the region and 8.3% to 62.5% of previously treated TB patients having MDR isolates [27]. Several reasons contribute to the rising drug resistance of TB in the UAE, including non-compliance with treatment, especially among patients who discontinue treatment prematurely [28]. Additionally, immigrants arriving from areas endemic to MDR TB, such as Southeast Asia, the Indian subcontinent, the former Soviet Union, and East Africa, may transmit the disease. Although effective pre-employment screening has helped control the situation, the potential for transmission remains [29–31].

Pulmonary TB's radiographic presentations vary widely, ranging from normal findings to Ghon's complex, lung cavitation, or a miliary pattern. Occasionally, non-tuberculous mycobacterial lung infections, such as those by *Mycobacterium kansasii* and *Mycobacterium abscessus*, are observed, especially in immunocompromised or cystic fibrosis patients [32].

36.4.2 Bacterial Infection

The rate of hospitalization due to community-acquired pneumonia (CAP) has been on the rise in the UAE. In a particular study, the most common microorganisms isolated from sputum cultures were *Haemophilus influenzae* (18.6%) and *Streptococcus pneumoniae* (10%). The overall mortality rate for CAP was 13%. In the case of hospital-acquired pneumonia (HAP), *Pseudomonas aeruginosa* emerged as the primary pathogen (in 50% of cases), with a higher mortality rate of 24% [33].

Pneumonia predominantly affects children under the age of 5 and adults over 65. According to WHO figures, 5% of deaths among children under 5 in the UAE are attributed to pneumonia. A study conducted at Sheikh Khalifa Medical City revealed a higher prevalence of pneumococcal disease among children in the UAE compared to the West, prior to the introduction of a vaccine targeting seven strains of pneumococcal bacteria known to cause pneumonia. The incidence rates of invasive pneumococcal disease and non-invasive pneumococcal disease were reported as 13.6/100,000 per year (95% CI 6.5–24.9) and 172.5/100,000 per year (95% CI 143.8–205.2), respectively. The total incidence of pneumonia in the UAE was estimated at 186.0/100,000 per year (95% CI 156.2–219.9) [34].

A multicenter, prospective, observational study aimed to delineate the treatment of community-acquired pneumonia (CAP) in outpatients in the Gulf region. This study also compared treatment approaches with the 2007 IDSA/ATS guidelines. Analyzing 641 patients from 41 medical sites, the study found that CAP diagnosis was broadly aligned with the IDSA/ATS guidelines. However, deviations in antibiotic prescriptions were observed: fluoroquinolones were excessively prescribed (88.2% for patients with comorbidities and 91% for those without), while macrolides were underused in patients without comorbidities. The study concluded that adhering to these guidelines generally improved the management of CAP. Yet, the overuse of fluoroquinolones might prompt the rapid emergence of resistance, emphasizing the importance of judicious antibiotic use based on patient comorbidities and the severity of community-acquired pneumonia [35].

36.4.3 COVID-19 Pandemic

COVID-19, caused by the severe acute respiratory syndrome coronavirus 2 (SARS-CoV-2), has resulted in a significant global impact. As of May 29, 2020, the worldwide figures indicated 609 million cases with 6.52 million deaths. The data, including new cases, deaths, recoveries, active cases, and critical cases, continue to be regularly updated on various platforms to offer current information on the state of COVID-19. The prevalence of the virus has yet to show signs of diminishing, persisting with an ongoing increase in reported cases and fatalities [36].

Amid this global crisis, the UAE government has proactively implemented stringent measures to control the spread of COVID-19, exhibiting success in reducing both morbidity and mortality. The country has been particularly notable for its comprehensive screening, diagnosis, treatment, and for remarkably low mortality rates, both from COVID-19 and associated non-COVID-19 illnesses. This reflects the provision of optimal treatment and evidence-based management of COVID-19 cases in the UAE [36].

As part of its screening and early detection strategy, the UAE conducted 213,615 tests per 1 million people, totaling 2.11 million tests for a population of approximately 9,878,576. This extensive screening, amounting to more than 20% of the population, enabled the timely identification, isolation, and quarantine of positive cases [36].

The UAE has conducted approximately 187,515,834 COVID PCR tests, representing the highest number of tests per million people compared to global data [37]. This extensive screening program aimed to promptly identify, isolate, and treat cases before the disease could progress.

In comparison with other developed nations, the UAE has demonstrated notable differences in the handling and control of the COVID-19 pandemic. With extensive screening, strict control measures, and high compliance, the incidence, prevalence, morbidity, mortality, and daily case counts have been effectively managed, resulting in a noticeable flattening, and even a decline, in the pandemic curve [36].

In statistical comparison, the UAE shows an average of 100,622 COVID-19 cases per 1 million people, with a total of 2342 deaths, or 231 per 1 million people, including cases directly associated with COVID-19 or its complications. The success in managing the pandemic in the UAE can be attributed to a multi-faceted approach involving government institutions, the health sector, private companies, social organizations, and public support. This synchronized effort, under the directives of various higher authorities, including the Ministry of Health and Prevention (MOHAP), Dubai Health Authority (DHA), and Health Authority of Abu Dhabi (HAAD), involved adherence to scientific guidelines endorsed by the World Health Organization and international and local experts. The UAE's low mortality rates due to COVID-19, compared to global figures, are a result of the extensive and timely efforts made by the government. Mass vaccination efforts have been initiated, with coverage reaching nearly 99% of the population (9.79 million), with approximately 24.9 million doses administered [36].

36.4.4 Asthma in the UAE

Asthma in the UAE: Severe asthma exacerbations directly correlate with uncontrolled asthma, encompassing factors such as medication noncompliance and exposure to environmental triggers. Utilizing questionnaires from the European Community Respiratory Health Survey (ECRHS) and data pooled from the AIRGNE (UAE) study, this study aimed to assess these determinants within the general population through a cross-sectional evaluation of a random sample of 1,229 participants. Among these individuals, 62.97% were male, 20.01% were UAE nationals, and the mean age was 32.9 years (±14.1) [38].

The prevalence of individual respiratory symptoms from the ECRHS questionnaire varied from 8 to 10% among all participants, with those aged 20–44 years exhibiting a lower prevalence of all symptoms ($P < 0.05$). These findings highlight specific persistent environmental factors, combined with nonadherence to controller medications, as significant contributors to uncontrolled asthma. This results in exacerbations, increased morbidity and mortality, and elevated healthcare costs in the UAE. Another study aimed to determine the prevalence of asthma in the UAE and identify factors, such as environmental, occupational, housing, patient, and physician perceptions, that contribute to asthma exacerbations and their resultant health impacts. While exact data regarding asthma prevalence in adults and children are unavailable, the ISAAC asthma center in the UAE reported a 13% prevalence of physician-diagnosed asthma [39].

Within the survey, 10.1% of asthma patients displayed allergic disorders, a notable risk factor for asthma development. Environmental, occupational, and housing factors contributing to allergies and asthma were found to be highly prevalent in the UAE. Central air conditioning or window units were the primary cooling sources in most homes, though the cleanliness of AC ducts remained uncertain for many households. Approximately 7% reported visible mold in their homes, while over half lived near construction or industrial sites, exposing them to fine dust and air pollution. Specific sensitizing aeroallergens from the desert exacerbated asthma, leading to unscheduled emergency room visits and hospitalizations. Sudden exposure to dust and sandstorms triggered acute severe asthma in uncontrolled asthmatics [40, 41].

Contributing factors include low parental education, low birth weight or prematurity, a family history of asthma, smoking, and exposure to indoor and outdoor allergens like house dust mites and pollen [42]. A notable proportion of surveyed patients were smokers, including users of shisha (water pipe) and passive smokers, which contribute to asthma exacerbations. The recorded level of annoyance from outdoor air pollution indicated a high level of air pollution in the UAE, prompting some individuals to change residences [43, 44]. The genetic aspect of asthma, along with varying environmental influences like microorganism exposure, pollutants, indoor and outdoor allergens, and diet, significantly influences susceptible individuals' disease development. Many asthma patients in the survey had pets and carpets at home, exposing them to allergens, dust, and dust mites, potentially triggering allergic asthma exacerbations [45]. Considering these findings, it is strongly recommended that patients receive education regarding environmental control measures to prevent asthma exacerbations.

36.4.5 Smoking-Related Lung Disease and COPD in the UAE

Despite the 2009 federal law prohibiting smoking in public places, encompassing the use of Midwakh and shisha, smoking remains a significant health concern in the UAE. The prevalence of tobacco smoking in the UAE, although lower than in many Middle Eastern countries, continues to be an issue, particularly among young Emiratis. This trend indicates an impending rise in smoking-related health conditions in the years to come. In 2009, approximately 1.72% of adult females and 18.7% of adult males were reported to smoke, based on the World Bank's 2010 report [46].

The Dubai Household Health Survey (DHHS), involving 5000 households, showed that 17.2% of Dubai residents smoke, with men five times more likely to smoke than women. Furthermore, a third of Dubai's population is exposed to smoking risks, either directly or as passive smokers. The DHHS highlighted that individuals in the lowest income and education brackets are nearly twice as likely to smoke compared to those in the highest income and education strata [47].

Startlingly, some individuals in Dubai begin smoking as early as 10 years of age for boys and 13 years of age for girls. Thirteen percent of Dubai smokers start before completing secondary school, with one in every five Emirati men in Dubai commencing smoking by the time they finish secondary school [44]. Among UAE nationals, the prevalence of smoking is notably lower, at 8.6%. Most male smokers in Dubai smoke daily (18.1%), while only 3% smoke occasionally. Female smokers in Dubai represent 3% who smoke daily and 1% who smoke occasionally [48].

Passive smoking is also prevalent among non-smoking residents in Dubai, with approximately 17% exposed in their homes and 62% in the workplace. Men are disproportionately more exposed to passive smoking compared to women [49].

In Abu Dhabi, the Weqaya population-based screening program conducted between 2008 and 2010 found smoking prevalence to be over 24% among males and only 1% among females. The prevalence was highest among males aged 20–39 years. The preferred smoking method remains cigarettes (78%), followed by midwakh (15%) and shisha (6.8%), though the popularity of shisha smoking has increased over the last three decades [49]. A Health Authority Abu Dhabi (HAAD) study in schools revealed that 25% of students had tried smoking before the age of 10. The home environment and exposure to parental smoking behaviors significantly influenced young individuals to take up smoking at an early age [50]. Another HAAD study in schools indicated that nearly half of the smoking students were Emiratis, with 15.7% starting before the age of 12 and 67% between 13 and 15 years. Approximately 21% of students had parents who smoked at home. Although efforts have been made to regulate tobacco sales, enforcement of these regulations is not consistent. Despite this, the prevalence of smoking in the UAE remains relatively lower compared to many other countries. These findings underscore the need for stronger measures to address and prevent the rise of smoking-related issues, particularly among the younger population [51].

36.5 Lung Cancer in the UAE

Lung cancer stands among the top five malignancies in the UAE based on accessible cancer registry data. The most prominently identified modifiable risk factor for these cancers is smoking [52]. The distribution of smokers in the UAE is estimated to be 0.8% among females and 24.3% among males [53]. Although there are various methods of inhaling smoke used worldwide, cigarette smoking (77.4%) remains the most prevalent form of smoking in the UAE, followed by midwakh, shisha, and cigars [54]. Notably, 7% of males and 3% of females reportedly smoke shisha, also known as hubbly-bubbly or hookah, which has a significant carcinogenic effect—its consumption is estimated to equate to the impact of smoking one hundred cigarettes [55]. The midwakh, originating from Arabia, is a small pipe in which a mixture of aromatic leaf and bark herbs is blended with dokha and smoked [56]. In comparison, the traditional Western tobacco pipe typically has a larger bowl than the midwakh pipe. To load the midwakh, a bowl is dipped into a container holding dokha flakes [57]. Iran and the UAE serve as the primary producers of midwakh. Dokha, similar to other smoking methods, exerts acute effects on blood pressure and respiratory rates. However, due to its use in tobacco blends, it is suspected to contain a notably high level of carcinogens [53].

36.6 High Prevalence of Obesity and Consequences of Sleep-Related Breathing Disorders

The UAE stands as 18th on the list of the world's most overweight nations, with approximately 68.3% of its citizens estimated to be overweight, signifying a significant prevalence of obesity within the country [58]. According to the latest available data from the World Health Organization (WHO), 67% of Emirati men and 72% of Emirati women are categorized as overweight [59]. Furthermore, approximately 39.9% of women and 25.6% of men in the UAE are classified as obese, ranking seventh and ninth globally, respectively. A study on national nutrition conducted by the Ministry of Health in the UAE revealed that about 33% of married women were overweight, and 38% were considered obese [4]. Among married men, 40.3% were found to be overweight, but only 15.8% were classified as obese. Overall, approximately 20% of the population grapples with obesity, surpassing the rates of obesity observed in the United States. Notably, a 2010 obesity conference in Abu Dhabi reported that 71% of the Emirati adult population was classified as obese. In a recent survey conducted in Abu Dhabi, 35% of the population was identified as obese, while 32% were categorized as overweight [59].

Overweight and obesity have surged to alarming levels in the Middle East and the UAE over the past decade, becoming a major health concern that fosters the development of other chronic conditions like hypertension (HTN), diabetes (DM), and sleep-related breathing disorders (SRBD). This upsurge has been predominantly attributed to urbanization and the sedentary lifestyle prevalent in the region. Research has indicated that expatriate workers are significantly more prone to obesity after spending time in the UAE, influenced by sedentary living conditions, the local climate, and dietary habits. A wellness survey conducted among 700 lay individuals in the UAE revealed that 38% of respondents identified themselves as overweight or obese. Among these individuals, 82% acknowledged that being overweight negatively impacts their health and day-to-day activities, yet many did not take steps to address their weight issues, suggesting potential barriers such as inadequate education, time constraints, low motivation, and other undefined factors. Additionally, more than 72% of healthcare professionals believed that the leading cause of obesity in the UAE is a sedentary lifestyle, coupled with insufficient awareness about the consequences of being overweight. This was followed by concerns regarding high-calorie Western diets, cultural and genetic predispositions, and the impact of the region's climate [60]. The prevalence of obesity in the UAE reflects the health and economic costs associated with the sedentary lifestyle among both Emiratis and expatriates, compounded by the influence of a diet abundant in Western-style fast food [61].

A recent study in Dubai focused on sleep disorders among 1200 participants attending primary healthcare (PHC) clinics, revealing that approximately 24% of males and 21% of females in the UAE may experience sleep-related disorders, primarily linked to Obstructive Sleep Apnea Hypopnea Syndrome (OSAHS). Another study, conducted in a PHC setting in Dubai, aimed to assess the prevalence of symptoms and the risk of OSAHS while exploring the relationship between obesity and OSAHS. The findings showed that 20.9% of patients attending PHC clinics were at high risk of developing OSAHS, with 22.9% being males and 19.5% being females [62, 63].

36.6.1 Sleep Services in the UAE

Following an extensive internet search to ascertain the status of sleep medicine services in Middle Eastern countries, limited available data have impeded a comprehensive understanding of the landscape. Although specifics regarding the state of sleep medicine services in the UAE were not found, extrapolating from similar socioeconomic contexts, ethical considerations, and medical issues in the region, it is plausible to assume that the status mirrors that of other Middle Eastern countries.

Presently, sleep medicine services in the UAE are still in their infancy. Despite an estimated 7–10% population prevalence of obstructive sleep apnea (OSA) in the UAE, there remains a significant need for more dedicated sleep laboratories and a greater number of trained physicians and technicians. As of now, there are only eight specialized sleep labs, each accommodating a single bed. These labs are predominantly situated in tertiary-level hospitals and are overseen by certified sleep physicians. However, the shortage of qualified sleep technicians persists, with most sleep studies conducted by respiratory therapists. The number of sleep tests performed annually ranges from 1500 to 2000 [60].

While a few companies offer home sleep tests, their focus is often skewed toward selling expensive positive airway pressure (PAP) machines like CPAP and BIPAP, primarily driven by financial motives. As a consequence, patients are inclined to seek diagnosis and treatment in their home countries, reflecting personal experiences observed in a major tertiary hospital in the UAE.

Alarmingly, there is limited awareness among both physicians and the general public regarding sleep apnea. Signs and symptoms of OSA are often considered part of daily life by patients, many of whom have adapted to living with these issues for years without understanding their significance or the risks associated with untreated sleep apnea.

36.7 Conclusion

The field of respirology and sleep medicine in the United Arab Emirates has rapidly emerged as one of the most dynamic specialties, boasting advanced technology and a cadre of highly skilled healthcare professionals in conventional pulmonology, interventional pulmonology, and sleep medicine services. Numerous cutting-edge public and private healthcare facilities now offer extensive pulmonary and sleep-related services, aiming to deliver cost-effective, quality-focused healthcare to the community. This development also seeks to position the UAE as a central hub for medical tourism in the Middle East and worldwide.

Conflicts of Interest The authors have no conflicts of interest to declare.

References

1. Abdul Jabbar Beg M. The Middle East in the twentieth century: a chronology of events. Cambridge; 2006.
2. Ziskind B, Halioua B. Tuberculosis in ancient Egypt. Rev Mal Respir. 2007;24:1277–83.
3. Zimmerman MR. Pulmonary and osseous tuberculosis in an Egyptian mummy. Bull N Y Acad Med. 1979;55:604–8.
4. Handwerk B. Egypt's "King Tut Curse" Caused by Tomb Toxins? http://news.nationalgeographic.com/news/2005/05/0506_050506_mummycurse.html. Accessed January 2010.
5. Smith RD. Avicenna and the canon of medicine: a millennial tribute. West J Med. 1980;133:367–70.
6. Alsowaidi S, Abdulle A, Bernsen R. Prevalance and risk factors of asthma among adolescents and their parents in Al-Ain. Respiration. 2010;79(2):105–11.
7. Khadadah M, Mahboub B, Al-Busaidi NH, et al. Asthma insights and reality in the Gulf and the near East. Int J Tuberc Lung Dis. 2009;13:1015–22.
8. Lestringant GG, Bener A, Frossard PM, et al. A clinical study of airborne allergens in The United Arab Emirates. Allerg Immunol (Paris). 1999;31:263–7.
9. Ezeamuzie CI, Al-Ali S, Khan M, et al. IgE-mediated sensitization to mould allergens among patients with allergic respiratory diseases in a desert environment. Int Arch Allergy Immunol. 2000;121:300–7.

10. Al-Kubaisy W, Ali SH, Al-Thamiri D. Risk factors for asthma among primary school children in Baghdad, Iraq. Saudi Med J. 2005;26:460–6.
11. Sattar HA, Mobayed H, Al-Mohammed AA, et al. The pattern of indoor and outdoor respiratory allergens in asthmatic adult patients in a humid and desert newly developed country. Eur Ann Allergy Clin Immunol. 2003;35:300–5.
12. Al Zabadi H, El Sharif N. Risk factors for asthma severity among emergency rooms attendees. Palestine Pulm Pharmacol Ther. 2009;22:208–13.
13. Rubin E, Weisbrod GL, Sanders DE. Pulmonary alveolar proteinosis. Relationship to silicosis and pulmonary infection. Radiology. 1980;135:35.
14. Miller RR, Churg AM, Hutcheon M, Lam S. Pulmonary alveolar proteinosis and aluminium dust exposure. Am Rev Respir Dis. 1984;130:312.
15. Gunen H, Hacievliyagil SS, Yetkin O, et al. Prevalence of COPD: first epidemiological study of a large region in Turkey. Eur J Intern Med. 2008;19:499–504.
16. Al Zaabi A, Asad F, Abdou J, et al. Prevalence of COPD in Abu Dhabi, United Arab Emirates. Respir Med. 2011;105(4):566–70.
17. Karcaaltincaba D, Kandemir O, Yalvac S, et al. Cigarette smoking and pregnancy: results of a survey at a Turkish women's hospital in 1,020 patients. J Obstet Gynaecol. 2009;29:480–6.
18. Waked M, Salameh P, Aoun Z. Water-pipe (narguile) smokers in Lebanon: a pilot study. East Mediterr Health J. 2009;15:432–42.
19. Al-Damegh SA, Saleh MA, Al-Alfi MA, et al. Cigarette smoking behavior among male secondary school students in the Central region of Saudi Arabia. Saudi Med J. 2004;25:215–9.
20. Maziak W, Ward KD, Afifi Soweid RA, Eissenberg T. Tobacco smoking using a waterpipe: a re-emerging strain in a global epidemic. Tob Control. 2004;13(4):327–33.
21. Komus N, Albayrak S, Ellidokuz H, et al. Occupational and environmental exposures and relations with pulmonary health. Tuberk Toraks. 2008;56:275–82.
22. Madanat H, Barnes MD, Cole EC. Knowledge of the effects of indoor air quality on health among women in Jordan. Health Educ Behav. 2008;35:105–18.
23. Hawamdeh A, Kasasbeh FA, Ahmad MA. Effects of passive smoking on children's health: a review. East Mediterr Health J. 2003;9:441–7.
24. Ekici A, Ekici M, Kurtipek E, et al. Obstructive airway diseases in women exposed to biomass smoke. Environ Res. 2005;99:93–8.
25. https://www.tbonline.info/posts/2011/10/24/uae-threat-deportation-increases-spread-tb/
26. Abbadi S, El Hadidy G, Gomaa N, et al. Strain differentiation of Mycobacterium tuberculosis complex isolated from sputum of pulmonary tuberculosis patients. Int J Infect Dis. 2009;13:236–42.
27. Multidrug and extensively drug-resistant TB (M/XDR-TB)-2010 GLOBAL REPORT ON SURVEILLANCE AND RESPONSE-WHO/HTM/TB/2010.322.
28. Samman Y, Krayem A, Haidar M, et al. Treatment outcome of tuberculosis among Saudi nationals: role of drug resistance and compliance. Clin Microbiol Infect. 2003;9:289–94.
29. Al-Hajjaj MS, Al-Kassimi FA, Al-Mobeireek AF, et al. Progressive rise of Mycobacterium tuberculosis resistance to rifampicin and streptomycin in Riyadh, Saudi Arabia. Respirology. 2001;6:317–22.
30. Chemtob D, Leventhal A, Weiler-Ravell D. Tuberculosis in Israel – main epidemiological aspects. Harefuah. 2002;141(226–32):316.
31. Farnia P, Masjedi MR, Mirsaeidi M, et al. Prevalence of Haarlem I and Beijing types of Mycobacterium tuberculosis strains in Iranian and Afghan MDR-TB patients. J Infect. 2006;53:331–6.
32. Wilder-Smith A, Foo W, Earnest A, Paton NI. High risk of Mycobacterium tuberculosis infection during the Hajj pilgrimage. Trop Med Int Health. 2005;10:336–9.
33. Al-Muhairi S, Zoubeidi T, Ellis M, et al. Demographics and microbiological profile of pneumonia in United Arab Emirates. Monaldi Arch Chest Dis. 2006;65:13–8.
34. Howidi M, Muhsin H, Rajah J. The burden of pneumococcal disease in children less than 5 years of age in Abu Dhabi, United Arab Emirates. Ann Saudi Med. 2011;31(4):356–9. https://doi.org/10.4103/0256-4947.83214.

35. Mahboub B, Niederman MS, Zaabi AAL, Vats M. Real-life management of outpatients with community-acquired pneumonia in the Gulf region and comparison with IDSA/ATS 2007 practice guidelines: a multicenter, prospective, observational study. EC Pulmonology and Respiratory Medicine. 2019;8(9):685–98.
36. https://www.worldometers.info/coronavirus/
37. https://covid19.ncema.gov.ae/en
38. Khadadah M, Mahboub B, Al-Busaidi NH, Sliman N, Soriano JB, Bahous J. Asthma insights and reality in the Gulf and the near East. Int J Tuberc Lung Dis. 2009;13(8):1015–22.
39. Al-Maskari F, Bener A, Al-Kaabi A, Al-Suwaidi N, Norman N, Brebner J. Asthma and respiratory symptoms among school children in United Arab Emirates. Allerg Immunol. 2000;32(4):159–63.
40. Lestringant GG, Bener A, Frossard PM, et al. A clinical study of airborne allergens in The United Arab Emirates. Allerg Immunol. 1999;31(8):263–7.
41. Ezeamuzie CI, Al-Ali S, Khan M, et al. IgE-mediated sensitization to mould allergens among patients with allergic respiratory diseases in a desert environment. Int Arch Allergy Immunol. 2000;121(4):300–7.
42. Waness A, EL-Sameed YA, Mahboub B, et al. Respiratory disorders in the Middle East: a review. Respirology. 2011;16(8):755–66.
43. Al-Kubaisy W, Ali SH, Al-Thamiri D. Risk factors for asthma among primary school children in Baghdad, Iraq. Saudi Med J. 2005;26(3):460–6.
44. Sattar HA, Mobayed H, Al-Mohammed AA, et al. The pattern of indoor and outdoor respiratory allergens in asthmatic adult patients in a humid and desert newly developed country. Eur Ann Allergy Clin Immunol. 2003;35(8):300–5.
45. Braman SS. The global burden of asthma. Chest. 2006;130(1, supplement):4S–12S.
46. Shafey O, Eriksen M, Ross H, Mackay J. The tobacco atlas. 3rd ed. American Cancer Society; 2009.
47. Mandil A, BinSaeed A, Ahmad S, Al-Dabbagh R, Alsaadi M, Khan M. Smoking among university students: a gender analysis. J Infect Public Health. 2010;3:179–87.
48. Trading Economics. Smoking prevalence; males (% of adults) in the United Arab Emirates. http://www.tradingeconomics.com/united-arab-emirates/smokingprevalence-males-percent-of-adults-wb-data.html. Accessed July 2013.
49. Dubai Health Authority. Dubai Household Health Survey 2009. Dubai Health Authority statistics released May, 2011.
50. Akl EA, Gunukula SK, Aleem S, et al. The prevalence of waterpipe tobacco smoking among the general and specific populations: a systematic review. BMC Public Health. 2011;11:244. https://doi.org/10.1186/1471-2458-11-244.
51. Nina Muslim. Gulfnews: teenagers resort to Arabic pipe for a high. 2006. http://gulfnews.com/news/gulf/uae/general/teenagers-resort-to-arabic-pipe-for-ahigh-1.235759. Accessed 10 Aug 2011.
52. Health Authority Abu Dhabi. Health Statistics 2011. http://www.haad.ae/HAAD/LinkClick.aspx?fileticket=JY0sMXQXrOU%3d&tabid=1243. Accessed July 2013.
53. Al-Houqani M, Ali R, Hajat C. Tobacco smoking using Midwakh is an emerging health problem – evidence from a large cross-sectional survey in the United Arab Emirates. PLoS One. 2012;7(6):e39189.
54. Aden B, Karrar S, Shafey O, Al Hosni F. Cigarette, water-pipe, and Medwakh smoking prevalence among applicants to Abu Dhabi's pre-marital screening program, 2011. Int J Prev Med. 2013;4(11):1290–5.
55. British Heart Foundation, Shisha. https://www.bhf.org.uk/heart-health/risk-factors/smoking/shisha. Accessed 1 July 2020.
56. Vupputuri S, Hajat C, Al-Houqani M, Osman O, Sreedharan J, Ali R, Crookes AE, Zhou S, Sherman SE, Weitzman M, et al. Midwakh/dokha tobacco use in the Middle East: much to learn. Tob Control. 2016;25(2):236–41.

57. Jayakumar M, Jayadevan S, Ranade AV, Mathew E. Prevalence and pattern of dokha use among medical and allied health students in Ajman, United Arab Emirates. Asian Pac J Cancer Prev APJCP. 2010;11(6):1547–9.
58. http://www.forbes.com/2007/02/07/worlds-fattest-countriesForbeslife-cxls0208worldfat.html
59. Gulf News. http://gulfnews.com/leisure/health/the-true-cost-ofobesity-in-the-uae-1.1044866. http://middleeasthospital.com/Mar2011lo.pdf
60. Mahboub B, Afzal S, Alhariri H, Alzaabi A, Vats M, Soans A. Prevalence of symptoms and risk of sleep apnea in Dubai, UAE. Int J Gen Med. 2013;6:109–14.
61. Zawya. https://www.zawya.com/story/GCCcounts cost of obesity-ZAWYA20141026052935/
62. http://www.me-oto.com/en/SiteRoot/MediaZone/IndustryNews/sleep-related/
63. Mahboub B, Safarainni B, Alhariri H, Vats M. Sleep breathing disorders in female population of Dubai, UAE. Health. 2013;5(12):2091–6.

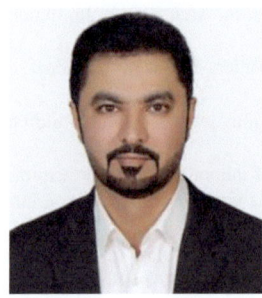

Bassam Mahboub is the program director of care model innovation at Dubai Health Authority and Assistant Dean at the College of Medicine, Sharjah University. He is a graduate of UAE University, Al Ain. He is American board-certified in internal medicine, allergy and clinical immunology, and pulmonology from the University of Toronto. He also has a master's in Business Administration from Wolverhampton University.

Dr. Mahboub is a consultant pulmonologist and the head of pulmonary medicine at Rashid Hospital under the Dubai Health Authority, UAE. He is also the head of the Emirates Allergy and Respiratory Society. Besides, he holds the position of associate clinical professor, faculty of medicine, at Sharjah University and is an associate research fellow at the Meakins Respiratory Research Centre at McGill University, Canada. Dr. Mahboub's areas of interest are health innovation and respiratory care, as well as translation research in airway diseases.

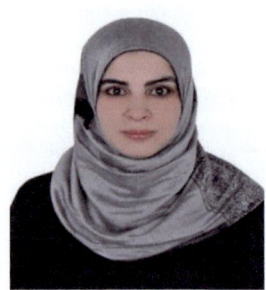

Dr. Laila Salameh is an accomplished medical researcher and healthcare professional. With a diverse educational background, including a PhD in Molecular Medicine and Translational Research from the University of Sharjah, an MPH from the United Arab Emirates University, and a Bachelor of Science in Nursing from the University of Jordan, Dr. Laila Salameh has demonstrated a commitment to academic excellence.

Throughout their career, Dr. Laila Salameh has made significant contributions to the medical field, notably pioneering a new lab methodology applying RNA linear amplification on archival formalin-fixed paraffin-embedded tissues. Recognized for excellence, Dr. Laila Salameh has received prestigious awards such as the "Best Researcher Award" from the Dubai Health Authority and the European Respiratory Society (ERS) award for the best abstract among allied health professionals.

With a history of professional roles ranging from expert thesis reviewer to lecturer and specialist nurse at Rashid Hospital, DAHC, Dr. Laila Salameh continues to drive progress in medical research and health care, showcasing a passion for improving patient outcomes and advancing the field.

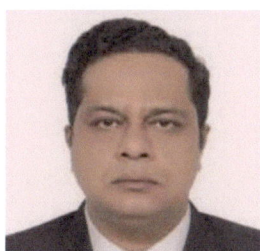

Dr. Mayank Vats is a senior specialist, interventional pulmonologist, pulmonologist, intensivist, and sleep physician at Rashid Hospital and Dubai Hospital. He developed the interventional pulmonology department at Rashid Hospital. Before coming to the United Arab Emirates, he was a consultant in respiratory medicine, critical care medicine, and sleep medicine at Escorts Heart Institute and Apollo Hospital, New Delhi, India, a tertiary-level care hospital in India. Dr. Vats's interest is to utilize his professional knowledge and interpersonal skills in order to provide the highest degree of patient care and satisfaction. Having worked in busy tertiary-level teaching hospital and specialty corporate hospitals as a consultant, he has been exposed to the complete spectrum of respiratory, critical care, and sleep medicine.

Open Access This chapter is licensed under the terms of the Creative Commons Attribution 4.0 International License (http://creativecommons.org/licenses/by/4.0/), which permits use, sharing, adaptation, distribution and reproduction in any medium or format, as long as you give appropriate credit to the original author(s) and the source, provide a link to the Creative Commons license and indicate if changes were made.

The images or other third party material in this chapter are included in the chapter's Creative Commons license, unless indicated otherwise in a credit line to the material. If material is not included in the chapter's Creative Commons license and your intended use is not permitted by statutory regulation or exceeds the permitted use, you will need to obtain permission directly from the copyright holder.

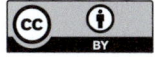

The Radiology Practice in the UAE in the Past, Present, and Future

37

Usama Albastaki

37.1 Introduction

Radiology was invented incidentally in 1895 by Wilhelm Rontgen while he was experimenting with fluorescent light and black cardboard [1]. The world recognized the greatness of his achievement, and he was awarded the first Nobel Prize in physics in 1901 [2]. The application of radiology in medicine was recognized very early, and Rinehart Hospital in Germany installed the first X-ray machine in 1897 [3]. Rontgen never used his right to patent the invention, choosing instead to keep it open for humans to innovate in the field [4].

As the United Arab Emirates (UAE) was united in 1971, the installation of the radiology department in its hospitals was early. Rashid Hospital, established in 1972, had a radiology department with two X-ray labs from day one [5]. Al Jazeera Hospital had a radiology department in the early 1970s, with radiologists and radiographers hired to cover its needs. One of the earliest radiologists in the main hospital of the Ministry of Health in Abu Dhabi was Dr. Naela Allamaki from Oman [6].

This chapter explains the role of the radiology department in the hospital, the different types of radiology departments in various hospitals, and the authorities of the UAE. We will go through the history of radiology in the UAE based on interviews with pioneering radiology practitioners who have witnessed the early days of radiology in this country and are still active in practice. As radiology is always associated with medical education, it is essential to track the history of radiology education in the UAE, including radiology residency programmes, radiographer

---

U. Albastaki (✉)
Department of Medical Imaging, Dubai Health, Dubai, United Arab Emirates

Mohammad Bin Rashid University of Medicine (MBRU), Dubai, United Arab Emirates

Radiology Society of the Emirates (RSE), Dubai, United Arab Emirates
e-mail: umalbastaki@dha.gov.ae

© The Author(s) 2025
H. O. Al-Shamsi (ed.), *Healthcare in the United Arab Emirates*,
https://doi.org/10.1007/978-981-96-0523-1_37

training, and the different conferences held annually in the UAE or international conferences previously hosted. We cannot mention the sensitive practice of radiology without mentioning the role of the Federal Authority for Nuclear Regulation (FANR), which supervises radiation-protection guidelines. Then we will explore the possibilities of evolving in the future to have the basic structures that are required for a practice equivalent to that of the modern world.

37.2 General Rules of Radiology Departments

Brady et al. [7], in an important article published last year, pointed out that the current rules of radiology in health care are as follows.

37.2.1 Prevention of Diseases

Radiology screening and monitoring programmes are expanding. In addition to the role that radiology plays in screening for breast cancer [8], prostate cancer [9], lung cancer [10], and colon cancer [11], it is widely used in our society to screen for chronic diseases with poor outcomes if not discovered early, such as multiple sclerosis [12] and Crohn's disease [13]. Many centres in the UAE have started to use it for screening for familial cardiomyopathy [14]. National breast cancer screening guidelines have been well established by the Ministry of Health and Prevention (MOHAP), the Department of Health—Abu Dhabi (HAAD), and the Dubai Health Authority (DHA) [15]. There are large campaigns during the Pink Month of October to encourage ladies to undergo mammograms [16].

With the rising science of radiogenomics [17, 18], there will be more rules in radiology for the prevention of diseases through the use of 'predictive imaging biomarkers'. These biomarkers will be used to identify the disease, grade it, and monitor the response to treatment. It is without a doubt that the practice of radiology is shifting from qualitative assessment of diseases to quantitative assessment, which will increase accuracy in diagnosis and exclude bias in assessment [19].

Radiology is even used to reassure people that illness does not exist. Different modalities of radiology are used to rule out pathologies and confirm for the clinician the absence of disease. Different guidelines and protocols are set to optimize imaging for these reasons [7].

37.2.2 Detection of Diseases

The detection of disease is achieved through a population-based screening programme, as mentioned in the section on prevention of disease. It helps in identifying abnormalities causing the clinical presentation of patients [7].

37.2.3 Diagnosis

It helps in staging or grading diseases such as tumours and disc hernias. Radiology facilitates management decision-making [20], and it can even directly guide biopsy procedures. It is vital in designing clinical decision pathways, as almost all international guidelines rely on imaging to support further decisions concerning patient management [7].

37.2.4 Delivery and Monitoring of Therapy

Different radiology modalities are used to assess the patient's response to treatment. The use of imaging biomarkers will support early disease detection and the expected response to treatment, resulting in a reduction in aggressive treatment and a shift towards more focused therapies. Biomarkers are vital in follow-ups and are the products of large clinical trials, emphasizing the importance of research in radiology practice [21].

Intervention radiology is widely used in managing different pathologies, such as brain new infarct management, or as part of a management plan, such as chemoembolization of tumours. It advantages over surgery in that it is minimally invasive and results in faster recovery [7].

37.2.5 Prognosis

Radiology is used to confirm the response to treatment, which might, in such cases, result in the complete healing of the pathology [7].

37.2.6 Others

(a) The modern practice of teleradiology connects small hospitals to large hospitals. It has even aided in establishing diagnostic centres in rural areas, which send images to larger, specialized centres for highly qualified radiologists to interpret.
(b) The modern radiology department should show quality in the services provided. This is achieved through what are called non-interpretive activities, such as teaching residents, radiographers, or even non-radiologist residents, interns, and medical students, who are mandated to have some knowledge of radiology to succeed in their medical practice [22].
(c) Radiologists should be able to communicate with patients, the public, the medical community, and other stakeholders [23].

37.3 Different Types of Radiology Departments in the UAE

The structures of radiology departments differ across health authorities. Adjustments were made according to the needs of each authority.

SEHA has established a breakthrough in Abu Dhabi since its introduction in 2007. Khalifa Hospital in Abu Dhabi recruited different subspecialties according to the hospital's clinical specialties. Al Mafraq Hospital followed the same model, and so does Sheikh Shakhbout Medical City today.

In Dubai, the Dubai Health Authority bases its practice on general radiologists and their 24/7 availability. Due to the expansion of interventional radiology, interventional radiologists were recruited in both Rashid and Dubai hospitals, and they now handle a high number of cases. A few different subspecialties started in Rashid Hospital in the early 2010s, and breast imaging was introduced in Dubai Hospital.

The Ministry of Health and Prevention (MOHAP) considered reducing the costs of services and the possibilities of enhancing them, so they privatized certain radiology services [24].

In addition, private hospitals in the UAE have their own radiology departments that follow the rules of the local authority. Even small diagnostic centres spread across the UAE provide services that may be unavailable in major hospitals, such as open MRI. These differ in pricing according to the quality of the services.

The departments are required to follow the rules of the local authorities. They must have a valid license with the FANR after confirming that they are following UAE standards in radiation protection. Each radiology unit in the country must be licensed by FANR; the vendor usually applies for the license.

37.4 History of Radiology in the UAE

Hamid Kazim [6] started his journey as the first Emirati radiology practitioner when he applied to study at King's College in London in 1964. He was trained in the different radiology modalities at the time and performed interventional procedures. He was a master at performing carotid studies and encephalograms. He gained extensive clinical and leadership experience working with pioneers such as Dr. David Bernestien at Paddington Neurosurgery Hospital. After three months of training, Dr. Bernestien told him that he was confident enough to work independently as an interventional radiology practitioner. He worked in multiple hospitals as a locum in London and even worked with Sir Majdi Yaqoub, who became his friend and met him every time the professor visited Dubai.

In 1979, Kazim decided to go back home. He joined the old Al Qasimi Hospital, which was managed by the British Allied Medical Group. The hospital had only a portable X-ray unit. A year later, the hospital's ownership was transferred to the Ministry of Health. He joined the main hospital in Abu Dhabi and was later assigned to the newly built Al Jazeera Hospital as head of the department. He was appointed head of the federal radiology department from 1982 to 2005 [6].

The Department of Federal Radiology of the Ministry of Health was:

- Supervising workflow in all hospitals, as the number of hospitals had increased at that time from 3 to 10.
- In charge of designing the departments, planning the rooms, and choosing and installing the different radiology units.
- Initiating the application of radiation dose monitoring, as every radiology staff member had a dosimeter, which was collected regularly and sent to the UK to be read monthly. This included collecting dosimeters for the Department of Health in Dubai (currently the DHA).
- Inspection of private clinics' radiology departments.
- Responsible for submitting regular reports to the higher leadership about the functionality and needs of radiology departments.
- Also, fulfilling the current role of FANR is ensuring radiation safety for both patients and staff [6].

In the beginning, the departments started with conventional X-ray labs and then added CT. Kazim was trained to operate it in the UK. He was the first to operate a CT scanner at Edinburgh Hospital in Cambridge in 1971. The first CT installed in the Ministry was at Al Jazeera Hospital in 1983. This was a four-slice CT, and Dr. Marwa Shafeeq from Egypt, who was trained in the UK, was recruited to operate it. The first ultrasound was installed in 1982, and the first MRI in 2001. Both were introduced at Al Jazeera Hospital [4].

Dr. Hani Afifi [5] joined Rashid Hospital in Dubai in 1981, nine years after it was established. He remembered Dr. Medhat Gharib as one of the pioneers of radiology practice in Dubai and the UAE. The Department of Radiology at Rashid Hospital consisted of two X-ray labs, and within the same year, they installed the first CT unit in the UAE. It was a single slice scanner, mainly used for CT brain examinations. The department was also managing an X-ray lab at Al Maktoum Hospital.

In 1983, the CT was replaced by a four-slice CT. The department made a breakthrough by bringing in Acuson's highest-standard ultrasound system in the early 1980s. In 1986, Dubai Hospital was established and was initially managed by the radiology department of Rashid Hospital. As the workflow in the hospital increased, establishing an independent radiology department was mandated. The radiology department at Rashid Hospital also managed the radiology department of Latifa Hospital until the 1990s.

The first hospital-based closed MRI unit was installed in 1997. The first MRI in the UAE was an open MRI, installed at the MEDIC diagnostic centre, owned by Abdulrahman Falaknaz. Dr. Afifi remembers the early days when interventional procedures were performed in conventional X-ray labs. He recalled an incident in the mid-80s involving a patient at a Dubai Hospital who had just delivered but presented with unexplained continuous vaginal bleeding. The vascular surgeons were consulted but could not intervene due to limited resources. Dr. Afifi performed a pelvic angiography, which revealed large ruptures and an arteriovenous malformation. He repaired it, and the patient survived [5].

In the 1990s, Dr. Amina Belhoul showed interest in radiology during her internship, then she was trained in Ireland and joined the department as the first Emirati female radiologist. Dubai city was growing, and so was the hospital population. The department had to set up 500 pages of policies and guidelines to make the workflow smooth [5].

The central department of Rashid Hospital radiology was technically supervising the other DHA radiology departments. This pushed even the department to think further about growing and encouraging many junior doctors to be further educated in radiology. In 2005, another milestone was reached when the trauma centre at Rashid Hospital was launched. The requirement for having 24/7 full radiology services of CT, X-ray, MRI, and ultrasound was fulfilled with the continuous availability of radiologists in the hospital. In the same year, the hospital installed the first picture archiving and communication system in the country (PACs). It offered a shared archive of all radiology images accessible at all DHA locations. The department also developed criteria for evaluating the staff to ensure that they provide the best care for the patients [5].

Shefa Alnakhi [25] was the first Emirati radiographer. She was sponsored by the Ministry of Education to study medical sciences and applied radiology sciences in Kuwait. After 4 years of a rich journey, including clinical attachments at the large hospitals of Kuwait, she joined the Department of Health and Medical Services in Dubai in 1987.

She was assigned to work with with Dr. Hani at Rashid Hospital. Later, she felt responsible for fulfilling the requirements of the newly established Al Wasl Hospital (currently Latifa Hospital) by being trained to perform sonographic studies for obstetrics and gynaecology exams. She helped develop the department further to reach today's standards and was gradually promoted to become the director of clinical support services in the hospital. She felt highly supported by the hospital management to promote the services in the department that provide dedicated care to women and children [25].

The radiology departments of the DHA were meeting regularly early on to discuss common issues and decide on centralized policies across the DHA under the umbrella of the medical imaging committee (Table 37.1).

Table 37.1 The pioneers of radiology in the UAE, according to the interviewee [5, 6, 25]

First Emirati radiology practitioner	Hr. Hamid Kazim—Ministry of Health
First Emirati radiologist	Dr. Ahmed Ali Albar—Zayed Military Hospital
First Emirati female radiologist	Dr. Amina Belhoul—Rashid Hospital
First Emirati radiographer	Shefa Alnakhi—Rashid Hospital/Latifa (Alwasl previously) Hospital
First radiology full residency programme	Tawam Hospital (UAE university)—2006
First CT in UAE	Rashid Hospital—1981
First MRI in UAE	MEDIC Diagnostic Center—Dubai (early or mid-1980s)

37.5 Radiology Education in the UAE

37.5.1 Residency and Radiology Education

Rashid Hospital considered radiology education very early, starting with the building of its conference room. Dr. Hani established a radiology education programme in the Medical College for Women in Dubai. A film library was established in the conference room and was available for all who were willing to learn [5].

The first national residency programme started at the UAE university. The Arab Board recognized Tawam Hospital as a training centre for the Arab Board in 2006. The other later recognized centres were Khalifa Hospital, Rashid Hospital, and Cleveland Clinic Abu Dhabi. The biggest residency programme today is in Rashid, with 24 residents. In 2012, one of the residents in the Dubai residency programme, Dr. Ahmad Saadat, received a prestigious award for the best-presented case from the American Institute of Radiologic Pathology (AIRP).

In 2021, a committee was formed to launch the Emirati Board of Diagnostic Radiology. This initiative will be carried out in alliance with the American Accreditation Council for Graduate Medical Education (ACGME) for the accreditation of the involved hospitals as training centres. The programme is expected to last 5 years and will be highly recognized locally.

37.5.2 Radiography

Hamid was the first chairman of the radiology advisor committee of the radiology college at Dubai Women's College when it was established, from 1994 to 2005. The first batch consisted of 16 Emirati female radiographers who graduated in 1996 [6]. Dr. Hani was one of the teaching staff members, giving a weekly lecture. The radiographers were rotating clinically in the DHA hospitals [5]. Shifa gave introductory lectures to the students and even to the parents to explain the importance of radiographers' work and that they are safer than commonly expected. The Women's Technology College curriculum was discussed with pioneers such as Shifa before implementation [25]. The authorities were encouraging more Emiratis to join the career of radiography through the career fairs held in multiple emirates annually [6, 25].

37.5.3 Radiology Conferences

Hamid Kazim founded the Total Radiology Conference in 1995 as part of the Arab Health Annual Exhibition. Twenty-five radiologists attended the first conference, held in March each year until the current date [6].

The annual radiology meeting in the UAE (ARM) is the official meeting of the Radiology Society of the Emirates (RSE), which started in 2015. It has enriched the radiology society of this country since it was launched, as it invites at least two speakers who are well-known pioneers in radiology every year. The society is cooperating with prominent radiology institutes around the world to ensure the high quality of the conference.

The Pan Arab Intervention Radiology Conference (PAIRS) has been held in Dubai since 2006. It is led by Dr. Aiman Alsibaei, a consultant in interventional radiology at Rashid Hospital. In 2016, it attained a Dubai International Centre license, making it more globally recognized. The organization today, in addition to its leading conference, organizes many workshops in different cities within the Arab World to raise the standards of interventional radiology practice.

37.6 Role of FANR

The Federal Authority for Nuclear Regulation (FANR) was established in 2009. Its function is to regulate radiation-related activity in the country, including medical radiation. Hospitals and medical centres undergo regular inspections by FANR to confirm that they are following the standards to ensure the safety of patients and staff. It is impossible to legally function as a radiation-related facility in the UAE without permission from FANR [26].

FANR works closely with local health authorities to ensure practice safety. It ensures that these authorities are conducting radiation protection courses for non-radiologists working closely with radiation, such as operation theatre staff in hospitals and dentists.

FANR should license each radiology unit available in the medical equipment market in the country before it is cleared for use in medical practice. Stringent measures are followed to ensure the safety of these units [26].

Recently, FANR has expanded its role by establishing a medical application group with representatives from each authority. The group's primary goal is to develop national diagnostic reference levels (DRLs) within the coming years, replacing the current option of using other countries' DRLs [26].

DRLs are radiation dose ranges that FANR will establish for each radiology exam, with minimum and maximum doses to ensure that images are obtained in good quality within acceptable radiation levels that will not harm the patient. They will be developed for each radiology exam.

In addition, the group is working closely with the Royal College of Radiologists in London to set up referral guidelines for each clinical indication to ensure the safe practice of radiology in the country [26].

37.7 Future of Practice

The practice of medicine is turning towards patient-valued care [27, 28], and the same is true for radiology [7]. In this section, we will mention how radiology is reaching patient-value care and what has been achieved or is expected to be achieved in radiology practice in the UAE to reach that.

According to Brady et al. [5], to reach patient-valued care:

1. Engage directly with the referral, understand their practice and needs, and develop a high standard of communication to reach that.

We should support the development of evidence-based referral guidelines to ensure that the referrals are strongly grounded in the fundamental values of the patients. FANR, in cooperation with RSE, will develop Emirati guidelines that will be mandated for use in both public and private sectors, and that will be evidence-based.

2. Understand the varying needs of referrals.

One step to fulfilling this is to have 24/7 services. Currently, the DHA hospitals: Rashid in Dubai and Hatta hospitals have 24/7 services, as radiology specialists are physically in the hospital 24/7 [5, 6]. In Abu Dhabi, specialists are available until 12 a.m., and then residents provide coverage for the rest of the night until 7 a.m. [5]. There is a presence of subspecialty experts: they exist in Khalifa Hospital, Sheikh Shakhbout Medical City, and Cleveland Clinic Abu Dhabi, and Rashid Hospital in Dubai, which also offers some subspecialty services.

There is also the presence of multidisciplinary input through multidisciplinary meetings (MDTs). The MDTs exist in a wide range of major hospitals in the country.

3. Ensuring that the radiology department staff works as a team.

This should be encouraged within the radiology department of any hospital.

4. Structuring the radiology department's work plan to meet the referee's needs.

This would be achieved by protecting time for the MDTs.

5. Utilizing available resources and tools.

New modality units have massive capabilities with the current evolution of computer sciences. The radiologists and radiographers are to be aware of that and use the capabilities of these units to the maximum to ensure the best care for the patients, providing up-to-date and varied exams.

Use of AI. Many hospitals are currently using AI to improve the quality of the images, help radiologists make specific measurements, or reduce workloads.

6. Engaging directly with the patients and answering their queries.

This is different from the old practice when the radiologist's main job was reporting.

7. Optimize information exchange.

This is done through fast reporting. Most of the radiology departments of the major hospitals in the country have PACS systems, which make images available to be reviewed not only by the radiologist within the same hospital but also by those using the same network. DHA started with PACS in 2005, making images available through the network.

8. Constant quality monitoring and promoting a culture of constant quality improvement.

JCI mandated that each radiology department have a quality officer, which exists in all JCI-accredited hospitals. Continuous quality improvement is also part of their role.

9. Experiment with research to improve the practice.

Each JCI-accredited department has multiple KPIs monitored and is then mandated to develop an improvement plan. This is mainly based on experimental projects.

There are many steps needed to reach the radiology practice of tomorrow. The UAE radiology departments have shown the capability to reach that based on their continuous improvement and the resources available to do so, as described above.

37.8 Conclusion

Radiology has been well established in the UAE, in the Health Authority of Abu Dhabi and the Dubai Health Authority. In this chapter, we met pioneers motivated to elevate the standard of practice in the country. The leadership of both authorities has recognized the importance of radiology in the general practice of medicine and encouraged innovation. The establishment of FANR has added to the practice in the UAE. All the elements exist for the practice to align with the developed world's practice of radiology (Fig. 37.1).

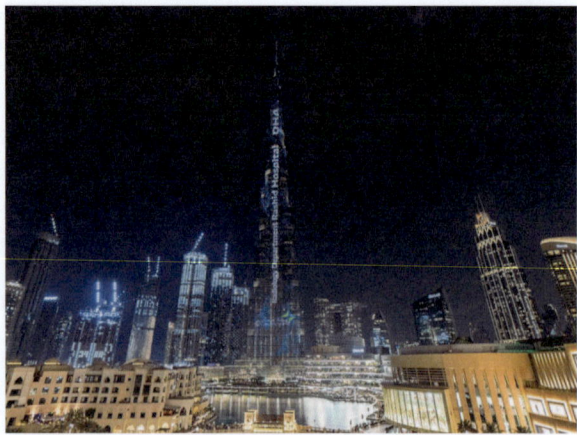

Fig. 37.1 In 2020, the year of COVID, the radiology department of the Rashid Hospital was awarded the Shaikh Hamdan Bin Rashid award as the best government medical department in the UAE

Acknowledgement I would like to acknowledge the following for the support provided to me throughout the writing of this chapter:

- Hamid Kazim, the Director of the Federal Radiology Department of the Ministry of Health between 1982 and 2005.
- Dr. Hani Afifi, the Head of the Radiology Department at the Rashid Hospital between 1981 and 2010.
- Shefa Alnakhi, the current Director of the Clinical Support Services at Latifa Hospital, and the first radiographer in the UAE.
- Dr. Abdullah Alremaithi, the President of the Radiology Society of the Emirates (RSE), and a consultant radiologist at Zayed Military Hospital.
- Dr. Talib Almansoor, Deputy President of the RSE; Assistant Dean of Clinical Affairs in the College of Medicine and Health Sciences at the UAE University, and Assistant Professor of Radiology, College of Medicine and Health Sciences, UAE University.

Conflicts of Interest The author has no conflicts of interest to declare.

References

1. Thomas AM, Banerjee AK. The history of radiology. OUP Oxford; 2013.
2. Chodos A. This month in physics history. November 8, 1895: Roentgen's discovery of X-rays. APS Phys. Am Phys Soc. 2001;19(10). Available in https://www.aps.org/publications/apsnews/200111/history.cfm. Accessed 17/07/2022.
3. Hodges PC. An autobiographical sketch. Perspect Biol Med. 1973;17(1):16–66.
4. Guy JM, Rønne P, Nielsen ABW. Development of the X-ray tube, with a description of the collection in the medical history museum, University of Copenhagen (book review). Bull Hist Med. 1990;64(2):354.
5. Afifi H interview. History of radiology in DHA [Personal interview, 15th July]. Dubai. 2022.
6. Kazim H interview. History of radiology in the Ministry of Health [Personal interview, 10th July]. Dubai. 2022.
7. Brady AP, Bello JA, Derchi LE, Fuchsjäger M, Goergen S, Krestin GP, Lee EJ, Levin DC, Pressacco J, Rao VM, Slavotinek J. Radiology in the era of value-based healthcare: a multisociety expert statement from the ACR, CAR, ESR, IS3R, RANZCR, and RSNA. Can Assoc Radiol J. 2021;72(2):208–14.
8. Feig SA, D'orsi CJ, Hendrick RE, Jackson VP, Kopans DB, Monsees B, Sickles EA, Stelling CB, Zinninger M, Wilcox-Buchalla P. American College of Radiology guidelines for breast cancer screening. AJR Am J Roentgenol. 1998;171(1):29–33.
9. Sciarra A, Barentsz J, Bjartell A, Eastham J, Hricak H, Panebianco V, Witjes JA. Advances in magnetic resonance imaging: how they are changing the management of prostate cancer. Eur Urol. 2011;59(6):962–77.
10. Huo J, Shen C, Volk RJ, Shih YCT. Use of CT and chest radiography for lung cancer screening before and after publication of screening guidelines: intended and unintended uptake. JAMA Intern Med. 2017;177(3):439–41.
11. Stracci F, Zorzi M, Grazzini G. Colorectal cancer screening: tests, strategies, and perspectives. Front Public Health. 2014;2:210.
12. Kalb R, Beier M, Benedict RH, Charvet L, Costello K, Feinstein A, Gingold J, Goverover Y, Halper J, Harris C, Kostich L. Recommendations for cognitive screening and management in multiple sclerosis care. Mult Scler J. 2018;24(13):1665–80.

13. Bruining DH, Bhatnagar G, Rimola J, Taylor S, Zimmermann EM, Fletcher JG. CT and MR enterography in Crohn's disease: current and future applications. Abdom Imaging. 2015;40(5):965–74.
14. Bluemke DA. MRI of nonischemic cardiomyopathy. AJR Am J Roentgenol. 2010;195(4):935.
15. Taher J, El Sebelgy M. The national guidelines for breast cancer screening and diagnosis. 2014.
16. Kharaba Z, Buabeid MA, Ramadan A, Ghemrawi R, Al-Azayzih A, Al Meslamani AZ, Alfoteih Y. Knowledge, attitudes, and practices concerning breast cancer and self examination among females in UAE. J Community Health. 2021;46(5):942–50.
17. Lubner MG. Reflections on radiogenomics and oncologic radiomics. Abdom Radiol. 2019;44(6):1959.
18. Rizzo S, Savoldi F, Rossi D, Bellomi M. Radiogenomics as association between non-invasive imaging features and molecular genomics of lung cancer. Ann Transl Med. 2018;6(23):447.
19. Pinker K, Shitano F, Sala E, Do RK, Young RJ, Wibmer AG, Hricak H, Sutton EJ, Morris EA. Background, current role, and potential applications of radiogenomics. J Magn Reson Imaging. 2018;47(3):604–20.
20. Lysack JT, Hoy M, Hudon ME, Nakoneshny SC, Chandarana SP, Matthews TW, Dort JC. Impact of neuroradiologist second opinion on staging and management of head and neck cancer. J Otolaryngol Head Neck Surg. 2013;42(1):1–7.
21. O'Connor JP, Aboagye EO, Adams JE, Aerts HJ, Barrington SF, Beer AJ, Boellaard R, Bohndiek SE, Brady M, Brown G, Buckley DL, Tozer GM, van Herk M, Walker-Samuel S, Wason J, Williams KJ, Workman P, Yankeelov TE, Brindle KM, McShane LM, Jackson A, Waterton JC. Imaging biomarker roadmap for cancer studies. Nat Rev Clin Oncol. 2017;14:169–86.
22. Brady AP. Measuring consultant radiologist workload: method and results from a national survey. Insights Imaging. 2011;2(3):247–60.
23. Brady A, Brink J, Slavotinek J. Radiology and value-based health care. JAMA. 2020;324(13):1286–7.
24. The Ministry of Health reduced the waiting time by renewing the machines and partnering with the private sector. Albayan. News and reports. 23rd May 2016. https://www.albayan.ae/across-the-uae/news-and-reports/2016-05-23-1.2645220. Accessed 10th July 2022.
25. AlNakhi S interview. Meeting the first radiographer in the UAE [Personal interview, 18th July]. Dubai. 2022.
26. Federal Authority of Nuclear Regulation. Radiation safety (FANR-RG007). Version 1. https://www.fanr.gov.ae/en/Documents/FANR_RG007%20ver1.pdf. Accessed 1st July 2022.
27. Porter ME, Teisberg EO. Redefining health care: creating value-based competition on results. Harvard Business Press; 2006.
28. Porter ME. What is value in health care. N Engl J Med. 2010;363(26):2477–81.

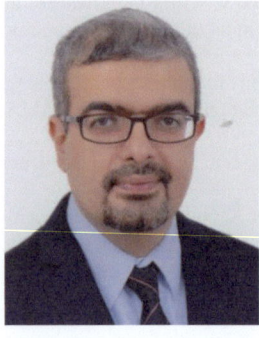

Dr. Usama Albastaki is currently the chair of medical imaging in Dubai Health. He was the Director of the Diagnostic Imaging Department of the Dubai Health Authority/Dubai Academic Health Corporation. He got his Swedish Board certification in Diagnostic Radiology in 2009. He is also a Clinical Associate Professor of Radiology at Mohammad Bin Rashid University of Medicine (MBRU). He is the General Secretary of the Radiology Society of the Emirates and Chairman of the medical application group of the FANR. He is a current member of the quality global steering group of the Royal College of Radiologists in London (RCR). He is Co-chairman of the Global RCR Congress in Dubai and the annual radiology meeting in the UAE.

Open Access This chapter is licensed under the terms of the Creative Commons Attribution 4.0 International License (http://creativecommons.org/licenses/by/4.0/), which permits use, sharing, adaptation, distribution and reproduction in any medium or format, as long as you give appropriate credit to the original author(s) and the source, provide a link to the Creative Commons license and indicate if changes were made.

The images or other third party material in this chapter are included in the chapter's Creative Commons license, unless indicated otherwise in a credit line to the material. If material is not included in the chapter's Creative Commons license and your intended use is not permitted by statutory regulation or exceeds the permitted use, you will need to obtain permission directly from the copyright holder.

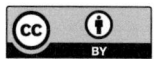

Postmortem Imaging in the UAE

Muhammad Al Shirawi

38.1 Introduction

The United Arab Emirates (UAE) is a federal country consisting of seven states. Each state has its own rules and regulations under the federal government. Abu Dhabi is the capital and largest state of the UAE. In this chapter, we focus on Abu Dhabi because of its governmental efforts in establishing and introducing the postmortem (PM) imaging facility in both forensic and natural death investigations. These efforts are not only limited to providing PM services, but they also extend to investing in human resources by ensuring a high level of competency in both educational and training strategic plans in a such a rare field in the Arab world. Currently, there are a number of competent local physicians who are highly qualified in both forensic pathology and radiology. It is worth mentioning that Dr. Nayef Al Janaahi, a fellow of the Royal College of Radiologists (UK), is the first Emirati licensed consultant in forensic radiology for the Department of Health–Abu Dhabi [1]. He commenced a 10-month Forensic Radiology placement at the Victorian Institute of Forensic Medicine in Australia (VIFM) in May 2016 [2, 3]. To the best of our knowledge, Dr. Essa Saeedi and Dr. Khamis Almazrouei are the first two Emirati board-certified forensic pathologists from the Royal College of Pathologists of Australasia (RCPA) with formal fellowship training and expertise in PM imaging. They commenced a long-term placement in Forensic Pathology Services at the VIFM in 2015. These placements at the VIFM were supported by the Government of the UAE [2].

In general, the Public Prosecution, the Centre of Forensic and Digital Sciences, the Department of Health–Abu Dhabi (DoH), and Abu Dhabi Police GHQ are the main elements of the forensic and natural death investigations in Abu Dhabi. The modern Central Morgue of Abu Dhabi is under the Department of Health–Abu Dhabi (DoH)

M. Al Shirawi (✉)
Forensic Pathology Services, Victorian Institute of Forensic Medicine (VIFM), Melbourne, VIC, Australia

and is well prepared for PMCT services in terms of construction, facilities, and equipment [1]. After the approval of the budget by the Executive Council of Abu Dhabi in 2017 [4], digital autopsy was established, and the first case reported during the COVID-19 pandemic in 2019 proved to be a major advantage for the health facility of the Government of Abu Dhabi [1, 3].

Before exploring the field of forensic radiology, i.e., postmortem imaging, let us shed some light on the population and its background in the UAE, which has a huge influence on introducing such a field to the multicultural population of the UAE.

38.2 Population, Crude Death Rate, and Culture of Abu Dhabi

According to the Statistics Centre of Abu Dhabi, the population of Abu Dhabi reached 3,789,860 people in 2023, indicating an increase of 83% compared to 2011. The census data indicates that the number of males accounts for 67% of the total population, while females represent 33% of the total population of Abu Dhabi (the median age of the Abu Dhabi population is 33 years). In 2018, the crude death rate was 1.2 deaths per 1000 population [5]. In the UAE, there are approximately 200 nationalities. Although multicultural, Islamic culture is dominant [6].

38.3 Islamic Teachings Support PM Imaging Service

According to Islamic teachings, the human body (alive or dead) must be respected. Burying without autopsy is considered a way of respecting humans in the Muslim and other communities. However, exceptions can be made, and permission to breach those religious teachings is given in certain conditions and circumstances with specific limitations. A forensic autopsy is one of these examples of breaching Islamic teachings in order to find out the cause of death in criminal or forensic cases. Avoiding or limiting classic autopsy is a major target in the Muslim community [7].

Consequently, this has empowered the early introduction of PM imaging services in Abu Dhabi. The introduction of this service facility marked a significant milestone in the field of forensic medicine and improved their common practice as it was more welcomed culturally and preferred over classic autopsy from both cultural and religious perspectives.

38.4 Main Stakeholders for the Introduction of PMCT Services in Abu Dhabi

- *Public Prosecution (Attorney General)*: under UAE Law No. 23 of 2006, it plays its role in criminal cases through investigation, indictment, dismissal, or referral, if needed, to the competent court [8].
- *AD Police GHQ*

- *Centre for Forensic and Digital Sciences* (Department of Justice)
- *Mortuary Staff*
- *Government Hospitals* (DoH)
- *IT teams and CT machine providers*

38.5 Working Hours at the Mortuary of Abu Dhabi

The working hours at the Central Mortuary of Abu Dhabi are from 7:00 a.m. to 03:00 p.m., Monday to Friday. Currently, the mortuary is reachable 24 hours a day if needed (e.g., for handling deceased bodies) [9].

38.6 Importance of PMCT Service

Besides the cultural and religious advantages of PMCT, the introduction of PMCT services into the field of postmortem in both forensic and natural death investigations expands the role of radiology in forensic autopsy. Postmortem imaging (forensic radiology) is now integrated with forensic autopsy. PMCT services have became common practice in various institutions in many countries, such as the UK, Australia, Switzerland, and Japan. It allows viewing of anatomy without dissection, specifically via 3-D reconstruction or digitization facilities. This facility may guide the forensic pathologist (before starting the dissection) by visualizing injuries in difficult or poorly accessible skeletal areas. Noninvasive or minimally invasive techniques can be applied to several areas where a specific finding may not be visible in a routine autopsy. In addition, PMCT can detect subtle, occult, or hazardous injuries and diseases that could be hard to detect without PM imaging. This PMCT service could also work as a triage tool, alerting forensic pathologists to adequate safety and environmental measures, e.g., deaths of pulmonary tuberculosis (Tb) or COVID-19. Moreover, PMCT helps forensic pathologists to decide which techniques to apply in terms of limited or complete autopsy. It adds findings to the external and internal examinations and toxicology [10, 11]. Currently, it is reported that PMCT exceeds the standards set and meets both families' and coroners' needs for its efficiency, time, and cost [12].

38.6.1 Scope of Practice

According to the College of Radiographers (CoR) and Institute of Forensic Radiographers (IAFR) guidelines:

(a) *Nonfatal injuries investigation*: by supporting individual(s) investigation of injuries involving nonaccidental injuries, nonfatal motor vehicle accidents, assaults, medical negligence, compensation claims, injuries in custody, torture, or systematic human rights abuses.

(b) *Forensic evidence location*: such as hidden foreign bodies, including ingested material, human and non-human narcotic packing, and ballistic materials.
(c) *Cause of death*: by supporting the investigations of suspicious or nonexplained deaths, e.g., RTA, suicide, homicide, and sudden infant death syndrome.
(d) *Human identification*: by providing supporting evidence that aids in confirming, determining, or eliminating the identification of both living and deceased cases via dental or other anatomical structures, or determining other biological profiles. These evaluations can be done using skeletal structures, DICOM viewers for 3D reconstructions, or personal effects, e.g., jewelry [13, 14].

38.6.2 Personnel

Personnel play an essential role by accessing the forensic radiology service, making case referrals, setting up a call-out system, providing semi- or permanent services (based on budgets and workloads), and assisting in the planning, organization, and training. This helps maintain a high standard of quality-assured crime lab facilities and overall quality assurance [13].

38.6.3 Senior Forensic Radiographer

The role of the senior forensic radiographer, who has received additional forensic training, is essential and collaborates closely with both forensic radiologists and pathologists. This radiographer working in forensic imaging should develop additional skills and be ready to work in challenging cases that are different from routine clinical cases. In the forensic institutions that accommodate forensic imaging, forensic technical imaging is performed by experienced registered radiographers. State registration or certification provides both quality and professionalism, specifically when using X-ray images as evidence in court. The radiographer needs to be familiar with almost all imaging types, equipment, and techniques and ready to work on duties where the forensic radiologist or pathologist may not be available. In addition, the forensic radiographer may perform some administrative procedures, e.g., filing radiographs, ordering or maintaining supplies, and computer operations. A competent forensic radiographer should be able to deal with some postmortem procedures such as PMCT angiography and ventilation. Child abuse, pediatric deaths, and forensic odontology and anthropology are additional skills for a competent forensic radiographer [13].

38.6.4 Forensic Radiologist/Necro-radiologist

A competent forensic radiologist (also known as a necro-radiologist), in collaboration with the forensic pathologist, plays a chief role in postmortem imaging services. A forensic radiologist should check and ensure appropriate imaging protocols, personnel, and necessary equipment is available. The forensic radiologist should ensure that postmortem imaging is designed and managed to standard levels [13]. An excellent integration between the forensic pathologist and necro-radiologist is mandatory and must be maintained thoroughly to ensure the quality of optimal PM practice.

38.6.5 Medical Radiation Physicist

Radiation exposure is hazardous. In diagnostic CT, radiation dose must be maintained within certain limits to avoid both short- and long-term complications. However, the radiation dose used in PM imaging is significantly higher than the diagnostic dose. Therefore, mortuary staff should take measures and precautions to protect themselves from direct and scattered radiation [13, 15]. Any X-ray equipment, including CT scanners, must be tightly regulated, monitored, calibrated, and controlled. The ionizing radiation equipment must be operated safely. The radiation dose to workers in the morgue must be monitored, kept as low as possible, and must not exceed safety limits. The forensic physicist must ensure all of these, as well as routine quality assurance, radiation protection, and dose monitoring [16, 17].

38.6.6 Postmortem Imaging Protocol

A written postmortem imaging protocol must be provided and available to staff. It must cover all types of X-rays and PMCT modalities in the institution and be specific, accurate, and appropriate according to the policies. It should be arranged in consultation with those who have a key role in the PMCT service. The forensic radiologists and pathologists, senior radiographers, morgue managers, public prosecution, police forensic coordinators, child protection, and elderly care teams are the most important key elements. It is important to address the need for adequate and proper consent in certain procedures, especially in high-profile public cases. The protocols should maintain confidentiality and the continuity of evidence [13].

38.6.7 Confidentiality

It is a legal right and must be maintained and provided at the highest professional conduct levels and standards, although forensic cases are always considered to be sub judice. Therefore, these forensic cases should never be discussed outside the mortuary or with anyone who is not directly involved, especially if the investigations have not yet been completed [13].

38.6.8 Health and Safety

It is important to apply the local or international policies of health and safety as in other hospitals, morgues, and the medical examiner's offices. This is to achieve best practices regarding infection and hazardous substance control, deceased care and handling, and manual handling. Guidance should be provided to forensic technicians, radiographers, and radiologists. Health and safety policies should provide appropriate precautions that minimize cross-infection and distress. Appropriate personal protective equipment (PPE) must be provided, accessible, and always worn during procedures. Rather than merely minimizing the risk of infection, the personal protective equipment prevents or limits the contamination of forensic evidence [13].

38.6.9 Radiation Protection

The policies on radiation protection should mainly provide guidance to forensic radiologists, radiographers, technicians, and others working in postmortem imaging. Advice from a qualified forensic radiation physicist's advice must be taken while setting up or changing the service. A forensic physicist plays a significant role in many jurisdictions regarding radiation procedures and equipment. Specific room arrangements need to be made for postmortem imaging and pathological specimens. The main purpose is to minimize the risk of radiation exposure to keep radiation doses as low as reasonably achievable. There are some measures that need to be taken to achieve and maintain safe X-ray equipment use, including a plan for radiation protection and rules and regulations in the radiation working area. Providing leaded protective doors, screens, walls, and personal protective equipment is a crucial safety measure [13, 16].

38.6.10 Referral Pathways

As in clinical CT services, each postmortem imaging request must be recognized, justified, and approved. The request form (electronic or paper) should provide details of the referral person and the circumstances of death, as well as subsequent external examinations. All referral pathways must be clearly traced and identified. To establish a proper referral system, the legal referral list and eligibility under the law must be discussed in detail with the stakeholders. In some countries, such as the UK, coroners and forensic pathologists may refer cases [13]. It is also permissible for forensic odonatologists, anthropologists, and crime scene police officers to refer specific cases according to the law of the UAE [8]. It is always encouraged that the referrals provide enough clinical and forensic details and discuss the cases with a forensic radiologist before starting the PMCT procedure in order to achieve the most appropriate modality and optimal image quality [13].

38.6.11 Legal Aspects

The medicolegal aspects in the field of forensics are extremely important in order to provide competent work. We also strongly suggest that the chief medical examiner and other stakeholders arrange courses and introductory lectures for mortuary staff, including radiographers, radiologists, and technicians. This will raise their knowledge and understanding of the importance of forensic evidence is and its value in the legal process, mainly regarding the nature and continuity of evidence [10].

38.6.12 Records

As in current clinical and forensic practices, all image data must be stored securely, and all measures must be taken in order to prevent unauthorized data release. This should protect the evidence in a court of law [13]. Records must be stored in compliance with the relevant local and national guidelines, including:

1. Identity of any radiographer and witness
2. Identity or role of any other individuals present
3. Date, time, and location of the examination
4. Subject and examination identifiers
5. Numbers and types of projections
6. Any retained evidence and its location
7. Handover details for the transfer of evidence with names and signatures

Each mortuary staff member should form their own formal evidence records and maintain them at the standard level [10, 13].

38.7 Education and Training

Staff education and training, mainly in forensic practice radiography/radiology, are essential for their competency and high performance. They need regular continuing medical education (CME), also known as continuing professional development, in order to ensure that they maintain relevant and up-to-date knowledge [13].

According to the strategic plan of Abu Dhabi, the scholarships for postgraduate training in forensic pathology and radiology have already been planned and granted. Currently, there are a couple of qualified competent forensic pathologists and radiologists, four of whom received their training from the Victorian Institute of Forensic Medicine (VIFM) in Australia, where PMCT service is a common practice [2, 4]. We strongly recommend ongoing governmental support to those physicians who are interested in this field, as well as support for international training if sufficient budget is available. Those local competent forensic physicians are encouraged to establish a national training program in PM imaging.

38.7.1 Suggestive Time Frame for PMCT Training

2–4 weeks for administrative and portal staff
3–6 months for radiographers
9–12 months for radiologists and pathologists

38.8 Staff Welfare

It is the responsibility of the employer to protect the physical and psychological health of employees. A risk assessment for forensic examinations should be conducted due to their potentially distressing nature [13].

38.9 Quality Assurance

A program for quality assurance must cover all forensic imaging aspects, as well as any investigation procedures at the crime lab, including standards of competence, qualifications, recruitment, policies, X-ray equipment maintenance records, radiation protection certification, etc. [13].

38.10 DICOM Viewer

This program is useful and widely used. We recommend the DICOM Viewer, which plays a significant role in the field of postmortem radiology. Basically, DICOM provides a standard means of exchanging information between users of imaging equipment. It produces, stores, displays, sends, queries, processes, retrieves, and prints medical images, as well as manages related workflows. It permits the integration of medical imaging devices such as scanners, servers, workstations, printers, network hardware, and PACS from multiple manufacturers. The major impact of DICOM is on PACS because it can serve many interfacing applications. New software programs incorporate artificial intelligence, which can be highly sensitive in detecting pathologic and/ or forensic abnormalities [18–20].

38.11 Modalities of Postmortem Imaging

The field of radiology has been revolutionized by the newer imaging methods that have been incorporated into forensic studies. PMCT is one of the new radiology modalities and stands for postmortem computed tomography. In order to achieve the best results from the PMCT, some methods have been introduced to enhance the scope of postmortem imaging, such as contrast angiography and ventilated PMCT. It has been reported that, in the absence of autopsy, an isolated PMCT may only determine a diagnosis or cause of death in 28–41% of cases. However, this diagnosis may become accurate up to 60% if detailed circumstances of death are considered in conjunction with PMCT results. This percentage could reach 92% in natural deaths due to cardiovascular events, such as myocardial infarction [13, 21–24].

38.11.1 Contrast Angiography

By contrast administration, PMCT sensitivity is significantly increased, which improves image quality. By enhancing the tissues and the vascular lamina, the structures can be shown without superimposition. It displays perfusion and vessel occlusion in a significant way. Both perfusion and occlusion are important postmortem findings, mainly in cardiac and cerebral diseases. Therefore, PMCT angiography (PMCTA) now plays a significant role as a supplement to postmortem biopsies [13]. Rutty et al. also showed in 2017 that PMCTA can detect the cause of death in 92% of coronial cases in a prospective study with 6% major discrepancies when compared to the gold standard autopsy [21].

Basically, as with any contrast medium used in CT scans, both oily and water-soluble media can be administered intravenously (i.e., so-called positive contrast). However, air has also been reported in specific coronary artery assessments in PMCT investigation (i.e., so-called negative contrast) [21–24].

38.11.1.1 Indications for PMCTA
1. Unexplained death
2. Ballistic cases
3. Trauma
4. Perinatal cases [13]

38.11.1.2 Challenges in PMCTA
The most common challenges in PMCT angiography are as follows:

1. *Contrast stasis*: Due to the absence of cardiovascular circulation.
2. An almost empty or collapsed vascular system, or one that may be air-filled, requires a larger quantity of contrast liquid compared to a regular clinical CT.
3. *Time*: Increasing postmortem delay is proportional to the chance of rapid contrast leakage and the use of water-soluble preparations, which may lead to massive edema.
4. Challenges in interpreting PMCTA findings. This is due to artifacts, clots, filling defects, and layering.
5. PMCTA influence on different examinations is not fully understood yet [25].

38.11.1.3 Whole Body Techniques
Multiphase PMCTA implementation in both natural and unnatural cause-of-death investigations is useful and has become routine practice. The use of whole-body PMCTA has increased in the last few years. This has become a routine medicolegal investigation in conjunction with the conventional autopsy in many centers. Unless there is a large PM occlusion in the vascular system, this technique visualizes the whole body's vascular system (mainly the head, thorax, and abdomen). The development of three distinct contrasts (arterial, venous, and dynamic) is useful for accurate interpretation. In Switzerland, whole-body PMCTA was reported using a roller

pump, while automated CPR techniques were reported in other centers, e.g., UK and Japan [24].

Various CT scanners can be used in a whole body PMCT, such as a Toshiba Aquilion CXL 128 slice scanner (120 kVp, 300 mA, and 128 × 0.5-mm slice thickness, matrix 512 × 512). Reconstruction: head and neck: 1-mm. Chest, abdomen, pelvis, and legs: 2-mm slices [26].

38.11.1.3.1 CPR Techniques

Due to the absence of cardiovascular circulation, PMCTA with cardiopulmonary resuscitation (CPR) techniques was introduced mainly to examine the whole body vascularity. It creates an external mechanism to produce circulation. This artificially produced circulation is essential for the whole body's transport of contrast medium [7, 11]. CPR by using the Lucas machine is described as an adequate technique and helps to avoid high radiation doses for healthcare providers [24].

38.11.1.3.2 Accessing the Vascular System

Injecting contrast through the vascular system is essential. It can be approached by finding suitable access via the neck, axillary, femoral, or other upper or lower extremity vessels. However, sometimes the minor neck invasiveness may be noticed by the next of kin and cause potential troubles. Small vessels are found to be problematic in cannulation. The axillary vessels are preferable, fast, and considered the best option. Access can be achieved by the insertion of a T-shaped cannula, with a caliber between 16F (arterial) and 20F (venous), which permits complete perfusion [13, 24, 27].

An automatic pump injector via extremity venous access (most likely the cubital fossa) is also reported and found to be useful in sustaining enough contrast throughout the scan period [27].

38.11.1.4 Targeted Techniques

A targeted or limited study technique has been developed and found to be helpful in investigating unexplained natural or sudden death cases, especially when an autopsy is not preferable or required. Cardiac and peripheral angiographies are two examples of targeted PMCTA. However, there are some limitations in diagnosing intraplaque pathology and plaque hemorrhage [25].

38.11.1.4.1 Cardiac Angiography

Method

Contrast administration must be immediate and continuous, just before and during the scan period. This helps maintain significant vessel lumen distension. A modified 14-Ch Foley urinary catheter is advanced down to the ascending aorta. Raising the body under the mortuary block is helpful and found to be useful in positioning the catheter. After approximately 20 cm of catheter insertion, particularly if no resistance is felt, the catheter is most likely to advanced sufficiently [13, 25].

This could be achieved by:

1. Right axillary artery insertion, aiming to position the tip of the catheter above the aortic valve, adjacent to the coronary ostia.
2. Neck dissection, access via the left common carotid artery has a higher success rate than the right. Just above the medial aspect of the left clavicular head is the incision place of choice.
3. Balloon inflation is required to prevent back contrast flow [13, 25].

Precaution
1. Vein dissection may lead to significant blood loss.
2. Avoid catheter advancement into the descending aorta.

In certain suspicious coronary artery diseases, two arterial phases are recommended: supine and prone. This provides sufficient ventral aortic root filling (in the supine) as well as sufficient right coronary artery perfusion [13].

Positive Contrast and Air (Negative Contrast)
Substances alter the X-ray beam attenuation by either increasing or decreasing, and are known as contrast agents. Positive contrast agents appear white because they increase beam attenuation. Gas and fat appear black and are of low attenuation on PMCT. Air is simply known as negative contrast. In the UK, Oxford and Leicester apply targeted coronary PMCTA. The deliberate use of both negative (air) and positive contrasts was developed by the Leicester Group. This improves the study of coronary filling defects. Nevertheless, both Oxford and Leicester techniques identify significant ischemic heart diseases adequately [24].

Compared to positive contrast, air contrast provides additional details for assessing small myocardial vessels. A maximum volume of 400 ml can be injected using standard CT pump injectors, which is considered a limitation. Another disadvantage is time, requiring about five extra minutes per case [27].

Usage of a Medrad Stellant Pump Injector System
The uses of a Medrad stellant pump injector system (Medrad UK Ltd., UK) for targeted PMCTA are as follows:

- One to two syringes can be used to load the pump.
- A connector tube is used to link the pump and syringes to the catheter.
- Injected volume and rate are set as follows: likely 6 ml/s for 300 ml of air and 3 ml/s for 150 ml of fluid contrast.
- Firstly, air contrast: an air syringe of 150 ml is connected via T-connector tubing to both syringes. Five milliliter of air must be advanced out as a precaution.
- Forty-eight seconds is the ideal injecting time.
- Water-soluble iodinated contrast media injection runs after air.
- The use of 150 ml of 1:10 diluted Urografin® (Bayer Healthcare) is reported.
- Advance plunger: To get rid of air and fill the contrast within the connector tube.
- The Foley catheter is attached to the connector tubes. A plastic connector of choice is a double Christmas tree connector or a double reducing connector [27].

38.11.1.4.2 Peripheral Angiography

The most common indications of peripheral angiography are

1. Arterial trauma
2. Signs of vascular injury, e.g., extravasation
3. Bone or soft tissue injury
4. DVT which is limited due to venous valve function [13]

38.11.1.5 Ventilation Technique

In PMCT, the lungs appear densely opaque. Thus, the interpretation of the imaging is extremely nondiagnostic due to normal postmortem changes or internal lividities [28].

In order to get reasonable diagnostic images, lung expansion is successfully achieved. This is achieved by ventilated postmortem computed tomography (VPMCT). It improves the detection of pulmonary diseases by lowering the density or ground glass attenuation of the dependent parts. Consequently, the pulmonary pathologic changes—for example, consolidations, pulmonary nodules, and septal thickening—become clearer for detection [26, 29].

An endotracheal tube, a larynx mask, or a continuous positive airway pressure (c-PAP) mask are required for VPMCT. In order to have good PMCT image quality, both preliminary non-VPMCT and VPMCT of 40 mbar (40.8 cm H_2O) are recommended. Segmentation software can be used to measure lung volumes. Postmortem ventilation at 40 mbar has been chosen because it induces dramatic lung unfolding. This is found to be a mean volume increase of 1.32 L. 40 mbar has been chosen as a standard in VPMCT due to the reduction of internal livores [29].

Back in 2014, the previous work of Germerott et al. was expanded by the PMCT research group in Leicester. They used a Dräger Savina 300 ventilator (Dräger, UK) in positive end-expiratory pressure (PEEP) mode with a constant 40 cm H_2O (equivalent to 40 mbar) of pressure. PEEP mode on the ventilator simulates clinical inspiratory lung imaging [30].

A breathhold can be achieved by using a certain setting in a spontaneous–continuous positive airway pressure ventilator. This maintains continuous airway pressure [26].

Surgical tracheostomy airways may be used in ventilation if present from the antemortem period.

Definitive airway insertion may be performed in two ways: orally or through a tracheostomy. An endotracheal tube or cuffed tracheostomy tube would produce good sealing throughout the ventilation period. Blind or direct vocal cord visualization may be applied in oral insertion [26].

A standard tracheostomy tube or shortened ET tube may be used with a tracheostomy incision. The insertion of a shortened endotracheal tube (ETT) through a tracheostomy is the easiest technique. Direct laryngeal visualization is a useful alternative if blind intubation fails. A fiber optic laryngoscope can be easily applied in nonstiff cases. An Airtraq optical laryngoscope may be applied if tooth gap is present and is found to be more useful than the traditional laryngoscope. If needed, intubation with a Bougie endotracheal tube (ET) tube and Magill intubation forceps may be used. A photo/video borescope with a 5.5-mm detachable camera improves vocal cord visualization in difficult cases. The bore diameter of 5.5 mm is another option to introduce the borescope down [26]. An 8.0-mm-diameter endotracheal tube provides an adequate "air seal" [28].

38.11.1.5.1 Devices Used in Ventilation
1. Home care ventilator: Draeger, Hemel Hempstead, UK
2. Pertrach Cric/tracheostomy device: Portex® Blue Line Ultra®
3. A *Dräger Savina 300* ventilator [26, 28, 30]

38.11.1.5.2 Challenges
1. Key problem: Head and neck rigor causing difficult intubation.
2. Balloon rupture (major technical problem).
3. Inadequate balloon sealing (minor technical problem).
4. Inadequate lung expansion.
5. Gastric distension.
6. Failure to maintain 40 mbar ventilation pressure.
7. Apparent diminished heart diameter.
8. Inadequate positioning of ETT and esophageal intubation.
9. Surgical emphysema.
10. Pneumothoraces, new or enlarged [26, 28–30].

38.12 Overall Limitations of PMCT

Despite all advantages of the PMCT in investigating the cause of death in both forensic and natural death investigations, there are some limitations. Due to the PM changes such as autolysis and putrefaction, the image quality of PMCT degrades as the PM interval increases. Hence, the diagnostic ability of the PM imaging is directly proportional to the level of decomposition and the PM interval. Several unique artifacts can potentially mimic or mask underlying disease processes. These artifacts, if not well recognized, may lead to misdiagnosis or false interpretations. Subluxation at the craniocervical and atlanto-axial articulations, hematocrit formation, pulmonary lividity, and pseudo-subarachnoid hemorrhage are examples of artifacts that are commonly seen in PM imaging and could be easily misdiagnosed by an inexperienced physician [31].

38.13 Advanced PM Imaging Modality

We also recommend considering PM-MRI for the purpose of having comprehensive PM facilities and for its significant applications in PM investigations including child abuse, strangulation, organ lesions, and skeletal age estimation [10].

38.14 Conclusion

The PM imaging service has already been perfectly planned, founded, and applied in Abu Dhabi, the capital of the UAE. This facility has excellent cultural and religious acceptance. The operation of the PM imaging service is ready for advanced technique updates and is almost fully established. In order to achieve high-quality image standards, infection control, and radiation protection in the working environment, standard operating procedures and appropriate policies and protocols are arranged with the stakeholders, as they would be applied in crime lab facilities [13]. Artifacts in PM imaging are challenging and can easily mislead an inexperienced radiologist [31].

Conflicts of Interest   The author has no conflicts of interest to declare.

References

1. Abu Dhabi Media Office. Department of Health Abu Dhabi introduces virtual autopsy for mortuary investigations. Abu Dhabi Media Office. February 29, 2024. https://www.mediaoffice.abudhabi/en/health/department-of-health-abu-dhabi-introduces-virtual-autopsy-for-mortuary-investigations/.
2. 2015–16 VIFM annual report. 2016. https://www.vifm.org/wp-content/uploads/VIFM-Annual-Report-2015-16.pdf [cited 01 July 2024].
3. Alhamoodi M. Naif Al Janahi is the first Emirati consultant doctor in "digital anatomy" [In Arabic]. Aletihad News Center. 2022 [cited 13 October 2023].
4. 474 M Dirhams for 8 AD Police new constrictive buildings in Abu Dhabi [Internet]. Wam. 2019 [cited 24 December 2019]. Available from: http://wam.ae/ar/details/1395302727438.
5. Statistical Year of Abu Dhabi 2023/Population and Demography [Internet]. Scad.gov.abudhabi. 2024 [cited 01 July 2024]. Available from: https://scad.gov.ae/web/guest/w/statistics-centre-abu-dhabi-reports-results-of-abu-dhabi-census-2023.
6. Population and demographic mix – The Official Portal of the UAE Government [Internet]. Government.ae. 2019 [cited 24 December 2019]. Available from: https://government.ae/en/information-and-services/social-affairs/preserving-the-emirati-national-identity/population-and-demographic-mix.
7. Almasad M, Alshuwaier M. The forensic decisions of the Great Fiqh Scholars [Arabic version]. 2003. [online] Repository.nauss.edu.sa. Available at: https://repository.nauss.edu.sa/handle/123456789/51523. Accessed 24 Dec 2019.
8. Prosecution [Internet]. Adjd.gov.ae. 2019 [cited 24 December 2019]. Available from: https://www.adjd.gov.ae/EN/Pages/Prosecution.aspx.
9. Mortuary Services FAQs [Internet]. Health Authority of Abu Dhabi. 2019 [cited 24 December 2019]. Available from: https://www.haad.ae/haad/tabid/1468/Default.aspx.
10. Grabherr S, Baumann P, Minoiu C, Fahrni S, Mangin P. Post-mortem imaging in forensic investigations: current utility, limitations, and ongoing developments. Res Rep Forensic Med Sci. 2016;6:25–37.
11. Levy AD, Harcke HT Jr, Mallak CT. Essentials of forensic imaging : a text-atlas. Baton Rouge: CRC Press LLC; 2010.
12. Robinson C, Deshpande A, Richards C, Rutty G, Mason C, Morgan B. Post-mortem computed tomography in adult non-suspicious death investigation—evaluation of an NHS based service. BJR|Open. 2019;1(1):20190017.
13. Thali MJ, Viner MD, Brogdon BG. Brogdon's forensic radiology. Baton Rouge: CRC Press LLC; 2010.

14. Applications of Radiography for Forensic Purposes | Society of Radiographers [Internet]. Sor.org. 2019 [cited 24 December 2019]. Available from: https://www.sor.org/learning/document-library/guidance-radiographers-providing-forensic-radiography-services/3-applications-radiography-forensic.
15. Goldman LW. Principles of CT: radiation dose and image quality. J Nucl Med Technol. 2007;35(4):213–25.
16. Mustapha ZP, Allisy-Roberts J. Williams Farr's physics for medical imaging. 2nd ed.; 2008. 978-0-7020-2844-1, 207 pp, p. e158-e.
17. Huda W. Review of radiologic physics. Lippincott Williams & Wilkins; 2010.
18. Mildenberger P, Eichelberg M, Martin E. Introduction to the DICOM standard. Eur Radiol. 2002;12(4):920–7.
19. Bankman I. Handbook of medical image processing and analysis. Elsevier; 2008.
20. Mustra M, Delac K, Grgic M, editors. Overview of the DICOM standard. 2008 50th international symposium ELMAR, 10–12 September 2008.
21. Rutty GN, Morgan B, Robinson C, Raj V, Pakkal M, Amoroso J, et al. Diagnostic accuracy of post-mortem CT with targeted coronary angiography versus autopsy for coroner-requested post-mortem investigations: a prospective, masked, comparison study. Lancet. 2017;390(10090):145–54.
22. Grabherr S, Djonov V, Yen K, Thali MJ, Dirnhofer R. Postmortem angiography: review of former and current methods. Am J Roentgenol. 2007;188(3):832–8.
23. Ross S, Spendlove D, Bolliger S, Christe A, Oesterhelweg L, Grabherr S, et al. Postmortem whole-body CT angiography: evaluation of two contrast media solutions. Am J Roentgenol. 2008;190(5):1380–9.
24. Rutty GN. Essentials of autopsy practice: advances, updates and emerging technologies. London: Springer; 2013.
25. Grabherr S, Grimm J, Heinemann A. Atlas of postmortem angiography. Cham: Springer; 2016.
26. Rutty GN, Biggs MJP, Brough A, Robinson C, Mistry R, Amoroso J, et al. Ventilated post-mortem computed tomography through the use of a definitive airway. Int J Legal Med. 2015;129(2):325–34.
27. Robinson C, Barber J, Amoroso J, Morgan B, Rutty G. Pump injector system applied to targeted post-mortem coronary artery angiography. Int J Legal Med. 2013;127(3):661–6.
28. Arthurs OJ, Guy A, Kiho L, Sebire NJ. Ventilated postmortem computed tomography in children: feasibility and initial experience. Int J Legal Med. 2015;129(5):1113–20.
29. Germerott T, Flach PM, Preiss US, Ross SG, Thali MJ. Postmortem ventilation: a new method for improved detection of pulmonary pathologies in forensic imaging. Legal Med. 2012;14(5):223–8.
30. Rutty GN, Morgan B, Germerott T, Thali M, Athurs O. Ventilated post-mortem computed tomography – a historical review. J Forensic Radiol Imaging. 2016;4:35–42.
31. Sutherland T, O'Donnell C. The artefacts of death: CT post-mortem findings. J Med Imaging Radiat Oncol. 2018;62(2):203–10. https://doi.org/10.1111/1754-9485.12691.

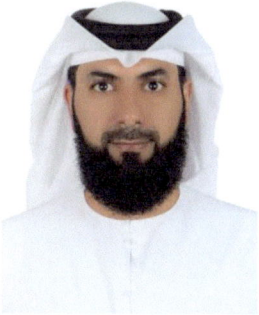

Dr. Muhammad Al Shirawi is an Emirati-registered medical expert/physician specializing in postmortem imaging and artificial intelligence (AI) in forensic death investigation. He founded his path in medicine by joining the medical school at the Royal College of Surgeons in Ireland (RCSI) in 2001. After his graduation from RCSI in June 2008, he joined the medical staff of Waterford University Hospital, where he showed his interest in radiology. In 2010, he was selected for a certain training program in forensic radiology. In order to achieve this goal, Dr. Al Shirawi was among those who joined the training course in virtopsy (virtual autopsy) at the University of Zurich in 2014. In 2015 and 2018, he was employed and joined the radiology staff at Alfred

Hospital in Australia. In 2021, he obtained an MSc in postmortem imaging for natural and forensic death investigations from the University of Leicester (UK). In May 2024, he joined the Victorian Institute of Forensic Medicine in Melbourne (Australia) as an International Fellow in Postmortem Radiology.

Since 2008, Dr. Al Shirawi has obtained several medals and badges of appreciation and excellence, including six first-class medals. Also, he received three awards for creative ideas in the field of his career in Abu Dhabi.

Open Access This chapter is licensed under the terms of the Creative Commons Attribution 4.0 International License (http://creativecommons.org/licenses/by/4.0/), which permits use, sharing, adaptation, distribution and reproduction in any medium or format, as long as you give appropriate credit to the original author(s) and the source, provide a link to the Creative Commons license and indicate if changes were made.

The images or other third party material in this chapter are included in the chapter's Creative Commons license, unless indicated otherwise in a credit line to the material. If material is not included in the chapter's Creative Commons license and your intended use is not permitted by statutory regulation or exceeds the permitted use, you will need to obtain permission directly from the copyright holder.

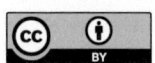

Evolution of Surgery in the UAE

39

Sara Al Bastaki, Zakir K. Mohamed, Nahla Al Mansoori, Ali Al Hassani, Zialyazan Sabbagh, and Hisham Hurreiz

39.1 Introduction

The father of modern surgery, Ambroise Pare, said: "There are five duties of surgery: to remove what is superfluous, to restore what has been dislocated, to separate what has grown together, to reunite what has been divided, and to redress the defects of nature" [1]. This definition of surgery holds well even today, some 500 years after Ambroise Pare's famous words.

S. Al Bastaki (✉)
President of Emirates Society of Colon & Rectal Surgery (ESCRS), Dubai, UAE

Consultant Colorectal Surgeon, Mediclinic City Hospital & Airport Road, Dubai/Abu Dhabi, UAE

Emirates Medical Association, EMA, Dubai, UAE

Z. K. Mohamed
Vice President of Emirates Society of Colon & Rectal Surgery (ESCRS), regional medical director at NMC healthcare, Dubai, UAE

Regional Medical Director & Consultant Colorectal Surgeon, NMC Healthcare, Dubai, UAE

N. Al Mansoori
Head of Department Plastic and reconstructive Surgery, Health Point/M42, Abu Dhabi, UAE

A. Al Hassani
Head of Department of General Surgery, Sheikh Khalifa Medical City, Abu Dhabi, UAE
e-mail: ahasani@seha.ae

Z. Sabbagh
Trauma Medical Director, NMC Royal Hospital, Abu Dhabi, UAE

H. Hurreiz
Consultant General Surgeon, Sheikh Khalifa Medical City, Abu Dhabi, UAE
e-mail: hhurreiz@seha.ae

© The Author(s) 2025
H. O. Al-Shamsi (ed.), *Healthcare in the United Arab Emirates*,
https://doi.org/10.1007/978-981-96-0523-1_39

The journey of modern healthcare in the United Arab Emirates (UAE) started with Al Maktoum Hospital opening in Dubai in 1951. In the 1970s, it became the first hospital to have a surgical department in the city. The unit consisted of 12 male surgical beds and 12 beds for women and children.

"We were doing all kinds of surgeries except thoracic surgery," Dr. Abd Al Nabi Al Redha, the first Emirati surgeon and the director of Rashid Hospital from 1982 to 2002, revealed. Furthermore, he was one of only two surgeons leading the surgical department at Al Maktoum Hospital, alongside one anesthetist and one house officer. The two surgeons were receiving patients who needed surgical intervention not only from the Northern Emirates but also from other Gulf Cooperation Council (GCC) areas such as Oman, and these were managed successfully.

Sheikh Hamdan bin Rashid Al Maktoum, may his soul rest in peace, had a clear vision and determination to develop the healthcare sector. Hence, in the early 1970s, he encouraged and supported the youth to become physicians by providing scholarships. Four of those Emirati doctors who benefited from this program were Dr. Abd Al-Nabi Al Redha, Dr. Saeed Jaffar, Dr. Mirza Ali, and Dr. Abdulla Al Khayat. All four were sent to the UK to pursue their postgraduate studies. On his return, Dr. Abd Al Nabi introduced major surgeries such as Heller myotomies, gastrectomies, and Whipple surgeries.

In 1973, Rashid Hospital opened its doors to further expand in surgical services. The surgical workforce later grew with the addition of two more surgeons to the existing team. Soon, there were 25 to 30 beds in both the men's and women's wards of Rashid Hospital. It also became the main center for trauma in the region.

For the first three decades after the hospital was established, general surgeons were still managing most of the subspecialty cases, that included urology, vascular surgery, and neurosurgery, as was the practice in most parts of the world.

As subspecialties started to evolve in the late 1970s, Rashid Hospital added neurosurgery, urology, and orthopedics departments, along with other subspecialties. Dr. Ahmed Kazim, the first Emirati orthopedic surgeon, joined Rashid Hospital in 1977, while upper and lower GI endoscopy procedures began in 1975 at the same hospital.

It was a time for expansion, and at the start of the 1980s, Latifa and Dubai Hospital began operations. Consequently, some subspecialties, such as obstetrics and gynecology, moved from Rashid to Latifa Hospital. Meanwhile, Dubai Hospital built a thoracic surgery department and recruited a thoracic surgeon. General surgeons were now able to focus their practice on visceral and endocrine surgeries.

In the early 1990s, the first laparoscopic cholecystectomy was performed at Rashid Hospital by Dr. Abdul Nabi. He trained two consultants in minimally invasive surgery, and in turn, they trained another two consultants. Soon after, a training program was rolled out at the hospital to train future surgeons.

39.2 Women in Surgery

The entry of women surgeons was a challenge, especially in the early days when women had to literally swim against the tide to navigate their way to success and build a career in a male-dominated field. This myth was soon shattered by Dr. Houriya Kazim, the first Emirati woman surgeon.

Despite the challenges, Dr. Kazim, a doctor on a mission, pushed forward to overcome all odds and succeed, not only in her own practice but also in laying the foundation and blueprint for the success of all female surgeons in the UAE. According to the author's knowledge, her pioneering role created a path for others to follow. It was a milestone. Since then, there has been no looking back for women surgeons in this progressive city, where they have a very strong and unique presence with professional skills that match the best in the world.

Surgery continues to evolve in the UAE, and procedures once considered "lengthy" and "larger" have now come to be regarded as "day cases" and "minimal." Based on the author's knowledge and experience, subspecialties became more focused, and centers of excellence were established. Open, conventional surgeries decreased significantly in favor of minimally invasive surgery. Robotics is now becoming more prominent in all surgical fields.

With changes in lifestyle, there has been and will be an inevitable increase in the prevalence of colon and rectal cancers. Dr. Sara Al Bastaki, the first Emirati-certified colorectal woman surgeon, founded the Emirates Society of Colon and Rectal Surgery in the UAE. The Society aims to educate and exchange experiences to promote a culture of excellence, best practices, and quality care, both locally and internationally. These distinguished efforts by society have significantly improved cancer screening, early detection, quality of treatment, and survival rates for many patients.

In this chapter, we will cover many striking topics in all aspects of surgery, taking you with us on our evolutionary journey in the UAE through the years.

39.3 Breast Cancer Care in the UAE

Surgery for diseases of the breast is a sensitive topic the world over. In this part of the world, because of certain cultural norms, breast cancer surgery has often become more complex than it really is. Young women diagnosed with breast cancer find their lives virtually grinding to a halt, though they can lead a normal life after successful treatment. Therefore, apart from proper surgery for breast cancer, it is of utmost importance to sensitize the general population about breast cancer as a disease that is, like any other, treatable.

Now let us look at the history of breast cancer surgery in the UAE. Until the late 1990s, surgery for breast cancer was part of the general surgical domain. Thereafter, it became a subspecialty in itself in the developed world. Dr. Houriya Kazim recalls how it was almost by chance that she ended up in a subspecialty breast surgery training program after her surgical training in the 1980s in the UK.

A stressful interview at one of the UK's leading centers for oncology, the Royal Marsden Hospital in London, was followed by an unexpected offer of a job to a young, unassuming Arab doctor. This offer forced Dr. Kazim to choose the first specialty that was shown to her in a list. Thus, it happened that she chose to specialize in breast cancer.

Dr. Kazim moved back to the UAE in 1998 after completing her advanced training in breast cancer surgery. She then tried to convince multiple hospitals to set up a dedicated breast cancer service. Finally, she succeeded and started this department at Dubai's Welcare Hospital in 1999. She followed this up by setting up the Friends of Cancer Patients charity and the Brest Friends charity in 2000 at the same hospital.

Dubai's super-specialty Rashid Hospital was also working towards a dedicated breast cancer service, which took a couple of years to bear fruit. In 2004, the hospital set up its first breast cancer program and flagged off its social awareness campaign alongside its Pink program under Dr. Rolf Hartung and Dr. Zaid Al Mazem. They were subsequently joined by Dr. Esaaf Hasan Ghazi, who now heads the unit in Dubai Hospital and is another pioneer Emirati woman breast surgeon. The southern emirates of Abu Dhabi and Al Ain also saw similar trends with the setting up of their first breast cancer units in 1999, spearheaded by Dr. Mouza Al Ameri, another Emirati surgeon. According to the author's knowledge, these milestones marked the true beginning of organized breast cancer care in the UAE, with Emirati women surgeons playing a central role.

The recognition of breast surgery as a subspecialty came about as a result of two fundamental changes in how services were delivered, namely "one-stop" or triple testing model and the MDT (Multidisciplinary Team) approach to treatment. The one-stop clinic concept presented an anxious patient with the facility of having a suspicious breast mass examined by an expert doctor, followed by radiology imaging and a biopsy, if needed, all on the same day. This was then followed by another appointment to discuss biopsy results, if necessary.

The concept of the one-stop clinic gave a sense of reassurance to a large proportion of the women who would visit the clinic with concerns about their health. They were diagnosed on the same day with the MDT approach, ensuring the right treatment. Regular auditing of the unit's performance against a set of established standards was another reassuring factor for these women.

In the 1990s, the focus of cancer treatment evolved to include reconstructive surgery. This was a significant development as it helped to give women the confidence of a normal appearance, which is very important for the rehabilitation of patients. Breast oncoplastic surgery is now the purview of a dual-trained physician who treats cancer and is also trained in plastic surgery. This treatment has now become the norm in the UAE and can be considered a landmark in breast cancer surgery, placing the Emirates on par with the developed world.

Surgeons vividly recall the early challenges of breast cancer screening programs. The local population was hesitant to come forward for a physical examination. Cultural challenges were a roadblock and prevented the communication of the importance of breast self-examination to young women. Moreover, there were legal challenges in developing the required teaching materials. The confiscation of self-breast examination videos and literature by customs officers, who mistook these teaching aids as explicit content, is an example of the lack of awareness of breast cancer among officials. Developing such material in a culturally sensitive way took a lot of creative thinking by the early pioneers in this field.

The advent of the Pink campaign and Brest Friends helped take the initiative forward. Latifa Hospital's dedicated Center for Cancer Awareness promoted the interaction and education of women in the community. The facility is run by cancer survivors who have now become champions of cancer eradication. This success is a testimonial to the efforts of all the clinicians who have helped transform the landscape of breast surgery in the UAE. Based on author's observation and knowledge, these efforts are critical in shaping culturally appropriate breast cancer awareness programs that continue to benefit the UAE population today.

39.4 Evolution of Trauma Care in the UAE

As 10% of the world's oil was discovered in the UAE in the early 1960s, its development was assured. The UAE has since diversified its economy to become a major industrial, tourism, trade, and financial hub. The population has multiplied, mainly due to the immigration of expatriate workers. According to the last census, the UAE's population in 2010 was estimated at 8.19 million and is expected to double by 2029 [2, 8].

As part of the modernization program of the country, a wide network of roads was established, resulting in a significant rise in the use of high-speed vehicles. As the economy continues to expand year after year, it must be matched with a robust labor force to fill critical jobs across multiple industries. Despite the implementation of a standardized approach to managing occupational health and safety (OHS) risks, work accidents have risen.

In order to address this problem, it became critical to establish trauma centers to manage the rising incidence of accidents [4].

Moreover, the phenomenal increase in the number of motor vehicles, keeping pace with development, has resulted in a near epidemic of traumatic injuries and deaths due to road traffic crashes (RTCs). In addition to work accidents and road accidents, domestic accidents have also risen.

The combination of these three categories of accidents has placed a tremendous burden on the healthcare system and, to a significant extent, on the economy as well. In fact, trauma-related injuries have become the leading cause of disability and the second highest cause of death in the UAE [2].

39.5 Trauma Care

Trauma patients in the UAE are younger than those in North America, reflecting differences in demographics. The median age of trauma patients in the UAE is 30 years, compared with 37 years in North America [3]. Major trauma injuries have the potential to lead to prolonged disability or, eventually, death. Major trauma injuries can be classified as blunt and penetrating and may be caused by falls, road accidents, or injuries caused by machines in factories [2].

In the UAE, most trauma patients sustain blunt mechanisms of injury, as penetrating trauma is rare. According to the World Health Organization, residents of the UAE, with 32 deaths per 100,000 population, are seven times more likely to die in a car crash than citizens of the United Kingdom (4 deaths per 100,000 inhabitants) [5]. Since the 1980s, motor vehicle crashes have been the second most common cause of death in the UAE after cardiovascular diseases. This figure has been increasing steadily. The authorities are introducing more stringent highway safety laws and have plans to impose stricter fines for speeding. These measures are expected to limit the danger of road accidents [4].

Sheikh Khalifa Medical City and Mafraq Hospital in Abu Dhabi, Tawam and Al Ain Hospital in Al Ain, and Rashid Hospital Trauma Center in Dubai are now designated as regional trauma hospitals [6].

In the beginning, trauma care in the UAE was based on individual initiative within the facility. Each hospital's trauma unit worked closely with divisions like general surgery, emergency, and orthopedics. Now, trauma has become more specialized with the creation of a separate division of trauma and acute care, which has its own trauma committee, overseeing trauma care locally, and launching a trauma registry.

The first local trauma registry was started in Al Ain Hospital in 2003 after two years of preparation by the Trauma Group [5]. The studied variables included age, gender, nationality, mechanism and location of injury, method of transportation, physiological and anatomical severity markers, Injury Severity Score (ISS), New Injury Severity Score (NISS), Glasgow Coma Scale (GCS), ICU admission, length of hospital stay, and clinical outcome [6, 7].

The Abu Dhabi Health Authority introduced the Abu Dhabi Trauma Initiative in 2009, and one of its important achievements was the launch of the Trauma Registry in 2014 [4, 6].

Dubai Health Authority's (DHA) Trauma and Emergency Centre at Rashid Hospital was featured in 2011 as one of the top 10 among more than 300 trauma centers that form the biggest poly trauma registry in Germany [11].

To optimize the outcome of initial resuscitation performed on severely injured patients, trauma care should be delivered only by qualified and trained providers following the guidelines of the Advanced Trauma Life Support® (ATLS) course developed by the ACS, which is regarded as the gold standard for care in trauma resuscitation. The ATLS program was first established in 2004 [12]. Participants trained under the Introduction to ATLS program significantly improved their trauma care services [4]. Physicians from different specialties were able to speak the same language and provide the best protocol for trauma management to their patients.

The trauma care system has gradually moved from the individual center initiative developed in Abu Dhabi's SKMC, Mafraq, and SSMC Hospital; Al-Ain's Tawam and Al Ain Hospital; Rashid Hospital in Dubai; and Al-Qasimi Hospital in Sharjah; as well as other hospitals in the North Emirates to the newer trauma system initiative led by the Department of Health Abu Dhabi, Dubai Health Authority, and the Ministry of Health.

A trauma system for the Emirate of Abu Dhabi is being developed, with plans to extend it to the whole of the UAE over the next decade [10]. The Abu Dhabi Trauma Initiative (2009–2016) led to the formation of the Trauma Committee at the Department of Health (DOH). This project viewed trauma care more holistically and began with extensive guidelines on how to prevent accidents and, of course, focused on treatment modalities from the time of injury through rehabilitation. The initiative follows guidelines provided by the Committee on Trauma of the American College of Surgeons [9].

Several success stories have already left a mark: the introduction of injury prevention programs, efficient prehospital response, the launch of a trauma registry, and the development of Trauma Centre of Excellence, such as Sheikh Shakhbout Medical City (SSMC), among other programs.

With the development of healthcare facilities, trauma care in the UAE has undergone tremendous change, especially with the implementation of advanced diagnostic and therapeutic technology that has significantly improved the outcomes of trauma management.

The accessibility of different diagnostic tools in UAE hospitals, such as FAST (Focused Assessment with Sonography in Trauma) and whole-body trauma CT scans, has played a major role in the early recognition of life-threatening conditions.

Trauma care has remarkably benefited from the introduction of efficient resuscitation and hemorrhage control, including the massive transfusion protocol (MTP), using hemostatic compounds, different minimally invasive tools like angiographic embolization of bleeding, and endovascular procedures.

The establishment of angiosuites in large centers in the UAE made procedures like embolization of bleeding vessels in trauma feasible. These have been widely used to control bleeding in serious injury cases like retroperitoneal bleeding, uncontrolled hemorrhage in pelvic fractures, liver injury, splenic injury, and stenting of large bleeding vessels.

Trauma centers, once established, led to a reduction in the number of open surgeries performed to control bleeding. The presence of a well-equipped ICU, particularly a surgical ICU, facilitated the implementation of advanced conservative treatment for spleen, liver, kidney, and lung injuries.

Laparoscopy, vacuum-assisted closure devices, and organ support have been widely adopted in trauma management.

Trauma care has come a long way in a comparatively short period of time in the UAE. It is now considered advanced, both in terms of its specialized training programs and systems of care.

39.6 The Evolution of Minimally Invasive Surgery in the UAE

Rapid growth and development in the healthcare system in the UAE since its union have been mirrored by an equally rapid evolution in healthcare technology and innovation.

Minimally invasive surgery was first introduced in Abu Dhabi at the old Jazeera Hospital when the first laparoscopic cholecystectomy was performed in November 1991 by an Emirati team with help from Dr. John Saunders from Edinburgh; the surgery was supported by Olympus. In Dubai, the first laparoscopic cholecystectomy was performed at Rashid Hospital. Laparoscopic surgery gradually became more popular and was introduced in other hospitals in the UAE, with Saqer Hospital in Ras Al Khaimah starting laparoscopic cholecystectomies in late 1998.

More general surgeons soon developed an interest in laparoscopy during that period, with many traveling abroad for further training and returning to establish minimally invasive units. In addition, they trained junior colleagues back in the UAE, and the number of surgeons well-versed in laparoscopic surgery grew steadily. This led to an exponential rise in the number of cases performed, with new procedures such as laparoscopic appendectomies and hernia operations being added.

The UAE made giant strides in the adoption of laparoscopic procedures in the Gulf, ahead of other countries in the Middle East. By the late 1990s, many more medical facilities in Abu Dhabi, Dubai, and the northern Emirates were performing laparoscopy regularly, with laparoscopic cholecystectomy becoming routine. The road had been paved for the introduction of laparoscopy in other specialties, and gynecologists also began using diagnostic laparoscopy techniques with help from their general surgery colleagues before performing them independently, widening the scope to include operations such as laparoscopic hysterectomy and surgery to remove tubes and ovaries.

By the beginning of the new century, minimally invasive surgery was well established in the UAE, with most major government and private hospitals having dedicated laparoscopic theatres. Major pharmaceutical companies also invested heavily in minimally invasive technology, alongside continued medical education and training of surgeons. Medical professionals also raised public awareness about the benefits of minimally invasive surgery over traditional open surgery.

Soon, the scope of laparoscopy was extended to include procedures such as arthroscopy, sclerotherapy, and laser treatment for varicose veins; laser hemorrhoidectomy; video-assisted anal fistula surgery (VAAFT); minimally invasive thyroidectomy; and minimally invasive surgery for pilonidal disease, which has become routine over the last couple of years, as well as other surgical subspecialties. In author's point of view, the rapid adoption of minimally invasive surgery across the Emirates reflects the UAE's commitment to innovation and training, with outcomes now comparable to international benchmarks.

Worldwide, laparoscopic techniques were being used to treat obesity-related issues, and it was not long before the technique was adopted in the UAE for performing laparoscopic bariatric surgeries. The prevalence of obesity and obesity-related diseases in the UAE is among the highest in the world, and in 2004, the first major laparoscopic bariatric operation was performed in Abu Dhabi, followed by another in Dubai in the same year [20]. The common procedures performed were laparoscopic sleeve gastrectomy and laparoscopic Roux-En-Y gastric bypass.

Prior to the introduction of these two procedures, a few private clinics in Abu Dhabi and Dubai were already performing laparoscopic adjustable gastric band surgery with varying results. Bariatric surgery quickly became very popular and attracted both media and public attention, not only because of its significantly superior results but also due to its sometimes potentially fatal complications. The increase in the number of these procedures led the authorities to act quickly, and new legislation was soon introduced by the Department of Health (DOH) in Abu Dhabi, the Dubai Health Authority (DHA), and the Ministry of Health (MOH) to regulate bariatric services in the country [12].

High-volume centers now exist in Abu Dhabi, Dubai, and Sharjah, both in the public and private sectors, where bariatric procedures such as sleeve gastrectomies, gastric bypass, laparoscopic adjustable gastric band, single anastomosis duodenal-ileal bypass (SADI), and single-anastomosis stomach-ileal bypass (SASI) were pioneered in Sharjah's Qasimi Hospital and have become established bariatric procedures worldwide. In addition to their clinical contributions, these centers are hubs of significant research activity, with numerous publications and presentations at international forums.

In 2018, Dubai hosted the highly successful 23rd World Congress of the International Federation for the Surgery of Obesity and Metabolic Disorders (IFSO), the largest and most important global bariatric conference [13]. This success in bariatric surgery was followed by the introduction of major laparoscopic resections in colorectal surgery in large centers as well as the establishment of single incision laparoscopic surgery (SILS) for a number of procedures such as appendectomy, cholecystectomy, hernia operations, and sleeve gastrectomy. In 2016, Tawam Hospital performed the first laparoscopic pancreatico-duodenectomy in the UAE. The unit has also performed laparoscopic gastrectomies for cancer in addition to launching the first bariatric fellowship in the country [21].

Laparoscopic pediatric surgery was initiated in Abu Dhabi in 2001 in collaboration with the pediatric surgical unit at Sheikh Khalifa Medical City (SKMC). In the same year, the first laparoscopic pediatric adrenalectomy was performed. Laparoscopic appendectomy and Nissen fundoplication were introduced thereafter.

By 2011, the unit was also performing laparoscopic hernia repair in children. In the same year, neonatal minimally invasive surgery was introduced at SKMC, with the team performing procedures such as thoracoscopic lung lobectomies and laparoscopic diaphragmatic hernia repair. Laparoscopic pediatric urology was introduced in 2014. The unit now performs pediatric urological procedures, including surgery for undescended testes, pyeloplasty, and ureteric re-implantation laparoscopically. It has emerged as a national and regional training center in the field. Many other pediatric surgical units in the country followed in the footsteps of SKMC.

Another major innovation in the field of minimally invasive surgery was the introduction of the Da Vinci robot in surgical practice. In 2014, the Ministry of Health and Prevention introduced its first robot to perform cardiac catheterizations at Al Qassimi Hospital in Sharjah [14]. The robot was upgraded in 2018 to carry out more complex cardiac catheterizations. Cleveland Clinic Abu Dhabi performed the first robotic hysterectomy in the UAE in 2018 [15].

The following year, the Ministry of Health and Prevention launched the robotic surgery program in gynecology and obstetrics. The launch came in the wake of the successful use of the robot in heart surgeries and its ability to access complicated parts of the human body. Al Qassimi Hospital was also the first in the UAE to use the Da Vinci robot to perform six successful bariatric operations in 2016 [22]. Many hospitals in the UAE have now invested in sophisticated robots to perform complex surgical procedures in gynecology, bariatrics, colorectal surgery, urology, and other specialties.

39.7 Plastic Surgery in the UAE

It was not until the mid-1980s that plastic surgery took off in the UAE. In the early years, cases that required plastic surgery, such as general trauma cases and burns, were handled by general surgeons, with some of the more complex cases being sent abroad, primarily to India and Germany.

By the early 1980s, the concept of plastic surgery had evolved in the region with the establishment of the Plastic Surgery Society (Gulf Plast) in Kuwait and Bahrain. The UAE was represented unofficially by Dr. Ali Al Numairi, who started off as a general surgeon, but whose interest in plastic surgery took him to Lyon in France [16]. He finally received his official plastic surgery certification only later in the 1990s. In 1993, he set up the Emirates Plastic Surgery Society. In 1996, he established the Gulf Speciality Hospital, Dubai's first specialized hospital for plastic surgery and laser surgery. He was among the first plastic surgeons from the Emirates to specialize in the field.

Also among the early pioneers was Dr. Khalil Saab [17], the current medical director and head plastic surgeon at the European Medical Center's Department of Aesthetic Surgery. In the mid-1980s, Dr. Saab operated from a small clinic in Dubai, which later became the foundation for Al Noor Hospital. At around the same time, Dr. Wang and Dr. Saleh Saad Kadhim were managing plastic surgery cases at Rashid Hospital in Dubai, while Dr. Hasan Fikki was making a name for himself in Abu Dhabi.

The late 1980s, 1990s, and onwards were a period of rapid growth in healthcare infrastructure in the UAE. Initially, a number of expatriate doctors were recruited, chief among them Dr. Ashok Govila, who became chief of plastic surgery at Mafraq Hospital in Abu Dhabi in 1993, and Dr. Sabet Salahia in Dubai in 1999, who later emerged as one of the main pillars of the CosmeSurge hospital group. Prof. Ashok Gupta started his practice in Dubai in 2000 and was awarded the H.H. Sheikh Hamdan International Award for Humanitarian Medical Services in 2010.

By the year 2000, our own Emirati doctors had also returned home with top qualifications from European and American universities to offer their services to hospitals that were being set up all over the Emirates. Among them were H.H. Sheikh

Dr. Saqer Almalla, Dr. Qassim Ahli, Dr. Marwan Al Zarouni, Dr. Zuhair Al-Fardan, and Dr. Buthainah Al Shunnar.

It was only in 1999 that the entire scenario began to change. The specialty became more specific and subspecialized, and with a team of well-qualified surgeons and state-of-the-art equipment, it was at last possible to treat complex cases that included microsurgery at our own Emirates' hospitals. All of a sudden, complicated microsurgeries were possible, such as those that helped salvage upper and lower extremities that would have otherwise been amputated. Dr. Thabet Salahia, along with Dr. Amna Belhoul, performed the first abdominoplasty in 1999. In 2002, Dr. Mark Hill and Dr. Khalid Alawadi performed the first microsurgical hand reimplantation and salvage. In the authors' observation, this period marked the true turning point when Emirati plastic surgeons established themselves as leaders in advanced reconstructive techniques, reducing dependence on treatment abroad and laying the foundation for the UAE's modern plastic surgery practice.

With their advanced, state-of-the-art services in plastic surgery, modern hospitals soon became household names for people looking for both reconstructive and cosmetic surgery. A Dubai Health Authority (DHA) report now states that the number of plastic surgeons in the Emirates is among the highest in the region, with 50 specialists per million people [23].

Over the next decade, plastic surgery in the UAE became more specific, and the demand for reconstructive surgery rose until it surpassed that for cosmetic surgery. The UAE now offers advanced plastic surgery including regenerative surgery using adipose stem cells for reconstruction. Post-burn and oncological resections and anti-aging treatments, orthoplastic and oncoplastic reconstructive surgery, genital reconstructive surgery, pediatrics congenital reconstructive surgery, and upper- and lower-extremity surgery are now available in the Emirates.

The concept of microsurgery allowed for more complex cases, including free flap tissue transfer for trauma cases, oncological reconstructive procedures, and supermicrosurgery for lymphovenous anastomosis to treat lymphedema.

Today, only a handful of patients are sent abroad for treatment, as almost all kinds of reconstructive procedures, including complex procedures involving the upper and lower extremities, are skillfully performed in the Emirates.

Most of the important hospitals in Dubai, Sharjah, and Abu Dhabi now have thriving departments of plastic surgery that offer life-saving correctional procedures, in addition to the ever-popular cosmetic and aesthetic surgery options aimed at improving a person's appearance. The demand for surgical procedures of the latter kind has been on the rise ever since 2000, as people now opt for anti-aging treatments as well as correctional plastic surgery for birth defects. A regular inflow of patients is now also seeking body-contouring and fat-reduction surgeries [18].

To the UAE's credit, many women doctors also began leaving a mark in the history of the Emirates' plastic surgery practice. Dr. Buthainah Al Shunnar became the first American board-certified plastic surgeon to perform free flap reconstructive surgery in 2002 with her team. In 2019, Dr. Nahla Almansoori became the first German Board-certified plastic surgeon to perform a lymphovenous anastomosis and lymph node transplant in the UAE, along with visiting surgeon Prof. J.P. Hong. In the authors' knowledge, these pioneering contributions by Emirati women surgeons not only advanced the practice of reconstructive surgery in the UAE but also set new benchmarks for female representation in a traditionally male-dominated specialty.

Dr. Sahar Al Kazzaz is another woman who made her mark in the field of plastic surgery. She earned a subspecialty degree in aesthetic surgery from the University of London's Queen Mary and Westfield College and became the first woman to receive an Appreciation Award in 2004 from the Emirates Plastic Surgery Society [19].

39.8 Conclusion

The UAE has recorded significant development in the complex field of surgery during the past few decades. However, its medical fraternity is not resting on its laurels but is constantly striving to enhance its skills in sync with the latest medical and technological developments, keeping pace with international standards.

Conflicts of Interest The authors have no conflicts of interest to declare.

References

1. https://hekint.org/2020/02/10/ambroise-pare-standard-bearer-for-barber-surgery-reform/amp/
2. United Arab Emirates. 2013. http://en.wikipedia.org/wiki/United_Arab_Emirates#cite_note-36
3. Regional Health Systems Observatory: United Arab Emirates: health system profile. EMRO, WHO. 2006. https://rho.emro.who.int/ar/per-country-uae
4. Fares S, Irfan FB, Corder RF, et al. Emergency medicine in The United Arab Emirates. Int J Emerg Med. 2014;7:4. https://doi.org/10.1186/1865-1380-7-4.
5. Trauma system developments reduce mortality in hospitalized trauma patients in Al-Ain City, United Arab Emirates, despite increased severity of injury David O. Alao, Arif Alper Cevik, Hani O. Eid, Zia Jummani & Fikri M. Abu-Zidan. https://doi.org/10.1186/s13017-020-00327-y
6. Shaban S, Ashour M, Bashir M, El-Ashaal Y, Branicki F, Abu-Zidan FM. The long-term effects of early analysis of a trauma registry. World J Emerg Surg. 2009; https://wjes.biomedcentral.com/articles/10.1186/1749-7922-4-42
7. Grivna M, Eid HO, Abu-Zidan FM. Epidemiology, morbidity and mortality from fall-related injuries in The United Arab Emirates. Scand J Trauma Resusc Emerg Med. 2014;22:51. https://doi.org/10.1097/MD.0000000000026258.
8. The Prospect Group: Healthcare in the United Arab Emirates (UAE). 2012. http://www.theprospectgroup.com/healthcare-in-the-united-arab-emirates-uae-81878
9. Griffiths JL, Estipona A, Waterson JA. A framework for physician activity during disasters and surge events. Am J Disaster Med. 2011;6(1):39–46. https://doi.org/10.1186/1865-1380-7-4.
10. Dubai centre features among top 10 in poly trauma registry In 2011, Rashid Hospital's Trauma and Emergency Centre became the first in the Middle East region to be included in this registry. https://www.khaleejtimes.com/health/dubai-centre-features-among-top-10-in-poly-trauma-registry
11. Alao DO, Cevik AA, Eid HO, et al. Trauma system developments reduce mortality in hospitalized trauma patients in Al-Ain City, United Arab Emirates, despite increased severity of injury. World J Emerg Surg. 2020;15:49. https://doi.org/10.1186/s13017-020-00327-y.

12. https://www.dha.gov.ae/uploads/112021/5aab17ca-d943-4ee3-a894-7f5dd6302397.pdf
13. https://ifso2018.com
14. https://www.emirates247.com/news/robot-cardiac-surgery-in-uae-s-al-qassimi-hospital-2014-09-06-1.561984
15. https://www.thenationalnews.com/uae/first-uae-robotic-surgery-performed-on-hysterectomy-patient-in-abu-dhabi-1.716530
16. https://en.wikipedia.org/wiki/Ali_Al_Numairy
17. https://emc.ae/profile/drkhalilsaab-plastic-surgeon-dubai/
18. https://www.asterhospital.com/blog/the-best-plastic-surgeons-in-dubai/
19. https://www.novomed.com/specialist/doctor/dr-sahar-al-kazzaz/
20. Mamdouh H, Hussain HY, Ibrahim GM, et al. Prevalence and associated risk factors of overweight and obesity among adult population in Dubai: a population-based cross-sectional survey in Dubai, The United Arab Emirates. BMJ Open. 2023;13(1):e062053. https://doi.org/10.1136/bmjopen-2022-062053.
21. https://www.thenationalnews.com/uae/health/abu-dhabi-doctors-break-ground-with-pancreatic-cancer-surgery-1.149050
22. https://gulfnews.com/uae/health/al-qasimi-hospital-performs-first-robotic-bariatric-surgery-1.1929070
23. https://gulfnews.com/amp/uae/health/dubai-is-the-new-beverly-hills-of-the-middle-east-heres-why-1.69023909

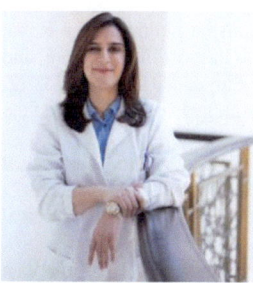

Sara Al Bastaki is a colorectal surgeon from the UAE. She completed her medical schooling at the Royal College of Surgeons of Ireland (RCSI). She continued her surgical residency program in Germany and subsequently completed her 3-year fellowship in colorectal surgery between Germany and London. She joined Sheikh Khalifa Medical City, Abu Dhabi, as a consultant colorectal surgeon, and in addition to that, she was elected president of the Emirates Society of Colon and Rectal Surgery (ESCRS).

Dr. Sara was appointed as Division Head of General Surgery in Sheikh Khalifa Medical City, Abu Dhabi. Since November 2023 Dr Sara Joined Mediclinic City Hosptial in Dubai and Mediclinic airport Road in Abu Dhabi. She chaired to establish clinical certificate in Robotic Surgery under the umbrella of NIHS.

Dr. Al Bastaki is specialized in laparoscopic surgery for benign and malignant colorectal diseases, management of low rectal cancer like TATME/TAMIS, and proctology.

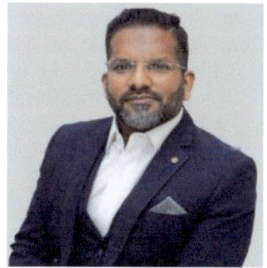

Dr. Zakir K. Mohamed is the Chief of Staff and Consultant Colorectal Surgeon at Mediclinic Parkview Hospital and the Vice President of the Emirates Society of Colorectal Surgeons.

He was Consultant Colorectal Surgeon at United Lincolnshire NHS Trust, following higher surgical training and CCT from Newcastle Deanery with Fellowships of the Royal College of Surgeons of England and Edinburgh.

He also served as an associate colorectal consultant at the University of Hong Kong and as a consultant at King Fahad Specialist Hospital, Dammam, before moving to the UAE.

His areas of interest are minimally invasive surgery for Colorectal Cancers and IBD, HIPEC, and PIPAC. He is also an Adjunct Associate Professor of Surgery at MBRU.

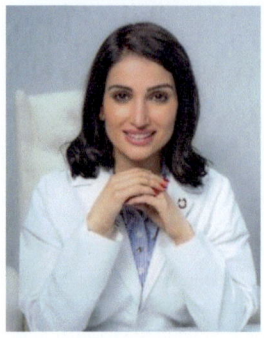

Dr. Nahla Al Mansoori is the head of plastic and reconstructive surgery at Healthpoint (MUBADALA), Abu Dhabi, UAE. She achieved her Bachelor of Medicine, Bachelor of Surgery, and Bachelor of Obstetrics at the Royal College of Surgeons in Ireland. She holds a German Board Fachartz residency in plastic and aesthetic surgery. She completed her clinical fellowship in breast micro-reconstructive surgery fellowship in Zurich, Switzerland, at the same time, she did a master's degree at the European School of Microsurgery in surgical oncology, reconstructive, and aesthetic breast surgery. She also did lymphedema fellowships in Japan and South Korea. Her specialties include breast aesthetic and reconstructive surgery, lymphedema, lipedema surgery, and body contouring procedures post-massive weight loss. Dr. Al Mansoori is the founder of the Emirates Lymphedema Framework Group in the UAE.

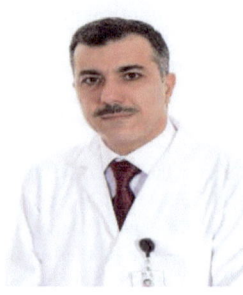

Ali Al Hassani Following completion of his MBChB at Baghdad University in 1991, Dr. Al Hassani became a fellow of the Iraqi Commission of Medical Specialization (FICMS) before being certified by the Arab Board in General Surgery (CABS) in 2001. He is a member of the Royal College of Surgeons of Edinburgh (MRCSEd) and a Fellow of the Royal College of Surgeons in Ireland (AFRCSI). Dr. Al Hassani is also a Fellow of the Royal College of Physicians and Surgeons of Glasgow FRCS(Glasg) and a Fellow of the American College of Surgeons (FACS). In 2012, he received a fellowship in surgical oncology from Detroit Medical Centre/Wayne State University, USA.

He is currently working as a consultant general surgeon at Sheikh Khalifa Medical City in Abu Dhabi, where he specializes in general and gastrointestinal surgery. He is also the surgical trauma team leader and gastrointestinal endoscopist.

Dr. Al Hassani is a member of the Society of American Gastrointestinal and Endoscopic Surgeons (SAGES) and the American Society for Surgery of the Alimentary Tract (SSAT), as well as a member of the Iraqi Surgeon Society (ISS), the UAE Medical Association (EMA), the International Society of Surgery (SSI), the Jordanian Medical Association (JMA), the Emirates Society of Laparoendoscopic Surgeons (ESLES), and member of International Federation of Obesity and Metabolic Disorder (IFSO).

Dr. Al Hassani is the Director of the Abu Dhabi Advances Trauma Life Support course, ATLS, and the instructor and co-director of both the Basic Surgical Skills (BSS) and Care of Critically Ill Surgical Patient CcRISP courses by the Royal College of Surgeons of England at Sharjah University.

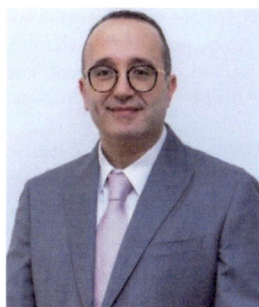

Dr. Zialyazan Sabbagh is the Chair of the Trauma Committee at Sheikh Khalifa Medical City, Abu Dhabi. He graduated from Rostov State Medical University in 1997 (Russian Federation), then joined the surgical residency program at RSMU, based at the Rostov Oncological National Center, for 5 years, for which he guaranteed a certificate of registration and a Ph.D. in general and oncological surgery in 2001 and 2002, respectively. Dr. Sabbagh moved to Syria and worked as an attending surgeon at MOH Damascus until 2004. Dr. Sabbagh was appointed to Mafraq Hospital in the UAE as a senior specialist in trauma and acute care surgery for 12 years. Currently, Dr. Sabbagh is working as a senior general surgeon specialist with consultant privileges at SKMC; he specializes in general, laparoscopic, and gastrointestinal surgery; and he also has special interest in open and laparoscopic repair of abdominal wall hernias. In addition to that, he is the Chair of the Trauma Committee at SKMC.

Dr. Sabbagh is a member of the following:

- The UAE Medical Association, Emirates Society of Colon and Rectal Surgery.
- The European Hernia Society.
- He is an instructor in the ATLS course.
- Dr. Sabbagh has several publications on oncology and trauma surgery.

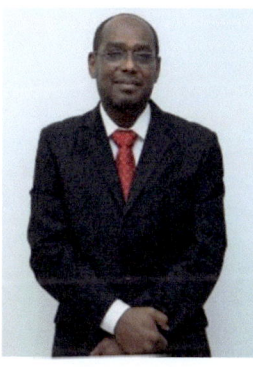

Dr. Hisham Hurreiz graduated from the University of Khartoum, Sudan, in 1995. In 2000, he was awarded the Fellowship of the Royal College of Surgeons in Ireland. He joined the higher surgical training program in the Northern Ireland deanery and obtained his FRCS(Gen) and CCT in general surgery, after which he completed a post-CCT fellowship in benign upper GI and laparoscopic surgery at Colchester Hospital. He then completed another fellowship in bariatric and metabolic surgery at the North of the Tyne Bariatric Unit in Newcastle. In addition to his surgical training, he obtained an MSC in clinical education from Queen's University Belfast.

Dr. Hurreiz then joined the Southern Trust, where he worked as a consultant general and upper GI surgeon in Daisy Hill Hospital until 2016, when he moved to Abu Dhabi to start a new job as a consultant general and bariatric surgeon in Al Ain Hospital. He joined SKMC in 2020. He has many publications in peer-reviewed medical journals and presentations at international meetings.

- Dr. Hurreiz holds an adjunct academic post at the UAE University.
- He is a member of the European Association of Endoscopic and Laparoscopic Surgeons (EAES), the British Association of Upper Gastrointestinal Surgeons of Great Britain and Ireland (AUGIS), the International Federation for Surgery of the Obesity (IFSO), the European Hernia Society, the British Obesity and Metabolic Surgery Society (BOMSS), and the Association of Laparoscopic Surgeons of Great Britain and Ireland.

Open Access This chapter is licensed under the terms of the Creative Commons Attribution 4.0 International License (http://creativecommons.org/licenses/by/4.0/), which permits use, sharing, adaptation, distribution and reproduction in any medium or format, as long as you give appropriate credit to the original author(s) and the source, provide a link to the Creative Commons license and indicate if changes were made.

The images or other third party material in this chapter are included in the chapter's Creative Commons license, unless indicated otherwise in a credit line to the material. If material is not included in the chapter's Creative Commons license and your intended use is not permitted by statutory regulation or exceeds the permitted use, you will need to obtain permission directly from the copyright holder.

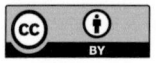

Infectious Disease in the UAE Health System

40

Ahmed Abdul Kareem AlHammadi,
Fatima Ali Salem Khalfan Al Dhaheri,
Huda Sulaiman Al Dhanhani, and Jens Thomsen

40.1 History of Infectious Diseases in the UAE

The United Arab Emirates (UAE) is a multinational country with an estimated total population of 9.89 million people, which grew by 5 million between 2000 and 2010. The population is projected to reach 10 million by 2033 [1]. Abu Dhabi, the capital of the UAE and the largest city in the country, has a high expatriate population, reported by the Department of Health Statistics in 2009 to constitute 78.8% of the total population [2].

A. A. K. AlHammadi (✉)
Infectious Diseases, Al Rahba Hospital, SEHA, PureHealth, Abu Dhabi, UAE

Department of Medicine, United Arab Emirates University, Al Ain, UAE

Transplant Infectious Diseases, Emirates Organ Transplant Center, Dubai, UAE

Emirates Infectious Disease Society, Emirates Medical Association, Dubai, UAE
e-mail: ahhammadi@seha.ae

Fatima Ali Salem Khalfan Al Dhaheri
Transplant Infectious Diseases, Emirates Organ Transplant Center, Dubai, UAE

Emirates Infectious Disease Society, Emirates Medical Association, Dubai, UAE

Sheikh Khalifa Medical City, SEHA, PureHealth, Abu Dhabi, UAE

United Arab Emirates University, Al Ain, UAE
e-mail: Fatimaald@uaeu.ac.ae

H. S. Al Dhanhani
Sheikh Khalifa Medical City, SEHA, PureHealth, Abu Dhabi, UAE
e-mail: hdhanhani@seha.ae

J. Thomsen
Khalifa University, Abu Dhabi, UAE

Abu Dhabi Public Health Center (ADPHC), Abu Dhabi, UAE
e-mail: jtw.thomsen@web.de

© The Author(s) 2025
H. O. Al-Shamsi (ed.), *Healthcare in the United Arab Emirates*,
https://doi.org/10.1007/978-981-96-0523-1_40

Before the union of the UAE in 1971, the first recorded infectious disease outbreak in the country dated back to the eighteenth century on Delma Island, west of Abu Dhabi. Delma Island, a major pearl diving hub, was plagued by smallpox, believed to have originated from pearl traders from India. It was reported that the population of the island, which ranged from several hundred to a few thousand, perished, with only 15 survivors [3].

Smallpox, a member of the poxviruses, genus Orthopoxvirus, and species variola virus, had a case fatality rate as high as 30% and an estimated global mortality of more than 300 million prior to its eradication [4]. Smallpox was eradicated successfully worldwide in 1980, and the last outbreak reported in the UAE occured in 1971 (Table 40.1). A mass vaccination program was one of the major strategies implemented to combat smallpox in the country, with a survey conducted in 1971 demonstrating that 95% of the population living in the emirates of Abu Dhabi and 85–90% of adults and school-aged children living in Dubai were vaccinated against smallpox [5].

After the formation of the country, the UAE government issued federal law No. 27 on November 7, 1981, addressing the prevention of communicable diseases. The 1981 law defined communicable diseases as those transmitted to others by human beings, animals, insects, food, and substances contaminated by microbes and toxins. The 1981 law also enforced penalties for violators of the law [6].

Table 40.1 Reported cases of smallpox in the UAE, 1957–1978

Year	Number of cases	Location
1957	0	No particulars available
1958	0	Dubai and Sharjah
1959	0	No particulars available
1960	0	Dubai
1961	0	Dubai, Al Ain, Abu Dhabi
1962	17	
1963	0	
1964	0	
1965	0	
1966	0	
1967	10	
1968	2	
1969	0	
1970	18	
1971	30	
1972	0	
1973	0	
1974	0	
1975	0	
1976	0	
1978	0	

Source: WHO communication of smallpox eradication [5] "Used with permission from author"

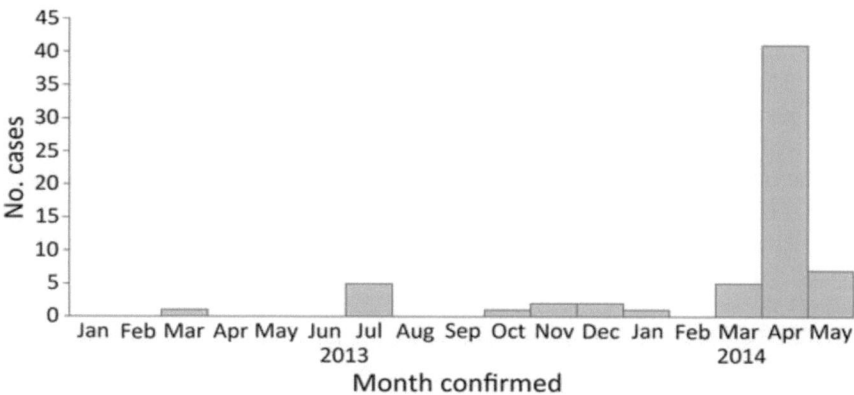

Fig. 40.1 Epidemiologic curve showing confirmed cases of Middle East respiratory syndrome coronavirus (MERS-CoV) infection, Abu Dhabi, United Arab Emirates, January 1, 2013–May 9, 2014 ($N = 65$). (*Source*: Response to Emergence of Middle East Respiratory Syndrome Coronavirus, Abu Dhabi, United Arab Emirates [7])

First reported in 2013, the Middle East Respiratory Syndrome-Related Coronavirus (MERS-CoV) is a zoonotic infection most commonly transmitted from dromedary camels [7]. In response to the emergence of MERS-CoV in October 2012 in Saudi Arabia and its subsequent report in 27 counties, with a mortality rate of 35% [8], the UAE initiated the MERS-CoV surveillance system in January 2013, and a total of 1586 cases were reported (Fig. 40.1) [7, 9]. As a result of the MERS-CoV epidemic, the UAE issued federal law No. 14 on November 20, 2014, combating communicable diseases. The 2014 law provided a broader definition and inclusion of diseases compared to the 1981 law and thus introduced more effective and broad measures to tackle communicable diseases. This law was later used to guide measures for managing the COVID-19 pandemic [6].

On a similar front, the national vaccination program has significantly reduced the burden of vaccine-preventable diseases in the country. The targets of the national vaccination program include diphtheria, tetanus, pertussis, tuberculosis, poliomyelitis, measles, mumps, rubella, chickenpox, hepatitis B, *Haemophilus influenzae* type B, *Streptococcus pneumoniae*, and *rotavirus*. The national vaccination program succeeded in interrupting polio transmission, and the country declared itself polio-free in 2000. The UAE, however, mirroring global emerging threats, has experienced a high incidence of measles since 2010 due to the growing anti-vaccine movement [8, 10].

The UAE is considered a low-burden and low-risk country for malaria. The total number of confirmed cases increased from 1,760 cases in 2003 to 5,165 cases in 2012, with all these cases imported from outside the UAE [11]. The UAE was declared malaria-free in 2007 with no reported local transmission, and post-elimination strategies have focused on surveillance of imported cases with prompt detection and treatment, while sustaining its malaria-free status in the country through active monitoring of mosquito breeding sites [10].

Tuberculosis is another important infectious disease that has a very low incidence rate (2 cases per 100,000) and a mortality rate of 0.7 per 100,000 in the UAE. The treatment success rate for new and relapsed cases registered in 2012 was 76%, and only 1.7% of new cases had drug-resistant tuberculosis. There has not been any incidence of drug resistance in previously treated patients [12].

The UAE is also considered a low-burden country for human immunodeficiency virus (HIV) infection. The National HIV/AIDS Prevention and Control Program was established in 1985, with updated laws and decrees issued in 2010 to protect the rights of patients living with HIV and to reduce the stigma surrounding the disease [13].

The UAE has also focused its efforts on the eradication of neglected tropical diseases at home and abroad. The UAE has helped support the Carter Foundation's guinea worm eradication program for the past 30 years, with the goal of making it the second human disease to be eradicated after smallpox [14]. The UAE itself was declared free of guinea worm (dracunculiasis) in 1998 [15].

40.2 Antimicrobial Resistance

Antimicrobial resistance (AMR) is the ability of a microorganism to resist the action of one or more antimicrobial agents. AMR has become a major threat to public health worldwide, including in the Middle East and the Gulf region. AMR impacts human health due to increased length of stay, treatment failures, and significant human suffering and deaths, as well as leading to increased healthcare costs and indirect costs. Globally, an estimated 700,000 deaths annually are currently attributable to antimicrobial resistance, and this number is expected to increase to 10,000,000 deaths by 2050, with an associated estimated loss to global gross domestic product of up to USD 100 trillion per year [16]. Without effective antibiotics, the success of major surgery and cancer chemotherapy would be compromised [17].

The Gulf Cooperation Council (GCC) region has continued to report an increase in isolated extended-spectrum β-lactamase-producing bacteria, carbapenemase-producing bacteria, pan-drug-resistant Gram-negative bacilli, as well as multidrug-resistant (MDR) tuberculosis. Furthermore, most of the multi-drug Carbapenem-*K. pneumoniae* infections from the GCC countries were found to be OXA-48 producers and were associated with hospital outbreaks and mortality. This trend of observed AMR was linked to the deaths of 60–90% of patients with ventilator-associated pneumonia, 40% of patients in a tertiary hospital, and 20% of pediatric hematology-oncology patients [18].

40.3 Antimicrobial Stewardship in the UAE

The UAE is known to have high international travel and a large expatriate population due to the booming tourism in the country. This mobility of the population has also been suggested as an important factor in AMR globalization. Like other areas in the world, the misuse of antimicrobials is one of the main factors associated with AMR; 20–50% of antimicrobial prescriptions are considered inappropriate. This was also shown by the increase in retail trends in the GCC region to 38–788 defined daily doses (DDD) per 1,000 population in 2015 in Saudi Arabia, the UAE, and Kuwait compared to a previous range of 27–844 DDD per 1,000 population in the year 2000 [18].

Antimicrobial Stewardship Programs (ASPs) have been the most important intervention to combat the rise in antimicrobial resistance. ASPs are defined as multiple strategies to improve the proper utilization of antimicrobials, aiming to reduce the side effects and costs related to antimicrobial prescriptions. This can be achieved through proper selection of the medication, duration, dosage, and route of administration. The main intervention strategies in ASPs are prospective auditing and feedback, pre-authorization, restriction of certain antimicrobials, promoting early de-escalation or early switch of the route from parenteral to oral therapy, as well as dose optimization, and other helpful interventions through education of healthcare providers and utilization of computerized models in medication monitoring and ordering. A significant drop in the length of stay in hospitals and antimicrobial consumption (DDDs/1000 inpatient days) was observed after the adoption of the ASP practices, as demonstrated in multiple studies [19].

In addition to the traditional ASP interventions, the utilization of rapid diagnostic tests as an ASP intervention has been reported at a quaternary care hospital in the UAE through the utilization of a multiplex PCR-based blood culture identification panel (BCID), which has proven to enable significantly earlier rationalization of empirical antibiotics to the proper agent [20].

The Department of Health Abu Dhabi (DoH), which is the regulatory authority of the healthcare sector in the emirate of Abu Dhabi in the UAE, mandated the implementation of ASPs in all hospitals and large healthcare centers within the emirate of Abu Dhabi in March 2016 and published a standard and guideline for healthcare facilities focusing on ASP [21].

Likewise, in GCC countries, the ASPs in the UAE were mainly led by ID physicians, with clinical pharmacists as co-chairs in government hospitals in Abu Dhabi. A qualitative cross-sectional study across nine hospitals in the emirate of Abu Dhabi, including both private and government hospitals, reported that the lack of skilled professionals in ASP programs, particularly clinical pharmacists, was one of the barriers to hospital-wide ASP optimization [19], which is similar to international surveys of comparable programs, which reported lack of time (66%), financial resources (63%), and information technology issues (61%), as major barriers to ASP implementation [22].

40.4 Emerging Antimicrobial Resistance in the UAE

AMR surveillance is important for better understanding the local epidemiology of antimicrobial resistance, detecting emerging resistance trends, predicting trends of antimicrobial resistance, developing antibiotic usage guidelines for common infections, and informing antimicrobial stewardship programs.

AMR surveillance has been established in the UAE since 2010. First at a subnational (Emirate) level (Abu Dhabi Emirate, HAAD, now: DoH), the system was expanded to the national level in 2015, led by the Ministry of Health and Prevention (MOHAP), in collaboration with the UAE Ministry of Presidential Affairs (MOPA), Dubai Health Authority (DHA), Department of Health Abu Dhabi (DoH), and Abu Dhabi Public Health Center (ADPHC).

As of September 2022, the UAE AMR surveillance system relies on a network of 318 surveillance sites (87 hospitals and 231 centers/clinics) that are served by 44 clinical microbiology laboratories across all seven Emirates of the UAE.

40.5 Current Levels and Trends of AMR in the UAE

A large body of scientific literature, as well as evidence from the UAE National AMR Surveillance System, has demonstrated that AMR is widespread and continuing to increase in clinical settings in the UAE; see, e.g., [16, 17, 23, 24]. Table 40.2 summarizes current (2020) levels of AMR among common pathogens in the UAE.

Table 40.2 Current levels of AMR among relevant and priority pathogens in the UAE, percentage resistant isolates (%R), UAE, 2020 [16]

Priority[a]	Organism	Antibiotic or antibiotic class	N (isolates)	% Resistant isolates
Priority 1: Critical	*Acinetobacter* spp.	Carbapenems (IPM or MEM)	1,772	21.9
	Pseudomonas aeruginosa	Carbapenems (IPM or MEM)	7,322	14.5
	Enterobacterales (all)	Carbapenems (IPM or MEM)	43,085	4.0
	Escherichia coli	Carbapenems (IPM or MEM)	26,335	1.0
	Klebsiella pneumoniae	Carbapenems (IPM or MEM)	10,760	4.8
	Enterobacterales (all)	Ceftriaxone/Cefotaxime (ESBL)[b]	33,273	27.6/25.0
	Escherichia coli	Ceftriaxone/Cefotaxime (ESBL)[b]	19,103	33.0/30.3
	Klebsiella pneumoniae	Ceftriaxone/Cefotaxime (ESBL)[b]	7,544	29.0/23.0
Priority 2: High	*Enterococcus faecium*	Vancomycin (VRE)[c]	338	8.9
	Staphylococcus aureus	Oxacillin (MRSA)[d]	14,103	35.1
	Salmonella spp. (non-typh.)	Fluoroquinolones (ciprofloxacin)	149	5.4
	Neisseria gonorrhoeae	3rd-generation cephalosporins	245	1.2
	Neisseria gonorrhoeae	Fluoroquinolones (ciprofloxacin)	272	90.0
Priority 3: Medium	*Streptococcus pneumoniae*	Penicillin (oral)	442	13.8
	Streptococcus pneumoniae	Penicillin (meningitis)	442	45.5
	Streptococcus pneumoniae	Penicillin (non-meningitis)	442	3.2
	Haemophilus influenzae	Ampicillin	723	30.7
	Shigella spp.	Fluoroquinolones (ciprofloxacin)	45	20.0

[a] Based on: (WHO, 2017), (Tacconelli, et al., 2018). [b]ESBL: Extended-spectrum beta-lactamase producer (based on resistance to ceftriaxone and/or cefotaxime), [c]VRE: Vancomycin-resistant *Enterococcus faecium*, [d]MRSA: Methicillin (oxacillin)-resistant *S. aureus*.

Tables 40.3, 40.4, and 40.5 summarize AMR trends observed for Gram-negative bacteria, Gram-positive bacteria, *Candida albicans*, and *Mycobacterium tuberculosis* in the UAE during the period 2010–2020.

Table 40.3 AMR trends, UAE, 2010–2020: Gram-negative bacteria [16]

Antibiotic class/substance	Escherichia coli	Klebsiella pneumoniae	Salmonella spp. (non-typhoid) [a]	Pseudomonas aeruginosa	Acinetobacter spp. [a]
Aminopenicillins (Ampicillin)	↓	n/a	↑↑	R	R
Amoxicillin/Clavulanic acid	↑	↑↑	→	R	R
Piperacillin/Tazobactam	↓	↓	→	↓	↓↓
3rd-/4th-gen. cephalosporins	↑↑/↑↑	↑↑/↑↑	→	→/→	↓↓/↓↓
Carbapenems (IPM/MEM)	<1 %R	→/↑	→ (<1%R)	→/→	↓↓/↓↓
Fluoroquinolones (Ciprofloxacin)	↑	↑↑	→	→	↓↓
Aminoglycosides (Gentamicin)	↓	↑	n/a	↓	↓↓
Trimethoprim/sulfamethoxazole	↓	↑ (n.s.)	↓	R	↓↓
Multidrug resistance (≥ 3 classes)	→	↑↑	→	↓	↓↓

↓/↑/→: decreasing/increasing/horizontal trend of percentage resistant isolates (%R), R: intrinsically resistant, n/a: not applicable, n.s.: not significant
[a] Salmonella spp. (non-typhoid), and Acinetobacter spp.: Trend is for 2014-2020 only.

Table 40.4 AMR trends, UAE, 2010–2020: Gram-positive bacteria [16]

Antibiotic class/substance	Staphylococcus aureus	Streptococcus pneumoniae	Enterococcus faecalis	Enterococcus faecium
Beta-lactam antibiotics	↑↑ (OXA)	↓ (PEN)/↑ (CTX)	→ (AMP)	→ (AMP)
Macrolides (Erythromycin)	↑↑	↑↑	n/a	n/a
Lincosamides (Clindamycin)	↑↑	→ (33%R)	n/a	n/a
Aminoglycosides (Gentamicin)	↑	n/a	↑↑	↑↑
Fluoroquinolones (Levo/Moxi))	↑↑/↑↑	↑/↑	↑ (LVX)	→
Glycopeptides	→ (0 %R)	→ (0 %R)	→ (<1 %R)	↓↓ (VRE)
Trimethoprim/sulfamethoxazole	↑	↑	R	R
Multidrug resistance (≥ 3 classes)	↑↑	↑↑	↑	↑↑

↓/↑/→: decreasing/increasing/horizontal trend of percentage resistant isolates (%R), R: intrinsically resistant, n/a: not applicable, n.s.: not significant, AMP: Ampicillin, CTX: Cefotaxime (non-meningitis breakpoints), LVX: Levofloxacin, OXA: oxacillin, PEN: penicillin, VRE: Vancomycin-resistant *Enterococcus faecium*.

Table 40.5 AMR trends, UAE, 2010–2020: *Candida albicans* and *Mycobacterium tuberculosis* [16].

Antibiotic class/substance	Candida albicans
Triazoles	
Fluconazole	↑
Voriconazole	↑
Polyenes	
Amphotericin B	↑, then ↓
Echinocandins	
Caspofungin	↓
Micafungin	↓

Antibiotic class/substance	M. tuberculosis
Rifampin	↑
Ethambutol	→ (<2%R)
Isoniazid	→
Pyrazinamide	↓
Streptomycin	No data
Multidrug resistance (RIF+INH)	↑ (3.2%)

↓/↑/→: decreasing/increasing/horizontal trend of percentage resistant isolates (%R)

40.6 Multidrug Resistance (MDR, XDR, and PDR)

Multi drug resistance (MDR) is antimicrobial resistance shown by a species of microorganism to at least one antimicrobial drug in three or more antimicrobial categories. Extensively drug-resistant (XDR) is the nonsusceptibility of a bacterial species to all antimicrobial agents except in two or fewer antimicrobialcategories. Within XDR, pandrug-resistant (PDR) is the nonsusceptibility of bacteria to all antimicrobial agents in all antimicrobial categories [25].

As of 2020, an average of 35% of common pathogens in the UAE were shown to be MDR, 4.6% XDR, and 0.7% PDR (Table 40.6, Fig. 40.2).

Between 2010 and 2020, multidrug resistance has overall increased in the UAE, in particular for clinically relevant Enterobacterales (*K. pneumoniae*), all Gram-positive pathogens under enhanced surveillance, and *M. tuberculosis*.

During the same period, the prevalence of multidrug resistance decreased for common non-lactose-fermenting bacteria such as *P. aeruginosa* and *Acinetobacter* spp.

Table 40.6 MDR, XDR, and PDR Summary, UAE, 2020 [16]

Organism	Number of isolates	MDR	Possible XDR	Possible PDR
Escherichia coli	29,139	12,882 (44.2%)	809 (2.8%)	8 (0%)
Klebsiella pneumoniae	12,208	4,171 (34.2%)	1,213 (9.9%)	225 (1.8%)
Salmonella spp. (non-typhoidal)	1,182	91 (7.7%)	20 (1.7%)	0 (0%)
Pseudomonas aeruginosa	7,933	1,276 (16.1%)	785 (9.9%)	93 (1.2%)
Acinetobacter sp.	1,929	450 (23.3%)	394 (20.4%)	147 (7.6%)
Staphylococcus aureus	14,131	5,625 (39.8%)	25 (0.2%)	0 (0%)
Streptococcus pneumoniae	691	260 (37.6%)	7 (1.0%)	1 (0.1%)
Enterococcus faecalis	4,210	271 (6.4%)	47 (1.1%)	1 (0.1%)
Enterococcus faecium	349	148 (42.4%)	29 (8.3%)	1 (0.3%)
Mycobacterium tuberculosis	791	25 (3.2%)	25 (3.2%)	3 (0.4%)
Total	72,563	25,199 (34.7%)	3,354 (4.6%)	479 (0.7%)

MDR: Multidrug resistance, XDR: Extensive drug resistance, PDR: Pan-drug resistance.

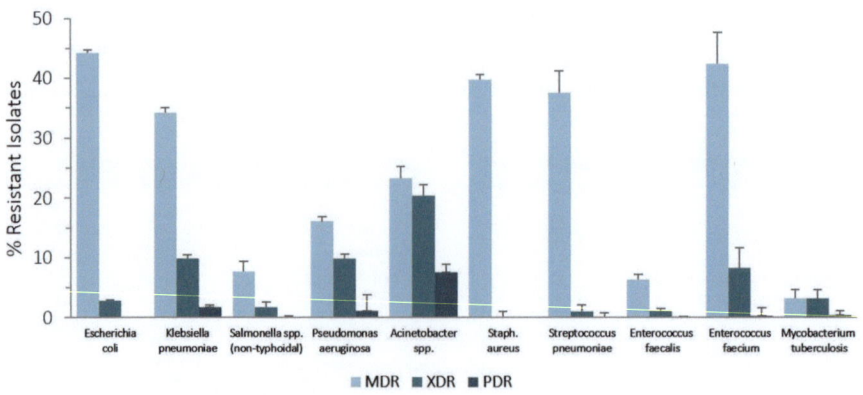

Fig. 40.2 MDR, XDR, and PDR Summary, UAE, 2020 [16]

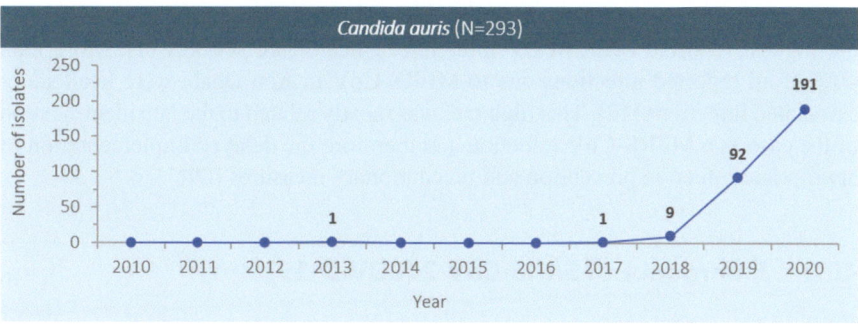

Fig. 40.3 *Candida auris*: number of isolates reported in the UAE, by year [16]

40.7 Other Emerging Resistance Trends

Candida auris is a new and emerging, often multidrug-resistant yeast that is able to cause candidiasis in humans, including invasive candidiasis (fungemia). It has been associated with hospitalized patients with weakened immune systems and has caused outbreaks in healthcare settings [26]. In the UAE, it has been emerging since 2017 [27].

The number of reported isolates of *Candida auris* in the UAE increased between 2010 and 2020 from 0 to 191 (Fig. 40.3).

40.8 Emerging and Re-emerging Infections in the UAE

Abu Dhabi, being the largest city in the UAE, has a high expatriate population; according to 2009 DOH statistics, 78.8% of the population were noncitizens [2].

The UAE shared its experience in dealing with multiple emerging and re-emerging infections. The Department of Health reported in 2011 the emerging H1N1, and in 2009 pandemic experience in the emirates of Abu Dhabi, where 2806 patients were reported and 26 patients (0.9%) died from confirmed pandemic (H1N1) 2009 infection [2].

The Middle East Respiratory Syndrome Coronavirus (MERS-CoV) was first reported in November 2013 as an infection associated with severe respiratory symptoms and renal failure, the majority of which were linked to the Arabian Peninsula, while other European and African countries reported imported cases. A study from the UAE investigated the positive rate of camel serum for neutralizing antibodies against MERS-CoV. Six hundred fifty-one samples were tested in 2003 and 2013, and the majority (632/651, 97.1%) tested positive, indicating that camels had antibodies against MERS-CoV since at least 2003, when 151 serum samples were collected and tested. This suggested that dromedary camels from the UAE were infected with MERS-CoV or a closely related virus, probably years prior to the identification of the first human MERS-CoV cases [28].

According to the WHO, the UAE, Korea, and the Kingdom of Saudi Arabia had the highest reported MERS-CoV infection in healthcare settings [7]. More than 40% of all reported infections due to MERS-CoV in Abu Dhabi were healthcare-associated infections [12]. This high rate was mostly related to the late identification of the case as a MERS-CoV infection and therefore the delayed implementation of appropriate infection prevention and precautionary measures [29].

40.9 Emergence of SARS-CoV-2 (COVID-19)

As a response to the global pandemic of COVID-19, the UAE managed the pandemic with high efficiency; the case fatality rate related to COVID-19 was only 0.3%, which was lower than in developed countries, and the case recovery rate was 89%. Moreover, the UAE led the global testing for COVID-19 through very active surveillance, as the number of tests conducted per 1,000 people was the highest in the UAE compared to other developed nations (Fig. 40.4).

The UAE was one of the countries that hosted Phase 3 clinical trials of the COVID-19 vaccine, including the Phase 3 trial of the inactivated SARS-CoV-2 vaccine, BBIBP-CORV. Given the promising results of vaccine effectiveness, with a seroconversion rate of 92.8%, the UAE Ministry of Health and Prevention (MOHAP) granted an emergency use authorization (EUA) for the inactivated SARS-CoV-2 vaccine, BBIBP-CORV, to healthcare workers on the frontline in September 2020, with the aim of protecting high-risk individuals [31].

More recently, the UAE encountered the global outbreak of the mpox virus, which is a closely related virus to smallpox. It belongs to the genus Orthopox of the family Poxviridae. Hence, the name mpox comes from its discovery in monkeys, and the first human case was reported in 1970 in the Democratic Republic of the Congo, after which it spread to multiple African countries and beyond the African

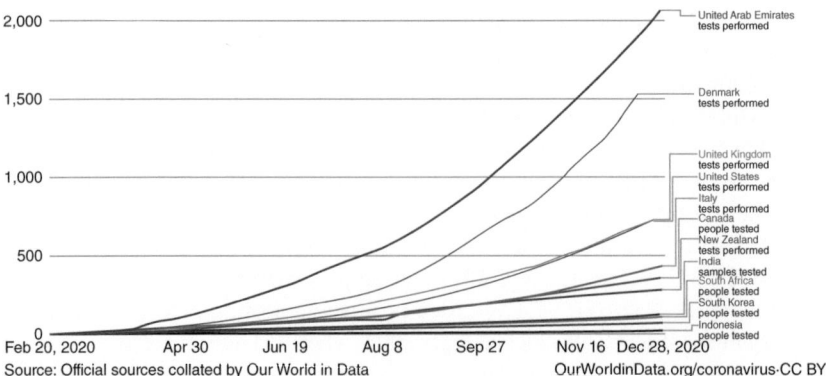

Fig. 40.4 The number of tests conducted per 1000 people in the UAE and other countries as of December 2020. (*Source*: Response to COVID-19 pandemic in the UAE [30] "Used with permission from author")

continent. Mpox incidence can be as high as 50 per 10,000 to as low as 0.64 per 100,000 Mpox has two distinctive genotypes, the Congo type and the West African type, with Cameroon marking the geographical division between the two types, where both genetic types exist. The central African type has a significantly higher mortality rate compared to the West African type, and the known case fatality ratio in Africa was reported to be as high as 10% [32].

Since the beginning of January 2022, cases of mpox have been reported to the WHO, resulting in a total of 58,285 laboratory-confirmed cases and 480 probable cases, including 22 deaths, as of September 13, 2022. The UAE reported 17 cases and no deaths from the beginning of the outbreak until July 2022, which has been considered a global health emergency [33].

40.10 The COVID-19 Response in the UAE

On January 29, 2020, the UAE was the first country to report COVID-19 in the region, implementing immediate public health measures that ensued to ensure effective control over the outbreak that not long after emerged into a global pandemic. Early during the pandemic, the mandatory use of masks came into effect in March 2020. Emergency response systems were activated and steered by the National Emergency Crisis and Disasters Management Authority (NCEMA), which announced mass health measures and educational campaigns to educate the public about COVID-19 signs and symptoms, screening, quarantine, isolation, and when they needed to present to COVID-19 assessment centers for evaluation, workup, and treatment.

Furthermore, large-capacity field hospitals were established, and rapid drive-through centers were provided across the emirates to facilitate effective screening of suspected cases, providing an efficient way to identify cases and track outbreaks. Areas with hotspots were identified and extensively targeted for screening by tracing confirmed contacts, such as in labor camps and industrial areas where workers tend to be crowded.

By November 2021, 100% of the UAE's population had been vaccinated with at least one dose of COVID-19 vaccines approved under the EUA. In addition, with over 186 million tests conducted, the UAE was able to diagnose and manage over 1 million confirmed cases of COVID-19 with a mortality rate of only 0.24%, making it one of the lowest in the world [34]. Very early in the pandemic, the healthcare system was prepared and alerted with protocols and clinical pathways to manage COVID-19 at all stages and severity. All necessary diagnostics, COVID-19 therapies, face masks, vaccines, and monoclonal antibodies used for the prevention of severe outcomes and hospitalizations were utilized and widely provided.

Smart technology platforms were used to effectively communicate with the public and ease their transition into the pandemic. The Al Hosn system was used to monitor vaccination status and ensure safe access and entry into closed public areas. The UAE was one of the first countries to adopt remote e-learning for students in schools and universities as well as remote working systems to ensure the safety and health of their employees while work was carried out from home.

For the first time in its history, the UAE launched a major Phase III vaccine clinical trial in July 2020 using inactivated BBIBP-CorV "Sinopharm" and was successful in recruiting more than 44,000 volunteers. Given the promising results of vaccine effectiveness, with a seroconversion rate of 92.8%, the UAE MOHAP granted an EUA for the inactivated SARS COV-2 vaccine, BBIBP-CorV, to healthcare workers on the frontlines in September 2020, with the aim of protecting high-risk individuals [31].

This was soon followed by a Phase II/III clinical trial in December 2020 that involved the use of the Gam-COVID-Vac combined adenovirus vector vaccine "Sputnik V," which also recruited 1,000 subjects [35]. Later on, multiple Phase II and Phase III clinical trials were conducted as well. Multiple publications from the UAE aided and supported the emergency use authorization of these vaccines around the world [36–40]. Studies looked at the immunogenicity, safety, and efficacy of such vaccines and were among the first to be conducted globally. They also examined new generation recombinant Sinopharm vaccines, as well as a Phase II clinical trial investigating the efficacy of combining two adenovirus-vectored vaccines, such as Gam-COVID-Vac "Sputnik V" and AZD1222 "AstraZeneca" COVID-19 vaccines, in 100 subjects.

The UAE has participated actively in providing global medical aid around the world. In 2021, the UAE provided 25% of the syringes and needles required for UNICEF's and COVAX's global initiatives. In addition, the UAE started a global initiative called the "HOPE Consortium" [41], bringing together leading public and private industry partners to facilitate the delivery of more than 18 billion doses of COVID-19 vaccines around the world and building a capacity to store more than 11 million vaccine doses at ultra-cold temperatures of −80 °C.

The COVID-19 pandemic was a significant opportunity to bring together different organizational entities to collaborate and establish nationwide COVID-19 research groups. One main group was the national COVID-19 Research Committee, which included members from the Ministry of Health and Prevention (MOHAP), ADPHC, and DHA. Three main subcommittees were formed, including epidemiology, diagnostics, and therapeutic subcommittees. The Institutional Review Board (IRB) committee was very active, meeting weekly to expedite and facilitate approval of proposals and actively reviewing hundreds of COVID-19-related research proposals, maintaining a timely online registry to provide research status and avoid duplication of research and efforts.

Noteworthy, due to concerns about COVID-19 pathogenesis and severity, especially for immunocompromised hosts, solid organ transplantation programs took a serious hit, and their numbers declined worldwide. As vaccinations were introduced and the pathogenesis of the disease became better understood, programs came forward to cautiously resume their transplantation programs. The UAE was one of the first countries worldwide, and the first in the Middle East and North Africa (MENA) region, to use organs from COVID-19-infected donors. Organs procured and transplanted included two kidneys and one liver, which were transplanted successfully to three recipients with excellent outcomes. In order to effectively and safely utilize solid organs from COVID-19-positive donors, a protocol was rapidly developed to evaluate COVID-19 donors and recipients, involving a multidisciplinary team.

Moving forward, more than 25 million doses of the COVID-19 vaccine have been administered, and most adults have now been vaccinated with at least one or two booster doses. While other countries are still struggling with the aftermath of the pandemic and lacking adequate programs for mass vaccination, the UAE has become a hub for international summits and conferences. In over 182 days between October 1, 2021, and March 31, 2022, Dubai EXPO 2020 recorded over 24 million visitors. The UAE has also been actively performing genotype sequencing to monitor the emergence and distribution of different strains of COVID-19. This helped to effectively target treatment and vaccination efforts, better plan required booster doses, and contribute to the global understanding of the emergence of different strains.

40.11 Conclusion

The UAE is a multinational country with a high expatriate population, contributing to the diversity of infectious diseases in the country. Given strong public health measures, the UAE today is a low- burden and low-risk country for global threats like tuberculosis and malaria. On the other hand, AMR has emerged in the UAE, mirroring global trends resulting from the misuse of antimicrobials. The country established AMR surveillance in 2010, starting in Abu Dhabi and expanding nationally in 2015. Finally, the UAE's response to the current COVID-19 pandemic has been robust, resulting in a mortality rate of only 0.24%.

Conflicts of Interest The authors have no conflicts of interest to declare.

References

1. United Arab Emirates Population 2022 (Live) 2022. Available from: https://worldpopulationreview.com/countries/united-arab-emirates-population
2. Khan G, Al-Mutawa J, Hashim MJ. Pandemic (H1N1) 2009, Abu Dhabi, United Arab Emirates, May 2009–March 2010. Emerg Infect Dis. 2011;17(2):292–5.
3. Saeed SA. Abu Dhabi Book Fair 2021: how did the UAE handle pandemics and plagues in the past? 2021 May 25, 2021.
4. Henderson DA. The eradication of smallpox--an overview of the past, present, and future. Vaccine 2011;29 Suppl 4:D7–D9.
5. World Health Organization. Report to the Global Commission For Certification of Smallpox Eradication. Available from: http://apps.who.int/iris/bitstream/handle/10665/68250/WHO_SE_78.118.pdf?sequence=1&isAllowed=y. Accessed.
6. History of federal law no 14 for the year 2014 on combating the communicable diseases 2022. Available from: https://www.legal500.com/developments/thought-leadership/history-of-federal-law-no-14-for-the-year-2014-on-combating-the-communicable-diseases/

7. World Health Organization. Middle East respiratory syndrome 2022. Available from: https://www.emro.who.int/health-topics/mers-cov/mers-outbreaks.html
8. National policy of vaccination in UAE 2022. Available from: https://u.ae/en/information-and-services/health-and-fitness/combatting-communicable-diseases
9. Al Hosani FI, Pringle K, Al Mulla M, Kim L, Pham H, Alami NN, et al. Response to Emergence of Middle East Respiratory Syndrome Coronavirus, Abu Dhabi, United Arab Emirates, 2013–2014. Emerg Infect Dis. 2016;22(7):1162–8.
10. World Health Organization. Regional Office for the Eastern Mediterranean. United Arab Emirates health profile 2015. World Health Organization. Regional Office for the Eastern Mediterranean 2022. 2016. Available from: https://apps.who.int/iris/handle/10665/253775
11. Malaria in the Eastern Mediterranean Region 2013. Cairo: World Health Organization Regional Office for the Eastern Mediterranean; 2014 2022. Available from: applications.emro.who.int/dsaf/emropub_2014_EN_1778.pdf?ua=1
12. WHO global tuberculosis database 2014. Geneva: World Health Organization; 2014 2015. Available from: http://www.who.int/tb/country/data/profiles/en
13. UNAIDS Middle East and North Africa regional report on AIDS 2011. Geneva: Joint United Nations Programme on HIV/AIDS (UNAIDS); 2011 2022. Available from: www.unaids.org/sites/default/files/media_asset/JC2257_UNAIDS-MENA-report-2011_en_1.pdf
14. UAE carter foundation 2022. Available from: https://www.cartercenter.org/news/upcoming_events/promo/uae-and-carter-center.html
15. Global health observatory data repository: Neglected tropical diseases. Geneva: World Health Organization; 2015 2022. Available from: http://apps.who.int/gho/data/node.main.A1629?lang=en
16. National AMR Surveillance Report. Annual report 2019. Dubai: Ministry of Health and Prevention; 2019.
17. Al-Kaabi M, Tariq W, Hassanein A. Rising bacterial resistance to common antibiotics in Al Ain, United Arab Emirates. EMHJ. 2009:479–84.
18. Alghamdi S, Shebl NA, Aslanpour Z, Shibl A, Berrou I. Hospital adoption of antimicrobial stewardship programmes in Gulf Cooperation Council countries: a review of existing evidence. J Glob Antimicrob Resist. 2018;15:196–209.
19. Ababneh MA, Nasser SA, Rababa'h AM. A systematic review of Antimicrobial Stewardship Program implementation in Middle Eastern countries. Int J Infect Dis. 2021;105:746–52.
20. Nasef R, El Lababidi R, Alatoom A, Krishnaprasad S, Bonilla F. The impact of integrating rapid PCR-based blood culture identification panel to an established antimicrobial stewardship program in the United Arab of Emirates. Int J Infect Dis. 2020;91:124–8.
21. Hamdan, S. and El-Dahiyat, F. Implementation and evaluation of an antimicrobial stewardship program across nine hospitals in the United Arab Emirates: a qualitative study. J Pharm Pract Res. 2020;50:124–31.
22. Doernberg SB, Abbo LM, Burdette SD, Fishman NO, Goodman EL, Kravitz GR, et al. Essential resources and strategies for antibiotic stewardship programs in the acute care setting. Clin Infect Dis. 2018;67(8):1168–74.
23. Sonnevend A, Blair I, Alkaabi M, Jumaa P, Al Haj M, Ghazawi A, et al. Change in meticillin-resistant Staphylococcus aureus clones at a tertiary care hospital in The United Arab Emirates over a 5-year period. J Clin Pathol. 2012;65(2):178–82.
24. Sonnevend A, Abdulrazzaq N, Ghazawi A, Thomsen J, Barathan G, Makszin L, et al. The first nationwide surveillance of carbapenem-resistant Enterobacterales in The United Arab Emirates – increased association of Klebsiella pneumoniae CC14 clone with Emirati patients. IJID. 2022;120:103–12.
25. Magiorakos A-P, Srinivasan A, Carey R, Carmeli Y, Falagas M, Giske C. Multidrug-resistant, extensively drug-resistant and pandrug-resistant bacteria: an international expert proposal for interim standard definitions for acquired resistance. Clin Microbiol Infect. 2012;18(3):268–81.
26. Schelenz S, Hagen F, Rhodes J, Abdolrasouli A, Chowdhary A, Hall A, et al. First hospital outbreak of the globally emerging Candida auris in a European Hospital. Antimicrob Resist Infect Control. 2016;5:35.

27. Alatoom A, Sartawi M, Lawlor K, AbdelWareth L, Thomsen J, Nusair A, et al. Persistent candidemia despite appropriate fungal therapy: first case of Candida auris from The United Arab Emirates. IJID. 2018;70:36–7.
28. Meyer B, Müller MA, Corman VM, Reusken CB, Ritz D, Godeke GJ, et al. Antibodies against MERS coronavirus in dromedary camels, United Arab Emirates, 2003 and 2013. Emerg Infect Dis. 2014;20(4):552–9.
29. Hunter JC, Nguyen D, Aden B, Al Bandar Z, Al Dhaheri W, Abu Elkheir K, et al. Transmission of Middle East respiratory syndrome coronavirus infections in healthcare settings. Abu Dhabi Emerg Infect Dis. 2016;22(4):647–56.
30. Al Hosany F, Ganesan S, Al Memari S, Al Mazrouei S, Ahamed F, Koshy A, et al. Response to COVID-19 pandemic in the UAE: a public health perspective. J Glob Health. 2021;11:03050.
31. Al Kaabi N, Oulhaj A, Al Hosani FI, Al Mazrouei S, Najim O, Hussein SE, et al. The incidence of COVID-19 infection following emergency use authorization of BBIBP-CORV inactivated vaccine in frontline workers in The United Arab Emirates. Sci Rep. 2022;12(1):490.
32. Ahmed M, Naseer H, Arshad M, Ahmad A. Monkeypox in 2022: a new threat in developing. Ann Med Surg (Lond). 2022;78:103975.
33. Organization WH. Multi-country outbreak of monkeypox, External situation report #4-24 August 2022 2022. Available from: https://www.who.int/publications/m/item/multi-country-outbreak-of-monkeypox%2D%2Dexternal-situation-report%2D%2D4%2D%2D-24-august-2022
34. NCEMA. UAE CORONAVIRUS (COVID-19) UPDATES 2020. Available from: https://covid19.ncema.gov.ae/en
35. Ahmed A.K. AlHammadi, Amna H.Alzaabi, Haneen B. Choker, Ahmed A. Ibrahim, Asma Bin Ishaq, Ahmed E. Mahboub, Reem S. Al Dhaheri, Mohamed N. Alzaabi, Timothy A. Collyns, Gehad ElGhazali, Stefan Weber, Basel K. Al-Ramadi, A phase II/III, randomized, double-blind, placebo controlled trial to evaluate immunogenicity and safety of the Gam-COVID-Vac combined vector vaccine in the prophylactic treatment for SARS-CoV-2 infection in the United Arab Emirates, Vaccine: X, Volume 25, 2025, 100698. https://doi.org/10.1016/j.jvacx.2025.100698.
36. Al Kaabi N, Zhang Y, Xia S, Yang Y, Al Qahtani MM, Abdulrazzaq N, et al. Effect of 2 inactivated SARS-CoV-2 vaccines on symptomatic COVID-19 infection in adults: a randomized clinical trial. JAMA. 2021;326(1):35–45. https://doi.org/10.1016/j.jvacx.2025.100698.
37. Mahmoud S, Ganesan S, Al Kaabi N, Naik S, Elavalli S, Gopinath P, et al. Immune response of booster doses of BBIBP-CORV vaccines against the variants of concern of SARS-CoV-2. J Clin Virol. 2022;150-151:105161.
38. Al Kaabi N, Oulhaj A, Ganesan S, Al Hosani FI, Najim O, Ibrahim H, et al. Effectiveness of BBIBP-CorV vaccine against severe outcomes of COVID-19 in Abu Dhabi, United Arab Emirates. Nat Commun. 2022;13(1):3215.
39. Kaabi NA, Yang YK, Du LF, Xu K, Shao S, Liang Y, et al. Safety and immunogenicity of a hybrid-type vaccine booster in BBIBP-CorV recipients in a randomized phase 2 trial. Nat Commun. 2022;13(1):3654.
40. Kaabi NA, Yang YK, Zhang J, Xu K, Liang Y, Kang Y, et al. Immunogenicity and safety of NVSI-06-07 as a heterologous booster after priming with BBIBP-CorV: a phase 2 trial. Signal Transduct Target Ther. 2022;7(1):172.
41. HOPE CONSORTIUM 2022. Available from: https://hopeconsortium.com/

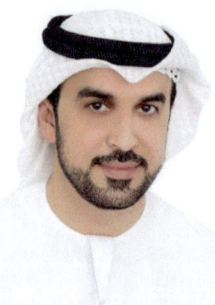

Dr. Ahmed Abdul Kareem Al Hammadi graduated from UAE University in 2009. He received his American Board of Internal Medicine certification in 2015. He completed an infectious disease fellowship at the University of Massachusetts Medical School, Worcester, MA, in 2015–2016 and at the University of Texas Health Sciences Center at Houston, McGovern Medical School, Houston, TX, in 2016–2017. He is certified by the American Board of Internal Medicine—Infectious Disease Subspecialty, 2017. Dr. AlHammadi completed a fellowship in transplantation infectious diseases at McGovern Medical School, Houston, TX, and the University of Texas MD Anderson Cancer Center, 2018–2019.

Dr. Ahmed is currently the consultant for infectious diseases at Al Rahba Hospital, SEHA, PureHealth. He is also the president of the Emirates Infectious Diseases Society. He is also a member of many medical societies, such as the ACP, IDSA, and EMA.

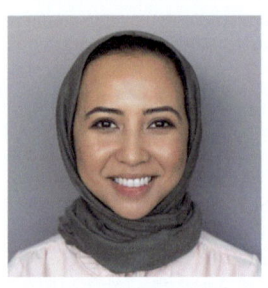

Dr. Fatima Ali Salem Khalfan Al Dhaheri is a pediatric infectious disease faculty member with expertise in infectious diseases in immunocompromised hosts. Dr. Al Dhaheri received her medical degree in 2013 from the United Arab Emirates University (UAEU) (honors) and completed her pediatric residency training at the Children's National Medical Center in Washington, DC, an affiliate of the George Washington School of Medicine (2015–2017). She then completed her infectious diseases fellowship and sub-fellowship training in immunocompromised infectious diseases at Boston Children's Hospital in Boston, an affiliate of Harvard Medical School (2017–2020). Dr. Al Dhaheri also completed a 2-year program at the Harvard Catalyst Academy for clinical and translational research. Dr. Al Dhaheri is currently an assistant professor in the Department of Pediatrics, in the College of Medicine and Health Sciences at UAEU, a consultant physician in Sheikh Khalifa Medical City, and a contributing expert in transplant infectious diseases at the Emirates organ transplant center. Dr. Al Dhaheri is also a core member of the Emirates Infectious Disease Society (EIDS), serving as Vice President of the Emirates Medical Association.

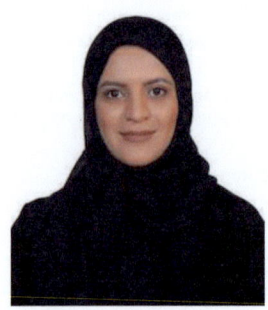

Dr. Huda Sulaiman Al Dhanhani is a pediatric infectious disease consultant working at SKMC. She graduated from UAE University in 2009 and completed her residency training in pediatrics in 2014. Dr. Huda perused further training in pediatric infectious disease and completed the international fellowship of PID from the Royal College of Physicians of Ireland in 2018. She joined SKMC as a consultant in pediatric infectious disease in 2021, and she is a member of multiple committees in SEHA, such as the infectious disease and infection control committee, the antimicrobial stewardship committee. Dr. Huda is interested in ASP programs, OPAT, bone and joint infectious, and infections in special hosts.

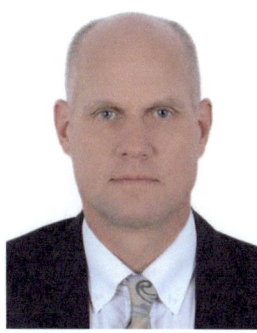

Dr. Jens Thomsen Consultant, Clinical Microbiology and Infectious Disease Epidemiology, Medics Labor AG, Bern, Switzerland Associate Clinical Professor (adjunct), Dept. Public Health and Epidemiology, Khalifa University, Abu Dhabi, United Arab Emirates International Consultant for AMR Surveillance, WHO Dr. Thomsen is a consultant in clinical microbiology and infectious disease epidemiology with 30+ years of professional experience in clinical medicine, microbiology, infection control, and public health. Dr. Thomsen holds also a Master of Public Health degree (MPH) from Emory university, Atlanta, as well as a Master of Business Administration (MBA) and Master of Science in Healthcare Management (MSc) from Swiss Business School, Zürich, Switzerland. Furthermore, he holds professional certificates in hospital infection prevention and control (BAEMI), and antibiotic stewardship (ABS expert, DGI). Dr. Thomsen joined the Department of Health (DoH) in Abu Dhabi in 2007 and served there as a section head for occupational and environmental health until 2019. From 2019 until 2023 he was then holding the position of section head, environmental health at the Abu Dhabi Public Health Center (ADPHC). From 2010 to 2023 he was in charge of establishing, implementing, and leading the Abu Dhabi Emirate and the UAE National AMR Surveillance program, in the capacity of Chair, National AMR surveillance sub-committee (MoHAP). He was also a founding member of the UAE Higher Committee on AMR and the National Sub-Committee for Antibiotic Stewardship (MoHAP). In other roles, Dr. Thomsen served as the founding board member and President of the Emirates Society of Clinical Microbiology (ESCM), as an adjunct associate clinical professor for epidemiology and public health at Khalifa University, Abu Dhabi, UAE, as the GLASS national focal point for AMR surveillance for the UAE, and several times as a temporary consultant for AMR for the World Health Organization (WHO).

Open Access This chapter is licensed under the terms of the Creative Commons Attribution 4.0 International License (http://creativecommons.org/licenses/by/4.0/), which permits use, sharing, adaptation, distribution and reproduction in any medium or format, as long as you give appropriate credit to the original author(s) and the source, provide a link to the Creative Commons license and indicate if changes were made.

The images or other third party material in this chapter are included in the chapter's Creative Commons license, unless indicated otherwise in a credit line to the material. If material is not included in the chapter's Creative Commons license and your intended use is not permitted by statutory regulation or exceeds the permitted use, you will need to obtain permission directly from the copyright holder.

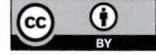

Sports Medicine and Rehabilitation in the UAE

41

Mahesh Cirasanambati and Sabahat A. Wasti

41.1 Introduction to Sports Medicine and Rehabilitation

Sports medicine is an emerging branch of medicine. However, it is considered elitist, purely because of misconceptions and a lack of awareness of its availability even for school and club-level sportspersons. It deals with physical fitness and the treatment and prevention of sports-related injuries.

This branch of medicine requires wide-ranging expertise, and the major components of sports medicine include the following:

- General medical knowledge
- Orthopaedic principles
- Sports nutrition
- Body biomechanics
- Exercise physiology
- Sports rehabilitation, along with an understanding of the general principles of rehabilitation
- Sports psychology

This field of medicine aims to help people engage in sports safely and effectively to attain their training goals [1].

This field of medicine has gained a lot of importance in recent times in the Middle East. The youth here rarely engage in the required physical activities and often fail to attain or maintain the desired level of physical fitness. There may be too

M. Cirasanambati (✉)
Physical Medicine and Rehabilitation, Burjeel Medical City, Abu Dhabi, United Arab Emirates
e-mail: mahesh.c@himmah.rehab

S. A. Wasti
Cleveland Clinic Abu Dhabi, Abu Dhabi, United Arab Emirates

© The Author(s) 2025
H. O. Al-Shamsi (ed.), *Healthcare in the United Arab Emirates*,
https://doi.org/10.1007/978-981-96-0523-1_41

much reliance on technology for training, and the general lifestyle is also not conducive to acquiring the correct fitness status prior to or during sporting activities [2].

Over the past two to three decades, rehabilitation medicine has evolved into a branch of medicine that deals with delivering the right interventions in order to achieve the best functional outcomes for patients with varied injuries and impairments. It facilitates optimal functional, vocational, and social outcomes in line with recipients' values and wishes. It also aims to facilitate autonomy (the ability to make choices and decisions), and the freedom from pain and distress. The aim of all rehabilitation is to minimize the impact of impairments due to disease or injury, and it does so with focused attention to understanding the nature of each impairment and its potential to result in disability.

Although the youngest medical specialty, rehabilitation medicine is rapidly gaining favour as a vital component of almost all clinical management protocols. As the trend towards specialized and condition-specific rehabilitation has grown, there has been an emergence of different fields of specialized rehabilitation, including neurorehabilitation, musculoskeletal and orthopaedic rehabilitation, pain rehabilitation, cardiac rehabilitation, pulmonary rehabilitation, paediatric rehabilitation, cancer rehabilitation, post-critical illness rehabilitation, transplant rehabilitation, and sports rehabilitation.

Rehabilitation is typically effective when delivered by a multidisciplinary team. This team should include a physician trained in rehabilitation, a physiotherapist, an occupational therapist, a speech and language therapist, a trained rehabilitation nurse, and other supportive disciplines such as psychologists, nutritionists, social workers, and case managers. It is imperative that all individual members of the team have specialist training in rehabilitation medicine and sports medicine.

According to Prof. Michael Barnes [3], one of the pioneers in rehabilitation medicine who has played a key role in establishing neurological rehabilitation programmes in the United Kingdom, rehabilitation is an active and dynamic process through which a disabled person is helped to acquire knowledge and skills to maximize their physical, psychological, and social functioning. This process can be conveniently broken down into three key areas:

- Approaches that reduce disability.
- Approaches designed to acquire new skills and strategies that will maximize activity.
- Approaches that help to alter the environment, both physical and social, so that a given disability carries minimal resulting handicap.

Furthermore, it is imperative that rehabilitation teams aim to limit the potential of impairments to result in disability and cause a person to remove themselves from their prior activity status.

The expense of rehabilitation is significant and beyond the scope of this chapter. We will mostly limit our discussion of rehabilitation to sports injury rehabilitation (SIR) and will only refer to other areas of specialized rehabilitation where they become relevant in the context of SIR.

41.2 Sports Injury Rehabilitation

In this section, we will focus on the following:

1. The history of sports therapy and rehabilitation
2. The role of rehabilitation in sports injuries
3. The principles of sports injury rehabilitation
4. Rehabilitation services in the United Arab Emirates (UAE)

41.2.1 The Brief History of Sports Therapy and Rehabilitation

The development of various elements of treatment for sports injuries dates back to the Greeks and Romans. In Roman times, valuable athletes were well cared for and received considerable attention for their injuries. As the number of injuries increased, the need for a better understanding of the mechanisms of injuries and their treatments also grew. This prompted better education in the science of sports-related body mechanics and the risk of injury. At that time, the main focus was to reduce the number of injuries to athletes. Subsequently, a lot of work in this context was done by Ibn e Sina (Avicenna) [4]. He initiated the process of rehabilitation interventions, including those for muscle pain, through the introduction of therapeutic massage. In the thirteenth century, Santorio Santorius [5], an Italian physician, studied the effects of activities on pulse rate and temperature, and was the first to explain how these could be modified through rest and nutrition after activities. In the sixteenth century, Gerolamo Mercuriale [6], another Italian physician, published *De Arta Gymnastica* in 1569, essentially the first text that focused on the effects of exercise on the human body. In the seventeenth century, Bernardino Ramazzini [7] studied the body movements and posture of athletes. Ramazzini is referred to as the Father of Sports Medicine.

Formal setups for sports activity-related medical and surgical issues started in the twentieth century, when committees were established to examine the impact of athletic activity on motion and posture, and how these could be optimized for everyone to facilitate better performance and reduce injury. Specific societies were formed, and the rehabilitation fraternity began to become formally involved in the care of patients with sports injuries. In the twenty-first century, the sciences of sports medicine and rehabilitation have drawn closer, and now the care of athletes is the domain of both.

Considering the UAE's interest in sports, data from YouGov's report, the Global Sports Media Landscape, reveals that just over two-thirds of global consumers (67%) follow sports regularly through TV or digital platforms. When analysed by country, the UAE has the highest proportion of 'sport engagers' (89%), defined as those who engage with sports they regularly follow (in the last 30 days); the only other country equalling this is Indonesia (89%). Other Asian markets reporting high levels of sports engagement include India (85%), Hong Kong (83%), and China (79%). Comparatively, European countries and America register lower levels of engagement [8]. This clearly shows a high interest in sports among the UAE population, highlighting the importance of not only developing high-end sports facilities but also equally responsive sports health facilities.

Since the formation of the UAE in 1971, the political leadership has given full attention to the growth, welfare, and institutionalisation of the sports sector in view of the significant role it plays in the development and advancement of the nation. Establishing and maintaining sports clubs falls under the scope of social development services.

The UAE is keen on providing the necessary support for sports in the country through the construction of many modern sports facilities, such as football (soccer) stadiums, car-racing tracks, golf courses, and training centres throughout the country, to serve professionals and beginners. Achieving a cohesive society and a preserved identity is one of the six pillars of the national agenda, in line with Vision 2021. One of the KPIs to measure such achievement is the number of medals won in the Olympic and Paralympic championships in various sports [9].

Accordingly, the National Sports Strategy 2031 of the UAE was formed; it aims to enhance community sports, competitive sports, and the overall sports system in the UAE. Its objective is to promote sustainable growth and prosperity in the country's sports sector.

By 2031, the National Sports Strategy will implement 17 initiatives to achieve several goals, which include the following:

- Increasing the proportion of people practising diverse sports to 71% of the population
- Developing sports professionals
- Discovering talented athletes in schools
- Upgrading the sports education methodology
- Enhancing regulations governing the sports sector

The strategy seeks to strengthen the UAE's participation in various international tournaments, including the Olympic Games, and to establish a global identity for Emirati sports [9].

The efforts to develop sports professionals align with those of the UAE National Olympic Committee, which focuses on preparing professional athletes for major regional and international competitions [9].

The national strategy prompted the development of facilities and bodies that will regulate and enhance participation in their respective sports. The current regulatory bodies in the UAE are shown in Table 41.1 [9].

41.2.2 Role of Rehabilitation in Sports Injuries

An analysis of injuries conducted by a study of around 6363 adolescents in the UAE identified injuries in the past 12 months, and socio-demographic, behavioural, and sensory data noted that 18% experienced injury; the three top causes were

Table 41.1 Current regulatory bodies in the UAE [9]

Federations in UAE	
UAE Football Association	UAE Cycling Federation
UAE Cricket Board	UAE Tennis federation
UAE Falcons Federation	UAE Volleyball Association
Emirates Aerosports Federation	UAE Equestrian and Racing Federation
UAE Ice Sports Federation	UAE Chess Federation
UAE Handball Federation	UAE Basketball Association
UAE Table Tennis Association	UAE Padel Association
Emirates Weightlifting Federation	UAE Billiard and Snooker Association
UAE Wrestling Federation	UAE Rugby Federation
UAE Archery Federation	UAE Karate Federation
UAE Sports for All Federation	UAE Boxing Association
UAE Wrestling & Judo Federation	Emirates Bodybuilding & Fitness Federation
United Arab Emirates Taekwondo Federation	UAE Fencing Federation
UAE Jiu-Jitsu and Mixed Martial Arts Federation	Emirates Bowling Federation
Emirates Motorsports Organization	UAE Swimming Federation
UAE Triathlon Association	UAE Muay Thai & Kickboxing Federation
Emirates Canoe & Rafting Federation	Emirates Golf Federation
UAE Darts Association	UAE Police Sports Federation
Emirates Arabian Horse Society	UAE Sports Arbitration Center
UAE Marine Sports Federation	Emirates Women's Sports Federation
UAE Badminton Federation	UAE Sports Federation for Polo
UAE Federation of Roller Skating Sports	
Sports Councils	
Abu Dhabi Sports Council	
Sharjah Sports Council	
Dubai Sports Council	
Committees	
National Olympic Committee	
UAE Pro League	
UAE Paralympic Committee	

accidental falls (38%), being struck by an object or person (18%), and motor vehicle injuries (13%). Most injuries happened around a sportsperson's home or the surrounding area. This study clearly identifies the need for public health policies and education programmes that reduce injuries among the UAE adolescent population [10].

The current model of sports injury management is based on a multidisciplinary approach. The team includes a sports medicine physician with a good understanding of rehabilitation principles after sports-related injuries, a sports/MSK-trained physiotherapist, a strength training and conditioning coach, a sports psychologist, a sports nutritionist, and a sport-specific coach. The athlete is indeed the most important member of this team.

For SIR to be successful, it is essential that the treating team has a full understanding of the basic principles of rehabilitation as well as possesses specific knowledge of an injured athlete's sport. The treating team should direct the rehabilitation interventions based on the biomechanical and physiological aspects of care, specific to the athlete's sport, with the aim of returning him or her to play the sport. The need for sport-specific rehabilitation necessitates that the teams delivering rehabilitation have sport-specific rehabilitation training. This, however, has training and resource implications, and therefore we find that mostly generic sports rehabilitation teams provide even sport-specific SIR programmes.

The main aim of all sport rehabilitation is to have the athlete return to playing sport, and in pursuing this alongside physical rehabilitation, psychosocial support and readjustments are necessary. Injury time is often a very disruptive time for an athlete, and comprehensive care is necessary to prevent maladaptive emotional and psychological responses. It is necessary to engage appropriate psychologists and social workers and enact family (parents and spouses) support in the rehabilitation programmes. However, even with the best available surgical, medical, and rehabilitation services and support, some athletes may not return to playing sports completely or to the level they were playing at prior to injury. In such cases, the goal of rehabilitation interventions must be to have the athlete return to a gainful level of functioning and help him or her adjust to this altered status. It is also important that, alongside improvement of function, the athlete is trained in acquiring skills to engage in gainful employment, preferably within the area of his or her sport, for example, to become a trainer, commentator, etc.

41.2.3 Principles of Sports Injury Rehabilitation

The key principles or practice parameters of sports injury rehabilitation are as follows [11]:

- Determination and documentation of the pre-injury status of the athlete:
  - Level at which the athlete was participating in his or her sport
  - Age and years of playing
  - Previous history of injuries and time out of play
  - Where he or she is playing and the protocols for fitness and training for his team or club
- Athlete Assessment:
  - Type of injury.
  - Treatments undertaken
  - Functional status
  - Training and exercise restrictions that are still recommended by the surgical team
  - Associated medical issues
  - Preferred return-to-play time as per athlete or his or her club/employers

- Treatment Planning:
  - The main objective of all treatment plans is to return to sports, most likely incrementally, to the pre-injury level.
  - Prevent secondary reinjury
  - The above goal should be determined by the pre-injury physical status of the athlete
  - The goals and timeline should be clearly charted
  - Secondary deconditioning must be prevented during the injury period
  - Exercise and training programmes should be designed to restore strength, power, and endurance
  - Safe return-to-sport parameters must be clearly defined and discussed with the athlete, his or her coach, and employers
  - The transition from rehabilitation to competitive sport must be well planned and incrementally intensified
  - The programme will depend on the individual athlete's sport and his or her role as a team member in team sports

41.2.4 Episodes of Rehabilitation in Sports

- Regular training to prevent injury
- Before each game
- Preventive measures to avoid worsening immediately after an injury
- After acute surgical interventions to maintain function and begin prevention of secondary deconditioning
- In the short term, to overcome the effects of injury and acute interventions, start loading, strengthening, and restoring power
- Medium term to start non-competitive sport training
- Long term return to competitive sport

41.3 Rehabilitation Provisions in the UAE

In the last 15 years, rehabilitation services in the UAE have increased exponentially, but mostly this increase has been generic and to a certain degree in the fields of neurorehabilitation and long-term care. The development of specialized domains of rehabilitation such as amputee rehabilitation, pain rehabilitation, cancer rehabilitation, paediatric rehabilitation, cardiac rehabilitation, pulmonary rehabilitation, and even structured musculoskeletal rehabilitation is relatively lacking, and their availability is somewhat restricted. Furthermore, even in the field of neurorehabilitation, there is very limited availability of specialized brain injury, spinal cord injury, rehabilitation for neurodegenerative disorders, and even stroke rehabilitation [12].

Sport rehabilitation, too, is not readily available to all athletes, and where it is provided, the quality of rehabilitation is rather suboptimal due to the fact that it is not sport-specific and the practice is not standardized across providers. There are some specialized and well-equipped sports rehabilitation facilities, but these are expensive and accessible only to high-end athletes. Also, with the increase in sporting competitions, there is a drive to improve sports rehabilitation in the UAE. There is a drive to increase the availability of rehabilitation at the school level and to improve both the quantity and quality of post-sport injury rehabilitation [12].

Overall, the growth of the sports medicine industry in the UAE has a great future, with the support of the government's proactive policies and increased investment in this sector. With these initiatives, there has been a great demand for such high-end services, which is establishing the UAE to be the world hub for sports medicine and rehabilitation [12].

41.4 Conclusion

Sports medicine has evolved into a specific specialty in medicine that bridges rehabilitation and orthopaedics to deliver the best treatments to athletes after they sustain injuries. Rehabilitation is an integral component of sports medicine, and its availability so far in the UAE is relatively restricted. There need to be a concerted effort on the part of sports organizations and healthcare providers to meet the shortfall. Also, there must be a mechanism to oversee established and new sports rehabilitation facilities for quality, efficacy, and efficiency. Minimum standards and parameters must be set to ensure high-quality sports rehabilitation.

Conflicts of Interest The authors have no conflicts of interest to declare.

References

1. Snook GA. The history of sports medicine. Part I. Am J Sports Med. 1984;12(4):252–25.
2. Sibai AM, Nasreddine L, Mokdad AH, et al. Nutrition transition and cardiovascular disease risk factors in Middle East and North Africa countries: reviewing the evidence. Ann Nutr Metab. 2010;57(3–4):193–203.
3. Barnes M. Principles of Neurological rehabilitation. J Neurol Neurosurg Psychiatry. 2003;74(s4) PG 3–7
4. Hajar R. The Air of History (Part V) Ibn Sina (Avicenna): the great physician and philosopher. Heart Views. 2013;14(4):196–201.
5. Britannica T. Editors of Encyclopaedia. "Santorio Santorio". Encyclopedia Britannica, March 25, 2022. https://www.britannica.com/biography/Santorio-Santorio
6. Ford E. The de arte gymnastica of mercuriale. Aust J Physiother. 1955;1(1):30–2.
7. Franco G, Franco F. Bernardino Ramazzini: the father of occupational medicine. Am J Public Health. 2001;91(9):1382. https://doi.org/10.2105/AJPH.91.9.1382.
8. August 24th, 2023, YouGov 2023 Sports Report: The Global Sports Media Landscape. Accessed on 02/12/2023 at https://business.yougov.com/content/47055-2023-sports-report
9. Accessed online on 02/12/2023 at https://u.ae/en/about-the-uae/culture/sports-and-recreation
10. Barakat-Haddad C, Siddiqua A. Injuries among adolescents in The United Arab Emirates. Inj Prev. 2013;20:121–7.

11. Kumar P, Sharma JP. Assessment of the status of injury knowledge prevention and management at various levels of sports persons. Int J Physiol Nutrit Phys Educ. 2017;2:505–7. https://doi.org/10.22271/journalofsport.2017.v2.i2i.253.
12. The UAE: Sports rehabilitation destination and science hub, article accessed online on 02/12/2023 at https://lexsportiva.blog/2019/12/20/uae/

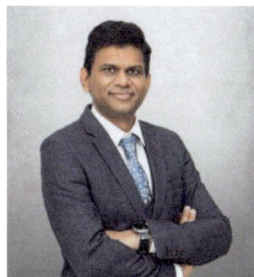

Dr. Mahesh Cirasanambati has completed his MRCS, Board Certification (CCT) in Physical Medicine and Rehabilitation from the UK and is also a Diplomate of Sports and Exercise Medicine from the UK. He has worked as a consultant and director of rehabilitation medicine in the UK and the MENA region for more than nine years. He was also chair of the Musculoskeletal Special Interest Group of the British Society of Rehabilitation Medicine. He is interested in training and research and is currently director of the Center for Advanced Rehabilitation Training and Education, UK (CARTE-UK). He also works as a sports and exercise medicine consultant for several Premier League football and rugby clubs in the UK. He specializes in the rapid rehabilitation of sports injuries using a combination of high-end interventions and the most advanced rehabilitation techniques. He has a broad clinical practice that includes neurological problems, brain injury rehabilitation, stroke, spinal cord injury rehabilitation, chronic pain, including neuromodulation with spinal cord stimulators and intrathecal pain pumps, musculoskeletal and joint problems, paediatrics, sports injuries, and spasticity management with nerve blocks and Botox treatments. He is currently Chief of Rehabilitation for Burjeel Holdings. He leads a skilled multidisciplinary team of physiotherapists, occupational therapists, speech and language therapists, psychologists, dieticians, nutrition specialists, and advanced-skilled rehabilitation nurses.

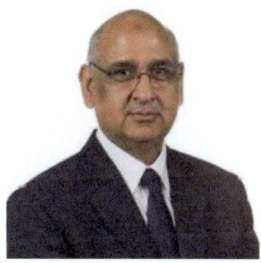

Dr. Sabahat A Wasti received his bachelor's degree in medicine and surgery from Khyber Medical College, Peshawar, Pakistan, and then moved to the United Kingdom for postgraduate studies in 1984. After obtaining membership of the Royal College of Ireland, he completed rehabilitation medicine training at Leeds Teaching Hospital. He then became a Consultant in Rehabilitation Medicine at Sheffield Teaching Hospitals, Sheffield, UK, where he served for nearly nine years before moving to the United Arab Emirates to take up the position of Senior Consultant in Physical Medicine and Rehabilitation at Sheikh Khalifa Medical City in 2007.

He has served in both the public and private sectors in the UAE and spearheaded the development of rehabilitation services in both. He served as a British Society of Rehabilitation representative in the Consensus Reference Group for Multiple Sclerosis Guidelines, commissioned by the National Institute of Clinical Excellence.

Dr. Wasti is recognized for promoting the cause of neurorehabilitation in particular and is widely respected by his peers. He is well known for his views on cultural and ethical variances and their implications of these on neurorehabilitation.

He currently serves as Regional VP, WFNR (Gulf Region), Chair of Service Development SIG and Co-Chair of Ethics SIG, WFNR. He has also served as Chair of several conferences and frequently delivers invited lectures.

Open Access This chapter is licensed under the terms of the Creative Commons Attribution 4.0 International License (http://creativecommons.org/licenses/by/4.0/), which permits use, sharing, adaptation, distribution and reproduction in any medium or format, as long as you give appropriate credit to the original author(s) and the source, provide a link to the Creative Commons license and indicate if changes were made.

The images or other third party material in this chapter are included in the chapter's Creative Commons license, unless indicated otherwise in a credit line to the material. If material is not included in the chapter's Creative Commons license and your intended use is not permitted by statutory regulation or exceeds the permitted use, you will need to obtain permission directly from the copyright holder.

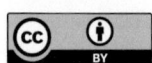

Oral Health in the UAE: Current Status Within Global and Regional Perspectives

42

Nabeel H. Alsabeeha 🄳, Mohammed A. Al Shalabi, Nada O. Al Shamsi, Shaikha A. AlSamahi, and Manal A. Awad 🄳

42.1 Introduction

Oral health is an essential component of the overall state of health and well-being, yet a universal definition of it did not exist until very recently. In 2016, the World Dental Federation (FDI) introduced a definition and a structured framework for oral health that aimed to bring attention to the wider dimensions of oral health, including care and support for patients and increasing community awareness [1]. The definition is multifaceted and describes oral health as the ability to speak, smile, smell, taste, touch, chew, swallow, and convey a range of emotions through facial expressions with confidence and without pain, discomfort, or disease of the craniofacial complex [2]. Oral diseases with the greatest global burden affect more than 3.5 billion people worldwide [3]. Of these, dental caries is the most prevalent, affecting the permanent dentition of nearly two billion people and the primary teeth of 550

N. H. Alsabeeha
Department of Restorative Dentistry, College of Dentistry, Ajman University, Ajman, United Arab Emirates
e-mail: dr.nabeel@yahoo.com; n.alsabeeha@ajman.ac.ae

M. A. Al Shalabi
Private Practice, Abu Dhabi, United Arab Emirates
e-mail: m.alshalabi@arabiansmca.ae

N. O. Al Shamsi (✉)
Burjeel Cancer Institute, Burjeel Medical City, Abu Dhabi, United Arab Emirates

S. A. AlSamahi
Department of Dental Services, Emirates Health Services, Dubai, United Arab Emirates
e-mail: shaikha.abdulla@ehs.gov.ae

M. A. Awad
Department of Orthodontics, Pediatric and Community Dentistry, College of Dental Medicine, University of Sharjah, Sharjah, UAE
e-mail: awad@sharjah.ac.ae

© The Author(s) 2025
H. O. Al-Shamsi (ed.), *Healthcare in the United Arab Emirates*,
https://doi.org/10.1007/978-981-96-0523-1_42

million children around the globe. Periodontal diseases, on the other hand, affect 14% of the world's adult population [4], while oral cancer remains a global health concern with a prevalence rate between 4 and 22 cases per 100,000 [5]. Orofacial clefts, which include cleft lip and/or palate, are common birth defects with global prevalence rates between one in 1500 births [6] or 0.3 to 0.45 per 1000 births [7]. Although a global trend toward a declining incidence of orofacial clefts has been observed, these conditions remain prevalent in many regions of the world [6, 7]. Another oral disease burden is "Noma," which mainly affects underprivileged populations and particularly targets children between the ages of 6 and 12 years [8]. While relatively rare in the Middle East, "Noma" remains a major oral health concern in the sub-Saharan African region, where an estimated 14,000 new cases are reported every year, with an approximate 90% mortality rate [9].

The association between general health and oral health is multifaceted and complex. Noncommunicable diseases such as cardiovascular diseases, diabetes mellitus, and cancer share common risk factors with oral diseases such as dental caries, periodontal diseases, and oral cancer, with obesity and smoking being risk factors of interest [10, 11]. While a cause-and-effect relationship remains controversial, the association between these conditions and oral health has been widely accepted [11].

In this chapter, the oral health status of the United Arab Emirates (UAE) population is described within global and regional settings, focusing on oral diseases with the greatest impact on the UAE community. The influence of noncommunicable diseases and conditions such as diabetes, cardiovascular diseases, obesity, and smoking on the oral health in the UAE will also be briefly discussed.

42.2 Dental Caries

It is estimated that 60–90% of school-aged children and nearly 100% of adults worldwide have tooth decay [12]. This makes dental caries the most common, yet preventable, chronic disease and a global public health challenge.

The global prevalence of childhood caries (i.e., caries in children under 6 years of age) varies widely, with the lowest prevalence reported in some Western countries, such as Sweden, Italy, and the USA [13]. The observed reduction has been mainly due to changes in living conditions, the implementation of healthy lifestyles, the effective use of fluoride, enhanced self-care practices, and the establishment of preventive oral care programs [13]. Conversely, a higher prevalence of dental caries has been reported in the Middle East, where many countries are still undergoing economic transition or have healthcare systems that are still developing [14–16].

In the UAE, several studies reported a high prevalence of dental caries ranging from 74% to 83% among 4- to 5-year-olds, and the severity of caries (measured by the number of decayed, missing, and filled teeth index (dmft)) ranged from as low as 1.7 to as high as 10.9 [17–19]. These considerable variations in the estimates could be attributed to factors such as the relatively small sample sizes used in many studies, the difference in indices used to measure dental caries, as well as variations in the age of the children surveyed. On the other hand, studies conducted among school-age children and adolescents aged 7–18 years old provided additional evidence of the severity of dental caries in the UAE. These studies reported DMFT scores that ranged from 1.48 to 3.19 [20, 21], with the decay component accounting for the majority of the DMFT values.

42.2.1 Determinants of Dental Caries

Several determinants and associated risk factors for dental caries have been discussed in the literature [22–27]. These have been classified into individual, parental, and environmental factors. Children's oral health is influenced by factors related to the children themselves, their families, and society [26]. Parental variables directly associated with children's oral health include sociodemographic characteristics, oral health behaviors, cognitions, and anxiety [22, 26, 27]. With this in mind, a caries risk assessment should not only focus on dental caries and associated dietary and oral hygiene habits but should also examine the associated familial risk factors.

Studies on dental caries conducted in the UAE [20, 21, 28–30] mainly assessed the impact of different known risk factors, such as children's dietary habits, frequency of tooth brushing, number of visits to the dentist, and parental socioeconomic levels, in a statistical manner, assuming an additive model that evaluated the additional contribution of each risk factor to dental caries. High consumption of sucrose, sweet drinks, high sugar intake between meals, and frequent snacking were all associated with dental caries [17, 29]. Moreover, socioeconomic factors such as income and parental education level were also found to be linked to dental caries [28]. However, understanding the contribution of each of the factors in a conceptual model that has previously been tested and takes into account the complexity of the relationship between different risk factors is needed [22]. Additionally, a clear understanding of the pathways that could lead to a decrease in the incidence of tooth decay among children in the UAE is also needed. For example, a comprehensive framework that delineates the relationships that dental caries and dental visit behaviors share with individual factors (e.g., oral health behaviors) and parental characteristics (e.g., parental socioeconomic status, family structure, oral health behaviors, and parenting style) may help policymakers, dental professionals, and community-based preventive programs design strategies that can improve children's oral health in the UAE. Understanding the mediating role of parents and the environment in children's dental caries and oral health behaviors is also necessary.

42.2.2 Directions for Effective Prevention

Despite the availability of free dental services for UAE nationals, dental caries continues to be a public health burden. This indicates that an in-depth assessment of the factors that contribute to suboptimal oral health among children in the UAE is still needed. Unless there is a clear understanding of the underlying causes of the relatively high prevalence of tooth decay, planned clinical or educational preventive approaches will not achieve a long-term reduction in the incidence of dental caries. Moreover, understanding the impact of culture and behavioral factors may be helpful in deciding whether a community-based or individual-based preventive approach would be more effective [31]. Therefore, policies that take into account the complexity of dental caries as a chronic disease should be considered. For example, in addition to the positive steps of increasing taxes on sugary drinks, stronger regulation of the advertising and promotion of sugary foods and drinks targeting children, and the promotion of appropriate exposure to fluoride in toothpaste and drinking water are equally needed. Moreover, the integration of oral health into national and community health programs is essential. There is also an urgent need to change the current approach to dealing with dental caries from a treatment-dominated, high-technology intervention to a preventive approach that addresses the determinants of this disease in the UAE [32].

42.3 Periodontal Diseases

Periodontal diseases are a group of inflammatory conditions that affect the supporting structures of the teeth and are generally categorized into gingivitis and periodontitis [33]. Gingivitis is the earliest form of periodontal disease in which the inflammation is limited to the gingiva but may extend further, resulting in the destruction of the dental attachment apparatus and the occurrence of periodontitis [34]. Clinical attachment loss and pocket depth are the measures used to clinically diagnose periodontitis, and a combination of these measures is usually used to assess its severity [35].

There is an evident lack of up-to-date data on the prevalence of periodontitis in the adult Arab population overall. Information from a review paper by Al-Harthi et al. [36] showed that more than one-third of missing permanent teeth in the adult Arab population were lost because of periodontitis. Moreover, periodontitis accounted for a greater number of tooth losses among individuals aged over 40 years than any other contributing factor. To date, there are no large-scale epidemiological studies in the UAE from which the prevalence of periodontal disease can be estimated. Much of the published literature on periodontal disease consists of cross-sectional studies conducted to assess the relationship between periodontal disease and various risk factors [37–41].

42.3.1 Risk Factors and Systemic Association

In the last two decades, significant developments have occurred in the understanding of the initiation and progression of periodontal diseases. This includes understanding the importance of the immune system and the inflammatory response of the host, as well as the recognition that periodontal disease is a multifactorial condition influenced by genetic and environmental risk factors [42, 43].

42.3.1.1 Periodontal Disease and Smoking

Cigarette smoking has long been associated with periodontal disease and tooth loss. Studies have shown that smoking has a causal effect on periodontitis [44, 45]. A positive relationship has also been observed between the number of cigarettes smoked and the severity of periodontal disease [46]. This is because tobacco smoking can affect the microbial ecology of the oral cavity through immunosuppression, oxygen deprivation, antibiotic effects, and other possible mechanisms [44]. Moreover, the loss of beneficial oral species due to smoking can lead to pathogen colonization and ultimately to the progression of periodontitis [47]. In the UAE, it was reported that smoking in general, as well as the exclusive use of cigarettes and dokha was associated with significant alterations in the oral microbiome structure and relative taxa abundances [48]. It was also found that nonsmokers, when compared to all smoking groups combined, had significantly lower levels of periodontal disease, as assessed by pocket depth and clinical attachment loss. Although in recent years many studies have been conducted on the adverse effects of "shisha" and "dokha" smoking [49–52], fewer studies have examined the association between these forms of tobacco and periodontal disease. Such studies are essential to our understanding of the impact of "shisha" on oral health and severity of periodontal diseases in the UAE population.

42.3.1.2 Periodontal Diseases and Diabetes Mellitus

There are approximately 537 million adults between the ages of 20 and 79 living with diabetes worldwide, and this number is projected to increase to 643 million in 2030 and to 783 million in 2045 [53]. In the UAE, recent data estimate the prevalence of diabetes among adults at 12.3%, with a total count of 990,900 cases [54].

The association between diabetes mellitus and periodontal disease has been extensively researched, and a strong link has been clearly demonstrated. Diabetes has been identified as an important host risk factor for periodontal disease in large epidemiological studies [55–59]. Landmark studies relating periodontitis to type 2 diabetes mellitus showed increased prevalence and incidence of periodontal disease in those individuals who also had type 2 diabetes compared to those who did not [59]. In a recent systematic review and meta-analysis of 15 cohort studies, Stöhr et al. [58] showed that there was a positive bidirectional association between periodontal disease and diabetes mellitus. For patients with diabetes, the data indicated a 24% higher incidence of periodontal disease and that the relative risk of developing diabetes mellitus was elevated by 26% among patients with periodontitis. Conversely, improved periodontal health with conventional periodontal therapy has been shown to result in better glycemic control in diabetic patients [60, 61], including older adults with uncontrolled type 2 diabetes mellitus [62].

In the UAE, epidemiological studies investigating the association between periodontal diseases and diabetes mellitus are scarce, and the results are inconclusive [38, 39, 41]. For example, Awad et al. [41] found no association between clinical attachment loss and individuals with type 2 diabetes, while Khalifa et al. [38] reported clinical attachment loss of 3 mm in 23% of their diabetic cohort. On the other hand, Al-Rawi and Al-Marzooq [39] failed to draw any correlation between blood glucose levels and periodontal pathogen levels in diabetic and nondiabetic obese patients. With currently limited information, the interplay between diabetes and periodontal diseases in the UAE population remain to be explored with large-scale, longitudinal studies and sustained long-term support. These studies are essential, not only to help draw up constructive preventive plans specific to the UAE population but also to enhance the role of dentists, as healthcare providers, in the overall management of diabetic patients. Raising public awareness about how good periodontal health can help improve diabetic control should also be addressed as part of a sustained community-driven oral health promotion [63].

42.3.1.3 Periodontal Disease and Cardiovascular Diseases (CVDs)

There is a wealth of information on a strong but independent association between CVDs and periodontal diseases [64]. Bacteremia and elevated systemic inflammatory biomarkers observed in periodontitis have been causally linked to CVDs in several studies [65, 66]. The comorbid existence of periodontitis and CVDs has been shown to result in significantly higher mortality rates among the CVD population [67]. Higher risks of developing atherosclerotic CVD [68] and myocardial infarction [69] have also been demonstrated in patients with periodontitis compared to those without periodontal disease. Genetic analyses of large data sets have identified shared genetic risk factors among patients with coronary heart disease and patients with periodontitis [70]. On the other hand, improvements in periodontal health with routine dental prophylaxis [69] and professional oral hygiene maintenance at least once a year have been shown to reduce the risk of CVDs by 14% [71]. Additionally, intensive periodontal therapy has been shown to result not only in improvements in periodontal health but also in a correlated improvement in endothelial function in patients with periodontitis [72]. These reports support the notion that periodontitis is a modifiable nontraditional risk factor in the development of CVDs and that periodontal therapy can have positive impacts on the CVD risk profile of patients with periodontitis [64].

Cardiovascular disease is a leading cause of global mortality, responsible for nearly one-third of all deaths reported worldwide [73]. In the UAE, the estimated incidence rate for major CVDs stands at 12.7 per 1,000 people per year [74], with a mortality rate of 84 deaths per 100,000 as of 2021 [75]. Known risk factors include abdominal obesity, dyslipidemia, hypertension, diabetes, and smoking, especially among young adults [76]. Population-based studies looking into the association between periodontitis and CVDs are still lacking in the UAE, and, hence, exploration of this area of research is imperative given the burden of CVDs and periodontal diseases among the UAE population. Nevertheless, extrapolation of findings from international studies to the local UAE setting is possible given the commonality of the disease processes and risk factors between CVDs and periodontal diseases across a wide spectrum of world populations.

42.4 Malocclusion and Facial Traits

Malocclusion is an irregularity of the teeth or a mal-relationship of the dental arches beyond what is considered normal [77]. Not all malocclusions require treatment, and specific guidelines have been established to determine treatment priorities based on dental health and aesthetic indications [78]. Malocclusion has been linked to an increased risk of developing dental caries, periodontal disease, temporomandibular joint disorders, and oro-dental trauma [79]. Malocclusion is the third oral disease burden after dental caries and periodontal diseases, and hence a major global health issue [80]. The global prevalence of malocclusion among school-age children is estimated to be between 43% and 78% [81], and the associated aesthetic, functional, and emotional impacts, as well as the decrease in the overall quality of life, are well documented in the literature [82, 83]. The severity of these impacts increases with the severity of malocclusion, particularly in younger age groups [84].

Malocclusion, associated facial traits, and common dental anomalies among the UAE population have been presented in limited cross-sectional studies [85–89]. An early study conducted at Ajman University provided interesting insights into malocclusion traits in the UAE population [85]. The sample of that study was composed of 300 children between the ages of 9 and 12 who attended regular dental check-ups at the university dental clinics. Based on the Index of Orthodontic Treatment Needs (IOTN), crowding was the most prevalent trait observed, at 38.3%. This was followed by increased overjet, crossbite, impacted teeth, and open bite with 32%, 19%, 11.3%, and 9.3%, respectively. The observation of the prevalence of crowding as the main dental anomaly is not surprising, considering that early extraction of deciduous teeth, as a result of the high DMFT rate in the UAE, is the main contributor to this occurrence. This observation was a reflection of a global trend of crowding being the most common type of malocclusion observed [86]. Other cross-sectional studies analyzed the cephalometric measurements of Emirati samples and compared these measurements with those of Caucasian populations [87]. The findings showed some significant differences, with the Emirati population having reduced ANB values, indicating a degree of mandibular retrognathia, along with increased lower anterior and posterior face height. These findings suggest that a Class II skeletal base is more common in the UAE population compared with Caucasian populations. Another interesting finding reported in that study was the common norm of a reduced inter-incisal angle among the Emirati population, indicating more protruded maxillary and mandibular incisors. Similar facial norms were also reported in neighboring GCC populations, indicating a shared gene pool resulting in such phenotype expression [88].

Gender differences influencing the soft tissue profiles of indigenous Emirati adults were also investigated in a recent cross-sectional study by Abutayyem and associates [89]. In that study, cephalometric analyses of 176 participants with normal occlusion showed that men had a greater soft tissue profile and H-angle compared to women. These findings underline the need for a rational prescription of orthodontic treatment that takes into account gender variation in soft tissue norms among Emiratis [89].

Currently, there is a paucity of research on malocclusion and dental anomalies in the UAE, and more nationwide, large-scale, and well-funded studies are urgently needed. Based on findings from such research, the orthodontic treatment needs of the UAE population can be more objectively assessed, and appropriate healthcare policies for management can be implemented.

42.5 Oral Cancer

Oral cancer is a major global disease burden with high mortality rates and debilitating impacts on the general health and well-being of affected individuals. There is a paucity of information and inconsistency in reporting oral cancer at the global and regional levels [90–92]. It is reported that nearly 450,000 new cases of oral cancer are diagnosed every year worldwide, and only 40–50% of these cases survive for five years from the time of diagnosis [92]. In 2020, cancer of the lip and oral cavity accounted for 2% of all new cases of cancer reported worldwide, with an overall mortality rate of 1.8% [93]. These numbers are projected to multiply over the next two decades, with anticipated global incidence and mortality rates of 900,000 and 450,000, respectively [94].

In Arab countries, the incidence of oral cancer (oral cavity and oropharynx combined) was estimated in 2018 at an age-standardized incidence rate (ASR) of 2.4, with 3500 deaths reported [90]. In the UAE, the number of new malignant oral cancer cases (lip, oral cavity, and pharynx combined) increased from 94 in 2011 to 151 in 2017, parallel to an increase in the overall number of new cancer cases [95] (Fig. 42.1). The relatively steady increase over time is consistent with a global trend of an increased number of oral cancer cases reported in developing and developed

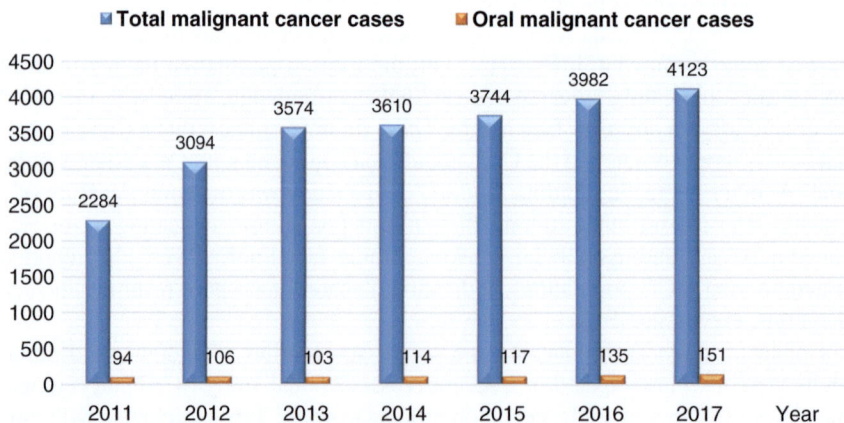

Fig. 42.1 Malignant oral cancer cases relative to total malignancies in the UAE across the period from 2011 to 2017. (*Source*: Data extracted from the National Disease Registry Center, The Statistics and Research Dept., Ministry of Health and Prevention. https://smartapps.moh.gov.ae/ords/f?p=105:511)

countries [92]. In the 2017 National Cancer Registry report of the UAE, oral cancer ranked as the eighth-most common malignant lesion of all sites, accounting for 3.66% of the total number of malignant cancer cases reported. Data retrieved from the Global Cancer Observatory (GCO) report of 2020 [5] estimated the number of new cases of oral cancer in the UAE at 125, which included 82 cases of the lip and oral cavity, 32 of the nasopharynx, and 11 cases of the oropharynx. The combined incidence rate was 2.6% of the total 4807 cancer cases reported for the year 2020. The number of deaths resulting from oral cancer was 61 cases out of the total 1896 deaths reported from all cancer sites, with a mortality incidence rate of 3.2%. When compared to other Arab countries, the UAE had the lowest ASR oral cancer incidence rate of 1.0 (34 cases) and the third-lowest ASR mortality rate of 0.8 (27 cases) as of 2018 [90]. Between 2018 and 2040, however, the incidence and mortality rates of oral cancer in the UAE are expected to increase as a result of population growth and associated demographic changes [90].

Population-based studies on oral cancer in the UAE remain very scarce. In one multicenter retrospective study [96], the authors examined the records of four major hospitals. Information on 992 oral lesions was retrieved, and out of these, 147 were found to be malignant, revealing a malignancy rate of 14.8%. Of the malignancies identified, oral squamous cell carcinoma (OSCC) was the most prevalent (77%), followed by mucoepidermoid carcinoma of the salivary gland. The most common sites of OSCC were the tongue (51.9%), the buccal mucosa (19.48%), and the lip (11.6%). These results seem to be in agreement with those reported globally for common malignancies of the oral cavity and salivary glands [91]. When compared to other Arab countries, the prevalence of oral cancer varies greatly, primarily because of the regional differences and associated sociocultural behaviors and habits of the population, and the manner of reporting oral cancer within the cancer registry of each country. Nevertheless, a prevalence ranging between 2% and 18% was reported in one systematic review of 19 studies from 10 Arab countries [97]. The most common oral cancer sites reported in that study were the tongue, floor of the mouth, and lower lip. In line with the UAE-based study, squamous cell carcinoma was the most prevalent malignant lesion [97].

42.5.1 Etiology and Associated Risk Factors

The etiology of oral cancer in the UAE and the GCC countries, in general, is multifactorial. Smoking, a sedentary lifestyle with lack of physical activity, dietary, genetic, and environmental factors, and alcohol consumption were risk factors associated with the progression of oral cancer [98]. Smoking, in particular, is an emerging health concern among UAE nationals aged 18 years and older, with a prevalence rate of 24.3% and 0.8% among males and females, respectively [51]. Common forms of tobacco use reported were cigarette smoking (77.4%), "midwakh" (15.0%), waterpipe (6.8%), and cigar smoking (0.66%). The use of "Midwakh" is particularly alarming because of its growing popularity among younger age groups and its frequency of use, which can be up to 12 times per day. In another report, the UAE ranked second highest in the GCC region in the prevalence of tobacco smoking among adults, with a rate of 34.9% in males and 1.6% in females [99]. The corresponding relative risk estimate for oral cancer (lip and oral cavity) among these tobacco smokers was 3.34%. When the pharynx and nasopharynx sites are included, the relative risk for the development of cancer increases to 12% overall [99].

The overall incidence and mortality rates of oral cancer in the UAE remain low when compared to the global average and other Arab countries. Changing demographics caused by continued population growth and economic prosperity, and the inflow of expatriate workers of diverse cultures and ethnicities, however, may change the oral cancer landscape in the UAE over time [90]. Prevention and increased awareness at the societal and healthcare professional levels are paramount measures to curb the anticipated increase in new oral cancer cases [100]. Furthermore, early detection utilizing emerging state-of-the-art diagnostics cannot be overemphasized in this context [101]. Supporting nationwide population-based oral cancer studies and establishing a national oral cancer registry are essential requirements for better oral cancer data collection and reporting in the UAE.

42.6 Obesity

Obesity is the excessive accumulation of fat to a level that impairs the health of adults or children. An adult with a body mass index (BMI) of 30 Kg/m^2 or greater is considered obese; for a child between the ages of 5 and 19, a BMI more than 2 standard deviations above the WHO growth reference would be considered obese [102]. Obesity is a global epidemic with a rate that has nearly tripled since 1975 and is still on the rise among adults and children worldwide. As of 2016, approximately 13% of the world's adult population was obese, while 18% of children aged 5 to 19 were either obese or overweight [102]. Evidence indicates that 55% of obese children will continue to be obese adolescents, with 80% of these adolescents eventually becoming obese in adulthood [103].

The prevalence of obesity in the GCC countries is alarming, with these countries falling into the top 40 countries with the highest rates of obesity [104]. Between 2017 and 2018, the prevalence of obesity among adults aged 18 years and older in the UAE was estimated at 27.8%, and for the 5- to 17-year-old age group, it was 17.35% [105]. When looking across the period from 2000 to 2018, no clear trend in the prevalence of obesity could be established. However, the obesity estimates remained high across the entire period, ranging from 21.5% in 2000 to 27.8% in 2018 for adults and from 13% to 17.7% in 2019 for children and adolescents, respectively [106].

42.6.1 Associated Risk Factors

The rapid economic growth and development and changes in lifestyle experienced over the past decades have been linked to the increased prevalence of obesity in the

UAE [107]. A sedentary lifestyle with reduced physical activity, the increased consumption of refined carbohydrates and energy drinks, and diets rich in saturated fats are all causative factors implicated in the increased prevalence of obesity among the youth and adults in the UAE [108]. For example, dietary habits such as fast-food consumption, frequent snacking between breakfast and lunch, and refined sugar intake in the form of chocolates and sweet drinks have been associated with an increased risk of obesity in school-age children to varying degrees [109]. Lifestyle habits such as watching TV for more than four hours a day, a lack of physical exercise, and smoking have also been associated with increased risks of obesity among UAE adolescents [110]. Other factors, such as a family history of obesity and lower educational attainment among mothers, have also been associated with an increased risk of obesity among school-age children and adolescents [111]. Socioeconomic variables allowing access to household help, preference for car use over walking, cultural and environmental barriers to outdoor activities, and reliance on indoor amusement have all contributed to the prevalence of obesity among the UAE population [112].

42.6.2 Obesity and Oral Health

The association between obesity and oral health has been described in several cross-sectional studies and reviews, and positive links to several diseases and conditions have been established. Among these are dental caries, periodontal diseases, tooth erosion, xerostomia, dentinal hypersensitivity, poor compliance with dental care, as well as the number of teeth present in the mouth [113–117].

Locally, the association between obesity and the DMFT index was investigated in one cross-sectional study of 803 school-age children in the Emirate of Sharjah [20]. Despite a significant positive correlation between BMI and DMFT scores, a strong correlation between obesity and dental caries among these children was not established. However, soft drink consumption was found to be a strong predictor of the risk of developing obesity and dental caries. These findings confirm earlier results linking carbonated drinks to an increased risk of obesity among adolescent females in the UAE [118]. Moreover, dietary habits, a known risk factor for the development of obesity, have been associated with the increased severity of dental caries in preschool children [29, 119]. Snacking three or more times per day [119], for example, and sugary food consumption [29] were found to significantly increase the caries risk in these young children.

42.6.3 Obesity Control Measures

The current state of obesity calls for effective preventive and interventional strategies to reverse the trend of the obesity epidemic in the UAE. These strategies should, with time, reflect improved general and oral health outcomes in the UAE population. For example, comprehensive awareness campaigns, counseling services, interventional programs, and outpatient health-promotion clinics are recommended to improve the health of the UAE population [37]. Other measures would include increasing parental awareness of the risks associated with childhood obesity and the importance of implementing healthy lifestyle choices such as avoiding processed and high-fat fast food, engaging in regular exercise, and actively participating in school-based sports activities [120].

42.7 Conclusion

The status of oral health in the UAE remains under-explored with a paucity of comprehensive research efforts. This is despite the pivotal developments that shaped its landscape in the country over the past decades (Fig. 42.2). Current findings suggest a relatively high prevalence of dental caries in the UAE population, while the prevalence of periodontal disease requires further exploration. These conditions are compounded by the prevalence of chronic health conditions such as cardiovascular diseases and diabetes mellitus, with obesity and smoking as modifiable risk factors of significance. Effective preventive strategies require strengthening the health information system and upscaling the existing oral health programs. The UAE Vision 2021 has prioritized the reduction of diabetes, cardiovascular diseases, and obesity rates among the main target areas, with multisector health policies and initiatives put into action. The formulation of a national oral health policy, however, remains imperative in light of the current status of oral health. That policy must be formulated as an integral part of the national health agenda and include clear objectives and defined key performance indicators. The rollout of tax levies on tobacco, energy drinks, and soft drinks was an important measure, and its positive impacts on

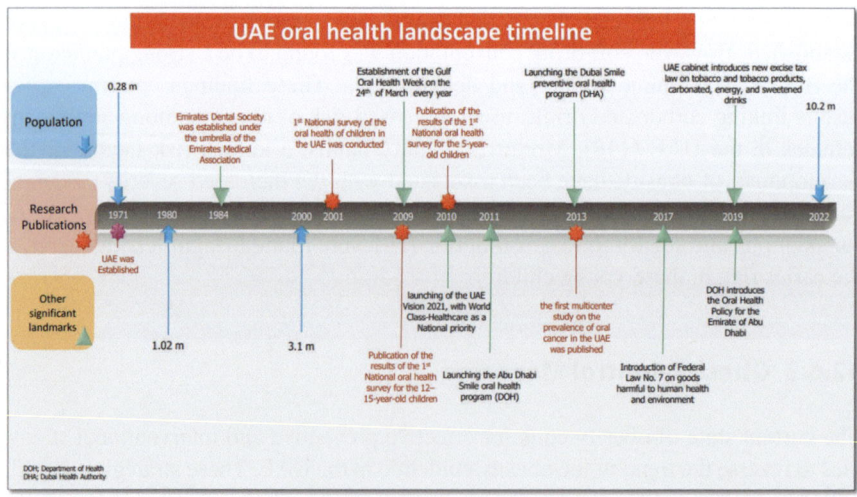

Fig. 42.2 UAE Oral health Landscape Timeline. (Created by Authors, Sources: [121–131])

general and oral health need to be reinforced with continuous awareness campaigns and nationally driven epidemiological studies. The diverse nature of the UAE community presents challenges when addressing the oral health status of the population. Yet, it provides a uniquely rich environment to explore multiple areas of research opportunity and the chance to test the impacts of various cultural models on the status of oral health in the UAE.

Conflicts of Interest The authors have no conflicts of interest to declare.

References

1. Glick M, Williams DM, Kleinman DV, Vujicic M, Watt RG, Weyant RJ. A new definition for oral health developed by the FDI world dental federation opens the door to a universal definition of oral health. Br Dent J. 2016;221(12):792–3.
2. FDI. FDI's definition of oral health. 2016. https://www.fdiworlddental.org/fdis-definition-oral-health. Accessed 23 Apr 2022.
3. WHO. Oral health. 2020. https://www.who.int/news-room/fact-sheets/detail/oral-health. Accessed 30 May 2022.
4. Roth G. Global Burden of Disease Collaborative Network. Global Burden of Disease Study 2017 (GBD 2017) results. Seattle, United States: Institute for Health Metrics and Evaluation (IHME), 2018. Lancet. 2018;392:1736–88.
5. GCO. Cancer incidence and mortality statistics worldwide and by region. Global Cancer Observatory. 2020. https://gco.iarc.fr/today/data/factsheets/cancers/1-Lip-oral-cavity-fact-sheet.pdf. Accessed 30 May 2022.
6. WHO. Birth defects surveillance: a manual for programme managers. 2020. https://apps.who.int/iris/bitstream/handle/10665/337425/9789240015395-eng.pdf. Accessed 30 May 2022.
7. Salari N, Darvishi N, Heydari M, Bokaee S, Darvishi F, Mohammadi M. Global prevalence of cleft palate, cleft lip and cleft palate and lip: a comprehensive systematic review and meta-analysis. J Stomatol Oral Maxillofac Surg. 2021;123(2):110–20.
8. Petersen PE, Bourgeois D, Ogawa H, Estupinan-Day S, Ndiaye C. The global burden of oral diseases and risks to oral health. Bull World Health Organ. 2005;83:661–9.
9. WHO. Information brochure for early detection and management of Noma. WHO Regional Office for Africa. 2016. https://apps.who.int/iris/bitstream/handle/10665/254579/978-929023354-1-eng.pdf. Accessed 5 June 2022.
10. Bennett JE, Stevens GA, Mathers CD, Bonita R, Rehm J, Kruk ME, Riley LM, Dain K, Kengne AP, Chalkidou K. NCD countdown 2030: worldwide trends in non-communicable disease mortality and progress towards sustainable development goal target 3.4. Lancet. 2018;392(10152):1072–88.
11. Dörfer C, Benz C, Aida J, Campard G. The relationship of oral health with general health and NCDs: a brief review. Int Dent J. 2017;67:14–8.
12. CDA. Oral health: a global perspective. 2017. https://www.cda-adc.ca/stateoforalhealth/global/#:~:text=Worldwide%2C%20the%20most%20common%20oral,of%20adults%20have%20tooth%20decay. Accessed 29 May 2022.
13. Anil S, Anand PS. Early childhood caries: prevalence, risk factors, and prevention. Front Pediatr. 2017;5:157.
14. El Tantawi M, Folayan MO, Mehaina M, Vukovic A, Castillo JL, Gaffar BO, Arheiam A, Al-Batayneh OB, Kemoli AM, Schroth RJ. Prevalence and data availability of early childhood caries in 193 United Nations countries, 2007–2017. Am J Public Health. 2018;108(8):1066–72.

15. Elamin A, Garemo M, Mulder A. Determinants of dental caries in children in the Middle East and North Africa region: a systematic review based on literature published from 2000 to 2019. BMC Oral Health. 2021;21(1):1–30.
16. Çolak H, Dülgergil ÇT, Dalli M, Hamidi MM. Early childhood caries update: a review of causes, diagnoses, and treatments. J Nat Sci Biol Med. 2013;4(1):29.
17. Kowash MB. Severity of early childhood caries in preschool children attending Al-Ain Dental Centre, United Arab Emirates. Eur Arch Paediatr Dent. 2015;16(4):319–24.
18. Kowash MB, Alkhabuli J, Dafaalla S, Shah A, Khamis A. Early childhood caries and associated risk factors among preschool children in Ras Al-Khaimah, United Arab Emirates. Eur Arch Paediatr Dent. 2017;18(2):97–103.
19. El Nadeef M, Hassab H, Al Hosani E. National survey of the oral health of 5-year-old children in The United Arab Emirates. East Mediterr Health J. 2010;16(1):51–5.
20. Khadri FA, Gopinath VK, Hector MP, Davenport ES. Evaluating the risk factors that link obesity and dental caries in 11–17-year-old school going children in The United Arab Emirates. Eur J Dent. 2018;12(02):217–24.
21. Al Mashhadani SS, Al Khoory T, Saleh N, Fargali K, Mathew R, Al Qasem N. National survey of the oral health status of school children in Dubai, UAE. EC Dental Sci. 2017;8:48–58.
22. Buldur B. Pathways between parental and individual determinants of dental caries and dental visit behaviours among children: validation of a new conceptual model. Community Dent Oral Epidemiol. 2020;48(4):280–7.
23. Vanobbergen J, Martens L, Lesaffre E, Bogaerts K, Declerck D. Assessing risk indicators for dental caries in the primary dentition. Community Dent Oral Epidemiol. 2001;29(6):424–34.
24. Poulton R, Caspi A, Milne BJ, Thomson WM, Taylor A, Sears MR, Moffitt TE. Association between children's experience of socioeconomic disadvantage and adult health: a life-course study. Lancet. 2002;360(9346):1640–5.
25. Fontana M. The clinical, environmental, and behavioral factors that foster early childhood caries: evidence for caries risk assessment. Pediatr Dent. 2015;37(3):217–25.
26. Fisher-Owens SA, Gansky SA, Platt LJ, Weintraub JA, Soobader M-J, Bramlett MD, Newacheck PW. Influences on children's oral health: a conceptual model. Pediatrics. 2007;120(3):e510–20.
27. Lee CY, Ting CC, Wu JH, Lee KT, Chen HS, Chang YY. Dental visiting behaviours among primary schoolchildren: application of the health belief model. Int J Dent Hyg. 2018;16(2):e88–95.
28. Al-Hosani E, Rugg-Gunn A. Combination of low parental educational attainment and high parental income related to high caries experience in pre-school children in Abu Dhabi. Community Dent Oral Epidemiol. 1998;26(1):31–6.
29. Elamin A, Garemo M, Gardner A. Dental caries and their association with socioeconomic characteristics, oral hygiene practices and eating habits among preschool children in Abu Dhabi, United Arab Emirates—the NOPLAS project. BMC Oral Health. 2018;18(1):1–9.
30. Ahmad SH, Petrou MA, Alhumrani A, Hashim R, Splieth C. Prevalence of molar-incisor hypomineralisation in an emerging community, and a possible correlation with caries, fluorosis and socioeconomic status. Oral Health Prev Dent. 2019;17(4):323–7.
31. Lagerweij M, Van Loveren C. Declining caries trends: are we satisfied? Curr Oral Health Rep. 2015;2(4):212–7.
32. Watt RG, Daly B, Allison P, Macpherson LM, Venturelli R, Listl S, Weyant RJ, Mathur MR, Guarnizo-Herreño CC, Celeste RK. Ending the neglect of global oral health: time for radical action. Lancet. 2019;394(10194):261–72.
33. Könönen E, Gursoy M, Gursoy UK. Periodontitis: a multifaceted disease of tooth-supporting tissues. J Clin Med. 2019;8(8):1135.
34. Highfield J. Diagnosis and classification of periodontal disease. Aust Dent J. 2009;54:S11–26.
35. Page RC, Eke PI. Case definitions for use in population-based surveillance of periodontitis. J Periodontol. 2007;78:1387–99.
36. Al-Harthi LS, Cullinan MP, Leichter JW, Thomson WM. Periodontitis among adult populations in the Arab world. Int Dent J. 2013;63(1):7–11.

37. Malik M, Bakir A. Prevalence of overweight and obesity among children in The United Arab Emirates. Obes Rev. 2007;8(1):15–20.
38. Khalifa N, Rahman B, Gaintantzopoulou MD, Al-Amad S, Awad MM. Oral health status and oral health-related quality of life among patients with type 2 diabetes mellitus in The United Arab Emirates: a matched case-control study. Health Qual Life Outcomes. 2020;18(1):1–8.
39. Al-Rawi N, Al-Marzooq F. The relation between periodontopathogenic bacterial levels and resistin in the saliva of obese type 2 diabetic patients. J Diabetes Res. 2017;2017:1.
40. Hashim R, Akbar M. Gynecologists' knowledge and attitudes regarding oral health and periodontal disease leading to adverse pregnancy outcomes. J Int Soc Prevent Commun Dent. 2014;4(Suppl 3):S166.
41. Awad M, Rahman B, Hasan H, Ali H. The relationship between body mass index and periodontitis in Arab patients with type 2 diabetes mellitus. Oman Med J. 2015;30(1):36.
42. Kornman KS. Mapping the pathogenesis of periodontitis: a new look. J Periodontol. 2008;79:1560–8.
43. Genco RJ, Borgnakke WS. Risk factors for periodontal disease. Periodontology 2000. 2013;62(1):59–94.
44. Nociti FH Jr, Casati MZ, Duarte PM. Current perspective of the impact of smoking on the progression and treatment of periodontitis. Periodontology 2000. 2015;67(1):187–210.
45. Valles Y, Inman C. Peters B types of tobacco consumption and the oral microbiome in The United Arab Emirates Healthy Future (UAEHFS) Pilot Study. Sci Rep. 2018;8(1):11327.
46. Grossi SG, Zambon JJ, Ho AW, Koch G, Dunford RG, Machtei EE, Norderyd OM, Genco RJ. Assessment of risk for periodontal disease. I. Risk indicators for attachment loss. J Periodontol. 1994;65(3):260–7.
47. Wu J, Peters BA, Dominianni C, Zhang Y, Pei Z, Yang L, Ma Y, Purdue MP, Jacobs EJ, Gapstur SM. Cigarette smoking and the oral microbiome in a large study of American adults. ISME J. 2016;10(10):2435–46.
48. Al Kawas S, Al-Marzooq F, Rahman B, Shearston JA, Saad H, Benzina D, Weitzman M. The impact of smoking different tobacco types on the subgingival microbiome and periodontal health: a pilot study. Sci Rep. 2021;11(1):1–16.
49. Ramôa CP, Eissenberg T, Sahingur SE. Increasing popularity of waterpipe tobacco smoking and electronic cigarette use: implications for oral healthcare. J Periodontal Res. 2017;52(5):813–23.
50. Fakhreddine HMB, Kanj AN, Kanj NA. The growing epidemic of water pipe smoking: health effects and future needs. Respir Med. 2014;108(9):1241–53.
51. Al-Houqani M, Ali R, Hajat C. Tobacco smoking using Midwakh is an emerging health problem–evidence from a large cross-sectional survey in The United Arab Emirates. PLoS One. 2012;7(6):e39189.
52. Awan KH, Siddiqi K, Patil S, Hussain QA. Assessing the effect of waterpipe smoking on cancer outcome-a systematic review of current evidence. Asian Pac J Cancer Prev. 2017;18(2):495.
53. IDF.Diabetes facts and figures. 2021. https://www.idf.org/aboutdiabetes/what-is-diabetes/facts-figures.html. Accessed 16 June 2022.
54. IDF. IDF MENA Members. United Arab Emirates. 2022. https://idf.org/our-network/regions-members/middle-east-and-north-africa/members/49-united-arab-emirates.html. Accessed 16 June 2022.
55. Ryan ME, Carnu O, Kamer A. The influence of diabetes on the periodontal tissues. J Am Dent Assoc. 2003;134:34S–40S.
56. Taylor GW, Burt BA, Becker MP, Genco RJ, Shlossman M, Knowler WC, Pettitt DJ. Severe periodontitis and risk for poor glycemic control in patients with non-insulin-dependent diabetes mellitus. J Periodontol. 1996;67:1085–93.
57. Demmer RT, Holtfreter B, Desvarieux M, Jacobs DR Jr, Kerner W, Nauck M, Völzke H, Kocher T. The influence of type 1 and type 2 diabetes on periodontal disease progression: prospective results from the Study of Health in Pomerania (SHIP). Diabetes Care. 2012;35(10):2036–42.

58. Stöhr J, Barbaresko J, Neuenschwander M, Schlesinger S. Bidirectional association between periodontal disease and diabetes mellitus: a systematic review and meta-analysis of cohort studies. Sci Rep. 2021;11(1):1–9.
59. Nelson RG, Shlossman M, Budding LM, Pettitt DJ, Saad MF, Genco RJ, Knowler WC. Periodontal disease and NIDDM in Pima Indians. Diabetes Care. 1990;13(8):836–40.
60. Kıran M, Arpak N, Ünsal E, Erdoğan MF. The effect of improved periodontal health on metabolic control in type 2 diabetes mellitus. J Clin Periodontol. 2005;32(3):266–72.
61. Stewart JE, Wager KA, Friedlander AH, Zadeh HH. The effect of periodontal treatment on glycemic control in patients with type 2 diabetes mellitus. J Clin Periodontol. 2001;28(4):306–10.
62. Promsudthi A, Pimapansri S, Deerochanawong C, Kanchanavasita W. The effect of periodontal therapy on uncontrolled type 2 diabetes mellitus in older subjects. Oral Dis. 2005;11(5):293–8.
63. Eldarrat AH. Awareness and attitude of diabetic patients about their increased risk for oral diseases. Oral Health Prev Dent. 2011;9(3):235.
64. Sanz M, Marco del Castillo A, Jepsen S, Gonzalez-Juanatey JR, D'Aiuto F, Bouchard P, Chapple I, Dietrich T, Gotsman I, Graziani F. Periodontitis and cardiovascular diseases: consensus report. J Clin Periodontol. 2020;47(3):268–88.
65. Schenkein HA, Loos BG. Inflammatory mechanisms linking periodontal diseases to cardiovascular diseases. J Periodontol. 2013;84:S51–69.
66. Tonetti MS, Van Dyke TE, workshop* wgotjEA. Periodontitis and atherosclerotic cardiovascular disease: consensus report of the Joint EFP/AAPWorkshop on Periodontitis and Systemic Diseases. J Periodontol. 2013;84:S24–9.
67. Sharma P, Dietrich T, Ferro CJ, Cockwell P, Chapple IL. Association between periodontitis and mortality in stages 3–5 chronic kidney disease: NHANES III and linked mortality study. J Clin Periodontol. 2016;43(2):104–13.
68. Dietrich T, Sharma P, Walter C, Weston P, Beck J. The epidemiological evidence behind the association between periodontitis and incident atherosclerotic cardiovascular disease. J Periodontol. 2013;84:S70–84.
69. Lee Y-L, Hu H-Y, Chou P, Chu D. Dental prophylaxis decreases the risk of acute myocardial infarction: a nationwide population-based study in Taiwan. Clin Interv Aging. 2015;10:175.
70. Schaefer AS, Bochenek G, Jochens A, Ellinghaus D, Dommisch H, Güzeldemir-Akçakanat E, Graetz C, Harks I, Jockel-Schneider Y, Weinspach K. Genetic evidence for PLASMINOGEN as a shared genetic risk factor of coronary artery disease and periodontitis. Circul Cardiovas Genet. 2015;8(1):159–67.
71. Park S-Y, Kim S-H, Kang S-H, Yoon C-H, Lee H-J, Yun P-Y, Youn T-J, Chae I-H. Improved oral hygiene care attenuates the cardiovascular risk of oral health disease: a population-based study from Korea. Eur Heart J. 2019;40(14):1138–45.
72. Tonetti MS, D'Aiuto F, Nibali L, Donald A, Storry C, Parkar M, Suvan J, Hingorani AD, Vallance P, Deanfield J. Treatment of periodontitis and endothelial function. N Engl J Med. 2007;356(9):911–20.
73. GBD. GBD 2016 Causes of Death Collaborators. Global, regional, and national age-sex specific mortality for 264 causes of death, 1980–2016: a systematic analysis for the Global Burden of Disease Study 2016. 2016. https://www.thelancet.com/journals/lancet/article/PIIS0140-6736(17)32152-9/fulltext. Accessed 16 June 16 2022.
74. Al-Shamsi S, Regmi D, Govender RD. Incidence of cardiovascular disease and its associated risk factors in at-risk men and women in The United Arab Emirates: a 9-year retrospective cohort study. BMC Cardiovasc Disord. 2019;19(1):1–9.
75. UAE Vision 2021. Number of deaths from cardiovascular diseases per 100,000 people. 2018. https://www.vision2021.ae/en/national-agenda-2021/list/card/number-of-deaths-from-cardiovascular-diseases-per-100-000-population. Accessed 21 June 2022.
76. Radaideh G, Tzemos N, Ali TM, Eldershaby Y, Joury J, Abreu P. Cardiovascular risk factor burden in The United Arab Emirates (UAE): the Africa Middle East (AfME) cardiovascular epidemiological (ACE) study sub-analysis. Int Cardiovasc Forum J. 2017; 11.

77. Jacobson A. The dental aesthetic index. Am J Orthod Dentofacial Orthop. 1987;92(6):521–2.
78. Brook PH, Shaw WC. The development of an index of orthodontic treatment priority. Eur J Orthod. 1989;11(3):309–20.
79. Houston W. Walther's orthodontic notes. 4th ed. Berkeley: Stonebridge Publishers; 2000.
80. Dos Santos RR, Nayme JG, Garbin AJ, Saliba N, Garbin CA, Moimaz SA. Prevalence of malocclusion and related oral habits in 5-to 6-year-old children. Oral Health Prev Dent. 2012;10(4):311–8.
81. Dimberg L, Arnrup K, Bondemark L. The impact of malocclusion on the quality of life among children and adolescents: a systematic review of quantitative studies. Eur J Orthod. 2015;37(3):238–47.
82. Alrashed M, Alqerban A. The relationship between malocclusion and oral health-related quality of life among adolescents: a systematic literature review and meta-analysis. Eur J Orthod. 2021;43(2):173–83.
83. Baskaradoss JK, Geevarghese A, Alsaadi W, Alemam H, Alghaihab A, Almutairi AS, Almthen A. The impact of malocclusion on the oral health related quality of life of 11–14-year-old children. BMC Pediatr. 2022;22(1):1–6.
84. Simões RC, Goettems ML, Schuch HS, Torriani DD, Demarco FF. Impact of malocclusion on oral health-related quality of life of 8-12 years old schoolchildren in southern Brazil. Braz Dent J. 2017;28:105–12.
85. Abu-Fanas A, Hashim R, Al-Ali S. Orthodontic treatment needs among 9-12 years old children in the Emirate of Ajman, United Arab Emirates. J Adv Oral Res. 2015;6(3):39–42.
86. Cenzato N, Nobili A, Maspero C. Prevalence of dental malocclusions in different geographical areas: scoping review. Dent J. 2021;9(10):117.
87. Al Zain T, Ferguson DJ. Cephalometric characterization of an adult Emirati sample with class I malocclusion. J Orthodontic Sci. 2012;1(1):11.
88. Aldrees AM. Lateral cephalometric norms for Saudi adults: a meta-analysis. Saudi Dental J. 2011;23(1):3–7.
89. Abutayyem H, Alshamsi A, Quadri MFA. Soft tissue cephalometric norms in Emirati population: a cross-sectional study. J Multidiscip Healthc. 2021;14:2863.
90. Kujan O, Idrees M, Farah CS. Oral and oropharyngeal cancer in arab nations. In: Metzler JB, editor. Handbook of healthcare in the Arab world. Ismail Laher; 2019. p. 1–24.
91. García-Martín JM, Varela-Centelles P, González M, Seoane-Romero JM, Seoane J, García-Pola MJ. Epidemiology of oral cancer. In: Oral cancer detection. Springer; 2019. p. 81–93.
92. Ren ZH, Hu CY, He HR, Li YJ, Lyu J. Global and regional burdens of oral cancer from 1990 to 2017: results from the global burden of disease study. Cancer Commun. 2020;40(2–3):81–92.
93. Sung H, Ferlay J, Siegel RL, Laversanne M, Soerjomataram I, Jemal A, Bray F. Global cancer statistics 2020: GLOBOCAN estimates of incidence and mortality worldwide for 36 cancers in 185 countries. CA Cancer J Clin. 2021;71(3):209–49.
94. Ferlay J, Ervik M, Lam F, Colombet M, Mery L, Piñeros M, Znaor A, Soerjomataram I, Bray F. Global cancer observatory: cancer today. Lyon; 2018. International Agency for Research on Cancer
95. Ministry of Health and Prevention (MOHAP). The Statistics & Research Dept. – National Disease Registry Section. 2017. https://smartapps.moh.gov.ae/ords/f?p=105:511. Accessed 22 June 2022.
96. Anis R, Gaballah K. Oral cancer in the UAE: a multicenter, retrospective study. Libyan J Med. 2013;8(1):21782.
97. Al-Jaber A, Al-Nasser L, El-Metwally A. Epidemiology of oral cancer in Arab countries. Saudi Med J. 2016;37(3):249.
98. Alqahtani WS, Almufareh NA, Al-Johani HA, Alotaibi RK, Juliana CI, Aljarba NH, Alqahtani AS, Almarshedy B, Elasbali AM, Ahmed HG. Oral and oropharyngeal cancers and possible risk factors across Gulf Cooperation Council countries: a systematic review. World J Oncol. 2020;11(4):173.
99. Al-Zalabani AH. Cancer incidence attributable to tobacco smoking in GCC countries in 2018. Tob Induc Dis. 2020;18:18.

100. Alfano MC, Horowitz AM. Professional and community efforts to prevent morbidity and mortality from oral cancer. J Am Dent Assoc. 2001;132:24S–9S.
101. Chattopadhyay I, Panda M. Recent trends of saliva omics biomarkers for the diagnosis and treatment of oral cancer. J Oral Biosci. 2019;61(2):84–94.
102. Organization WH. Obesity and overweight. 2021. https://www.who.int/news-room/fact-sheets/detail/obesity-and-overweight#:~:text=%2Fm2).-,Adults,than%20or%20equal%20to%2030. Accessed 22 June 2022.
103. Simmonds M, Llewellyn A, Owen CG, Woolacott N. Predicting adult obesity from childhood obesity: a systematic review and meta-analysis. Obes Rev. 2016;17(2):95–107.
104. Global Obesity Observatory. World obesity data tables. 2022. https://data.worldobesity.org/tables/. Accessed 29 May 2022.
105. Gulf News. MoHAP sharpens focus on nutrition in UAE ahead of world obesity Day. 2022. Gulf News, 03 March 2022.
106. Global Obesity Observatory. World obesity. United Arab Emirates. 2022. https://data.worldobesity.org/country/united-arab-emirates-225/. Accessed 29 May 2022.
107. ALNohair S. Obesity in gulf countries. Int J Health Sci. 2014;8(1):79.
108. Razzak HA, El-Metwally A, Harbi A, Al-Shujairi A, Qawas A. The prevalence and risk factors of obesity in The United Arab Emirates. Saudi J Obesi. 2017;5(2):57.
109. Bin Zaal A, Musaiger A, D'Souza R. Dietary habits associated with obesity among adolescents in Dubai, United Arab Emirates. Nutr Hosp. 2009;24(4):437–44.
110. Musaiger A, Lloyd O, Al-Neyadi S, Bener A. Lifestyle factors associated with obesity among male university students in The United Arab Emirates. Nutrit Food Sci. 2003;33(4):145147.
111. Moussa M, Skaik M, Selwanes S, Yaghy O, Bin-Othman S. Factors associated with obesity in school children. Int J Obes Relat Metab Disord. 1994;18(7):513–5.
112. Rajan PB. The growing problem of obesity in the UAE. Academicus Int Sci J. 2018;9(18):106–13.
113. Linden G, Patterson C, Evans A, Kee F. Obesity and periodontitis in 60–70-year-old men. J Clin Periodontol. 2007;34(6):461–6.
114. Morita I, Okamoto Y, Yoshii S, Nakagaki H, Mizuno K, Sheiham A, Sabbah W. Five-year incidence of periodontal disease is related to body mass index. J Dent Res. 2011;90(2):199–202.
115. Östberg A-L, Bengtsson C, Lissner L, Hakeberg M. Oral health and obesity indicators. BMC Oral Health. 2012;12(1):1–7.
116. Sheiham A, Steele J, Marcenes W, Finch S, Walls A. The relationship between oral health status and Body Mass Index among older people: a national survey of older people in Great Britain. Br Dent J. 2002;192(12):703–6.
117. Suvan J, D'Aiuto F. Assessment and management of oral health in obesity. Curr Obes Rep. 2013;2(2):142–9.
118. Mahmood M, Saleh A, Al-Alawi F, Ahmed F. Health effects of soda drinking in adolescent girls in The United Arab Emirates. J Crit Care. 2008;23(3):434–40.
119. Hashim R, Williams SM, Murray Thomson W. Diet and caries experience among preschool children in Ajman, United Arab Emirates. Eur J Oral Sci. 2009;117(6):734–40.
120. AlBlooshi A, Shaban S, AlTunaiji M, Fares N, AlShehhi L, AlShehhi H, AlMazrouei A, Souid AK. Increasing obesity rates in school children in United Arab Emirates. Obes Sci Pract. 2016;2(2):196–202.
121. UAE population figures (1971, 1980, 2000, 2022): https://www.worlddata.info/asia/arab-emirates/populationgrowth.php#google_vignette
122. 1984 (Establishment of the Emirates Dental Society): Personal communication, Emirates Dental Society Board).
123. 2001 (1st National Survey of the oral health of children in the UAE was conducted): El Nadeef MAI, Hassab H, Al Hosani E. National survey of the oral health of 5-year-old children in the United Arab Emirates. East Mediterranean Health J. 2010;16(1):51–5.
124. 2009 (Establishment of the Gulf Oral Health Week): https://saudigazette.com.sa/article/530810/BUSINESS/Unified-Gulf-Week-starts-to-boost-oral-and-dental-health-program

125. 2009 (publication of the results of the 1st National Oral Health Survey of the 12–15 year-old-children): El Nadeef MAI, Al Hussani E, Hassab H, Arab IA. National survey of the oral health of 12-and 15-year-old schoolchildren in the United Arab Emirates. East Mediterranean Health J. 2009;15(4):993–1004.
126. 2010 (publication of the results of the 1st National Oral Health Survey for the 5-year-old children): El Nadeef MAI, Hassab H, Al Hosani E. National survey of the oral health of 5-year-old children in the United Arab Emirates. East Mediterranean Health J. 2010;16(1):51–55.
127. 2010 (launching the UAE vision 2021): https://uaecabinet.ae/en/details/prime-ministers-initiatives/vision-2021
128. 2011 (launching of the Abu Dhabi Smile Oral Health, DOH): https://www.prlog.org/11753716-abu-dhabi-smiles-oral-health-promotion-program-launched-in-abu-dhabi-global-citynews.html
129. 2013 (launching of the Dubai Smile Preventive Oral Health Program, DHA): https://capp.mau.se/bank-of-ideas/united-arab-emirates-my-smile-tooth-brushing-program-for-schoolchildren-in-dubai-uae/
130. 2013 (The first multicenter study on the prevalence of oral cancer in the UAE was published): Anis R, Gaballah K. Oral cancer in the UAE: a multicenter, retrospective study. Libyan J Med. 2013;8(1):2017, 2019: https://u.ae/en/information-and-services/finance-and-investment/taxation/excise-tax#:~:text=Consumers%20will%20need%20to%20pay,human%20health%20or%20the%20environment.&text=Under%20the%20UAE%20Federal%20Decree,excise%20goods%20into%20the%20UAE
131. 2017 (Introduction of Federal Law No 7 on goods harmful to human health and environment), 2019 (UAE cabinet introduces new excise tax law on tobacco and tobacco products, carbonated, energy, and sweetened drinks): https://u.ae/en/information-and-services/finance-and-investment/taxation/excise-tax#:~:text=Consumers%20will%20need%20to%20pay,human%20health%20or%20the%20environment.&text=Under%20the%20UAE%20Federal%20Decree,excise%20goods%20into%20the%20UAE

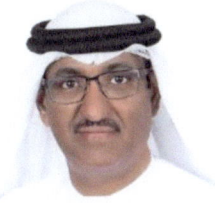

Dr. Nabeel Alsabeeha is a highly respected dental professional with a distinguished career spanning over 25 years in clinical practice, academia, and research. He earned his Doctor of Dental Medicine degree from the University of the East in the Philippines, followed by a master's degree in Prosthodontics from the University of Glasgow in 2005. In 2010, Dr. Alsabeeha completed his clinical PhD in Implant Prosthodontics at the Sir John Walsh Research Institute, University of Otago, New Zealand. Dr. Alsabeeha is a member of the Royal College of Physicians and Surgeons of Glasgow, UK, a Fellow of the International Team of Implantology (ITI), and a member of the Council of Scientific Affairs of the National Institute of Health Specialties (NIHS) of the UAE.

For over 25 years, Dr Alsabeeha served as a consultant prosthodontist in the Ministry of Health and Prevention and later with the Emirates Health Services in the UAE, where he played a pivotal role in enhancing the quality of dental care in the country.

Currently, Dr. Alsabeeha is a full-time Professor of Prosthodontics at the Department of Restorative Dentistry, College of Dentistry, Ajman University, UAE. In his current role, he remains actively committed to advancing the field of prosthodontics, with particular interest in addressing the dental needs of the elderly population, alongside his continued contributions to scientific research and dental education.

Throughout his career, Dr. Alsabeeha has authored over 45 peer-reviewed publications in renowned journals, covering wide areas of prosthodontics, implantology, and oral health education. His contributions to the dental community have earned him widespread recognition, culminating in the prestigious Medal of Excellence, awarded by the Prime Minister of the UAE during the 2019 Government Excellence Awards.

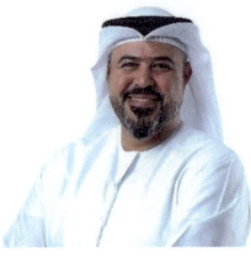

Dr. Mohammed Al Shalabi is a highly experienced consultant orthodontist with vast expertise in the field. He earned his BDS degree from the University of Glasgow, UK, in 2004, followed by a master's degree in orthodontics from Cardiff University, UK. In 2010, he obtained membership in orthodontics from the Royal College of Surgeons of Edinburgh, UK. From 2012 to 2019, Dr. Mohammed served as the Director and Head of the Orthodontic Department at Al-Ain Dental Center in Abu Dhabi, UAE. During his tenure, he played a pivotal role in establishing the orthodontic residency program in Abu Dhabi. Recently, he transitioned to private practice, assuming the role of a consultant orthodontist at Al-Arabi Medical Center in Al-Ain and the 360 Center in Dubai. Dr. Mohammed is recognized as an expert in the management of orthognathic malformation, cleft lip, and other oral defects and a pioneer in the use of clear aligners in the UAE.

Dr. Nada O. Al Shamsi possesses a rich and diverse background in dentistry, with over 15 years of experience in the field. She earned her Doctor of Dental Surgery degree from Ajman University of Science and Technology in 2005. She subsequently obtained a master's degree in orthodontics from the Jordan University of Science and Technology, Jordan. To further expand her scope of expertise, she completed a diploma in implant dentistry from Sharjah University in 2012 and a master's degree in Business Administration (MBA) from Abu Dhabi University in 2018. Dr. Alshamsi served as an orthodontist at the Ministry of Health and Prevention from 2006 to 2012 before moving to the Ambulatory Health Services in Abu Dhabi, where she continued her dedicated services. At present, Dr. Alshamsi serves as an orthodontist at Burjeel Hospital, Abu Dhabi, where she adeptly oversees orthodontic cases of diverse complexity, with a distinct focus on preventive, interceptive, and corrective orthodontics, including surgical cases. Dr. Alshamsi's unwavering commitment is devoted to the transformation of smiles, a process she believes significantly boosts the self-esteem and confidence of her patients.

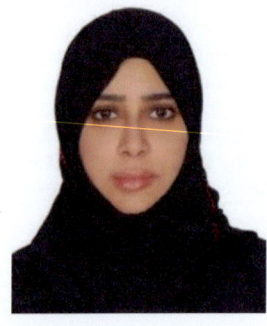

Dr. Shaikhah AlSamahi obtained her bachelor's degree in dental surgery from Ajman University in 2004, followed by a master's degree in endodontics from Jordan University of Science and Technology in 2009. In 2020, Dr. AlSamahi completed her PhD in endodontics from the University of Otago, New Zealand. Currently, she is a full-time consultant endodontist at Emirates Health Services and an adjunct faculty member in the master's program in Endodontics at the University of Ajman, UAE. Dr. AlSamahi has a special interest in pulpal biology, focusing on studying the relationship between systemic health, particularly diabetes type 2, and dental pulp. Her research work in this area has

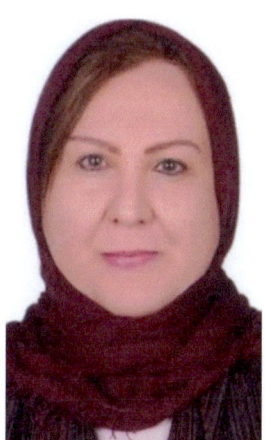

been presented at numerous international conferences and published in several international dental journals.

Manal A. Awad is a Professor of Dental Public Health and the Chair of the Department of Orthodontics, Pediatric and Community Dentistry, University of Sharjah, UAE. She obtained her BDS degree from the University of Alexandria, Egypt; her master's degree in dental public health from the University of Alberta, Canada; and her PhD in clinical epidemiology from McGill University, Canada. Prof. Awad's research is in the field of population health, with a focus on the assessment of therapies for chronic oral conditions, particularly tooth loss. Prof. Awad's area of expertise is in the use of patient-based outcomes and quality of life measurements in the assessment of therapies. She has made a significant contribution to the understanding of the impact of implant-supported prosthesis on the quality of life of edentulous patients (with colleagues in Canada, the United Kingdom, and Germany). She received many grants to support her research studies, including industrial support. Professor Awad is the former President of the International Association of Dental Research, UAE Section. She has also provided many years of service as a member of the editorial board for international scientific journals, including the prestigious *Journal of Dental Research*. Currently, she is an academic editor of the *International Journal of Dentistry*.

Open Access This chapter is licensed under the terms of the Creative Commons Attribution 4.0 International License (http://creativecommons.org/licenses/by/4.0/), which permits use, sharing, adaptation, distribution and reproduction in any medium or format, as long as you give appropriate credit to the original author(s) and the source, provide a link to the Creative Commons license and indicate if changes were made.

The images or other third party material in this chapter are included in the chapter's Creative Commons license, unless indicated otherwise in a credit line to the material. If material is not included in the chapter's Creative Commons license and your intended use is not permitted by statutory regulation or exceeds the permitted use, you will need to obtain permission directly from the copyright holder.

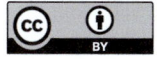

Early Childhood Caries (ECC) in the UAE

43

Anas AlSalami , Manal AlHalabi, Mawlood Kowash, Iyad Hussein, and Mohammed Mansour

43.1 Introduction

Early childhood caries (ECC), previously known as nursing bottle caries and baby-bottle tooth decay, continues to be a prevalent and serious chronic condition affecting children and remains a public health concern [1].

The burden of this disease on the child, the family, and society, including its impact on quality of life, is significant [2]. Oral health is crucial to maintaining oral functions, including eating, speech development, and a positive self-image. Hence, the most suitable way to manage this preventable disease is by adopting preventive measures that can reduce the chances of a child developing it [1].

ECC is characterized by the presence of one or more decayed, missing (due to decay), or filled tooth surfaces in any primary tooth of a child aged 71 months or younger. The detection of any smooth-surface caries in children under the age of three is considered severe early childhood caries (S-ECC). In children aged 3–5 years, the presence of one or more cavitated, missing (due to decay), or filled smooth surfaces in primary maxillary anterior teeth or a decayed, missing, or filled score of ≥ 4 (at age 3), ≥ 5 (at age 4), or ≥ 6 (at age 5) surfaces, is indicative of S-ECC [1].

ECC initially manifests as white-spot lesions in the upper primary incisors located along the gingival margin. If the disease progresses, complete crown

---

A. AlSalami (✉) · M. AlHalabi · M. Kowash · I. Hussein
Hamdan Bin Mohammed College of Medicine, Mohammed Bin Rashid University of Medicine and Health Sciences (MBRU), Dubai Health, Dubai, United Arab Emirates
e-mail: anas.alsalami@dubaihealth.ae; Manal.Halabi@dubaihealth.ae; mawlood.kowash@dubaihealth.ae; iyad.hussein@dubaihealth.ae

M. Mansour
Chair of Oral Health, Dubai Health, Dubai, United Arab Emirates
e-mail: mmahmed@dubaihealth.ae

© The Author(s) 2025
H. O. Al-Shamsi (ed.), *Healthcare in the United Arab Emirates*,
https://doi.org/10.1007/978-981-96-0523-1_43

destruction can occur with the involvement of the vital tooth pulp structures and the surrounding periodontal tissues and bone.

There are several factors that can pose a risk to the development and progression of ECC, including microbiological, dietary, and environmental factors. These factors are linked to structural enamel hypoplasia, oral colonization by cariogenic bacteria (especially *Mutans streptococci* [MS]), and acid production by these bacteria present in the dental plaque surrounding the teeth. This acid, over time, can reduce the mineral content of the tooth structure, leading to demineralization [3]. In addition, saliva plays a regulatory role and can be either a protective or risk factor, depending on its flow and composition [4].

ECC is a prevalent dental condition that arises due to several factors. Inadequate feeding habits, including excessive consumption of sugary foods and drinks, play a significant role in the development of ECC. Family socioeconomic status and insufficient parental education can also contribute to the condition, as families may not have access to proper dental health education or resources. Additionally, the limited availability of dental healthcare can make it difficult for families to seek preventive or restorative care for their children's teeth, leading to an increased risk of ECC.

When dealing with ECC, the usual method of restorative care often involves sedation or general anesthesia, which can be very expensive and pose potential health risks. Additionally, there is a high likelihood of the lesions recurring after the procedure [5]. The prevention and cessation of disease progression are critical objectives in healthcare. Effective implementation of chronic disease management, careful monitoring, and judicious intervention are key strategies that recent studies have emphasized as essential for achieving these goals [1].

43.2 Prevalence and Severity of ECC in the UAE

Several factors affect the prevalence and severity of ECC worldwide. One of those factors is the geographic region; children living in rural and deprived areas tend to have poorer oral health, primarily due to inadequate exposure to fluoride and poor access to dental services. Socioeconomic status is another factor; children from low-income families are at a higher risk of developing ECC as they depend on a high-sugar diet that is more available and affordable [6].

A Global Burden of Disease study in 2019 estimated that 2 billion people suffer from caries in permanent dentition, while 520 million in primary (milk) dentition [7]. Hence, ECC poses a worldwide public health concern, as it is considered one of the most common diseases affecting children.

The prevalence of ECC differs globally. A systematic review of 37 studies conducted in various countries, 20 in Asia, 7 in Europe, 6 in South America, 2 in the Middle East (Saudi Arabia and Turkey), 1 in Oceania (Australia), and 1 in Africa (Sudan), showed a wide range of prevalence (23–90%) and mean decayed, missing, and filled teeth (dmft) scores (0.9–7.5). Of the 37 studies, 26 scored higher than 50% of ECC [8].

ECC prevalence is relatively lower in Western countries [9] compared to countries in the Middle East and MENA regions. For example, in Saudi Arabia, the prevalence of ECC was 62–84%, with a mean dmft score of 3.0–7.1 [10]. Likewise, in the United Arab Emirates (UAE), the prevalence ranged from 74.1% to 83% in 4- to 5-year-olds with a dmft of 3.07–10.9 [11–13].

In 1998, Al-Hosani et al. [14] studied the prevalence of ECC in the Emirate of Abu Dhabi and reported the following: 41.5%, 78.5%, and 88% for the age groups 2, 4, and 5 years old, respectively. Unfortunately, several recent studies reported the same higher prevalence of ECC in the UAE. Hashim et al. [15] examined 1297 children aged 5 and 6 years in the Ajman emirate and reported 72.9% and 80% prevalence rates, respectively. El Nadeef et al. [11] examined 1340 5-year-old children as part of the first national survey of children's oral health in the UAE, and the prevalence rate was found to be 83%. In 2015, Kowash, in a convenience sample of 176 Al Ain preschool children aged 2–5 years old, found that the prevalence rate of dental caries was 99.4% [12]. In a sample of 540 preschool children in the Emirate of Ras Al-Khaimah, the reported prevalence was 74.1%, and the mean dmft was 3.07 [13].

Elamin et al. [16] studied 186 children aged 18 months to 4 years with a mean age of 2.46 years in seven Abu Dhabi nurseries. The prevalence of ECC was 41%, and the mean dmft was 1.70 (±2.81). There was a very low care index (CI = f/dmf × 100 = 0.65%), which means that most teeth had open cavities and fewer restored teeth (mean decayed component (dt) of 1.68 ± 2.80 and mean filled component (ft) of 0.02 ± 0.19). Previous studies in Al Ain [12] and Ras Al-Khaimah [13] also reported low care indexes of 6.4% and 3.8%, respectively.

A systematic review conducted by Al-Bluwi [17] included 11 studies that reported high prevalence and mean dmft ranges in preschool children (72.9–95% and 5.1–8.4, respectively). Another recent systematic review by Al Anouti et al. [18] reported that the prevalence range in the UAE was 22–99.4%, and the dmft range was 3.07–10.9. These wide ranges were reported because the included cross-sectional studies used WHO criteria for caries diagnosis but with different sampling techniques and inclusion criteria. Table 43.1 summarizes most of the UAE-published prevalence studies in preschool children.

It is clear that in the UAE, especially in the Abu Dhabi emirate, children demonstrate high and alarming levels of dental caries, although the average family income of the population is high and dental health services are free for Emiratis. The ECC prevalence is among the highest in the world, with higher caries scores in higher-income families. The underlying causes include the availability of high-sugar foods and drinks, which are given freely to children by affluent parents and extended family members, poor oral hygiene, and a lack of regular dental visits.

Table 43.1 UAE ECC studies on the prevalence and mean dmft in preschool children

Author	Year	Sample (n)	Study type	Age (years)	Mean dmft (±SD)	Prevalence (%)
Al-Hosani et al. [14]	1998	217	Cross-sectional	2	–	41.5
Al-Hosani et al. [14]	1998	204	Cross-sectional	4	–	78.5
Al-Hosani et al. [14]	1998	219	Cross-sectional	5	8.4	88
El-Nadeef et al. [11]	2010	1340	Cross-sectional	5	5.1	83
Hashim et al. [15]	2010	518	Cross-sectional	5	4.0 (±4.1)	72.9
Hashim et al. [15]	2010	518	Cross-sectional	6	4.9 (±4.3)	80
Al-Bluwi [17]	2014	–	Systematic review	4–6	5.1–8.4	72.9–95
Kowash et al. [12]	2015	176	Cross-sectional	2–5	10.9	99.4
Kowash et al. [13]	2017	540	Cross-sectional	3–6	3.07 (±0.14)	74.1
Amal Elamin [16]	2018	186	Cross-sectional	1.5–4	1.70 (±2.81)	41
Al Anouti et al. [18]	2021	54–24,220	Systematic review	–	3.07–10.9	22–99.4

43.3 Etiology of ECC

There are several factors that can influence the development of dental caries, including exposure to fluoride, salivary composition, and salivary flow. Additionally, the consumption of dietary sugars can have a significant impact on the presence of caries in dentin. The early stages of dental caries involve alterations within the complex biofilm, which are reversible and can be halted at any point. By being aware of these key factors and taking steps to maintain good oral hygiene, individuals can help prevent the onset and progression of dental caries [19].

It is important to differentiate between dental caries and ECC. Dental caries typically affects areas with plaque buildup, while ECC mainly affects the front teeth of the upper jaw that have not yet been affected by decay. There are various factors that can contribute to ECC, but prolonged breastfeeding or bottle use is often considered a major risk factor. Despite this, using a bottle at bedtime is not the sole cause of early childhood caries development. However, it is believed to increase the risk of developing caries [20].

The development of carious lesions is influenced by several factors, including the interplay between cariogenic microorganisms, fermentable carbohydrates, and vulnerable tooth surfaces. However, the specific factors that trigger the onset of caries may vary among different populations. Early childhood caries is most strongly linked to bottle use during sleep and a diet high in sugar. Furthermore, numerous risk factors may contribute to ECC, including elevated *Mutans streptococcus* (MS) levels and inadequate oral hygiene practices [21, 22]. Over time, dental caries develops due to the interplay of acid-producing bacteria and various host factors, such as teeth and saliva.

There are various factors that can impact tooth susceptibility to dental caries. These may include immunological factors, reduced saliva production, immature enamel, and defects in tooth tissues. It is important to note that susceptibility can also vary from surface to surface and from person to person, depending on factors such as tooth morphology, vulnerable areas that promote plaque buildup, and tooth positioning [23–25]. Dental caries tends to affect certain areas more than others, such as enamel pits and fissures, proximal enamel smooth surfaces, cervical margins, and exposed root surfaces due to gingival recession. Additionally, restored areas with deficient or overhanging margins can be particularly vulnerable to recurrent caries.

Maintaining ideal oral health requires a proper ecological balance, and saliva plays an important role in this process. Saliva's buffering capacity, secretion rate, ion composition (specifically calcium and phosphate), and cleansing action aid in counteracting the factors that lead to the development and progression of cavities. The oral immune system present in saliva, both specific and nonspecific, also plays a significant role in reducing the impact of cariogenic bacteria [26].

There is compelling evidence to suggest that fermentable carbohydrates, including sucrose, fructose, and glucose, are integral to the onset and progression of dental caries [27]. Sucrose is considered the most significant cariogenic food as it has the ability to convert noncariogenic or anti-cariogenic foods into forms that can cause tooth decay [28–30].

Frequent consumption of fruit juices and carbonated beverages has been linked to ECC in children. This is because fruit juices, which are naturally high in sugar (fructose), are also intrinsically acidic. Similarly, carbonated drinks may have an acidic pH and contain sugar-sweetened formulas (often fructose), both of which can significantly lower plaque pH and initiate the carious process [31].

Milk can be human breast, cow's milk, or formula. As recommended by the WHO, children should be breastfed until 24 months of age [32], argue that the prolonged exposure of teeth to daytime or nighttime breastfeeding is associated with a risk of ECC. According to reports, the American Dental Association (ADA) suggests that mothers should start weaning their children from breastfeeding after their first birthday [22]. In addition, the American Academy of Paediatric Dentistry (AAPD) strongly recommends restricting the use of baby bottles to up to 1 year and avoiding extended periods of breastfeeding [33].

It is important to note that children under 3 years of age have the highest incidence of ECC, which can be attributed to improper nursing habits like prolonged bottle-feeding and the use of sweetened pacifiers during bedtime [34]. Some experts believe that bottle-feeding can cause tooth decay, especially if a child is allowed to fall asleep while sucking on a bottle [34].

ECC has been reported to be associated with prolonged bottle-feeding, falling asleep with a bottle, and taking a bottle at nighttime [35, 36]. Du and coworkers observed a fivefold higher risk of developing rampant caries in children who were bottle-fed compared to those who were breastfed [37]. In contrast, Tsai and coworkers found that there was no direct relationship between bottle-feeding at night and dental caries, nor between a sugary drink in a bottle and dental caries in children [38].

According to the AAPD guidelines, it is advisable to introduce infants to drinking from a cup at 6 months of age. Additionally, bottle-feeding should be discouraged after the child turns 1 year old [39].

Consuming sweet foods, especially between meals, can cause a drop in pH levels that can persist over time. This can lead to demineralization of the teeth because there is not enough time for the pH levels to return to normal. The decrease in pH levels occurs during the fermentation of carbohydrates, mainly due to sucrose, which promotes an increase in *Mutans Streptococci* and *Lactobacilli* and a decrease in *Streptococcus sanguinis* proportions. Consequently, it can be concluded that acid production resulting from sucrose metabolism can disrupt the balance of the microbial community [40]. An imbalance in the oral microbiome can lead to increased growth of cariogenic species, which in turn can cause demineralization of a healthy biofilm. Sucrose is a fermentable carbohydrate that can contribute to this imbalance and has been found to exhibit higher cariogenicity than other carbohydrates [41]. Studies have unequivocally demonstrated that tooth decay in children is a direct result of excessive sugar intake and frequent snacking [41, 42].

Mothers play a crucial role in their children's oral health. As primary caregivers, they have a significant impact on what their child eats and how they eat. When mothers lack knowledge about proper feeding practices and oral hygiene maintenance, or neglect to seek professional dental care, it can put their child at a higher risk of developing caries compared to other children who receive better care. Additionally, beliefs that primary teeth are unimportant or that a child is not predisposed to caries can lead to early ECC and place a child at an increased risk of developing dental caries [43].

In a 3-year clinical trial conducted on preschool children, the frequency of tooth brushing was found to have a significant correlation with their experience of caries [44]. Individuals who reported that they brushed their teeth more than one time each day exhibited a 20% reduction in the progression of dental caries when compared to those who brushed their teeth less than once per day. The frequency of brushing and rinsing occurred had a considerable effect, with over 50% of the variance in caries increment between both groups being attributable to this factor [45]. Furthermore, based on a systematic review conducted in 2012 regarding the use of fluoride toothpaste, incorporating twice-daily use of fluoridated toothpaste alongside regular brushing resulted in a 14% reduction in caries [46].

Moreover, a cross-sectional study carried out in 2002 revealed that Flemish children who brushed their teeth less than once a day were at a higher risk of developing tooth decay and cavities [47]. The current recommendation for optimal oral hygiene is to brush teeth for at least 2 minutes, twice daily—once in the morning and once in the evening. It is advised to abstain from consuming any food or drink or from rinsing the mouth immediately after brushing to ensure maximum effectiveness of the cleaning process [48].

Extensive research has indicated that the utilization of toothpaste containing fluoride can lead to a notable reduction in the incidence of fresh dental cavities [49, 50]. This effect increases with higher concentrations of fluoride [51]. During the initial phases of tooth development, the introduction of fluoride can yield beneficial outcomes. This can be achieved through a variety of sources, including water, beverages, food, salt, fluoride supplements, or dental products [52]. Ensuring appropriate fluoride dosages are provided is vital to mitigating the risk of fluorosis, especially during infancy and toddlerhood. Emphasizing the importance of fluoridation is essential [53].

According to a study conducted by Nazzal et al. in 2016, it is recommended that children with a higher risk of tooth decay use toothpaste with a fluoride concentration of over 1000 ppm. Additionally, it is advised to spit out any excess toothpaste without rinsing after brushing [54].

There is a widely accepted recommendation among pediatricians and dentists in numerous countries to initiate tooth brushing with toothpaste containing fluoride upon the emergence of the first tooth [50, 55, 56]. According to research findings, the initiation of tooth brushing at an early age has been linked to a reduction in the prevalence of tooth decay among children [57].

43.4 Prevention of ECC

43.4.1 Individual-Based Intervention Content

The risk of oral disease among the pediatric population remains to this day, despite various preventive interventions. The impact of poor oral hygiene on a child's well-being is a major concern. The effects are not limited to the teeth but also extend to overall health. Oral diseases can significantly reduce children's quality of life, leading to speech impairment, poor nutrition, reduced school performance, and low self-esteem. Neglecting oral hygiene can result in infections and pain, which can escalate into more serious complications such as swelling, abscesses, malocclusion, and loss of space for future adult teeth if not treated promptly. The fortunate aspect of oral disease is that it is mostly preventable, and by following simple measures and recommendations, it can be eliminated [9].

Establishing a child's dental home is a critical step in ensuring the lifelong maintenance of oral health. To accomplish this, it is essential to begin preventive measures before the child reaches 12 months of age. This approach fosters a long-term relationship between the dentist and the patient, which encompasses all aspects of oral healthcare, including comprehensive, accessible, coordinated, and family-centered care. The dental home approach includes anticipatory guidance, preventive, acute, and comprehensive oral health care, with referral to dental or medical specialists when necessary. By implementing this approach, children's oral health can be ensured the attention and care it deserves [1, 3].

The risk of developing dental disease varies among children and may change over time. Therefore, assessing each child's risk for dental caries and identifying specific risk factors regularly allows for the effective delivery of individualized oral health preventive measures. For instance, high-caries-risk groups (children who nurse with a bottle at night, children with special health care needs, children from low socioeconomic groups, children with low exposure to fluoride, and children with a history of dental caries in mother/caregiver/sibling) will require more frequent dental visits and additional preventive interventions compared to low-caries-risk children (those who are caries-free or have well-controlled caries, have good oral and dietary habits, are highly motivated, and attend their dental appointments regularly) [58].

Multiple measures can be taken to prevent dental disease, including plaque removal through toothbrushing, limiting sugar in the diet, optimizing fluoride exposure in dentifrices and the water supply, applying fissure sealants, and regular dental checks with radiographs when appropriate [20].

43.4.2 Fluoride

The use of fluoride-containing preparations, such as toothpaste, gels, varnishes, and rinses, can provide significant benefits in preventing the development of dental caries, particularly in areas without water fluoridation. The incorporation of fluoride helps increase the tooth structure's resistance to demineralization, facilitates remineralization, and reduce the cariogenic potential of dental plaque. In recent years, fluoride varnish has gained popularity as a topical agent, particularly among preschool children and individuals with special healthcare needs. The American Academy of Pediatrics (AAP) recommends fluoride varnish application for children up to 5 years of age. However, healthcare providers must be mindful of the risk of ingesting too much fluoride in young children, as it can cause fluorosis [59].

43.4.3 Plaque Control/Toothbrushing

Effective and supervised toothbrushing with fluoridated toothpaste is important for preventing dental and periodontal disease. It is recommended to use a pea-sized amount of fluoridated toothpaste for children over 3 years of age and a smear-sized amount for children under 3. As the spaces between teeth start closing, dental floss is indicated. Moreover, children with special healthcare needs may require additional assistance because of their potential motor and cognitive challenges [60].

43.4.4 Diet

Sugar intake and frequency play a significant role in the occurrence of dental caries. Sugar decreases the pH in the mouth, which leads to the demineralization of enamel.

If sugar is consumed frequently, the salivary buffering action will not be sufficient to neutralize and remineralize the enamel and prevent further breakdown, which leads to dental caries. The risk of dental caries can be lowered through diet by minimizing the amount and frequency of sugar-containing foods and drinks, especially at bedtime, and by consuming sugar-containing foods and drinks with main meals rather than between meals. Moreover, parents and caregivers must be educated about bottle-feeding and the importance of avoiding it at night or while the child is sleeping [61].

43.4.5 Fissure Sealants

The long-term benefit of caries reduction from the use of sealants on teeth has been proven over the years, and they should be considered for all children with deep pits and fissures. While most sealants are applied to permanent teeth, there are instances where primary teeth can also benefit from them. Sealants fill the pits and fissures on the occlusal surfaces of posterior teeth. For some patients, the anatomy of their pits and fissures is such that it is deep and can trap food, which puts them at risk for fissure caries [59].

43.4.6 Community-Based Intervention Content

Community-based programs and initiatives for oral health promotion create a healthy environment that lowers the risk of dental caries in children [62]. Some examples of these programs include the following:

- Community water fluoridation to optimize the fluoride level in the water has been shown to be a cost-effective way to prevent dental caries and reduce the burden on the healthcare system.
- School-based programs that screen children for caries risk and devise nationwide plans and strategies to provide preventive interventions such as prenatal and postnatal counseling, fluoride varnish application, and sealants.
- Dental educational programs targeting caregivers, dental and medical healthcare providers, teachers, and school nurses emphasizing training the trainers on ways to combat oral disease.
- For some of these community programs to be effective, strong collaboration is often required with private and government healthcare and educational systems, as well as policymakers and regulators [62, 63].

43.5 Treatment of ECC in the UAE

43.5.1 Introduction

The high prevalence of ECC/S-ECC in the UAE [12, 13, 15, 17, 18] has increased the need and demand for professional care for such children, especially those who are underprivileged and require a high level of care [64]. The treatment of children's ECC must follow internationally recognized evidence-based guidelines (such as those provided by the AAPD) [33], and the provision of globally recognized treatment modalities for ECC/S-ECC is widely available in the UAE, whether through conventional restorative methods or minimally invasive approaches [65, 66].

There is evidence that UAE children's quality of life (QoL) improves at the patient and family level when specialists provide care in pediatric dentistry [67]. In the UAE, the general treatment of pediatric dental patients is mainly carried out by specialists in the field but is also provided by general dental practitioners (GDPs), specialists in pediatric dentistry who are based in private clinics and hospitals, government-based clinics and hospitals, and university-teaching hospitals and clinics [68].

Although expert pediatric dental care is needed to manage ECC, it is well known that the condition affects the general health and well-being of the child [12, 69]. Thus, it is imperative that all those caring for the health of children, especially pediatricians [70], are involved in the management of such patients as well. The treatment of patients with comorbidities, who are at high risk of dental caries compared to healthy children [71], is usually reserved for multidisciplinary specialist children's hospitals [72]. Unfortunately, some pediatricians lack awareness about ECC in the UAE [70], and thus supportive educational courses are required for this group and other healthcare professionals. It is essential to highlight that many children may not have access to dental care due to health inequalities related to costs. In addition, many children are "not brought in" by their caregivers due to possible dental neglect or a lack of education [73]. As such, UAE children who have ECC or S-ECC must have access to such treatment as part of their overall needs and rights, and efforts must focus on reaching out to the caregivers of such children, especially mothers, to educate them about the importance of prevention.

43.5.2 Treatment of ECC/SECC

The range of treatment offered for patients varies from primary caries prevention in the first instance to complete dental exodontia. On the other side of the spectrum, many children are brought in for dental treatment when it is too late, and there is pain or sepsis. Dental extractions are the only treatment option for severe and extensive tooth destruction.

Adequate treatment requires a thorough clinical examination and adequate radiographs (bitewings and/or periapical radiographs) to tailor the patient's treatment plan.

The spectrum of care for the treatment of care for ECC/S-ECC in the UAE is outlined in Table 43.2 and illustrated in Fig. 43.1.

Table 43.2 Treatment of ECC/SECC in the UAE

Treatment of ECC/SECC in the UAE		Notes
No care	This is dental neglect when the child patient is not brought to receive dental care	Dental care inequalities need to be reduced
Chronic disease management [74]	Combination of Temporizing open cavities with intermediate restorative materials Extensive prevention (toothbrushing, flossing) Diet advice Fluoride varnish application Silver diamine fluoride	This is a new concept of managing disease in very young children (6 months to 3 years), delaying active treatment until the child is older
Biological nonrestorative care (minimally invasive or noninvasive) [65, 66]	Prevention only	Toothbrushing Flossing Fluoride varnish	As above but for younger/older children
	Silver diamine fluoride (SDF)	The use of SDF 38% to arrest the carious lesion immediately	Causes clear black staining
	Interim therapeutic restorations	Placement of restorative materials, such as glass ionomers, in deep cavities close to the pulp	Helps diagnose the pulp status of a tooth Will need subsequent definitive treatment
	Anterior GIC strip crowns	Using preformed celluloid crowns with GIC cement	
	Atraumatic restorative technique (ART)	Gentle excavation of caries and placement of GIC or IRM	
	SMART	Coupling ART with SDF as above	
	Nonrestorative caries treatment	Using a high speed to open up a cavity to make itself cleansable with a toothbrush	Some caries removal Can be used for posterior and anterior teeth
	The Hall Technique [68, 75, 76]	Used for the non-pulpally involved asymptomatic carious primary molar non-near exfoliation	No caries removal Uses elastomeric orthodontic separators (EOSs) to create space
	The Modified Hall Technique [77]	As mentioned above, it is used for non-pulpally involved asymptomatic carious primary molar non-near exfoliation	Involves the drill to open up mesial and distal spaces No EOSs are used

(continued)

Table 43.2 (continued)

Treatment of ECC/SECC in the UAE			Notes

Full restorative care in the dental chair	*Quadrant dentistry*: Dividing the mouth into four quadrants and treating several teeth in one appointment	Topical anesthesia
		Local anesthesia
		Rubber dam isolation
			Anterior teeth [78, 79]:
			  Composites
			  Strip crowns
			  Zirconia crowns

	This is conducted in the dental chair with a reasonably cooperative child over multiple appointments		*Posterior teeth*:
			  Composites
			  Preformed metal crowns
			  Zirconia crowns

			Pulp therapy may be involved in any of the teeth, such as
			  Indirect pulp cap
			  Direct pulp cap
			  Pulpotomy (Ferric sulfate, Formocresol, MTA)
			  Pulpectomy (Metapex)

Full restorative care in the dental chair with sedation [80]	This is conducted in the dental chair in an *anxious* but cooperative child over multiple appointments	Inhalation sedation (nitrous oxide/oxygen -N_2O) or Oral sedation
		Intravenous sedation
			Anterior teeth [78, 79]:
			  Composites
			  Strip crowns
			  Zirconia crowns

			Posterior teeth:
			  Composites
			  Preformed metal crowns
			  Zirconia crowns

			Pulp therapy may be involved in any of the teeth, such as
			  Indirect pulp cap
			  Direct pulp cap
			  Pulpotomy (Ferric sulfate, Formocresol, MTA)
			  Pulpectomy (Metapex)

Full restorative care in the operating room (OR) [67, 72]: Hospital setting	Full mouth care comprehensive oral rehabilitation (COR)
	Anterior and posterior teeth restored in one session
	Close collaboration with the anesthetists and pediatricians required
		General anesthesia	*Anterior teeth* [78, 79]:
			  Composites
			  Strip crowns
			  Zirconia crowns

			Posterior teeth:
			  Composites
			  Preformed metal crowns
			  Zirconia crowns

			Pulp therapy may be involved in any of the teeth, such as
			  Indirect pulp cap
			  Direct pulp cap
			  Pulpotomy (Ferric sulfate, Formocresol, MTA)
			  Pulpectomy (Metapex)

Extraction of solitary teeth			May involve fitting of space maintainers
Full dental clearances			

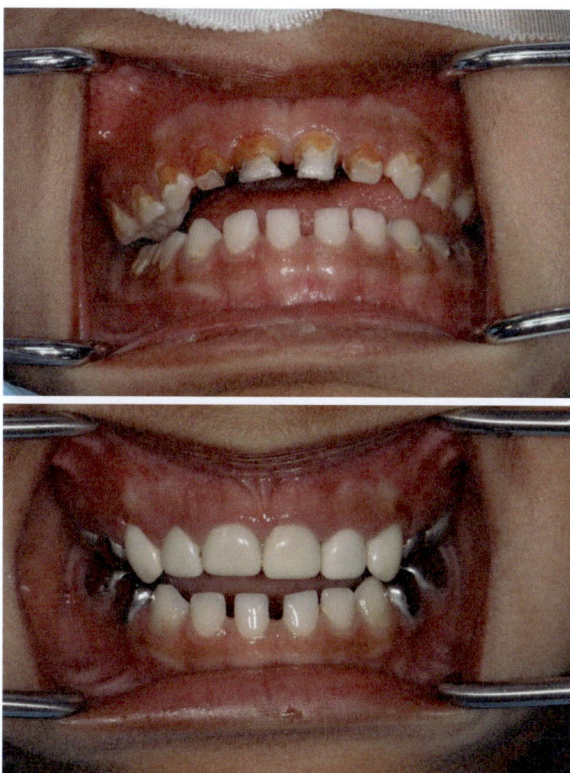

Fig. 43.1 The top photo shows a preoperative photograph of SECC, and the bottom picture shows a postoperative photograph after complete oral rehabilitation under general anesthesia

43.6 Conclusion

Early childhood caries (ECC) is a chronic oral health condition that affects primary teeth. It is caused by a combination of factors, including frequent consumption of fermentable carbohydrates in liquid form, on-demand breast- or bottle-feeding, oral colonization by cariogenic bacteria, inadequate oral hygiene, and suboptimal parenting practices. ECC is a prevalent issue among children and poses a significant public health concern in both developed and developing countries. The condition can cause discomfort, disfigurement, and a decreased quality of life for affected children, potentially impacting their future dental health.

Treating ECC can be costly and time-intensive and may require complete dental rehabilitation under general anesthesia by a pediatric dentist. However, ECC can be prevented through education for the parents of young children and for pregnant mothers. Dental health messaging should aim to alter the behavior of caregivers and parents by being practical, culturally sensitive, and considerate of their socioeconomic status.

In order to effectively manage ECC, it is crucial to have a comprehensive understanding of the biological process of tooth decay and the protective mechanisms that come into play. Consistent follow-up and long-term preventive strategies are imperative to monitor active lesion restorations. By prioritizing prevention and early intervention, the impact of ECC on children's health and well-being can be significantly minimized.

Conflicts of Interest The authors have no conflicts of interest to declare.

References

1. American Academy of Pediatric Dentistry. Policy on early childhood caries (ECC): classifications, consequences, and preventive strategies. Pediatr Dent. 2018;40(6):60–2. PMID: 32074852.
2. Zaror C, Matamala-Santander A, Ferrer M, Rivera-Mendoza F, Espinoza-Espinoza G, Martínez-Zapata MJ. Impact of early childhood caries on oral health-related quality of life: a systematic review and meta-analysis. Int J Dent Hyg. 2022;20(1):120–35. https://doi.org/10.1111/idh.12494. Epub 2021 May 26. PMID: 33825317.
3. Tinanoff N. Introduction to the conference: innovations in the prevention and management of early childhood caries. Pediatr Dent. 2015;37(4):198–9.
4. Hicks J, Garcia-Godoy F, Flaitz C. Biological factors in dental caries: role of saliva and dental plaque in the dynamic process of demineralization and remineralization (part 1). J Clin Pediatr Dent. 2003;28(1):47–52. https://doi.org/10.17796/jcpd.28.1.yg6m443046k50u20. PMID: 14604142.
5. Berkowitz RJ, Amante A, Kopycka-Kedzierawski DT, Billings RJ, Feng C. Dental caries recurrence following clinical treatment for severe early childhood caries. Pediatr Dent. 2011;33(7):510–4.
6. Otero G, Pechlaner G, Gurcan EC, Liberman G. The neoliberal diet and inequality in the United States. Soc Sci Med. 2015;142:47–55.
7. Global Burden of Disease Collaborative Network. Global burden of disease study 2019 (GBD 2019). Seattle: Institute of Health Metrics and Evaluation (IHME); 2020. Available from http://ghdx.healthdata.org/gbd-results-tool.
8. Chen KJ, Gao SS, Duangthip D, Lo ECM, Chu CH. Prevalence of early childhood caries among 5-year-old children: a systematic review. J Investig Clin Dent. 2019;10(1):e12376. https://doi.org/10.1111/jicd.12376. Epub 2018 Nov 30. PMID: 30499181.
9. Anil S, Anand PS. Early childhood caries: prevalence, risk factors, and prevention. Front Pediatr. 2017;5:157. https://doi.org/10.3389/fped.2017.00157.
10. Al Agili DE. A systematic review of population-based dental caries studies among children in Saudi Arabia. Saudi Dent J. 2013;25:3–11. https://doi.org/10.1016/j.sdentj.2012.10.002.
11. El-Nadeef MA, Hassab H, Al-Hosani E. National survey of the oral health of 5-year-old children in the United Arab Emirates. East Mediterr Health J. 2010;16:51–5. https://doi.org/10.26719/2010.16.1.51.
12. Kowash M. Severity of early childhood caries in preschool children attending Al-Ain Dental Centre, United Arab Emirates. Eur Arch Paediatr Dent. 2015;16(4):319–24.
13. Kowash M, Alkhabuli J, Dafaalla S, Shah A, Khamis A. Early childhood caries and associated risk factors among preschool children in Ras Al-Khaimah, United Arab Emirates. Eur Arch Paediatr Dent. 2017;18(2):1–7.
14. Al-Hosani E, Rugg-Gunn A. Combination of low parental educational attainment and high parental income related to high caries experience in pre-school children in Abu Dhabi. Community Dent Oral Epidemiol. 1998;26(1):31–6.
15. Hashim R, Williams S, Thomson W, Awad M. Caries prevalence and intra-oral pattern among young children in Ajman. Community Dent Health. 2010;27(2):109–13.

16. Elamin A, Garemo M, Gardner A. Dental caries and their association with socioeconomic characteristics, oral hygiene practices and eating habits among preschool children in Abu Dhabi, United Arab Emirates – the NOPLAS project. BMC Oral Health. 2018;18(1):104. https://doi.org/10.1186/s12903-018-0557-8. PMID: 29884158; PMCID: PMC5994070.
17. Al-Bluwi GS. Epidemiology of dental caries in children in the United Arab Emirates. Int Dent J. 2014;64:219–28. https://doi.org/10.1111/idj.12114.
18. Al Anouti F, Abboud M, Papandreou D, Haidar S, Mahboub N, Rizk R. Oral health of children and adolescents in the United Arab Emirates: a systematic review of the past decade. Front Oral Health. 2021;2:744328. https://doi.org/10.3389/froh.2021.744328. PMID: 35048059; PMCID: PMC8757796.
19. Ripa LW. Nursing caries: a comprehensive review. Pediatr Dent. 1988;10(4):268–82.
20. Lam PPY, Chua H, Ekambaram M, Lo ECM, Yiu CKY. Risk predictors of early childhood caries increment-a systematic review and meta-analysis. J Evid Based Dent Pract. 2022;22(3):101732. https://doi.org/10.1016/j.jebdp.2022.101732. Epub 2022 Apr 29. PMID: 36162891.
21. Begzati A, Berisha M, Mrasori S, et al. Early childhood caries (ECC)—etiology, clinical consequences and prevention. In: Emerging trends in oral health sciences and dentistry. InTech; 2015. p. 31–63.
22. Syed S, Nisar N, Mubeen N. Early childhood caries: a preventable disease. Dent Open J. 2015;2(2):55–61.
23. Berkowitz RJ. Cause, treatment and prevention of early childhood caries. J Can Dent Assoc. 2003;69:304–7.
24. Congiu G, Franca P. Early childhood caries (ECC) prevalence and background factors: a review. Oral Health Prev Dent. 2014;12(1):71–7. https://doi.org/10.3290/j.ohpd.a31216.
25. Seow WK. Biological mechanism of early childhood caries. Community Dent Oral Epidemiol. 1998;26(Supplement 1):8–27.
26. Kleinberg I. Etiology of dental caries. J Can Dent Assoc. 1979;45(12):661–8.
27. White GE. Diet, dental caries and other degenerative diseases. J Oral Biol. 2015;2(2):1–6.
28. Tinanoff N. Association of diet with dental caries in preschool children. Dent Clin N Am. 2005;49:725–37.
29. Zafar S, Harnekar SY, Siddiqi A. Early childhood caries: etiology, clinical considerations, consequences and management. Int Dent S Afr. 2009;11(4):24–37.
30. Zaki NAA, Dowidar KML, Abdelaziz WEE. Assessment of the Healthy Eating Index-2005 as a predictor of early childhood caries. Int J Paediatr Dent. 2015;25(6):436–43. https://doi.org/10.1111/ipd.12150.
31. Roberts G, Cleaton-Jones PE, Fatti P, et al. Pattern of breast and bottle feeding and their association with dental caries in 1 to 4 year old South African children. 2. A case control study of children with nursing caries. Community Dent Health. 1994;11:38–41.
32. World Health Organization. Dentition status and criteria for diagnosis and coding (caries). In: Oral health surveys. Basic methods. 4th ed. Geneva: WHO; 1997. p. 39–44.
33. American Academy of Pediatric Dentistry. Chicago. In: Pediatric restorative dentistry. AAPD; 2022. https://www.aapd.org/globalassets/media/policies_guidelines/bp_restorativedent.pdf. Accessed 30 Sept 2022.
34. Congiu G, Campus G, Sale S, Spano G, Cagetti M, Luglie P. Early childhood caries and associated determinants: a cross-sectional study on Italian preschool children. J Public Health Dent. 2014;74(2):147.
35. Hallett KB, O'Rourke PK. Social and behavioural determinants of early childhood caries. Aust Dent J. 2003;48(1):27–33.
36. Hallett KB, O'Rourke PK. Pattern and severity of early childhood caries. Community Dent Oral Epidemiol. 2006;34:25–35.
37. Du M, Bian Z, Guo L, Holt R, Champion J, Bedi R. Caries patterns and their relationship to infant feeding and socio-economic status in 2–4-year-old Chinese children. Int Dent J. 2000;50(6):385–9.

38. Tsai AI, Chen C-Y, Li L-A, Hsiang C-L, Hsu K-H. Risk indicators for early childhood caries in Taiwan. Community Dent Oral Epidemiol. 2006;34:437–45.
39. American Academy of Pediatric Dentistry. Guideline on infant oral health care. Pediatr Dent. 2014;36(6):141–6.
40. Layakumar H, Chandra M. Management of early childhood caries – a perpetual challenge to clinician. J Oral Health Community Dent. 2011;5(1):4–11.
41. Paes Leme AF, Koo H, Bellato CM, Bedi G, Cury JA. The role of sucrose in cariogenic dental biofilm formation—new insight. J Dent Res. 2006;85(10):878–87.
42. Rosenblatt A, Zarzar P. Breast-feeding and early childhood caries: an assessment among Brazilian infants. Int J Paediatr Dent. 2004;14:439–45.
43. Tiwari T, Albino J, Batliner TS. Challenges faced in engaging American Indian mothers in an early childhood caries preventive trial. Int J Dent. 2015;2015:179189. https://doi.org/10.1155/2015/179189.
44. American Academy of Pediatric Dentistry. Policy on early childhood caries (ECC): classifications, consequences, and preventive strategies. Pediatr Dent. 2014;37(6):50–2.
45. American Academy of Pediatric Dentistry. Guideline on caries-risk assessment and management for infants, children, and adolescents. Pediatr Dent. 2014;36(6):127–35.
46. Armfield J, Spencer A, Roberts-Thomson K, Plastow K. Water fluoridation and the association of sugar-sweetened beverage consumption and dental caries in Australian children. Am J Public Health. 2013;103(3):494–500.
47. American Academy of Pediatric Dentistry. Guideline on fluoride therapy. 2015. http://www.aapd.org/media/Policies_Guidelines/G_fluoridetherapy.pdf.
48. European Academy of Pediatric Dentistry. Guidelines on the use of fluoride in children: an EAPD policy document. Eur Arch Paediatr Dent. 2009;10:129–35.
49. Gülzow HJ, Hellwig E. Fluoride treatment for caries prevention. Guideline of the German association for dental, oral and maxillofacial health. 2007. http://www.dgzmk.de/uploads/tx_szdgzmkdocuments/Fluoridierungsmassnahmen_Langversion.pdf.
50. Wagner Y, Heinrich-Weltzien R. Pediatricians' oral health recommendations for 0- to 3-year-old children: results of a survey in Thuringia, Germany. BMC Oral Health. 2014;14(5):14–44. https://doi.org/10.1186/1472-6831-14-44.
51. Wong MC, Glenny AM, Tsang BW, Lo EC, Worthington HV, Marinho VC. Topical fluoride as a cause of dental fluorosis in children. Cochrane Database Syst Rev. 2010;20(1):CD007693.
52. Moynihan P, Petersen PE. Diet, nutrition and the prevention of dental diseases. Public Health Nutr. 2004;7:201–26.
53. Edelstein BL, Crall JJ. Best practice approach: prevention and control of early childhood tooth decay. The Association of State and Territorial Dental Directors; 2011. p. 1–37.
54. Nazzal H, Duggal MS, Kowash MB, Kang J, Toumba KJ. Comparison of residual salivary fluoride retention using amine fluoride toothpastes in caries-free and caries-prone children. Eur Arch Paediatr Dent. 2016;17(3):165–9.
55. American Academy of Pediatrics. A pediatric guide to children's oral health. Elk Grove: American Academy of Pediatrics; 2009.
56. Bottenberg P, Van Melckebeke L, Louckx F, Vandenplas Y. Knowledge of Flemish paediatricians about children's oral health – results of a survey. Acta Paediatr. 2008;97:959–63.
57. Chesters RK, Pitts NB, Matuliene G, et al. An abbreviated caries clinical trial design validated over 24 months. J Dent Res. 2002;81:637–40.
58. Kotha SB. Prevalence and risk factors of early childhood caries in the Middle East region: a systematic review. J Popul Ther Clin Pharmacol. 2022;29(3):e43–57. https://doi.org/10.47750/jptcp.2022.937. PMID: 36196937.
59. Rashed T, Alkhalefa N, Adam A, AlKheraif A. Pit and fissure sealant versus fluoride varnish for the prevention of dental caries in school children: a systematic review and meta-analysis. Int J Clin Pract. 2022;2022:8635254. https://doi.org/10.1155/2022/8635254. PMID: 36263239; PMCID: PMC9553663.
60. Goff SL, Gahlon G, Geissler KH, Dick AW, Kranz AM. Variation in current guidelines for fluoride varnish application for young children in medical settings in the United States.

Front Public Health. 2022;10:785296. https://doi.org/10.3389/fpubh.2022.785296. PMID: 35309203; PMCID: PMC8930922.
61. Davies GM, Davies RM. Delivering better oral health--an evidence-based toolkit for prevention: a review. Dent Update. 2008;35(7):460–2, 464. https://doi.org/10.12968/denu.2021.35.7.460. PMID: 18853715.
62. Ogenchuk M, Graham J, Uswak G, Graham H, Weiler R, Ramsden VR. Pediatric oral health: community-based participatory research. BMC Pediatr. 2022;22(1):93. https://doi.org/10.1186/s12887-022-03153-0. PMID: 35168600; PMCID: PMC8845330.
63. de Silva AM, Hegde S, Akudo Nwagbara B, Calache H, Gussy MG, Nasser M, Morrice HR, Riggs E, Leong PM, Meyenn LK, Yousefi-Nooraie R. Community-based population-level interventions for promoting child oral health. Cochrane Database Syst Rev. 2016;9(9):CD009837. https://doi.org/10.1002/14651858.CD009837.pub2. Update in: Cochrane Database Syst Rev. 2016;12:CD009837. PMID: 27629283; PMCID: PMC6457580.
64. Al Salami A, Al Halabi M, Hussein I, Kowash M. Oral health status of preschool children of incarcerated mothers in United Arab Emirates prison nurseries and oral health knowledge and attitudes of their caregivers. Eur Arch Paediatr Dent. 2018;19(4):255–66.
65. Al Halabi M, Kowash M, Hussein I. Hybrid child-friendly biological primary molar restorative alternatives to general anaesthesia. Dent Update. 2018;45:728–41.
66. Al-Halabi M, Salami A, Alnuaimi E, Kowash M, Hussein I. Assessment of paediatric dental guidelines and caries management alternatives in the post COVID-19 period. A critical review and clinical recommendations. Eur Arch Paediatr Dent. 2020;21(5):543–56.
67. Alantali K, Al-Halabi M, Hussein I, El-Tatari A, Hassan A, Kowash M. Changes in preschool children's oral health-related quality of life following restorative dental general anaesthesia. Br Dent J. 2020;229(10):670–6. https://doi.org/10.1038/s41415-020-2335-7. Epub 2020 Nov 27. PMID: 33247261.
68. Binladen H, Al Halabi M, Kowash M, et al. A 24-month retrospective study of preformed metal crowns: the Hall technique versus the conventional preparation method. Eur Arch Paediatr Dent. 2021;22(1):67–75.
69. Al Ayyan W, Al Halabi M, Hussein I, Khamis AH, Kowash M. A systematic review and meta-analysis of primary teeth caries studies in Gulf Cooperation Council States. Saudi Dent J. 2018;30(3):175–82.
70. Aburahima N, Hussein I, Kowash M, Alsalami A, Al Halabi M. Assessment of paediatricians' oral health knowledge, behaviour, and attitude in the United Arab Emirates. Int J Dent. 2020;2020:7930564.
71. Mansoor D, Al Halabi M, Khamis AH, Kowash M. Oral health challenges facing Dubai children with autism spectrum disorder at home and in accessing oral health care. Eur J Paediatr Dent. 2018;19(2):127–33.
72. Abdo M, Al Halabi M, Hussein I, et al. Characteristics of pediatric dental treatment provided under general anesthesia in Dubai, United Arab Emirates: a retrospective analysis. Int J Dent. 2022;2022:9900775.
73. Al Hashmi R, Hussein I, Kowash M, Welbury R, Al-Halabi M. Child maltreatment in Dubai and the northern United Arab Emirates: dental hygienists and assistants' knowledge. Eur Arch Paediatr Dent. 2021;22(4):651–8.
74. Ng MW, Fida Z. Dental hygienist-led chronic disease management system to control early childhood caries. J Evid Based Dent Pract. 2016;16(Suppl):20–33.
75. Abu Serdaneh S, AlHalabi M, Kowash M, et al. Hall technique crowns and children's masseter muscle activity: a surface electromyography pilot study. Int J Paediatr Dent. 2020;30(3):303–13.
76. Innes NP, Evans DJ, Stirrups DR. The Hall Technique; a randomized controlled clinical trial of a novel method of managing carious primary molars in general dental practice: acceptability of the technique and outcomes at 23 months. BMC Oral Health. 2007;7:18.
77. Elamin F, Abdelazeem N, Salah I, Mirghani Y, Wong F. A randomized clinical trial comparing Hall vs conventional technique in placing preformed metal crowns from Sudan. PLoS One. 2019;14(6):e0217740.

78. Salami A, Walia T, Bashiri R. Comparison of parental satisfaction with three tooth-colored full-coronal restorations in primary maxillary incisors. J Clin Pediatr Dent. 2015;39(5):423–8.
79. Walia T, Salami AA, Bashiri R, Hamoodi OM, Rashid F. A randomised controlled trial of three aesthetic full-coronal restorations in primary maxillary teeth. Eur J Paediatr Dent. 2014;15(2):113–8.
80. Halabi MA, Hussein I, Salami A, et al. A study protocol of a single-center investigator-blinded randomized parallel group study to investigate the effect of an acclimatization visit on children's behavior during inhalational sedation in a United Arab Emirates pediatric dentistry postgraduate setting as measured by the levels of salivary Alpha Amylase and Cortisol. Medicine (Baltimore). 2019;98(35):e16978.

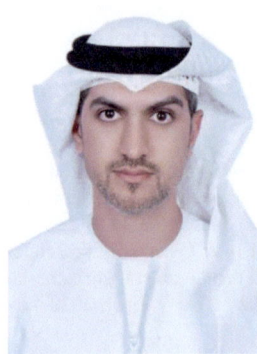

Dr. Anas AlSalami is an assistant professor and program director of the Master of Science in Pediatric Dentistry at Hamdan Bin Mohammed College of Dental Medicine, MBRU. He has been a consultant in pediatric dentistry with a special interest in the oral health of children with special needs at Dubai Dental Hospital and AlJalila Children's Hospital since 2017. Dr. Al Salami is a member of the Royal College of Surgeons of Edinburgh, UK, and Ireland. He received his Ph.D. in dental public health from Queen's University Belfast, UK. He has been in academia and research since he obtained his D.D.S. degree and has published over 30 articles in scientific journals of international repute. In 2017, he published his first book, *Oral Health of Children of Incarcerated Mothers at UAE Jail Nurseries*. Since 2015, he has been a volunteer pediatric dentist at the UAE Red Crescent Medical Center. Dr. Al Salami has received multiple awards, including the IADR Hutton Award and the DHCC Excellence Award in 2018. He is a member of the National Institute of Health Specialties (NIHS) Scientific Committees of the Emirati Board for Pediatric Dentistry and Dental Internship Programs in the UAE. Recently, he has been appointed as an Associate Designated Institutional Official at Dubai Health (DH).

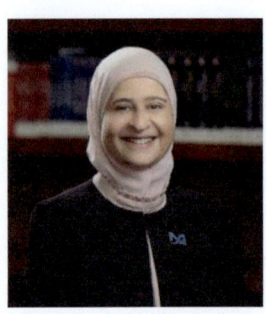

Dr. Manal AlHalabi obtained her dental degree from the University of Jordan in Amman and her Certificate of Specialty Training in Pediatric Dentistry and Master of Oral Biology from the University of Maryland at Baltimore in the USA. She is certified by the American Board of Pediatric Dentistry. Dr. Manal is the Dean and Professor of Pediatric Dentistry at Hamdan Bin Mohammed College of Dental Medicine, Mohammed Bin Rashid University of Medicine and Health Sciences. She is also a founding executive board member of the Emirates Pediatric Dentistry Club of the Emirates Dental Association. Dr. Manal is an appointed member of the Educational Committee of the International Association of Paediatric Dentistry and the Standardized Records Committee of the International Association of Dental Traumatology. Her experience includes academic positions with Boston University and the University of Maryland, as well as private clinical practice in the USA and the UAE. Her research interests include dental education, the oral health of patients with special needs, traumatic dental injuries, and biological caries management in primary teeth. Dr. Manal has numerous publications in internationally renowned, high-impact professional journals.

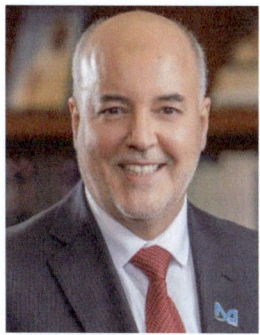

Dr. Mawlood Kowash received his Dental Degree (BDS) from Libya in 1985 and his master's and Ph.D. in Pediatric Dentistry from the University of Leeds, UK, in 1993 and 1999, respectively. He became a fellow of the Royal College of Dentists of Canada in 1998 and a fellow of the Royal College of Physicians and Surgeons of Glasgow and the Royal College of Surgeons of Edinburgh in 2015 and 2019, respectively. Currently, Dr. Kowash is working at MBRU as a professor and consultant in pediatric dentistry in Dubai, UAE.

Dr. Kowash is an examiner for the Royal College of Edinburgh MFDS Part 2 and has served as an external examiner for pediatric dentistry regionally and internationally. He has over 60 publications in peer-reviewed journals, and he is a reviewer for several international peer-reviewed journals.

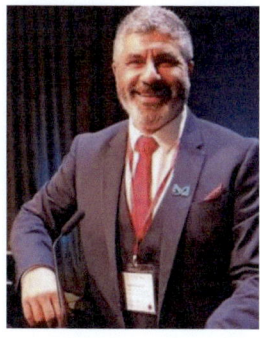

Iyad Hussein has been a consultant in pediatric dentistry and an associate professor at Mohammed Bin Rashid University of Medicine and Health Sciences (MBRU), Dubai Dental Hospital, and AlJalila Speciality Children's Hospital in Dubai, United Arab Emirates (UAE) since 2014. He is British and has been on the UK's "Specialist in Paediatric Dentistry" list since 2001. He has 32 years of experience in his discipline and is also a member of the Faculty of Dentistry of the Royal College of Physicians and Surgeons of Glasgow. Iyad received his pediatric dentistry (MDentSci) training at Leeds Dental Institute, England, after obtaining a DDS from Damascus University, Syria. He worked for the UK's NHS hospital for pediatric dentistry and adult oral and maxillofacial surgery services in Leeds, Halifax, Bradford, Dewsbury, Huddersfield, and Airedale in England. Following that, he moved to Scotland (UK) to work at Dundee Dental Hospital and School, where he taught dentistry to undergraduates and postgraduates for 16 years. Iyad has 40+ scientific publications in high-impact dental journals. His interests are in dental caries, dental anxiety, special needs, sedation, dental trauma, and child protection.

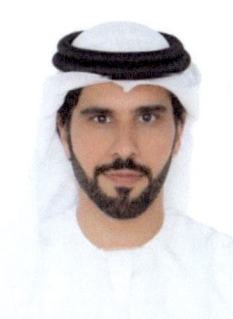

Dr. Mohammed Mansour is an American Board-Certified Pediatric Dentist with a sub-specialty in craniofacial deformities. He obtained his pediatric dentistry and master of science degrees at Tufts University, USA. He then pursued his interest in cleft lip and palate and obtained a fellowship in Craniofacial at the Institute of Reconstructive Plastic Surgery at NYU.

From 2011 to 2015, Dr. M. Mansour was appointed as an adjunct assistant clinical professor in the Department of Pediatric Dentistry at Tufts University and New York University.

Dr. M. Mansour is passionate about research and has authored two chapters in a cleft lip palate atlas book and multiple journal publications. Dr. Mansour has been invited to speak at various conferences locally and internationally, including as a keynote speaker at the American Academy of Pediatric Dentistry Annual National Meeting, a keynote speaker at the College of Diplomates of the American Academy of Pediatric Dentistry, the American Academy of Cleft Lip and Palate, and the International Congress on Cleft Lip and Palate.

Open Access This chapter is licensed under the terms of the Creative Commons Attribution 4.0 International License (http://creativecommons.org/licenses/by/4.0/), which permits use, sharing, adaptation, distribution and reproduction in any medium or format, as long as you give appropriate credit to the original author(s) and the source, provide a link to the Creative Commons license and indicate if changes were made.

The images or other third party material in this chapter are included in the chapter's Creative Commons license, unless indicated otherwise in a credit line to the material. If material is not included in the chapter's Creative Commons license and your intended use is not permitted by statutory regulation or exceeds the permitted use, you will need to obtain permission directly from the copyright holder.

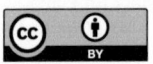

Safeguarding Children in UAE Healthcare Settings

44

Louise Cremonesini, Asrar Rashid, David Cremonesini, Sara Al Marri, and Teresa Quinn

44.1 Safeguarding Children in UAE Healthcare Settings

Child abuse represents a global public health concern; it happens in every corner of the world. In many instances, it takes place in settings where children should feel safest; at school, in their family homes, and online. In most cases, children are abused by people they are familiar with or who are known to their families [1].

All children, regardless of where they are in the world, should be entitled to a life free from violence and abuse. Article 19 of the United Nations Convention on the Rights of the Child [2] clearly states that "governments must do all they can to

---

L. Cremonesini (✉)
Clinical Training, Orbis International, London, United Kingdom
e-mail: louise.cremonesini@orbis.org

A. Rashid
CCST Pediatrics and Pediatric Intensive Care (UK), and Pediatric Services Head of Department Pediatric Intensive Care, NMC Royal Hospital,
Abu Dhabi, United Arab Emirates
e-mail: asrar.rashid@nmc.ae

D. Cremonesini
Asthma and Allergy, Mediclinic Parkview Hospital, Dubai, United Arab Emirates
e-mail: David.Cremonesini@mediclinic.ae

S. Al Marri
Medical Affairs, Al Jalila Children's Specialty Hospital, Dubai, United Arab Emirates
e-mail: Sara.almarri@ajch.ae

T. Quinn
Mubadala Health, Abu Dhabi, United Arab Emirates

Teresa Quinn Consulting & Coaching, Dubai, United Arab Emirates
e-mail: tquinn@mubadalahealth.ae

© The Author(s) 2025
H. O. Al-Shamsi (ed.), *Healthcare in the United Arab Emirates*,
https://doi.org/10.1007/978-981-96-0523-1_44

ensure that children are protected from all forms of violence, abuse, neglect, and bad treatment by their parents or anyone else who looks after them" [2].

44.2 Prevalence

It is difficult to gauge the scale of violence and abuse in the United Arab Emirates (UAE) due to the scarcity of published population-based epidemiological data. Instead, it is helpful to look at global statistics generated by the World Health Organization (WHO) [3]. International evidence tells us that almost half of the world's children have experienced some form of abuse, with 20% of women having experienced sexual abuse in childhood, compared to almost 8% of men. The WHO also examines data pertaining to domestic abuse or intimate partner violence, something known to have a profound effect on children. They report that 30% of ever-partnered women across the globe will be subjected to intimate partner violence at some point in their lifetime [4].

It is with this understanding of the global context that our work in the UAE begins.

44.3 Child Maltreatment and UAE Federal Law

In 1959, the United Nations created the Declaration of the Rights of the Child; following this, in 1989, the General Assembly adopted the Convention on the Rights of the Child [2]. The purpose of this convention is to establish universal criteria for a child's well-being and protection. All nations that signed the convention are then tasked with adhering to its specific elements [5]. It has established certain standards with the intention of promoting children's well-being and protecting them from abuse and neglect [5].

The UAE is a country dedicated to ensuring the welfare of all children and protecting the universal rights of those under the age of 18. The government of the UAE established Federal Law No. 3 concerning Child Rights (Wadeema's Law) in June 2016 [6]. It was named following a serious case of child abuse and neglect that resulted in the death of that child [8].

The death of Wadeema was a pivotal moment that shaped current child protection legislation. It led to the enactment of extraordinarily comprehensive and immediate child protection laws and legislation in the UAE. Every authority in the UAE was tasked with ensuring that the best interests of all children, citizens and non-citizens, were upheld.

In 2018, His Highness Sheikh Mohammed bin Rashid Al Maktoum, Prime Minister, established Cabinet Resolution No. 52 of 2018, governing the Executive Regulations of Federal Law No. 3 of 2016 on the Child Rights Law (Wadeema) [6]. His Highness emphasized the importance of naming this law after Wadeema to remind all people of the heinous acts that parents might commit against their children [7].

The law emphasizes that all children, citizens, and expatriates, must have appropriate living standards, access to health services and education, and equal access to critical services and resources without prejudice. Wadeema's law addresses seven key rights: basic rights, family rights, health and medical rights, social rights, cultural rights, the right to education, and the right to protection. Thus, it emphasizes the child's rights to protection, shelter, security, education, freedom from all forms of abuse, access to proper nourishment, and an environment that encourages development in all fields [7].

If any violation of these rights is identified, it becomes mandatory to report it to the legal entities in all emirates. Following the establishment of Wadeema's law [6], several entities were created across the emirates to protect the best interests of the child. These entities have developed child protection mechanisms, making child protection and safeguarding a legal obligation for all members of UAE's society. They have also established hotlines and platforms to encourage all individuals, including children and organizations, to report any concerns or suspicions that a child may be subjected to any form of mistreatment or deprivation of rights.

Wadeema's Law (2016) highlighted the role of the child protection specialist (CPS). This is a person with a specific responsibility to preserve the rights of the child and to protect him or her within the limits of their competencies [6]. Since the establishment of this law, many Emiratis in the social support sector have shown interest in working as child protection specialists to support the government's efforts. They have developed skills in child protection and in the early detection of child abuse cases to protect the best interests of the child.

44.4 Defining Child Abuse and Child Maltreatment

Any form of maltreatment or intentional harm to a child under the age of 18 is considered child abuse. Child abuse can take many forms, but there are four distinct, internationally recognized categories, as defined by the Ministry of Interior (MOI), of the UAE in 2018 [8].

44.4.1 Sexual Abuse

Sexual abuse can be defined across two separate elements: contact abuse and non-contact abuse. Contact abuse refers to instances where an abuser makes physical contact with the victim, here, a child may be forced or persuaded to engage in sexual activity, which may be penetrative or non-penetrative in nature. Examples of this include touching the genitals or rape. Non-contact sexual abuse may include exposure to pornography, being forced to pose for sexually explicit pictures, or being forced to watch others engage in sexual activities. Non-contact abuse can happen online or in person [8].

44.4.2 Neglect

Neglect happens when a child's needs are persistently not met. Those needs can be psychological, physical, or emotional. Failing to meet such needs may result in the child being at risk of significant harm. Neglect can be intentional or unintentional; either way, the outcome can be extremely damaging to the child. Some examples might be the infant who rolls off the bed and sustains a head injury due to a lack of supervision, or the child who repeatedly suffers an accidental injury. When we consider educational neglect, it might be a child who is simply not taken to school regularly. A persistent lack of access to education can have a significant impact on a child's learning and ability to achieve the best outcomes [8].

44.4.3 Emotional Abuse

Emotional abuse is a pattern of behavior or a way of being that damages a child's sense of self and affects their ability to develop emotional well-being. A lack of emotional well-being can impact a child's whole life, the way they react to stressful situations, and the way they interact with those around them. Some examples might be a caregiver or parent withholding emotional warmth and love, or a child who is persistently insulted and made to feel worthless. Emotional abuse can also be experienced in homes where intimate partner violence, substance misuse, or complex parental mental health problems exist [8].

44.4.4 Physical Abuse

Physical abuse is the purposeful physical harming of a child, or the willful, neglectful failure to prevent physical injury or suffering. Physical abuse can take many forms; examples may include punching, slapping, or hitting a child with hands or objects; purposeful burning with cigarettes or hair straighteners; or deliberate poisoning. Fabricated illness also falls under the category of physical abuse.

Child abuse often encompasses more than one category at a time. One could argue that an emotional impact is experienced with all forms of abuse [8].

44.5 Consequences of Child Abuse

Child abuse can cause immediate and catastrophic physical injuries, but equally concerning are the lifelong and often intergenerational effects created by the experience of child abuse.

So far, we have a limited understanding concerning the long-term effects of different forms of abuse. Much of the research on long-term effects is concentrated on those who have been sexually abused. Strathearn et al., however, examine the effects of four types of abuse on the long-term cognitive, psychological, addiction, and health outcomes of children assessed at ages 14 and 21 [9]. They focus particularly on the long-term impact of emotional abuse and neglect, a rather sparse area of research previously. In a cohort of 7,214 children, more than half reported experiencing two or more types of abuse. This was of particular note with emotional abuse and neglect. This combination was found in 59% of cases. Those children that expereinced both emotional abuse and neglect demonstrated markedly lower cognitive funtioning at ages 14 and 21, alongside negative long-term educational outcomes. confounding factors, such as sex, birth weight, and breastfeeding, were adjusted for. In particular, reading ability seemed to be significantly associated with abuse and neglect [9].

From a mental health perspective, emotional and physical abuse were strongly linked to externalizing and internalizing behavioral issues. Emotional abuse and neglect were linked to a long list of problems at age 21, including anxiety, post-traumatic stress disorder (PTSD), depression, experiencing intimate partner violence, and psychosis. When examining the mental health outcomes for those who had suffered sexual abuse in a single form, issues experienced included clinical depression, lifetime PTSD, and intimate partner violence. Physical abuse was linked with internalizing and externalizing behavioral issues, intimate partner violence, PTSD, and depressive disorders [9].

Substance abuse has long been associated with a significant risk for children who have experienced abuse [10]. Strathearn et al.'s findings concur with this view; overall, they identified that emotional abuse and neglect were linked with all categories of substance use and addiction at ages 14 and 21. Notably, children who had been exposed to physical or sexual abuse were linked with fewer substance abuse outcomes. Interestingly, emotional abuse demonstrated significant injecting drug usage, but only in young male adults.

Every form of abuse was linked with an early first experience of sexual intercourse and an increased prevalence of teenage pregnancy. This finding correlates with a large-scale study from Fortin Langelier et al. in 2019, which examined the correlation between sexual abuse and teenage pregnancy [11].

In terms of physical health, a reduction in adult height at age 21 was linked with all abuse types except sexual abuse. Alongside height reduction, physical abuse was linked with a high-fat diet, thus creating an obesogenic picture [12].

This important study demonstrates that child abuse leads to adverse outcomes across all cognitive, psychological, and health outcomes. Given the magnitude of the effects, it is worth considering how such exposure may affect the next generation of children. Emerging research looks at the effects of parents' childhood abuse experiences and how this impacts their own offspring, highlighting the need for specific intervention and support from clinicians in order to break the cycle of abuse [12].

44.5.1 Brain Development

Children who have positive experiences in childhood tend to develop healthy brains. Conversely, those children who live with stress and adversity are at risk of suboptimal brain development and harm to brain function. Bick and Nelson describe how a child's experience of child abuse can be associated with a reduction in brain size and volume, which, in turn, may impact the function of the amygdala, hippocampus, and orbitofrontal cortex [13]. The great news is that our brains continue to develop until well into adulthood, and the chance of reversing the damage is possible.

44.6 The Importance of Safeguarding Children

The term "safeguarding" covers all aspects of assistance for a child or young person, which ensures they flourish in a life that is free from harm, thus allowing them to retain independence, achieve optimal well-being, and ensure the best outcomes. Safeguarding children's work is focused on the prevention of abuse and neglect; the need for early intervention cannot be underestimated.

44.6.1 The Role of Healthcare Organizations

Healthcare organizations, whether they are government or private entities, all have an obligation to offer appropriate care to their patients and appropriate training to their staff. According to UAE Federal Law 3/2016, they have a responsibility to ensure the safety of suspected or reported child abuse or neglect victims through the provision of an integrated and multidisciplinary system of care, consistent with the national legislation in the UAE [6].

Alongside legal requirements, we also have a moral obligation to support the most vulnerable members of our society. All front-facing healthcare professionals are in an advantageous position to assess, identify, and report abuse due to their ability to directly observe most assessment criteria instead of having to rely on self-reporting measures. Pediatricians are particularly well-placed, as they often have a continued relationship with a family throughout its lifespan.

44.7 The Vision for All Healthcare Providers Within the UAE

All healthcare settings, large or small, should place strong emphasis on implementing the legal framework of the Child Rights Law within their organization [6], with the goal of ensuring safety for children and young people. In doing so, they will also enable their staff to practice safely, with compassion and a focus on supporting the community and the welfare of children and young adults.

44.7.1 Aims of a Healthcare Safeguarding Service

To work in partnership with government bodies, including the Department of Health (DOH), Family Care Authority (FCA), and Early Childhood Authority (ECA), to share expertise and provide strategic leadership to advance safeguarding practice across the Middle East and North Africa (MENA) region.

To build an effective governance assurance framework across facilities that demonstrates clear accountability for safeguarding children.

To work to ensure that staff feel empowered to act when they see or suspect a safeguarding issue by leading a culture of speaking up, and ensuring that all staff, regardless of role or seniority, receive the appropriate level of training based on local standards.

To develop safeguarding training based on the best international evidence, while also accounting for the nuances of cultural relativism, taught by well-qualified, credible facilitators who have experience working in the region.

To ensure that patients are protected by overarching organizational safeguarding policies that are embedded and reflect a clear, evidence-based approach, enabling staff to do the "right thing."

To develop informatics systems that are available to be reviewed by the Department of Health or Dubai Health Authority and that demonstrate safeguarding activity, capacity, and the statutory requirements as set out in Federal Law No. 3/2016 [6].

44.8   UAE Safeguarding: A New Era in Pediatrics

Safeguarding children in the UAE from a hospital perspective brings many challenges. First, there is a merger of cultures, languages, and processes. When developing guidelines and policies for child protection, this needs to be done in such a way that it incorporates local nuances, including the involvement of child protection services. As child protection processes continue to be formalized in the UAE, policies and processes are evolving to help support the physicians on the ground delivering care. The physician must deal with cultural and social processes to deliver the best care within the current healthcare framework. Policies need to be standardized across organizations, and consistency is needed around when to report and how to report. Currently, most child protection concerns are seen in government settings. However, as the infrastructure grows and child protection hubs are created, a unified approach across both the public and private sectors will be required. In all settings, physicians should feel supported in their child protection practice.

The development of pediatric practice in the UAE has occurred against the backdrop of an emerging economy. This has attracted physicians trained in different health systems to the shores of the UAE. Such health systems vary in their child protection structures, and thus, doctors vary with respect to their experience in this area of work. Indeed, a historical landmark in the UAE was the decision taken by His Highness Sheikh Mohammed bin Rashid Al Maktoum in supporting the government to introduce the Child Rights Law (Wadeema's Law), where the sanctity of the child is a core testament. The law is there to protect children first and foremost, but also to protect health professionals when tasked with making a decision about reporting. The child should be the key focus of that decision, and doctors and employers should understand the law's guidance on when to do this [6].

In healthcare operations, one cannot predict the moment when a situation arises requiring the safeguarding process to be enacted. Child abuse may be suspected in many environments, such as a hospital or clinic, including the emergency room, pediatric clinic, pediatric ward, pediatric theatre, or hospital waiting room; it may be present anywhere in a hospital. This means that anybody working for a healthcare organization who might encounter a child needs a minimum level of training to understand when safeguarding concerns for a child are present. This means training healthcare workers on safeguarding is paramount and should be at a level appropriate for their level of interaction with children. This should be standardized across all sectors and, in time, become a requirement of any organization that treats children. More crucially, such training should be relevant to the local population and environment, so it links with local services, enabling professionals to understand how reporting concerns are dealt with.

44.9 The Case of Suspected Non-accidental Injury

An important aspect of caring for children with non-accidental injuries (NAI) is the ability to ensure 24/7 supervision in a place of safety. Until child protection services can understand the degree of risk, the case also needs to be managed in partnership with key people within the organization. The child then needs to be managed in a place where they can be in constant view of the healthcare team. With many hospital rooms being single rooms, this is a challenge. Therefore, on arrival, it may be best to consider admitting the child to a high-dependency area where they can be closely monitored.

The initial arrival of the child and the situation may well be emotionally charged, as an event may have triggered the admission. In such cases, the support of the family is important, but the support of the medical team also needs to be considered. It is prudent, therefore, that a child protection plan be drawn up, including the mobilization of hospital security to ensure the safety of all parties concerned. The involvement of the most senior doctor may be useful in this scenario to ensure the best treatment is undertaken, and all the relevant tests are performed to rule out diagnoses that may mimic the signs of non-accidental injury. Full documentation is key, particularly at the first contact with medical professionals. Here, all details, including timing, signs, and symptoms, as well as the family's interpretation of incidents and key information, are valuable for medical report writing. The senior doctor should aim for a thorough examination and detailed record of findings, laboratory, and clinical examinations with appropriate documentation of the same. Height and weight measurements and their recording are also key and must not be forgotten.

Given the complexity of non-accidental injuries, multidisciplinary team involvement should be activated as soon as possible. This should also involve the legal and governance teams of the hospital organization, along with key doctors, including those representing hospital administration. Ideally, liaison with the regional safeguarding support services should also be undertaken at the earliest possible time.

44.9.1 Importance of Prevention

In many cases, incidences of child abuse are never reported by the victim. Despite this, services such as healthcare, the judiciary, and social services are tasked with dealing with the consequences suffered by victims throughout their lives [5]. If we look to other countries that record cost data, we can see the significant financial burden that is associated with the short- and long-term treatment of child abuse and neglect. In comparison, the figures are comparable to the cost of other substantial public health challenges such as coronary artery disease and diabetes.

The prevention of child abuse is a complex undertaking and one that requires a multisectoral approach; the causal factors need to be addressed simultaneously and across different entities. This requires the appropriate human capital, motivation, commitment, and, finally, adequate funding.

44.10 Conclusion

It is not one person's role to keep children safe, but as healthcare professionals, we have unique access to children, young people, and their families, often at times of heightened vulnerability. Hence, we are in a good position to identify children and young people who may be at risk of significant harm. As raising awareness and education continue to gather momentum in the region, we will undoubtedly begin to see more child protection cases coming through our hospital and clinic doors.

One's ability to demonstrate professional kindness, empathy, sensitivity, and compassion to all parties concerned should not be underestimated. This is undoubtedly one of the most difficult situations any family will ever face, and the support of a healthcare professional is imperative. This approach will also increase the likelihood of parental engagement.

As the United Arab Emirates positions itself as a global healthcare leader, the importance of protecting children has never been more critical. Much has been done in a short space of time to embed federal law and processes and to develop national infrastructure, motivated by the passion of healthcare leaders to create safe environments for our children. With the continued support of our esteemed leadership, we will together strive to make the UAE a place where our children can thrive without fear of abuse or violence.

Conflicts of Interest The authors have no conflicts of interest to declare.

References

1. UNICEF. 2022. Available at https://www.unicef.org/child-protection.
2. UN General Assembly, Convention on the Rights of the Child, 20 November 1989, United Nations, Treaty Series, vol. 1577, p. 3. Available at: https://www.refworld.org/docid/3ae6b38f0.html.

3. World Health Organization. Global status report on preventing violence against children 2020. World Health Organization 2020; 2020. Available at https://www.who.int/publications/i/item/9789240004191.
4. World Health Organization. Violence against women prevalence estimates, 2018: global, regional and national prevalence estimates for intimate partner violence against women and global and regional prevalence estimates for non-partner sexual violence against women. Geneva: World Health Organization; 2021. Available at https://www.who.int/publications/i/item/9789240022256.
5. Nadan Y, Spilsbury JC, Korbin JE. Culture and context in understanding child maltreatment: contributions of intersectionality and neighborhood-based research. Child Abuse Negl. 2015;41:40–8. Available at https://pubmed.ncbi.nlm.nih.gov/25466427/.
6. United Arab Emirates Government. Ministry of Justice. E-Justice portal Federal Law No. 3 of 2016 On Child Rights (Wadeema's Law). Available from: https://u.ae/en/information-and-services/justice-safety-and-the-law/children-safety/childrensrights.
7. Al Khoori A, Salem O. Wadeema's law renamed child rights law'. In The National; 2013. Available at https://www.thenationalnews.com/uae/government/wadeemas-law-renamed-child-rights-law-1.334198.
8. Ministry of Interior. United Arab Emirates; 2018. Available at https://www.moi-cpc.ae/en/CHILD.PROTECTION.DIMENSION.aspx.
9. Strathearn L, Giannotti M, Mills R, et al. Long-term cognitive, psychological, and health outcomes associated with child abuse and neglect. Pediatrics. 2020;146(4). Available at https://pubmed.ncbi.nlm.nih.gov/32943535/.
10. Dube SR, Felitti VJ, Dong M, Chapman DP, Giles WH, Anda RF. Childhood abuse, neglect, and household dysfunction and the risk of illicit drug use: the adverse childhood experiences study. Pediatrics. 2003;111(3):564–72. Available at https://pubmed.ncbi.nlm.nih.gov/12612237/.
11. Fortin-Langelier E, Daigneault I, Achim J, Vézina-Gagnon P, Guérin V, Frappier J-Y. A matched cohort study of the association between childhood sexual abuse and teenage pregnancy. J Adolesc Health. 2019;65(3):384–9. Available at https://www.sciencedirect.com/science/article/pii/S1054139X19301351.
12. Greene CA, Haisley L, Wallace C, Ford JD. Intergenerational effects of childhood maltreatment: a systematic review of the parenting practices of adult survivors of childhood abuse, neglect, and violence. Clin Psychol Rev. 2020;80:101891. Available at https://europepmc.org/backend/ptpmcrender.fcgi?accid=PMC7476782&blobtype=pdf.
13. Bick J, Nelson CA. Early adverse experiences and the developing brain. Nueropsychopharmacology. 2016;41:177–96. Available at https://pubmed.ncbi.nlm.nih.gov/26334107/.

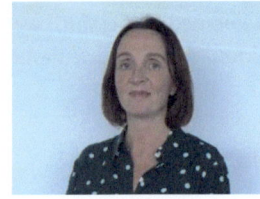

Louise Cremonesini is a dedicated and motivated senior nurse with over 30 years of experience in clinical services, nurse education, and safeguarding. She holds a master's degree in Safeguarding Vulnerable Children and Families and a BA (Hons) in Public Health.

Louise has worked in the UK in both the national health service (NHS) and private sectors as a child protection lead. She has extensive experience dealing with children who have been subjected to child abuse or who are at risk of significant harm. Louise also has experience working with victims of domestic abuse in the UK and the United Arab Emirates.

She has previously worked for Mubadala Healthcare in the UAE as their senior manager for safeguarding across its assets. Louise is the subject matter expert for all matters relating to safeguarding children and vulnerable adults. Mubadala Health is the first healthcare organization in the UAE to mandate safeguarding education for all of their staff. Safeguarding practices are well embedded across the organization. Louise is an ardent advocate for children's rights, enhancing the lives of children and supporting parents in their role. Currently, Louise is working with Orbis International as a Clinical Training Consultant.

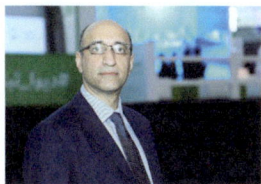

Dr. Asrar Rashid   serves as the Chairman of Pediatric Services at NMC Royal in Khalifa City and is the Head of the Pediatric Critical Care Department. His professional qualifications include a Fellowship from the Royal College of Paediatrics and Child Health, and he has been trained in the UK, the USA, and Australia. He is currently pursuing a PhD in artificial intelligence. In addition to his professional roles, Dr. Asrar actively contributes to charitable efforts. As the volunteer director of child health for the NGO, Midland Doctors, he oversees a hospital in North Pakistan. He has initiated and manages a malnutrition program and is responsible for the operations of a secondary care hospital. In recognition of his substantial charity contributions, Dr. Asrar was honored with an invitation to meet Her Royal Highness Queen Elizabeth at Buckingham Palace in 2008.

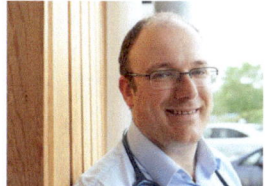

Dr. David Cremonesini   is trained and qualified in pediatrics and allergy in the UK. He studied at Oxford University before going to St. Georges in London to complete his medical training. David has a wide range of clinical experience and has worked as a pediatrician since 1997. David completed his certificate of completion of specialist training (CCST) in the Oxford Deanery and went on to be a consultant, first in the West Midlands and then in Cambridgeshire. David has worked at Royal Brompton Hospital, London, specializing in breathing problems, and in 2018, he graduated from the University of Southampton with a master's degree in Allergy.

From a child protection perspective, David has been exposed to a wide range of child abuse cases while being a pediatric consultant on call in the UK. This enabled him to build up comprehensive experience in managing such cases and also develop an appreciation of the importance of a multi-disciplinary approach to safeguarding children. David currently works as a pediatric consultant at Mediclinic Parkview Hospital in Dubai.

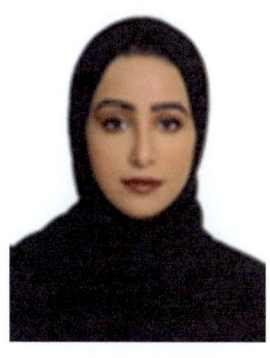

Sara Al Marri has been a specialized child protection social worker since 2016. She recently graduated from the University of Kent in the United Kingdom with a master's degree in Advanced Child Protection. Currently, Al Marri is a social worker within the Child Protection Committee at Dubai Academic Health Corporation. Through her leading role, Al Marri evaluates allegations of neglect and physical, sexual, and emotional abuse in order to facilitate protection for children across governmental healthcare facilities in Dubai. She liaises with the other local authorities in the UAE within the child protection field to promote, support, and safeguard the well-being of all children in need. Al Marri is dedicated to the protection of vulnerable children from any harm as well as to the promotion of child mental well-being.

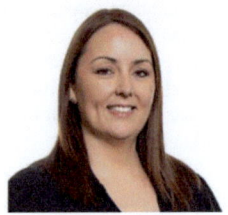

Teresa Quinn is a dynamic and forward-thinking Senior Director of Clinical Operations, with many accomplishments in pioneering and shaping clinical programs across Ireland and the Middle East. Teresa has an unwavering dedication to enhancing patient outcomes through the optimization of care delivery systems, embracing innovation and technology, and orchestrating transformative healthcare initiatives across the diverse landscape.

Teresa has a passion for population health and is dedicated to protecting vulnerable individuals in society. She has an unwavering commitment to pushing the boundaries of what is possible in healthcare and advocating for those whose voices are often unheard. Teresa leads with heart, and her passion for leading and creating change spans a spectrum of services catering to vulnerable populations, including championing the development of safeguarding services in line with national priorities and advocating for equity and policy change for those who are marginalized.

Teresa's educational journey has equipped her with the knowledge and skills to effect positive change in healthcare. Her credentials include BSc—Nursing, PGD—Public Health, MSc—Chronic Disease Management, and MBA—International Health Care Leadership. Her commitment to lifelong learning ensures that she is at the forefront of healthcare trends, driving meaningful change.

Open Access This chapter is licensed under the terms of the Creative Commons Attribution 4.0 International License (http://creativecommons.org/licenses/by/4.0/), which permits use, sharing, adaptation, distribution and reproduction in any medium or format, as long as you give appropriate credit to the original author(s) and the source, provide a link to the Creative Commons license and indicate if changes were made.

The images or other third party material in this chapter are included in the chapter's Creative Commons license, unless indicated otherwise in a credit line to the material. If material is not included in the chapter's Creative Commons license and your intended use is not permitted by statutory regulation or exceeds the permitted use, you will need to obtain permission directly from the copyright holder.

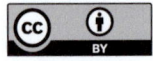

Genetic Diseases in the UAE

45

Mode Al Ojaimi, Rabah Almahmoud,
Bashar J. Banimortada, Abduljalil Alragheb,
and Ayman W. El-Hattab

45.1 Introduction

The United Arab Emirates (UAE) with a total area of 83,600 square kilometers is a Middle Eastern country located in Southwest Asia along the southern border of the Arabian Gulf. The country consists of seven Emirates that were united in 1971, with Abu Dhabi being both the capital and the largest emirate. The population currently stands at 9.77 million, which has nearly doubled over a 10-year period. The annual growth rate is 1.2%. The UAE nationals make up only 11% of the total population. The remaining 89% of the population is made up of expatriates from different parts of the world. Due to the high percentage of immigrants, males account for 72% and females 28% of the total population. In addition, a significant proportion of the population in the UAE belongs to the 25–54- year age group, with over 6.29 million (69.9%), followed by children and young adults at 2.57 million (26.9%) [1].

M. Al Ojaimi
College of Medicine, University of Sharjah, Sharjah, United Arab Emirates

Pediatrics Department, University Hospital Sharjah, Sharjah, United Arab Emirates

Pediatrics and Adolescent Medicine Department, American University of Beirut, Beirut, Lebanon

Department of Pediatrics and Adolescent Medicine, Keserwan Medical Center, Keserwan, Lebanon
e-mail: ma717@aub.edu.lb

R. Almahmoud · B. J. Banimortada · A. Alragheb
College of Medicine, University of Sharjah, Sharjah, United Arab Emirates
e-mail: ralmahmoud@sharjah.ac.ae; u19105685@sharjah.ac.ae; A.Abduljalil90@outlook.com

A. W. El-Hattab (✉)
College of Medicine, University of Sharjah, Sharjah, United Arab Emirates

Genetics and Rare Disease Center, Burjeel Medical City, Abu Dhabi, United Arab Emirates
e-mail: ayman.elhattab@burjeelmedicalcity.com

© The Author(s) 2025
H. O. Al-Shamsi (ed.), *Healthcare in the United Arab Emirates*,
https://doi.org/10.1007/978-981-96-0523-1_45

Analysis of mitochondrial DNA (mtDNA) sequencing of Emirati women indicated that gene flow from Africa is evident in the UAE population, as shown by the presence of haplogroups U6, M1, and L. Around 17% of the population can be traced back to an Eastern origin, characterized by the haplotypes: U and M Indian (12%). Additionally, Asian and Eurasian western haplogroups (R, J, and K) represent approximately 11–15% of the population [2].

Consanguinity originates from the Latin term "consanguinitatem," which means "of the same blood" or having a shared ancestry with another individual. It refers to the practice of marriage between individuals who have common biological ancestors, extending up to second cousins. This definition of consanguinity is employed because it is believed that the genetic impact in marriages involving couples with a lesser degree of relatedness would only exhibit marginal variations compared to those observed in the general population. Due to the sharing of common alleles, consanguineous marriages have been associated with a higher incidence of autosomal recessive conditions [3]. Like many Arabian countries, consanguineous marriages are widely prevalent in the UAE. One study found the rate to be as high as 50%, of which 26% are first-degree cousins [4, 5]. These high rates have been linked to a higher incidence of autosomal recessive diseases [6]. Furthermore, autosomal dominant disorders due to de novo mutations are relatively common secondary to advanced paternal age, which is also common in the UAE [51].

This chapter presents the common genetic diseases in the UAE, which include inborn errors of metabolism, neurodevelopmental disorders, hemoglobinopathies, genetic skin disorders, inherited skeletal dysplasias, inherited lung diseases, inborn errors of immunity, hereditary hearing loss, and genetic diseases of the eye.

45.2 Inborn Errors of Metabolism

Inborn errors of metabolism are inherited, heterogeneous biochemical disorders that occur secondary to mutations in the genes responsible for encoding enzymes or transporters of metabolic pathways. The main mode of inheritance is autosomal recessive, but X-linked inheritance occurs in some cases [7]. In the UAE, they are highly prevalent due to elevated consanguinity rates. The estimated birth prevalence is 75/100,000 [8], and the clinical manifestations vary greatly due to the ethnic diversity of the population [9]. To date, over 40 metabolic disorders have been identified in this country [8–10] (Table 45.1).

Phenylketonuria is the predominant inborn error of metabolism observed in the UAE, occurring at an incidence of approximately 1 in 14,000 individuals [9]. It is autosomal recessive and caused by biallelic pathogenic variants in the *PAH gene*. No predominant mutation for PKU has been identified in the UAE population to date [10]. Isovaleric acidemia is an autosomal recessive inborn error of leucine metabolism caused by isovaleryl-CoA dehydrogenase's deficiency, which results from biallelic pathogenic variants in *IVD*. A study examining the clinical and molecular features of five unrelated Emirati families with isovaleric acidemia revealed four novel mutations in *IVD* with p.R395Q present in two families. This study also reported an exceptional case involving a 17-year-old female who was homozygous for the p.R392H mutation but was clinically asymptomatic. These

Table 45.1 Inborn errors of metabolism in the UAE [8–10]

Disease	MIM#	Gene	MIM#	Mode of inheritance	Main clinical presentation
Alkaptonuria	203500	HGD	607474	AR	Dark urine, pigmentation of connective tissue, joint and spine arthritis, and destruction of the cardiac valves
Arginase deficiency	207800	ARG1	608313	AR	Triad of hyperammonemia, encephalopathy, and respiratory alkalosis
Asparagine synthetase deficiency	615574	ASNS	108370	AR	Developmental delay, seizures, progressive encephalopathy, microcephaly, and cerebral atrophy
Biotinidase deficiency	253260	BTD	609019	AR	Cutaneous and neurologic abnormalities
Canavan disease	271900	ASPA	608034	AR	Severe intellectual disability, blindness, megalocephaly, hypotonia, atonia of neck muscles, hypotonia, hyperextension of legs, flexion of arms, and death by 18 months on average
Carbamoyl phosphate synthetase deficiency	237300	CPS1	608307	AR	Triad of hyperammonemia, encephalopathy, and respiratory alkalosis
Carnitine–acylcarnitine translocase deficiency	212138	SLC25A20	613698	AR	Neurologic abnormalities, cardiomyopathy and arrhythmias, skeletal muscle damage, and liver dysfunction
Cerebellar hypoplasia and mental retardation	224050	VLDLR	192977	AR	Intellectual disability, congenital nonprogressive cerebellar ataxia, disequilibrium, and cerebellar hypoplasia
Fructose-1,6-bisphosphatase deficiency	611570	FBP1	229700	AR	Hypoglycemia, metabolic acidosis on fasting, hyperventilation, apnea, and ketosis
Fucosidosis	230000	FUCA1	612280		Developmental delay, failure to thrive, seizures, short stature, hearing loss, skeletal anomalies, skin anomalies, and distinctive facial features
Glutaric aciduria type 1	231670	GCDH	608801	AR	Progressive movement disorder that usually begins in the first year of life

(continued)

Table 45.1 (continued)

Disease	MIM#	Gene	MIM#	Mode of inheritance	Main clinical presentation
Glycogen storage disease type Ia	232200	G6PC	613742	AR	Severe hypoglycemia, and hepatomegaly in first year of life
GM1 gangliosidosis	230500	GLB1	611458	AR	Neurodegeneration and skeletal abnormalities
Hereditary fructose intolerance	229600	ALDOB	612724	AR	Recurrent vomiting, abdominal pain, and fatal hypoglycemia
Hypophosphatasia with mental retardation syndrome type 4	615716	PGAP3	611801	AR	Intellectual disability, developmental delay, seizures, and distinctive facial features
I-Cell disease	252500	GNPTAB	607840	AR	Developmental delay, short stature, cardiomegaly, and skeletal abnormalities
Isovaleric acidemia	243500	IVD	607036	AR	Severe neonatal ketoacidosis leading to death
Leigh disease	256000	MTATP6	516060	Mito	Developmental delay, developmental regression, hypotonia, ataxia, dystonia, ocular anomalies, and abnormal brain imaging
Mannosidosis alpha	248500	MAN2B1	609458	AR	Intellectual disability, motor abnormalities, hearing impairment, skeletal abnormalities, immune deficiency, and coarse facial features
Mannosidosis beta	248510	MANBA	609489	AR	Developmental delay, intellectual disability, hyperactivity, mild bone disease, and coarse facial features
Medium chain acyl-CoA dehydrogenase deficiency	201450	ACADM	607008	AR	Intolerance to prolonged fasting, recurrent episodes of hypoglycemic coma with medium-chain dicarboxylic aciduria, impaired ketogenesis, and low plasma and tissue carnitine levels
Methylmalonic acidemia, cblB type	251000	MMAB	609058	AR	Developmental delay, hypotonia, lethargy, failure to thrive, cardiomyopathy, genitourinary anomalies, and gastrointestinal anomalies

Disease	OMIM	Gene	Gene OMIM	Inheritance	Clinical features
Methylmalonic aciduria and homocystinuria, cblC type	277400	MMACHC	609831	AR	Intellectual disability, developmental delay, failure to thrive, seizures, hypotonia, tremors, cognitive and neurologic regression, microcephaly, ocular anomalies, renal anomalies, hematologic abnormalities, and distinctive facial features
Mevalonic aciduria	610377	MVK	251170	AR	Developmental delay, progressive cerebellar ataxia, febrile seizures, hepatosplenomegaly, lymphadenopathy, arthralgia, skin rash, and distinctive facial features
Mitochondrial deoxyribonucleic acid depletion 2	609560	TK2	188250	AR	Childhood onset of muscle weakness, and depletion of mtDNA in skeletal muscle
Mitochondrial deoxyribonucleic acid depletion 3	251880	DGUOK	601465	AR	Onset in infancy of progressive liver failure and neurologic abnormalities, hypoglycemia, and increased lactate in body fluids
Mucopolysaccharidosis type III A	252900	SGSH	605270	AR	Intellectual disability, behavioral abnormalities, and distinctive features
Mucopolysaccharidosis type III B	252920	NAGLU	609701	AR	Progressive neurodegeneration, behavioral abnormalities, mild skeletal anomalies, and shortened life span
Mucopolysaccharidosis type III C	252930	HGSNAT	610453	AR	Developmental delay, behavioral abnormalities, learning disability, skeletal anomalies, and distinctive features
Multiple mitochondrial dysfunctions syndrome 3	615330	IBA57	615316	AR	Intellectual disability, developmental regression, hypotonia, seizures, microcephaly, ocular anomalies, musculoskeletal anomalies, distinctive features, and abnormal neuroimaging

(continued)

Table 45.1 (continued)

Disease	MIM#	Gene	MIM#	Mode of inheritance	Main clinical presentation
Neonatal diabetes mellitus	176730	ISN	618858	AR, AD	Chronic hyperglycemia due to severe nonautoimmune insulin deficiency diagnosed in the first months of life
Phenylketonuria	261600	PAH	612349	AR	Intellectual disability, behavioral anomalies, seizures, peripheral neuropathy, microcephaly, ocular anomalies, skin anomalies, and blond hair
Pompe disease	232300	GAA	606800	AR	Cardiomyopathy and muscular hypotonia
Propionic acidemia	606054	PCCA	232000	AR	Intellectual disability, seizures, growth impairment, pancreatitis, cardiomyopathy, and basal ganglia lesions
Pyruvate dehydrogenase E1-alpha deficiency	312170	PDHA1	300502	XLD	Developmental delay, tremor, movement abnormalities, difficulty in swallowing, and drooling
Sandhoff disease	268800	HEXB	606873	AR	Developmental delay, growth delay, ocular anomalies, macrocephaly, and distinctive facial features
Tay-Sachs disease	272800	HEXA	606869	AR	Developmental delay, paralysis, dementia, blindness, and early death
Tyrosinemia type 1	276700	FAH	613871	AR	Progressive liver disease, and secondary renal tubular dysfunction leading to hypophosphatemic rickets
Wilson disease	277900	ATP7B	606882	AR	Neurologic and hepatic abnormalities
Zellweger syndrome	614862	PEX6	601498	AR	Hypotonia, seizures, ocular anomalies, feeding difficulties, and distinctive craniofacial features

findings underscore the diverse range of mutations and clinical manifestations associated with isovaleric acidemia in the UAE [11]. Propionic acidemia is a hereditary metabolic disorder characterized by an autosomal recessive inheritance pattern. It is caused by mutations in the genes encoding propionyl-CoA carboxylase, namely, *PCCA* or *PCCB*. The disorder manifests in two forms: a neonatal-onset form and a late-onset form that occurs in older children and adults. The late-onset form is less prevalent and typically milder in severity. In a recent study, a newly identified homozygous frameshift variant, c.2158_2159insT (p.Glu720Valfs*14), was reported in the last exon of *PCCA*. This variant was associated with a severe presentation of the disease in a newborn Emirati female. Other commonly observed inborn errors of metabolism in the Emirati population include biotinidase deficiency, tyrosinemia type 1, glycogen storage disease type Ia, mitochondrial DNA depletion, and glutaric aciduria type 1 [8].

45.3 Neurodevelopmental Disorders

Neurodevelopmental disorders are characterized by impaired cognition and developmental delays. They affect >3% of children worldwide. Their prevalence in the UAE is unknown; however, a recent study investigated the spectrum of these disorders among Emirati patients [12]. The main reported conditions in the studied population were developmental delay, cognitive impairment, autism spectrum disorder, attention deficit hyperactivity disorder, and epilepsy associated with abnormalities in other organ systems. Seventy percent of patients with a positive molecular diagnosis had a history of consanguinity. Microarray results were positive in 11% of those affected, with microduplication or microdeletions in chromosome 15 being the most common abnormality, followed by microdeletions in chromosome 22. Approximately 39% of studied cases had a positive molecular test (68% had genetic diseases and 42% had inborn errors of metabolism). Autosomal recessive diseases accounted for 48% (96% of which were caused by homozygous mutations), autosomal dominant diseases accounted for 35% (84% of which were de novo), and X-linked disorders accounted for 10%. This high frequency of autosomal dominant disorders with de novo mutations is attributed to the advanced paternal age prevalent in the UAE [12].

The most frequently reported autosomal recessive disorders were, respectively, mucopolysaccharidosis type 3, biotinidase deficiency, and mannosidosis (alpha and beta), while the most frequently reported autosomal dominant diseases were consecutively neurofibromatosis type 1, Kabuki syndrome, and Cowden syndrome. The most commonly reported X-linked disorders were Rett syndrome and pyruvate dehydrogenase E1-alpha deficiency (Table 45.2).

Table 45.2 Neurodevelopmental disorders in the UAE [12]

Disease	MIM#	Gene	MIM#	Mode of inheritance	Main clinical presentation
Aicardi-Goutieres syndrome	610333	RNASEH2A	606034	AR	Developmental delay, seizures, spasticity, intrauterine growth retardation, microcephaly, respiratory anomalies, gastrointestinal anomalies, distinctive facial features, pancytopenia, and abnormal neuroimaging
Angelman syndrome	105830	UBE3A	601623	AD	Intellectual disability, developmental delay, behavioral abnormalities, and distinctive features
Arboleda-Tham syndrome	616268	KAT6A	601408	AD	Intellectual disability, speech delay, microcephaly, cardiovascular malformations, and gastrointestinal anomalies
Asadollahi-Rauch syndrome	616789	MED13L	608771	AD	Intellectual disability, behavioral abnormalities, ataxia, cardiac anomalies, and distinctive features
Axonal Charcot–Marie–Tooth disease type 20	614228	DYNC1H1	600112	AD	Developmental delay, learning disabilities, peripheral neuropathy, and weakness
Baraitser–Winter syndrome 1	243310	ACTB	102630	AD	Intellectual disability, epilepsy, microcephaly, sensorineural deafness, musculoskeletal anomalies, distinctive features, and abnormal brain imaging
CACNA1-associated seizure disorder	617106	CACNA1A	601011	AD	Intellectual disability, seizures, axial hypotonia, peripheral hypertonia with hyperreflexia, tremor, ataxia, and abnormal eye movements
CADASIL syndrome	125310	NOTCH3	600276	AD	Developmental delay, seizures, hypotonia, leukoencephalopathy, cerebral arteriopathy, and subcortical infarcts
CEBALID syndrome	618774	MN1	156100	AD	Developmental delay, intellectual disability, structural brain abnormalities, and distinctive features
CHARGE syndrome	214800	CHD7	608892	AD	Intellectual disability, and congenital anomalies including choanal atresia, malformations of the heart, inner ear, and retina
Coffin-Siris syndrome 1	135900	ARID1B	614556	AD	Intellectual disability, skeletal anomalies, cardiovascular malformation, and distinctive features
Cohen syndrome	216550	VPS13B	607817	AR	Intellectual disability, microcephaly, progressive retinopathy, truncal obesity, intermittent congenital neutropenia, and distinctive facial features

Congenital insensitivity to pain and anhidrosis	256800	NTRK1	191315	AR	Intellectual disability, developmental delay, behavioral abnormalities, autonomic dysfunction, pain insensitivity, temperature insensitivity, anhidrosis, ocular anomalies, skeletal anomalies, and skin anomalies
Cornelia de Lange syndrome 4	614701	RAD21	606462	AD	Intellectual disability, holoprosencephaly, short stature, skeletal anomalies, distinctive features, and abnormal brain imaging
Cortical dysplasia with other brain malformations-2	615282	KIF5C	604593	AD	Intellectual disability, developmental delay, behavioral anomalies, seizures, absent speech, macrocephaly, fetal akinesia, and abnormal brain imaging
Cowden syndrome type 1	158350	PTEN	601728	AD	Developmental delay, macrocephaly, gait abnormalities, hamartomas, increased carcinoma risk, immunologic anomalies, and abnormal brain imaging
DEGCAGS syndrome	619488	ZNF699	609571	AR	Developmental delay, cardiovascular malformations, gastrointestinal anomalies, skeletal anomalies, and urogenital anomalies
Developmental and epileptic encephalopathy 2	300672	CDKL5	300203	XLD	Intellectual disability, developmental delay, seizures, motor abnormalities, movement abnormalities, sleep disturbance, gastrointestinal anomalies, and distinctive features
Developmental and epileptic encephalopathy 64	618004	RHOBTB2	607352	AD	Intellectual disability, developmental delay, seizures, and movement abnormalities
Developmental delay, cerebellar atrophy, ataxia, and epilepsy	618170	ADPRHL2	610624	AR	Developmental regression, autistic spectrum disorder, seizures, peripheral neuropathy, hearing loss, ocular anomalies, muscular anomalies, and abnormal brain imaging
Developmental delay with variable intellectual impairment and behavioral abnormalities	618430	TCF20	603107	AD	Intellectual disability, behavioral abnormalities, and distinctive facial features

(continued)

Table 45.2 (continued)

Disease	MIM#	Gene	MIM#	Mode of inheritance	Main clinical presentation
Desanto-Shinawi syndrome	616708	WAC	615049	AD	Developmental delay, behavioral abnormalities, ocular anomalies, and distinctive features
Dias-Logan syndrome	617101	BCL11A	606557	AD	Developmental delay, microcephaly, asymptomatic persistence of fetal hemoglobin, and distinctive facial features
Early infantile epileptic encephalopathy type 4	612164	STXBP1	602926	AD	Developmental delay, spasticity, quadriplegia, infantile seizures, and abnormal brain imaging
Gould syndrome 1	175780	COL4A1	120130	AD	intellectual disability, seizures, hemiplegia, spasticity, pyramidal signs, migraine with/without aura, central facial palsy, ocular anomalies, hematologic anomalies, and abnormal brain imaging
GRACILE syndrome	603358	BCS1L	603647	AR	Failure to thrive, cholestasis, aminoaciduria, iron overload, lactic acidosis, and early death
Heart defect, cleft palate and intellectual disability	600987	MEIS2	601740	AD	Developmental delay, microcephaly, cardiovascular malformations, skeletal anomalies, and distinctive facial features
Holoprosencephaly type 7	610828	PTCH1	601309	AD	Developmental delay, seizures, macrocephaly, pan hypopituitarism, distinctive features, and abnormal brain imaging
Hypomyelinating leukodystrophy type 6	612438	TUBB4A	602662	AD	Developmental delay, cognitive regression, learning difficulties, seizures, gait anomalies, movement abnormalities, and abnormal brain imaging
Hypomyelinating leukodystrophy type 10	616420	PYCR2	616406	AR	Developmental delay, postnatal progressive microcephaly, and hypomyelination on brain imaging
Idiopathic generalized epilepsy 15	618357	RORB	601972	AD	Intellectual disability, developmental delay, and seizures

Intellectual developmental disorder with cardiac defects and dysmorphic facies	618316	TMEM94	618163	AR	Intellectual disability, developmental delay, seizures, cardiovascular malformations, skeletal anomalies, and distinctive facial features
Joubert syndrome 5	610188	CEP290	610142	AR	Developmental delay, hypotonia, ataxia, oculomotor apraxia, neonatal breathing abnormalities, and abnormal neuroimaging
Joubert syndrome type 6	610688	TMEM67	609884	AR	Developmental delay, hypotonia, ataxia, oculomotor apraxia, neonatal breathing abnormalities, abdominal anomalies, and abnormal neuroimaging
Joubert syndrome type 21	615536	CSPP1	611654	AR	Developmental delay, hypotonia, ataxia, oculomotor apraxia, sensorineural hearing loss, neonatal breathing abnormalities, abdominal anomalies, genitourinary anomalies, and abnormal neuroimaging
Kabuki syndrome type 1	147920	KMT2D	602113	AD	Developmental delay, behavioral abnormalities, learning disability, hypotonia, microcephaly, skeletal anomalies, and distinctive features
KBG syndrome	148050	ANKRD11	611192	AD	Intellectual disability, developmental delay, seizures, microcephaly, macrodontia, skeletal anomalies, and distinctive features
Leber congenital amaurosis type 2	204100	RPE65	204100	AR	Developmental delay, retinal dystrophy, vision loss, and nystagmus
Mental retardation type 21	615502	CTCF	604167	AD	Intellectual disability, developmental delay, behavioral abnormalities, hypotonia, microcephaly, feeding difficulties, cardiovascular abnormalities, cryptorchidism, ocular anomalies, and distinctive features
Mental retardation type 23	615761	SETD5	615743	AD	Intellectual disability, developmental delay, behavioral abnormalities, ocular anomalies, and distinctive features
Mental retardation type 36	615286	ADAT3	615302	AR	Intellectual disability, developmental delay, behavioral abnormalities, failure to thrive, seizures, endocrine anomalies, distinctive facial features, and abnormal neuroimaging
Mental retardation type 57	618050	TLK2	608439	AD	Developmental delay, behavioral abnormalities, hypotonia, gastrointestinal anomalies, and distinctive features

(continued)

Table 45.2 (continued)

Disease	MIM#	Gene	MIM#	Mode of inheritance	Main clinical presentation
Myhre syndrome	139210	SMAD4	600993	AD	Intellectual disability, microcephaly, short stature, skeletal anomalies, cardiovascular malformations, and distinctive facial features
Myopathy with extrapyramidal signs	615673	MICU1	605084	AR	Learning disabilities, early onset proximal muscle weakness, progressive extrapyramidal signs, and abnormal brain imaging
Native American myopathy	255995	STAC3	615521	AR	Congenital myopathy, scoliosis, malignant hyperthermia, and myopathic facies
Neurodegeneration with ataxia, dystonia, and gaze palsy, childhood-onset	617145	SQSTM1	601530	AR	Cognitive regression, ataxia, hearing loss, ocular anomalies, movement abnormalities, dysarthria, dystonia, and abnormal brain imaging
Neurodegeneration with brain iron accumulation 5	300894	WDR45	300526	XLD	Developmental delay, progressive dystonia, parkinsonism, extrapyramidal signs, dementia, and abnormal brain imaging
Neurofibromatosis type 1	162200	NF1	613113	AD	Intellectual disability, learning disability, Lisch nodules in the eye, fibromatous tumors of the skin, and cafe-au-lait spots
Neurodevelopmental disorder coarse facies and mild distal skeletal abnormalities	618505	KDM6B	611577	AD	Intellectual disability, developmental delay, behavioral abnormalities, hypotonia, genitourinary anomalies, and distinctive features
Neurodevelopmental disorder with dysmorphic facies and variable seizures	619264	EMC10	614545	AR	Intellectual disability, developmental delay, behavioral abnormalities, failure to thrive, ocular anomalies, skeletal anomalies, genitourinary anomalies, distinctive facial features, and abnormal neuroimaging

Neuropathy, hereditary sensory and autonomic type V	608654	NGF	162030	AR	Intellectual disability, self-mutilation, insensitivity to pain and temperature, peripheral neuropathy, immunologic anomalies, skin anomalies, and skeletal anomalies
Nonsyndromic hearing loss type 53	609706	COL11A2	120290	AR	Pre-lingual, profound, and non-progressive hearing loss
Noonan syndrome type 1	163950	PTPN11	176876	AD	Short stature, cardiovascular malformations, and distinctive features
Okur-Chung Neurodevelopmental syndrome	617062	CSNK2A1	115440	AD	Intellectual disability, developmental delay, behavioral abnormalities, delayed to absent speech, cardiovascular anomalies, immunologic anomalies, skeletal anomalies, and distinctive features
Omodysplasia type 2	164745	FZD2	600667	AD	Developmental delay, seizures, and distinctive features
Pitt-Hopkins syndrome	610954	TCF4	602272	AD	Intellectual disability, epilepsy, encephalopathy, autonomic dysfunction, intermittent hyperventilation, and distinctive features
Primary microcephaly type 1	251200	MCPH1	607117	AR	Intellectual disability, short stature, microcephaly, and abnormal brain imaging
Primary microcephaly type 5	608716	ASPM	605481	AR	Intellectual disability, developmental delay, seizures, microcephaly, congenital hearing loss, distinctive facial features, and abnormal neuroimaging
Pseudo-TORCH syndrome 1	251290	OCLN	602876	AR	Developmental delay, failure to thrive, seizures, spasticity, ocular anomalies, apneas, abdominal anomalies, genitourinary anomalies, distinctive facial features, and abnormal neuroimaging
Retinal arterial macroaneurysms and supravalvular pulmonic stenosis	614224	IGFBP7	602867	AR	Ocular anomalies and cardiovascular malformations
Rett syndrome	312750	MECP2	300005	AD	Developmental delay, hypotonia, spasticity in lower extremities, and distinctive features

(continued)

Table 45.2 (continued)

Disease	MIM#	Gene	MIM#	Mode of inheritance	Main clinical presentation
Rubinstein-Taybi syndrome 1	180849	CREBBP	600140	AD	Intellectual disability, microcephaly, postnatal growth retardation, skeletal anomalies, and distinctive features
Sanjad Sakati syndrome	241410	TBCE	604934	AR	Intellectual disability, short stature, seizures, and hypoparathyroidism
Schuurs-Hoeijmakers syndrome	615009	PACS1	607492	AD	Intellectual disability, developmental delay, seizures, cardiovascular malformations, genitourinary anomalies, and distinctive facial features
Skraban-Deardorff syndrome	617616	WDR26	617424	AD	Intellectual disability, developmental delay, seizures, and distinctive features
Sotos syndrome	117550	NSD1	606681	AD	Intellectual disability, seizures, overgrowth, acromegaly, and distinctive features
Spastic paraplegia type 52	607243	AP4S1	614067	AR	Intellectual disability and spasticity
Stankiewicz-Isidor syndrome	617516	PSMD12	604450	AD	Intellectual disability, developmental delay, behavioral disorders, cardiovascular malformations, urogenital anomalies, and distinctive features
Stuve-Wiedemann syndrome	601559	LIFR	151443	AR	Episodic hyperthermia, feeding difficulties, skeletal anomalies, respiratory distress, and early death
Suleiman-El-Hattab syndrome	618950	TASP1	608270	AR	Intellectual disability, developmental delay, behavioral abnormalities, hypotonia, microcephaly, feeding difficulties, and distinctive features
Temtamy syndrome	218340	C12ORF57	615140	AR	Intellectual disability, multiple congenital anomalies, seizures, ocular anomalies, distinctive features, and abnormal brain imaging
Wiedemann-Steiner syndrome	605130	KMT2A	159555	AD	Intellectual disability, developmental delay, behavioral abnormalities, short stature, hairy elbows, and distinctive features
Wooly hair	278150	LPAR6	609239	AR	Hair shaft disorders that are characterized by fine and tightly curled hair

45.4 Hemoglobinopathies

45.4.1 Beta Thalassemia

Beta Thalassemia is a major health concern in the UAE, as the national population has an elevated carrier rate of 8.5% [13]. This has led the government to launch a premarital screening program in 2011 [13]. A study examining the frequency of the beta thalassemia pathogenic variants among nationals in the UAE showed that c.92+5G>C (IVS1-5G>C) is the most common, accounting for 53% of the variants [14]. This mutation is known to be common in the Indian subcontinent and was suggested to have originated from migration from areas like Baluchistan, which is an area located today between Iran, Pakistan, and Afghanistan [5].

45.4.2 Alpha Thalassemia

A neonatal screening study found that 49% of the tested neonates had at least one alpha-globin gene mutation, which is one of the highest prevalence rates globally [15]. The most prevalent mutation is the poly A1 mutation, which accounts for nearly 50% of all α-thalassemia mutations [15]. It is important to mention that the Arabs of the Gulf do not exhibit α-globin gene deletion in cis (−α, αα). In other words, they exhibit deletional mutations involving one of the α-globin genes (−α, αα) or two deletions in trans (−α, −α), in addition to the normal genotype (αα, αα) [16].

45.4.3 Sickle Cell Disease

The incidence of sickle cell trait in the UAE is estimated at around 0.8% on the national neonatal screening program [17]. The disease has a milder severity in the UAE, similar to the eastern region of Saudi Arabia. This was further assessed by genetic studies, which showed that 68% of the patients have the Indian/Saudi Arabian haplotype (31/31), which has a higher level of fetal hemoglobin. Nevertheless, 8% of patients were found to be homozygous for the Bantu haplotype (20/20), suggesting that these patients originate from Africa [18, 19].

45.5 Genetic Skin Disorders

Genetic skin disorders include blistering disorders, keratosis, ectodermal dysplasia, and other congenital disorders that follow the Mendelian inheritance pattern. We hereby present common genetic skin disorders reported in the UAE. They mainly follow an autosomal recessive inheritance.

- *Mal de Meleda disease* is a rare genetic disorder that is seen frequently in the UAE due to homozygous mutations in the *SLURP1 gene*. It is primarily characterized by congenital palmoplantar/skin keratosis, perioral erythema, abnormal nails, and brachydactyly [20].
- *Ehlers-Danlos syndrome VIA* (kyphoscoliotic type) is a disorder of the connective tissues secondary to pathogenic variants in *PLOD1*, leading to lysyl hydroxylase deficiency. Affected patients present with skin hyperextensibility, joint hypermobility, tissue fragility, muscle hypotonia, scoliosis, and scleral fragility. Several UAE families have been reported with this condition [21].
- *Congenital ichthyosis* is a heterogeneous group of autosomal recessive diseases characterized by abnormal keratinization, which leads to abnormal scaling of the skin over the entire body. A study conducted in the UAE reported cases of congenital ichthyosis due to mutations in three genes: *ABCA12, ALOX12B,* and *TGM1* [22].
- *Junctional epidermolysis bullosa* is a blistering disease of the skin and mucus membranes. The prevalent type in the UAE is the non-Herlitz type, which is less severe and is caused by pathogenic variants in *LAMB3* [23].
- *Restrictive dermatopathy* is a rare disorder caused by biallelic pathogenic variants in *ZMPSTE24*. Two children belonging to two distantly related families in the UAE were reported to have a founder mutation in *ZMPSTE24*. Affected patients have lethal contractures of all their joints, translucent skin, tightly adherent skin, erosions occurring at flexure sites, superficial vessels, hyperkeratosis, and distinctive facial features [24].
- *Setleis syndrome* is a rare disorder characterized by bitemporal skin or preauricular lesions and distinctive facial features. Two cases with *TWIST2* mutations were described in the UAE from a consanguineous Omani family [25].

45.6 Inherited Skeletal Dysplasias

The estimated prevalence of skeletal dysplasias in the UAE is 9.5 per 10,000. They are mainly inherited as autosomal recessive, with a birth prevalence of 4.7/10,000 births, followed by de novo dominant variants (2.6/10,000) [6]. Common skeletal dysplasias in the UAE are briefly discussed here.

- *Stuve-Wiedmann syndrome* is inherited as an autosomal recessive disorder. Affected patients present with skeletal anomalies such as bowing of the long bones, along with feeding difficulties, respiratory distress, episodic hyperthermia, feeding difficulties, and distinctive craniofacial anomalies. Its estimated prevalence in the UAE is approximately 0.5 per 10,000 births [26]. A Molecular workup unveiled a founder mutation (c.653_654insT) within *LIFR* [27].
- *Aarskog-Scott syndrome* is a rare X-linked syndrome caused by pathogenic variants in *FGD1,* with one novel variant found in two affected Emirati brothers. Common features include short stature, skeletal anomalies, genital anomalies, and distinctive facial features [28].

- *Ellis-van Creveld syndrome* is an autosomal recessive skeletal dysplasia secondary to biallelic pathogenic variants in either *EVC1 or EVC2* [29]. Main features include skeletal anomalies (short limbs or ribs, postaxial polydactyly, dysplastic teeth or nails) and congenital cardiac defects. Six children with Ellis-van Creveld syndrome from four families in the UAE were reported. Affected children had the main clinical features of this syndrome and different mutations in *EVC1 or EVC2*, highlighting the molecular heterogeneity observed in UAE patients affected by this syndrome and eliminating the possibility of a common founder effect [30].
- *Geleophysic dysplasia* is a rare autosomal recessive disease caused by biallelic pathogenic variants in *ADAMTSL2*. It is characterized by severe short stature, skeletal anomalies manifesting as short hands or feet and joint contractures, in addition to tight skin. Two children with geleophysic dysplasia from two consanguineous Arab families residing in the UAE were described. They showed two novel homozygous variants in *ADAMTSL2* [31].
- *Raine syndrome* is a rare autosomal recessive disease caused by pathogenic variants in *FAM20C*. It mainly presents as microcephaly, exophthalmos, hypoplastic nose, midfacial hypoplasia with choanal atresia, generalized osteosclerosis, and brain calcifications. In the UAE, several affected children from four families were described as having *FAM20C* mutations [32].
- *Thanatophoric dysplasia* is an autosomal dominant syndrome caused by monoallelic pathogenic variants in *FGFR3*. It is a severe dwarfism syndrome that is lethal during the perinatal period. In the UAE, two affected and unrelated children with this syndrome were reported, and both had the same mutation in *FGFR3* [33].
- *Dyggve-Melchoir-Clausen syndrome* is a rare autosomal recessive disease caused by pathogenic variants in *DYM*. It is characterized by progressive spondyloepimetaphyseal dysplasia, short-trunk dwarfism, microcephaly, and impaired intellectual development. It was reported in two Arab families living in the UAE who had homozygous pathogenic variants in *DYM* [34].
- *Wollcott-Rallison syndrome* is a rare autosomal recessive disease caused by biallelic pathogenic variants in *EIF2AK3*. It is characterized by childhood-onset insulin-dependent diabetes mellitus and the later onset of multiple epiphyseal dysplasias. Two children from the same Omani origin family were reported in the UAE. Both had a homozygous mutation in *EIF2AK3* [35].

45.7 Inherited Lung Diseases

Cystic fibrosis (CF) is an autosomal recessive disorder caused by biallelic pathogenic variants in *CFTR*, with ΔF508 being the most prevalent variant worldwide [36]. In the UAE, its estimated incidence is approximately 1 in 15,000 live births [37]. Few studies are available from the UAE regarding the genetics of cystic fibrosis. Unlike in European and western countries, the most common mutation in the UAE is p.S549R (28%), followed by ΔF508 (23%). Due to the high prevalence of consanguinity in the UAE, a high rate of homozygosity is observed, with only 13% of the patients being heterozygous for cystic fibrosis mutations [38].

Affected patients present in early infancy with small airways and interstitial lung diseases. A study was conducted in the UAE to determine the pathogenic variants associated with these disorders. It identified variants in two genes linked to dysfunction in the metabolism of surfactants (*CSF2RB* and *ABCA3*), two genes associated with pulmonary fibrosis (*SFTP* and *MUC5B*), one gene associated with alpha-1-antitrypsin deficiency (*SERPINA1*), and one gene associated with bronchiectasis (*SCNN1B*) [39].

45.8 Inborn Errors of Immunity

Human inborn errors of immunity (IEI), previously known as primary immunodeficiency disorders, are a heterogeneous group of immune dysfunctions that result in specific impairments of normal immune function and regulation. Affected patients exhibit heightened vulnerability to infections, autoimmune and autoinflammatory conditions, atopy, lymphoproliferation, and an increased risk of malignancies. More than 400 gene defects leading to different phenotypes have been identified [40]. A recent study evaluated 162 patients with IEI in the UAE. Of these, 152 were children; two-thirds were Emirati nationals; 38% of the cases were familial; and 64% had consanguineous parents. Twenty percent had immunodeficiencies affecting both humoral and cellular immunity; 38% had combined immunodeficiencies with syndromic features; 16% had mainly antibody deficiencies; 4% had immune dysregulation; and 8% had congenital phagocyte defects. Genetic testing was done for 82% of cases with an elevated diagnostic yield (93%). The main mode of inheritance was autosomal recessive (61% of IEI), followed by autosomal dominant, then X-linked recessive [40].

45.9 Hereditary Hearing Loss

Hearing loss is the most prevalent sensory defect, affecting 1 in 1,000 newborns, with at least 50% of cases having a genetic etiology [41]. Genetic forms are classified as non-syndromic or syndromic depending on whether the hearing loss is accompanied by additional manifestations. Eighty percent of non-syndromic types are autosomal recessive, with only 20% being autosomal dominant. Mitochondrial forms and X-linked inheritance have also been reported [42]. Based on the latest statistics from the Hereditary Hearing Loss homepage, a total of 124 non-syndromic hearing loss genes have been reported, including 51 autosomal dominant, 78 autosomal recessive, and 5 X-linked. The *GJB2 gene* is the most common and is globally associated with non-syndromic hearing loss. At least 90 pathogenic variants in this gene have been recognized as responsible for autosomal recessive non-syndromic hearing loss. The c.35delG truncating mutation accounts for most of the *GJB2* pathogenic variants [43]. In a study assessing the occurrence of *GJB2* mutations in 50 unrelated individuals from the Emirates who had non-syndromic hearing loss, mutations in *GJB2* were detected in 12 cases (24%). Specifically, the c.35delG mutation was observed in 6 cases (12%), highlighting its prominence as the most commonly observed causative mutation in the UAE [44].

Mutations in *MTRNR1*, which encodes the mitochondrial 12S rRNA, have been documented as causing hearing loss. The contribution of this mutation to hearing loss was studied in 74 unrelated patients in the UAE with no *GJB2* mutations, who underwent *MTRNR1* sequencing. Two known deafness variants (m.669 T>C and m.827A>G) were detected in two unrelated deaf patients. Therefore, the contribution of mitochondrial mutations in this gene was calculated at 2.7%. The results of this study suggested that both variants m.827A>G and m.669 T>C, should be considered as part of the molecular diagnosis for individuals with hearing loss in the UAE [45].

45.10 Genetic Disorders of the Eyes

Inherited eye diseases encompass a diverse range of disorders affecting 1 in every 1,000 people worldwide, with over 400 genes identified as responsible for these conditions [46]. The mode of inheritance can be autosomal recessive (65%), autosomal dominant (25%), X-linked (5%), or mitochondrial (1%) [47]. Common genetic eye diseases in the UAE include Stargardt disease, retinitis pigmentosa, and achromatopsia (Table 45.3).

A study reported the genetic outcomes of 91 patients from 74 unrelated UAE families affected by syndromic or non-syndromic inherited eye diseases. Seventy-eight percent of the families reported consanguinity, and the ethnicity of the families was Arab in 74%. Autosomal recessive inheritance was seen in 74% of the cases (72% involving homozygous variants), with autosomal dominant accounting for 8% and X-linked accounting for 3%. Sixty-two pathogenic variants were recognized in 40 genes linked to various inherited eye diseases. The most common was the *ABCA4* gene, identified in 12 families, followed by *MERTK* and *RP1* in 3 families each, and then *CNGB3*, *RS1*, and *USH2A* in 2 families each. Another study evaluated 71 patients with childhood-onset retinal disease in the UAE and revealed mutations in *ABCA4* (in 14 individuals), *KCNV2* (in 8 individuals), *CRB1* (in 6 individuals), and *CNGA3* (in 5 individuals) [49]. The *ABCA4* variant c.5882G>A (p.Gly1961Glu) has been identified in several families, indicating that this variant is a founder mutation in the UAE [50].

Table 45.3 Genetic eye diseases in the UAE [49, 50]

Disease	MIM#	Gene	MIM#	Mode of inheritance	Main clinical presentation
Achromatopsia 2	216900	*CNGA3*	600053	AR	Nystagmus, photophobia, reduced visual acuity, color blindness, decreased foveolar thickness
Achromatopsia 3	262300	*CNGB3*	605080	AR	
Cone-rod dystrophy 3	604116	*ABCA4*	601691	AR	Reduced visual acuity, impairment of the central visual field, color vision deficits, maculopathy
Retinal cone dystrophy 3B	610356	*KCNV2*	607604	AR	Photophobia, reduced color vision, and central scotomata
Retinitis pigmentosa 1	180100	*RP1*	603937	AR	Night blindness, constricted visual fields, decreased visual acuity, abnormal retinal examination, and abnormal electroretinogram
Retinitis pigmentosa 12	600105	*CRB1*	604210	AR	
Retinitis pigmentosa 19	601718	*ABCA4*	601691	AR	
Retinitis pigmentosa 39	613809	*USH2A*	608400	AR	
Retinoschisis 1	312700	*RS1*	300839	XLR	Retinal dystrophy leading to schisis of the neural retina, and reduced visual acuity
Rod-cone dystrophy	613862	*MERTK*	604705	AR	Childhood onset, progressive degeneration of rod and cone photoreceptors in a rod-cone pattern of dysfunction
Stargardt disease 1	248200	*ABCA4*	601691	AR	Reduced visual acuity, macular degeneration, and central retinitis pigmentosa

45.11 Conclusion

Genetic disorders, namely, autosomal recessive ones, are common in the UAE due to the high prevalence of consanguineous marriages. There are new variants, as discussed above, that are peculiar to the Emirati population and are associated with novel genotypes and phenotypes. Many genetic characteristics and disorders specific to the Emiratis remain uncovered. More studies are required to reveal more details regarding these genetic diseases. Prevention programs that incorporate screening for these disorders when feasible, along with genetic counseling, should be implemented nationwide to reduce the burden of these disorders.

Conflicts of Interest The authors have no conflicts of interest to declare.

References

1. United Arab Emirates (UAE) Population Statistics 2022 | GMI [Internet]. Official GMI Blog. 2022 [cited 2022 Oct 31]. Available from: https://www.globalmediainsight.com/blog/uae-population-statistics/.
2. Aljasmi FA, Vijayan R, Sudalaimuthuasari N, Souid AK, Karuvantevida N, Almaskari R, et al. Genomic landscape of the mitochondrial genome in the United Arab Emirates native population. Genes (Basel) [Internet]. 2020 [cited 2022 Sep 20];11(8):876. Available from: https://www.ncbi.nlm.nih.gov/pmc/articles/PMC7464197/.
3. Woods CG, Cox J, Springell K, Hampshire DJ, Mohamed MD, McKibbin M, et al. Quantification of homozygosity in consanguineous individuals with autosomal recessive disease. Am J Hum Genet. 2006;78(5):889–96.
4. Bener A, Abdulrazzaq YM, Al-Gazali LI, Micallef R, Al-Khayat AI, Gaber T. Consanguinity and associated socio-demographic factors in The United Arab Emirates. Hum Hered. 1996;46(5):256–64.
5. Al-Gazali LI, Bener A, Abdulrazzaq YM, Micallef R, Al-Khayat AI, Gaber T. Consanguineous marriages in The United Arab Emirates. J Biosoc Sci. 1997;29(4):491–7.
6. Abouelhoda M, Sobahy T, El-Kalioby M, Patel N, Shamseldin H, Monies D, et al. Clinical genomics can facilitate countrywide estimation of autosomal recessive disease burden. Genet Med. 2016;18(12):1244–9.
7. Sanjurjo P, Baldellou A, Aldámiz-Echevarría K, Montejo M, García JM. Inborn errors of metabolism as rare diseases with a specific global situation. An Sist Sanit Navar. 2008;31(Suppl 2):55–73.
8. Al-Shamsi A, Hertecant JL, Al-Hamad S, Souid AK, Al-Jasmi F. Mutation spectrum and birth prevalence of inborn errors of metabolism among Emiratis. Sultan Qaboos Univ Med J [Internet] 2014 [cited 2022 Sep 14];14(1):e42–9. Available from: https://www.ncbi.nlm.nih.gov/pmc/articles/PMC3916276/.
9. Ali BR, Hertecant JL, Al-Jasmi FA, Hamdan MA, Khuri SF, Akawi NA, et al. New and known mutations associated with inborn errors of metabolism in a heterogeneous Middle Eastern population. Saudi Med J. 2011;32(4):353–9.
10. Ben-Rebeh I, Hertecant JL, Al-Jasmi FA, Aburawi HE, Al-Yahyaee SA, Al-Gazali L, et al. Identification of mutations underlying 20 inborn errors of metabolism in The United Arab Emirates population. Genet Test Mol Biomarkers [Internet] 2012 [cited 2022 Sep 14];16(5):366–71. Available from: https://www.ncbi.nlm.nih.gov/pmc/articles/PMC3354585/.
11. Hertecant JL, Ben-Rebeh I, Marah MA, Abbas T, Ayadi L, Ben Salem S, et al. Clinical and molecular analysis of isovaleric acidemia patients in The United Arab Emirates reveals remarkable phenotypes and four novel mutations in the IVD gene. Eur J Med Genet. 2012;55(12):671–6.
12. Saleh S, Beyyumi E, Al Kaabi A, Hertecant J, Barakat D, Al Dhaheri NS, et al. Spectrum of neuro-genetic disorders in The United Arab Emirates national population. Clin Genet. 2021;100(5):573–600.
13. Saffi M, Howard N. Exploring the effectiveness of mandatory premarital screening and genetic counselling programmes for β-thalassaemia in the Middle East: a scoping review. Public Health Genomics. 2015;18(4):193–203.
14. Baysal E. Molecular basis of β-thalassemia in The United Arab Emirates. Hemoglobin. 2011;35(5–6):581–8.
15. El-Kalla S, Baysal E. Alpha-thalassemia in The United Arab Emirates. Acta Haematol. 1998;100(1):49–53.
16. Higgs DR, Weatherall DJ. The alpha thalassaemias. Cell Mol Life Sci. 2009;66(7):1154–62.
17. Al Hosani H, Salah M, Osman HM, Farag HM, El Assiouty L, Saade D, et al. Expanding the comprehensive national neonatal screening programme in The United Arab Emirates from 1995 to 2011. EMHJ – East Mediterr Health J, 2014;20(1):17–23 [Internet]. 2014 [cited 2022 Sep 28]. Available from: https://apps.who.int/iris/handle/10665/118617.
18. Baysal E. Hemoglobinpathies in United Arab Emirates. Hemoglobin. 2001;25:247–53.

19. Baysal E. Molecular heterogeneity of beta-thalassemia in The United Arab Emirates. Community Genet. 2005;8(1):35–9.
20. Eckl KM, Stevens HP, Lestringant GG, Westenberger-Treumann M, Traupe H, Hinz B, et al. Mal de Meleda (MDM) caused by mutations in the gene for SLURP-1 in patients from Germany, Turkey, Palestine, and The United Arab Emirates. Hum Genet. 2003;112(1):50–6.
21. Giunta C, Randolph A, Al-Gazali LI, Brunner HG, Kraenzlin ME, Steinmann B. Nevo syndrome is allelic to the kyphoscoliotic type of the Ehlers-Danlos syndrome (EDS VIA). Am J Med Genet A. 2005;133A(2):158–64.
22. Bastaki F, Mohamed M, Nair P, Saif F, Mustafa EM, Bizzari S, et al. Summary of mutations underlying autosomal recessive congenital ichthyoses (ARCI) in Arabs with four novel mutations in ARCI-related genes from The United Arab Emirates. Int J Dermatol. 2017;56(5):514–23.
23. Nakano A, Lestringant GG, Paperna T, Bergman R, Gershoni R, Frossard P, et al. Junctional epidermolysis bullosa in the Middle East: clinical and genetic studies in a series of consanguineous families. J Am Acad Dermatol. 2002;46(4):510–6.
24. Sander CS, Salman N, van Geel M, Broers JLV, Al-Rahmani A, Chedid F, et al. A newly identified splice site mutation in ZMPSTE24 causes restrictive dermopathy in the Middle East. Br J Dermatol. 2008;159(4):961–7.
25. Al-Gazali LI, Al-Talabani J. Setleis syndrome: autosomal recessive or autosomal dominant inheritance? Clin Dysmorphol. 1996;5(3):249–53.
26. Al-Gazali LI, Bakir M, Hamid Z, Varady E, Varghes M, Haas D, et al. Birth prevalence and pattern of osteochondrodysplasias in an inbred high risk population. Birth Defects Res A Clin Mol Teratol. 2003;67(2):125–32.
27. Dagoneau N, Scheffer D, Huber C, Al-Gazali LI, Di Rocco M, Godard A, et al. Null leukemia inhibitory factor receptor (LIFR) mutations in Stuve-Wiedemann/Schwartz-Jampel type 2 syndrome. Am J Hum Genet. 2004;74(2):298–305.
28. Hamzeh AR, Saif F, Nair P, Binjab AJ, Mohamed M, Al-Ali MT, et al. A novel, putatively null, FGD1 variant leading to Aarskog-Scott syndrome in a family from UAE. BMC Pediatr. 2017;17(1):31.
29. D'Asdia MC, Torrente I, Consoli F, Ferese R, Magliozzi M, Bernardini L, et al. Novel and recurrent EVC and EVC2 mutations in Ellis-van Creveld syndrome and Weyers acrofacial dyostosis. Eur J Med Genet. 2013;56(2):80–7.
30. Ali BR, Akawi NA, Chedid F, Bakir M, Ur Rehman M, Rahmani A, et al. Molecular and clinical analysis of Ellis-van Creveld syndrome in The United Arab Emirates. BMC Med Genet. 2010;11:33.
31. Ben-Salem S, Hertecant J, Al-Shamsi AM, Ali BR, Al-Gazali L. Novel mutations in ADAMTSL2 gene underlying geleophysic dysplasia in families from United Arab Emirates. Birth Defects Res A Clin Mol Teratol. 2013;97(12):764–9.
32. Al-Gazali LI, Jehier K, Nazih B, Abtin F, Haas D, Sadagahatian R. Further delineation of Raine syndrome. Clin Dysmorphol. 2003;12(2):89–93.
33. Simsek M, Al-Gazali L, Al-Mjeni R, Bayoumi R. Improved diagnosis of a common mutation (R248C) in the human growth factor receptor 3 (FGFR3) gene that causes type I Thanatophoric dysplasia. Clin Biochem. 2003;36(2):151–3.
34. El Ghouzzi V, Dagoneau N, Kinning E, Thauvin-Robinet C, Chemaitilly W, Prost-Squarcioni C, et al. Mutations in a novel gene Dymeclin (FLJ20071) are responsible for Dyggve-Melchior-Clausen syndrome. Hum Mol Genet. 2003;12(3):357–64.
35. Brickwood S, Bonthron DT, Al-Gazali LI, Piper K, Hearn T, Wilson DI, et al. Wolcott-Rallison syndrome: pathogenic insights into neonatal diabetes from new mutation and expression studies of EIF2AK3. J Med Genet. 2003;40(9):685–9.
36. Jih KY, Li M, Hwang TC, Bompadre SG. The most common cystic fibrosis-associated mutation destabilizes the dimeric state of the nucleotide-binding domains of CFTR. J Physiol. 2011;589(Pt 11):2719–31.
37. Frossard PM, Lestringant G, Girodon E, Goossens M, Dawson KP. Determination of the prevalence of cystic fibrosis in The United Arab Emirates by genetic carrier screening. Clin Genet. 1999;55(6):496–7.

38. Shafiq I, Shabeer S, Haider Uzbeck M, Zoumot Z, Abuzakouk M, Saeed WA. Genetic and clinical demographics of adult cystic fibrosis patients in a Middle Eastern population. Turk Thorac J [Internet] 2021 [cited 2022 Sep 20];22(4):279–83. Available from: https://www.ncbi.nlm.nih.gov/pmc/articles/PMC8975356/.
39. Alsamri MT, Alabdouli A, Alkalbani AM, Iram D, Tawil MI, Antony P, et al. Genetic variants of small airways and interstitial pulmonary disease in children. Sci Rep [Internet]. 2021 [cited 2022 Oct 7];11:2715. Available from: https://www.ncbi.nlm.nih.gov/pmc/articles/PMC7851163/.
40. Shendi HM, Al Kuwaiti AA, Al Dhaheri AD, Al-Hammadi S. The spectrum of inborn errors of immunity in the United Arab Emirates: 5 year experience in a tertiary center. Front Immunol [Internet]. 2022 [cited 2022 Sep 13];13:837243. Available from: https://www.ncbi.nlm.nih.gov/pmc/articles/PMC8841332/.
41. Marazita ML, Ploughman LM, Rawlings B, Remington E, Arnos KS, Nance WE. Genetic epidemiological studies of early-onset deafness in the U.S. school-age population. Am J Med Genet. 1993;46(5):486–91.
42. Morton NE. Genetic epidemiology of hearing impairment. Ann N Y Acad Sci. 1991;630:16–31.
43. Chan DK, Chang KW. GJB2-associated hearing loss: systematic review of worldwide prevalence, genotype, and auditory phenotype. Laryngoscope. 2014;124(2):E34–53.
44. Tlili A, Al Mutery A, Kamal Eddine Ahmad Mohamed W, Mahfood M, Hadj Kacem H. Prevalence of GJB2 mutations in affected individuals from United Arab Emirates with autosomal recessive nonsyndromic hearing loss. Genet Test Mol Biomarkers. 2017;21(11):686–91.
45. Mohamed WKE, Arnoux M, Cardoso THS, Almutery A, Tlili A. Mitochondrial mutations in non-syndromic hearing loss at UAE. Int J Pediatr Otorhinolaryngol. 2020;138:110286.
46. Stone EM. Genetic testing for inherited eye disease. Arch Ophthalmol. 2007;125(2):205–12.
47. Al-Gazali L, Hamamy H, Al-Arrayad S. Genetic disorders in the Arab world. BMJ. 2006;333(7573):831–4.
48. Méjécase C, Kozak I, Moosajee M. The genetic landscape of inherited eye disorders in 74 consecutive families from the United Arab Emirates. Am J Med Genet C Semin Med Genet [Internet]. 2020 [cited 2022 Sep 24];184(3):762–72. Available from: https://www.ncbi.nlm.nih.gov/pmc/articles/PMC8432150/.
49. Khan AO. Phenotype-guided genetic testing of pediatric inherited retinal disease in the United Arab Emirates. Retina. 2020;40(9):1829–37.
50. Khan AO. Homozygosity for a novel double mutant allele (g1961e/l857p) underlies childhood-onset abca4-related retinopathy in the united arab emirates. Retina. 2020;40(7):1429–33.
51. Acuna-Hidalgo R, Veltman JA, Hoischen A. New insights into the generation and role of de novo mutations in health and disease. Genome Biol. 2016;17:1–9.

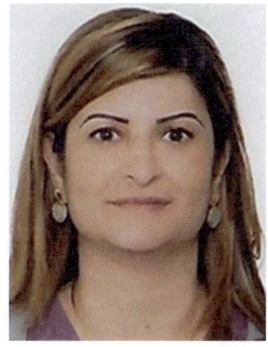

Mode Al Ojaimi MD, is an American Board-Certified Pediatrician from the State University of New York and holds an Executive Master's in Business Administration from the University of Balamand, Lebanon. She is currently Clinical Assistant Professor of Pediatrics at American University of Beirut and Deputee Central Medical Officer for Pediatric Affairs at Keserwan Medical Center. Dr Ojaimi was an Assistant Professor of Pediatrics at the University of Sharjah, co-coordinator of the pediatrics rotation, and consultant in pediatrics at the University Hospital Sharjah. She is the founder and previous director of the Balamand Medical Simulation Center. She served as the Chair of the Pediatrics Department at Family Medical Center-Lebanon for 4 years. She has been running her own private pediatric practice in North Lebanon for the last 23 years. Her research interests are mainly clinical and molecular genetics, and clinical pediatrics, in addition to academic assessments and curricular development.

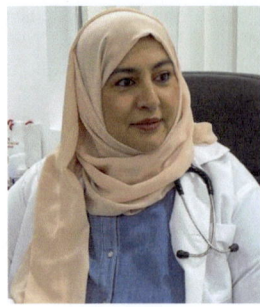

Dr. Rabah Almahmoud is a UAE national Consultant pediatrician and pediatric hematologist with clinical experience spanning over 16 years. She has a vast understanding and skill set in the diagnosis, treatment, and management of childhood cancers and blood-related disorders.

Academically, Dr. Rabah is affiliated with the College of Medicine, University of Sharjah, as an Assistant Professor of Pediatrics. She is a recipient of numerous awards, including the Rashid Award for Academic Excellence in 2008 and the Award of Excellence in Fellowship in Hematology and Oncology in 2011 in Toronto, Canada.

Dr. Rabah has conducted numerous medical research projects in the fields of pediatrics, pediatric hematology, and oncology, which have been published in various international medical journals. She has also actively participated in numerous local and international conferences and symposia.

Dr. Rabah is an active member of various medical associations, including the Emirates Hematology Group and the Thalassemia Research Committee.

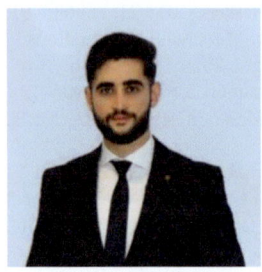

Bashar J. Banimortada is a fourth-year medical student at the University of Sharjah who aims to bridge the gap between research and clinical practice. He is actively engaged in a diverse array of research projects and has delivered numerous presentations at prestigious conferences. He aspires to make a lasting impact in the field of medicine, leaving an unforgettable legacy built on passion, research, and a dedication to improving healthcare practices.

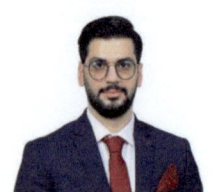

Abduljalil Alragheb a passionate fourth-year medical student at the University of Sharjah, discovered his calling for medicine early on while growing up in a family of healthcare professionals in Syria. His academic journey has been marked by outstanding achievements, including multiple excellence scholarships at the university, excelling in international exams and contributing to several peer-reviewed publications. Abduljalil's dedication to patient care has been fortified through his extensive clinical and research experiences in genetics, community health, and vaccinations. His deep desire for learning, unwavering commitment to patient well-being, and exceptional qualities make him a promising future physician.

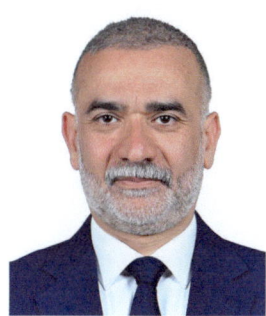

Dr. Ayman W. El-Hattab is Consultant Clinical Genetics and the Director of the Genetics and Rare Disease Center at Burjeel Medical City in Abu Dhabi, United Arab Emirates. He is also a Professor at the College of Medicine, University of Sharjah; the Founder and President of the MENA Organization for Rare Diseases; and Consulting Editor for GeneReviews, University of Washington, Seattle, USA. Professor Ayman El-Hattab has conducted many clinical research projects, and he has more than 120 publications, several book chapters, and many presentations at scientific conferences. Dr. El-Hattab's research fields include chromosomal abnormalities, metabolic disorders, neurogenetic diseases, novel gene and syndrome discoveries, and mitochondrial diseases.

Open Access This chapter is licensed under the terms of the Creative Commons Attribution 4.0 International License (http://creativecommons.org/licenses/by/4.0/), which permits use, sharing, adaptation, distribution and reproduction in any medium or format, as long as you give appropriate credit to the original author(s) and the source, provide a link to the Creative Commons license and indicate if changes were made.

The images or other third party material in this chapter are included in the chapter's Creative Commons license, unless indicated otherwise in a credit line to the material. If material is not included in the chapter's Creative Commons license and your intended use is not permitted by statutory regulation or exceeds the permitted use, you will need to obtain permission directly from the copyright holder.

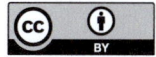

The Historical Perspectives, Present Status, and Future Prospects of Pharmaceutical Services in the UAE

46

Asim Ahmed Elnour , Adel Sadeq ,
and Mariam Al Qahtani

About This Chapter

This chapter encompasses historical perspectives, present status, and future prospects of pharmaceutical services in the United Arab Emirates (UAE). We have described the major landmark events that have evolved over the last 50 years in developing pharmaceutical services (clinical pharmacy, hospital pharmacy, ambulatory pharmacy, and community pharmacy), the pharmaceutical industry (agents, companies, and manufacturing facilities), and regulatory affairs.

This chapter consists of two main sections. The first section describes the versatile pharmaceutical services in the UAE (historical perspectives, present status, and future prospects). We have summarized hospital and clinical pharmacy services, narcotics, intravenous admixtures (drug admixtures, fluid hyper-alimentation, and parenteral nutrition), oncology, automated pharmacy services, drug information services and pharmacovigilance, pharmaceutical agencies, companies, and industries, as well as regulatory affairs.

The second section emphasizes the recent advancements in pharmaceutical services, such as the pharmacist initiative for immunization in the Abu Dhabi emirate (pharmacist as immunizer), tele-pharmacy and artificial intelligence in pharmaceutical services, pharmacist prescribing, and innovative research in the pharmacy profession.

A. A. Elnour (✉)
Program of Clinical Pharmacy, College of Pharmacy, Al Ain University, Abu Dhabi Campus, Abu Dhabi, United Arab Emirates

AAU Health and Biomedical Center, Al Ain University, Abu Dhabi, United Arab Emirates
e-mail: asim.ahmed@aau.ac.ae

A. Sadeq · M. Al Qahtani
Sheikh Khalifa Medical Centre (SKMC), Abu Dhabi, United Arab Emirates
e-mail: adel.sadeq@aau.ac.ae

© The Author(s) 2025
H. O. Al-Shamsi (ed.), *Healthcare in the United Arab Emirates*,
https://doi.org/10.1007/978-981-96-0523-1_46

Dedication

This chapter is dedicated to all pharmacists at every level in the UAE who have served in the past and those who are currently serving the Emirates community. We also extend our message to the future generation of pharmacists, who will build upon the achievements in the pharmacy profession and take over as leadership professionals. We are very indebted to many pharmacists who have worked hard throughout the last 50 years to the current modern pharmacy practice and continue to provide the highest quality pharmaceutical services to the Emirates community. We thank all former and current pharmacists for the esteemed professionalism, dedication, respect, and enthusiasm demonstrated throughout the past five decades across the pharmaceutical field in the UAE.

46.1 The Pharmaceutical Services in the UAE

46.1.1 The Historical Perspective, Present Status, and Future Prospects of Pharmaceutical Services in the UAE

The pharmaceutical services in the United Arab Emirates (UAE) have witnessed tremendous transformational changes throughout the last 50 years since the emirate's union in 1971. Commencing from 1971, the national day of the formation of the union of the seven emirates, the late Sheikh Zayed Bin Sultan Al Nahyan (may Allah have all his mercy upon him), the founder of the UAE, declared the first pharmaceutical services law, referred to as Federal Law Number (5) of 1974, on practicing the pharmaceutical profession and trading in medicine. This was followed by the Federal Law of 1983 on the pharmaceutical profession and institutions. However, this followed the Federal Law Number (1) of 1972 and the laws amending it on the jurisdictions of ministries and powers of ministers after approval from the provisional constitution [1].

In the years prior to the union of the seven emirates, a mini-healthcare center opened in 1943 in the Al Ras area of Dubai. This was followed by the launch of the Al Maktoum Hospital in 1951 by the Ruler of Dubai, Sheikh Saeed bin Maktoum (may Allah have all his mercy upon him) [1]. The turning point in the healthcare sector in the Abu Dhabi emirate was in 1960, when the late Sheikh Zayed and Sheikh Shakhbout invited Pat and Marian, leaders of the American mission, to open a clinic in Al Ain city in the Abu Dhabi Emirate [2], which was named the Oasis Hospital (Al Ain city), while being called by locals the "Kennedy Hospital." Another milestone was the opening of a small outpatient department in Abu Dhabi in 1966, followed a year later by the appointment of Dr. Philip Horniblow to develop a national health service. In 1968, Sheikh Zayed opened a new hospital called the Central Hospital in the Abu Dhabi capital of the UAE [3].

The Corniche Hospital is a leading tertiary women's (maternal) and newborn healthcare facility that has served the community in the Abu Dhabi emirate for 40 years as a long-standing maternal hospital. The armed forces and the police administration have contributed largely to the growth of health services in the

UAE. The medical services delivered by the extensive infrastructure of facilities, such as Zayed Military Hospital and police medical clinics have served the Emirate community throughout the entire UAE. These facilities provide high-quality and specialized healthcare services [3].

Currently, there are more than 40 public hospitals, compared to 7 in the early 1970s. The Ministry of Health (MOH) is undertaking a multimillion-dollar program to expand healthcare facilities and hospitals, medical centers, and a trauma center in the seven emirates. A trauma unit (143 beds) opened in Abu Dhabi with a state-of-the-art project as the first home healthcare program in the UAE. A new multi-level facility, namely, Al Ain Hospital, with more than 800 beds, is located in Al Ain, with new dimensions of buildings surrounded by a resort atmosphere. This parallels the development of Dubai Healthcare City (DHCC) and Dubai Hospital Free Zone (2010), with a global vision of international standards, and advanced healthcare with an academic medical training center [4].

Recently, the UAE reported an increase in medical tourism [5].

The turning point in 2001 saw Abu Dhabi leading the way in using national electronic health models and medical record systems with the establishment of the General Authority for Health Services (GAHS). GAHS, encompassing major hospitals (e.g., Al Ain, Al Jazeera, Corniche, Mafraq, Madinat Zayed, and Tawam), was followed by the launch of Health Authority Abu Dhabi (HAAD) during the period from 2002 to 2006. HAAD is responsible for regulating healthcare facilities, licensing, inspection, and developing health policies. This was followed by the restructuring and introduction of Abu Dhabi Health Services Company (SEHA) in managing government-owned healthcare facilities (2006–2007). SEHA operates 46 ambulatory healthcare centers, 13 hospitals, 3 or more maternal and child health centers, 3 specialized dental centers, 1 center for autism, and 5 specialized facilities including rehab, a blood bank, and an herbal center [6].

The opening of the Sheikh Khalifa Medical City (SKMC) as a complex that demonstrates a high-quality health services in the Abu Dhabi capital provided high-level medical care with diverse medical specialties. SEHA established a restructured framework of all health services in the Abu Dhabi Emirate with a more sophisticated expansion of health services that encompasses specialized ambulatory health services and joint ventures with international healthcare stakeholders such as Cleveland, Imperial College, and Mayo Clinics [6].

The Abu Dhabi Healthcare Summit in 2005 at the Emirates Palace, Abu Dhabi witnessed the government's international vision of signing contracts with a dozen highly reputable international healthcare stakeholders as a milestone in health services in the Abu Dhabi Emirate. Sheikh Nahyan Bin Mubarak represented the government at this summit. During this period, another turning point was the introduction of insurance programs (January 2006), in which all residents of Abu Dhabi were covered by new comprehensive health insurance programs, with costs shared between employers and employees [7].

The private sector has grown tremendously, from individually owned hospitals to group-owned hospitals, to internationally driven hospitals such as American Hospital, Saudi German Hospital, Cleveland Medical Clinic (a world-class hospital), Cromwell Hospital, Imperial College Diabetes Center, and multinational healthcare entities. Recently, further advancement has occurred in the private healthcare sector with more state-of-the-art hospitals such as Bareen International Hospital, Burjeel, Danat Al Emarat, LifeLine Hospitals, Medeor, Mediclinic, New Medical Center, and Royal Hospitals with more specializations, e.g., sports medicine, women's hospitals. Most hospitals nowadays embrace innovative technology such as artificial intelligence, telemedicine, telehealth, and telepharmacy.

In Dubai, the historical Al Maktoum, Rashid, Al Baraha, Alwasal, Al Amal, and Dubai hospitals have provided the basis of healthcare services offered by the Dubai Health Authority (DHA) with diverse medical specialties. The northern emirates (Ajman, Sharjah, Umm Al Quwain, Ras Al Khaimah, and Al Fujairah) have been a part of the growth in government healthcare facilities, with Khalifa (Ajman), Al Kuwaiti, Al Qassimi (Sharjah), Saqr (Ras Al khaimah), Umm Al Quwain, and Fujairah hospitals at the top of the list. The private sector for healthcare facilities in the northern emirates has seen substantial growth throughout the years. In all of the above-mentioned hospitals, pharmaceutical services have grown tremendously with the digitalization of most services. The UAE government embraces the philosophy that a healthy population is key to any country's growth.

Historically, in the early 1960s, the first UAE national pharmacist licensed was Dr. Abdulrahman Almahmeed, who graduated from the School of Pharmacy at the American University of Beirut in 1961. Then he spent 1 year in hospital pharmacy at University College London (UCL) in 1962 and was the first UAE national registered by the Ministry of Health (MOH) as a pharmacist; thereafter, in 1967, he opened his first pharmacy in Abu Dhabi and became its pharmaceutical agent [8].

The pharmaceutical services in the UAE have grown enormously from traditional services to more specialized patient-care, individualized, and continuum-of-care programs. A remarkable milestone started in 1996 at the Abu Dhabi Hilton Hotel, where International Hospital Pharmacy Day was held by key speakers from the United Kingdom (e.g., Saint James Hospital-London), under the auspices of the Ministry of Health, UAE. Another step forward was achieved with the development of health authorities across the UAE during the years 2000–2006 [9].

Huge transformational changes were undertaken with the introduction of Abu Dhabi Health Services Company (SEHA) public joint services in 2007. Further advancements in pharmaceutical services were accomplished, such as unit-dose dispensing, intravenous clean rooms, clinical pharmacy services at the ward level, reconciliation, discharge counseling, and the implementation of medication safety practices. Additional pharmaceutical services are offered via the development of committees such as the pharmacy and therapeutic committee, infection control, drug utilization evaluation, logistics/supply, procurement/purchasing, and medication safety committees.

A breakthrough milestone was the international accreditation programs that reviewed all pharmaceutical practices and services with more standards and performance indicators. This was coupled with specialty pharmaceutical services with satellite pharmacies, on-call, 24-h operating services, discharge medications, counseling, reconciliation, medication reviews, electronic medication orders, quality control, consultations, clinical pharmacists' interventions, clinical pharmacy rounds, specialty services (oncology, unit-dose dispensing, intravenous admixture, parenteral nutrition, neonatal, geriatric, nursing home, etc.), and implementation of quality measures, audits, and reports. The pharmacists have worked very hard throughout the years to attain high standards in pharmaceutical services, with more board specialties, certified pharmacotherapists, master's degrees in clinical pharmacy, continuing pharmacy education, and pharmacy practice training programs. Private pharmaceutical services have evolved more with the development of chain pharmacies, internet pharmacies, counseling and consulting kiosks, electronic waiting services, and areas for consumers. The interface of electronic medical records (e.g., Cerner™), insurance programs, and supply services has marked the delivery of pharmaceutical services. The licensing of new pharmacists is set at a very high international standard, and multinational data-flow operations attract expert global pharmacy candidates.

46.1.2 The Hospital and Clinical Pharmacy Services

46.1.2.1 Unit Dose Distribution System (UDDS), Medication Reviews, and Ward Services

The pharmaceutical services at hospitals in the UAE commenced an early phase of the unit dose distribution system (UDDS) for pharmaceuticals. UDDS is a pharmacy-coordinated service of stocking, distribution, dispensing, surveillance, regulation, and monitoring of pharmaceuticals, which has now transformed into more sophisticated, organized, and automated settings. In the UDDS, the pharmaceuticals are distributed in single-unit packages and dispensed in ready-to-administer form, with not more than a 24-h continuous supply of deliverable doses to all patient-care clinical areas. The UDDS provided safe, effective, and economical utilization of hospital budgets. Furthermore, UDDS resulted in a minimization of total costs relevant to medication-related services, staff, medication reimbursement from insurance, improved drug inventories, and facilitated computerization and automation. In the hospitals within the UAE, all pharmaceuticals are ordered, verified, reviewed, monitored, delivered, and documented via the electronic health information system (HIS). The pharmacy UDDS services provided a structured evaluation of a patient's pharmaceuticals with the aim of optimizing their utility and safety and improving clinical and humanistic outcomes [9].

46.1.2.2 Narcotic Pharmaceutical Services

The UAE countersigned several international conventions on narcotics and psychotropic substances, as the conventions' aim is to ensure their appropriate use, ensure their safe handling, and limit their diversion for illicit use. This standard applies to healthcare providers (facilities and professionals) and pharmaceutical facilities licensed by the Department of Health (DOH) to store, distribute, prescribe, dispense, administer, and handle narcotics, psychotropics, and semi-controlled medications throughout the UAE. As part of the pharmaceutical registration process by the Ministry of Health and Prevention (MOHAP), the mode of dispensing is determined by semi-controlled drugs (SCDs), controlled drugs (CDs), and narcotics [10].

- *Semi-controlled substances (SCD)*: Substances or drugs that are not categorized as narcotic or psychotropic substances. However, they should be controlled within the country because their misuse could harm public health.
- *Controlled substances and products*: Products and substances in medical and commercial circulation require controlling actions. Such products include: (1) toxic substances and plants, (2) prohibited veterinary substances, (3) narcotic and psychotropic substances, whether in the form of raw materials or incorporated into a medical product, and (4) hazardous medical products.
- *Narcotic and psychotropic substances (CD)*: Medical and therapeutic products and others containing any active substances controlled according to Federal Law Number 14 for the year 1995 and its amendments.

Registration of Narcotic and Psychotropic Medicinal Products
The pharmacists within the pharmaceutical facilities use the psychotropic drug registry book maintained within the pharmacy and pharmaceutical warehouses/stores. The narcotics drug register book for wards and clinical departments is used by the nursing staff to document narcotic stock received from the pharmacy and details of administration to end-users. The narcotics registry for stores and pharmacies is used by the pharmacist in charge to document the narcotic purchases and details of dispensing to end-users [10].

All narcotics and psychotropic pharmaceutical products in both inpatient and outpatient settings are prescribed electronically through the unified platform system.

- *Narcotics*: Only a specialist or consultant may prescribe narcotics for a maximum duration of 30 days.
- *Psychotropic Medicinal Products*: Only a HAAD-licensed physician can prescribe a psychotropic for an outpatient in the emirate of Abu Dhabi. CD psychotropics, formerly known as ' Registered Prescription (RP) ' or ' Group 4' drugs, have unique requirements. All healthcare operators authorized to prescribe and dispense narcotics and controlled drugs are required to keep a record in the MOHAP Controlled Drug Registration Book. Each respective register must be complete, legible, and accurate, with the prescription number and patient identifier. Controlled and narcotic drug prescriptions must be kept for 5 years, while semi-controlled drugs must be kept for 2 years from the last refill.

46.1.2.3 Oncology Pharmaceutical Services
The Department of Pharmaceutical Services at the UAE hospitals is devoted to providing high-quality, evidence-based, and patient-centered pharmaceutical care to patients that aligns with international standards. The oncology pharmaceutical services provided encompass procurement, preparation, dispensing, monitoring, and patient-centered follow-up of all cytotoxic pharmaceuticals. Many innovative

technologies are used to raise the bar in the delivery of oncology medications (hood-driven cytotoxic preparations, etc.) [11].

46.1.2.4 Automated Pharmaceutical Services

A. *Automated Robotics Pharmaceutical Services in the UAE*

The UAE has strong beliefs that the use of technology in the pharmaceutical field will redefine the industry and enhance health outcomes. Implementing automated robotics technology will aid in shifting the pharmacists' role perceptions from transaction-based business to healthcare provision.

B. *Robotic Pharmaceuticals in Al Fujairah Hospital*

In early 2017, MOHAP declared the launch of the first outpatient robotic pharmacy automation at Al Fujairah Hospital. The robotic pharmacy is fully equipped with automated robots and reliable software tools that maximize the efficiency and safety of drug dispensing. It handles all the drug dispensing services, including digital scanning, robotic sorting of medications, mobile e-prescription using the ID verification system, e-transactions, and finally robotic dispensing [12].

C. *The Smart Pharmacy (The Dubai Health Authority [DHA])*

Starting in 2017, the DHA has been launching robot-operated pharmacies all across Dubai, including the Nad Al Hamar Primary Healthcare Center, Rashid, Latifa, and Dubai hospitals. This project, known as "Smart Pharmacy," operates via a robot that stores up to 35,000 medications, prepares an average of 12 prescriptions per minute, and dispenses 8,000 medicines in an hour. It is also equipped with smart cold chain management that alarms the pharmacists if the storage temperature exceeds the safe limit. With this initiative, the DHA aims to eliminate medication errors, reduce the waiting time for patients, and increase pharmacist-dedicated time to properly explain medication information to patients [13].

D. *The Sheikh Khalifa Medical City (SKMC) Smart Pharmacy*

The first and largest smart pharmacy in Abu Dhabi, launched in 2018, is in SKMC, which utilizes artificial intelligence to prepare, dispense, and control pharmaceuticals. The artificially intelligent robot serves an average of 800 prescriptions per day, placing pharmacists in an excellent position to not only play a more primary role in treating illness but also enable them to provide additional preventive care and guidance to patients. The SKMC Smart Pharmacy is also equipped with full qualitative and quantitative safety measures, such as a 24-h alarm system for any temperature changes or malfunction errors [14].

46.1.2.5 Intravenous Fluid/Drug Admixtures and Parenteral

The improvement of intravenous fluid/drug admixture and parenteral nutrition (PN) practices in the UAE has shown tremendous growth in the last 30 years. Historically, intravenous fluid and drug admixture and parenteral nutrition were carried out in the clinical areas by nursing staff within the nursing team delivering them. However, the pharmacists' takeover began in the early 1990s with the development of sterile rooms at the central pharmacies. Moreover, sophisticated fluid and drug admixtures and PN pharmaceutical services have been introduced by pharmacists in inpatient pharmacies and in clinical areas with the growth of satellite pharmacies. By the year 2010, almost all hospitals had fully assumed command in delivering fluid and drug admixtures and PN pharmaceutical services from clean rooms with a full 24 h/week of services to the clinical areas. The development of technology has enabled the creation of clean rooms that are mobile, self-contained, transparent, modular, and custom-made. The cleanrooms in the UAE have undergone a conversion to sophisticated designs [14].

There are three types of intravenous fluids: isotonic, hypotonic, and hypertonic. The solutions used for infusion therapy are 0.9% normal saline (NS, 0.9 NaCl, or NSS), half-strength sodium chloride (0.45%), 3.0% sodium chloride (23.5% and 27.5% with restricted indication), dextrose (5%, 10%, etc.), Lactated Ringer, and others. Normal saline infusion is used for extracellular fluid replacement (e.g., dehydration, hypovolemia, hemorrhage, sepsis), treatment of metabolic alkalosis in the presence of fluid loss, and mild sodium depletion. Crystalloid solutions remain by far the most common, largely due to the overwhelming presence of normal saline in most hospital and healthcare settings. The best-known name is normal saline, sometimes called 0.9% normal saline (NS) or 0.9 sodium chloride (NaCl). The common drugs administered via intravenous infusion include: chemotherapy drugs (e.g., doxorubicin, vincristine, cisplatin, and paclitaxel), antibiotics (e.g., vancomycin, meropenem, and gentamicin), antifungals (e.g., anidulafungin, Caspufungin, micafungin, and amphotericin B), dopamine, dobutamine, and pain relief medications (e.g., paracetamol, hydromorphone, meperidine, morphine, and others) [15–18].

46.1.2.6 Drug Information Services and Pharmacovigilance

Pharmacovigilance is defined as the science and activities relating to the detection, monitoring, assessment, understanding, and prevention of adverse effects or any other drug-related adverse event. An adverse event (AE) is any untoward medical occurrence in a patient or clinical investigation subject administered a pharmaceutical product that does not necessarily have a causal relationship with the treatment (Fig. 46.1) [19].

Historically, the federal Ministry of Health (MOH) in the UAE commenced early reporting of adverse drug reactions (ADRs). However, a turning point was the introduction of medication safety programs, e.g., MedSafe®, by health authorities in the early 2000s, when a new era of medication safety practices emerged. Further advancements occurred in ADR and medication errors (MEs) reporting by clinical pharmacists in 2005 and onward. In December 2007, the UAE health authorities,

Fig. 46.1 Milestone in drug information and pharmacovigilance services in the UAE

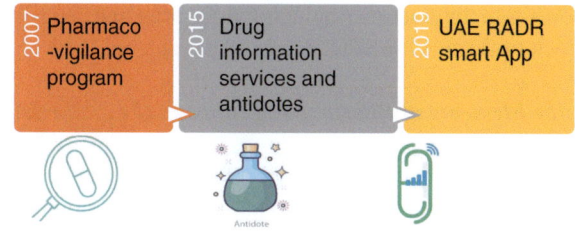

after holding the first pharmacovigilance conference, recommended that high-standard pharmacovigilance services be launched in the UAE. The Health Authority of Abu Dhabi (HAAD) took the initiative to launch and implement pharmacovigilance services in the Abu Dhabi emirate. This step facilitated the sharing of drug safety information among different healthcare facilities in the UAE and linked the country with other international drug safety bodies. The HAAD pharmacovigilance center was established as a reporting system for ADRs and MEs. The pharmacovigilance center had many functions, including collecting ADR and ME reports, assessing their quality of documentation and causality, advising health professionals and consumers on drug safety, investigating risk factors, and communicating drug safety data to national and international authorities [20].

In 2015, the Department of Health established the Drug Information Services (DIS) and Antidote Service (a prior service established in the early 2000s by HAAD). This service is available for public and healthcare professionals' use to enable them to achieve the most benefit and avoid unnecessary adverse events arising from the use of medications by providing precise, accurate, and up-to-date information in a timely manner in response to inquiries related to any medication or medical product. This service is free of charge, available during governmental operating hours (from 7:00 a.m. to 03:00 p.m.), and can be reached on the toll-free number 800–424 [20].

In January 2019, MOHAP launched "UAE RADR," a first-of-its-kind smart app on pharmacovigilance that promotes patients' safety and provides drug safety information. This useful smart application is used for regulating the process of reporting medication side effects, errors, and ADRs, and for analyzing data in a fast and precise manner to accelerate the process of decision-making and enhance preventive measures, and fight against the phenomenon of fake drugs. This initiative combines knowledge and skills with developed technology, aiming to consider benchmarks and become acquainted with the international trends used in shaping policies, making decisions, providing information, and providing evidence that contribute to updating drug items in the drug formulary [20].

Through pharmacovigilance services, healthcare professionals can report any suspected ADR, MEs, and adverse event following immunization (AEFI) experienced from any drug products within the stipulated timeframe as defined in Department of Health (DoH) policies, even if reporters are not certain that a particular medicinal product was the cause. Unintended adverse effects, drug abuse, overdose, interaction (including drug-drug and drug-food interactions), and unusual lack of therapeutic efficacy are all considered to be reportable suspected ADR [20].

Key Elements of Pharmacovigilance in the National Drug Policy

- Establishment of national pharmacovigilance systems for the reporting of adverse events, including national and, if appropriate, regional pharmacovigilance centers.
- Development of legislation or regulation for medicine monitoring.
- National policy development (to include costing, budgeting, and financing).
- Continuing education of healthcare providers on safe and effective pharmacotherapy.
- Provision of up-to-date information on adverse reactions to professionals and consumers.
- Monitoring the impact of pharmacovigilance through process indicators and outcomes [20].

Pharmacovigilance's Major Aims

The aim is to initiate early detection of safety issues, detection of increases in frequency, identification of risk factors, quantification of risks, and prevention of patients from being unnecessarily affected.

Risk Management

Risk management is the discipline within pharmacovigilance that is responsible for signal detection and the monitoring of the risk-benefit profile of drugs. Other key activities within the area of risk management are the compilation of risk management plans (RMPs) and aggregate reports such as the Periodic Safety Update Report (PSUR), Periodic Benefit-Risk Evaluation Report (PBRER), and the Development Safety Update Report (DSUR).

ADRs have various definitions, but according to the World Health Organization (WHO), an ADR is "a response to a drug that is noxious and unintended and occurs at doses normally used in humans for the prophylaxis, diagnosis, or therapy of disease, or for modification of physiological function." ADRs can occur at any time when using medications, and to maintain patients' safety, these adverse reactions should be appropriately reported to the concerned parties, namely pharmacovigilance centers. One of the most well-known pharmacovigilance centers in the world is the Uppsala Monitoring Centre (UMC) in Sweden, which is an independent center for drug safety and scientific research whose main aim is to guide the safe and effective use of medicines [21].

Underreporting of ADRs has placed a heavy financial burden on healthcare resources in Middle Eastern countries and worldwide. Optimum pharmacovigilance practice needs to be developed to ensure that data are collected and used in the right way and for the right purpose. Pharmacovigilance should be proactive in monitoring its possible consequences [22–26].

46.1.2.7 Medication Reconciliation

Medication reconciliation is defined as a formal process in which the pharmacist ensures that the patient's own (home) medication has been reviewed on admission, reconciled consistently during transitions of care, and reconciled again on discharge from the point of care. It encompasses a systematic review of all medications a patient is receiving to ensure that any addition, change, or discontinuation is appropriately commissioned. Medication reconciliation is a component of overall therapy management, which informs and permits clinicians to make the most appropriate therapeutic decisions for the patient [27].

The Importance of Medication Reconciliation
Medication reconciliation is very important since an incomplete medication history for the patient can lead to adverse effects. Therefore, the implementation of medication reconciliation is crucial to avoid mishaps in patients' medication histories. Medication reconciliation prevents the omission of regularly used medications, dosing and frequency errors, adverse drug reactions (ADRs), duplications, and drug-drug interactions. Medication reconciliation occurs in the following healthcare settings: acute care (inpatient) and long-term care settings, nursing homes, outpatient settings, including family practice settings, community pharmacies, ambulatory/specialist clinics, and in the home (e.g., home care services). Medication reconciliation involves reconciling medications on admission (medication history), medication reconciliation during transitions of care (internal healthcare facility transfer or long-term care setting), and finally reconciling all medication lists on discharge (all discrepancies resolved) [27].

46.1.3 The Pharmaceutical Agencies, Companies, and Industries in the UAE

46.1.3.1 The Pharmaceutical Agencies, Companies, and Industries

Pharmaceutical companies and industries are key players in the global economy. They improve patients' quality of life and health by developing new medicines and by boosting pharmaceutical drug manufacturing. The UAE government has provided numerous opportunities for drug design and production locally. Moreover, many UAE-based companies are experiencing enormous growth worldwide. The need for products manufactured in these industries has become inevitable in many countries to avoid medicine shortages (Figs. 46.2, 46.3, and 46.4).

The pharmaceutical industries are located in different regions in the UAE, including the Jebel Ali Free Zone, Dubai Science Park, Dubai Healthcare City, Ras Al-Khaimah, Abu Dhabi-Saniya, etc. In line with the Abu Dhabi Vision and Dubai Industrial Strategy 2030, the UAE is focusing on the pharmaceutical sector to make it a regional pharmaceutical manufacturing hub. The UAE is one of the highest-value pharmaceutical markets with a higher per capita medicine consumption [28, 29].

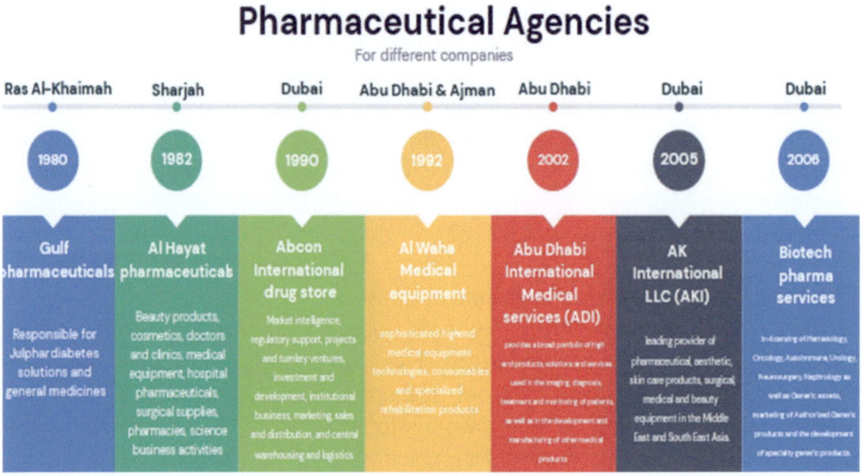

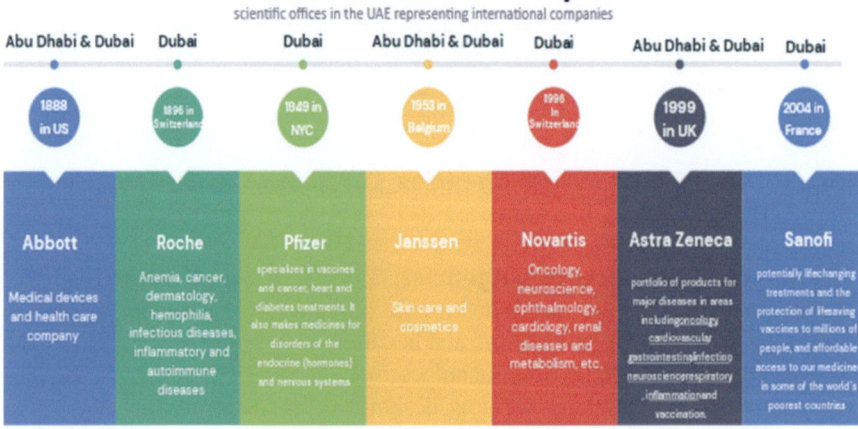

Fig. 46.2 Examples of some pharmaceutical agencies in the UAE

Fig. 46.3 Examples of some pharmaceutical companies in the UAE

46.1.3.2 Regulatory Affairs: Pharmaceutical Product Registration in the UAE

Registration of the Manufacturing Facility

In order to register any pharmaceutical products in the UAE, the manufacturing facility should follow cGMP regulations and be completely registered in the UAE. If the facility is registered with any stringent authority (e.g., the United States Food and Drug Administration [FDA]), the European Medicines Agency (EMA) audit will be waived and exempted [30].

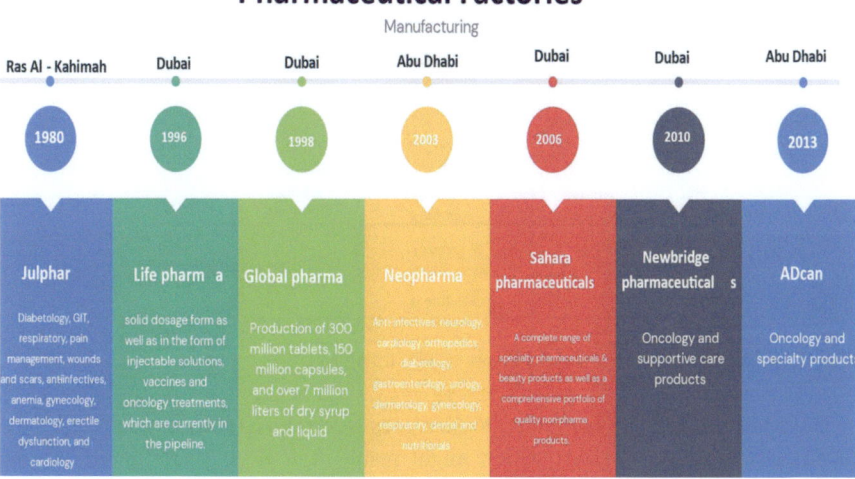

Fig. 46.4 Examples of pharmaceutical factories in the UAE

Active Substance
Since 2008, MOHAP, the UAE has been completely following the ICH (International Council for Harmonization) guidelines, which clearly state that the active pharmaceutical ingredients used in the manufacturing of the requested products for registration are either certified by EDQM (European Directorate for the Quality of Medicines and HealthCare) and have a CEP (Certificate of Suitability) or approved by the USFDA. Otherwise, the complete Drug Master File (DMF), including open and restricted parts, is shared with the authorities for their evaluation and approval [31].

Product Development
UAE falls globally under Zone IV, which means that all products should be developed and tested under stability conditions of 30 °C ± 2 °C/65% RH ± 5% RH (Relative Humidity) for the long term and should be stable [32].

Dossier Submission
Dossiers in eCTD formatting submitted to MOHAP evaluation contain all five modules for innovator products and M1, M2, and M3 for the generics, and the modules are as follows [33] (Fig. 46.5):

- Module 1: Administrative information and prescribing information. This module is regional, and all applicants are requested to strictly adhere to the checklist (Appendix 2).
- Module 2: Common Technical Document summaries.
- Module 3: Quality.
- Module 4: Nonclinical.
- Module 5: Clinical study reports.

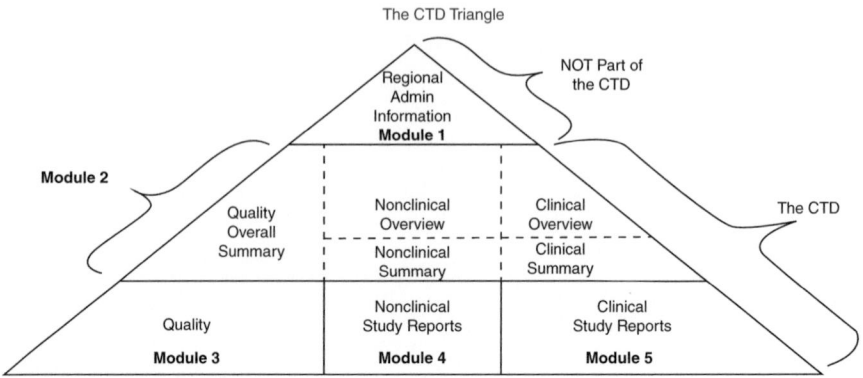

Fig. 46.5 The common technical document (CTD) triangle [33]

Post-submission, the complete dossier goes through rigorous evaluation by the technical teams in MOHAP, which might result in some queries that should be answered by the applicants in order to proceed with the registration process to acquire Product Marketing Authorization (PMA) Approval. The complete flow chart in Appendix 3 demonstrates the procedures.

Post-Approval Activities
(a) *Minor Variations*: After launching the products on the market, as the life cycle of the pharmaceutical product continues, companies have the right to file variation applications with MOHAP and obtain approval as per the published guidelines.
(b) *Renewal Process*: All the registered products are, by law, subject to the renewal process every 5 years from the date of registration [33].

46.2 Recent Advancements in Pharmaceutical Services

46.2.1 Pharmacists' Initiative for Immunization in the Abu Dhabi Emirate

Many professionals in the medical field are required to know how to administer vaccines. However, for a long time, a pharmacist's skill set and job specifications did not include this ability. In 1994, immunization by pharmacists finally became official and formalized by the Washington State Pharmacists Association, which trained fifty pharmacists in vaccine administration. Almost three decades later, the UAE made the leap, introducing vaccinations in pharmacies for the first time [34].

The initiative targeted select pharmacies, including Al Manara Pharmacy in Yas Mall and Al Thiqa Al Almyiah Pharmacy on Zayed the First Street, both of which are located in the Abu Dhabi Emirate [34]. Another three pharmacies, located in three different locations but belonging to the same Al Ain pharmacy retail chain, were granted licensure for the service in Al Ain city [34]. The document detailing the specifics of the new licensure was effective and published as of February 2022, titled "DOH Standard on Administration of Vaccines in Outpatient Pharmacies." The Department of Health (DOH) declared that outpatient pharmacies contain a designated section for the administration of vaccines as long as they obtain the necessary licensure and authorization. The licensure is granted to qualified pharmacies upon completion of a course designated by the DOH for administering vaccines [34]. Pharmacists involved were granted the pharmacy vaccinator title after completing the required course [34]. The training was not limited to the technical skills required for vaccine administration and included cardiopulmonary resuscitation (CPR) training as well as instructions on what to do in case a patient experiences an allergic reaction to the vaccine. The two weeks of training included theory and practice conducted in hospitals [34].

Pharmacies licensed to conduct vaccinations provided areas for registration, vaccination, and observation. Currently, in-house vaccinations are offered by some pharmacies, such as Burjeel and Al Thiqa pharmacies in Abu Dhabi. The immunization services provided by pharmacists received overwhelming acceptance from the local community and enthusiasm toward pharmacists as vaccinators, which increased the recruitment of more pharmacists. In the future, many pharmacies are expected to join in administering vaccines, not just those limited to pandemics, promising a welcome growth in pharmacists' extended professional roles (Fig. 46.6).

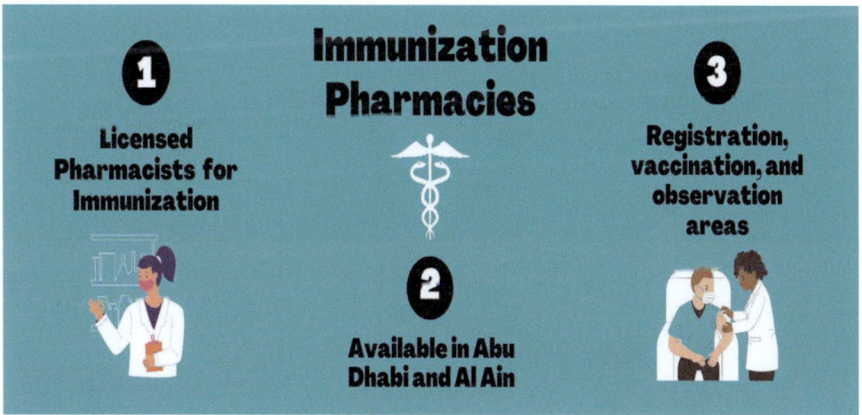

Fig. 46.6 Immunization pharmacies in the UAE

46.2.2 The Tele-Pharmacy and Artificial Intelligence in Pharmaceutical Services

46.2.2.1 Tele-Pharmacy

Tele-pharmacy is one of the key areas of healthcare under telemedicine. Tele-pharmacy is defined as "the delivery of pharmacy care provided by registered pharmacists and pharmacies using telecommunications technology for clients at a distance." The services include prescribing and dispensing medications, medical products, herbals, food supplements, cosmetic products, formulary compliance, patient counseling, medicine therapy management, automated packaging, and labeling systems (Fig. 46.7). Telemedicine, which also includes tele-pharmacy, has drawn more attention during the pandemic as these services decreased the likelihood of COVID-19 transmission by limiting in-person contact.

During the COVID-19 pandemic, several countries expanded the role of community pharmacists to serve customers through telecommunication tools. One of the first countries in the Middle East and North Africa (MENA region) to employ these services was the United Arab Emirates (UAE). The authorities responsible for regulating telemedicine in the UAE include the Department of Health Abu Dhabi (DOH) for the emirate of Abu Dhabi, the Dubai Health Authority (DHA) for the emirate of Dubai, the Dubai Healthcare City Authority (DHCA) in Dubai healthcare city, and the UAE Ministry of Health and Prevention (MOHAP) for the northern emirates [35]. After obtaining approval from the health authority designated, pharmacies in the UAE can offer tele-pharmacy services. Using telecommunication tools like phone, email, videoconferencing, websites, social media, and messaging applications, the community pharmacies in the UAE provide the following: managing mild ailments, dispensing and delivering prescribed and over-the-counter medications, counseling, general health information, selling cosmetic and other health products, providing services for patients with chronic diseases, and other relevant pharmaceutical services. Internationally, pharmacists have done substantial work on

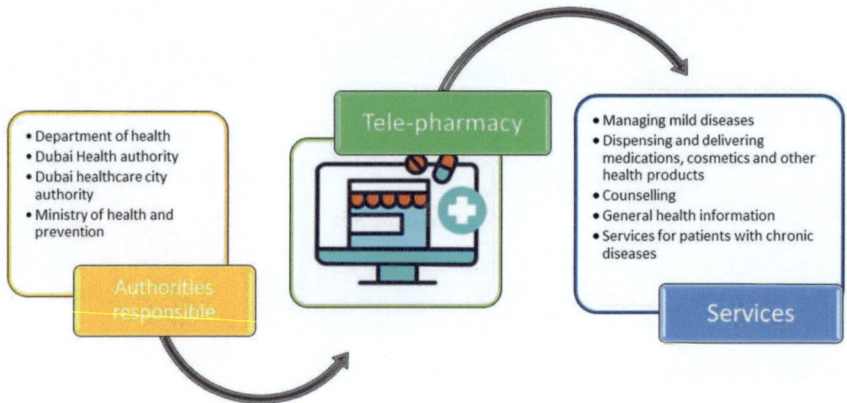

Fig. 46.7 The management of tele-pharmacy in the UAE

tele-pharmacy, improving pharmaceutical care at different clinical wards and units in many hospitals. Future research is warranted in the UAE to explore the value of pharmacist-delivered tele-pharmacy services.

Recent advancements in telemedicine services in the UAE include merging with Metaverse to expand traditional services. Dubai's Medcare Women and Children Hospital is the first in the country to adopt this change. Two more hospitals, Medcare Hospital Al Safa and Medcare Orthopedics and Spine Hospital, will soon enter the metaverse [36]. There is a dearth of studies on tele-pharmacy, which could contribute to enhancing pharmaceutical care services and be used in conjunction with traditional clinical area-based direct patient care across different levels of pharmacy care (intensive care unit, neonatal, emergency unit, etc.).

46.2.2.2 Artificial Intelligence

The policy of the Department of Health (DOH) that governs the use of artificial intelligence (AI) in healthcare defines the term as "the mimicking of human thought processes and cognition to solve complex problems automatically" [37].

The utilization of various technologies by pharmacies in the fields of research, industry, and retail has grown over the past two decades as a means of overcoming the rising demand for prescriptions, drug monitoring, patient counseling, and other aspects of pharmaceutical care. An example is the use of automated dispensing systems. The use of AI assists in optimizing clinical pharmacy services and can predict and evaluate the risks and outcomes of therapy. In addition, AI reduces the costs and time of treatment [38].In the UAE, Aster Hospital has employed AI to better serve patients and reduce medication errors (MEs) in various ways, including barcoded medication administration (BCMA), specimen collection systems, chatbots for diagnostic support and suggestive care, symptom analysis, and speech-to-text functionality that helps clinicians make accurate documentation of patient information and treatment [39].

Cleveland Clinic Abu Dhabi uses the advanced stroke interventional technology, the ARTIS Icono, which enables neuro-thrombectomy procedures for ischemic stroke to be performed more quickly and precisely [40]. Recently, a patient risk profile feature was added to the Malaffi provider portal. This feature displays predicted risk scores for each patient, indicating the likelihood of developing acute events such as heart attack or stroke, as well as chronic conditions like diabetes, hypertension, congestive heart failure, chronic kidney disease, and others [41].

46.2.3 The Pharmacist Prescribing, De-prescribing, and Research in Pharmacy

46.2.3.1 Pharmacists' Prescribing

Pharmacists' prescribing is a practice that has been implemented in a few countries around the world, with the main objective being to improve patient clinical outcomes while preserving patient safety. Other objectives include saving both patient and physician time, improving access to pharmaceuticals, and better utilizing the professional skills of pharmacists [42]. There are different models of pharmacist prescribing, such as dependent prescribing, based on a formal agreement where the physician delegates the prescribing to the pharmacist regarding specific medications (Fig. 46.8). Independent prescribing is performed based on the pharmacist's own decisions regarding what to prescribe and to whom, without any agreement with other practitioners. Emergency pharmacist prescribing is beneficial to fill major gaps among physicians or nurses. By providing pharmaceutical care, such as verifying prescriptions for clinical appropriateness, pharmacists in the emergency department can identify and intervene to assist in minimizing MEs. A few Gulf countries have taken steps toward pharmacist prescribing. A sequential explanatory mixed-methods study was done in Qatar, which explored the pharmacists' aspirations, readiness, facilitators, and barriers with regard to implementing pharmacist prescribing (pharmacists, $n = 554$) with a response rate of 62.8% ($n = 348$). The results showed that pharmacists were greatly aspired to and ready to be prescribers [43]. In 2020, in Saudi Arabia, a cross-sectional survey study was conducted on hospital pharmacists about views, prescribing, legislation, and barriers to implementing prescribing. The survey results showed the great confidence of pharmacists to prescribe. However, the pharmacists expressed that lack of prescribing training, limited resources, health providers' practice culture, and pharmacists' competency were key barriers [44]. Currently, other pharmacy colleges are taking initiative steps toward pharmacists' prescribing in the UAE. Another area is *de-prescribing*, a process that supports the patient in minimizing or discontinuing medications that may no longer be needed or may have harmful effects. Further research is highly needed in these areas [45].

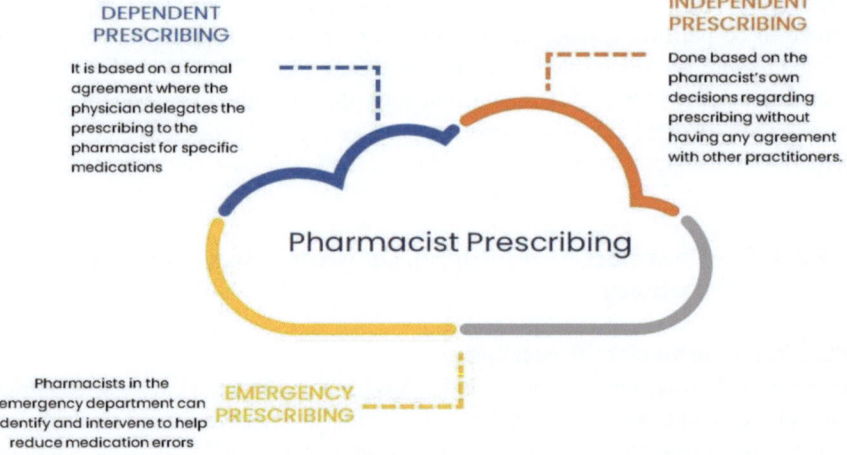

Fig. 46.8 Models of pharmacist prescribing

46.2.3.2 Research in the Pharmacy Field

Pharmacists in the UAE have started conducting research and publishing it in peer-reviewed journals at their healthcare facilities, postgraduate studies (master's and Doctor of Philosophy [PhD]), and at pharmacy colleges. There is also research conducted by hospital pharmacists in organizations such as SEHA, DOH, DHA, and the Ministry of Health in the Northern Emirates, which has increased in the last 20 years. Currently, pharmacists in the UAE are conducting extensive research in all sectors of the pharmacy profession, embracing all aspects of disease management, vaccinations, public health, hazardous pharmaceuticals, pharmacoepidemiology, pharmacoeconomics, pharmacogenomics, pharmacovigilance (post-marketing surveillance), and pharmacoinformatics (drug information and literature review). Further, pharmacists are conducting research in digital health, artificial intelligence in pharmacy, tele-pharmacy, and virtual and simulation pharmacy-based studies. Moreover, pharmacists research experimental and clinical pharmacology, anticancer, pharmaceutical technology (drug formulations and drug delivery systems), drug regulatory affairs, drug modeling, and medicinal chemistry. Nevertheless, the colleges of pharmacy embrace a plethora of educational research, the use of innovative technology in pharmacy education, simulation, virtual reality, and curriculum development.

46.3 Conclusion

The pharmaceutical industry in the UAE has grown tremendously throughout the last 50 years. The advancement of technology has been well recognized in the delivery of pharmaceutical care to the community. Pharmacists in the UAE strive daily to achieve and expedite quality care and patient satisfaction.

Acknowledgments We would like to acknowledge the supportive work contributed by the following pharmacy students (in alphabetical order): Aya Chayeb, Ahmed Isameldin Abdu, Dana Al Bek, Fariha Mostafiz, Khawla Abou-Hait, Lana Bustanji, Monia Aljumah, Nadia Sarfnaz, Nosayba Al-Damook, Nour Dhabbagh, Nour Juma, Razan Elmubarak, Rahma Elshcrif, Sara Alblooshi, Zainab Abdulnasser, Yukta Sughand, and Zayed Al Katheeiri.

Conflicts of Interest The authors have no conflicts of interest to declare.

Appendices

Appendix 1: Abbreviations

Full form	Abbreviations
Adverse drug reactions	ADR
Automatic dispensing machines	ADM
Automated drug cabinets	ADC
Adverse event	AE
Adverse reaction	AR
Al Ain University	AAU
Adverse event following immunization	AEFI
Barcoded medication administration	BCMA
Beyond use date	BUD
Controlled drugs	CD
Current Review of Clinical and Experimental Pharmacology Journal	CCREP
Cardiopulmonary resuscitation	CPR
Department of health	DOH
Dubai Healthcare City	DHCC
Dubai Healthcare City authority	DHCA
Drug Information services	DIS
Dubai health authority	DHA
Development safety update report	DSUR
Food and Drug Administration	FDA
Emergency department	ED
European medicine agency	EMA
High-efficiency particulate air	HEPA
Health information system	HIS
Intensive care unit	ICU
Intravenous	IV
Health authority Abu Dhabi	HAAD
General Authority for Health Services	GAHS
Identity document	ID
Intensive care unit	ICU
Medication errors	MEs
Middle East and North Africa	MENA
Ministry of health	MOH
Ministry of Health and prevention	MOHAP
New Emirates Medical Journal	NEMJ
National Institute for Occupational Safety and Health	NIOSH
Over the counter	OTC
Operation room	OR
Periodic safety update report	PSUR
Risk management plans	RMPs
Periodic benefit-risk evaluation report	PBRER
Abu Dhabi health services company	SEHA

(continued)

Full form	Abbreviations
Semi-controlled drugs	SCD
Sheikh Khalifa Medical City	SKMC
Total parenteral nutrition	TPN
Uppsala monitoring Centre	UMC
Unit dose distribution system	UDDD
United Arab Emirates	UAE

Appendix 2: Module 1—Administrative Information and Prescribing Information. This Module is Regional, and All Applicants are Requested to Strictly Adhere to the Below Checklist [Appendix 2]

1.0	Cover letter
1.1	Comprehensive table of content (M1)
1.2	Application form
1.3	Product information
1.3.1	Prescribing information (SPC)
1.3.2	Container labeling
1.3.3	Patient information leaflet
1.3.4	Artwork (Mockups)
1.3.5	Samples
1.4	Information about the expert
1.4.1	Quality
1.4.2	Nonclinical
1.4.3	Clinical
1.5	Environmental risk assessment
1.5.1	Non-genetically modified organism (Non-GMO)
1.5.2	GMO
1.6	Pharmacovigilance
1.6.1	Pharmacovigilance system
1.6.2	Risk management plan
1.7	Certificates and documents
1.7.1	GMP certificate
1.7.2	CPP or free sales
1.7.3	Certificate of analysis—Drug substance/finished product
1.7.4	Certificate of analysis—Excipients
1.7.5	Alcohol-content declaration
1.7.6	Pork—Content declaration
1.7.7	Certificate of Suitability to monographs of the European pharmacopoeia (CEP)
1.7.8	The diluents and coloring agents in the product formula
1.7.9	Patent information
1.7.10	Letter of access or acknowledgment to DMF

(continued)

1.8	Pricing
1.8.1	Price list
1.8.2	Other related documents
1.9	Response to questions

Appendix 3: Flow Chart [33]

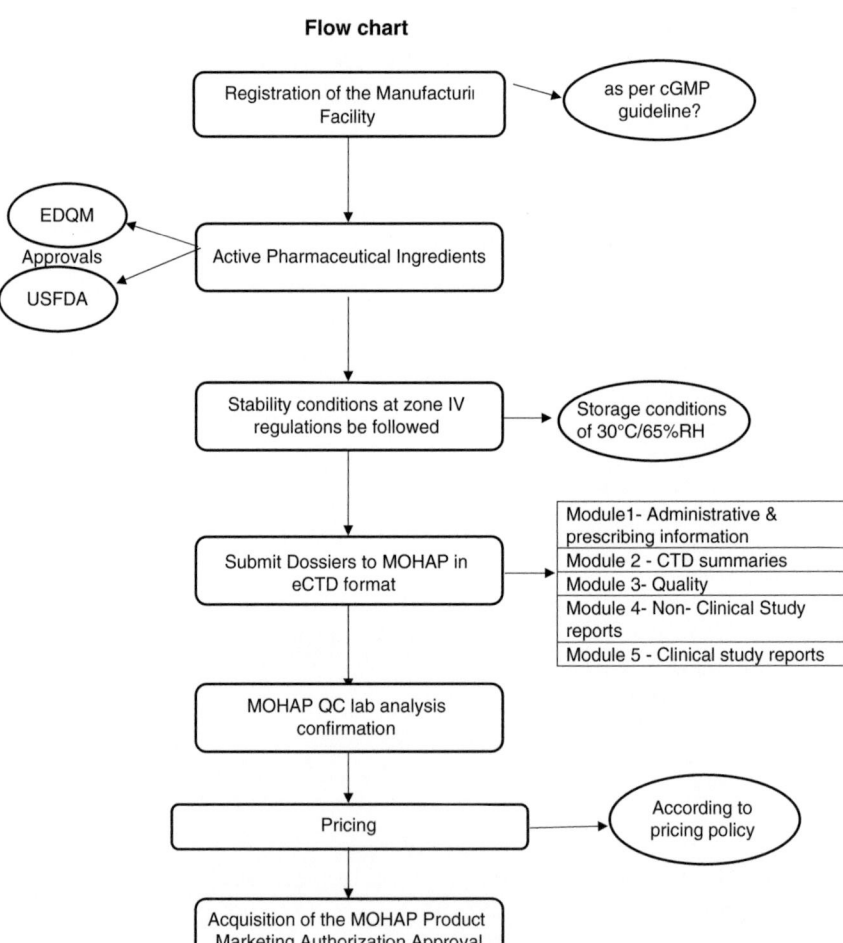

References

1. "Our History – Dubai Health Authority" Archived 2013-03-24 at the Wayback Machine. https://en.wikipedia.org/wiki/Healthcare_in_the_United_Arab_Emirates. Accessed Nov 2022.
2. "Oasis Hospital History" Archived 2014-02-09 at the Wayback Machine. https://en.wikipedia.org/wiki/Healthcare_in_the_United_Arab_Emirates. Accessed Nov 2022.
3. Beshyah S, Beshyah A. Central Hospital of Abu Dhabi: forty years of service to the community (1968–2008); Kazi, Nazir Mohammad, early days of health service in Abu Dhabi, United Arab Emirates: a personal perspective. Ibnosina J Med Biomed Sci. 2013;5(2):99–108. [1]. https://en.wikipedia.org/wiki/Healthcare_in_the_United_Arab_Emirates. Accessed Nov 2022.
4. United Arab Emirates country profile. Library of Congress Federal Research Division (July 2007). This article incorporates text from this source, which is in the public domain. https://en.wikipedia.org/wiki/Healthcare_in_the_United_Arab_Emirates. Accessed Nov 2022.
5. Bulatovic I, Iankova K. Barriers to medical tourism development in The United Arab Emirates (UAE). Int J Environ Res Public Health. 2021;18:1365.
6. https://www.seha.ae/. Accessed 10 Dec 2022.
7. https://adtt.dct.gov.ae/wp-content/uploads/2022/08/Knowledge-Bank.pdf. Accessed 15 Dec 2023.
8. https://www.citypharmacy.com/board-of-directors/. Accessed 15 Dec 2023.
9. Unpublished author own sources as participant in the event.
10. Department of health (DOH). Standard for the management of narcotics, psychotropic and semi controlled medicinal products. file:///C:/Users/asim.ahmed/Downloads/Standard-for-the-Management-of-Narcotics-and-Controlled-Medicinal-Products%20(1).pdf. Accessed 5 Oct 2022.
11. Diwas and Padilla. Chemotherapy preparation in Cleveland Clinic Abu Dhabi. Oncology Pharmacy Practitioners ISOPP. Chemotherapy Preparation in Cleveland Clinic Abu Dhabi Oncology Pharmacy Practitioners ISOPP. 2020. https://www.isopp.org/communication/oncology-pharmacy-news/2020/chemotherapy-preparation-cleveland-clinic-abu-dhabi. Accessed 3 Oct 2022.
12. https://fgs.futuregategroup.com/news/the-future-robotic-pharmacy-operating-now-for-first-time-in-fujairah-hospital-uae/. Accessed Oct 2022.
13. https://www.zawya.com/en/press-release/dha-launches-5th-smart-pharmacy-for-dispensing-and-prescribing-medication-ta3z7mfa. Accessed 8 Oct 2022.
14. https://www.uaebarq.ae/en/2018/11/27/artificial-intelligence-in-the-uaes-pharmacies/. Accessed 10 Oct 2022.
15. Hignett S, Otter ME, Keen C. Safety risks associated with physical interactions between patients and caregivers during treatment and care delivery in home care settings: a systematic review. Int J Nurs Stud. 2016;59:1–14.
16. Liu HC, Zhang LJ, Ping YJ, Wang L. Failure mode and effects analysis for proactive healthcare risk evaluation: a systematic literature review. J Eval Clin Pract. 2020;26(4):1320–37.
17. Micheletta F, Ferrara M, Bertozzi G, Volonnino G, Nasso M, La Russa R. Proactive risk assessment through failure mode and effect analysis (FMEA) for perioperative management model of oral anticoagulant therapy: a pilot project. Int J Environ Res Public Health. 2022;19(24):16430. https://doi.org/10.3390/ijerph192416430.
18. Persson J, Johansson G, Arvidsson I, Östlund B, Holgersson C, Persson R, Rydenfält C. A framework for participatory work environment interventions in home care – success factors and some challenges. BMC Health Serv Res. 2022;22(1):345. https://doi.org/10.1186/s12913-022-07710-2.
19. https://www.who.int/teams/regulation-prequalification/regulation-and safety/pharmacovigilance. Accessed 21 Oct 2022.
20. https://www.doh.gov.ae/en/. Accessed 23 Oct 2022.
21. https://who-umc.org/. Accessed 10 Nov 2022.

22. The 4th Annual Meeting of the European Society of Pharmacovigilance (ESOP): 1996 Sep 18–20; Lisbon. https://link.springer.com/article/10.2165/00002018-199921060-00001. Accessed Dec 2022. (Cross Reference).
23. Rawlins MD. Spontaneous reporting of adverse drug reactions. Br J Clin Pharmacol. 1988;26:1–11. https://doi.org/10.1111/j.1365-2125.1988.tb03356.x.
24. Parretta E, Rafaniello C, Magro L, et al. Improvement of patient adverse drug reaction reporting through a community pharmacist-based intervention in the Campania region of Italy. Expert Opin Drug Saf. 2014;13(suppl 1):S21–9.
25. HAAD Pharmacovigilance launching program, e-paper, Citeseerx.ist.psu.edu. 2022. [online] Available at: https://citeseerx.ist.psu.edu/viewdoc/download?doi=10.1.1.560.3911&rep=rep1&type=pdf. Accessed 18 Oct 2022.
26. https://www.doh.gov.ae/en/research/Dashboard/DIS-and-Antidote. [Accessed 20 Sept 2022]. http://wam.ae/en/details/1395302735346. Accessed 21 Sept 2022.
27. https://www.ncbi.nlm.nih.gov/books/NBK2648/. Accessed 8 Dec 2022.
28. Top 10 Pharma Brand/Companies in the UAE 2022 – Fast read info [Internet]. Fast read Info. 2022. Available from: https://www.info.fastread.in/top-10-pharma-brand-in-uae/. Accessed 25 Oct 2022.
29. Some Abu Dhabi pharmacies allowed to provide Covid-19 vaccines and PCR tests [Internet]. The National News. 2022. Available from: https://www.thenationalnews.com/uae/health/2022/07/29/some-abu-dhabi-pharmacies-allowed-issue-covid-19-vaccines-and-pcr-tests. Accessed 3 Dec 2022.
30. https://mohap.gov.ae/en/services/registration-of-a-conventional-pharmaceutical-product. Accessed 6 Sept 2022.
31. https://mohap.gov.ae/. Accessed 19 Sept 2022.
32. https://mohap.gov.ae/. Accessed 26 Sept 2022.
33. https://www.ich.org/page/ctd. Accessed 26 Nov 2022.
34. UAE: Inside pharmacy offering Covid-19 vaccine in Abu Dhabi [Internet]. Khaleej Times. 2022. Available from: https://www.khaleejtimes.com/health/uae-inside-pharmacy-offering-covid-19-vaccine-in-abu-dhabi. Accessed Nov 2022.
35. The regulation of telehealth in the UAE during COVID-19 – Al Tamimi & Company Retrieved from: https://www.tamimi.com/law-update-articles/the-regulation-of-telehealth-in-the-uae-during-covid-19/. Accessed 14 Oct 2022.
36. Dubai's Medcare Women & Children Hospital becomes first UAE healthcare facility to enter Metaverse | Markets – Gulf News. Retrieved from https://gulfnews.com/business/markets/dubais-medcare-women%2D%2Dchildren-hospital-becomes-first-uae-healthcare-facility-to-enter-metaverse-1.1665545606216. Accessed 13 Oct 2022.
37. Artificial Intelligence In Healthcare Sector In UAE – New Technology – United Arab Emirates (mondaq.com). https://www.mondaq.com/new-technology/770170/artificial-intelligence-in-healthcare-sector-in-uae. Accessed 05 Nov 2022.
38. Artificial intelligence (AI) and its relevance to pharmacy practice. https://www.linkedin.com/pulse/artificial-intelligence-ai-its-relevance-pharmacy-abiola-oluwagbemiga. Accessed 05 Nov 2022.
39. How Aster Hospitals UAE is transforming into a smart hospital – HMA (hospitalmanagementasia.com) Retrieved from https://www.hospitalmanagementasia.com/tech-innovation/how-aster-hospitals-uae-is-transforming-into-a-smart-hospital/. Accessed 05 Nov 2022.
40. UAE: Cleveland Clinic brings lifesaving, AI tech for treating stroke (zawya.com). Retrieved from https://www.zawya.com/en/business/healthcare/uae-cleveland-clinic-brings-lifesaving-ai-tech-for-treating-stroke-untbps3l. Accessed 05 Nov 2022.
41. https://malaffi.ae/. Accessed 13 Dec 2022.
42. Dat TV, Tu VL, Quan NK, Minh NH, Trung TD, Le TN, et al. Telepharmacy: a systematic review of field application, benefits, limitations, and applicability during the COVID-19 pandemic. Telemed J E Health. 2022;29:209. https://doi.org/10.1089/tmj.2021.0575.
43. Stewart D, Pallivalapila A, Thomas B, et al. A theoretically informed, mixed-methods study of pharmacists' aspirations and readiness to implement pharmacist prescribing. Int J Clin Pharm. 2021;43(6):1638–50.

44. Ajabnoor AM, Cooper RJ. Pharmacists' prescribing in Saudi Arabia: cross-sectional study describing current practices and future perspectives. Pharmacy. 2020;8(3):160.
45. Elnour AA, Raja NS, Abdi F, Mostafiz F, Elmubarak RI, Khalil AM, Hait KA, Alqahtani MM, Dabbagh N, Abdulnasser Z, Albek D. Protocol for systematic review and meta-analysis of randomized controlled trials, cost-benefit analysis and interrupted time-series interventions on pharmacist's prescribing. Pharm Pract. 2022;20(3):1–9.

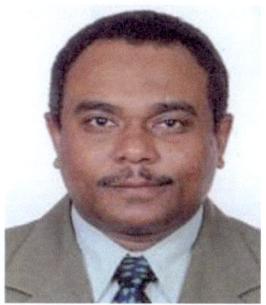

Asim Ahmed is currently working at the College of Pharmacy at Al Ain University, Abu Dhabi campus (UAE). He is the author or co-author of more than 120 papers (with 1590 citations in Google Scholar h-index 20 and 800 in SCOPUS h-index 14) that represent publications in international peer-reviewed journals and conference presentations. He is an editor, editorial board member, and reviewer for a variety of international peer-reviewed journals in the fields of pharmacy, clinical pharmacy, medicine, nursing, clinical pharmacology, and toxicology. For instance, he is the Editor-in-Chief of the *Pharmacy Practice* (Granada, Spain) Journal. He is an associate editor of the *New Emirates Medical Journal* (*NEMJ*) under the Emirates Medical Association (EMA), an editorial board member for the *International Journal of Clinical Pharmacy* (*IJCP*), a former editor for *Medicine* (Baltimore, USA), and an executive editor for *Current Reviews in Clinical and Experimental Pharmacology Journal* (*CCREP*). He serves as a consultant for the Association of Arab Universities and a referee for the inclusion of journals in the Scopus database. He recently led a group of Sudanese professors in free teaching, training, and research.

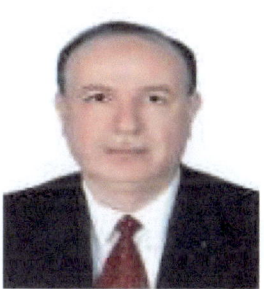

Professor Adel is a well-known professor of clinical pharmacy with immense expertise. He is the first PhD holder in Clinical Pharmacy in the UAE. He was the former director of pharmacy at Alain Hospital. He is director of clinical training and professor of the postgraduate master's program in clinical pharmacy. He is regarded as the father of clinical pharmacy in the UAE.

He serves as an Associate Professor, Program of Clinical Pharmacy, College of Pharmacy, Al Ain University, Al Ain Campus, United Arab Emirates.

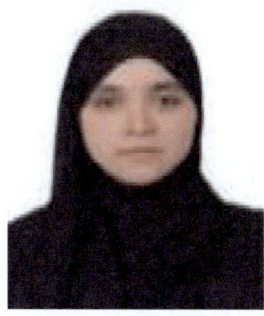

Dr. Mariam Al Qahtani is a dynamic UAE clinical pharmacist with outstanding performance in patient care, intravenous fluid services, parenteral nutrition, and oncology services. She serves in a reputable, prestigious hospital in Abu Dhabi as a Pharmacist at the Sheikh Khalifa Medical Complex (SKMC), Abu Dhabi, United Arab Emirates.

Open Access This chapter is licensed under the terms of the Creative Commons Attribution 4.0 International License (http://creativecommons.org/licenses/by/4.0/), which permits use, sharing, adaptation, distribution and reproduction in any medium or format, as long as you give appropriate credit to the original author(s) and the source, provide a link to the Creative Commons license and indicate if changes were made.

The images or other third party material in this chapter are included in the chapter's Creative Commons license, unless indicated otherwise in a credit line to the material. If material is not included in the chapter's Creative Commons license and your intended use is not permitted by statutory regulation or exceeds the permitted use, you will need to obtain permission directly from the copyright holder.

Clinical Nutrition Specialty in the UAE

47

Rayan Daoud and Raisa Alktebi

47.1 Introduction

Since ancient times, people have been interested in nutrition as they recognized how important food is to preserving health. Hippocrates, the father of medicine, stressed the value of a balanced diet for overall health and held the view that food served as the first medicine in ancient Greece [1]. Ancient Chinese medicine also placed a strong emphasis on the therapeutic value of food, with "food therapy" serving as a central concept in traditional Chinese medicine [2].

Nutrition research advanced further in the twentieth century with the identification and separation of several vitamins and minerals as well as their physiological functions. Recommended Dietary Allowances (RDAs), which set standards for the amounts of essential nutrients needed for optimal health, were first introduced in the United States in the 1940s [3]. The significance of diet in preventing chronic diseases, including cancer, diabetes, and heart disease, became more prominent in the second half of the twentieth century [4].

Today, nutritional science continues to advance and evolve, with a growing focus on personalized nutrition and the role of the gut microbiome in human health.

47.2 General Overview of Nutrition

Nutrition is the process of ingesting and utilizing nutrients from food components. Food produces energy and provides materials for bodily tissues and processes. Carbohydrates (sugars and starches), lipids, and proteins all provide calories. Minerals, vitamins, and dietary fiber are additional nutrients. A varied diet offers an appropriate supply because different foods contain varying levels of these elements.

R. Daoud (✉) · R. Alktebi
Emirates Medical Association/Emirate Clinical Nutrition Society,
Dubai, United Arab Emirates

© The Author(s) 2025
H. O. Al-Shamsi (ed.), *Healthcare in the United Arab Emirates*,
https://doi.org/10.1007/978-981-96-0523-1_47

Supplemental nutrition, which some individuals need, cannot make up for a poor diet. Water intake must always be adequate. Malnutrition and illness can be caused by inadequate dietary intake or absorption [5].

Through the diagnosis, treatment, and identification of any nutrition-related problems, the nutrition care plan seeks to enhance the patient's nutritional status. There are multiple steps in this procedure, including diagnosis, intervention, monitoring, and evaluation, in addition to an assessment of nutrition. The particular needs and health status of the patient will determine the plan's objectives and specific interventions.

47.3 Nutrition Background and Regulations in the UAE

Nutrition has gained attention in the United Arab Emirates (UAE) over the past few years due to the growing interest among people in leading healthier lives. The country has taken measures to promote healthy eating habits among its residents, including awareness campaigns, policy implementations, and support for nutrition research.

To encourage healthier food choices, the Dubai Municipality launched a campaign called "Eat Healthy, Live Healthy." This initiative aims to inspire individuals and families to adopt healthier eating habits. The campaign includes programs such as nutrition awareness initiatives for school students, promoting healthier cafeteria options at workplaces, and offering nutritious catering services for events [6].

Throughout the years, the UAE has instituted a number of nutrition-related laws and standards in an effort to encourage a healthy diet and lower the incidence of illnesses linked to undernourishment. The UAE government has implemented Federal Law No. 10 of 2015, among other important measures, to control food product manufacturing, importation, and distribution throughout the nation. The use of particular ingredients and nutritional information is covered by the standards for food labeling, packaging, and advertising that are outlined in this regulation [7].

The UAE government has introduced a number of programs to encourage physical exercise and a healthy diet among its people, including the Food-based Dietary Guidelines [8], the Nutrition Labelling Policy [9], and the National Nutrition Strategy for 2022–2030 [10]. These regulations seek to increase public awareness, impart knowledge, and provide individuals with the ability to make wise decisions about their diet and way of life.

The UAE is dealing with a number of nutrition-related issues, including chronic diseases, undernutrition, overnutrition, and micronutrient deficiencies, according to review research by Al Sabbah et al. [11]. The study draws attention to the opportunities that have gone unnoticed, as well as the gaps and difficulties in resolving these issues. The report recommends that further research be conducted on the nutrition situation in the UAE with a focus on obesity, diabetes, and malnutrition.

Data on the state of nutrition in the UAE, including the prevalence of anemia, diabetes, obesity, overweight, wasting, and stunting in various age groups and genders, are included in the Global Nutrition Report [12]. The report also demonstrates the United Arab Emirates' progress in meeting the World Health Organization's global nutrition targets.

The National Nutrition Guidelines [13], introduced by the UAE in 2019 in partnership with the Food Security Office, aim to enhance food safety protocols, addressing health issues, and optimizing nutrition frameworks. The guidelines are intended to prevent diseases related to nutrition, encourage healthy eating, and lessen health inequalities in the community.

Additionally, the UAE has food-based dietary guidelines [14], which offer helpful guidance on how to consume a varied, balanced diet that satisfies the population's nutritional needs and preferences. The food pyramid model, which shows the suggested serving sizes and quantities of several food groups, forms the foundation for the guidelines.

In general, there are a lot of programs in the UAE that aim to enhance nutrition in a variety of contexts and encourage wholesome eating habits. Numerous organizations, including businesses, schools, healthcare facilities, and the community, are realizing the value of a healthy diet and are acting to provide access to nutritious food and educate the public about it. Examples of these programs, starting in schools in the UAE, aim to promote a healthy diet and fight childhood obesity. It is mandatory for schools to serve wholesome meals and restrict access to unhealthy food options. Programs like the School Garden Project and the Healthy Students Program encourage youngsters to eat healthily and raise awareness of the value of nutrition [15].

Second community programs are planned to encourage UAE citizens to eat healthily. The Abu Dhabi Public Health Centre (ADPHC) has initiated the SEHHI program, which was formerly known as "Weqaya." The program's objectives are to increase access to healthy food options and promote nutritious food choices in Abu Dhabi by making it easier to identify nutritious foods and ingredients in food outlets, restaurants, cafes, healthcare facilities, hotels, and grocery stores and supermarkets throughout the Emirate [16].

47.4 Food Services and Catering in a Healthcare Setting: A Short Review

In recent years, catering and food services for healthcare facilities have grown in significance. Healthcare facilities can benefit from new sales-building opportunities from food catering, as the industry is focused on cost reduction and increasing its bottom line. Acute care facilities, as well as senior living facilities, might benefit from healthcare catering. There are two subcategories within these segments: internal and external catering. For healthcare operators, internal catering is the simplest and most popular option for serving personnel, patients, and/or residents. Opportunities for external catering can be as simple as promoting community spaces to neighborhood groups, offering your center's food for meetings, serving supper to the neighborhood Red Hat Society, or having clients pick up the catering.

When creating catering menu options for healthcare facilities, there are some gastronomic factors that must be taken into account. These include what goes well on the menu, what is portable, and what caters to the unique requirements of patients, residents, and guests. Operators in the healthcare foodservice industry are well-suited to providing meals that fulfill these specifications [17].

In health settings, particularly hospitals, where patients need nourishing meals to aid in their recovery, food services and catering are essential. Offering wholesome and enticing food options is crucial for patients' general health and may aid in their recovery.

In addition to food quality, it is critical to ensure that food is prepared and served in a safe, hygienic manner. Guidelines for the proper handling and storage of food in healthcare institutions are provided by the Centers for Disease Control and Prevention (CDC).

Finally, incorporating patients in the process of creating the menu and providing customized meals for individuals with particular dietary requirements or preferences can enhance the patient-centered approach to nutrition treatment [18].

47.5 Nutrition and Diet Research in the UAE

In a nation like the UAE, where rapid changes in the economy and society have affected dietary habits and lifestyles, nutrition plays a critical role in overall health and well-being. However, information about the state of nutrition in the UAE, its obstacles, and its prospects for improvement is not well updated or comprehensive.

Al Sabbah et al. [11] carried out one of the most recent research projects that sought to evaluate the nutritional status in the UAE. Upon analyzing published data spanning from 2010 to 2022, they discovered that the UAE faces numerous nutrition-related issues, including underweight, overweight, obesity, micronutrient deficiencies, and chronic diseases linked to nutrition. They also drew attention to the opportunities that have gone unexplored, as well as the gaps and difficulties that still exist in resolving these issues.

47.6 Future Demands of Clinical Dietitians and Nutritionists in the UAE Healthcare Setting

Nutrition professionals who support well-being, prevent and treat illness, and enhance population, group, and individual health professionals who apply the science of food are known as dietitians and nutritionists. In the UAE, these individuals must hold a bachelor's degree in nutrition or a closely related discipline and have completed an internship or supervised practice program [10]. The nutrition and dietetics team provides assessment, planning, implementation, and evaluation of nutritional interventions for various conditions, such as diabetes, obesity, cardiovascular disease, renal disease, gastrointestinal disorders, food allergies, and malnutrition [19, 20]. The UAE healthcare system offers nutrition and dietetics services in both acute and community settings, such as hospitals, clinics, schools, and workplaces.

Nearly 40% of adults in the UAE are overweight, and over 25% are obese, according to the UAE National Nutrition Survey, which also indicates that obesity and overweight are highly prevalent in the country. This places a strain on the healthcare system and emphasizes the need for interventions that are nutrition-focused [21].

Overall, it is anticipated that, due to the increased emphasis on preventive healthcare and the prevalence of health conditions, the need for dietitians in the UAE will only grow in the future.

47.7 Conclusion

Many chronic and noncommunicable diseases, including obesity, diabetes, hypertension, heart disease, stroke, cancer, and osteoporosis, can be avoided or postponed by adhering to healthy eating and physical activity guidelines. In the UAE, these illnesses are the primary causes of mortality and disability and are also highly prevalent and costly. Therefore, nutrition and preventive medicine are vital for the health of the UAE's population and the development of the country.

Conflict of Interest The authors have no conflicts of interest to declare.

References

1. Hippocrates. On ancient medicine.
2. Wu H, Wu E. The role of traditional Chinese medicine in the management of chronic diseases: a narrative review. Int J Gen Med. 2012;5:723–30. https://doi.org/10.2147/IJGM.S33473.
3. National Academies of Sciences, Engineering, and Medicine. Dietary reference intakes for sodium and potassium. National Academies Press (US); 2019. https://www.ncbi.nlm.nih.gov/books/NBK545442/.
4. Hu FB. The Mediterranean diet and mortality-olive oil and beyond. N Engl J Med. 2003;348(26):2595–6. https://doi.org/10.1056/NEJMe030070.
5. https://www.britannica.com/science/nutrition.
6. Dubai Municipality launches health and food safety campaign (thenationalnews.com).
7. Federal law on food safety | The Official Portal of the UAE Government.
8. https://www.fao.org/nutrition/education/food-dietary-guidelines/regions/countries/united-arab-emirates/en/.
9. https://www.hw.gov.ae/en/news/to-promote-healthy-lifestyle-and-wellbeing-in-the-uae-national-program-for-happiness-and-wellbeing-launches-nutrition-labelling-policy.
10. https://gulfnews.com/uae/uaes-new-nutrition-strategy-and-rules-all-you-need-to-know-1.92333541.
11. https://www.mdpi.com/2072-6643/15/2/363.
12. Global Nutrition Report | Country Nutrition Profiles – Global Nutrition Report.
13. UAE launches National Nutrition Guidelines | UAE – Gulf News.
14. Food-based dietary guidelines – United Arab Emirates (fao.org).
15. Dubai sets guidelines for healthy school meals, Guidelines and requirements for food & nutrition in schools in Dubai (dm.gov.ae).

16. Abu Dhabi Public Health Centre launches SEHHI program to promote healthier food choices Across Abu Dhabi (adphc.gov.ae).
17. https://gfs.com/en-us/ideas/build-your-healthcare-operations-bottom-line-food-catering/.
18. Centers for Disease Control and Prevention. Guidelines for environmental infection control in health-care facilities: recommendations of CDC and the Healthcare Infection Control Practices Advisory Committee (HICPAC). (https://www.cdc.gov/infectioncontrol/pdf/guidelines/environmental-guidelines-P.pdf.
19. https://u.ae/en/about-the-uae/strategies-initiatives-and-awards/strategies-plans-and-visions/health/national-nutrition-strategy-2030.
20. https://academic.oup.com/nutritionreviews/article/80/5/1027/6370473.
21. Prevalence of overweight and obesity in United Arab Emirates Expatriates: the UAE National Diabetes and Lifestyle Study - PubMed (nih.gov).

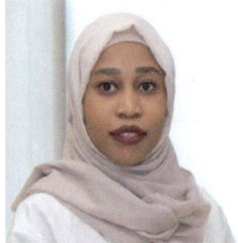

Rayan Ali Mahmoud Daoud qualified as a clinical dietitian with a master's in science degree in human nutrition and dietetics and then followed it up with a large portfolio of additional training and certifications in aspects of the clinical specialization. She also holds DOH and DHA licenses, allowing her to work as a clinical dietician. She has membership in the Emirates Medical Association/Emirates Clinical Nutrition Society and is the chairperson of the media and public relations committee. She has over 12 years of experience in the UAE and abroad.

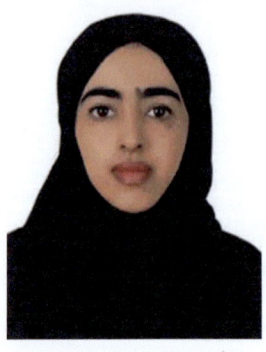

Raisa Shutait Alktebi is a clinical dietitian. She holds a master's degree in diabetes management, a bachelor's in clinical nutrition and dietetics from Sharjah University, and a postgraduate diabetes diploma from Cardiff University. She has been working as a clinical dietitian at Hatta Hospital, Dubai Health, since 2015 until recently. Member of the Emirates Medical Association (EMA), General Secretary of the Emirates Clinical Nutrition Society

- Provide diabetes education to help patients understand their condition and how to manage it effectively.
- Provide in-patient medical nutrition therapy for: pediatric, gynecology, intensive care patients, tube-feeding patients, and diabetic patients.
- Part of a multidisciplinary team for obesity management.
- Part of a multidisciplinary team for NCD management.
- Part of the BFHI (Baby Friendly Hospital Initiative).

Open Access This chapter is licensed under the terms of the Creative Commons Attribution 4.0 International License (http://creativecommons.org/licenses/by/4.0/), which permits use, sharing, adaptation, distribution and reproduction in any medium or format, as long as you give appropriate credit to the original author(s) and the source, provide a link to the Creative Commons license and indicate if changes were made.

The images or other third party material in this chapter are included in the chapter's Creative Commons license, unless indicated otherwise in a credit line to the material. If material is not included in the chapter's Creative Commons license and your intended use is not permitted by statutory regulation or exceeds the permitted use, you will need to obtain permission directly from the copyright holder.

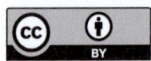

Alternative Medicine in the UAE

Khawla Mohamed Saeed binfraish Alkindi
and Kheireddine Youssef Chatra

48.1 Introduction

Traditional folk medicine is one of the ancient phenomena of the Arabian Peninsula, as Arabian doctors from antiquity believed in the efficacy of this form of treatment. The knowledge of this form of medicine has gradually developed from one generation to the next until it formed what is now called alternative medicine, which the Arabs documented in their travels and encyclopedias about medicinal plants and their benefits.

Alternative medicine in the United Arab Emirates has gone through several historical stages, as it moved in the past from traditional medicine laden with paganism and heresy, which is mostly inherited from the medical heritage of neighboring peoples, to traditional Islamic medicine, whose method follows the Prophet's guidance. Over time, this medicine was intertwined with human experience, and with this rich medical heritage, the Emiratis, like many others, have professionalized the practice of alternative medicine and certain health practices that contributed significantly to treating many diseases rampant at the time. What can be historically recorded is that Emirati women, in particular, excelled in this profession, demonstrating leadership and expertise.

According to the goals of this study, we seek to answer questions on the characteristics of alternative medicine, such as: How did medical and health life develop in Emirati society? What are the most important manifestations and advantages of this medical and health culture? What methods of herbal medicine and folk medical practices have been inherited in the Emirati environment?

K. M. S. b. Alkindi (✉) · K. Y. Chatra
Department of History and Islamic Civilization, University of Sharjah, Sharjah, United Arab Emirates
e-mail: U21103978@sharjah.ac.ae; kchatra@sharjah.ac.ae

© The Author(s) 2025
H. O. Al-Shamsi (ed.), *Healthcare in the United Arab Emirates*,
https://doi.org/10.1007/978-981-96-0523-1_48

Let us conclude our study by examining the feasibility of paying attention to folk medicine and determining whether it has an integral role in contemporary medical life in the United Arab Emirates.

48.2 The Nature of Alternative Medicine

Medicine has been defined as follows: "The treatment of body and soul, medicine embodies kindness, and a doctor is a companion.,. who is a clever man among men, skilled in his knowledge... A therapist is one who practices medicine yet does not know it well. It is said that a man—that is, an enchanted man—is treated."[1] It is also said that: "One who has medicine is a scholar, and through medicine, they know where to put their lightness."[2] Medicine in the history of Islamic civilization is defined as: "A science through which the conditions of the human body are understood, what is true and what goes away from health... to preserve health and restore it when lost."[3] Ibn Khaldun also defined it as: "An art that looks at the human body in terms of sickness and health, so its practitioner seeks to preserve health and cure disease with medicines and food."[4]

The term *alternative medicine*, or *complementary medicine*, in the historical context of the United Arab Emirates, refers to "knowledge, skills, and practices based on theories, beliefs, and experiences inherent in different cultures, which are used to maintain health and prevent, diagnose, treat, or improve the conditions of those affected by physical and mental illnesses."[5] Thus, it constitutes an inherited asset: "for all traditional ideas and views about disease and treatment and all behavior and practices related to the prevention and treatment of disease, regardless of the formal system of scientific medicine."[6] It can also be thought of as "a wide variety of treatments and practices which may vary greatly from country to country and region to

---

[1] Abi al-Fadl Ibn Manzur, (1999), Lisan al-Arab, Beirut, Revival of Heritage House, vol. 3, 3rd edition, p. 133. For expansion, see: The Arabic Language Academy (2004), Intermediate Lexicon, Cairo, Orient International Library, p. 549.

[2] Al-Khalil bin Ahmed Al-Farahidi, (2003), Al-Ain book, ed. Abd al-Hamid al-Hindawi, Beirut, Dar al-Kutub al-Ilmiyya, vol. 3, i 1, p. 34.

[3] Muhammad Habash, (1996), Muslims and the Sciences of Civilization, Damascus, House of Knowledge, p. 27.

[4] Ibn Khaldoun (Abdul Rahman), (2002), Diwan Al-Mubtada, Volume 2, Murr. Sohail Zakar, Beirut, Dar Al-Fikr for printing, p. 650, for expansion see: - Muhammad Ali Al-Thanawy, (1991), Scouts Encyclopedia of Terminology of Arts and Sciences, Volume 2, T. Ali Dahrouj, Beirut, Library of Lebanon Publishers, p. 41.

[5] Bakr Al-Mahasneh, Folk Medicine from Nature practiced by some natural or genetic healers, Al-Khaleej Newspaper, Publishing date 27/3/2014. Date of visit: 07/06/2019.
http://www.alkhaleej.ae/supplements/page/a635932e-964a-46bb-902c-ee4754b8d1ca

[6] Imad Naji Rashid, (2004), Medicinal Herbs and Plants treatment, Cultural Journal, p. 65, Amman. p. 303.

region…whether they are explicable or not."[7] Alternative medicines are used interchangeably with traditional medicine in some countries.[8]

From all of the above, we can define alternative medicine as: "a holistic medicine that looks at the human body as a single unit, treating the diseases that afflict it on this basis, through the use of many therapeutic practices that primarily depend on activating the human body's organs using natural substances or by adopting some spiritual path."[9]

Alternative medicine, then, "includes a wide range of treatments and practices that differ in different countries and regions,"[10] as it looks at the human body as a whole. It includes spiritual, social, physical, and mental dimensions, is closely related to the life and culture of certain groups of people, and may "depend on its methods on the laws of nature and natural matter, such as natural medicine."

"Although each of these medical forms may have its own characteristics and share with folk medicine some of these salient features that distinguish it from modern medicine, at the same time, it represents the focus of interest in it and works to increase its popularity."[11] Many conferences, including the São Paulo Conference held in Brazil in 1985 AD, confirm that this form of medicine is not linked to magic and sorcery but is a set of therapeutic methods developed to save man, and he is the faithful ally of contemporary medicine."[12] Among the terms associated with alternative medicine are the following:

- *Complementary medicine*: A set of healthcare practices that do not fall within the traditions of the country and do not fall within the main healthcare system.[13]

---

[7] World Health Organization, (2009), Sixty-second World Health Assembly, Document C 62/8, p. 1 - See also: - Abd al-Razzaq Salih Mahmoud, (2005), Traditional Medicine in the city of Mosul, a social study, unpublished master's thesis, University of Mosul, Iraq, pg. (7–8) - a group of authors, (2010), The Facilitated Arabic Encyclopedia, Volume 4, The Modern Library, Beirut, p. 2143.

[8] Ghazi Hanoun Al-Darji, (2017), criminal responsibility arising from the practice of folk medicine, Beirut, Al-Halabi Human Rights Publications, p. 27, for expansion see: -
Rahmatullah, M., Jahan, R., Azam, F. S., Hossan, S., Mollik, M. A. H., & Rahman, T. (2011). Folk medicinal uses of Verbenaceae family plants in Bangladesh. African Journal of Traditional, Complementary and Alternative Medicines, P8.

[9] The World Health Organization website,
https://www.who.int/topics/traditional_medicine/definitions/ar/.

[10] Mohamed El-Gohary, (1983), The Scientific Study of Popular Beliefs, Volume 1, Cairo, House of Culture, p. 93.

[11] Roquia Mellah, (2012), Spiritual Therapy by Writing Al-Awafaq, an unpublished master's thesis, specializing in Sociology, Oran University, pp. 52–53.

[12] Jarroys Vermont, (1996), Traditional Medicine and its Fields, Syria, Alaa El-Din House, p. 11–12.
Sheikh, S., & Furnham, A. (2000). A cross-cultural study of mental health beliefs and attitudes towards seeking professional help. Social Psychiatry and Psychiatric Epidemiology, PP(326–334)
http://www.pathways2promise.org/wp-content/uploads/2017/01/A-Cross-Cultural-Study-of-Mental-Health-Beliefs-and-Attitudes-Towards-Seeking-Professional-Help-1.pdf.

[13] The World Health Organization website,
https://www.who.int/topics/traditional_medicine/definitions/ar/

- *Ethnomedicine*: The study or comparison of traditional medicine based on biologically active compounds in plants and animals and practiced by different ethnic groups, especially those with little access to Western medicine, as well as interdisciplinary ethnomedical research applying medicinal and anthropological methods across diverse contexts.[14]
- *Physiatry*: A system that uses natural remedies to help the body heal, including many treatments, such as herbs, massage, acupuncture, exercise, and nutritional counseling. In the modern era, natural medicine combines traditional therapies with modern science.[15]
- *Integrative medicine*: A system of treatment that integrates all therapeutic traditional and non-traditional methods within a framework that focuses on health and the therapeutic relationship, closely tied to the lives and cultures of specific groups of people, with methods that may draw on the laws of nature and natural materials.[16]
- *Traditional medicine*: Medicine that does not depend on modern medicines and methods in university curricula, but rather depends on means and medicines derived from cultural heritage passed down from generation to generation, and this form of medicine may be practiced today or used by some doctors themselves, while in the past it was practiced by individuals unaffiliated with medicine, such as perfumers and barbers.[17]

As for the position of modern medicine on alternative medicine and traditional treatment, since ancient times, medicinal herbs have been of great importance due to their curative properties to overcome pain and treat diseases, and until this day, we still rely on the healing properties of plants in many medicines. In the 18th century, scientists began to further their research on the components of plants and the extraction of chemicals in the preparation of medicines, then "the matter developed to the manufacture of these materials in laboratories, thinking that understanding the actions of the active ingredients in plants is sufficient to benefit from them in the treatment of diseases, as in the beginning these medicines showed strong effectiveness against diseases, but this effectiveness began to weaken over time, as happened with antibiotics. Over the years, the body has become resistant to these antibiotics, which has made them lose their effectiveness, in addition to the appearance of some

---

[14] See website:
https://stringfixer.com/en/Ethnopharmacy

[15] The Website of Sotor: https://sotor.com/%D9

[16] Consumer Guide (MSD) website:
https://www.msdmanuals.com/en/home/%D8

[17] The Arabic Encyclopedia (2005), Chapter (Al-Sadat - The Ottomans), Volume 12, Syria, Al-Salhani Institution for Printing and Publishing, pg. 466.
Palincas, L. A., Kabongo, M. L., & Surfnet Study Group. (2000). the use of complementary and alternative medicine by primary care patients. Journal of Family Practice; 49(12), 1121–1132.

negative effects of some of these drugs. The reason for this is biomedicine is concerned only with the active parts and components in plants."[18]

> This has led to the need to return to herbal medicine, as it is concerned with the use of entire plants, and scientific research has shown that the active components of many herbs interact in complex ways to produce the therapeutic effect of the drug as a whole.[19]

48.3 The Evolution of Alternative Medicine, Traditional Health, and Preventive Habits in the Emirati Society

Historically, "man tried to use on his own many of the substances that he found scattered in the environment around him, in order to change and modify his behavioral and emotional states."[20] Throughout history, man has used many herbs, plants, stones, and minerals, among many other examples.[21] In the East, people used tea and opium, and in the West, they used tobacco, coffee, and wine. Each of these materials has been welcomed, respected, and appreciated by every cultural environment in which it was raised, but every civilization has also developed the broad lines that regulate the circulation of these materials. There is a long history of folk remedies for some diseases, often based on the availability of herbs in these areas, showing their medical impact on physical, psychological, and behavioral conditions.

There are "ancient sources of medicines found in all the peoples of the ancient world…in China, ancient Egypt, the Greeks, the Ptolemies, the Romans, and the Arabs."[22] The ancient Chinese knew medicinal herbs and medicinal plants, and their scientists always experimented to see the effect of medicines on themselves without first trying them on animals. This is evident in the approach of the founder of Chinese pharmacology.

---

[18] Beal, M. W. (1998). Women's use of complementary and alternative therapies in reproductive health care. Journal of Nurse-Midwifery. PP 224–234.

[19] Ayman Al-Husseini, (2005), Encyclopedia of Folklore and Alternative Therapy, Egypt, Family Library, p. 19.

Tada, T. Toward. (2004). The philosophy of CAM: super system and epidemiological sciences. Evidence-based Complementary and Alternative Medicine. P5.

[20] In ancient civilizations, herbs recorded in the papyri were discovered, and the most important discoveries were juniper herb, onions, and garlic. These herbs were used for many treatments for the body for a long time, and after that, they also discovered the poppy and ginger. In the second century AD, the Chinese scientist Shen Nong developed a curriculum for medical materials called the *Classic of Material Medica*, consisting of more than 400 therapeutic medicines from plants and medicinal herbs. See. Aladdin Hosni, previous reference, p. 1.

Hussain, S. A., Saeed, A., Ahmed, M., & Qazi, A. Contemporary role and future prospects of medicinal plants in the health care system and pharmaceutical industries of Pakistan. URL http://www.telmedpak.com/ doctors' articles. [accessed on 6/12/2013].

[21] Eisenberg D. Et al. Trends in alternative medicine use in the United States, 1990–1997. The Journal of the American Medical Association, 1998, P 280.

[22] Yassin El-Gamal, (2008), Black Seed Therapy, Egypt, Modern Arab Center, p. 9. And also: - Ragheb Al-Sirjani, (2008), The Story of Medical Sciences in Islamic Civilization, Iqra for Publishing and Distribution Association, Cairo, pg. (16–18).

Chen Tong (22nd century BC) wrote the famous Chinese pharmacology book *Ben Cao* and discovered the effect of *Shang Chang*, a tonic and sweaty *Ephedra* plant. We now extract the substance ephedrine from it. The ancient Chinese also divided plant drugs into three categories: sweet to nourish the muscles, salty to nourish the veins, and bitter to nourish the body. They gave great importance to single medicines, avoided compound medicines, and later exchanged medical information with Muslims.[23]

In ancient Egypt, priests monopolized the practice of medicine and pharmacology in special institutes attached to temples that were called *Bir Ankh*, meaning "houses of life." In these institutes, sciences and medicinal plants were taught in terms of their qualities, cultivation, and the most appropriate times for collecting medicinal compounds from them. The Egyptians used to prepare their medicines from wild plants grown in Egypt and surrounding countries. They had many missions, including those ordered by Queen Hatshepsut, to roam the surrounding countries gathering medicinal and aromatic plants and then bring them back and plant them in Egypt. Imhotep is considered one of the most famous doctors and pharmacists from ancient Egypt in the 30th century BC.[24] The Greeks benefited from the heritage of the ancient Egyptians, Babylonians, and other peoples of the ancient world through their influence regarding treatment with single medicines in particular, as well as compounds in general. They considered the snake a symbol of life, wisdom, and healing, "just as the Egyptians took the cobra snake as their symbol."[25]

As for the Arabs in the era of ignorance, medicine was primitive, as it was limited to experiences and spells inherited between individuals. Most of it was confined to ironing with fire, eradicating rotten limbs, and treating with honey or soaking with botanical herbs. However, the situation changed after the spread of Islam, as "Arab medicine derived its first elements from the prophetic medicine, which contained honorable hadiths that scholars took care of and made them a basis for treatment."

---

[23] Falkenberg T. Towards a global atlas of traditional/ complementary and alternative medicine utilization: Provisional indicators for monitoring traditional, complementary and alternative medicine use. In: Proceedings of WKC International Consultative Meeting Global Information on Traditional Medicine/Complementary and Alternative Medicine Practices and Utilization, WHO Collaborating Centre, Kobe, Japan, 19–21 September 2001.

[24] Ragheb Al-Sarjani, previous source, p.p. (11–14). Also reviews: - Ali Ammar, History of Folk Medicine ... Evolution and Diversity, a study published on the website of the Al-Nour Center for Studies.

http://www.alnoor.se/article.asp?id=260954

[25] Abdullah, A.A. Trends and challenges of traditional medicine in Africa. Afr. J. Tradit. Complement. Alternate. Med. 2011, 8, PP 115–123.

Ragheb Al-Sirjani, a previous source, pg. (21–23). p.p. (23–26) - Also review: - Muwaffaq Al-Din Abi Al-Abbas Al-Khazraji Ibn Abi Asaibah, (B.C), The Eyes of Doctors in Eye of news', ed. Nizar Rida, Al-Hayat Library Publications, Beirut, pg. (39–151).

The scholar Abdul Latif Al-Baghdadi, who died in 629 AH/1231 AD, wrote many useful compositions, the most important of which is "Forty Hadiths on Prophetic Medicine."[26]

As the Arab nation mixed with other peoples after the spread of Islam, Muslim scholars took an interest in translating medical books from Greek, Persian, and other languages into Arabic and devoted themselves to studying them. They were not satisfied only with transportation, but they added to the science of medicine additions that made Arabs and Muslims later the world's masters in this science and others. They were the first to establish medicine stores, or pharmacies, in Baghdad, the first to use alcohol to dissolve insoluble substances in water, and the first to use snack, camphor, nutmeg, cloves, and nigella in medicine. They were the first to reveal many of the secrets of these medicinal herbs that later became facts in science and technology,[27] and he who traces history finds it full of those interested in studying plants, herbs, and aromatic and medicinal oils.[28] "No one who studies the history of human civilization denies the influence of Ibn Sina, Ibn Tufail, Ibn al-Nafis, Ibn al-Haytham, al-Razi, and others in the science of medicine as well as their professorship of the world in it."[29]

When discussing the history of this form of medicine in the Emirates region, a link is apparent between the region's cultural heritage and its place within Arab-Islamic civilization, in addition to its ties with ancient non-Arab civilizations—whether through journeys in the region or historical trade relations that linked the people of the Arabian Gulf with civilizations of deep historical significance.

Since ancient times, the peoples of the Arabian Gulf have had relations with Indians, Persians, and even Africans. Many features and influences were brought from those countries to the societies of the Gulf. Over time, these influences became a tributary of popular culture in this region, including in the period of European colonialism (Portuguese, Dutch, and English) in the Gulf. The Arabs have also had an indirect influence on the local culture.

The distinctive social fabric of the region's population shaped medicine and the healing arts in the United Arab Emirates and the Arab Gulf, blending many experiences and forms of expertise through various crises. At certain periods, treatment methods appeared that were the product of intertwined cultures in the region, culminating in a medicine that reflected multiple human experiences.

Alternative medicine at this stage relied on cauterization, cupping, circumcision, casting, burial and raising, religious and magical medical prescriptions, and

---

[26] Ragheb Al-Sirjani, a previous source, pg. (26–28). The Islamic Organization for Education, Science and the Arts, Medical Schools in Islamic Civilization, (2011), Proceedings of the Symposium of Medical Schools in Islamic Civilization, Tripoli - Libya, Publications of the Islamic Organization for Education, Science and Arts, pg. (7–19). p. p. (153–167).

[27] Dzio Betika, (2001), Encyclopedia of Traditional Medicine, translated by Youssef Munir Ibrahim, Jordan, Radwan House, p. 53.

[28] Hosni, (2007), Alternative medicine in the treatment of some diseases, previous reference, p. 3–4. - Yahya Abdel Aziz Kahla, (B.T), Revival of Herbal Sciences and Pharmacology, Alexandria, Mansha'at Al Maaref, p. 56.

[29] Ibn Abi Asaibah, a previous source, pg. 161–183.

medicines composed of plants and herbs, in addition to therapeutic rituals accompanying each stage of treatment for various diseases.

The second stage of the development of medicine in the UAE was defined by missionary influence. The colonizing countries began "practicing missionary methods based on the establishment of many clinics and hospitals in the coastal cities before the emergence of the Union States that took advantage of the conditions of the region groaning under ignorance, poverty, and the spread of infectious diseases and pests, to achieve the Crusader goals by dominating the peoples of the region by Christianizing them and making them subject to Christian missionary teachings that began to appear in the form of clinics and medical hospitals on the coast of the Arabian Gulf."[30] The sources indicate that the emergence of modern medicine or missionary hospitals in the Emirates began in the year 1902 AD, when the doctor Sharon Thomas visited Sharjah and Dubai. In the memoirs of this doctor, he mentions his trip to the coastal Emirates by way of his missionary headquarters in Bahrain. In 1909, the doctor Paul Harrison arrived in Abu Dhabi, where he opened a clinic and treated several patients. "The American missionaries moved to Umm al-Quwain and Ras al-Khaimah, which were the goals of the American missionaries, since their arrival, focused on evangelism under the guise of providing medical and treatment services, but that attempt failed."[31] Soon after the discovery of oil, foreign doctors began to arrive to the place and contribute to the modernization of medicine. This included Philip Horniblau, who served as Director of Health in Abu Dhabi from 1966 to 1970 AD.

"The literature of Emirati alternative medicine has been rooted generation after generation in stories, tales, anecdotes, proverbs, and traditional sayings about cases of health and disease, the causes of symptoms of disease, the therapeutic value of cauterization, and the names of popular medical books for those interested in medicine or its professionals."[32] Much of the themes within folk literature involve recipes, treatment methods, types of disease, and their prevention. Among the most prominent are medical folk proverbs that contain therapeutic prescriptions, health advice, and medical experiences, such as the saying about eating unripe foods: "If a person eats green beans before they are ripe, paired with dates, he suffers pains and aches in his stomach."[33] Also therein are further expressions pertinent to human experience, such as: "health for free, sickness with money," "drinking on the wind is a medicine," and "drinking water is a remedy."

---

[30] Abdullah Ali Al-Tabour, (2008), Folk Medicine in the United Arab Emirates, Dubai, Bin Dasmal Press, p. 113.

[31] Rafia Ghobash and Maryam Sultan Lootah, (1997), Medicine in the United Arab Emirates, Evolution and Development, Publication of the Cultural Council, pg. (59–60); Khaled Al-Bassam, Caravans, "The Journeys of American Missionaries in the Cities of the Gulf and the Arabian Peninsula 1901–1926", 1993, p. 32

[32] Abu Dhabi Environment Network website:
https://www.abudhabienv.ae/news-3131.html/

[33] Abdullah Ali Al-Tabour, previous reference, p. 113.

When the Federation of the United Arab Emirates was established, the wise leadership paid attention to healthcare and sought to provide health services to citizens and residents. The efforts of the late Sheikh Zayed bin Sultan Al Nahyan (may Allah have mercy on him) stand out in this field since he assumed the presidency of the United Arab Emirates.[34]

In the context of alternative medicine investment, the United Arab Emirates has worked since its inception to develop this sector by encouraging those working in it. With the help of NGOs that sponsor this alternative heritage, along with an increase in development, the state has established several centers and clinics specialized in Arabic medicine and medicinal herbs. This includes but is not limited to the specialized center in Arab medicine and medicinal herbs in the UAE, which aims to use alternative therapeutic methods in the treatment of many diseases. This was opened in Abu Dhabi on January 23, 1989, and the Zayed Complex for herbal research and Traditional Medicine was established in 1996, with the goal of emphasizing the importance of using herbal and traditional medicines in the treatment of many diseases, as well as preserving the heritage of the ancestors and creating awareness among generations of young people in the Emirates about the importance of herbal medicine and related topics in light of Islamic law.[35]

Among the Emirati institutions sponsoring alternative medicine are the Institute of Prophetic Medicine and Medicinal Herbal Sciences in Sharjah, which was opened in 2002,[36] and Dr. Petra's Clinic for Alternative Medicine, which was opened in 2009 in Dubai Healthcare City, which implemented a pioneering legislative system in the region and in the world to ensure the provision of alternative medicine services.[37]

---

[34] Health services in the Emirates... From folk medicine to globalization, an article published on March 22, 2015. The weekly page provided by "Emirates Today", in cooperation with the "National Archives", affiliated to the Ministry of Presidential Affairs, to introduce the way of life in the Emirates before the union, during its early beginnings, and the great effort made by the founding fathers of the state for its establishment.
https://www.emaratalyoum.com/life/four-sides/2015-03-22-1.767537

[35] Ministry of Health of Abu Dhabi, see The Guide to Herbal and Traditional Medicine in the Health Care System, the publication of Zayed Herbal and Traditional Medicine Research Complex.

[36] The opening of the first Institute of Prophetic Medicine in the United Arab Emirates in Sharjah, the date of publication of the news is 8/9/2002.
https://www.albayan.ae/across-the-uae/2002-09-08-1.1378207

[37] The opening of alternative medicine clinic in Dubai Medical City, the date of publication of the news is 15/7/2009.
https://www.albayan.ae/across-the-uae/2009-07-15-1.453594

48.4 Traditional Medical Practices and Inherited Therapeutic Methods

> The traditional medical culture, besides having a societal privacy that distinguishes the character of the emirates from others, old historical ties and relationships are also considered to be another source of this culture, and everything related to health and healing. [38]

Therefore, we can identify three main sources of alternative medicine in the United Arab Emirates: the diversity of the environment, the multiplicity of aspects of social life, and the resilience of human and civilizational communication between the region and the world through the ages, given the geographical location and strategic importance of the region. This eventually led to the transfer of arts, medicines, drugs, herbs, and plants from other communities to the local United Arab Emirates markets at the request of certain perfume vendors and spice traders. The most recent of these sources is the Arab-Islamic heritage that has shaped the final form of alternative traditional medicine, and the human Emirati inherits this form of medicine from generation to generation. It is believed that the history of alternative medicine in the United Arab Emirates proves that it was the first step on the road to healing with modern medicine. If we look at people in the United Arab Emirates and the Persian Gulf in general, we see that this form of medicine has been passed down from one generation to the next by specialists who do not call themselves doctors but are experts in it. I also believe that alternative medicine is a form of medicine, but it does not rely on scientific theories, bases, or laboratory experiments, but rather on experiences and observations passed down from one generation to the next.

Traditional healing practices usually gain popularity based on the breadth of their acceptance within a society and the depth of its belief in them. The community of such practices exhibits a variety of characteristics and differs according to the forms of treatment it provides, the extent to which it can be maintained in the face of advanced modern medical practices, the nature and type of the disease, and the age, educational level, occupation, and social and cultural origins of the patients. From the above, it can be said that the community of traditional healers in Emirati society comprises several social groups concerned with this form of medicine and the medical profession.

Each group has a single specialty, and one therapist may combine several specializations—the most famous of which are *herbal therapy*,[39] *prophetic cautery therapy*,[40] and *cupping therapy*. The last of these involves the extraction and removal of excess or impure blood from the human body using an instrument to draw and

---

[38] Abdullah Ali Al-Tabour, op. cit., pp. (123–124). Ali Abdulaziz Al Sharhan, Transformations of the Popular Language, The Impact of Social Change in the United Arab Emirates, published by the Writers Union and the Emirates Writers, 1990, pp. (34–39).

[39] Mostafa Mahmoud, (2016), Popular Diseases and Therapies, Cairo, Al-Raya Top Publishing and Distribution, p. 18.

[40] Rafiah Ghobash - Maryam Sultan Lutah, (1997), Medicine in the United Arab Emirates, Growing up and Development, Abu Dhabi, Cultural Complex. pp. (36–37) - Abdullah Ali Al-Tabour, op. cit., p. 161.

collect blood in certain areas, such as the back of the head, the ankle, the calf, the thigh, under the chin, the back of the foot, or under the chest.[41] It should be noted that cupping therapy was not exclusively practiced by men; women in the United Arab Emirates have also excelled in it, the most prominent of whom in contemporary times being Ms. Zainab bint Qumber, a resident of Ras al-Khaimah, who practices cupping therapy on women.

Another method is *orthopedic therapy*, "which is based on the science of bone anatomy and on experience in treating it, a practice that has no doubt been based on scientific origins drawn from Arab and human experience in the field of the anatomy and treatment of bone diseases and accidents."[42]

One of the most important surgical operations that the UAE society has engaged in is the practice of circumcision. The most famous circumcision practitioners in the Emirates are Sheikh Darwish, the circumcision practitioner, and Sheikh Isa Barghouh, who comes from Ras Al Khaimah. The Abu Safard family, who inherited this complex profession from their ancestors, is also famous for circumcizing an important segment of the children of UAE families. "Often, the members performed the operations free of charge and considered it a gift from them to the parents of the circumcized child. It was first practiced in the family by Sheikh Ahmad Abu Safard and then passed on to his two sons, Ali and Hassan."[43]

The profession of the midwife, who supervises the delivery of pregnant women, has traditionally had the most bearing on the employment of alternative medicine in the *method of delivery* and pregnant women's healthcare in the UAE.[44] One of the best ways to treat women and help them have children was by the method of bagging. The midwife was able to determine the gender of the fetus by examining the pregnant woman. The treatment methods of the Emirati midwife are of particular interest in the area of post-delivery healthcare of the mother and fetus. They have innovated the most successful nutrition methods and tools and have devised methods that modern medicine has proven to be useful in maternal healthcare, such as putting a stone on a woman's abdomen after birth, as it is important to restore the uterus (the home of the fetus) to its natural place, as well as imposing hot-tasting foods, specifically pepper, on the mother to help clean a woman's abdomen. Traditional therapies have specialized in several areas, including gynecology, pregnancy and childbirth, herbal medicine, and surveying, which is meant to hand scan the patient's nerves and muscles—both mother and child—along with other useful medical practices.[45]

---

[41] Rafiah Ghobash - Maryam Sultan Lutah, op. cit., pp. (34–35) - Abdullah Ali Al-Tabour, op. cit., p. (194).

[42] Rafiah Ghobash - Maryam Sultan Lutah, op. cit., p. (33).

[43] Abdullah Ali Al-Tabour, op. cit., p. (178).

[44] Ibid., p. (194).

[45] Badria Muhammad Al-Shamsi, **Traditional Medicine… Treasures of Daily Life**, Emirates Today, on 12 / 4 / 2012, the link:
https://www.emaratalyoum.com/life/life-style/2012-04-12-1.475729

Traditional treatments include *Koran therapy (the profession of Islamic[46] jurist)*, *hot sand burial therapy (backfilling)*,[47] and *masseuse*, where massage is "a treatment for many diseases such as neck and back pain, spine and cervical pain, and vertebral dislocation." One of the most famous masseurs in Sharjah is Sheikh Saeed Abu Dukhan.[48] Other traditional treatments include amputation (cutting off part of the patient's body),[49] perforation (piercing of the female ear, which was usually the midwife's specialty),[50] and saltwater therapy.[51]

One of the most famous healing practices in the United Arab Emirates society, which has been innovative in diagnosing and describing the disease, is the use of the dried remains of camels to lift the tonsils, where the lifter uses droppings of camels for tonsils raising, the dressing of wounds and their treatment with salt in dressing wounds and treating them as a disinfectant and haemorrhagic reflux, or the use of gum Arabia as a holding or adhesive. Also, the treatment of anaemia, head pain, back and chest pain, etc., is also carried out by fading and the "vacillation" (cupping) method. They also used isolation for persons suffering from infectious diseases. Treatment methods varied from region to region, depending on the nature of the environment and the experiences of the people.[52]

Seasonal diseases, such as headaches, were treated with saffron, cloves, cardamom, roses, milk, and rose water, and ophthalmia was treated with the drug Murohush, while abdominal constipation (captivation) was treated with senna leaves, which were mixed with a little water and then drunk. A common disease in the UAE environment was influenza, which was treated with a mixture of herbaceous plants such as thyme and lame. These were soaked in hot water to make tea. Other diseases for which Emirati Traditional alternative medicine has been able to find the appropriate antidote include:

- *Scald disease*: A disease that affects divers in the sea, who were treated with a compound of medicines consisting of (peat, kurt, halili, turmeric).
- *Biliary disease (Bu saffar)*: Also known as jaundice; treated by cooking (Al-Jaddah).

---

[46] Mohamed Mahmoud Abdullah, (2009), **Quran medicine between food and medicine**, Alexandria, University Youth Foundation, p. 4 - Fawzi Abdel Rahman, (1984), **the study of Anthropology of medical practice in the Egyptian countryside**, Girls' College, Ain Shams University, p. 136, Abdullah Ali Al-Tabour, op. cit., pp. (236–237).

[47] Maher Hassan Mahmoud, (2010), **Herbal Medicine and Medicinal Plants Between Scientific Facts and Traditional Heritage**, Foundation of the World of Sports, p. 41- p. 222.

[48] Fawzia Diab, (2010), **Social Values and Traditions**, Beirut, Renaissance Arab Printing and Publishing House, p.-p. (41–43) - Abdullah Ali Al-Tabour, op. cit., p. 219.

[49] Rafiah Ghobash - Maryam Sultan Lutah, op. cit., p. 38.

[50] Abdullah Ali Al-Tabour, op. cit., p. 217.

[51] Ateya Salem, (2012), **Traditional medicine... Alternative Medicine**, Cairo, Shams Foundation Publishing and Distribution. P. 21.

[52] Ebtisam Al-Shaaeir, **Traditional medicine... Successful Experiences Pharmacy,** Al Bayan UAE newspaper, publication date 6/6/2010. Date of visit: 08/08/2019.
  https://www.albayan.ae/across-the-uae/2010-06-06-1.252376

- *Diabetes*: Treated with a mixture of pomegranate (peels) and alfalfa.[53]
- *Swelling of the breasts after childbirth*: Treated by the Emiratis with a mixture of roses and hot water.
- *Joint pain disease*: Treated by placing dates on the place of pain, massaging the joints with fat or oil, such as castor oil or olive oil, or massaging with rose water, ginger water, salt water, and milk.[54]
- *Eye disease*: Treated with mother's milk, especially in infants; roses and honey were used as a treatment for eye infections.[55]
- *Sciatica*: Treated by cauterization on the ankles or the site of pain, while abdominal swelling was treated by cauterization with two marks above it. It may also be treated by drinking ginger or thyme infusions.
- *Khaz Baz disease*: A contagious disease, treated using a medicine that consisted of red ochre and patience.
- *Toothache disease (molars)*: Treated by placing drops of *screw sweat* on a piece of cotton that is fixed inside the gap, and a small piece of amber is placed to fill the gap. The therapist may remove the teeth with a nylon floss called (prim floss) or use an iron tool such as the reel. After the dislocation, a piece of salt is placed to stop the bleeding.[56]
- *The disease of Umm al-Subayan*: Treated by cauterization, as its namesake was branded with two knives above and below the navel, and a third was used to brand him at the hairline on the head and the forehead. The patient may be treated with some medications consisting of Indian indigo, bitter parsnip, Sarakat Saleh, Arrayor, and a little kerosene.
- *Leap disease*: Symptoms are a state of tension, nausea, and convulsions, along with a nervous state, often from difficulty breathing. This disease is treated by labeling the patient with pads on the back of the neck.
- *The vertebra*: One of the diseases that causes severe pain due to exposure to infections in the abdomen, resulting in heaviness in the body and difficulty getting up. Also, the patient might have *mysir*, which is a stomachache. It can be treated with mop or trampling and, if not, with cauterization followed by placement of sutures above and below the navel.
- *Bubrigaa's disease (facial paralysis)*: Affects both men and women. For its treatment, the therapist prescribes a medicinal compound consisting of *ginger and nails* and a little water, then rubs the face of the patient. People in the past sometimes resorted to treating it with a drug called *Kast*.[57]

---

[53] United Arab Emirates Health Department official website: https://www.haad.ae/haad/tabid/1155/Default.aspx

[54] The official website of the Department of Health in the United Arab Emirates, https://www.haad.ae/haad/tabid/1155/Default.aspx.

[55] The official website of the Department of Health in the United Arab Emirates, https://www.haad.ae/haad/tabid/1155/Default.aspx

[56] Mohammed bin Rashid Al-Zaaki council website, http://www.dmi.ae/dubaizaman/program-detail.asp?PTID=159&PID=37478

[57] Abdullah Ali Al-Tabour, op. cit., p. 293.

- *Al-Mustajii disease*: A symptom of this serious disease involves abdominal swelling. It is usually cauterized, with a single poke on the right leg comb, and a poke on the left leg comb.
- *Measles*: Also known as hives, it appears in the form of a rash on a child's body. This disease affects children before the age of twelve. It can be treated by tagging the patient with a burnt sheep's tail and providing eggs for food.
- *Atrophic league disease*: The atrophic ligament was treated with cautery, whereby the patient was branded with a single poke under the nipple, which prevented the spread of the blood. Then the chest and respiratory arteries are compressed.[58]

This is a simple sample of the treatments given by traditional alternative medicine to the UAE community, some of which are still in place because of their medical efficacy and lack of side effects.

There is also an abundance of herbs used in traditional Emirati medicine. The nation's fertile soil and high mountains are an environment rich in medicinal plants used by the people for medicinal purposes and food. The most notable herbs and medicinal plants used by alternative medicine practitioners to treat numerous diseases are the Al-Salih herb, which is used to treat chest pain, the Geishum herb for constipation pain, the Al-Haramel herb for joint pain, abdominal inflammation, and headache, the Al-Milida herb for colic abdomen and cold, and (the maple plant) for rheumatoid pain. There is also the Al-Pinkie herb for diabetes, the Al-Muhtadi herb used as an appetizer, the Al-Suriyeh herb for fractures and muscle diseases, the Al-Futan herb for cough, cold, and stomach pain, and the Al-Hulul herb for treating constipation. Further, there is the Rumex vesicarius herb for long-term chronic diseases, serving also as a dewormer and diuretic, with many uses in the lives of the people from time to time.

There is also the Al-anzerot plant used to measure fractures, the plant of nail to treat nerves and muscle tightness, and the Elbow plant to treat scurvy and respiratory canal inflammation. Acacia Tortilis is used to treat colds, and floral grinders are used for skin and hair treatments. A blend of flowers and Acacia Tortilis leaves is also used for the treatment of smallpox, tuberculosis, measles, and other diseases.[59]

In fact, herbal medicine was the first step towards medication in modern medicine, and people in the Emirates and the Persian Gulf generally knew alternative medicine and passed it on from generation to generation through specialists who did not call themselves doctors but were familiar with it. This form of medicine is not based on a scientific theory, a scientific basis, or laboratory experience, but rather on

---

[58] Ibid., p. 295.

[59] Abu al-Fida Mohamed Izzat Mohamed Aref, (2005), The Secrets of treatment with Herbs, Food and Flowers, Cairo, Dar al-Fadilah, p. 215. See also the article: Traditional medicine is a cure from nature, published in Al Khaleej newspaper, on 27/3/2014.

See more at: https://www.alkhaleej.ae/%D9.

experience passed down from one generation to the next, although some types depend on some origins, such as fracture therapy.[60]

It is believed that the environment in the United Arab Emirates has created a large number of practitioners, both male and female, with extensive experience in the field of medicine and traditional medicine, who have a long legacy of traditional medicine and have gained great fame for treating many difficult cases. They are well-known throughout the country for utilizing natural materials found in the region, such as myrrh, bitter, rags, snorts, and other herbs and materials, whose usefulness in the appropriate treatment of diseases has been confirmed by repeated results.

One of the most popular scientists of medicine in the UAE is Sheikh Yousef Saeed Al-Mutalii, a cupping therapist licensed by the Ministry of Health. His nickname is "the cupping therapist Khor Fakan." He is the second Emirati to be licensed in the practice of cupping after Sheikh Yousef Al-Hammadi.[61]

One of the most famous women who mastered the traditional arts of alternative medicine in the contemporary Emirati community is Mrs. Hamama Al-Junaibi, from Al-Zaid. Despite her old age, she has "treated the patients and prescribed them appropriate medication from natural plants and herbal extracts. Her fame was probably derived from her distinction in cauterization, shaking, and wiping, in addition to her renown for the treatment of newborns. She also treats chronic diseases such as asthma, kidney and liver pain, infertility, diabetes, and hypertension, and she has extensive experience practicing gynecology, having delivered women and used traditional prescriptions for a long time."[62]

Maryam Salem al-Qaidi, from Ras al-Khaimah, is known for her treatment of many diseases prevalent in women by employing medical mixtures consisting mainly of herbs and wild plants gathered in the desert and mountains of the Emirates. In addition to these two women known for their treatment using traditional natural combinations, there was Halaweh Khamis Said (Um Said). Her father, from the Tuwaiyeh district of Fujairah, brought his experience to his people to treat them at a time when hospitals were not available.[63]

Another exceptional lady was Mrs. Halima bint Muhammad, a skilled woman of her profession who became famous in the region deriving the components of medical mixtures from wild herbs abundant in the rainy and spring seasons on the Fujairah and Kalba mountains.[64]

---

[60] The official website of the Department of Health in the United Arab Emirates, https://www.haad.ae/haad/tabid/1155/Default.aspx.

[61] Jamila Ismail, Youssef Al-Mutalii heals people's pain with "cups" of Healing, published on 4/7/2010. Date of visit: 30/06/2019.
https://www.albayan.ae/five-senses/2010-07-04-1.261844

[62] Bakr Al-Mohasanah, op. cit., p. 3.

[63] Ibid., p. 3.

[64] Ibid., p. 3.

48.5 Conclusion

1. The medical culture of the people of the Emirates is an ancient historical and cultural legacy that cannot be confined within a specific time frame or historical form. This results from the alternative medical culture's production from the age-old cultural, human, economic, religious, and ideological interaction between the people of the Emirates, who belong to the Arab-Islamic nations and culture, which is closely linked to many peoples and cultures throughout the world, which have been and continue to be an important source of historical relations.
2. One of the main reasons the members of the UAE community turn to alternative medicine is its status as a traditional occupation practiced by both men and women based on experience and self-experimentation. Its components were based on natural materials from agricultural, mountain, and wilderness areas, and relied on traditional methods and instruments of treatment, as well as the effectiveness and distinction of some methods of alternative medicine in the medical field. Another important reason is the reduction of cost in treatment it provides, in addition to the thriving trade in natural herbs and alternative medicines.
3. The history of the Emirates has been touched by many hands with extensive experience in the field of alternative medicine, both male and female, with long careers, during which they acquired a great reputation enabling them to treat many difficult cases.
4. Modern medicine is the epitome of the development of alternative medicine, yet it resorts to traditional medicine in providing its services.
5. The services offered by alternative medicine therapy share their systems with the concept of health for the individual, which is the ultimate achievement of happiness in all aspects of the spiritual, social, mental, and physical.

Second: Recommendations
1. We must not neglect either system of treatment. Some cases call for alternative medicine services, and others call for modern medicine, each of which is complementary to the other, according to the social and cultural composition of the Emirati community, the psychological factor of the patient, and even the factor of class.
2. We must establish other centers specializing in the field of alternative medicine, such as the Zayed Centre for Research of Herbs and Traditional Medicine, and the expansion of the revival of the findings of Arab and Muslim scientists in the field of medicine.
3. We must focus on the importance of traditional alternative therapies by assigning such importance to sulphur waterholes therapy, burial therapy, and orthopedic therapy. This indicates a need to maintain waterholes as sanatoriums, demonstrating their therapeutic benefits, as well as establishing special alternative physiotherapy clinics.

4. We must build a knowledge base within the United Arab Emirates to manage alternative medicine by developing an appropriate national policy for diversification in alternative medicine products, in the interest of practicing it alongside modern medicine.
5. We must promote comprehensive health coverage by integrating traditional and complementary medical services into healthcare and self-care services.

Conflicts of Interest The authors have no conflicts of interest to declare.

References

1. Abi al-Fadl Ibn Manzoor. Lisan Al-Arab "the Arab Tongue, vol. 3. 3rd ed. Beirut: Heritage Revival House; 1999.
2. Arabic Language Complex. Intermediate Lexicon. Cairo: East International Library; 2004.
3. Al-Khalil bin Ahmed Al-Farhidi, Kitab Al-Ain. "The Eye Book". Abdul Hamid Al-Hendawi, Beirut, Dar Al-Kotob Al-Ilmiyah, editors. "the Scientific Books House". Vol. 3, ed. 1, 2003 AD
4. Habash M. Muslims and civilization sciences. Damascus: Dar al-Marefa "the House of Knowledge; 1996.
5. Khaldoun I, Al-Rahman A. Diwan Al-Mobtadah, vol. 2. Suhail Zakar, Beirut: Dar al-Fikr Printing; 2002.
6. El-Thanwi MA. The Encyclopedia of the discovery of arts and sciences terminology, vol. 2. Ali Dahroj, Beirut: Lebanon Library Publishers; 1991.
7. Bakr Al-Mohasanah. Traditional medicine from nature practised by some natural therapists or genetics, Gulf Newspaper, published on 27/3/2014. Visit Date: 07/06/2019. http://www.alkhaleej.ae/supplements/page/a635932e-964a-46bb-902c-ee4754b8d1ca.
8. Rasheed IN. Medication with herbs and medicinal plants. Cult J. 2004;A65, Oman
9. World Health Organization. Sixty-second World Health Assembly, document vol. 62/8, 2009.
10. Mahmoud ARS. Traditional medicine in Mosul City, Social Study, Unpublished Master's Thesis, Mosul University, Iraq, 2005.
11. Collection of Authors. Accessible Arabic Encyclopedia, Mg4. Beirut: Modern Library; 2010.
12. al-Darji GH. Criminal liability arising from the practice of traditional medicine. Beirut: Halabi Rights Publications; 2017.
13. Rahmatullah M, Jahan R, Azam FS, Hossan S, Mollik MAH, Rahman T. Folk medicinal uses of Verbenaceae family plants in Bangladesh. Afr J Tradit Complement Altern Med. 2011;8:53.
14. World Health Organization website., https://www.who.int/topics/traditional_medicine/definitions/ar/.
15. El-Gouhari M. Scientific study of traditional beliefs, vol. 1. Cairo: House of Culture; 1983.
16. Mellah R. Spiritual therapy by writing Al-Awafaq, an unpublished master's thesis, specializing in sociology. Oran University; 2012.
17. Vermont J. Traditional medicine and its fields. Syria: Alaa El-Din House; 1996.
18. Sheikh S, Furnham A. Cross-cultural study of mental health beliefs and attitudes towards seeking professional help. Soc Psychiatry Psychiatr Epidemiol. 2000;35:326.
19. http://www.pathways2promise.org/wp-content/uploads/2017/01/A-Cross-Cultural-Study-of-Mental-Health-Beliefs-and-Attitudes-Towards-Seeking-Professional-Help-1.pdf.
20. 14. World Health Organization website., https://www.who.int/topics/traditional_medicine/definitions/ar/.
21. The website.: https://stringfixer.com/ar/Ethnopharmacy.
22. The website of Sotor.: https://sotor.com/%D9.
23. The Website Directory (MSD) Consumer Guidance. https://www.msdmanuals.com/ar/home/%D8

24. The Arab Encyclopedia. Bab (Sadat - Ottomans), vol. 12. Syria: Salhani Printing and Publishing Foundation; 2005.
25. Palinkas LA, Kabongo ML, Surfnet Study Group. The use of complementary and alternative medicine by primary care patients. J Fam Pract. 2000;49(12):1121.
26. Beal MW. Women's use of complementary and alternative therapies in reproductive health care. J Nurse Midwifery. 1998;43:224.
27. Husseini A. Encyclopedia of traditional medicine and alternative therapy. Egypt: Family Library; 2005.
28. Tada T. Toward the philosophy of CAM: super system and epidemical sciences. Evid Based Complement Alternat Med. 2004;1:5.
29. Hussain SA, Saeed A, Ahmed M, Qazi A. Contemporary role and future prospects of medicinal plants in the health care system and pharmaceutical industries of Pakistan. http://www.telmedpak.com/doctors' articles. [accessed on 6/12/2013. A. Eisenberg D et al. Trends in alternative medicine use in the United States, 1990–1997. The Journal of the American Medical Association, 1998, P 280.
30. Yassin al-Gamal. Black seed therapy. Egypt: Modern Arab Center; 2008.
31. Al-Sarjani R. Medical science story in Islamic civilization. Cairo: Read Foundation for Publishing and Distribution; 2008.
32. Falkenberg T. Towards a global atlas of traditional/ complementary and alternative medicine utilization: provisional indicators for monitoring traditional, complementary, and alternative medicine use. In: Proceedings of WKC international consultative meeting global information on traditional medicine/complementary and alternative medicine practices and utilization, WHO Collaborating Centre, Kobe, Japan, 19–21 September 2001.
33. Ammar A. The history of traditional medicine... development and diversity, a study published on the website. Al Noor Centre for Studies.
34. http://www.alnoor.se/article.asp?id=260954
35. Abdullah AA. Trends and challenges of traditional medicine in Africa. Afr J Tradit Complement Altern Med. 2011;8:115.
36. Mufaq Al-Din Abu al-Abbas al-Khazarji Ibn Abi Asaibah. The eyes of the doctors in the eyes of the news. Beirut: Nizar Reda, Publications of Life Library House.
37. The Islamic Organization for Education, Science and Arts, Medical Schools in Islamic Civilization. Symposium of medical schools in Islamic civilization. Tripoli-Libya: Islamic Organization for Education, Science and Arts publications; 2011.
38. Petika D. The Encyclopedia of traditional medicine, translation by Yousef Munir Ibrahim. Jordan: Dar Radwan; 2001.
39. Kallah YA. (B. T), Revival of Herbal Sciences and Pharmacy, Alexandria, Monchaat Al Maaref.
40. Al-Tabour AA. Traditional medicine in The United Arab Emirates. Dubai: Bin Dasmal Press; 2008.
41. Ghobash R, Lutah MS. Medicine in The United Arab Emirates, growing up and development. Abu Dhabi: Issuance of the Cultural Complex; 1997a.
42. Abu Dhabi Environment Network website.: https://www.abudhabienv.ae/news-3131.html.
43. UAE Health Services... From Traditional medicine to the world, article published on 22/3/2015. The weekly page presented by "Emirates Today", in cooperation with "the National Archives" of the Ministry of Presidential Affairs, to familiarize itself with the way of life in the UAE before the Union, during its early beginnings, and the great effort of the founding fathers of the State for its establishment. https://www.emaratalyoum.com/life/four-sides/2015-03-22-1.767537.
44. Ministry of Health of Abu Dhabi, see (The Guide to Herbal and Traditional Medicine in the Health Care System), the publication of Zayed Herbal and Traditional Medicine Research Complex.
45. The opening of the first Institute of Prophetic Medicine in the United Arab Emirates in Sharjah, the date of publication of the news is 8/9/2002. https://www.albayan.ae/across-the-uae/2002-09-08-1.1378207.

46. The opening of alternative medicine clinic in Dubai Medical City, the date of publication of the news is 15/7/2009. https://www.albayan.ae/across-the-uae/2009-07-15-1.453594.
47. Al-Sharhan AA. Dramatic language transformations, impact of social change in the UAE. Production of UAE Writers and Literature Federation; 1990.
48. Mahmoud M. Traditional diseases and treatments. Cairo: Al Raya Top for Publishing and Distribution; 2016.
49. Ghobash R, Lutah MS. Medicine in The United Arab Emirates, growing up and development. Abu Dhabi: The Cultural Complex; 1997.
50. Al-Shamsi BM. Traditional medicine… treasures of daily life, Emirates Today, on 12/4/2012, the link: https://www.emaratalyoum.com/life/life-style/2012-04-12-1.475729.
51. Abdullah MM, editor. Quran medicine between food and medicine. Alexandria: University Youth Foundation; 2009.
52. Rahman FA. The study of anthropology of medical practice in the Egyptian countryside. Girls' College, Ain Shams University; 1984.
53. Mahmoud MH. Herbal medicine and medicinal plants between scientific facts and traditional heritage. Foundation of the World of Sports; 2010.
54. Diab F. Social values and traditions. Beirut: Renaissance Arab Printing and Publishing House; 2010.
55. Salem A. Traditional medicine... alternative medicine. Cairo: Shams Foundation Publishing and Distribution; 2012.
56. Al-Shaaeir E. Traditional medicine... successful experiences pharmacy, Al Bayan UAE newspaper, publication date 6/6/2010. Date of visit: 08/08/2019. https://www.albayan.ae/across-the-uae/2010-06-06-1.252376.
57. United Arab Emirates Health Department official website. https://www.haad.ae/haad/tabid/1155/Default.aspx.
58. Mohammed bin Rashid Al-Zaaki council website., http://www.dmi.ae/dubaizaman/program-detail.asp?PTID=159&PID=37478.
59. Abu al-Fida Mohamed Izzat Mohamed Aref. The secrets of treatment with herbs, food and flowers. Cairo: Dar al-Fadilah; 2005.
60. Traditional medicine is a cure from nature, published in Al Khaleej newspaper, on 27/3/2014. https://www.alkhaleej.ae/%D9
61. Ismail J, Al-Mutalii Y. Heals people's pain with "cups" of Healing, published on 4/7/2010. Date of visit: 30/06/2019. https://www.albayan.ae/five-senses/2010-07-04-1.261844
62. Werner D. Who is not attended by a doctor, T: Mi Haddad. Beirut: Arab Scientific Research Foundation; 1981.

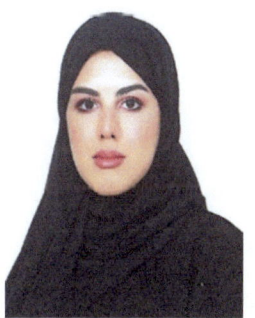

Khawla Mohammed Saeed bin Fresh ELKennedy PhD Student, Department of History and Islamic Civilization, University of Sharjah, Sharjah, United Arab Emirates.

In 2015, she obtained a bachelor's degree from the University of Sharjah, College of Arts and Humanities, Department of History and Islamic Civilization, History.

She obtained a master's degree in Islamic history and civilization. Her thesis is entitled "The History of Popular Medicine and Health Practices in Contemporary Emirati Society in 2020."

Among her research interests are the political, cultural, and social history of the Arab world (modern and contemporary periods). She has an article titled Medicine and Healthcare in Contemporary Emirati Society. It was published in the *University of Sharjah Journal for Humanities and Social Sciences* 1, no. 1 (2021): University of Sharjah Press, Sharjah, United Arab Emirates.

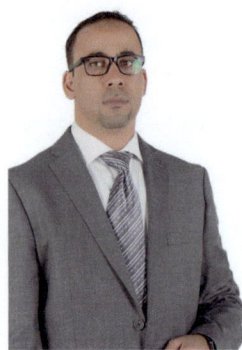

Kheireddine Youssef Chatra is a faculty member in the Department of History and Islamic Civilization, College of Arts, Humanities, and Social Sciences, at the University of Sharjah. He holds a doctorate in modern and contemporary history.

Among his research interests are the political, cultural, and social history of the Arab world (modern and contemporary periods), and he has authored or contributed to

numerous books, including *Algerian Students at the Zitouna Mosque* and *Algerian Immigrants to the Tunisian Countryside: Studies on the Intellectual and Civilizational Contributions of Algerian Elites in the Diaspora*.

Professor Kheireddine has published numerous scholarly articles in peer-reviewed journals, including "The Intellectual and Literary Legacy of Sheikh Muhammad bin Abdul Rahman Al-Disi and His Contributions to the Art of the Principles of Interpretation and Interpretation," a descriptive study.

He has also presented research papers at international conferences, including "The Intellectual Invasion of French Colonialism and Its Impact on Subjugating the Algerian Sahara," "Algeria's Relations with Eastern European Countries, 1959–1979," "The Algerian Personality and Its Civilizational Links with the Arab Levant," and "Recent Trends in Historical Studies and Their Social and Educational Uses," and "Epistemic Readings in Historical Research Methods and Rules for Heritage Investigation."

Open Access This chapter is licensed under the terms of the Creative Commons Attribution 4.0 International License (http://creativecommons.org/licenses/by/4.0/), which permits use, sharing, adaptation, distribution and reproduction in any medium or format, as long as you give appropriate credit to the original author(s) and the source, provide a link to the Creative Commons license and indicate if changes were made.

The images or other third party material in this chapter are included in the chapter's Creative Commons license, unless indicated otherwise in a credit line to the material. If material is not included in the chapter's Creative Commons license and your intended use is not permitted by statutory regulation or exceeds the permitted use, you will need to obtain permission directly from the copyright holder.

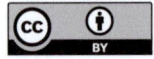

Artificial Intelligence in Healthcare in the UAE

49

Khalid Shaikh and Sreelekshmi Vivek

49.1 Introduction

The United Arab Emirates (UAE) has consistently been at the forefront of innovation, taking bold steps to integrate technology into various sectors, including healthcare. Despite initial skepticism from many, the UAE has wholeheartedly embraced smart technologies such as artificial intelligence, machine learning, and deep learning, revolutionizing the healthcare ecosystem and unlocking its true potential. Despite the buzz, the digital transformation of healthcare did not receive immediate acceptance initially. Yet, it stood firm and was ratified owing to its capacity to redesign the healthcare system.

Artificial intelligence (AI) is a field of computer science dedicated to enabling computer systems to perform tasks with human-like intelligence. It involves the ability of machines or computers to exhibit intellectual processes and human characteristics such as reasoning, learning from experience, and generalizing information. In the healthcare domain, AI plays a significant role in analyzing treatment techniques for various diseases and aiding in their prevention [1]. Its applications in healthcare encompass areas such as diagnostic processes, drug research, medicine, and patient monitoring in care centers. By utilizing electronic health records, AI helps gather historical data to facilitate disease prevention and diagnosis [1]. AI serves as a comprehensive tool that empowers humanity to integrate and analyze information, leveraging the resulting insights to enhance decision-making. Whether it is uncovering new connections in genetic codes or supporting surgery-assisting robots, AI is reshaping and revitalizing modern healthcare by enabling machines to predict, understand, learn, and take action [2]. One of the most promising applications of AI in healthcare is enhancing the diagnostic process, which has the potential

---

K. Shaikh (✉) · S. Vivek
Prognica Labs, Dubai, United Arab Emirates
e-mail: khalid@prognica.com; sreelekshmi@prognica.com

© The Author(s) 2025
H. O. Al-Shamsi (ed.), *Healthcare in the United Arab Emirates*,
https://doi.org/10.1007/978-981-96-0523-1_49

to significantly reduce the roughly 400,000 cases of preventable harm and 100,000 deaths that occur in hospitals each year [2].

49.2 The Genesis of AI in Healthcare: A New Era

In 1950, Alan Turing, a British polymath, published a paper outlining a method to evaluate the intelligence of a machine. He proposed that if a machine could engage in a conversation via a teleprinter and imitate a human to the extent that there were no discernible differences, it could be considered to be "thinking". Turing's groundbreaking paper was succeeded in 1952 by the Hodgkin-Huxley model, which depicted the brain as a network of neurons that communicate through electrical impulses. This model describes how individual neurons fire in binary pulses, either on or off. These significant developments, along with discussions held during a conference sponsored by Dartmouth College in 1956, played a pivotal role in catalyzing the concept of artificial intelligence [3].

In 1959, a significant paper was published by Robert Ledley and Lee Lusted in *Science*, highlighting the importance of reasoning processes in medical diagnosis and discussing the potential role of electronic computers. This publication is widely regarded as the pioneering work that initiated the field of medical informatics. Ledley and Lusted employed mathematical techniques such as Boolean algebra, Baye's theorem, and symbolic logic to aid in disease diagnosis. Another noteworthy advancement occurred in 1965 with the DENDRAL project at Stanford University, led by AI pioneer Edward Feigenbaum and Nobel Prize winner Joshua Lederberg. This project utilized rule-based and hypothesis-list approaches to identify unknown organic molecules based on the analysis of their mass spectrometry data [4].

Although the concept of AI was conceived in the 1950s, early models faced various limitations that hindered their widespread acceptance and application in medicine. However, in the early 2000s, the emergence of deep learning techniques helped overcome many of these limitations. With the ability to analyze complex data and engage in self-learning, AI has entered a new era in medicine. It can now be applied to clinical practice through the development of risk assessment models, enhancing diagnostic accuracy and improving workflow efficiency [5].

Over the past five decades, AI in Medicine (AIM) has undergone significant evolution. The introduction of machine learning (ML) and deep learning (DL) has expanded the scope of AIM, creating opportunities for personalized medicine that go beyond algorithm-based approaches. Predictive models have been developed for disease diagnosis and therapeutic response prediction and hold promise for preventative medicine in the future [5, 6]. The progressive growth and development of AI in medicine are chronicled below, organized by distinct time periods that mark transformative milestones.

49.2.1 The 1950s to 1970s

In the early stages of AI development, the primary focus was on creating machines capable of making inferences or decisions that were previously exclusive to humans. An important milestone occurred in 1961 when the first industrial robot arm, known as Unimate, manufactured by Unimation, was introduced on the assembly line at General Motors. Unimate specialized in automated die casting and operated by following step-by-step commands [5, 7]. Subsequently, in 1964, Joseph Weizenbaum introduced ELIZA, a program that utilized natural language processing. Eliza employed pattern matching and substitution techniques to simulate human conversation, although its communication was relatively superficial [5, 8]. This pioneering work laid the foundation for future chatbots and served as a framework for further advancements in AI communication.

In 1966, the development of Shakey marked a significant milestone in the field of robotics. Shakey, often referred to as "the first electronic person," was created at the Stanford Research Institute. Unlike previous robots, Shakey had the ability to interpret instructions and carry out more complex actions rather than simply following single-step commands [5, 9]. This breakthrough in robotics and AI showcased the potential for advanced mobility and decision-making in machines.

However, despite these engineering innovations, the adoption of AI in the medical field was relatively slow during this period. Nevertheless, this era was crucial for digitizing medical data, which later laid the groundwork for the future growth and utilization of AI in medicine (AIM). Notably, the development of the Medical Literature Analysis and Retrieval System and the PubMed search engine by the National Library of Medicine in the 1960s played a vital role in establishing a digital resource for the acceleration of biomedical research. Additionally, the creation of clinical informatics databases and medical record systems during this time formed the foundation for subsequent advancements in AIM [5, 10].

49.2.2 The 1970s to 2000s

The period that followed is commonly referred to as the "AI Winter," characterized by a decline in funding, interest, and significant developments in the field [5, 11]. Two major AI winters are recognized: the first occurred in the late 1970s due to perceived limitations of AI, and the second took place in the late 1980s, extending to the early 1990s, driven by the high costs associated with developing and maintaining expert knowledge databases [5]. Despite the reduced general interest during this time, collaboration among AI pioneers persisted.

In 1971, Saul Amarel established the Research Resource on Computers in Biomedicine at Rutgers University, which facilitated collaboration among experts in the field of AI. Additionally, Stanford University developed the Medical Experimental-Artificial Intelligence in Medicine time-shared computer system in 1973, enhancing networking capabilities for clinical and biomedical researchers across various institutions [5, 12]. These collaborations laid the groundwork for the first National Institutes of Health-sponsored AIM workshop, held at Rutgers University in 1975 [5, 10], representing an important milestone in the cooperative efforts of AIM pioneers.

During this period, one of the early prototypes that demonstrated the feasibility of applying AI to medicine was the development of a consultation program for glaucoma using the CASNET model [5, 13]. The CASNET model, consisting of three separate programs (model building, consultation, and database), employed a causal-associational network. It utilized disease-specific information to provide individualized advice to physicians on patient management [5, 13].

During the early 1970s, the development of an AI system called MYCIN introduced the concept of "backward chaining" [5, 14]. MYCIN relied on input from physicians regarding patient information and utilized a knowledge base consisting of approximately 600 rules. It was capable of generating a list of potential bacterial pathogens and providing antibiotic treatment recommendations tailored to the patient's body weight.

In 1986, the University of Massachusetts released DXplain, a decision support system that revolutionized the field. This program allowed for the input of symptoms and subsequently generated a differential diagnosis [5, 15]. DXplain also functioned as an electronic medical textbook, offering detailed disease descriptions and additional references.

By the late 1990s, there was a renewed interest in machine learning (ML), particularly within the medical community. These technological advancements, including MYCIN and DXplain, played a significant role in setting the stage for the modern era of AI in Medicine (AIM) [5].

49.2.3 From 2000 to 2020: Seminal Advancements in AI

In 2007, IBM developed a question-answering system called Watson, which gained recognition by winning first place on the television game show "Jeopardy!" in 2011, surpassing human participants [5, 16]. Unlike traditional systems that relied on forward reasoning, backward reasoning, or hand-crafted rules, Watson utilized a technology called DeepQA. This technology employed natural language processing and various searches to analyze unstructured data and generate probable answers. It offered advantages such as increased accessibility, easier maintenance, and cost-effectiveness [5, 16].

In 2017, Bakkar et al. successfully utilized IBM Watson to identify new RNA-binding proteins implicated in amyotrophic lateral sclerosis [5, 17]. This breakthrough, combined with advancements in computer hardware and software, led to the proliferation of digitalized medicine and rapid growth in AI in Medicine (AIM) [5]. Natural language processing (NLP) played a pivotal role in transforming chatbots from superficial communication, as seen with Eliza, to more meaningful and interactive conversation-based interfaces. This technology was integrated into Apple's virtual assistant, Siri, in 2011, and Amazon's virtual assistant, Alexa, in 2014. Additionally, specific chatbots like Pharmabot (developed in 2015 to provide medication education for pediatric patients and their parents) and Mandy (created in 2017 as an automated patient intake process for a primary care practice) further demonstrated the application of natural language processing in healthcare settings [5, 18, 19].

Deep learning (DL) represents a significant advancement in AI in medicine (AIM). In contrast to machine learning (ML), which relies on a predetermined set of features and human input, DL has the ability to autonomously classify data [5]. While DL was initially explored in the 1950s, its application to medicine was hindered by the challenge of overfitting.. Overfitting occurs when DL becomes excessively focused on a particular dataset, leading to difficulties in accurately processing new datasets. This issue stemmed from limited computing capacity and inadequate training data [5, 20]. However, these limitations were overcome in the 2000s due to the availability of larger datasets and significant improvements in computing power [5].

One particular DL algorithm applied to image processing is the convolutional neural network (CNN). CNNs simulate the interconnected behavior of neurons in the human brain and are primarily utilized for tasks such as image recognition. Composed of multiple layers, CNNs analyze input images to identify patterns and create specific feature maps. The combination of these features in the fully connected layers produces the final outcome [5, 20].

49.3 Role of AI in Healthcare

AI in healthcare refers to the application of AI or ML algorithms to replicate human cognitive abilities in the collection and comprehension of intricate medical and healthcare data. This is accomplished through the utilization of various techniques such as ML algorithms, computer vision, natural language processing, robotics, and deep learning. By employing these algorithms, AI can identify behavioral patterns and develop its own logic to generate precise outputs for end-users. Machine learning enables the extraction of valuable insights and predictions from large volumes of input data. Additionally, it provides guidance to experts on constructing alternatives to costly clinical trials [1].

The descriptions of AI technologies deployed in healthcare industries are as follows [1]:

- *Machine Learning (Neural Network and Deep Learning)*: In the healthcare field, machine learning technology is primarily utilized for precision medicine. This involves predicting the most effective treatment protocols for individual patients based on their unique characteristics and treatment context [1].
- *Natural Language Processing (NLP)*: Natural language processing plays a crucial role in creating, comprehending, and classifying clinical documents and published research. It aids in the analysis of unstructured clinical notes on patients and the generation of reports [1].

- *Robotics*: AI-powered physical robots are employed in various healthcare tasks. Surgical robots, for instance, assist surgeons by enhancing their visualization capabilities and facilitating tasks like suturing wounds. Robotic surgery is applied in procedures such as gynecologic surgery, prostate surgery, and head and neck surgery [1].
- *Rule-Based Expert Systems (RBES)*: Rule-based expert systems rely on a collection of if-then rules and are commonly used in the commercial sector, including electronic health records (EHR). Human experts and knowledge engineers create a set of rules that are then implemented in an easily understandable rule-based expert system. However, as knowledge domains evolve, the rules can become complex and time-consuming. Artificial intelligence is being employed to address this limitation in the healthcare sector [1].
- *Robotic Process Automation (RPA)*: Robotic process automation is utilized in the healthcare industry to automate repetitive tasks like updating patient records or billing. When combined with other technologies, RPA can also assist in data extraction [1].

AI plays a crucial role in revolutionizing healthcare by enabling disease prediction and prevention, drug research and manufacturing, disease treatments, surgery, and patient monitoring. With the ability to process and analyze massive amounts of data from various sources, AI technologies can detect diseases and provide valuable insights to guide clinical decisions. By effectively handling the vast volume of medical data, AI applications uncover hidden information within medical big data, leading to new discoveries and advancements. Additionally, these technologies contribute to identifying new drugs and improving health service management and patient care treatments [21].

49.4 Applications of AI in Healthcare

AI has experienced rapid expansion within the healthcare and associated research fields. There is a growing emphasis on conducting further studies and allocating investments toward AI applications in various healthcare sectors, including oncology, dermatology, radiology, screening, psychiatry, and drug interactions. The potential of AI in these areas is recognized, leading to increased support and resources being directed toward their development and implementation.

- *Radiology*:
  The utilization of artificial intelligence (AI) in the field of radiology has witnessed significant growth in recent years. AI is now being applied in various radiology domains to aid in disease detection and diagnosis using advanced imaging technologies like computerized tomography (CT) and magnetic resonance (MR) imaging. AI algorithms in radiology have demonstrated superior accuracy and recall rates in detecting pneumonia when compared to radiologists involved in clinical trials. Additionally, AI is being employed in oncology to identify key factors such as abnormalities and monitor changes over time. The

integration of AI in radiology not only reduces interaction time but also enables doctors to attend to a larger number of patients simultaneously, improving overall efficiency [1].In the context of breast cancer, one of the major challenges faced by healthcare professionals is the automated detection and classification of masses in breast mammogram images. In recent years, numerous researchers have proposed various solutions to address this issue. For instance, Prognica Labs has developed an algorithm utilizing deep neural networks for the unsupervised, annotation-free diagnosis of breast cancer across different categories as detailed in Figs. 49.1 and 49.2 [22].

The experimental results showed that the proposed algorithm provides up to 96% accuracy for the detection of breast cancer [22].*Screening*:

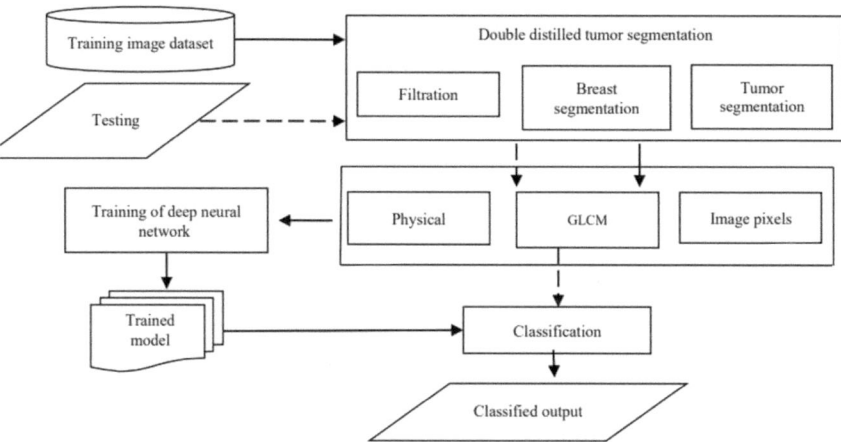

Fig. 49.1 Workflow of the proposed AI algorithm in mammograms for image analysis. (Image source Ref. [22])

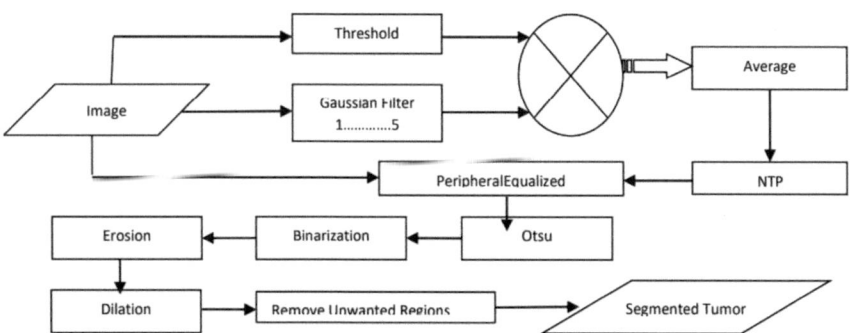

Fig. 49.2 Working flowchart of tumor segmentation from a mammogram image. (Image source Ref. [22])

AI is extensively utilized in the field of screening within the healthcare sector, particularly in the detection of skin cancer. Studies suggest that artificial intelligence systems can achieve higher accuracy in identifying skin malignancies [1]. Given the high prevalence of skin cancer, there is a growing need for timely diagnosis and continuous monitoring [23]. When implemented with appropriate regulations, AI can contribute to reducing the number of unnecessary biopsies by facilitating the detection and monitoring of skin cancer progression. Patients with skin cancer, along with their caregivers, can perform self-skin examinations (SSEs) following proper training. This approach also promotes teledermoscopy, which in turn leads to fewer medical consultations [23].

The integration of AI into smartphone applications can educate individuals on how to perform skin examinations and transmit the collected information to healthcare providers. To develop a new machine learning (ML) algorithm for skin cancer, each type of skin lesion is classified into categories such as benign or malignant or naevi and "melanoma." Deep learning algorithms are trained on a large dataset of images for each category and subsequently evaluated on new images. Although specialists can accurately diagnose cancer, their limited numbers necessitate the development of automated systems that can efficiently diagnose the disease, thereby saving lives and reducing the health and financial burdens on patients. ML holds great potential in this regard [23].

Likewise, the utilization of an AI algorithm called Google DeepMind has proven effective in detecting breast cancer at an early stage, surpassing the capabilities of human experts and enabling preventive interventions before the condition progresses to a severe stage. Additionally, the AI algorithm demonstrates improved accuracy in the detection of prostate cancer compared to human experts [1].

- *Psychiatry*:

AI in the field of psychiatry encompasses the use of computerized techniques and algorithms to assist in diagnosing, preventing, and treating mental illnesses. Current diagnostic approaches for psychiatric disorders heavily rely on physician-patient questionnaires, which often lack precision and fail to provide a reliable assessment of symptoms. However, the application of artificial intelligence (AI) to electronic medical databases and health records can overcome these limitations [25]. Existing AI applications in psychiatry include tools that support in psychiatric diagnoses, symptom tracking, prediction of disease progression, and psychoeducation. These AI-based interventions are delivered through various modalities, such as internet platforms, smartphone applications, and digital gaming. Examples of AI interventions in mental healthcare include chat and therapy bots that engage in conversational interactions to teach users coping strategies for emotional regulation and offer support to individuals with communication difficulties. Additionally, avatar therapy utilizes computer-generated images of faces to facilitate therapy, and advancements in digital psychiatry have introduced intelligent animal-like robots [26].

AI applications are being utilized to examine anxiety and depression, although they are currently in the proof-of-concept phase. Notably, a prominent company like Facebook has implemented screening measures for identifying suicidal ideation. However, the introduction of such applications has sparked discussions and concerns among healthcare professionals regarding professional standards, ethical considerations, and regulatory implications [1].

- *Primary Care*:

AI technologies, including predictive modeling, business analytics, and decision support systems, are gaining prominence in the field of primary care [1]. The application of artificial intelligence (AI) in primary care has been increasing, offering various advantages as the technology advances. AI can support primary care in several ways, including aiding in accurate diagnosis, providing decision support, and facilitating efficient management of patient records. By harnessing the power of AI, primary care providers can enhance patient outcomes and potentially lower healthcare costs [27].

- *Disease Diagnosis*:

AI technologies, including support vector machines, neural networks, and decision trees, are rapidly advancing in their ability to diagnose various diseases within the healthcare industry. These artificial intelligence techniques utilize Medical Learning Classifiers (MLCs) and leverage extensive electronic health records to effectively assist doctors in patient diagnosis [1].

The application of artificial intelligence in healthcare extends beyond diagnosis and encompasses a wide range of techniques, from machine learning to deep learning. These techniques play a vital role in disease diagnosis, drug discovery, and identifying patient risks. To achieve accurate disease diagnoses using artificial intelligence, multiple medical data sources are required, such as ultrasound, magnetic resonance imaging, mammography, genomics, computed tomography scans, and more. Additionally, artificial intelligence has greatly improved the patient experience within healthcare facilities and has expedited the process of preparing patients for continued rehabilitation at home [28].

Subasi, A. put forward a comprehensive framework for the detection of Alzheimer's disease utilizing artificial intelligence (AI) methods. The learning process involves optimizing the parameters of the model by utilizing a training dataset or previous experience. Learning models can serve two primary purposes: predictive, where they forecast future outcomes, and descriptive, where they gather data from various input sources and integrate them. Machine learning and deep learning involve two crucial stages: preprocessing the extensive input data and refining the model [28, 29].

Accurate disease diagnosis is of utmost importance for effective treatment planning and ensuring the overall well-being of patients. In this regard, AI offers a vast and diverse range of tools, including data analysis, algorithms, deep learning, neural networks, and insights. The field of AI is continuously evolving and adapting to meet the specific needs of the healthcare industry and its patients. It is crucial for medical professionals to have a comprehensive understanding of how AI can be utilized in disease diagnosis. This knowledge will contribute to the development of more refined and effective AI-based techniques in the future [28].

- *Drug Interaction*:
 In the healthcare industry, the utilization of AI algorithms for identifying drug-drug interactions (DDIs) can be enhanced through the application of NLP. In recent years, instances of polypharmacy have become prevalent in the treatment of multiple diseases. However, the occurrence of unwanted DDIs leading to unexpected adverse drug events (ADEs) remains a significant concern in multi-regimen therapies. With the ubiquity of artificial intelligence (AI), several AI prediction models have been developed to assist clinicians in making informed decisions regarding pharmacotherapy. Nevertheless, there are concerns about the reliability of AI models due to their opaque nature. To address this issue, it is crucial to construct AI models with explainable mechanisms, which can enhance their transparency. Explainable AI (XAI) promotes safety and clarity by elucidating the decision-making process in AI models, particularly in critical tasks like DDI predictions [30]. The overall workflow of traditional ML and DL for DDI prediction is depicted in Fig. 49.3.
- *Artificial Intelligence in Drug Discovery and Development*
 The application of artificial intelligence (AI) has facilitated the process of manufacturing new drugs, making it more efficient and time-saving as shown in Fig. 49.4 [1]. AI has gained significant traction in various sectors, including the pharmaceutical industry. Its involvement in the entire lifecycle of pharmaceutical product development, from initial research to patient treatment, holds great potential. AI can contribute to rational drug design, assist in decision-making processes, enable personalized medicine by identifying the most suitable therapy for individual patients, and effectively manage the vast amount of clinical data generated, which can be leveraged for future drug development endeavors [31].
- *Electronic Health Records (EHR)*
 Electronic health records (EHR) play a crucial role in the digitalization and development of the healthcare sector, and AI greatly assists in interpreting these records and providing up-to-date disease information. AI helps differentiate between similar diseases, such as myocardial infarction (heart attack), which are often treated by medical specialists. NLP has bridged the gap between these diseases and helps generate relevant prescription notes for future patients. It also aids in analyzing information entered by different physicians to ensure all pertinent details are captured for a specific disease [32].

Furthermore, AI algorithms can be applied to EHR to predict disease risks based on patients' historical data and their family history. Another algorithm follows a rule-based system, similar to the traditional human approach, where the machine predicts and makes decisions according to a predefined flowchart. By collecting and analyzing a vast amount of data, the machine creates new rule sets based on observations and arrives at a diagnosis. This approach facilitates data collection, identifies outstanding issues, and saves time compared with traditional alternatives. Studies have shown that predictive modeling of EHR can achieve up to 75% accuracy, leading to a doubling of online health records every five years [32].

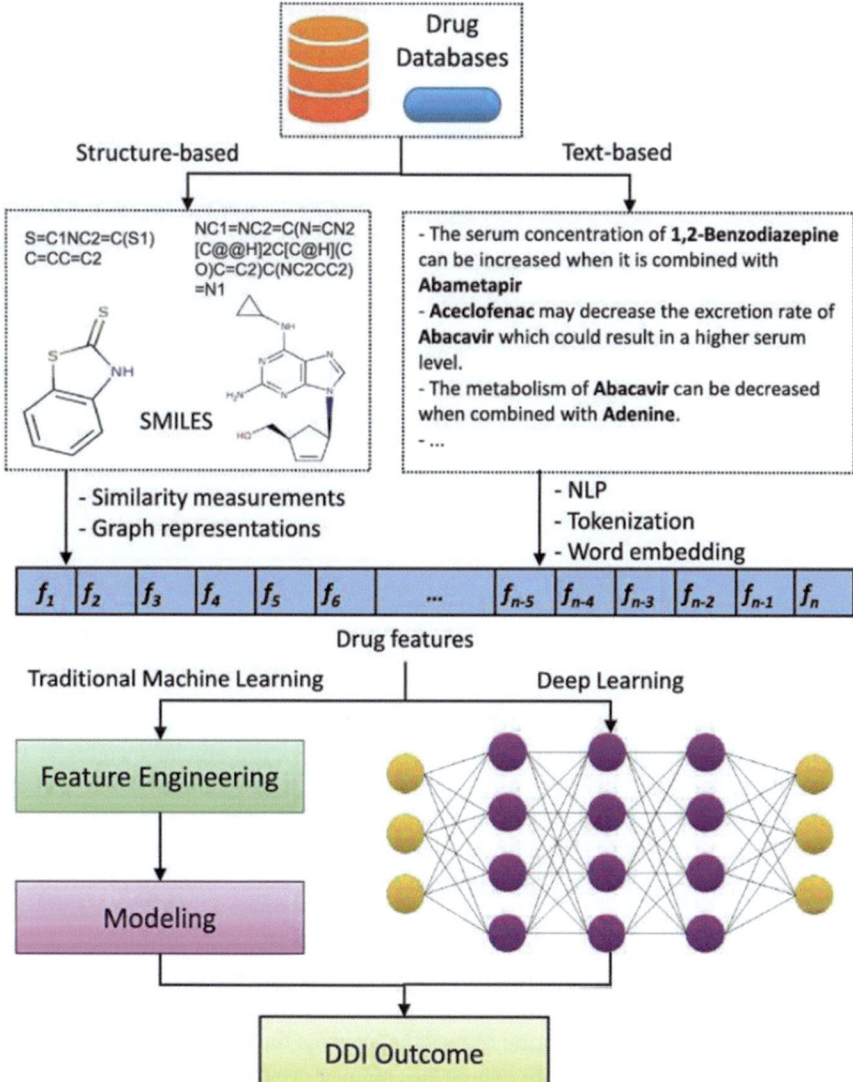

Fig. 49.3 Overall workflow of traditional ML and DL for DDI prediction. (Image source [30])

In addition, advancements in natural language processing (NLP) have resulted in the emergence of AI-powered medical transcription solutions, such as AI-powered voice assistants, which aid in converting medical audio recordings into text format [32].

Suki is an AI-powered voice assistant designed to alleviate the administrative workload of healthcare professionals. Dubbed "Alexa for Doctors," Suki enables clinicians to dictate voice notes during patient examinations, which are instantly transcribed and seamlessly integrated into the Electronic Health Record (EHR)

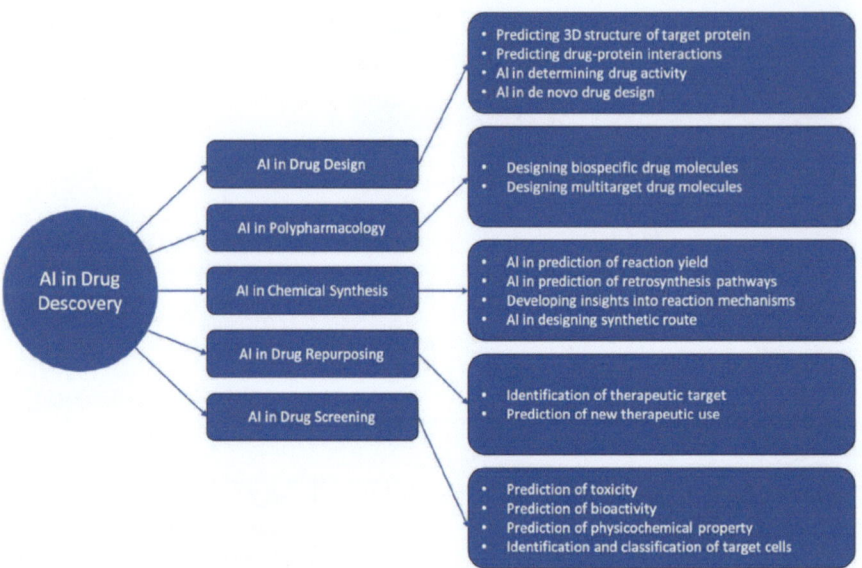

Fig. 49.4 Role of artificial intelligence (AI) in drug discovery. AI can be used effectively in different parts of drug discovery, including drug design, chemical synthesis, drug screening, polypharmacology, and drug repurposing. (Source: Adapted from [31])

system. Similar to how Alexa functions, doctors can also use voice commands to retrieve patient information from the system, providing crucial insights at the point of care. Suki claims that its digital assistant has significantly reduced the time physicians spend on documentation, with an average note-taking time reduction of 76% across users. Previously, it took over 13 minutes on average to complete a note, whereas now it only takes slightly over 3 minutes [32].

- *Digital Twin*
  Digital twin technology, initially introduced in the domains of production and engineering during the advent of Industry 4.0, has also made significant strides in the healthcare sector, representing a potentially transformative development. A digital twin refers to a digital replica that enables the modeling of the status of a physical system or asset. In healthcare, notable progress has been made in the creation of digital twins for both patients and medical devices. The digital twin of a patient is generated by transferring the individual's physical attributes and bodily changes into a digital environment. This technology presents innovative and comprehensive solutions for accurate diagnosis and the subsequent monitoring of treatment processes tailored to each patient, aligning with the fundamental principles of medicine. Simultaneously, the application of this technology is evident in personalized medicine research and the pharmaceutical industry, offering new possibilities for advancement [33].

Further details of AI applications in healthcare include the following [34]:

- AI-Powered Virtual Assistants: By 2022, chatbots driven by AI were expected to save approximately $8 billion annually across various sectors, including retail, e-commerce, banking, and, notably, healthcare. In the healthcare domain, AI-powered chatbots can aid physicians in diagnosing patients by engaging in a series of questions and providing recommendations based on the user's selected answers from a predefined set of choices.
- Robot-Mediated Explanation of Lab Results: Robots can take on the task of explaining lab results, relieving doctors of this responsibility and allowing them to focus on more critical aspects of patient care.
- AI-Assisted Surgery: AI assistance in surgical procedures can help reduce variations that may impact patient health and long-term recovery.
- Personalized AI-Powered Health Companions: Personal health companions equipped with AI can offer tailored medical assistance to track a patient's health, provide insights, and enhance the patient's understanding of any changes in their well-being.
- Cancer Detection Using Deep Learning: Deep learning algorithms are currently being applied in healthcare for the detection of cancer using gene expression data.
- AI in Pathology: AI-powered solutions have the potential to assist pathologists by streamlining their efforts and improving the accuracy of decision-making processes.
- AI-Enabled Detection of Rare Diseases: AI technologies can support healthcare providers in identifying rare diseases, employing techniques such as facial recognition software combined with machine learning to detect patterns in facial expressions and recognize potential indicators of rare diseases.
- Medication Management with AI: AI applications can facilitate autonomous confirmation of whether a patient is consistently adhering to their prescribed medication regimen.
- Health Monitoring with AI and Wearables: AI algorithms integrated with wearable devices enable the detection of exercise patterns and can send alerts if a routine is missed, promoting proactive health monitoring.

49.5 UAE Healthcare: The Beginning of the AI Revolution

The UAE is a trailblazer in global technology and medical innovation. It has positioned itself triumphantly as a global leader in embracing the Fourth Industrial Revolution (4IR). The UAE made history in 2017 by becoming the first country to appoint a dedicated Minister of State for Artificial Intelligence, Omar Bin Sultan Al Olama [35]. This strategic move by the UAE government reflects its commitment to driving technological advancements and innovation in the country. This development has had a significant impact on the healthcare sector, paving the way for new technological innovations.

Under the UAE's Vision 2021 [36], which focuses on achieving "world-class healthcare," the country has gained recognition for its exceptional healthcare ecosystem. The UAE has set remarkable benchmarks in combating the COVID-19 pandemic and is now facing the challenges posed by urbanization and the increasing burden of chronic diseases, which further emphasize the need for healthcare innovation.

A study on cancer care perspectives in Arab countries revealed disparities in cancer care burden in the UAE, influenced by factors such as gender, location, and other variables. Additionally, crises like conflict zones and the growing immigrant population have added strain to oncology care organizations and providers in several countries [37].

The Ministry of Health in the UAE has introduced new technologies that are revolutionizing the healthcare sector. For instance, innovative solutions like health monitoring pods have been implemented to detect early signs of illness and monitor individuals' health. The government also plans to launch an AI-enabled 24/7 video consultation service for global patients. Moreover, the Dubai Healthcare Authority (DHA) intends to utilize artificial intelligence for the treatment of diabetic retinopathy, a severe condition that can lead to permanent vision loss. Another groundbreaking innovation is the Healthcare and Innovative New Technology (HINT) neuroband, which can detect strokes in individuals [38].

The Ministry of Health has recently introduced the Enayati platform, an AI-based preventive healthcare system, as part of the country's National Agenda 2021. This platform has the ability to predict potential health risks and monitor health indicators. Equipped with sensors, the platform connects cardiac patients to healthcare authorities, providing real-time health data and triggering immediate actions in case of cardio-related issues [38].

Furthermore, the UAE government has made significant strides in the field of 3D printing in healthcare. Partnering with the additive manufacturing healthcare specialist firm Sinterex, the Dubai Health Authority (DHA) has established 3D printing labs in its hospitals. This initiative allows medical professionals to create patient-specific anatomical models, facilitating detailed preoperative analysis and enhancing patient communication. By utilizing these models, hospitals are projected to save over $3700 per surgery [39].

The workflow for 3D printing in healthcare begins with acquiring patient data, typically from CT or MRI scans. This data is then processed using medical image segmentation software to isolate the specific anatomical region of interest. The resulting digital model is converted into a 3D-printable file and produced using advanced 3D printers in the lab [39].

49.5.1 Virtual Hospitals and Telemedicine in the UAE

Du, a telecommunications company based in Dubai, has approached the Ministry of Health in the UAE with a proposal to introduce groundbreaking innovations that will revolutionize the healthcare industry. In January, Du signed a memorandum of understanding (MoU) with the Ministry of Health, outlining its plans to develop and provide intelligent healthcare services, which will include a telemedicine application [38].

The Dubai Health Authority (DHA) launched the "24/7 Doctor for Every Citizen" initiative in 2019, aligning with the directives of His Highness Sheikh Mohammed bin Rashid Al Maktoum, the Vice President and Prime Minister of the UAE and Ruler of Dubai [40].

The world's first telehealth-dedicated facility, an e-Hospital, is operated by the USA-based Mercy Virtual Care Centre. In Abu Dhabi, the Mubadala Telemedicine Centre offers telehealth services such as round-the-clock medical consultations over the phone. In 2019, Orient Insurance and Allianz Care introduced the country's inaugural telemedicine service for international health insurance customers [38].

Aster DM Healthcare and HealthHub, private healthcare units based in Dubai and owned by Al-Futtaim, have also launched their own video-conferencing consultation services. The Telecommunications Regulatory Authority (TRA) of the UAE has granted permission for companies to launch telemedicine solutions within the country. Okadoc, a platform for booking doctor appointments, expressed interest in launching telemedicine solutions in the second half of the year but expedited its plans due to the COVID-19 crisis, launching the solution in May. TruDoc 24x7 is another prominent telemedicine company in the UAE, providing subscribers with the ability to directly consult with doctors via video, phone, or live chat at any time and from anywhere in the world. Their services include specialist referrals, prescriptions, medicine deliveries, and telemonitoring. Wellness services offered by TruDoc 24x7 encompass access to wellness experts at any time, personalized nutrition and exercise plans, as well as programs for weight management, sleep disorders, and pregnancy [38].

49.5.2 Robotic Surgery in the UAE

Healthcare in the UAE has experienced a surge in demand for innovative robotic procedures in the Middle East. This growth is expected to continue as both the public and private healthcare sectors expand their spending and as patient awareness rises. The UAE government recognizes the importance of digital transformation and artificial intelligence in supporting long-term growth in the rapidly evolving healthcare landscape.

Surgeons who utilize robotic systems report improved accuracy, flexibility, and control during surgeries, surpassing conventional methods. These systems involve surgeons operating instruments attached to mechanical arms, providing them with a high-definition, three-dimensional view of the surgical site. The advancements in technology, including artificial intelligence, virtual reality, robotics, and the Internet of Things, have significantly influenced the healthcare sector. Over the past decade, research and development efforts have broadened the range of robotic applications, ranging from nurse robots and disinfecting robots to endoscopic systems, as well as more sophisticated devices like snake-like robots and nanobots capable of precise operations within the human body. The UAE has witnessed a noticeable increase in the adoption of robotics in healthcare.

One of the most advanced surgical technologies available is the da Vinci Surgical System, which has been implemented at Mediclinic City Hospital in Dubai, UAE. The da Vinci robotic surgery system is renowned worldwide for its cutting-edge capabilities in conducting laparoscopic surgery, providing patients with superior surgical experiences and outcomes. The hospital performed its inaugural robotic surgery in 2015 and, in 2018, accomplished the first robotic "Whipple" procedure for the treatment of pancreatic and duodenal tumors. With its minimally invasive approach, the da Vinci Surgical System offers both open surgery and laparoscopy alternatives [41].

In July 2020, a robot surgeon employed the da Vinci robotic surgical system to successfully remove a 5-kg tumor from a 44-year-old woman's ovaries at Sharjah's Al Qassimi Hospital for Women and Children. This complex surgery utilized advanced instruments and a high-definition 3D view of the surgical area, facilitated by the da Vinci system's capabilities. The Ministry of Health and Prevention (MoHAP) has performed over 135 active gynecological surgeries using the da Vinci robotic technique, with the assistance of visiting consultants. Minimally invasive surgery techniques are commonly employed in urology and gynecology [41].

Mediclinic International's subsidiary recently introduced the da Vinci Xi HD 4-arm robotic system at Dubai's Mediclinic City Hospital. Developed by Intuitive, this system is recognized as one of the most innovative laparoscopic surgical technologies available. It is part of the hospital's initiative to expand its comprehensive general surgery and laparoscopic surgery services. Additionally, Mediclinic City Hospital has pioneered robotic-assisted total or partial knee replacement surgery in the UAE, showcasing its commitment to robotics in healthcare [41].

At Abu Dhabi-based Sheikh Shakhbout Medical City (SSMC), the largest hospital in the UAE for serious and complex care, surgeons performed the first-ever robot-assisted surgery. SSMC is a joint venture between Mayo Clinic and Abu Dhabi Health Services Company (SEHA). The surgery was a part of the hospital's comprehensive robotic surgery program launch, aiming to enhance and enable minimally invasive procedures and improve clinical outcomes [41].

The Emirates Health Services Corporation is highly committed to incorporating new robotic technologies into surgical procedures and has made significant efforts to enhance its achievements in artificial intelligence. This aligns with the UAE government's strategic vision to establish the Middle East as a hub for the integration of AI into healthcare, particularly in the field of robotic surgery.

In 2014, the Ministry of Health and Prevention announced the introduction of the first robotic system for catheterization and cardiac surgery, utilizing computerized systems. The device was installed at Al Qasimi Hospital, where the first surgery using this technology took place in June 2014 [41].

In April 2019, the Ministry of Health and Prevention initiated the Gynecology and Obstetrics Robotic Surgeries Program. This program was launched following the successful application of robotics in heart surgery, as the robotic arm's precision and ability to reach complex areas of the human body proved beneficial [41].

The cost of robotic procedures can vary, and insurance coverage for such surgeries also varies. However, due to the continuous efforts of the UAE government, most insurances at Mediclinic City Hospital now cover laparoscopic surgeries. It is anticipated that insurers will further evaluate the benefits for patients and consider covering robotic procedures in the future. Despite the high cost of the da Vinci device, the Ministry of Health places special emphasis on strengthening the UAE's global leadership in terms of the number of accredited health facilities. Al Qassimi Hospital in Sharjah has received recognition as a center of excellence from the Joint Commission International (JCI). This achievement enhances the UAE's global leadership position in terms of the number of health facilities obtaining international JCI accreditation [41].

The notable accomplishments of Al Qassimi Hospital, one of the leading medical establishments under the Ministry of Health and Prevention, contribute to its growing reputation in the field of complex and unconventional medical procedures, including robotic cardiac procedures. The UAE ranks first globally in various key competitiveness studies, including the internationally accredited index of health facilities, which is effectively managed and monitored by the Ministry of Health in collaboration with health authorities [41].

MOHAP believes that the UAE has entered a new era of excellence in recent years, attaining advanced positions in various international metrics and reports. Recognizing the medical and therapeutic capabilities of robotic techniques, the Ministry of Health is keen to promote the adoption of these technologies in the UAE, as they are expected to bring about a transformative change in health and rehabilitation services [41].

49.5.3 First E-Hospital in the UAE and Further Developments

Mulk Healthcare, a healthcare company based in Sharjah, has announced the introduction of the first virtual hospital in the Middle East through their app. This innovative e-hospital app will provide a range of healthcare services, including medication delivery, appointment booking, consultations with medical specialists, health insurance approvals, diagnosis, and prescription services. Users can easily connect with over 2,000 medical specialists from various countries, including India, Pakistan, Thailand, the USA, the UK, and select European countries. With just a click, users can access initial consultations with doctors and receive post-hospital care, all from the convenience of their homes. The global telemedicine technologies market was valued at $17.8 billion in 2014, and it is anticipated to experience significant growth [38].

Additionally, the Dubai Health Authority (DHA) has developed the Tifli app, specifically designed for parents and expectant mothers seeking personalized, evidence-based content to guide them through the journey of pregnancy, childbirth, and parenthood. Through this app, users can connect with various DHA hospitals and doctors to seek clarification on their concerns. The application also enables users to monitor and track parameters such as weight, blood pressure, daily activity, and meditation, while also providing a search feature to find experienced doctors [38].

In early 2017, the Ministry of Health and Prevention (MoHaP) launched a robotic pharmacy at Al Fujairah Hospital's external clinics. The purpose of this robotic pharmacy is to minimize the risk of dispensing incorrect medications and reduce waiting times [42]. The DHA also introduced a robot-based smart pharmacy in 2018 to streamline the process of dispensing and prescribing medications. Patients can purchase their prescribed medications by scanning the barcode. The robotic system has a storage capacity of 35,000 medications and can dispense up to nine prescriptions per minute [38].

49.5.4 Smart Dubai Initiative

Smart Dubai, the government office responsible for transforming the UAE, has recently launched an AI-based solution aimed at enhancing healthcare services. This AI technology is specifically designed to assist doctors in monitoring patients' vital signs, including pulse, temperature, blood pressure, and other key indicators. In collaboration with the Dubai Health Authority (DHA) and IBM, Smart Dubai has developed this AI initiative as part of their AI Lab program. The long-term vision for this AI application is to provide advanced services that can significantly improve healthcare outcomes. During the proof-of-concept phase, the AI system was trained on patient data collected from various hospitals, such as Hatta Hospital, Latifa Hospital, and Dubai Hospital [38, 43].

The results of the proof-of-concept were remarkable, demonstrating that the AI technology achieved an accuracy rate of 90–98% in detecting deteriorating health conditions in patients within a timeframe of 1–20 hours. Additionally, the AI system will record vital information during emergency situations, such as a patient's worsening condition. These pilot features will enable the DHA and participating hospitals to gain valuable insights and enhance their understanding of the system's development [38, 43].

The successful pilot program highlights the potential of AI as an advanced system that can save lives by accurately collecting data and responding to patients' conditions appropriately. It also provides hospitals with insights into effectively managing resources, including doctors and nurses. By leveraging such technology, medical professionals can enhance their performance and focus on areas that require improvement. Moreover, the AI system provides complex insights to the medical staff, further supporting their decision-making process [38]. Smart Dubai's 2021 strategy aims to improve the quality of life for individuals by embracing technology and streamlining social, cultural, educational, and healthcare experiences within the emirate [43].

49.5.5 Strategic Partnerships in Healthcare AI

Like in every other sector, cross-pollination is important in the AI-driven healthcare sector. InHealth, a health technology company based in the UK, has joined forces with Saal, an Abu Dhabi-based AI company, to leverage the power of artificial intelligence and introduce state-of-the-art healthcare solutions at a reduced cost. This collaboration, announced in the latter part of 2019, aims to explore untapped areas and enhance healthcare services for residents in the UAE and the wider Middle East region. The partnership aligns with the UAE's vision of becoming a global tech hub, with the support of the country's private sector. Both companies will identify collaborative opportunities for joint AI initiatives, with Saal playing a significant role by providing AI-based healthcare tools for InHealth's extensive product portfolio. The joint initiatives will focus on improving patients' lifestyles and enhancing the quality of healthcare facilities [38].

Within Saal's portfolio, their innovative AI-based healthcare solutions assist patients through features such as symptom diagnosis checkers, lifestyle disease checkers, and medical image recognition. Patients can engage with Saal's health advisor in either English or Arabic, benefiting from advanced features like an AI chatbot interface capable of recognizing medical intent and handling indirect queries. This unique product greatly contributes to patient satisfaction. Saal also offers a specialized solution for hospitals and care centers known as the "no-show predictor," which boasts an impressive accuracy rate of nearly 80% in predicting patients' attendance for appointments [38].

Turning to inHealth's portfolio, their solutions are currently utilized by 17,000 end users across 4,500 pharmacies, hospitals, and clinics. The company develops a wide range of advanced cognitive solutions, products, and platforms to tackle real-life challenges in sectors such as public services, healthcare, education, and banking. One notable solution is the Health Information Exchange platform (HIE), which serves as the first unified platform solution for electronic prescription and medication dispensation [38].

In other collaborations within the healthcare sector, Abu Dhabi Health Services Company (SEHA) has signed a Memorandum of Understanding (MoU) with the Mohamed bin Zayed University of Artificial Intelligence (MBZUAI) to explore and introduce AI-driven solutions that address prominent healthcare challenges and enhance patient-centered services [44]. Mubadala Health, the healthcare unit of Abu Dhabi, has also entered into a preliminary agreement with G42 Healthcare to foster collaboration in the healthcare sector and seek innovative solutions for treating chronic diseases [45]. Additionally, AstraZeneca, a British-Swedish biotechnology and pharmaceutical multinational, has partnered with G42 Healthcare, one of Abu Dhabi's leading healthtech firms, to enhance research and diagnostic frameworks in the United Arab Emirates. Their collaboration will primarily focus on analyzing real-world data and conducting medical trials [46].

49.5.6 UAE's Launch of AI for Monitoring Vital Signs

At Arab Health 2019, the Ministry of Health in the UAE introduced Medopad, an AI-based smart application designed to remotely monitor the vital signs of the body. This innovative application has the potential to analyze patient information and provide predictive insights to detect life-threatening medical conditions. Developed with patients' needs in mind, Medopad is compatible with both iOS and Android devices. By collecting data through connected devices and supporting self-management through a dashboard, the application primarily gathers information related to daily activities like walking and running. By remotely analyzing, reviewing, and documenting patients' data and information, the application enables medical care teams to provide personalized care that suits each individual's needs. This AI-powered application also offers educational and awareness content for patients undergoing pre- and postoperative care, as well as those with conditions such as cancer, multiple sclerosis, kidney and heart diseases, chronic obstructive pulmonary disease (COPD), Parkinson's disease, and others [38, 41].

Additionally, the UAE has pioneered a research endeavor focused on monitoring vital signs using radar technology. This advancement aims to wirelessly monitor vital signs such as blood pressure and heart rate. Scientists envision the potential application of radar in public settings, such as airports, to monitor passenger health and prevent the spread of future pandemics [47].

49.5.7 The UAE's Ministry of Health's Recent Developments

In a collaborative effort, the Ministry of Health in the UAE has partnered with Pure Health, a prominent healthcare and medical supply company, to introduce an AI-based device aimed at assisting with irregular heartbeats and proactively preventing heart disease. This lightweight device, weighing 8 g, measures and monitors the heart's electrical signals through an electrocardiogram, offering a user-friendly solution for individuals with heart conditions to utilize anytime and anywhere. The results can be conveniently accessed through a companion smart app compatible with smartphones, desktops, and smartwatches. Furthermore, doctors have access to a dedicated website and a cloud portal where they can download and analyze patient records [38].

Additionally, the UAE's Ministry of Health has introduced a health information exchange system called Malaffi. This centralized platform is designed to enhance healthcare connectivity throughout the emirate of Abu Dhabi. It connects over 2000 public and private healthcare providers, catering to the healthcare needs of over three million individuals in the country. The implementation of Malaffi is expected to revolutionize healthcare delivery by streamlining services, reducing duplication, and enabling physicians to make faster and more efficient decisions. As a result, healthcare units are anticipated to experience improved quality of care and better patient outcomes. Reports suggest that the majority of the UAE's population is receptive to the deployment of AI systems in healthcare, indicating a willingness to embrace doctors who are adept at utilizing AI tools. This demonstrates a readiness for change among consumers in the UAE, even though many may not fully comprehend its full potential of AI in healthcare [38].

49.5.8 UAE Health Tech Start-Up Landscape

Artificial intelligence (AI)-based technologies are set to revolutionize the healthcare sector in the UAE by enabling a shift toward preventive medicine rather than solely relying on curative approaches [48]. The UAE's health technology domain is thriving, supported by abundant resources and a conducive infrastructure. The country is home to numerous successful health tech companies, with 405 health-tech startups recorded as of 2022 [49]. These include telemedicine platforms such as Okadoc, Altibbi, Insta Doctor, Health at Hand, Medcare, and TruDoc 24/7, as well as automated medical image analysis software like Prognica. Additionally, companies like DhonorHealthtech leverage blockchain solutions to facilitate safer and more streamlined organ donor matching and verification [50–52].

According to a report by Ken Research titled "UAE Health Tech Market Outlook to 2026: Driven by Increasing Demand for Faster Delivery & Convenience and Shifting Customer Behavior," the UAE health tech market offers various conveniences, including fast doorstep delivery of pharmaceutical products, convenient and instant teleconsultation services, and software products utilized by hospitals, pharmacies, and clinics. The market is experiencing significant growth due to factors such as the rise in chronic and lifestyle diseases, an aging population, increased private and public expenditure on healthcare, and a shift in consumer behavior during the pandemic [53].

The health tech industry in the UAE was expected to exhibit a double-digit compound annual growth rate (CAGR) between 2018 and 2021. The increasing trend of self-diagnosis among the population, improved affordability through online platforms with tax relaxations, and subscription-based benefits are further fueling the growth of the health tech market [53].

According to the report, the UAE's e-pharmacy market is predicted to experience a double-digit compound annual growth rate (CAGR) from 2022 to 2026, driven by technological advancements such as remote monitoring and data analytics to predict customer preferences and drug demand. The integration of fully virtual and near-virtual health solutions will bring care closer to home, offering increased convenience for patients to access healthcare services. The online consultation sector is expected to exhibit a significant double-digit CAGR from 2022 to 2026. Future trends in the market will be characterized by enhanced security services, big data analytics, and cloud computing, which are poised to dominate the industry. The market's growth, based on the gross transaction volume (GTV), is expected to expand at a double-digit CAGR between 2022 and 2026. Technologies such as mobile medical units, intermediaries, virtual reality (VR), artificial intelligence (AI), and blockchain are set to revolutionize the healthcare industry [53].

49.5.9 AI Policy by the Department of Health, Abudhabi (DOH)

The use of artificial intelligence (AI) in the healthcare sector of Abu Dhabi is governed by the AI Policy established in 2018. The Department of Health (DOH) recognizes the significant role of AI in healthcare and acknowledges the potential benefits it offers. The DOH supports and promotes the development, utilization, and adoption of customized AI technologies and software in healthcare within Abu Dhabi. It also prioritizes patient safety by minimizing potential risks associated with AI implementation [54].

The DOH aims to maximize the advantages of using AI in healthcare services, including enhanced efficiency, effectiveness, quality, sustainability, and accessibility. Simultaneously, it strives to minimize any potential risks to patient safety, treatment outcomes, and overall experience. The role of AI in healthcare service delivery is seen as a supportive technology that benefits various stakeholders, including healthcare regulators, providers, insurers, and practitioners [54].

Specifically, AI is utilized to enhance data analysis, draw conclusions, and support decision-making processes for healthcare regulators, providers, and insurers. It aids healthcare practitioners in improving the accuracy of diagnoses and prognoses, and in formulating and implementing appropriate treatment plans. Additionally, AI is encouraged to facilitate research and development (R&D) efforts focused on new treatments and precision medicine. The guiding principles for this AI policy are as follows [54]:

- Verifiability and Explainability: AI software should be capable of being verified and explained, enabling the identification of causes in the event of system failures.
- User Assistance and Supportive Technology: AI should support users by providing them with meaningful opportunities to make informed decisions using suggestions based on probabilities generated by AI.
- Safety and Security: AI systems must prioritize safety and security to prevent harm to users, their well-being, or the well-being of third parties. Ensuring the reliability and robustness of AI is essential.
- Privacy: Privacy considerations should be incorporated into AI to prevent the infringement of privacy rights for users or third parties.
- Ethics: The research and development of AI should uphold human dignity and respect individual autonomy.
- Accountability: Researchers and developers of AI should be accountable to users and other stakeholders. They should provide relevant explanations, disclose information, and maintain effective communication with stakeholders.

49.6 AI: A Game Changer in the Global Economy

The introduction of AI is anticipated to have a transformative impact on the global economy, presenting significant opportunities for value creation. By 2030, AI has the potential to contribute up to $15.7 trillion to the global economy, surpassing the combined current output of China and India. Out of this amount, approximately $6.6 trillion is projected to arise from increased productivity, while $9.1 trillion is expected to stem from consumer-related benefits [34, 55]. In the healthcare sector of the UAE, which ranks among the top 20 countries globally in terms of per capita healthcare expenditure ($1,200 or AED 4,400), there is a receptive environment for the integration of AI-based healthcare solutions. This is further evidenced by the implementation of AI policies by the major healthcare regulators in the Emirates of Dubai and Abu Dhabi, underscoring the UAE's commitment to harnessing the potential of AI in healthcare [34].

The global market size of AI in healthcare reached USD 10.4 billion in 2021 and is projected to grow at a compound annual growth rate (CAGR) of 38.4% from 2022 to 2030. This growth is driven by factors such as the expanding volume of patient health-related digital data, the increasing demand for personalized medicine, and the need to reduce healthcare costs. The growing global elderly population, changing lifestyles, and rising prevalence of chronic diseases have contributed to the increasing demand for early disease diagnosis and a better understanding of diseases in their initial stages. To achieve these objectives, healthcare systems are increasingly incorporating AI and machine learning algorithms, leveraging historical health datasets to accurately predict diseases in their early stages [56].

49.7 Conclusion

AI holds immense potential, ranging from streamlining processes to potentially saving lives. Despite the ethical and practical challenges, AI has demonstrated its promising integration into healthcare to enhance patient outcomes. Countries like the UAE are actively creating an environment conducive to fostering an agile and sustainable healthcare ecosystem by recognizing the productivity-enhancing capabilities of smart technologies. The UAE has introduced innovative development strategies, such as the Dubai Strategy Plan 2030, which emphasizes the importance of 3D printing technology [57]. Additionally, the Department of Health, Abu Dhabi (DoH), has implemented the Abu Dhabi Healthcare Information Security Strategy, which aims to establish a comprehensive and proactive framework to address current and future healthcare cybersecurity challenges in Abu Dhabi. This strategy maintains a focus on digital transformation, enabling technology, innovation, and the adoption of AI in the emirate's healthcare sector [58]. By embracing technology, the UAE continues to lead as a frontrunner in the Fourth Industrial Revolution (4IR).

Conflicts of Interest The authors have no conflicts of interest to declare.

References

1. Artificial Intelligence in Healthcare – JavaTpoint, Webpage – JavaTpoint. https://www.javatpoint.com/artificial-intelligence-in-healthcare#:~:text=AI%20is%20used%20in%20various%20areas%20of%20healthcare,electronic%20health%20records%20for%20disease%20prevention%20and%20diagnosis. Accessed on November 10.

2. 40 AI in Healthcare examples improving the future of medicine by Sam Daley, 40 AI in Healthcare Examples Transforming Medicine | Built In, Webpage – Built In. https://builtin.com/artificial-intelligence/artificial-intelligence-healthcare. Accessed on November 10.
3. A Brief History of Artificial Intelligence by Keith D. Foote on January 17, 2022, DATAVERSITY, Webpage. https://www.dataversity.net/brief-history-artificial-intelligence/. Accessed on November 10.
4. AI in Medicine and Healthcare – A Brief History & Implications for the Future by Krishnan Narayanan, Published on August 4, 2021. https://analyticsindiamag.com/ai-in-medicine-and-healthcare-a-brief-history-implications-for-the-future/#:~:text=The%20genesis%20of%20AI%20in%20medicine%20and%20healthcare,paper%20that%20launched%20the%20field%20of%20medical%20informatics. Accessed on November 10.
5. Kaul V, Enslin S, Gross SA. History of artificial intelligence in medicine. Gastrointest Endosc. 2020;92(4):807–12. ISSN 0016-5107, https://doi.org/10.1016/j.gie.2020.06.040, https://www.sciencedirect.com/science/article/pii/S0016510720344667.
6. Ruffle JK, Farmer AD, Aziz Q. Artificial intelligence-assisted gastroenterology—promises and pitfalls. Am J Gastroenterol. 2019;114:422–8.
7. Moran ME. Evolution of robotic arms. J Robot Surg. 2007;1:103–11.
8. Weizenbaum J. ELIZA—a computer program for the study of natural language communication between man and machine. Commun ACM. 1966;9:36–45.
9. Kuipers BF, Hart PE, Nilsson NJ. Shakey: from conception to history. AI Mag. 2017;38:88–103.
10. Kulikowski CA. Beginnings of artificial intelligence in medicine (AIM): computational artifice assisting scientific inquiry and clinical art—with reflections on present AIM challenges. Yearb Med Inform. 2019;28:249–56.
11. Greenhill AEB. A primer of AI in medicine. Tech Gastrointest Endosc. 2020;22:85–9.
12. Kulikowski CA. An opening chapter of the first generation of artificial intelligence in medicine: the first Rutgers AIM workshop, June 1975. Yearb Med Inform. 2015;10:227–33.
13. Weiss S, Kulikowski CA, Safir A. Glaucoma consultation by computer. Comput Biol Med. 1978;8:25–40.
14. Shortliffe EH, Davis R, Axline SG, et al. Computer-based consultations in clinical therapeutics: explanation and rule acquisition capabilities of the MYCIN system. Comput Biomed Res. 1975;8:303–20.
15. Amisha, Malik P, Pathania M, et al. Overview of artificial intelligence in medicine. J Family Med Prim Care. 2019;8:2328–31.
16. Ferrucci DL, Bagchi S, Gondek D, et al. Watson: beyond Jeopardy! Artif Intell. 2013;199–200:93–105.
17. Bakkar N, Kovalik T, Lorenzini I, et al. Artificial intelligence in neurodegenerative disease research: use of IBM Watson to identify additional RNA-binding proteins altered in amyotrophic lateral sclerosis. Acta Neuropathol. 135:227–47.
18. Comendador B, Francisco B, Medenilla J, et al. Pharmabot: a pediatric generic medicine consultant chatbot. J Autom Control Eng. 2015;3:137–40.
19. Ni L, Lu C, Liu N, et al. MANDY: towards a smart primary care chatbot application. In: Chen J, Theeramunkong T, Supnithi T, Tang X, editors. Knowledge and systems sciences. KSS 2017, Communications in computer and information science, vol. 780. Singapore: Springer.
20. Yang YJ, Bang CS. Application of artificial intelligence in gastroenterology. World J Gastroenterol. 2019;25:1666–83.
21. Secinaro S, Calandra D, Secinaro A, Muthurangu V, Biancone P. The role of artificial intelligence in healthcare: a structured literature review. BMC Med Inform Decis Mak. 2021;21(1):125. https://doi.org/10.1186/s12911-021-01488-9. PMID: 33836752; PMCID: PMC8035061.
22. Shaikh K, Krishnan S, Thanki R. Artificial intelligence in breast cancer early detection and diagnosis. Cham: Springer; 2021. https://doi.org/10.1007/978-3-030-59208-0.
23. Das K, Cockerell CJ, Patil A, Pietkiewicz P, Giulini M, Grabbe S, Goldust M. Machine learning and its application in skin cancer. Int J Environ Res Public Health. 2021;18(24):13409. https://doi.org/10.3390/ijerph182413409. PMID: 34949015; PMCID: PMC8705277.

24. An artificial intelligence tool that can help detect melanoma, MIT News, Megan Lewis | Institute for Medical Engineering and Science, Publication Date: April 2, 2021, Massachusetts Institute of Technology, Webpage. https://news.mit.edu/2021/artificial-intelligence-tool-can-help-detect-melanoma-0402. Accessed on November 23.
25. Fakhoury M. Artificial intelligence in psychiatry. Adv Exp Med Biol. 2019;1192:119–25. https://doi.org/10.1007/978-981-32-9721-0_6. PMID: 31705492.
26. Pham KT, Nabizadeh A, Selek S. Artificial intelligence and chatbots in psychiatry. Psychiatry Q. 2022;93(1):249–53. https://doi.org/10.1007/s11126-022-09973-8. Epub 2022 Feb 25. PMID: 35212940; PMCID: PMC8873348.
27. AI, The Use Of Artificial Intelligence In Primary Care, Rita, October 9, 2022, Surfactants, Webpage. https://www.surfactants.net/the-use-of-artificial-intelligence-in-primary-care/#:~:text=One%20way%20AI%20can%20be%20used%20in%20primary,symptoms%20that%20may%20point%20to%20a%20particular%20diagnosis. Accessed on November 23.
28. Kumar Y, Koul A, Singla R, Ijaz MF. Artificial intelligence in disease diagnosis: a systematic literature review, synthesizing framework and future research agenda. J Ambient Intell Humaniz Comput. 2023;14:1–28. https://doi.org/10.1007/s12652-021-03612-z. Epub ahead of print. PMID: 35039756; PMCID: PMC8754556.
29. Subasi A. Use of artificial intelligence in Alzheimer's disease detection. In: Artificial intelligence in precision health. London: Academic Press; 2020. https://doi.org/10.1016/B978-0-12-817133-2.00011-2.
30. Vo TH, Nguyen NTK, Kha QH, Le NQK. On the road to explainable AI in drug-drug interactions prediction: a systematic review. Comput Struct Biotechnol J. 2022;20:2112–23. https://doi.org/10.1016/j.csbj.2022.04.021. PMID: 35832629; PMCID: PMC9092071.
31. Paul D, Sanap G, Shenoy S, Kalyane D, Kalia K, Tekade RK. Artificial intelligence in drug discovery and development. Drug Discov Today. 2021;26(1):80–93. https://doi.org/10.1016/j.drudis.2020.10.010. Epub 2020 Oct 21. PMID: 33099022; PMCID: PMC7577280.
32. Electronic Health Records (EHRs): How AI is improving clinician use | Alldus, Webpage. https://alldus.com/blog/articles/electronic-health-records-ehrs-how-ai-is-improving-clinician-use/. Accessed on November 23.
33. TY – BOOK, Erol, Tolga, Mendi, Arif, Dogan, Dilara, 2020/10/22, 1, EP – 7c, T1 – The Digital Twin Revolution in Healthcare, https://doi.org/10.1109/ISMSIT50672.2020.9255249.
34. Impact of Artificial Intelligence (AI) in the UAE Healthcare & Global Economy, Webpage. https://middleeast.siliconindia.com/viewpoint/cxoinsights/impact-of-artificial-intelligence-ai-in-the-uae-healthcare-global-economy-nwid-16630.html. Accessed on November 15.
35. United Arab Emirates Ministry of Cabinet Affairs. https://www.moca.gov.ae/en/about/our-leadership/his-excellency-omar-bin-sultan-al-olama. Accessed on December 16.
36. Home, Webpage. https://www.vision2021.ae/en. Accessed on November 23.
37. Al-Shamsi HO, Abu-Gheida IH, Iqbal F, Al-Awadhi A. Cancer in the Arab world. Singapore: Springer Nature; 2022. https://doi.org/10.1007/978-981-16-7945-2_1.
38. The beginning of AI revolution in UAE healthcare – Global Business Outlook, Global Business Outlook, Webpage. https://www.globalbusinessoutlook.com/the-beginning-of-ai-revolution-in-uae-healthcare/. Accessed on November 11.
39. New DHA 3D printing lab for complex cases | Health – Gulf News, Gulf News, Health, Published on January 19, 2020, Webpage. https://gulfnews.com/uae/health/new-dha-3d-printing-lab-for-complex-cases-1.1579437700172. Accessed on November 11.
40. Doctor for Every citizen, Dubai Health Authority, Webpage. https://www.dha.gov.ae/en/services/details?id=86&segment=individual_services. Accessed on November 11.
41. Robotic Surgery Landscape In The UAE – DUPHAT, Webpage. https://duphat.ae/robotic-surgery-landscape-in-the-uae/#:~:text=Scenario%20in%20The%20United%20Arab%20Emirates. Accessed on November 15.
42. Robotics and AI applications – The Official Portal of the UAE Government, Webpage. https://u.ae/en/about-the-uae/digital-uae/robotics-and-ai-applications. Accessed on November 15.

43. Smart Dubai 2021 Strategy – The Official Portal of the UAE Government, About the UAE, Webpage. https://u.ae/en/about-the-uae/strategies-initiatives-and-awards/local-governments-strategies-and-plans/smart-dubai-2021-strategy. Accessed on November 12.
44. Abu Dhabi's SEHA and MBZUAI join forces to integrate AI in healthcare solutions | Healthcare IT News, Healthcare IT News, Webpage. https://www.healthcareitnews.com/news/emea/abu-dhabi-s-seha-and-mbzuai-join-forces-integrate-ai-healthcare-solutions#:~:text=Artificial%20Intelligence%20Abu%20Dhabi%E2%80%99s%20SEHA%20and%20MBZUAI%20join,technology%20sectors%2C%E2%80%9D%20in%20order%20to%20improve%20patient%20care. Accessed on November 12.
45. Abu Dhabi's Mubadala Health and G42 Healthcare agree to boost collaboration – G42 HealthCare, Webpage. https://www.g42healthcare.ai/latest-update/abu-dhabis-mubadala-health-and-g42-healthcare-agree-to-boost-collaboration/. Accessed on November 15.
46. G42 healthcare partners with AstraZeneca to improve research and diagnostics – Wi4, Webpage. https://nextdigitalhealth.com/g42-healthcare-partners-with-astrazeneca-to-improve-research-and-diagnostics/. Accessed on November 15.
47. Pioneering UAE research monitors vital signs by radar, The National News, Published on April 5, 2020. https://www.thenationalnews.com/uae/health/pioneering-uae-research-monitors-vital-signs-by-radar-1.1002005. Accessed on November 12.
48. Three tech innovations that are transforming UAE healthcare | UAE News, Webpage. https://gulfbusiness.com/three-tech-innovations-transforming-uae-healthcare/. Accessed on November 19.
49. HealthTech Startups in United Arab Emirates | Tracxn, Webpage. https://tracxn.com/explore/HealthTech-Startups-in-United-Arab-Emirates/#:~:text=There%20are%20389%20HealthTech%20startups%20in%20United%20Arab,platform%20for%20doctor%20appointment%20booking%20and%20doctor%20consultation. Accessed on November 19.
50. Telemedicine providers in UAE | Healthcare Business Club, Webpage. https://healthcarebusinessclub.com/articles/consumer/telemedicine-providers-in-uae/. Accessed on November 19.
51. Prognica Labs, Webpage. http://www.prognica.com/. Accessed on November 19.
52. Why Dubai's Healthcare Industry is Exciting for New Businesses, Webpage. https://blog.dmcc.ae/why-dubai-healthcare-industry-is-exciting-for-new-businesses. Accessed on November 19.
53. UAE Health Tech Market Future Outlook to 2026: Ken Research, Webpage. https://www.kenresearch.com/healthcare/general-healthcare/uae-health-tech-market-outlook-to-2026-/581657-91.html. Accessed on November 19.
54. Policies – Resources – Department of Health, DOH Webpage. https://www.doh.gov.ae/en/resources/policies. Accessed on November 19.
55. The potential impact of Artificial Intelligence in the Middle East – PwC Middle East, Webpage. https://www.pwc.com/m1/en/publications/potential-impact-artificial-intelligence-middle-east.html. Accessed on November 19.
56. Artificial Intelligence In Healthcare Market Size, Share, and Trends Analysis Report by Component (Software Solutions, Hardware, Services), by Application (Virtual Assistants, Connected Machines), by Region, and Segment Forecasts, 2022–2030, Report ID: GVR-3-68038-951-7, 2030, Webpage. https://www.grandviewresearch.com/industry-analysis/artificial-intelligence-ai-healthcare-market. Accessed on November 23.
57. 2021–2030 – The Official Portal of the UAE Government, Dubai 3D Printing Strategy, Webpage. https://u.ae/en/more/uae-future/2021-2030. Accessed on 24.
58. Department of Health – Abu Dhabi | News, Webpage. https://www.doh.gov.ae/en/news/DoH-develops-strategy-for-healthcare-information-security. Accessed on November 24.

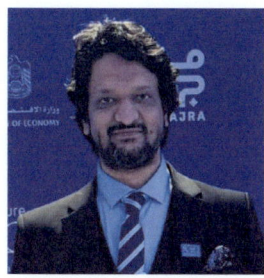

Khalid Shaikh is the founder and CEO of Prognica Labs, a healthcare technology company that specializes in developing AI-powered solutions for breast cancer detection and treatment.

Khalid Shaikh is a serial entrepreneur, author, technocrat, and business strategist. He is also a member of the HBR Advisory Council and has received numerous awards for his innovations and contributions to healthcare and public health.

In addition to his professional commitments, he also gives back to the aspiring entrepreneur community by serving as an advisor and mentor. He has published and lectured extensively on healthcare performance improvement, digitalization, and innovation.

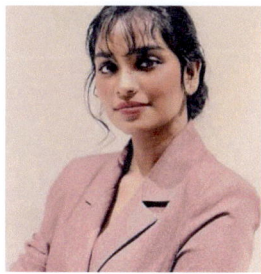

Dr. Sreelekshmi Bekal is an adept and well-mentored healthcare advocate dedicated to accessible top-tier care and AI-driven digital health innovation. Her propensity is "Healthcare for All," leveraging cutting-edge technologies and evidence-based research for healthcare transformation. She is a fervent proponent of multidisciplinary collaboration, policy shaping, and strategic healthcare reform. She is an accomplished public speaker, author, and leads generator with innovative thinking and relationship-building prowess.

Open Access This chapter is licensed under the terms of the Creative Commons Attribution 4.0 International License (http://creativecommons.org/licenses/by/4.0/), which permits use, sharing, adaptation, distribution and reproduction in any medium or format, as long as you give appropriate credit to the original author(s) and the source, provide a link to the Creative Commons license and indicate if changes were made.

The images or other third party material in this chapter are included in the chapter's Creative Commons license, unless indicated otherwise in a credit line to the material. If material is not included in the chapter's Creative Commons license and your intended use is not permitted by statutory regulation or exceeds the permitted use, you will need to obtain permission directly from the copyright holder.

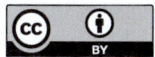

Artificial Intelligence in Radiology in the UAE

50

Ahmed ElSerafi and Mohammad Rawashdeh

50.1 Introduction

Artificial intelligence (AI), a term coined at the Dartmouth conference in 1956, has evolved into a distinct field of computer science [1, 2]. The increasing amount of data being fed to AI, as well as efforts directed toward its development, have allowed it to learn new algorithms and encompass a broad range of applications [3]. AI is already being used in manufacturing, transportation, space exploration, and healthcare [4]. Examples in healthcare include virtual assistants, laparoscopic surgery, robotic assistants for rehabilitation, medical imaging software, and wearable vital monitoring devices [5]. For AI algorithms to be effective, the training of neural networks is necessary to enable the ability to identify pathologies such as coronary artery disease, COPD, pneumothorax, cancers, stroke, or fractures, amongst a multitude of examples, which can present a real challenge even to experts [6]. Radiologists analyze and interpret medical images to detect, monitor, and analyze diseases [7]. The task of detecting, monitoring, and analyzing diseases in accordance with the experience and education of radiologists can be subjective. By integrating AI into clinical processes as a tool for assisting physicians, radiology assessments can be more reproducible and accurate [8].

In this chapter, we define terms commonly used in conjunction with AI in diagnostic imaging, present AI in the context of its applications in the United Arab emirates (UAE), provide an overview of the balance between AI threats and opportunities, and analyze the integration of AI into the radiological workflow.

A. ElSerafi (✉)
Faculty of Medicine, Canal University, Ismailia, Egypt

M. Rawashdeh
Faculty of Health Sciences, Gulf Medical University, Ajman, United Arab Emirates

Faculty of Applied Medical Sciences, Jordan University of Science and Technology, Irbid, Jordan
e-mail: dr.rawahdeh@gmu.ac.ae

50.2 Machine Learning Algorithms

Machine learning algorithms (ML) are a subset of AI that allow computers to mimic humans' output using a defined set of inputs, such as training data, learning graphs, and past experiences, without the intervention of humans [9]. ML possesses three essential aspects: task, experience, and performance [10]. Like humans, ML systems need to learn from accurate and sufficiently large training datasets in order to make accurate inferences from a large set of data [7]. ML techniques can be divided into four categories according to how they learn (Fig. 50.1).

50.2.1 Supervised Learning

Supervised learning involves developing a predictive model using labeled data, i.e., data with known outcomes, known as the "ground truth." In other words, supervised ML involves learning how to produce an output from a given input, with the help of another input-output sample [11]. Supervised learning is a task-driven ML technique in which the machine works to achieve a specific outcome from a particular set of data. Supervised machine learning can be used to resolve common tasks, including regression (relating to or predicting the value or classification label of the data) and classification [12]. In supervised ML, the algorithm is guided by the examples provided to find its own way to achieve a satisfying outcome. Under the supervision and correction of the operator, supervised ML predicts and solves problems until the machine attains a high level of accuracy in completing tasks [10].

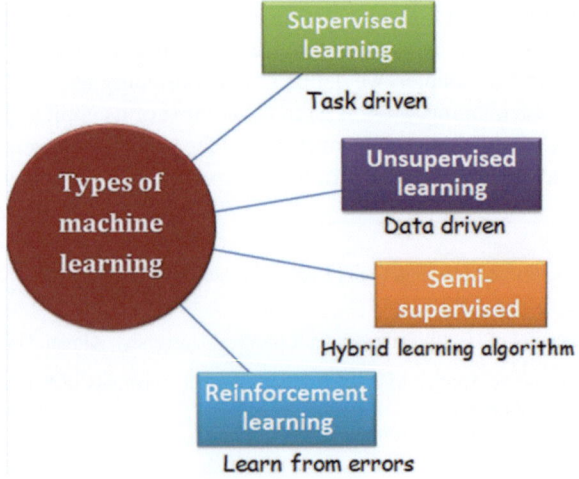

Fig. 50.1 Types of machine learning algorithms and their respective work mechanisms

50.2.2 Unsupervised ML

Data-driven learning is the most basic form of unsupervised machine learning. With unsupervised machine learning, data is unlabeled, and no instructions are given to the algorithm [13]. ML analyzes large data sets and determines the relationships and patterns among them before grouping the data according to those relationships and patterns [11, 12]. As a result of unsupervised ML, unlabeled data is labeled and organized in a way that describes its structure, enhancing the ML's ability to make decisions regarding the data sets. Over time, this refines the outcome of the unsupervised ML algorithm [14]. Unsupervised machine learning tasks include clustering (grouping) and dimensional reduction (refining the variables included in the search) [14].

50.2.3 Semi-Supervised ML

In semi-supervised learning, both unlabelled and labelled data types are used to solve problems. Semi-supervised ML works similarly to supervised ML in that it requires examples of a known dataset in order to learn and perform tasks accordingly. There will be a small amount of labeled data, and a considerable amount of unlabeled data so that the machine can learn from it and develop the ability to predict correctly [8, 13].

50.2.4 Reinforcement ML

Reinforcement machine learning is an environment-driven method of machine learning in which the machine aims to maximize its reward [14, 15]. Maximum rewards can be obtained when the machine decides the best action to take based on the current environmental conditions [14]. Because there is no supervision in reinforcement learning, the machine observes the environment and tries in a manner similar to a trial-and-error search [15]. As a result of reinforcement ML, the outcome is not only measured with immediate action but also with the delayed reward that may be obtained [15].

A reinforcement learning algorithm is a very dynamic and powerful algorithm with significant applications in autonomous self-driving cars and robot programming [15].

50.3 Deep Learning

Deep learning (DL) technology, introduced by Hinton and colleagues in 2006, is an important component of ML and has been described as a new learning model in AI [12]. DL has demonstrated significant advances in learning and problem-solving. Combining it with a central neural network (CNN) forms the core of the fourth industrial revolution (4IR) [12, 16]. By using deep learning (DL) models, feature extraction can be carried out entirely by the model on its own, with very little guidance from the programmer [16]. Therefore, DL mimics the way the human brain processes data and makes decisions about it [16]. Neural networks are like the backbone of DL; they are always used in conjunction with DL models and resemble layers of neurons in a brain [16]. The performance of DL is significantly influenced by the amount of data available; the more data available, the better the performance [16]. When data amounts are small, DL performance is considered poor [3, 12, 16]. Examples of DL applications include visual identification, cybersecurity, visual assistance, robotics, and healthcare [16].

50.4 AI Applications in the Healthcare System of the UAE

The incorporation of AI within the healthcare system of the UAE presents significant potential in alleviating the burden on healthcare workers, optimizing cost management, and enhancing patient care. Through the utilization of AI, healthcare practitioners can effectively handle costs and expenditures [17]. While the transition from a manual to an automated healthcare system has occurred, the challenge persists in programming and digitizing healthcare services to develop efficient AI systems [17].

A number of exceptionally useful applications have already been developed using AI, such as cancer detection and AI-guided chatbots, which significantly reduce the number of unnecessary visits to general practitioners and the costs to patients [17]. Developing chatbots using AI-based algorithms to interact with people instead of going directly to the doctor is an effective method of reducing healthcare costs. While AI chatbots will not diagnose or prescribe medicines for patients, they will provide guidance to patients on how to respond to minor health complaints [17]. Using chatbots is a fast and cost-effective method, as they are available 24 hours a day [17]. Robotic surgeries and virtual assistance with nurses are other AI applications in the healthcare sector [17]. The use of AI also extends to dentistry, as dental AI applications assist the dentist during the treatment procedure by predicting the success rate of the treatment if the treatment plan is followed. In addition, it can assist the dentist in identifying root fractures, detecting periapical lesions, and performing robotic-assisted endodontic procedures [18]. Therefore, the integration of AI in the UAE's healthcare system presents immense potential for alleviating pressure on healthcare workers, effectively managing costs, and enhancing patient care. While notable advancements like AI-based cancer detection and chatbots have streamlined patient interactions and reduced unnecessary visits, challenges persist in optimizing AI systems and digitizing healthcare services. Despite these technical hurdles, AI's diverse applications, from robotic surgeries to dental assistance, signify promising strides in revolutionizing healthcare delivery in the UAE.

50.5 Utilizing AI for Diagnostic Radiology Advancements in the UAE

The healthcare sector in the United Arab Emirates (UAE) has witnessed a substantial evolution in radiology, primarily due to the integration of AI applications [19]. These AI-powered technologies have fundamentally reshaped diagnostic imaging practices, offering a spectrum of functionalities ranging from image analysis to predictive analytics and workflow optimization [20]. Within radiological contexts, these innovations significantly enhance the precision and efficiency of interpreting a diverse array of medical images, encompassing modalities such as X-rays, MRIs, and CT scans [21]. Their capacity to enable early detection, precise characterization, and tailored treatment planning for various medical conditions underscores their potential to elevate patient care standards [22]. Moreover, these AI-driven solutions contribute to streamlining radiological workflows, resulting in reduced reporting times and improved operational efficiency across healthcare facilities in the UAE [22]. Radiology lends itself perfectly to the use of AI applications, particularly when it comes to reading images and generating reports [23]. With the very limited number of trained radiologists in practice, a dramatic strain is placed on the available readers. This heavy workload makes it necessary for radiologists to interpret a greater volume of images in a shorter period of time [24]. Research has shown that radiologists must read one image every 3–4 seconds to complete the required workload during an 8-hour working day [24].

In essence, the integration of AI applications has significantly transformed radiology within the UAE's healthcare landscape, showcasing immense potential in enhancing diagnostic precision and efficiency across various imaging modalities. As AI-driven technologies streamline workflows and enable early detection of medical conditions, they offer promising prospects for elevating patient care standards. However, the burgeoning reliance on AI in radiology must navigate critical challenges such as data governance, algorithm transparency, and the pressing need for ongoing professional education to ensure seamless and effective integration of AI within the radiological domain in the UAE. The demand for AI in radiology becomes increasingly pertinent, especially considering the limited number of trained radiologists and the escalating workload, necessitating rapid and accurate image interpretation to meet healthcare demands.

50.5.1 Radiographic Image Segmentation

One of the remarkable AI applications in radiology within the UAE lies in image segmentation and registration, employing Deep Learning (DL) algorithms to address tissue-related issues by utilizing intensity patches as inputs [25]. This technique facilitates the segmentation of diverse tissues, encompassing tumor tissues in the brain, cartilage, bone tissues, cellular membranes, and cellular mitosis. Despite the time-intensive nature of training AI software on intensity patches, advancements like full Convolutional Neural Networks (fCNNs) have emerged, enabling crowd segmentation akin to monitoring crowded videos, albeit resulting in lower-quality segmented images compared to the original input [25]. The integration of consecutive pooling and convolutional layers in fCNN often compromises image quality and reduces data dimensionality. However, recent advancements by Brosch et al. introduced a three-layer network consisting of convolutional and deconvolutional layers, showcasing improved accuracy in producing higher-quality segmented images, especially in localizing lesions [26, 27]. This signifies a significant stride in achieving more precise and detailed tissue segmentation within radiology applications in the UAE.

50.5.2 Radiomics and Radiogenomic

The term "radiomics" was introduced in 2016 by Gillies et al., who stated that radiographic images are not only images but also a valuable amount of data that, when analyzed quantitatively, can provide a wide range of quantitative features useful for research, hypothesis generation, and testing [27]. Moreover, they provide radiologists with diagnostic support tools to assist them in making the final diagnostic decisions [27]. The use of radiomics in conjunction with genomic data can enhance diagnostic decision support tools, a process known as radiogenomics. Radiogenomics has the potential to provide greater predictive, prognostic, and diagnostic capabilities than radiomics [27].

50.5.3 AI in Oncology Imaging in UAE's Healthcare System

The healthcare sector in the UAE has actively embraced technological advancements, particularly in AI, aimed at enhancing healthcare delivery. Oncology, as a pivotal domain within this sector, has experienced a substantial integration of AI-driven solutions, showing promising potential for more precise diagnostics, personalized treatment plans, and improved patient outcomes. Feedback from clinical radiologists indicates the potential utility of radiogenomics imaging in aiding oncology imaging. Existing research has compellingly demonstrated radiogenomics' ability to differentiate between cancerous and benign tissues in prostatic tumors [28]. This capability significantly enhances the prognosis for cancer patients by enabling early detection of tumor heterogeneity [29]. Moreover, the utilization of radiogenomics extends to evaluating patient prognosis in instances of lung cancer and glioblastoma [25]. However, advancing and expanding this decision-support tool necessitates concerted efforts from radiologists alongside continuous development of radiogenomic databases for future utilization [27].

Table 50.1 demonstrates the performance of AI applications in breast imaging, showcasing their effectiveness and potential impact within this specific domain.

Table 50.1 Sample of studies conducted to assess AI performance in breast cancer detection

Authors	Method used	Performance
Kozegar et al. [30]	Iterated segmentation	Sensitivity = 91%, False positive = 4.8
Carneiro et al. [31]	Fast CNN (CNN-F)	ROC = 0.91
Al-antari et al. [32]	YOLO	Detection accuracy = 98.96%, ROC = 0.948
Agarwal et al. [33]	Pat CNN	True positive rate = 0.98 ± 0.02, false positive rate 0.02

50.6 Artificial Intelligence Adoption in UAE's Radiology

A recent investigation conducted by Mohamed Abuzaid in 2022 and his colleagues examined radiologists' and radiographers' knowledge, perceptions, readiness, and challenges regarding the integration of AI into radiology practice in the UAE [34]. Researchers found that radiologists and radiographers lacked an understanding of AI fundamentals and knowledge of some aspects of AI integration into radiology [34]. However, it is worth noting that while AI adoption is on the rise, its full potential is not yet realized. There may be an absence of educational resources in the local area as a contributing factor. It may be possible to address this through the development of local educational resources by universities and continuing education centers in the United Arab Emirates, as well as by international professional societies [34]. Despite the UAE's relatively young workforce, it can recognize and implement international developments [34]. Through government support of healthcare improvement plans in the form of education and infrastructure, understanding and implementation of AI can be developed and optimized for the UAE healthcare system [34].

50.7 Limitations, Challenges, and Future Directions

While machine learning algorithms' capacity to handle vast, complicated, heterogeneous datasets is part of what makes them attractive, the success of their development depends on data that is clean, frequently annotated, sufficiently specified, and broad and sizable enough [35]. It might be challenging to gather and time-consuming to pre-process this amount of data [35]. Furthermore, the majority of machine learning research relies on data from a single modality [35]. Although multimodal imaging-based AI is still in its infancy, it has the potential to further advance the capacity for diagnosis and prediction [36]. The combination of demographics, clinicopathology, biochemistry, pathology, and imaging, among other data, may result in comprehensive and potent AI assessment tools, going beyond the use of imaging alone and imitating healthcare professionals' approaches [35]. Uneven mistake costs must be incorporated into models by radiologists who are interested in creating real-world application tools. This is crucial for cancer assessment [33]. Any algorithm must consider the impact of a false negative rather than only distinguishing between malignant and benign tumors [37]. Clinicians automatically minimize false negatives while tolerating increased false positive rates [37], and any ML model should be adjusted accordingly. Radiologists in the UAE who are interested in AI should familiarize themselves with worldwide guidelines on both the interpretation of AI research and the design of AI studies [37].

Explainability: These algorithms become unfathomably complicated through the fine-tuning of millions of connections (particularly in deep learning) [38]. Machine learning algorithms are frequently referred to as "black box" models since they produce a result without the user being aware of the decision-making process [36, 38]. Despite their superhuman abilities, humans find the lack of accountability that comes with using these technologies unpleasant [38]. Any gadget used in patient care needs to be reliable, especially for medical professionals [38]. Any reservations clinicians may have about new AI technologies will simply be exacerbated by a lack of explainability. Despite this moral conundrum, others contend that the "black box" should be ignored in favor of implementing this technology if it can be proven to improve patient care [38]. They draw attention to the fact that clinicians commonly rely on intuition and are frequently unable to articulate their thinking or the supporting data clearly and instantly for the various clinical judgments they make. However, the majority of AI ethicists advocate for the development of "explainable AI" due to legal, technological, patient-related, and clinician-related concerns [38]. Hyper-advanced AI may eventually be able to explain complicated and multidimensional correlations in data in a way that humans can understand them; in the meantime, explainable AI seems to be a crucial first step toward general adoption [38].

Privacy: The ability to access enormous amounts of data, typically retrospective, is necessary for the creation of high-functioning and trustworthy algorithms [36]. It is impractical to obtain consent from thousands or millions of patients, and although many images, sounds, and brain signal-related data may be easily anonymized, clinicopathological data makes anonymization more challenging [36]. Moreover, data that is ostensibly sufficiently anonymized can occasionally be traced back [36]. Confidentiality should be protected by strict rules that are universally followed. In particular, deep neural networks are vulnerable to "fragility." These networks are so complex that they can extract subtle information (features) from the input data [36]. Some of these patterns may provide superhuman levels of detection or diagnosis because they are invisible to humans [36]. However, the peculiarities of the training dataset may cause many other patterns to appear salient despite being irrelevant [36]. Therefore, seemingly slight and unimportant changes to the image or data can lead the algorithm to classify something incorrectly [38]. Adversarial training is one strategy to assist in combating this weakness, which will likely become more prevalent in the near future. In this approach, a second algorithm tests and trains the first one using samples that are intended to trick it, creating a more reliable model to guard against errors [38]. However, this strategy is inherently flawed, as algorithms may be strengthened in some areas while being weakened in others. In the end, our extensive and in-depth understanding of the universe enables us to view images as a collection of concepts in context, allowing us to avoid becoming sidetracked by petty or unimportant details [38].

Universalizability: Algorithms learn based on a specific set of unique parameters and signals when they are trained on a single data acquisition source, such as a particular ultrasound machine model [37, 38]. They might not be well-equipped to analyze data from a different source, such as data from various scanners or recording equipment [33]. ML may be more challenging when using multiple data sources [37, 38]. Researchers can, however, anticipate that in sufficiently large studies, an algorithm may be able to see through this noise and develop into a more general model with good accuracy, regardless of the equipment employed [37, 38]. However, it is acknowledged that the use of data with widely divergent acquisition parameters may result in signal changes that are not due to biology, reducing model effectiveness and restricting the generalizability of the algorithm [37, 38].

Involvement of patients and the public: While a complete comprehension of any new technology is not a requirement for use, patient confidence in the system is essential [37, 38]. Participating with the public during both the early and late stages of development will not only build trust but also ensure that their requirements as patients are met [37, 38]. The idea of AI assisting doctors rather than replacing them is related to public trust [37, 38]. In this regard, algorithms should, at least in the near future, be specific enough to leave a human clinician responsible for providing the majority of the care [37, 38].

Algorithm bias is still a challenge in applications of AI in the real world [38, 39]. Unfair, unethical, and unreliable outcomes can be produced by trained models that reflect systematic biases found in a dataset [38, 39]. These biases may be difficult to identify due to the aforementioned lack of explainability in DNNs, which highlights the concern surrounding the broad deployment of such systems [38, 39]. Outside of medicine, image assessment algorithms in cameras have shown data limitations and resulting bias by failing to distinguish faces with dark skin and misclassifying East Asian faces as blinking faces [39]. Outside of AI, racial and ethnic minorities are typically underrepresented in large research studies conducted in the industrialized world, which results in inadequate risk categorization, diagnoses, and management [39]. The fact that skin cancer detection algorithms perform substantially worse when detecting malignancies in darker skin is probably due to the data source's preponderance of photos with light skin [39]. Whatever the justification, creating and using algorithms that are less effective when applied to certain groups based on ethnicity or any other factor presents severe ethical concerns [39]. Biases in data can also produce unanticipated algorithmic quirks in other ways. In two significant image diagnostic investigations, the presence of a ruler or a chest drain, respectively, increased the likelihood of diagnosing skin cancer or pneumothorax [39]. These shortcomings jeopardize precision and confidence in sophisticated AI systems, even though their effects on social equality may be less severe [39].

50.8 Limitations, Challenges, and Future Directions in the Adoption of AI in the UAE

Artificial intelligence has emerged as a revolutionary technology in various industries, including healthcare. It has shown great potential in radiology, where it can assist radiologists in tasks such as image interpretation, diagnosis, and treatment planning. However, the implementation of AI in radiology in the UAE faces several challenges that need to be addressed for its successful integration and utilization. These challenges include a lack of standardized data collection and annotation, limited access to high-quality training datasets, concerns regarding data privacy and security, regulatory barriers, resistance from healthcare professionals, and the need for continuous education and training in AI technologies. Additionally, the UAE radiology community must be trained to critically analyze the possibilities, risks, and threats associated with implementing AI tools [40]. Furthermore, there should be a focus on developing rigorous data collection criteria and uniform global ethical guidelines for AI to establish its role in clinical practice [41]. Moreover, to ensure the responsible and effective use of AI in radiology, ethical and legal responsibilities for decision-making must remain with physicians. These challenges highlight the need for collaborative efforts between healthcare providers, AI developers, policymakers, and regulatory bodies to address the technological, ethical, and educational aspects.

50.9 Conclusion

Industries, healthcare, and even routine daily activities have all been transformed by artificial intelligence. AI uses machine learning algorithms to model human thought, decision-making, and behavior. Based on the learning process and the desired results, machine learning approaches can be divided into four groups: supervised learning, unsupervised learning, semi-supervised learning, and reinforcement learning. Deep learning, a branch of machine learning, has also been developed. AI is a fantastic tool in the healthcare industry for assisting with the care of the expanding population, which puts more strain on healthcare providers. Diagnostic radiology is one of the medical specialties with the greatest need for AI. One of the main difficulties in developing algorithms for AI is data availability. AI applications in diagnostic imaging have great potential, but they face many challenges. In the UAE, AI in radiology has revolutionized medical imaging by enhancing diagnostic accuracy and streamlining workflows. It enables early disease detection and empowers radiologists to offer personalized treatment plans. However, it is worth noting that while AI adoption is on the rise, its full potential is not yet fully realized. In this chapter, we have discussed different machine learning algorithms, their use in diagnostic radiology and healthcare, and their drawbacks.

Acknowledgments We express our profound appreciation to our research assistant, Daniah Kashabash, for her invaluable contributions to this research chapter. Daniah's unwavering dedication to preparing resources and creating graphs and tables has significantly enhanced the quality and presentation of our findings.

Conflicts of Interest The authors have no conflicts of interest to declare.

References

1. Moor J. The Dartmouth College artificial intelligence conference: the next fifty years. AI Mag [Internet]. 2006;27(4):87. Available from: https://ojs.aaai.org/index.php/aimagazine/article/view/1911
2. Trattner C, Jannach D, Motta E, Costera Meijer I, Diakopoulos N, Elahi M, et al. Responsible media technology and AI: challenges and research directions. AI Ethics. 2022;2(4):585–94. Available from: https://doi.org/10.1007/s43681-021-00126-4.
3. Yang YC, Islam SU, Noor A, Khan S, Afsar W, Nazir S. Influential usage of big data and artificial intelligence in healthcare. Comput Math Methods Med [Internet]. 2021;2021:5812499. Available from: https://doi.org/10.1155/2021/5812499.
4. Bye S. Artificial intelligence and its impact on everyday life [Internet]. University of York; 2022. Available from: https://online.york.ac.uk/artificial-intelligence-and-its-impact-on-everyday-life/.
5. Bohr A, Memarzadeh K. The rise of artificial intelligence in healthcare applications. In: Bohr A, Memarzadeh K, editors. Artificial intelligence in healthcare. San Diego: Elsevier; 2020. p. 25–60.
6. Lewis T. A brief history of artificial intelligence [Internet]. Live Science; 2021. Available from: https://www.livescience.com/49007-history-of-artificial-intelligence.html.
7. Lidströmer N, Aresu F, Ashrafian H. Basic concepts of artificial intelligence: primed for clinicians. In: Artificial intelligence in medicine. Cham: Springer International Publishing; 2022. p. 3–20.
8. Kicky G. How does artificial intelligence in radiology improve efficiency and health outcomes? Pediatr Radiol [Internet]. 2022;52(11):2087–93. Available from: https://doi.org/10.1007/s00247-021-05114-8.
9. Shearer C. The CRISP-DM model: the new blueprint for data mining. J Data Warehous. 2000;5(4):13–22. www.javatpoint.com.
10. Available from: https://www.javatpoint.com/basic-concepts-in-machine-learning.
11. Jiang T, Gradus JL, Rosellini AJ. Supervised machine learning: a brief primer. Behav Ther. 2020;51(5):675–87. Available from: https://doi.org/10.1016/j.beth.2020.05.002.
12. Sarker IH. Machine learning: algorithms, real-world applications and research directions. SN Comput Sci. 2021;2:160. https://doi.org/10.1007/s42979-021-00592-x.
13. National Human Genome Research Institute. Artificial intelligence, machine learning and genomics [Internet]. Genome.gov. [cited 2022 Dec 12]. Available from: https://www.genome.gov/about-genomics/educational-resources/fact-sheets/artificial-intelligence-machine-learning-and-genomics.
14. SAS Institute. A guide to the types of machine learning algorithms [Internet]. Sas.com. 2021 [cited 2022 Dec 13]. Available from: https://www.sas.com/en_gb/insights/articles/analytics/machine-learning-algorithms.html.
15. Diamantidis PVA. Reinforcement learning explained in 90 seconds [Internet]. Synopsys. 2021 [cited 2022 Dec 17]. Available from: https://www.synopsys.com/ai/what-is-reinforcement-learning.html.

16. Emmert-Streib F, Yang Z, Feng H, Tripathi S, Dehmer M. An introductory review of deep learning for prediction models with big data. Front Artif Intell. 2020;3:4. Available from: https://doi.org/10.3389/frai.2020.00004.
17. Rangaiah M. Artificial intelligence in healthcare: applications and threats [Internet]. Analyticssteps.com. [cited 2022 Dec 17]. Available from: https://www.analyticssteps.com/blogs/artificial-intelligence-healthcare-applications-and-threats.
18. Agrawal P, Nikhade P. Artificial intelligence in dentistry: past, present, and future. Cureus. 2022;14(7):e27405. Available from: https://doi.org/10.7759/cureus.27405.
19. Johnson KB, Wei WQ, Weeraratne D, et al. Precision medicine, AI, and the future of personalized health care. Clin Transl Sci. 2021;14(1):86–93. https://doi.org/10.1111/cts.12884.
20. Smith H, Downer J, Ives J. Clinicians and AI use: where is the professional guidance? J Med Ethics. 2024;50:437–41. https://doi.org/10.1136/jme-2022-108831.
21. Adams SJ, Henderson RDE, Yi X, Babyn P. Artificial intelligence solutions for analysis of X-ray images. Can Assoc Radiol J. 2021;72(1):60–72. https://doi.org/10.1177/0846537120941671.
22. Robinson A, Asaduzzaman M, Jena R, Naemi R. Simulation as a tool to model potential workflow enhancements in radiotherapy treatment pathways – a systematic review. J Appl Clin Med Phys. 2023;24:e14132. https://doi.org/10.1002/acm2.14132.
23. Waller J, O'Connor A, Rafaat E, Amireh A, Dempsey J, Martin C, et al. Applications and challenges of artificial intelligence in diagnostic and interventional radiology. Pol J Radiol. 2022;87(1):e113–7. Available from: https://doi.org/10.5114/pjr.2022.113531.
24. Hosny A, Parmar C, Quackenbush J, Schwartz LH, Aerts HJWL. Artificial intelligence in radiology. Nat Rev Cancer. 2018;18(8):500–10. Available from: https://doi.org/10.1038/s41568-018-0016-5.
25. Lee J-G, Jun S, Cho Y-W, Lee H, Kim GB, Seo JB, et al. Deep learning in medical imaging: general overview. Korean J Radiol. 18(4):570. Available from: https://synapse.koreamed.org/articles/1027354.
26. Brosch T, Tang LYW, Yoo Y, Li DKB, Traboulsee A, Tam R. Deep 3D convolutional encoder networks with shortcuts for multiscale feature integration applied to multiple sclerosis lesion segmentation. IEEE Trans Med Imaging. 2016;35(5):1229–39. Available from: https://doi.org/10.1109/TMI.2016.2528821.
27. Gillies RJ, Kinahan PE, Hricak H. Radiomics: images are more than pictures, they are data. Radiology [Internet]. 2016;278(2):563–77. Available from: https://doi.org/10.1148/radiol.2015151169.
28. Wibmer A, Hricak H, Gondo T, Matsumoto K, Veeraraghavan H, Fehr D, et al. Haralick texture analysis of prostate MRI: utility for differentiating non-cancerous prostate from prostate cancer and differentiating prostate cancers with different Gleason scores. Eur Radiol [Internet]. 2015;25(10):2840–50. Available from: https://doi.org/10.1007/s00330-015-3701-8.
29. Coroller TP, Grossmann P, Hou Y, Rios Velazquez E, Leijenaar RTH, Hermann G, et al. CT-based radiomic signature predicts distant metastasis in lung adenocarcinoma. Radiother Oncol [Internet]. 2015;114(3):345–50. Available from: https://doi.org/10.1016/j.radonc.2015.02.015.
30. Kozegar E, Soryani M, Minaei B, Domingues I. Assessment of a novel mass detection algorithm in mammograms. J Cancer Res Ther [Internet]. 2013;9(4):592–600. Available from: https://doi.org/10.4103/0973-1482.126453.
31. Carneiro G, Nascimento J, Bradley AP. Unregistered multiview mammogram analysis with pre-trained deep learning models. In: Lecture notes in computer science. Cham: Springer International Publishing; 2015. p. 652–60.
32. Al-Antari MA, Al-Masni MA, Choi M-T, Han S-M, Kim T-S. A fully integrated computer-aided diagnosis system for digital X-ray mammograms via deep learning detection, segmentation, and classification. Int J Med Inform [Internet]. 2018;117:44–54. Available from: https://doi.org/10.1016/j.ijmedinf.2018.06.003.
33. Agarwal R, Diaz O, Lladó X, Yap MH, Martí R. Automatic mass detection in mammograms using deep convolutional neural networks. J Med Imaging (Bellingham) [Internet]. 2019;6(3):1. Available from: https://doi.org/10.1117/1.jmi.6.3.031409.

34. Abuzaid MM, Elshami W, Tekin H, Issa B. Assessment of the willingness of radiologists and radiographers to accept the integration of artificial intelligence into radiology practice. Acad Radiol [Internet]. 2022;29(1):87–94. Available from: https://doi.org/10.1016/j.acra.2020.09.014.
35. Academy of Medical Royal Colleges. Artificial intelligence in healthcare. 2019. https://www.aomrc.org.uk/wp-content/uploads/2019/01/Artificial_intelligence_in_healthcare_0119.pdf.
36. Howard J. Artificial intelligence: implications for the future of work. Am J Ind Med [Internet]. 2019;62(11):917–26. Available from: https://blogs.cdc.gov/niosh-science-blog/2019/08/26/ai/.
37. Abuzaid MM, Elshami W, Kadhom M, McConnell J, Mc Fadden S. The changing concept of radiographer's role in UAE: an analysis of radiologists' opinions and acceptance. Radiography (Lond) [Internet]. 2022;28(4):1042–9. Available from: https://doi.org/10.1016/j.radi.2022.07.010.
38. Amann J, Blasimme A, Vayena E, Frey D, Madai VI, Precise4Q Consortium. Explainability for artificial intelligence in healthcare: a multidisciplinary perspective. BMC Med Inform Decis Mak [Internet]. 2020;20(1):310. Available from: https://doi.org/10.1186/s12911-020-01332-6.
39. Adamson AS, Smith A. Machine learning and health care disparities in dermatology. JAMA Dermatol [Internet]. 2018;154(11):1247–8. Available from: https://doi.org/10.1001/jamadermatol.2018.2348.
40. Alelyani M, Alamri S, Alqahtani MS, Musa A, Almater H, Alqahtani N, Alshahrani F, Alelyani S. Radiology community attitude in Saudi Arabia about the applications of artificial intelligence in radiology. Healthcare. 2021;9(7):834. https://doi.org/10.3390/healthcare9070834.
41. Lin X-F, Wang Z, Zhou W, Luo G, Hwang G-J, Zhou Y, et al. Technological support to foster students' artificial intelligence ethics: an augmented reality-based contextualized dilemma discussion approach. Comput Educ. 2023;201:104813.

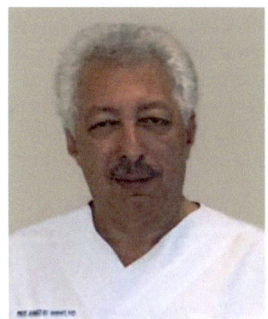

Prof. Ahmed ElSerafi, a prominent figure in radiology, who graduated from Ain Shams University, Cairo, in 1982. He joined the radiology department at the university's affiliated hospital and remained there until 1994. During this time, he achieved academic excellence, earning a Master of Science Degree in Radiology (MScR) in 1986 and a Doctorate Degree in Radiology (PhD) in 1990. Dr. ElSerafi's commitment to academic and professional growth was evident during his post-graduate training in the radiology departments of Cardiff University Hospital and Nevill Hall Hospital, Abergavenny, both located in Wales in the United Kingdom. In 1994, he took on the role of Lecturer in Radiology at Suez Canal University in Ismailia, Egypt. He later earned promotions to the position of Associate Professor in 1999 and Professor in 2004. His active involvement in the radiological community is reflective of his keen knowledge in the field and awareness of its advancements. He has been a member of key organizations, including the Egyptian Society of Radiology & Nuclear Medicine (ESRNM) since 1987, the Radiological Society of North America (RSNA) since 1994, Radiological Society of Emirates (RSE) since 2008, and the Korean Society of Radiology (KSR) since 2010. Dr. ElSerafi's leadership extends to directorship at the CAI Academy (Computer Aided Implantology Academy) in Egypt, a position held since 2019. Chairman of the Scientific Committee of the Emirates Radiology Society between 2012 and 2015. and has held the role of Secretary General of the Emirates Osteoporosis Society since 2013. His areas of specialist interest include computed tomography, ultrasonography, osteoporosis imaging, dental imaging, imaging informatics, and artificial intelligence, all underscored by published articles, thesis supervisions, and reviews. Presently, he holds the position of Professor of Radiology at Suez Canal University in Egypt, and serves as a Visiting Professor of Radiology at both Sharjah University and Gulf Medical University in the UAE, and fulfills the role of CEO at International Radiology Centre, and Meridian Healthcare, in the United Arab Emirates.

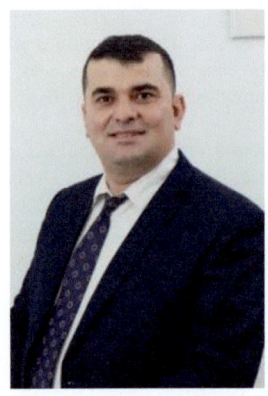

Dr. Mohammad Rawashdeh is a Professor and Associate Dean of Academics, as well as the program director in the Department of Medical Imaging Sciences at Gulf Medical University (GMU). He also holds a faculty position at Jordan University of Science and Technology (JUST). His academic experience includes serving as a lecturer at the University of Sydney and as Chairman of the Allied Medical Sciences department at JUST from 2017 to 2021. Dr. Rawashdeh earned his Ph.D. in Medical Imaging from the University of Sydney in 2014, he also holds Postgraduate Certificates in University Teaching and Learning, as well as University Research Supervision, earned in 2013. In 2011, he completed a Master of Diagnostic Radiography (Honours) also from the University of Sydney, following a Bachelor of Diagnostic Radiography from the Jordan University of Sciences and Technology in 2006. His research focuses on medical imaging perception, receiver operating characteristic (ROC) analysis, human performance, and radiation dose and image quality optimization. He has authored over 80 peer-reviewed articles and presented his work at prominent national and international imaging conferences. His research has significantly influenced clinical practices, national imaging guidelines, and international policy reports. In addition to his scholarly contributions, Dr. Rawashdeh has successfully supervised 20 higher-degree research students , all of whom have completed their degrees—demonstrating his dedication to academic mentorship and capacity building in the field of medical imaging.

Open Access This chapter is licensed under the terms of the Creative Commons Attribution 4.0 International License (http://creativecommons.org/licenses/by/4.0/), which permits use, sharing, adaptation, distribution and reproduction in any medium or format, as long as you give appropriate credit to the original author(s) and the source, provide a link to the Creative Commons license and indicate if changes were made.

The images or other third party material in this chapter are included in the chapter's Creative Commons license, unless indicated otherwise in a credit line to the material. If material is not included in the chapter's Creative Commons license and your intended use is not permitted by statutory regulation or exceeds the permitted use, you will need to obtain permission directly from the copyright holder.

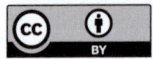

Health Media in the UAE

Bassam Darwish

51.1 Introduction

Media can generally be defined as a process aimed at conveying and communicating news, information, facts, and ideas about a particular issue or event to inform and define what is going on, or even to influence, modify, or change the behavior of individuals. It is also defined as the communication channels used to disseminate news, advertisements, and data; as a communication between a sender and receiver using a means or as the social means of communication with the public.

Specialized media is defined as a media format that is carried out through different media outlets, gives most of its attention to a certain area of knowledge, and relies on specialized information and facts. Health media, which is a type of specialized media, shares many characteristics with public media but is characterized by its focus and specialization in the health field, covering news, data, information, health statistics, and awareness programs to serve the public health of society as a whole.

The demand for health information has grown exponentially in the last few years. People are interested in food, diet, beauty, and related topics beyond just a basic level, and are also increasingly concerned about their health. This is reflected in the huge media coverage in magazines, newspapers, radio, television programs, and on the Internet.

There is no doubt that many patients enter the doctor's office with five questions in their minds, for example, about their health condition, and leave the office with even more questions, so they resort to search engines such as Google. However, they may not find the correct information, or the information may be incomplete, misleading, or promotional.

B. Darwish (✉)
Balsam Academy of Medical Education and Research, Dubai, United Arab Emirates
e-mail: bassam@balsamone.com

© The Author(s) 2025
H. O. Al-Shamsi (ed.), *Healthcare in the United Arab Emirates*,
https://doi.org/10.1007/978-981-96-0523-1_51

Since there are no studies in this field, we refer to a study conducted in the United States of America on the use use of the Internet to search for health information [1].

51.2 Consumers Seeking Health Information

In the past, the printed materials provided by medical centers and hospitals, in addition to health magazines and medical books, were the primary sources of health information. However, in the digital age, a large percentage of community members seek health information through the Internet, social networking sites, and YouTube.

And because the doctor and the medical team do not play their primary role in health awareness and in enabling the patient to manage their health life, and they do not give the patient enough time to listen to their medical story and explain their condition, for this reason, a section of patients leave the consultation without knowing how they will deal with their health condition or disease. So, they search through the Google search engine and receive a large number of sites from different sources, from which the average individual cannot know which one is reliable. Hence, the emphasis is on the importance of health media, which fills a large gap in health knowledge and its sources.

It should be noted that consumer use of the Internet for health information is large and growing. In 1997, nearly half of the Internet users in the USA sought health information. Recent estimates range from 60 to 100 million people doing so at least once a month.

The reasons for the growth of consumers looking for health information online include searching for service providers and prices, in addition to obtaining information on nutrition, obesity, and erectile dysfunction (ED), and searching for modern treatments or news that offers hope to terminally ill patients [2].

Hence, we say that although this problem is global, it is gaining more importance in our Arab world, and in the United Arab Emirates (UAE), due to the scarcity of trusted health information in Arabic compared to sources in English.

It is worth mentioning that the United Arab Emirates (UAE) government considers health as one of its most important strategic objectives, as confirmed by the National Agenda.

51.2.1 UAE Government Support of the Health Sector

Providing world-class healthcare is one of the six pillars of the UAE National Agenda, in line with Vision 2021.

For the year 2016, the UAE government allocated 7.9% of the budget, amounting to approximately AED 3.83 billion, to the health sector alone [3].

In 2017, the UAE government allocated 8.6% of the federal budget to the health sector, in addition to the significant spending by the local emirates. According to the Sustainable Economic Development Assessment (SEDA) scores from the Boston Consulting Group (BCG), healthcare standards in the UAE outperform regional and worldwide averages on multiple dimensions, such as well-being and education.

51.2.2 Public Health Protection

The UAE is keen to develop a preventive healthcare system that includes the provision of special vaccines, including the cervical cancer vaccine, and periodic examinations for the early detection of tumors such as breast, colorectal, and prostate, among others, in addition to blood pressure, diabetes, and other necessary tests.

Of course, such services require continuous health awareness, and this is a basic task that must be carried out by media, educational, social, and other institutions [4].

51.2.3 Media Institutions

In the United Arab Emirates, there are many governmental, private, local, Gulf, Arab, and international media institutions. In this field, Dubai Media City has attracted many international institutions such as CNN and BBC.

There are many newspapers published in different languages, in addition to radio and television channels, and large media and public relations companies that contribute to the creation and dissemination of news.

It should be noted that newspapers and magazines devote special pages to health, as well as radio and television programs that specialize in medical content or short medical segments.

But the question remains: does the above play a role in raising awareness, or not? We have many channels and media, but do we have dedicated health media?

51.3 The Health Journalism Award

In 2008, the General Secretariat of the Arab Journalism Award announced the creation of a new award to be added to the existing categories, which aims to activate the role of press institutions and their engagement in various medical issues, spread health awareness, and contribute to filling the noticeable shortage of specialized medical journalism at the level of the Arab world.

Maryam bin Fahad, Executive Director of the Dubai Press Club, said: "The launch of the Health Journalism Award comes within the framework of the modernization and development plan pursued by the Arab Journalism Award over the past seven cycles." Mariam bin Fahd added that the mission of the professional and ethical award encourages us to raise the level of specialized, creative journalistic work in light of the development of means of communication and informatics, so that press institutions can harness journalistic technologies in the service of health and medical publishing and be keen to publish everything that matters and serves this vital sector, as well as motivating journalists to participate in writing, perform their roles, and assume their responsibilities toward society.

She said that the award seeks to push the Arab press toward specialization in various fields, including the health and medical field, which is a serious attempt to improve the level of health and medical services in the Arab world by presenting and discussing topics related to the conditions of the medical sector.

According to Mariam bin Fahd, the Arab world suffers from the scarcity of specialized periodicals published in Arabic, or specialized pages for the dissemination of health culture. For this reason, the launch of the Health and Medical Journalism Award category came to contribute to encouraging journalists to write in this vital and very important sector in order to develop public awareness, introduce modern medical sciences, and follow up on the latest developments, innovations, and medical achievements [5].

On the other hand, Dubai Healthcare City launched a training course in health media in cooperation with Harvard Medical School, and this initiative did not continue despite its importance and the need for cadres specializing in health media.

Such initiatives need programs and messages to raise awareness of their importance.

Do media organizations play this role?

Do we have a media strategy in the health sector?

51.4 What Is Health Media?

The primary mission of various health-conscious media through radio and television programs, medical pages, and dedicated corners in print media is centered around empowerment, that is, enabling community members to manage their healthy lives, and not just publishing medical news, statistics, and updates in the field of medicine.

Through my long experience in the field of health media, I say that the main task is to convey the health message in a simplified way that can be understood and applied in our daily lives to change behavior in order to feel healthy. Health, according to the definition of the World Health Organization, does not mean the absence of disease but is a state of well-being and a balance between physical and psychological health [6].

Mass communications can play a vast role in health promotion, but they can never be effective alone without practical changes in behavior, regulations, and laws, and effective cooperation between various government institutions. In addition to that, the correct use of the media can dispel fears, remove rumors, correct misconceptions, and help members of society identify the specific risk factors that lead to diseases in order to stay away from them and prevent them.

Unfortunately, through the author's observation and follow-up of various radio programs and medical segments on television, as well as what is published in newspapers and magazines, the focus is almost entirety on treatment rather than prevention.

In addition to that, the media reports or press releases issued by official health institutions focus on disease, treatment, and modern devices, and do not focus on prevention and health awareness campaigns, the impact of which does not end with the publication of news about the campaign and some photos.

As we know, the cost of disease is very high, and the cost of preventing it is very low.

Behavior change cannot be achieved through the dissemination of such news alone, and those who follow the official statistics of pathological cases find that the incidence of obesity, diabetes, cancerous tumors, heart disease, and other diseases is increasing. Therefore, we must have an integrated media strategy to promote health among members of society. Additionally, we must take advantage of the critical role played by the National Emergency, Crisis, and Disaster Management Authority during the COVID-19 pandemic, where media messages contributed to the commitment of community members to the instructions that helped reduce COVID-19 infections and facilitated proper and correct handling of the disease, including adherence to isolation and medical instructions.

51.4.1 Knowledge Is the Foundation of Awareness

Public health institutions usually aim to provoke some kind of short- or long-term behavioral response from large numbers of people.

These institutions work with their strategic partners to provide community members with health information in a simplified manner so that this information can be used to help change behavior.

One of the strategic partners is the media, especially since the media plays a fundamental role in guiding public opinion and changing behavior according to a strategic action plan defined by goals and means of assistance.

It is useful to note that the media is a strategic partner in achieving the strategic goals of the UAE government, including improving health and quality of life. In order to achieve this goal (health and quality of life), the media must work to change behavior gradually by influencing public opinion, and this requires the provision of trained specialists in the field of health media.

It is very important that the message is clear and specific, with the selection of the appropriate media channels for the target segment of society.

As we know, many diseases are clinically silent and are discovered by chance when visiting the doctor or because of the progression of the disease and the occurrence of complications. That is why we say, "Early diagnosis is certain of the risks, and the cost of the disease is very high and the cost of preventing it is very low."

51.5 Health Awareness

Health education develops awareness, skills, and positive attitudes among community members toward health. It helps them perceive the concept of health as something precious, not a luxury or secondary. Health education requires skills, not just information, skills that help individuals make the right decisions using mindfulness to enjoy wellness and stay free from disease. That is, it involves health promotion, disease prevention, and disease management in the correct way in order to avoid complications.

Health awareness must be integrated into the teaching curriculum from a young age, because awareness in childhood means health and vitality in old age.

The media plays a vital role as the link between health workers and the larger public. Health authorities educate and entrust the media with essential health information, which is then relayed to the public in readily accessible formats through a variety of media channels. For instance, the National Emergency and Crisis Authority contributed to the delivery of health messages to all members of the community during the COVID-19 pandemic and strengthened the important role of credible media, including social media, which helped to fight rumors and correct misconceptions with accurate and necessary information.

It is worth mentioning that through various media such as radio and television, for example, we can send health messages so that they reach as many members of society as possible, and modern social media contributes to this area as well.

The mass media can empower populations to fight major causes of disease and emphasize the importance of prevention.

51.5.1 Health for Everyone

Health for everyone and through everyone, and for this, we must work together for health. This requires the availability of conviction and decision-making to modify behavior and provide support in order to sustain that change.

There is no doubt that different visual, audio, and written media can broadcast health awareness messages. However, to be effective, these messages must be customized for each of the target groups. Therefore, it is very useful for the health message to be designed in different ways to reach each target group.

In promoting health awareness campaigns through different media, there must be diversity in the production of health messages, in the form of videos and radio tips, and through the use of graphics, infographics, and flyers designed in an attractive way.

51.6 Roles of Media for Health Intervention

To illustrate the important role that different media can play, we mention smoking as a common health issue.

Although many people who smoke know about the dangers of smoking to their health, perhaps only a small percentage of them know about health programs that help and support those who want to quit smoking.

That is why we return to emphasizing the fundamental role of the media in promoting the concept of health in our daily lives.

For audience awareness to occur, the audience must be exposed to information (i.e., the intervention), attend to it, and remember it. Campaigns that fail to raise awareness generally do not achieve the necessary preconditions, that is, messages are not aired or distributed for the target audience to be exposed adequately, or messages are not constructed to capture attention and present information clearly.

That's why we say that many health awareness campaigns fail to achieve their goals.

Unfortunately, many health awareness campaigns are not evaluated to determine the extent of their impact, whether their messages have reached the target groups, and whether the messages are understandable.

In order to achieve the desired goals in the field of health awareness, it is necessary to design appropriate health messages that capture the public's attention in order to help change behavior [7].

51.7 The Media and Health Literacy

Health literacy is a term introduced in the 1970s that has become an increasingly important concept in public health. It refers to an individual's capacity for accessing, interpreting, and comprehending primary healthcare (PHC) information and care required for appropriate decision-making.

In the event that a person does not understand health information or understands it incorrectly, it means that he will not be able to make a sound decision regarding his health. From here, the concept of health literacy gains even more importance and requires significant and sustained efforts to enable the individual to manage his health effectively. This is a task that must be achieved through practical cooperation between health, educational, media, community, and other institutions [8].

51.8 Recommendations

For the various media to play their effective role in the field of health promotion and disease prevention, it is useful to work on studying the health reality and identifying strengths, weaknesses, challenges, and opportunities, and then design an action plan through brainstorming that combines medical and media cadres. In addition to this, training is essential to develop skills and ensure the optimal use of media to achieve these goals.

It should be noted that it is necessary to benefit from the success in managing the COVID-19 crisis in a different way, by investing in resources and knowledge to serve human beings.

Finally, we must establish a research center that specializes in health and to work to provide a health platform in Arabic that offers reliable health information in an understandable and applicable way for our daily lives.

Moreover, it is essential for the media to have an impact on the quality of health advertising. For example, it is not acceptable to talk about health while broadcasting an advertisement for energy drinks or junk food.

51.8.1 Knowledge First

Knowledge is the basis of awareness, and traditional and modern media are essential and quick sources of information, which may not always be used in the right way. Therefore, this information must be communicated in a correct and simplified way in order to be applied in our daily lives, and thus health becomes a way of life, through behavior change. The primary task lies in urging individuals to change their behavior, and each category of society requires a specific approach to communication. The message itself may need to be modified to reach each group in the right way. Note here that a large percentage of diseases suffered by members of society are related to behavior, and behavior change requires an integrated marketing process, with an impact on the emotional, psychological and other relevant aspects. It is not enough to talk about the importance of quitting smoking on May 31 or about breast cancer in October; there must be an integrated strategic plan for health awareness that focuses on behavior change and leverages the stories of patients who were able to control the diseases they suffer from by gradually changing their lifestyle.

51.8.2 Lessons Learned

The lessons learned from the coronavirus pandemic, despite its cruelty in many ways, undoubtedly highlight the need to concentrate on prevention and combat misinformation that spreads via social media and WhatsApp. These goals can be achieved by arming people with knowledge, facts, and health information supported by evidence, and credible sources, such as the National Authority for Disasters, Crises, and Emergencies, which operated with a well-thought-out plan and clear messaging, and collaborated with a variety of media institutions that have been instrumental in raising awareness of health issues, enabling community members to take care of their health and follow the guidelines.

Today, we hope that effective cooperation will be carried out between health and media institutions so that the media discourse, whether through newspapers and magazines, radio and television, or social media, contributes to achieving the objectives of the United Arab Emirates' strategy to maintain health, prevent diseases, and improve the quality of life.

This requires conducting training courses for workers in media institutions and health institutions so that the work of the health media department is not limited to the dissemination of news but also focuses on health and the delivery of health messages in an attractive and innovative way. It is no longer acceptable to continue our work in the old way in health media, especially when there are many technical means that can be used to promote the concept of health in our daily lives through various media.

51.9 Conclusion

The main problem that must be addressed by official institutions remains misinformation, which spreads very quickly through social media platforms without verifying the source or validity of the news or information. Misinformation is one of the most prominent concerns of official institutions, especially because misleading information contributes to public anxiety and fear, which in turn leads to confusion and misguides the public.

To meet these challenges, it is necessary to train and qualify media professionals specializing in health media and to foster effective cooperation between media institutions, healthcare experts, decision-makers, and policymakers.

Among the challenges faced by health media is that those in charge of preparing radio and television programs, as well as journalists working in newspapers, magazines, and digital platforms need guests and speakers, and these are often difficult to access. They are spokespersons and are therefore often selected from private health workers who speak according to their interests, rather than as required by the public interest.

It is essential to promote accurate information, critical thinking, and responsible participation; mitigate the impact of health misinformation; and protect public health and well-being.

Conflicts of Interest The author has no conflicts of interest to declare.

References

1. https://www.cdc.gov/nchs/products/databriefs/db66.htm#:~:text=Research%20has%20shown%20that%2074,specific%20medical%20condition%20or%20problem.
2. National Agenda 2021 (vision2021.ae).
3. https://u.ae/en/about-the-uae/strategies-initiatives-and-awards/strategies-plans-and-visions/strategies-plans-and-visions-untill-2021/vision-2021-and-health.
4. Types of media – The Official Portal of the UAE Government.
5. https://www.albayan.ae/across-the-uae/2008-11-11-1.69116.
6. https://iris.who.int/bitstream/handle/10665/350161/9789240038349-eng.pdf?sequence=1.
7. https://www.annualreviews.org/doi/pdf/10.1146/annurev.pu.10.050189.001145.
8. (PDF) The role of mass media communication in public health: The impact of Islamic Republic of Iran broadcasting health channel on health literacy and health behaviors (researchgate.net).

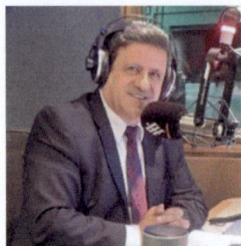

Dr. Bassam Darwish is a renowned figure in healthcare and medical marketing, with a prolific career spanning 33 books. He serves as the editor-in-chief of the "Health in Arabic" website, focusing on providing evidence-based health information to empower individuals and communities. Dr. Darwish is the host of the "Balsam" program on Noor Dubai Radio and TV, where he passionately advocates for health awareness and engages the audience on various health-related topics. His central mission is prevention and promoting healthier lifestyles.

Through his extensive writing, program hosting, and editorial work, Dr. Darwish has consistently demonstrated a commitment to improving healthcare and raising public awareness. His multifaceted contributions have made a significant impact on health awareness, and he remains dedicated to delivering reliable health information to foster a healthier and more informed society.

Open Access This chapter is licensed under the terms of the Creative Commons Attribution 4.0 International License (http://creativecommons.org/licenses/by/4.0/), which permits use, sharing, adaptation, distribution and reproduction in any medium or format, as long as you give appropriate credit to the original author(s) and the source, provide a link to the Creative Commons license and indicate if changes were made.

The images or other third party material in this chapter are included in the chapter's Creative Commons license, unless indicated otherwise in a credit line to the material. If material is not included in the chapter's Creative Commons license and your intended use is not permitted by statutory regulation or exceeds the permitted use, you will need to obtain permission directly from the copyright holder.

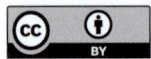

The Future of Healthcare in the UAE

52

Vivienne Mendonca and Humaid O. Al-Shamsi

52.1 Introduction

The dynamic and growing healthcare sector in the United Arab Emirates (UAE) is embracing new digital technologies and adopting data-driven decision-making to improve health outcomes [1]. The UAE's leadership is highly supportive of the healthcare sector and has invested in increasing capacity and quality, along with private investment and public-private partnerships. Investment in healthcare technology is expanding in line with the UAE's Vision 2025 and Digital Government Strategy, contributing to the goal of building a world-class healthcare system [2]. Digital healthcare technologies and data insights are being leveraged to improve preventive healthcare and to devise tailored therapies [1]. Over the last few decades, the UAE has undergone a transformation into a global healthcare and healthtech hub, empowered by the health strategies put forward by the UAE government.

V. Mendonca (✉)
Professional Medical Writer, Dubai, United Arab Emirates

H. O. Al-Shamsi
Burjeel Cancer Institute, Burjeel Medical City, Abu Dhabi, United Arab Emirates

Department of Medical Oncology, Dana-Farber Cancer Institute, Harvard Medical School, Boston, MA, United States

Harvard Medical School, Harvard University, Boston, MA, United States

College of Medicine, Ras Al Khaimah Medical and Health Sciences University, Al Juwais, Al Qusaidat, Ras Al Khaimah, United Arab Emirates

Gulf Medical University, Ajman, United Arab Emirates

Gulf Cancer Society, Alsafa, Kuwait

Emirates Oncology Society, Dubai, United Arab Emirates

College of Medicine, University of Sharjah, Sharjah, United Arab Emirates
e-mail: humaid.al-shamsi@medportal.ca

© The Author(s) 2025
H. O. Al-Shamsi (ed.), *Healthcare in the United Arab Emirates*,
https://doi.org/10.1007/978-981-96-0523-1_52

52.2 How the UAE Is Turning Challenges into Opportunities

Despite the many challenges currently facing the world, under the wise leadership of the country's rulers, the UAE continues to grow and develop. The UAE welcomes people from all over the world and is seen as a safe and attractive country in which to work, live in, and invest. During the COVID-19 pandemic, the UAE was a world leader in COVID-19 testing and vaccination rates [3] and ranked first for COVID-19 resilience [4]. As a global logistics hub, the UAE played a vital role in COVID-19 vaccine supply chain solutions. With continuing research and development, the UAE is working to be ready for new challenges and emerging diseases. Life expectancy in the UAE is increasing, but as in other countries, so is the burden of chronic diseases such as cardiovascular and musculoskeletal diseases and mental health issues [5]. Responding to the changing needs and expectations of its citizens and residents, the UAE's healthcare system is shifting its focus to holistic, personalized, and preventive care. Innovative technologies are being leveraged to provide integrated, value-based care to improve clinical outcomes and health indicators.

52.3 The UAE's Growing Healthcare Sector

Although oil was the initial driver of economic growth in the UAE, the country has diversified its economy into many sectors, including healthcare and innovation. Incredible developments in the healthcare sector in recent decades have been led by the vision and foresight of the UAE government, accompanied by significant financial investment. The federal budget for 2022–26 allocated AED 4.9 billion (8.4% of the total) to healthcare and community protection [1]. Among countries in the Gulf Cooperation Council (GCC), the UAE has the highest healthcare spending growth rate at a compound annual growth rate of 7.4% [6]. A strong private sector, in collaboration with government entities, is driving growth in healthcare infrastructure, capacity, and access to specialized care [7]. An accessible, innovative, future-ready healthcare system that supports healthy lifestyles is a key strategy for building a "Forward Society," one of the pillars of the "We the UAE 2031" vision [8].

The UAE healthcare system is well regulated, with mandatory health insurance coverage provided by the government for Emirati citizens, and mostly by employers for expat residents [9]. However, some gaps still need to be addressed to achieve 100% universal health coverage. The UAE is also fast becoming a regional and global hub for medical tourism [7]. Medical education and research and development (R&D) within the country are also growing. Life-science research and innovation are facilitated by many initiatives, such as the Dubai Science Park, the Department of Health's Research and Innovation Center, and the Al Jalila Foundation's multidisciplinary medical research center.

52.4 Digital Innovation for Health

Digital innovation is one of the key drivers of growth in the UAE's healthcare sector. This is demonstrated by a variety of initiatives aimed at improving healthcare provision and medical education.

52.4.1 Virtual Healthcare and Metaverse Platforms

In the UAE, there has been significant investment in telemedicine and virtual care services by public and private healthcare providers, as well as health insurance companies [10].

Metaverse platforms, using virtual and augmented reality, enable doctors to interact with patients from all over the world. The experience is much closer to in-person care than can currently be achieved with video consultations. In October 2022, Thumbay Group, a UAE-based healthcare and medical education organization, launched the world's first virtual hospital, which will provide an immersive healthcare experience in the metaverse. Virtual hospitals have great potential to enhance the patient's experience and enable wider access, overcoming geographical barriers [11].

52.4.2 Genome Sequencing and Precision Medicine

In a first-of-its-kind national project, the UAE is undertaking the genomic sequencing of one million Emirati volunteers to produce a reference genome specific to Emirati citizens. Launched in 2019 by the Department of Health in Abu Dhabi, the Emirati Genome Program is set to use advanced sequencing technology and artificial intelligence to help prevent or treat chronic diseases [12]. The results will provide valuable data on population health and eventually lead to the development of personalized gene therapy and precision medicine. The UAE Genomics Council will oversee and regulate the implementation, paying careful attention to issues of ethics, consent, education, and data protection [13].

52.4.3 Robotic-Assisted Surgeries

Robotic-assisted surgery is available in many hospitals across the UAE. It enables procedures to be performed more precisely and accurately, with fewer complications. More surgeries in the UAE are expected to utilize robotic and AI technologies in the future as investment in healthcare technologies expands [14]. The first robotic surgical training hub in the Middle East and Africa region has been launched through a strategic partnership between American Hospital Dubai and CMR Surgical. This will enable many surgeons to receive hands-on robotic surgical training, expanding the adoption of robotic-assisted technology in the region [15].

52.4.4 3D Printing and Simulation Technology

3D printing and simulation technologies are currently being used for many applications in surgery and medical education in the UAE. Dubai's 3D printing strategy, implemented in 2016, aims to make the UAE a global leader in 3D printing. Medical uses include prosthetics, surgical planning, and patient education [16]. As the technology develops, broader applications of 3D printing are predicted for the future. The Simulation Center at the United Arab Emirates University's College of Medicine and Health Sciences (CMHS) creates a realistic hospital experience for medical students to acquire clinical skills and confidence. This will encourage best practice and improve patient safety [17].

52.4.5 Health Information Exchange

As part of the ongoing digital transformation, the UAE is in the process of unifying existing electronic medical records databases to enable the reliable and secure exchange of health information. The "Riayati" unified medical records platform, launched by the Ministry of Health and Prevention (MOHAP) in 2021, will integrate with the "Malaffi" platform in Abu Dhabi, the "Nabidh" platform in Dubai, and the "Wareed" platform in the Northern Emirates [18]. Unifying digital medical records enhances care coordination and reduces duplication. Patients can securely access their own medical records and control permissions for access by public and private healthcare providers.

52.5 Future Opportunities and Challenges

52.5.1 Investing in the Future

The UAE, as a logistics, manufacturing, and innovation hub for the region, will continue to be a magnet for talent and investment. However, there is a need for more investment, especially for home-grown investors seeking to move into the healthcare innovation sector. Venture capital involves taking risks, and investors need to focus on opportunities and growth over the long term. The UAE has instituted a health technology assessment process to evaluate the value of proposed new technologies for healthcare [19]. To maximize the benefits of these new technologies, insurance coverage is required, which may require a review of the International Classification of Diseases (ICD) and Current Procedural Terminology (CPT) insurance codes.

52.5.2 Investing in the Workforce

The healthcare workforce in the UAE and the ability to recruit, train, and retain talent in the country are crucial. Further unifying medical licensing across the different authorities in the UAE will be beneficial. The future of healthcare will see growth in the use of artificial intelligence, machine learning, and automation. New competencies and skills will be required, including a need to invest in AI engineers, data scientists, and data governance experts. With the increasing popularity of the metaverse, virtual reality, and augmented reality, healthcare needs to catch up with other industries. This requires investment in both technology and training for healthcare professionals.

52.5.3 Ensuring Robust Regulation

Digital healthcare technologies produce large volumes of personal and sensitive data that require robust regulation to ensure biosecurity, cybersecurity, and data protection. Policies are also required to regulate access to data for research purposes. In the UAE, Federal Law No. 2 (Health Data Law, 2019), similar to HIPAA in the USA, regulates the use of information and communication technology (ICT) in the field of health [20]. As global health providers increasingly provide cross-border care, cooperation between states for the development of international regulation is vital.

52.6 Conclusion

The innovative and growing healthcare sector in the UAE is well placed to take advantage of new technologies and increasing digitization. With continued robust regulation and investment in research and development, the UAE is set to further establish itself as a hub for high-quality healthcare and innovation. The healthcare sector in the UAE is likely to witness a significant evolution of the entire health system, driven by strong government support for innovation and research.

Conflicts of Interest The authors have no conflicts of interest to declare.

References

1. Omnia Health, The future of UAE healthcare is preventive, predictive, and precision-led, https://insights.omnia-health.com/management/future-uae-healthcare-preventive-predictive-and-precision-led, Accessed 16 Oct 23.
2. UAE Government Portal, The UAE Digital Government Strategy 2025, https://u.ae/en/about-the-uae/strategies-initiatives-and-awards/strategies-plans-and-visions/government-services-and-digital-transformation/uae-national-digital-government-strategy, Accessed 16 Oct 23.
3. The Emirates News Agency (WAM), UAE continues to lead in global rankings for COVID-19 vaccination rates, https://wam.ae/en/details/1395302980184, Accessed 16 Oct 23.
4. The Emirates News Agency (WAM), UAE ranks first on Bloomberg's COVID Resilience Ranking https://www.wam.ae/en/details/1395302998502, Accessed 16 Oct 23.

5. US-UAE Business Council, The UAE Healthcare Sector, June 2021, http://usuaebusiness.org/wp-content/uploads/2019/01/2021-U.A.E.-Healthcare-Report.pdf, Accessed 16 Oct 23.
6. The Emirates News Agency (WAM), UAE's healthcare sector leads regionally, globally with scientific breakthroughs in 2023, https://www.wam.ae/en/details/1395303163635, Accessed 16 Oct 23.
7. KPMG, UAE Healthcare Perspectives (Sept. 2020) https://assets.kpmg/content/dam/kpmg/ae/pdf-2020/09/uae-healthcare-perspectives.pdf, Accessed 16 Oct 23.
8. We the UAE 2031, Forward Society, https://wetheuae.ae/en/pillar/forward-society, Accessed 16 Oct 23.
9. UAE Government Portal, Health Insurance, https://u.ae/en/information-and-services/health-and-fitness/health-insurance, Accessed 16 Oct 23.
10. Omnia Health, The boom of telehealth in UAE, https://insights.omnia-health.com/technology/boom-telehealth-uae-it-here-stay, Accessed 16 Oct 23.
11. UAE Set to Launch the First Metaverse Hospital, https://www.magazine.medicaltourism.com/article/uae-set-to-launch-the-first-metaverse-hospital, Accessed 16 Oct 23.
12. Department Of Health unveils world's most comprehensive Genome Program, Transforming health and well-being with genomics and Artificial Intelligence, the nation's leading strengths, https://www.doh.gov.ae/en/news/Department-Of-Health-unveils-worlds-most-comprehensive-Genome-Program, Accessed 13 Dec 2022.
13. UAE Government Portal, Research in the Field of Health, https://u.ae/en/information-and-services/health-and-fitness/research-in-the-field-of-health, Accessed 16 Oct 23.
14. Allocation Assist, Expansion of Robotic Surgery in Dubai, https://www.allocationassist.com/expansion-of-robotic-surgery-in-dubai/, Accessed 16 Oct 23.
15. American Hospital, News Center., https://www.ahdubai.com/news/american-hospital-dubai-sets-up-first-robotic-surgical-training-hub-for-mea, Accessed 16 Oct 23.
16. Arab Health Online, DHA: Embracing the Future of 3D Printing in Healthcare, https://www.arabhealthonline.com/magazine/en/latest-issue/Issue-6/DHA-Embracing-the-Future-of-3D-Printing-in-Healthcare.html, Accessed 16 Oct 23.
17. UAEU, Medical Simulation and Clinical Skills Center, https://www.uaeu.ac.ae/en/cmhs/simulation_center/, Accessed 17 Oct 23.
18. Gulf News, UAE launches unified medical records platform for all patients, https://gulfnews.com/uae/health/uae-launches-unified-medical-records-platform-for-all-patients-1.84167227, Accessed 16 Oct 23.
19. The British University in Dubai, Health Technology Assessment (HTA) Institutionalization in the UAE, https://bspace.buid.ac.ae/items/203b86c7-4a1e-4346-839c-59a8ec93bfde, Accessed 16 Oct 23.
20. UAE Government Portal, Data Protection Law, https://u.ae/en/about-the-uae/digital-uae/data/data-protection-laws#:~:text=Protection%20of%20health%20data%20and,UAE%2C%20including%20its%20free%20zones, Accessed 17/10/23.

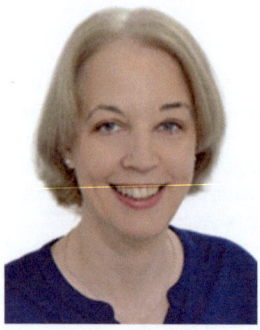

Vivienne Mendonca is a British dental surgeon and professional medical writer, based in Dubai. After graduating from the University of Liverpool in 1998, she worked for 12 years in general dental practice and the NHS Community Dental Service, as well as for 1 year in an Oral and Maxillofacial Surgery hospital department. She gained her MFDS from the Royal College of Surgeons of England in 2005 and her master's in public health with merit from the University of Liverpool in 2018. Her MPH dissertation research was published in The Cleft Palate-Craniofacial Journal in 2020. Vivienne enjoys researching and writing on a wide variety of medical and healthcare topics. Her experience of living and working in the UK, the USA, India, and the UAE has given her a broad insight into challenges and solutions in healthcare systems. Vivienne's writing is concise, clear, and tailored for the target audience. She is skilled in both scientific writing and explaining health information and research in plain language.

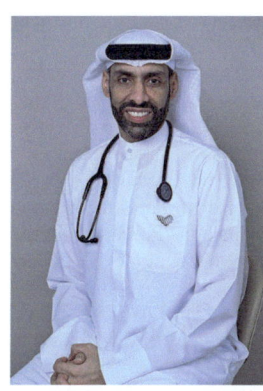

Professor Humaid Obaid Al-Shamsi is the Chief Executive Officer of Burjeel Cancer Institute in Abu Dhabi, UAE; President of the Emirates Oncology Society; Visiting Professor at Harvard Medical School at Harvard University; Visiting Scientist at Dana-Farber Cancer Center, Harvard Medical School, Boston, USA; Full Professor of Oncology at Ras Al Khaimah Medical and Health Sciences University; Ras Al Khaimah, UAE; an Adjunct Professor of Oncology at the College of Medicine, University of Sharjah; and Clinical Professor at Gulf University, Ajman, UAE. He is the first Emirati to be promoted as a professor in oncology in UAE history. He is also the Chairman for Colorectal Cancer in the MENA region, appointed by the prestigious National Comprehensive Cancer Network® in the USA. He is also the only member of the Lung Cancer Policy Network in the MENA region, which aims to advance lung cancer research and screening globally. He is the Chairman of the Oncology and Hematology Fellowship Training Program for the National Institute for Health Specialties in the United Arab Emirates. He is also the only member in the GCC in the WIN Consortium, which comprises organizations representing all stakeholders in personalized cancer medicine globally.

He is board-certified in both internal medicine and oncology from the UK, the USA (ABIM), the National Board of Physicians and Surgeons in the USA, and Canada (FRCPC). He has also been awarded the FRCP (Canada) in 2012, FRCP (London) in 2023, FRCP (Glasgow) in 2024, and FRCP (Edinburgh) in 2025. He is the only physician in the UAE with a subspecialty fellowship certification and training in gastrointestinal oncology and the first Emirati to complete a clinical post-doctoral fellowship in palliative care. He was an Assistant Professor at the University of Texas MD Anderson Cancer Center between 2014 and 2017. He has published more than 170 peer-reviewed articles in *JAMA Oncology, Lancet Oncology, Journal of Clinical Oncology, The Oncologist, BMC Cancer,* and many others. His area of expertise includes precision oncology and cancer care in the UAE. In 2016, he published with his group from MD Anderson in the *Journal of Clinical Oncology* a study describing a new distinct subgroup of colorectal cancer, NON-V600 BRAF-mutated colorectal cancer. In 2022, he published the first book about cancer research in the UAE and also the first book about cancer in the Arab world, both of which were launched at Dubai Expo 2020. *Cancer in the Arab World* has been downloaded more than 500,000 times in its first 2 years of publication and is the ultimate source of cancer data in the Arab region. He also published the first comprehensive book, *Cancer Care in the United Arab Emirates*, which is the first book in UAE history to document cancer care in the UAE, with many topics addressed for the first time. The book was also another success with over 100,000 downloads in the first 2 months of publication.

He is passionate about advancing cancer care in the UAE and the GCC and has made significant contributions to cancer awareness and early detection for the public using social media platforms. He engages actively with the public through awareness campaigns and serves on numerous national health committees, including with the UAE Ministry of Health and the Department of Health, Abu Dhabi.

He is considered the most followed oncologist in the world, with over half a million followers across his social media platforms (Instagram, Twitter, LinkedIn, and TikTok). In 2022, he was awarded the prestigious Feigenbaum Leadership Excellence Award from Sheikh Hamdan Smart University for his exceptional leadership and research, and he was also awarded the Sharjah Award for Volunteering. He was also named the Researcher of the Year in the UAE in 2020 and 2021 by the Emirates Oncology Society.

In May 2024, HH Sheikh Mansour bin Zayed Al Nahyan, Vice President of the United Arab Emirates, awarded him first place in the Emirati Talent Competitiveness Council (NAFIS) program for outstanding leadership in the private sector across all business and medical disciplines. In February 2025, he was awarded the *Sheikha Fatima bint Mubarak Family Award* for being a successful role model in UAE society.

As CEO of Burjeel Cancer Institute, he is leading the largest cancer network in the UAE with over 30 oncologists and hematologists and built the first pediatric bone marrow transplant program in the UAE. He secured the UAE's first European Society for Medical Oncology (ESMO) accreditation for a cancer center in the UAE at Burjeel Cancer Institute.

Besides his clinical and administrative duties, he is engaged in education and various levels of research training for medical trainees to enhance their clinical and research skills. He established the UAE's first hematology and oncology fellowship training program accredited by the UAE National Institute for Health Specialties at Burjeel Cancer Institute.

His mission is to advance cancer care in the UAE and the MENA region and make cancer care accessible to everyone in need around the globe.

Open Access This chapter is licensed under the terms of the Creative Commons Attribution 4.0 International License (http://creativecommons.org/licenses/by/4.0/), which permits use, sharing, adaptation, distribution and reproduction in any medium or format, as long as you give appropriate credit to the original author(s) and the source, provide a link to the Creative Commons license and indicate if changes were made.

The images or other third party material in this chapter are included in the chapter's Creative Commons license, unless indicated otherwise in a credit line to the material. If material is not included in the chapter's Creative Commons license and your intended use is not permitted by statutory regulation or exceeds the permitted use, you will need to obtain permission directly from the copyright holder.

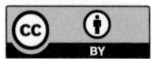

Index

A

Abu Dhabi, 2, 4, 11–13, 15, 25, 29, 33, 50, 56, 71, 101, 125, 139, 165, 175, 177, 180, 181, 183, 184, 186, 187, 194, 195, 204, 206–210, 218–220, 233, 241, 244, 246–248, 253, 255, 279, 296, 313, 340, 352, 353, 365, 367, 368, 374, 389–391, 397–399, 401, 415, 420, 423, 431, 432, 435, 441–447, 455, 457, 472, 489, 491, 492, 494, 495, 508, 509, 512, 515, 523, 545, 546, 548, 549, 552–554, 559–561, 569, 570, 583, 616, 629, 651, 681, 711, 738–740, 742, 743, 745, 747, 750–753, 756, 765, 776–778, 803, 804, 807–809, 811, 843
Abu Dhabi Public Health Center (ADPHC), 71–81, 83–87, 283, 285, 634, 640, 765
Adolescent medicine, 367, 368
Adults vaccination, 165–169, 263
Advanced nursing practice, 229
Advanced practice nursing (APN), 229, 230, 241–250, 267
Aging population, 268, 377, 415, 514, 531, 809
AI in diagnosis, 796, 797, 820
AI in Medicine (AIM), 790–793
AI in radiology, 591, 794, 795, 817–826
Air contrast, 605, 607
Al Ain, 3, 4, 33, 34, 39, 41, 42, 44, 45, 80, 175, 260, 266, 295–298, 318, 325, 363, 364, 367, 382, 398, 401, 415, 442, 475, 495, 524, 531, 534, 555, 616, 618, 738, 739, 751, 756
Alternative medicine, 262, 769–773, 778–780, 782–785
American missionaries, 2–5, 29, 35, 776
Antimicrobial resistance (AMR), 632–636, 641
Antimicrobial resistance emerging, 634
Antimicrobials, 532, 633, 636
Arab alternative medicine, 769, 770, 773, 775, 777, 778, 784
Arthritis, 507, 508, 510–514
Artificial intelligence (AI), 50, 66, 72, 74, 96, 117, 302, 368, 448, 462, 497, 740, 743, 752–753, 755, 789–811, 817, 819, 824–826, 843, 845
Asplenia, 167
Asthma, 183, 280, 567, 569, 573, 574, 783
Autosomal recessive disease, 712, 717, 726, 727
Awareness, 86

B

Bibliometric analysis, 201–211, 324
Biomechanisms, 468–469
Body mass index (BMI), 95, 259, 278–280, 307, 308, 317, 342, 507, 510, 527, 546, 666, 667
Bronchogenic carcinoma, 283, 383, 389, 414, 567, 568, 575, 584, 822
Buildings, 377

C

Cancer, 2, 11, 51, 58, 75, 94, 105–107, 165, 182, 183, 187, 207, 209, 241, 243, 259, 277, 283, 285, 341, 342, 344, 374, 381, 414, 415, 418–420, 424, 523, 615, 632, 648, 763, 795, 817, 833, 838
Cardiology, 58, 131, 139, 243, 320, 322–324, 561
Cardiometabolic risk factors, 318
Cardiovascular disease (CVD), 163, 243, 266
Care, 283

Centers for Disease Control and Prevention (CDC), 720
Challenges, 2, 4, 6–11, 17, 24, 27, 66, 85, 93, 103–104, 118, 134–135, 140–141, 156, 175, 176, 180, 181, 183, 186, 196, 197, 209, 218, 228–233, 245–247, 249, 254, 261, 265, 267–268, 294, 306–308, 325–326, 353–354, 366–368, 377–379, 394, 396, 404, 406–408, 418, 423, 424, 444, 446, 447, 458, 461, 469, 474, 486, 487, 492, 495–497, 513, 515, 521, 523, 552, 559–561, 570, 605, 609, 616, 658, 686, 705, 707, 793, 795, 802, 807, 811, 817, 820, 821, 823, 825, 826, 837, 839, 842, 844–845
Chatbots, 494, 753, 791, 792, 801, 807, 820
Child abuse, 600, 609, 699–704, 706, 707
Child health, 79, 131, 267, 364, 365, 367, 368, 739
Child protection, 366, 601, 700, 701, 705–707
Children vaccination, 167–171
Chronic care, 262, 263, 268
Chronic disease, 62, 74, 75, 78, 80, 86, 103, 109, 140, 176, 182, 183, 243, 253, 263, 268, 283, 285, 286, 349, 366, 374, 514, 528, 584, 658, 660, 680, 689, 710, 752, 763, 764, 766, 782, 783, 802, 807, 811, 842, 843
Chronic obstructive pulmonary disorder (COPD), 94, 259, 263, 569, 574–575, 808
Classification, 818, 844
Clinical characteristics, 294, 297, 404
Clinical impact, 246, 247
Clinical leadership, 194, 227, 249, 267, 707
Clinical nurse specialist, 229, 242–244, 246, 247, 402
Clinical pharmacy, 97, 737–741, 753, 761
Clinical practice, 104, 127, 149, 220, 231, 232, 286, 294, 297, 446, 477, 560, 790, 826
Collision, 467–478
Competency framework, 132
COVID-19, 65, 73–76, 84–87, 89, 90, 124, 140, 168–171, 173, 180, 186, 213, 215, 230, 257, 258, 261, 263–265, 286, 291, 306, 368, 374, 435, 446, 456–458, 461, 462, 474, 475, 485, 487, 493, 494, 496, 497, 527, 559, 567, 572, 598, 599, 631, 638–641, 752, 801, 803, 835–837, 842, 845
COVID response, 73–76, 85, 170, 180, 186, 258, 263, 265, 435, 446, 638, 639, 641
Critical illness, 456–459, 461, 648

D

DataFlow, 141–143, 148, 149
Death, 12, 17, 19, 40, 63, 73, 78, 79, 94, 95, 153–155, 158, 159, 163, 168, 176, 182, 183, 243, 254, 257–259, 280, 308, 313, 314, 317, 342, 343, 364, 367, 374, 381, 383, 390, 402, 416, 424, 457, 461, 467–477, 487, 529, 531, 555, 557, 558, 568, 571, 572, 597–600, 604–606, 609, 618, 632, 662, 664, 700, 714, 724, 790
Deep learning (DL), 789, 790, 793, 796, 797, 801, 819, 821, 824
Delivery care model, 59–60, 67
Dental caries, 60, 367, 657–660, 663, 667, 668, 681–684, 686–688
Dental restoration, 680, 681, 683, 690
Dental screening, 79
Department of Health (DoH), 6, 50, 56, 58, 71, 74, 76, 77, 101, 129, 131, 140–142, 144, 145, 148, 170, 180, 194, 202, 208, 218, 220, 248, 253, 261, 268, 282–285, 321, 352, 365, 368, 391, 432, 446, 456, 489, 490, 492, 523, 546, 584, 587, 588, 597, 619, 621, 629, 633, 637, 704, 705, 741, 745, 751–753, 756, 809–811, 842, 843
Department of Health Insurance, 282
Diabetes complications, 294–296, 298, 299, 302, 306
Diabetes epidemiology, 294–298
Diabetes mellitus (DM), 293, 297, 316, 339, 531, 546, 658, 661–662, 668, 716, 727
Diabetes pharmacotherapies, 299–301
Diabetes technology, 302–303
DICOM viewer, 604
Diet, 65, 95, 263, 278, 279, 283, 284, 287, 293, 299, 341, 390, 512, 573, 576, 667, 680, 682, 686–687, 689, 703, 763–766, 831
Digital innovation, 139, 843–844
Digital twin, 800
Disability-adjusted life years (DALYs), 73, 94, 95, 257, 258, 314, 316, 485, 487, 488
Disaster medicine, 442, 446–448
Disease, 3, 49, 51, 57, 76, 93–96, 103, 127, 131, 139, 163, 176, 192, 217, 253, 277, 294, 314–318, 341, 365, 393, 414–416, 443, 444, 457, 461, 507–515, 526, 547, 567, 584, 599, 615, 630–641, 648, 657, 679, 707, 711–730, 746, 763, 789, 817, 832, 842
Drug information, 744–746, 755, 756
Dubai, 2, 34, 56–61, 63–67, 85, 100, 124, 139, 166, 175, 194, 204, 218, 247, 279, 313, 316, 319, 322, 324, 325, 365, 415, 423,

Index

432, 436, 440, 507, 545, 570, 614, 630, 651, 738–740, 743, 747, 752, 753, 756, 764, 776, 777, 833, 842
Dubai health authority (DHA), 50, 56–64, 66, 67, 102, 105, 106, 117, 129, 131, 132, 140–144, 147–149, 164, 165, 168, 177, 180, 184, 185, 194, 195, 208, 219, 220, 254, 260, 261, 265, 267, 268, 307, 319, 322, 324, 341, 352, 375, 390, 391, 432, 456, 462, 489, 490, 514, 523, 527, 546, 570, 572, 584, 586, 588, 589, 591, 592, 619, 621, 623, 634, 640, 705, 740, 752, 755, 756, 802, 803, 805, 806

E

Early childhood caries (ECC), 679–688, 691
Early detection, 51, 71, 76, 79, 81, 87, 106, 183, 265, 283, 285, 286, 342, 357, 365, 390, 392–394, 556, 615, 666, 701, 821, 822, 833
Economic evaluation, 193, 197
Education, 2, 36, 74, 165, 183, 195, 196, 202, 218–221, 228, 229, 233, 241–243, 245, 249, 254, 256, 277, 299, 324, 335, 351, 376, 417, 441, 459, 476, 486, 510, 547, 567, 603, 617, 633, 649, 659, 680, 701, 741, 746, 755, 793, 817, 832
Elderly, 51, 75, 77, 168, 171, 263, 268, 373–379, 468, 514, 524, 601, 811
Emergency care, 101, 128, 323, 439, 440, 442, 444, 445, 448
Emirates, 1, 34, 49, 56–61, 63–67, 72, 99, 111, 123, 153, 175, 193, 201–204, 206, 209, 210, 218, 223, 225, 244, 246, 247, 253, 278, 313, 381, 431, 486, 507, 521, 534, 545, 567, 583, 597, 629, 649, 681, 700, 701, 711, 764, 769, 789, 821
Emirati society, 51, 374, 769, 773–777
End-of-life care, 356, 375
Epidemiological transition, 182, 257, 260, 263

F

Family medicine, 59, 128, 131, 260–263, 265–267
Federal Law, 82, 153, 156, 366, 377, 424, 489, 574, 630, 700–701, 704, 705, 707, 738, 742, 764, 845
First hospital, 33–38, 40–43, 45, 58, 246, 401, 432, 439, 446, 587, 614
Folk medicine, 769–771, 777
Food services, 765, 766
Future, 11, 25, 40, 44, 52, 64–67, 78, 84, 85, 104, 105, 134–135, 171, 175, 180, 195, 196, 230, 232, 233, 244, 248–249, 254, 261, 265, 268, 285, 286, 318, 355, 376, 378, 394–396, 407–408, 418, 446, 448, 456, 458, 461, 462, 492, 495–497, 515, 528, 531, 546, 547, 552, 559, 560, 583–593, 614, 654, 685, 691, 738–755, 766–767, 790, 791, 797, 798, 805, 808, 809, 811, 822, 824, 825
Future directions, 107, 112, 117–118, 217–220, 227–233, 294, 307–308, 325–326, 485–494, 496, 497, 823, 826

G

GCC emergency medicine, 440
GCC neurology, 545, 546, 554, 555
Genetic diseases, 365, 369, 555, 711–730
Genome sequencing, 843
Genomics, 81, 209, 365, 436, 556, 797, 843
Geriatric medicine, 373
Global Burden of Disease (GBD), 93–96, 259, 314, 316, 317, 553, 556, 557, 680
Guinea worm, 632
Gulf insurance, 181, 184, 194, 195, 197, 247, 377, 423, 491, 495, 546, 548, 739, 804, 805

H

Health, 1, 49–52, 56, 93, 99, 112, 124, 139, 155–157, 159, 175–177, 180–184, 186, 191–197, 201–211, 217, 219, 226, 228–232, 241–243, 245, 249, 278, 308, 335, 373, 381, 413, 455, 468, 471, 473, 485, 507, 522, 546–548, 597, 598, 616, 630–641, 650, 657–663, 665–668, 699, 725, 738, 763, 769, 789, 820, 831–834
Health awareness, 12, 18, 51, 489, 490, 497, 832–838
Health care, 1–29, 584
Health coverage, 100, 194, 495–496, 785, 842
Health economics (HE), 191–197
Health education, 18, 61, 79, 217, 534, 680, 835
Health financing, 100, 105, 192
Health in Abu, 776
Health information, 262, 268, 269, 435, 741, 752, 808, 831–833, 835–838, 844
Health information system (HIS), 62, 76, 668, 741, 756
Health insurance, 50, 60, 61, 99–107, 140, 176, 181, 184, 186, 194, 195, 197, 260, 261, 282, 307, 364, 376, 423, 491, 739, 803, 805, 842, 843
Health media, 831–839

Health outcomes, 93–95, 99, 253, 303, 357, 569, 702, 703, 743, 841
Health policy, 60, 61, 93, 104, 191–193, 257, 261, 264, 651, 668, 739
Health strategy, 63, 65, 96, 102, 182, 373, 489, 841
Health technology assessment (HTA), 192, 844
Healthcare, 34, 75, 112, 113, 115–118, 169, 175, 191, 208, 241, 294, 313, 335, 381, 415, 510–512, 521, 567, 607, 614, 632, 664, 680, 738, 765, 777, 789, 832, 839
Healthcare education, 111, 112, 115, 118, 132, 533
Healthcare financing, 60–61, 99, 181, 184, 194, 195
Healthcare history, 1–29
Healthcare modeling, 196, 197
Healthcare services, 2, 3, 5, 7–9, 11, 13, 14, 19–21, 24, 28, 29, 49, 50, 56–59, 64, 65, 94, 100, 130, 175, 176, 179–181, 185, 186, 192, 243, 253, 257, 262, 266, 359, 363–365, 374, 378, 423, 432, 489, 490, 514, 532, 739, 740, 802, 805–807, 809, 810, 820
Healthcare system, 56–61, 63–67, 94, 96, 99, 100, 105–107, 123, 139–140, 155, 175, 176, 185–187, 192, 193, 197, 217, 218, 228, 231, 241, 268, 282, 283, 307, 308, 320, 325, 326, 351, 355, 359, 373, 406, 408, 443, 446, 456, 458, 461, 485, 488, 490, 496, 523, 530, 532–534, 546–548, 559, 561, 620, 639, 767, 789, 802, 811, 820, 822, 823, 833, 841, 842
Heart failure, 301, 314, 316, 321, 324, 753
Heart transplant, 321
Hemoglobinopathies, 365, 712, 725
Hepatitis B immunity, 166
HIV, 77, 78, 166–169, 257, 533
Home care, 58, 374–375, 416, 490, 493, 609, 747
Hospice, 413–420, 422–425
Human immunodeficiency virus (HIV), 632
Hyperlipidemia, 80, 265, 277, 297, 301, 302, 318, 662
Hypertension (HTN), 80, 94, 265, 277, 301, 302, 318, 339, 367, 374, 529, 546, 547, 551, 576, 753, 767, 783

I

Inborn errors of immunity (IEI), 712, 728
Inborn errors of metabolism, 712–717
Incidence, 18, 95, 241, 294, 296–298, 307, 308, 314–316, 343, 367, 382, 383, 404, 407, 471–473, 477, 509, 523, 526–528, 530, 531, 533, 534, 557–559, 570–572, 617, 631, 632, 639, 658–662, 664–666, 683, 685, 712, 725, 727, 764, 835
Infant, 351
Infection, 27, 86, 163, 165–167, 169, 207, 528, 532, 533, 571, 602, 610, 631, 632, 637, 638, 740
Information dissemination, 833
Informed decisions, 561, 798, 810
Infrastructure, 2, 3, 8, 11, 14, 25, 39, 56, 58, 64, 85, 87, 104, 180, 263, 354, 373, 376, 404, 448, 473, 497, 557, 560, 567, 622, 705, 707, 739, 809, 823, 842
Injury, 94, 95, 258, 259, 443, 444, 447, 468–478, 535, 549, 551, 608, 618, 619, 648–654, 702, 706
Injury prevention, 367
Injury prevention policies, 77
Innovation, 57, 67, 71, 72, 74, 75, 81, 103–107, 111, 112, 115, 116, 195, 202, 204, 208–210, 286, 323, 367, 394, 469, 488, 492, 494, 497, 559, 592, 620, 621, 789, 791, 801, 802, 811, 821, 834, 842, 844, 845
Intensive care (IC), 6–7, 246, 247, 418, 455–462
International confederation of midwives, 351
International Obesity Task Force (IOTF), 280
Ischemic heart disease, 94, 258, 259, 314–317, 367, 607
Islamic alternative medicine, 769

J

Joint Commission International (JCI), 139, 177, 179, 185, 375, 805

K

Kanad Hospital, 33–43, 45
Kidney transplant, 319, 529, 530
Kuwaiti health services, 13–21
Kuwaiti health support, 14

L

Laboratory medicine, 431–436
Limited PMCT, 598
Long-term, 63, 64, 104, 105, 107, 141, 184, 187, 232, 241, 242, 265, 375–377, 496, 532, 597, 601, 653, 660, 662, 685, 687, 692, 702, 703, 707, 747, 749, 782, 801, 803, 806, 835, 844

Index

M

Machine learning, 66, 67, 96, 229, 789, 790, 792, 793, 796, 797, 801, 811, 818, 819, 823, 824, 826, 845
Malaria, 7, 10–12, 18, 21, 24, 26–28, 631, 641
Maternal and infant mortality rate, 183, 357
Maternal mortality rates, 351
Media impact, 834
Medical and health sciences research, 211
Medical college, 126, 589
Medical education, 112–114, 117, 124–135, 139, 144, 265–267, 366, 417, 418, 441, 493, 494, 583, 603, 620, 842–844
Medical liability, 153–159, 424, 457
Medical licensing, 140–142, 150, 845
Medical malpractice, 157, 159
Medical professionalism, 127, 132
Medical reimbursement, 103, 106, 134, 195, 197, 406, 423, 741
Medical simulation, 733
Medical skills, 242, 244, 266
Medical tourism, 66, 99, 104, 139, 176, 406–408, 524, 526, 527, 536, 560–561, 577, 739, 842
Medication reconciliation, 747
Medicine, 2, 28, 35, 124, 127, 203, 261, 264, 267, 378, 396, 415, 439, 442–443, 455, 460, 471, 494, 583, 598, 647, 648, 654, 738, 752, 769, 771, 779, 783, 784, 790, 792, 793, 843, 844
MENA neurology, 547–550, 555–557
Menopause, 340, 533
Menstrual health, 336–337
Mental health, 63, 79, 80, 86, 87, 209, 222, 231, 262, 265, 283, 298, 325, 335, 339, 341, 344, 345, 374, 485–497, 512, 703, 796, 842
Mental health strategies, 86
MERS-Cov, 631, 637, 638
Midwifery, 217, 219, 222, 227, 228, 231, 242, 244–246, 351–359
Midwifery practice, 351, 352, 354, 355, 357
Midwives, 355
Minimal invasive surgery, 321
Minister, 13, 52, 115, 376, 700, 801, 803
Ministry of Health (MOH), 22, 23, 39, 49–52, 57, 59, 100, 144, 180–181, 186, 253, 260, 317, 343, 365, 431, 440, 509, 523, 575, 583, 586–588, 619, 621, 739, 740, 744, 755, 756, 777, 783, 802, 804, 805, 807, 808
Ministry of Health and Prevention (MOHAP), 49–52, 56, 84, 129, 140–142, 148, 156, 163, 169, 170, 194, 209, 253, 261, 268, 285, 319, 324, 341, 344, 352, 374, 391, 396, 446, 456, 489, 490, 492, 514, 524, 546, 551, 572, 584, 586, 621, 622, 634, 638, 664, 742, 756, 804, 844
Misinformation, 85, 838, 839
Modern medicine, 6, 35, 363, 423, 568, 771, 772, 776, 778, 779, 782, 784, 785
Mpox, 638, 639
Musculoskeletal disorders, 507–509, 511

N

National Institute for Health Specialties (NIHS), 111–118, 130, 266, 405, 441, 515
Negative contrast, 605, 607
Neglected tropical diseases, 632
Neonatology, 368
Neural networks, 793, 795, 797, 820, 821, 824
Neurology medical tourism, 560–561
Newborn screening, 79, 81, 87, 365
Non-communicable diseases, 183, 186, 193, 241, 257, 258, 260
Nurse leaders, 228, 232, 233, 244, 247, 249
Nurse practitioner (NP), 242–247, 249, 250
Nursing, 20, 117, 217–220, 227–233, 241, 244, 245, 248, 354, 378, 741, 742, 744, 747
Nursing education, 219–227, 230–231, 241, 244
Nursing practice, 218, 219, 228–232
Nursing Shortage, 228–229
Nursing specialization, 229
Nutrition, 6, 17, 83–85, 129, 261, 262, 265, 283–285, 299–300, 339, 341, 353, 367, 394, 514, 575, 649, 685, 741, 744, 763–767, 779, 803, 832

O

Oasis Hospital, 3, 4, 34, 39, 42, 738
Obesity, 51, 84, 207, 241, 258, 263, 277–280, 283–287, 318, 324, 342, 367, 390, 404, 546, 547, 551, 575–577, 620, 658, 666, 667, 764–767, 835
Oral cancer, 658, 664–666
Oral hygiene, 659, 662, 681–685, 691
Organ donation, 529
Osteoporosis, 51, 80, 376, 468, 507, 509, 513–515, 767
Outpatient, 9, 10, 16, 17, 23, 25, 44, 45, 58, 175, 181, 246, 247, 321, 322, 365, 375, 376, 415, 423, 490, 491, 493, 514, 532, 668, 738, 742, 743, 747, 751

Outreach Programs, 74–75
Overweight, 65, 79, 241, 277–280, 283, 284, 286, 287, 300, 342, 390, 527, 546, 547, 575, 576, 666, 764, 766, 767

P

Palliative care (PC), 81, 100, 103, 127, 396, 401, 402, 414–425
Pathology, 125, 431–434, 436, 568–570, 585, 597, 603, 606, 801, 823
Patient-centered care, 262
Pediatric healthcare, 4, 41, 367
Pediatrics, 128, 131, 140, 267, 365, 366, 623, 705–706
People of Determination (POD), 74, 75, 86, 87, 489
Periodontal diseases, 658, 660–663
Pharmaceutical services, 738–755
Pharmacist immunization, 741
Pharmacists' prescribing, 753–755
Pharmacoeconomics, 196, 755
Pharmacovigilance services, 745
Pharmacy practice, 741
Plastic, 319, 535, 607, 616, 622–624
Plastic surgery, 622
Pleural diseases, 568
PMCT angiogram (PMCTA), 605–607
PMCT service, 599, 601, 603
Pneumonia, 168, 169, 457, 571, 632, 794
Point-of-care testing (POCT), 433
Policies, 60–62, 67, 71, 76, 78, 87, 101, 102, 105, 106, 117, 182, 195, 197, 211, 245, 256, 264, 282, 344, 345, 355, 357, 358, 376–377, 391, 418, 423, 443, 446, 486, 489–490, 497, 534, 588, 601, 602, 604, 610, 654, 664, 705, 745, 811, 845
Policymaking, 79, 209
Positive contrast, 605, 607
Postgraduate curriculum, 124
Postgraduate training, 114, 118, 418, 494, 603
Postmortem imaging, 597–610
Practice challenges, 294
Pregnancy, 79, 165, 169, 298, 338, 339, 342, 352–354, 356, 359, 533, 534, 569, 703, 779, 803, 805
Prehospital care, 445, 468, 477, 478
Prevention, 10, 49–52, 59, 61, 66, 72, 76, 79, 81, 83–87, 127, 165, 181, 183, 187, 230, 260–263, 265, 282–286, 296, 302, 317, 320, 324, 341, 367, 390, 392–396, 442–444, 447, 468, 469, 473, 476–478, 489, 496, 512, 514, 534, 550, 584, 619, 630, 632, 638, 639, 647, 653, 666, 680, 685–689, 692, 704, 707, 730, 744, 770, 776, 789, 794, 834, 836–838
Preventive care, 105, 253, 259, 262, 268, 376, 490, 842
Primary health care (PHC), 253, 254, 256–263, 265–267, 269, 376, 377, 435, 487, 491, 837
Primary source verification (PSV), 141, 142, 148, 149, 432
Private healthcare, 56, 58, 60, 140, 175, 176, 181, 249, 306, 375, 415, 559–561, 803, 808, 843, 844
Professional development, 111, 112, 115–118, 130, 132, 135, 227, 228, 232, 355, 357, 603
Professional Qualification Requirements (PQR), 141, 142, 144, 148, 242
Psychiatry, 129, 131, 365, 491–495, 794, 796
Public health, 4, 7, 10, 15, 24, 49, 51, 60, 61, 71–72, 76–79, 81, 85, 87, 102, 128, 129, 140, 156, 181, 186, 193, 195, 207, 209, 229, 257, 261, 263–265, 267, 284, 286, 294, 297, 303, 319, 342, 344, 345, 415, 443, 447, 458, 497, 528, 534, 570, 632, 639, 641, 651, 658, 679, 680, 691, 699, 707, 755, 831, 833, 835–837, 839
Publications, 11, 73, 87, 143, 202–208, 211, 265, 324, 390, 417, 476, 493, 494, 527, 557, 621, 640

Q

Quality, 283
Quality of care, 185, 186, 232, 242, 268, 319, 375, 557, 561, 808

R

Registers, 78, 81
Rehabilitation medicine and sports, 648
Reliability inside and outside, 170
Reliable information, 832
Religious tolerance, 40
Research productivity, 201–211
Residency programs, 117, 124, 127, 129, 266, 377, 418, 447, 494, 495, 583
Respiratory tract infections, 568
Responsible journalism, 833
Rheumatology, 131, 507–515
Road traffic, 467–478, 617
Robotics, 743, 791, 793, 803, 804, 820

S

Safeguarding, 700–707
SARS-CoV-2, 572, 638–639
Satisfaction, 63, 101, 185, 186, 232, 246, 247, 458, 460, 755
Schools, 14, 17, 18, 80, 128, 196, 218, 244, 260, 287, 297, 393, 417, 418, 475, 640, 765
Screening, 51, 78–81, 86, 87, 107, 181, 183, 187, 265, 278, 283, 284, 296, 298, 302, 318, 325, 326, 389–390, 393, 400, 406, 433, 488, 496, 509, 513, 514, 552, 556, 557, 571, 572, 574, 584, 639, 794, 796, 797, 800
Screening programs, 283
SEHHI, 84, 285, 765
Senior citizens, 283, 375, 377, 378
Significant, 394
Skeletal dysplasias, 712, 726, 727
Smallpox, 10, 13, 26, 27, 630, 638
Smoking, 51, 63, 263, 390, 391, 570, 574, 575, 661, 666, 836
Smoking-related lung disease, 574–575
Social media, 81, 220, 286, 390, 497, 530, 752, 838, 839
Specialty training, 112, 113, 116, 118, 130, 441, 448, 460
Sports medicine UAE, 647
Sports rehabilitation UAE, 647, 648, 654
Streptococcus Mutans, 683
Sugar, 277, 282, 284, 341, 391, 659, 667, 681–683, 686
Surgery, 17, 38, 57, 207, 320, 525, 585, 613, 615, 616, 620, 621, 623, 794, 804

T

Tele-pharmacy, 752, 753, 755
3D printing, 139, 802, 811, 844
Traditional medicine, 3, 58, 769, 771, 772, 774, 777, 778, 783, 784
Transplant, 165, 169, 399, 461, 529, 648
Trauma, 443, 444, 447, 468, 476–478, 605, 617–619, 623, 663, 739
Trauma System, 476–478
Trucial States, 2–4, 11–16, 18, 20–22, 24–26, 28, 29

Tuberculosis (TB), 77, 163, 567, 568, 570, 599, 632, 635, 641, 782

U

UAE economy, 193
UAE emergency medicine, 440, 441, 448
UAE health tech landscape, 809
UAE healthcare, 56, 57, 94, 104–107, 141, 148, 150, 241, 246, 262, 546, 700–707, 801–810
UAE healthcare system, 155, 227, 247, 546, 823, 842
UAE insurance, 103, 247
UAE medical licensing, 142–149
UAE neurology, 550–559
Undergraduate curriculum, 196, 418
United Arab Emirates (UAE), 1, 34, 49, 56, 111, 126, 130, 139, 141, 146, 163, 204, 206–207, 209, 325, 335, 341, 351, 363, 373, 402, 415, 431, 433, 467, 468, 470, 471, 475, 476, 478, 486, 489, 493, 507, 510, 521, 531, 545, 567–577, 597, 614, 629, 658, 701, 764, 765, 770, 775–781, 783, 785, 789, 821, 832, 833, 838, 841, 842, 844
The United Arab Emirates University (UAEU), 204
Urology, 521–536, 614, 621, 804

V

Vaccination, 9, 10, 18, 22, 27, 76, 77, 164, 165, 169–171, 258, 391, 400, 630, 631, 641, 750, 751, 755, 842
Ventilated PMCT (VPMCT), 604
Virtual hospital, 802–803, 805, 843

W

Whole-body PMCTA, 605
Women's health, 267, 336–340, 345
Workforce development, 262, 486
World Health Organization (WHO), 28, 59, 72, 93, 132, 140, 163, 217, 244, 253, 256, 260, 269, 278, 280, 338, 339, 401, 467, 571, 575, 765, 834